# WHO Classification of Tumours

# Paediatric Tumours

## Part B

WHO Classification of Tumours Editorial Board

**International Agency for Research on Cancer**

World Health
Organization

## Suggested citation

WHO Classification of Tumours Editorial Board. Paediatric tumours.
Lyon (France): International Agency for Research on Cancer; 2022.
(WHO classification of tumours series, 5th ed.; vol. 7).
https://publications.iarc.fr/608.

## Sales, rights, and permissions

Print copies are distributed by WHO Press, World Health Organization, 20 Avenue Appia, 1211 Geneva 27, Switzerland
Tel.: +41 22 791 3264; Fax: +41 22 791 4857; email: bookorders@who.int; website: https://whobluebooks.iarc.fr

To purchase IARC publications in electronic format, see the IARC Publications website (https://publications.iarc.fr).

Requests for permission to reproduce or translate IARC publications – whether for sale or for non-commercial distribution – should be submitted through the IARC Publications website (https://publications.iarc.fr/Rights-And-Permissions).

## Third-party materials

If you wish to reuse material from this work that is attributed to a third party, such as figures, tables, or boxes, it is your responsibility to determine whether permission is needed for that reuse and to obtain permission from the copyright holder. See *Sources*, pages 1037–1053. The risk of claims resulting from infringement of any third-party-owned component in the work rests solely with the user.

The contributors of all images in which the patient may be identifiable have affirmed that the appropriate informed consent has been obtained for the use of said images in this publication.

## General disclaimers

The designations employed and the presentation of the material in this publication do not imply the expression of any opinion whatsoever on the part of WHO or contributing agencies concerning the legal status of any country, territory, city, or area, or of its authorities, or concerning the delimitation of its frontiers or boundaries. Dotted and dashed lines on maps represent approximate border lines for which there may not yet be full agreement.

The mention of specific companies or of certain manufacturers' products does not imply that they are endorsed or recommended by WHO or contributing agencies in preference to others of a similar nature that are not mentioned. Errors and omissions excepted, the names of proprietary products are distinguished by initial capital letters.

All reasonable precautions have been taken by WHO to verify the information contained in this publication. However, the published material is being distributed without warranty of any kind, either expressed or implied. The responsibility for the interpretation and use of the material lies with the reader. In no event shall WHO or contributing agencies be liable for damages arising from its use.

First print run (5500 copies)

Updated corrigenda can be found at https://publications.iarc.fr

## IARC Library Cataloguing-in-Publication Data

Names: WHO Classification of Tumours Editorial Board.
Title: Paediatric tumours / edited by WHO Classification of Tumours Editorial Board.
Description: Fifth edition. | Lyon: International Agency for Research on Cancer, 2022. | Series: World Health Organization classification of tumours. | Includes bibliographical references and index.
Identifiers: ISBN 9789283245100 (pbk.) | ISBN 9789283245117 (ebook)
Subjects: MESH: Neoplasms. | Infant. | Child.
Classification: NLM QZ 275

The WHO classification of paediatric tumours presented in this book reflects
the views of the WHO Classification of Tumours Editorial Board that convened
via video conference from 31 August to 2 September 2020,
as well as subsequent consultation.

# The WHO Classification of Tumours Editorial Board

For the complete list of all contributors and their affiliations, see pages 1021–1036.

# WHO Classification of Tumours
## Paediatric Tumours

| | |
|---|---|
| Edited by | The WHO Classification of Tumours Editorial Board |
| IARC Editors | Subasri Armon |
| | Ian A. Cree |
| | Daphne de Jong |
| | Anil Felix Angelo Fonseca |
| | Daphne Fonseca |
| | Gabrielle Goldman-Lévy |
| | Dilani Lokuhetty |
| | B. Vishal Rao |
| | Valerie A. White |
| Epidemiology | Eva Steliarova-Foucher |
| Project Assistant | Asiedua Asante |
| Assistant | Anne-Sophie Bres |
| Production Editor | Jessica Cox |
| Technical Editing | Julia Slone-Murphy |
| Principal Information Assistant | Alberto Machado |
| Information Assistant | Catarina Marques |
| Layout | Meaghan Fortune |
| | Catarina Marques |
| Printed by | Omnibook |
| | 74370 Argonay, France |
| Publisher | International Agency for Research on Cancer (IARC) |
| | 150 Cours Albert Thomas |
| | 69372 Lyon Cedex 08, France |

# Contents

Please note that the contents of this volume have been split into two parts for publication in print: Part A (in the accompanying book) and Part B (in this book).

List of abbreviations    xiii

Foreword    xiv

PART A (IN ACCOMPANYING BOOK)

ICD-O topographical coding of paediatric tumours    1

ICD-O morphological coding: Introduction    5
   Haematolymphoid disorders    6
   CNS tumours    10
   Peripheral neuroblastic tumours    13
   Eye tumours    14
   Soft tissue and bone tumours    15
   Germ cell tumours    20
   Renal and male genital tumours    22
   Female genital tumours    23
   Breast tumours    24
   Digestive system tumours    25
   Endocrine tumours    27
   Head and neck tumours    28
   Thoracic tumours    29
   Skin tumours    30

TNM staging of paediatric tumours    31

1   Introduction to paediatric tumours    35

2   Haematolymphoid disorders    39
   Introduction    40
   Myeloid neoplasms
     Myeloproliferative neoplasms
      Chronic myeloid leukaemia (CML)    41
     Myelodysplastic/myeloproliferative neoplasms
      Juvenile myelomonocytic leukaemia    45
     Myelodysplastic syndromes
      Refractory cytopenia of childhood (childhood
        myelodysplastic neoplasm with low blasts)    48
      Myelodysplastic syndrome with excess blasts
        (childhood myelodysplastic neoplasm with
        increased blasts)    51
     Acute myeloid leukaemia (AML)
      AMLs defined by differentiation    53
      AMLs with defining genetic abnormalities    56
     Myeloid neoplasms and proliferations associated with
      antecedent or predisposing conditions
      Myeloid neoplasms associated with germline
        predisposition    62
      Myeloid proliferations associated with Down syndrome    66
   Mast cell neoplasia
     Mastocytosis    69
   Lymphoid neoplasms
     Precursor lymphoid neoplasms
      B-lymphoblastic leukaemia/lymphoma    75
      T- and NK-lymphoblastic leukaemia/lymphoma    80
     Mature B-cell neoplasms
      Primary mediastinal large B-cell lymphoma    83
      Diffuse large B-cell lymphoma NOS    86
      EBV-positive diffuse large B-cell lymphoma    89
      Large B-cell lymphoma with *IRF4* rearrangement    91
      Paediatric-type follicular lymphoma    93

      Paediatric nodal marginal zone lymphoma    96
      ALK-positive large B-cell lymphoma    99
      Lymphomatoid granulomatosis    101
      Plasmablastic lymphoma    103
      Mediastinal grey zone lymphoma    106
      Burkitt lymphoma    109
      High-grade B-cell lymphoma with 11q aberration    113
     Mature T/NK-cell neoplasms
      Peripheral T-cell lymphoma NOS    115
      Aggressive NK-cell leukaemia    117
     Primary cutaneous T-cell neoplasms
      Mycosis fungoides    119
      Primary cutaneous CD30-positive T-cell lym-
        phoproliferative disorders    123
      Subcutaneous panniculitis-like T-cell lymphoma    126
     Anaplastic large cell lymphoma
      ALK-positive anaplastic large cell lymphoma    129
     Hepatosplenic T-cell lymphoma
      Hepatosplenic T-cell lymphoma    133
     EBV-positive lymphoproliferative diseases of childhood
      Systemic EBV-positive T-cell lymphoma of childhood    135
      Hydroa vacciniforme lymphoproliferative disorder    138
   Hodgkin lymphoma
     Classic Hodgkin lymphoma    141
     Nodular lymphocyte-predominant Hodgkin
      lymphoma    145
   Histiocytic and dendritic cell neoplasms
     Langerhans cell histiocytosis and related disorders    148
   Immunodeficiency-associated lymphoproliferative disorders
     Primary immunodeficiency–associated lympho-
      proliferative disorders    154
     Posttransplant lymphoproliferative disorders    158
     HIV-associated lymphoproliferative disorders    163

3   CNS tumours    167
   Introduction    169
   Gliomas, glioneuronal tumours, and neuronal tumours
     Introduction    172
     Paediatric-type diffuse low-grade gliomas
      Diffuse astrocytoma, *MYB*- or *MYBL1*-altered    174
      Angiocentric glioma    177
      Polymorphous low-grade neuroepithelial tumour
        of the young    180
      Diffuse low-grade glioma, MAPK pathway–altered    183
     Paediatric-type diffuse high-grade gliomas
      Diffuse midline glioma, H3 K27–altered    187
      Diffuse hemispheric glioma, H3 G34–mutant    193
      Diffuse paediatric-type high-grade glioma,
        H3-wildtype and IDH-wildtype    196
      Infant-type hemispheric glioma    200
     Circumscribed astrocytic gliomas
      Pilocytic astrocytoma    202
      High-grade astrocytoma with piloid features    209
      Pleomorphic xanthoastrocytoma    213
      Subependymal giant cell astrocytoma    218
      Astroblastoma, *MN1*-altered    222
     Glioneuronal and neuronal tumours
      Ganglioglioma    225
      Desmoplastic infantile ganglioglioma / desmo-
        plastic infantile astrocytoma    230
      Dysembryoplastic neuroepithelial tumour    234

| | |
|---|---|
| Diffuse glioneuronal tumour with oligodendro- | |
| glioma-like features and nuclear clusters | 238 |
| Diffuse leptomeningeal glioneuronal tumour | 241 |
| Multinodular and vacuolating neuronal tumour | 245 |
| Ependymal tumours | |
| Introduction | 248 |
| Supratentorial ependymoma | 249 |
| Supratentorial ependymoma, ZFTA fusion–positive | 252 |
| Supratentorial ependymoma, YAP1 fusion–positive | 255 |
| Posterior fossa ependymoma | 257 |
| Posterior fossa group A (PFA) ependymoma | 260 |
| Posterior fossa group B (PFB) ependymoma | 263 |
| Spinal ependymoma | 265 |
| Spinal ependymoma, MYCN-amplified | 268 |
| Myxopapillary ependymoma | 271 |
| Choroid plexus tumours | |
| Choroid plexus papilloma | 274 |
| Atypical choroid plexus papilloma | 277 |
| Choroid plexus carcinoma | 279 |
| CNS embryonal tumours | |
| Medulloblastoma: Introduction | 282 |
| Medulloblastomas, molecularly defined | |
| Medulloblastoma, WNT-activated | 285 |
| Medulloblastoma, SHH-activated and | |
| TP53-wildtype | 288 |
| Medulloblastoma, SHH-activated and | |
| TP53-mutant | 291 |
| Medulloblastoma, non-WNT/non-SHH | 293 |
| Medulloblastomas, histologically defined | |
| Medulloblastoma, histologically defined | 295 |
| Other CNS embryonal tumours | |
| Introduction | 302 |
| Atypical teratoid/rhabdoid tumour | 303 |
| Cribriform neuroepithelial tumour | 308 |
| Embryonal tumour with multilayered rosettes | 310 |
| CNS neuroblastoma, FOXR2-activated | 314 |
| CNS tumour with BCOR internal tandem duplication | 317 |
| CNS embryonal tumour NEC/NOS | 320 |
| Pineal tumours | |
| Pineal tumours | |
| Introduction | 322 |
| Pineoblastoma | 323 |
| Melanocytic CNS tumours | |
| Introduction | 327 |
| Diffuse meningeal melanocytic neoplasms: | |
| Melanocytosis and melanomatosis | 328 |
| Tumours of the sellar region | |
| Introduction | 331 |
| Pituitary endocrine tumours | |
| Pituitary adenoma / pituitary neuroendocrine tumour | 332 |
| Pituitary blastoma | 341 |
| Craniopharyngiomas | |
| Adamantinomatous craniopharyngioma | 343 |
| **4  Peripheral neuroblastic tumours** | **349** |
| Introduction | 350 |
| Ganglioneuroma | 351 |
| Ganglioneuroblastoma, intermixed | 353 |
| Neuroblastoma | 356 |
| Ganglioneuroblastoma, nodular (and other | |
| composite neuroblastic tumours) | 363 |
| **5  Eye tumours** | **365** |
| Introduction | 366 |
| Conjunctival neoplasms | |
| Hamartomas | |
| Epibulbar choristoma | 367 |
| Epibulbar osseous choristoma | 369 |
| Phakomatous choristoma | 370 |
| Melanocytic neoplasms | |
| Conjunctival junctional, compound, and subepi- | |
| thelial naevi | 372 |
| Inflamed juvenile conjunctival naevus | 375 |
| Uveal neoplasms | |
| Diffuse choroidal neurofibroma and ganglioneuroma | 378 |
| Lisch nodule (iris hamartoma) | 381 |
| Retinal and neuroepithelial tumours | |
| Retinocytoma | 383 |
| Retinoblastoma | 385 |
| Medulloepithelioma | 392 |
| Optic nerve tumours | |
| Pilocytic astrocytoma and other gliomas of the | |
| optic nerve | 395 |
| **6  Soft tissue and bone tumours** | **397** |
| Introduction | 399 |
| Soft tissue tumours | |
| Adipocytic tumours | |
| Lipomatosis | 402 |
| Lipoblastoma/lipoblastomatosis | 405 |
| Liposarcoma | 408 |
| Fibroblastic and myofibroblastic tumours | |
| Fasciitis/myositis | 411 |
| Fibrodysplasia ossificans progressiva | 415 |
| Fibroma of tendon sheath | 417 |
| Gardner fibroma | 418 |
| Fibrous hamartoma of infancy | 420 |
| Lipofibromatosis | 422 |
| Inclusion body infantile digital fibromatosis | 424 |
| Juvenile hyaline fibromatosis | |
| (hyaline fibromatosis syndrome) | 426 |
| Fibromatosis colli | 428 |
| Calcifying aponeurotic fibroma | 430 |
| Sinonasal angiofibroma | 432 |
| Plantar/palmar fibromatoses | 435 |
| Dermatofibrosarcoma protuberans | 437 |
| Desmoid fibromatosis | 441 |
| EWSR1::SMAD3-rearranged fibroblastic tumour | 443 |
| Infantile fibrosarcoma | 445 |
| Paediatric NTRK-rearranged spindle cell neoplasm | 448 |
| Low-grade fibromyxoid sarcoma / sclerosing | |
| epithelioid fibrosarcoma | 451 |
| Inflammatory myofibroblastic tumour | 454 |
| Low-grade myofibroblastic sarcoma | 457 |
| So-called fibrohistiocytic tumours | |
| Fibrous histiocytoma | 459 |
| Plexiform fibrohistiocytic tumour | 462 |
| Tenosynovial giant cell tumour | 464 |
| Vascular tumours | |
| Capillary malformations | 466 |
| Venous malformations | 468 |
| Arteriovenous malformations | 471 |
| Intramuscular vascular anomalies | 474 |
| Lymphatic anomalies | 477 |
| Congenital haemangioma | 479 |
| Infantile haemangioma | 481 |
| Haemangioma of placenta | 483 |
| Lobular capillary haemangioma (pyogenic | |
| granuloma) | 485 |
| Epithelioid haemangioma | 487 |
| Tufted angioma and kaposiform haemangioen- | |
| dothelioma | 489 |
| Papillary intralymphatic angioendothelioma and | |
| retiform haemangioendothelioma | 492 |
| Pseudomyogenic haemangioendothelioma | 494 |
| Kaposi sarcoma | 497 |

| | |
|---|---|
| Epithelioid haemangioendothelioma | 500 |
| Angiosarcoma | 502 |
| Pericytic (perivascular) tumours | |
| Myofibroma and myopericytoma | 504 |
| Glomus tumour and glomuvenous malformation | 507 |
| Smooth muscle tumours | |
| EBV-associated smooth muscle tumour | 509 |
| Skeletal muscle tumours | |
| Rhabdomyoma | 511 |
| Rhabdomyosarcomas | 513 |
| Ectomesenchymoma | 517 |
| Gastrointestinal stromal tumour | |
| Paediatric gastrointestinal stromal tumour | 519 |
| Peripheral nerve sheath tumours | |
| Schwannoma | 522 |
| Neurofibroma | 525 |
| Perineurioma | 529 |
| Hybrid nerve sheath tumour | 531 |
| Granular cell tumour | 533 |
| Solitary circumscribed neuroma | 535 |
| Ectopic meningioma and meningothelial hamartoma | 537 |
| Benign triton tumour / neuromuscular choristoma | 539 |
| Malignant peripheral nerve sheath tumour | 541 |
| Tumours of uncertain derivation | |
| Intramuscular/juxta-articular myxoma | 545 |
| Superficial angiomyxoma | 547 |
| Deep angiomyxoma | 548 |
| Angiomatoid fibrous histiocytoma | 550 |
| Clear cell sarcoma of soft tissue | 552 |
| Alveolar soft part sarcoma | 554 |
| Extrarenal rhabdoid tumour | 556 |
| PEComa | 559 |
| Synovial sarcoma | 562 |
| Epithelioid sarcoma | 565 |
| Myoepithelial tumours of soft tissue | 569 |
| Phosphaturic mesenchymal tumour | 572 |
| Desmoplastic small round cell tumour | 574 |
| Undifferentiated sarcomas | 577 |
| Undifferentiated small round cell sarcomas of soft tissue and bone | |
| Ewing sarcoma | 579 |
| Round cell sarcoma with *EWSR1*::non-ETS fusions | 582 |
| *CIC*-rearranged sarcoma | 585 |
| Sarcoma with *BCOR* genetic alterations | 587 |
| Bone tumours | |
| Osteogenic tumours | |
| Subungual exostosis | 590 |
| Bizarre parosteal osteochondromatous proliferation | 592 |
| Osteoblastoma | 594 |
| Osteoid osteoma | 596 |
| Chondromesenchymal hamartoma of the chest wall | 598 |
| Osteosarcoma | 600 |
| Chondrogenic tumours | |
| Chondroblastoma | 608 |
| Osteochondroma | 611 |
| Chondromyxoid fibroma | 613 |
| Enchondroma and enchondromatosis | 616 |
| Chondrosarcoma | 618 |
| Mesenchymal chondrosarcoma | 623 |
| Other bone tumours | |
| Vascular tumours of bone | 625 |
| Aneurysmal bone cyst | 628 |
| Giant cell tumour of bone | 630 |
| Non-ossifying fibroma | 632 |
| Notochordal tumours | 634 |
| Simple bone cyst | 638 |

| | |
|---|---|
| Adamantinoma | 640 |
| Osteofibrous dysplasia | 642 |
| Fibrous dysplasia | 644 |

**PART B (IN THIS BOOK)**

| | | |
|---|---|---|
| **7** | **Germ cell tumours** | **647** |
| | Introduction | 648 |
| | Germ cell tumours | |
| | Non-invasive germ cell neoplasia | |
| | Intratubular germ cell neoplasia (male gonadal) | 649 |
| | Gonadoblastoma | 652 |
| | Germinoma-family tumours | |
| | Germinoma/dysgerminoma/seminoma | 655 |
| | Non-germinomatous germ cell tumours | |
| | Introduction | 661 |
| | Mature cystic teratoma | 663 |
| | Extragonadal teratoma | 666 |
| | Monodermal teratomas (female gonadal) | 668 |
| | Immature teratoma (female gonadal) | 671 |
| | Prepubertal-type testicular teratoma | 673 |
| | Postpubertal-type teratoma | 675 |
| | Embryonal carcinoma | 679 |
| | Yolk sac tumour | 681 |
| | Fetus in fetu | 684 |
| | Choriocarcinoma (non-gestational) | 686 |
| | Malignant mixed germ cell tumours | 688 |
| | | |
| **8** | **Renal and male genital tumours** | **691** |
| | Introduction | 692 |
| | Renal tumours | |
| | Nephroblastic and related tumours | |
| | Paediatric cystic nephroma | 695 |
| | Nephroblastoma | 697 |
| | Molecularly defined renal tumours | |
| | Renal cell carcinoma with MiT translocations | 702 |
| | *ALK*-rearranged renal cell carcinoma | 706 |
| | Eosinophilic solid and cystic renal cell carcinoma | 708 |
| | SMARCB1-deficient renal medullary carcinoma | 710 |
| | Metanephric tumours | |
| | Metanephric adenoma | 712 |
| | Metanephric adenofibroma | 714 |
| | Metanephric stromal tumour | 716 |
| | Mesenchymal renal tumours | |
| | Ossifying renal tumour of infancy | 718 |
| | Mesoblastic nephroma | 720 |
| | Clear cell sarcoma of the kidney | 722 |
| | Malignant rhabdoid tumour of the kidney | 725 |
| | Anaplastic sarcoma of the kidney | 727 |
| | Renal Ewing sarcoma | 729 |
| | Testicular tumours | |
| | Non–germ cell testicular tumours: Introduction | 731 |
| | Juvenile granulosa cell tumour of the testis | 732 |
| | | |
| **9** | **Female genital tumours** | **735** |
| | Non–germ cell tumours of the female genital tract: Introduction | 736 |
| | Ovarian tumours | |
| | Sex cord stromal tumours | |
| | Ovarian fibroma | 737 |
| | Sclerosing stromal tumour | 739 |
| | Juvenile granulosa cell tumour of the ovary | 741 |
| | Sex cord tumour with annular tubules | 743 |
| | Papillary cystadenoma | 745 |
| | Sertoli–Leydig cell tumour | 746 |
| | Gynandroblastoma | 749 |
| | Other ovarian tumours | |

| | | |
|---|---|---|
| Small cell carcinoma of the ovary, hypercalcaemic type | 751 | |
| Lower female genital tract tumours | | |
| Epithelial tumours | | |
| Mesonephric remnants and hyperplasia | 753 | |
| Müllerian papilloma | 755 | |
| Condyloma acuminatum | 757 | |
| Peritoneal tumours | | |
| Mesothelial tumours | | |
| Peritoneal inclusion cysts | 759 | |

## 10 Breast tumours — 761
| | |
|---|---|
| Introduction | 762 |
| Breast tumours | |
| Fibroepithelial tumours | 764 |
| Juvenile fibroadenoma | 767 |
| Juvenile papillomatosis | 770 |

## 11 Digestive system tumours — 773
| | |
|---|---|
| Introduction | 774 |
| Liver tumours | |
| Epithelial tumours | |
| Hepatoblastoma | 775 |
| Fibrolamellar variant of hepatocellular carcinoma | 781 |
| Paediatric hepatocellular carcinoma | 784 |
| Mesenchymal tumours unique to the liver | |
| Mesenchymal hamartoma | 790 |
| Calcifying nested stromal-epithelial tumour | 793 |
| Embryonal sarcoma of the liver | 795 |
| Hepatic congenital haemangioma | 797 |
| Hepatic infantile haemangioma | 800 |
| Hepatic angiosarcoma | 803 |
| Pancreatic tumours | |
| Epithelial tumours | |
| Pancreatoblastoma | 805 |
| Pancreatic acinar cell carcinoma | 809 |
| Solid pseudopapillary neoplasm | 812 |
| Gastrointestinal tumours | |
| Epithelial tumours | |
| Gastroblastoma | 816 |
| Appendiceal neuroendocrine tumours | 818 |

## 12 Endocrine tumours — 821
| | |
|---|---|
| Introduction | 822 |
| Thyroid tumours | |
| Thyroid epithelial tumours | |
| Follicular adenoma of the thyroid | 823 |
| Papillary thyroid carcinoma | 827 |
| Cribriform morular thyroid carcinoma | 834 |
| Medullary thyroid carcinoma | 837 |
| Spindle epithelial tumour with thymus-like elements | 841 |
| Parathyroid tumours | |
| Parathyroid endocrine tumours | |
| Parathyroid adenoma | 843 |
| Adrenal tumours | |
| Adrenocortical tumours | |
| Adrenal cortical tumours | 846 |
| Tumours of the adrenal medulla and extra-adrenal paraganglia | |
| Sympathetic paraganglioma | 851 |
| Parasympathetic paraganglioma (head and neck paraganglioma) | 854 |
| Phaeochromocytoma | 858 |
| Composite phaeochromocytoma/paraganglioma | 865 |
| Neuroendocrine neoplasms | |
| Neuroendocrine tumours | |
| Other neuroendocrine tumours | 867 |

## 13 Head and neck tumours — 873
| | |
|---|---|
| Introduction | 874 |
| Benign tumours | |
| Squamous papilloma and papillomatosis | 875 |
| White sponge naevus | 877 |
| Congenital granular cell epulis | 879 |
| Central giant cell granuloma | 881 |
| Odontogenic tumours | 883 |
| Ossifying fibroma | 888 |
| Sinonasal tract myxoma | 890 |
| Nasal dermoid cyst | 891 |
| Nasopharyngeal dermoid | 893 |
| Nasal chondromesenchymal hamartoma | 894 |
| Pleomorphic adenoma | 896 |
| Malignant tumours | |
| Mucoepidermoid carcinoma | 899 |
| Acinic cell carcinoma | 901 |
| Sialoblastoma | 903 |
| Nasopharyngeal carcinoma | 905 |
| NUT carcinoma | 908 |
| Melanotic neuroectodermal tumour of infancy | 910 |

## 14 Thoracic tumours — 913
| | |
|---|---|
| Lung tumours | |
| Fetal lung interstitial tumour | 914 |
| Congenital peribronchial myofibroblastic tumour | 916 |
| Pleuropulmonary blastoma | 918 |
| Heart tumours | |
| Cardiac rhabdomyoma | 922 |

## 15 Skin tumours — 925
| | |
|---|---|
| Introduction | 926 |
| Hamartomas | |
| Hamartomas | 927 |
| Epithelial neoplasms | |
| Squamous neoplasms | |
| Angiokeratoma | 932 |
| Epidermal naevi | 934 |
| Pilomatricoma | 938 |
| Melanocytic neoplasms | |
| Naevi | |
| Congenital naevi | 940 |
| Junctional, compound, and dermal naevi | 943 |
| Blue naevus | 945 |
| Spitz naevus | 947 |
| Pigmented spindle cell naevus (Reed naevus) | 950 |
| Melanoma | |
| Melanoma | 952 |

## 16 Genetic tumour syndromes — 957
| | |
|---|---|
| Selected tumour predisposition syndromes: Introduction | 958 |
| Syndromes predisposing primarily to neural tumours | |
| Neurofibromatosis type 1 | 962 |
| Neurofibromatosis type 2 | 966 |
| Tuberous sclerosis | 971 |
| Naevoid basal cell carcinoma syndrome (Gorlin syndrome) | 975 |
| Retinoblastoma syndrome | 979 |
| Syndromes predisposing primarily to endocrine tumours | |
| Von Hippel–Lindau syndrome | 981 |
| Hereditary phaeochromocytoma–paraganglioma syndromes | 984 |
| Syndromes predisposing primarily to Wilms tumours | |
| WAGR syndrome | 987 |
| Beckwith–Wiedemann and related overgrowth syndromes | 989 |

Syndromes predisposing primarily to gastrointestinal tumours
    Familial adenomatous polyposis    991
    Lynch syndrome    994
Other syndromes
    Xeroderma pigmentosum    999
    Rothmund–Thomson syndrome    1002
    Li–Fraumeni syndrome    1005
    *DICER1* syndrome    1008
    *BAP1* tumour predisposition syndrome    1012
    Constitutional mismatch repair deficiency syndrome    1014
    Rhabdoid tumour predisposition syndrome    1017

Contributors    1021

Declaration of interests    1034

IARC/WHO Committee for ICD-O    1036

Sources    1037

References    1055

Subject index    1177

Previous volumes in the series    1191

# List of abbreviations

2D, 3D — two-dimensional, three-dimensional
AIDS — acquired immunodeficiency syndrome
AJCC — American Joint Committee on Cancer
ALT — alternative lengthening of telomeres
AMT PET — α-[11C]methyl-L-tryptophan positron emission tomography
AR — androgen receptor
ATP — adenosine triphosphate
bp — base pair
BSRTC — Bethesda System for Reporting Thyroid Cytopathology
cAMP — cyclic adenosine monophosphate
cART — combination antiretroviral therapy
CAYA — childhood, adolescent, and young adult
ClinGen/GA4GH — Clinical Genome Resource / Global Alliance for Genomics and Health
CMV — cytomegalovirus
CNS — central nervous system
COG — Children's Oncology Group
CT — computed tomography
dMMR — mismatch repair–deficient
DNA — deoxyribonucleic acid
EBRT — external beam radiation therapy
EBV — Epstein–Barr virus
EC cell — enterochromaffin cell
ECL cell — enterochromaffin-like cell
EpSSG — European Paediatric Soft Tissue Sarcoma Study Group
ER — estrogen receptor
ESR — erythrocyte sedimentation rate
ETP — early T-precursor
FDA PET — 18F-fluorodopamine positron emission tomography
FDG PET — 18F-fluorodeoxyglucose positron emission tomography
FDOPA PET — 18F-L-dihydroxyphenylalanine positron emission tomography
FIGO — International Federation of Gynecology and Obstetrics
FISH — fluorescence in situ hybridization
FLAIR — fluid-attenuated inversion recovery
FNAB — fine-needle aspiration biopsy
GCB — germinal-centre B cell
GFAP — glial fibrillary acidic protein
H&E — haematoxylin and eosin stain
HBV — hepatitis B virus
HCV — hepatitis C virus
HHV — human herpesvirus
HIV — human immunodeficiency virus
HPF — high-power field
HPV — human papillomavirus
HRS cell — Hodgkin/Reed–Sternberg cell
HRS-like cell — Hodgkin/Reed–Sternberg–like cell
HSCT — haematopoietic stem cell transplantation
IARC — International Agency for Research on Cancer
ICD-11 — International Classification of Diseases, 11th revision

ICD-O — International Classification of Diseases for Oncology
Ig — immunoglobulin
INPC — International Neuroblastoma Pathology Classification
INRG — International Neuroblastoma Risk Group
InSiGHT — International Society for Gastrointestinal Hereditary Tumours
IPNHLSS — International Pediatric Non-Hodgkin Lymphoma Staging System
IRSG — Intergroup Rhabdomyosarcoma Study Group
ITD — internal tandem duplication
kb — kilobase
kDa — kilodalton
KSHV/HHV8 — Kaposi sarcoma–associated herpesvirus / human herpesvirus 8
lincRNA — long intervening/intergenic non-coding RNA
LP cell — lymphocyte-predominant cell
M:F ratio — male-to-female ratio
MALT lymphoma — extranodal marginal zone lymphoma of mucosa-associated lymphoid tissue
MIM number — Mendelian Inheritance in Man number
MITF — melanocyte-inducing transcription factor
MRI — magnetic resonance imaging
MSI — microsatellite instability
N:C ratio — nuclear-to-cytoplasmic ratio
NER — nucleotide excision repair
NK cell — natural killer cell
NMDAR — N-methyl-D-aspartate receptor
NOS — not otherwise specified
NSAID — non-steroidal anti-inflammatory drug
NSE — neuron-specific enolase
NWTS — National Wilms Tumor Study
Pap — Papanicolaou stain
PAS staining — periodic acid–Schiff staining
PASD — periodic acid–Schiff staining with diastase
PCR — polymerase chain reaction
PET — positron emission tomography
PHITT — Paediatric Hepatic International Tumour Trial
PR — progesterone receptor
PTGC — progressively transformed germinal centre
RT-PCR — reverse transcription polymerase chain reaction
SEER Program — Surveillance, Epidemiology, and End Results Program
SIOP — International Society of Paediatric Oncology
SNP — single-nucleotide polymorphism
SNV — single-nucleotide variant
SPM — second primary malignancy
SV — structure variant
TFH cell — T follicular helper cell
TKD — tyrosine kinase domain
TKI — tyrosine kinase inhibitor
TME — tumour microenvironment
TNM — tumour, node, metastasis
UICC — Union for International Cancer Control
UV — ultraviolet

# Foreword

The WHO Classification of Tumours, published as a series of books (also known as the WHO Blue Books) and now as a website (https://tumourclassification.iarc.who.int), is an essential tool for standardizing diagnostic practice worldwide. It also serves as a vehicle for the translation of cancer research into practice. The diagnostic criteria and standards that make up the classification are underpinned by evidence evaluated and debated by experts in the field. About 400 authors and editors participated in the production of this volume, and they give their time freely to this task. I am very grateful for their help; it is a remarkable international team effort of great significance to both patients and their doctors.

This volume of the fifth edition of the WHO Blue Books is in a sense a first edition: it is the first time that the WHO Classification of Tumours has included a separate volume on paediatric tumours. This has been a considerable challenge for all involved. The volume covers all the systems of the body and must be coordinated with the other volumes in the series, so it has taken nearly 2 years to produce. Along the way we have had many excellent scientific discussions, and I hope that the final product meets with your approval. Classifications evolve with time, and there will be an opportunity in the next edition to make changes on the basis of new evidence. It is important to note that the chapter on haematolymphoid disorders has been coordinated with a relatively early version of the forthcoming fifth-edition WHO Classification of Tumours *Haematolymphoid tumours* volume, and there may be some differences as a result of this, as well as differences in the paediatric equivalents of adult tumour types.

This volume, like the rest of the fifth edition, has been led by the WHO Classification of Tumours Editorial Board, composed of standing and expert members. The standing members, who have been nominated by pathology organizations, are the equivalent of the series editors of previous editions. The expert members for each volume, equivalent to the volume editors of previous editions, are selected on the basis of informed bibliometric analysis and advice from the standing members. The diagnostic process is increasingly multidisciplinary, and we are delighted that several radiology and clinical experts have joined us to address specific needs.

The most conspicuous change to the format of the books in the fifth edition is that tumour types common to multiple systems are dealt with together – so there are separate chapters on haematolymphoid disorders and germ cell tumours. There is also a chapter on genetic tumour syndromes. Genetic disorders are of increasing importance to diagnosis in individual patients, and the study of these disorders has undoubtedly informed our understanding of tumour biology and behaviour over the past decade.

We have attempted to take a more systematic approach to the multifaceted nature of tumour classification; each tumour type is described on the basis of its localization, clinical features, epidemiology, etiology, pathogenesis, histopathology, diagnostic molecular pathology, staging, and prognosis and prediction. We have also included information on macroscopic appearance and cytology, as well as essential and desirable diagnostic criteria. This standardized, modular approach makes it easier for the books to be accessible online, but it also enables us to call attention to areas in which there is little information, and where serious gaps in our knowledge remain to be addressed.

**Table A** Approximate number of fields per 1 mm² based on the field diameter and its corresponding area

| Field diameter (mm) | Field area (mm²) | Approximate number of fields per 1 mm² |
| --- | --- | --- |
| 0.40 | 0.126 | 8 |
| 0.41 | 0.132 | 8 |
| 0.42 | 0.138 | 7 |
| 0.43 | 0.145 | 7 |
| 0.44 | 0.152 | 7 |
| 0.45 | 0.159 | 6 |
| 0.46 | 0.166 | 6 |
| 0.47 | 0.173 | 6 |
| 0.48 | 0.181 | 6 |
| 0.49 | 0.188 | 5 |
| 0.50 | 0.196 | 5 |
| 0.51 | 0.204 | 5 |
| 0.52 | 0.212 | 5 |
| 0.53 | 0.221 | 5 |
| 0.54 | 0.229 | 4 |
| 0.55 | 0.237 | 4 |
| 0.56 | 0.246 | 4 |
| 0.57 | 0.255 | 4 |
| 0.58 | 0.264 | 4 |
| 0.59 | 0.273 | 4 |
| 0.60 | 0.283 | 4 |
| 0.61 | 0.292 | 3 |
| 0.62 | 0.302 | 3 |
| 0.63 | 0.312 | 3 |
| 0.64 | 0.322 | 3 |
| 0.65 | 0.332 | 3 |
| 0.66 | 0.342 | 3 |
| 0.67 | 0.352 | 3 |
| 0.68 | 0.363 | 3 |
| 0.69 | 0.374 | 3 |

The organization of the WHO Blue Books content now follows the normal progression from benign to malignant – a break with the fourth edition, but one we hope will be welcome.

The volumes are still organized by anatomical site (digestive system, breast, soft tissue and bone, etc.), and each tumour type is listed within a taxonomic classification that follows the format below, which helps to structure the books in a systematic manner:

**Site:** e.g. central nervous system

    **Category:** e.g. gliomas, glioneuronal tumours, and neuronal tumours

        **Family (class):** e.g. paediatric-type diffuse high-grade gliomas

            **Type:** e.g. infant-type hemispheric glioma

                **Subtype:** e.g. infant-type hemispheric glioma, NTRK-altered

The issue of whether a given tumour type represents a distinct entity rather than a subtype continues to exercise pathologists, and it is the topic of many publications in the literature. We continue to deal with this issue on a case-by-case basis, but we believe there are inherent rules that can be applied. For example, tumours in which multiple histological patterns contain shared truncal mutations are clearly of the same type, despite the differences in their appearance. Equally, genetic heterogeneity within the same tumour type may have implications for treatment. A small shift in terminology in the fifth edition is that the term "variant" in reference to a specific kind of tumour has been wholly superseded by "subtype", in an effort to more clearly differentiate this meaning from that of "variant" in reference to a genetic alteration.

Another important change in this edition of the WHO Classification of Tumours series is the conversion of mitotic count from the traditional denominator of 10 HPF to a defined area expressed in $mm^2$ {1484}. This serves to standardize the true area over which mitoses are enumerated, because different microscopes have high-power fields of different sizes. This change will also be helpful for anyone reporting using digital systems. The approximate number of fields per 1 $mm^2$ based on the field diameter and its corresponding area is presented in Table A.

We are continually working to improve the consistency and standards within the classification. In addition to having moved to the International System of Units (SI) for all mitotic counts, we have standardized genomic nomenclature by using Human Genome Variation Society (HGVS) notation. This includes the recent move in fusion gene notation to the separation of involved genes by a double colon (e.g. *BCR::ABL1*) {911}. We have also standardized our use of units of length, adopting the convention used by the International Collaboration on Cancer Reporting (https://www.iccr-cancer.org/) and the UK Royal College of Pathologists (https://www.rcpath.org/), so that the size of tumours is now given exclusively in millimetres (mm) rather than centimetres (cm). This is clearer, in our view, and avoids the use of decimal points – a common source of medical errors.

The WHO Blue Books are much appreciated by pathologists and of increasing importance to practitioners of other clinical disciplines involved in cancer management, as well as to researchers. The editorial board and I certainly hope that the series will continue to meet the need for standards in diagnosis and to facilitate the translation of diagnostic research into practice worldwide. It is particularly important that cancers continue to be classified and diagnosed according to the same standards internationally so that patients can benefit from multicentre clinical trials, as well as from the results of local trials conducted on different continents.

Dr Ian A. Cree

Head, WHO Classification of Tumours Programme
International Agency for Research on Cancer

December 2022

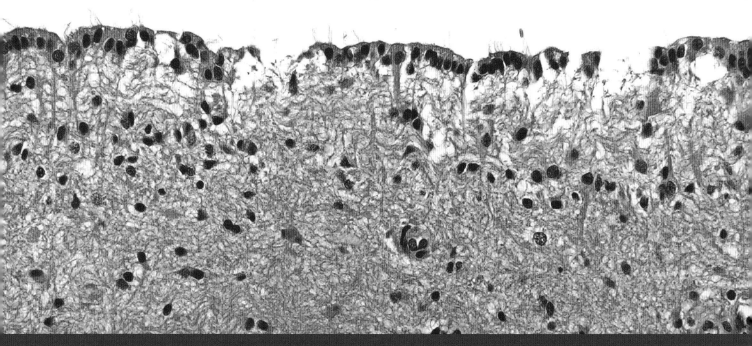

# 7

# Germ cell tumours

Edited by: Cheung AN, Moch H, Reyes-Múgica M, Srigley JR

Germ cell tumours
  Non-invasive germ cell neoplasia
    Intratubular germ cell neoplasia (male gonadal)
    Gonadoblastoma
  Germinoma-family tumours
    Germinoma/dysgerminoma/seminoma
  Non-germinomatous germ cell tumours
    Mature cystic teratoma
    Extragonadal teratoma
    Monodermal teratomas (female gonadal)
    Immature teratoma (female gonadal)
    Prepubertal-type testicular teratoma
    Postpubertal-type teratoma
    Embryonal carcinoma
    Yolk sac tumour
    Fetus in fetu
    Choriocarcinoma (non-gestational)
    Malignant mixed germ cell tumours

# Germm cell tumours: Introduction

Reyes-Múgica M
Looijenga LHJ
Oosterhuis JW
Srigley JR
Tsuzuki T

Germ cell tumours are a seemingly heterogeneous group of neoplasms occurring at various anatomical locations in both female and male patients, and affecting neonates, infants, adolescents, and (young) adults. From a developmental perspective, germ cell tumours appear to derive from cells across a continuum of maturation, from early embryonic cells to progressively maturing germ cells. Although predominantly localized in the gonads, they can also occur at extragonadal sites, particularly in patients aged < 6 years, usually along the midline of the body. This is explained by the migration of primordial germ cells during embryogenesis {5198}.

A crucial mechanism in the pathogenesis of germ cell tumours is the illicit activation (reprogramming) of the latent developmental programme of non-neoplastic germ cells, whereby migrating primordial germ cells may escape their normal fate of apoptosis. This explains why most germ cell tumours are benign. However, owing to genomic instability, they are prone to progression, most often towards yolk sac tumour and/or somatic-type malignancy. The only germ cell tumours that are malignant per se are the germinoma-family tumours and derived non-seminomas. Even these are rarely initiated by driver mutations. Their malignant behaviour is due to the ability of the late primordial germ cell, from which they are derived, to survive in the gonadal and defined extragonadal surrogate niches in the thymus and the midline of the brain. From there, they may progress to the known germinoma-family precursor lesions: germ cell neoplasia in situ of the testis, gonadoblastoma of the dysgenetic gonad/ovary, and a similar lesion in the thymus. Their progression is, by default, along the germinoma-family lineage, which subsequently, upon reprogramming, may give rise to non-seminomas.

Differentiating between teratomas with similar morphologies poses a diagnostic challenge, particularly in the ovary and testis. In uncertain cases, a germinoma family–derived malignant teratoma must be ruled out by molecular means.

# Intratubular germ cell neoplasia (male gonadal)

Looijenga LHJ
Oosterhuis JW
Stoneham SJ

## Definition
Germ cell neoplasia in situ (GCNIS) is the common precursor of seminoma and non-seminoma, which are type II testicular germ cell tumours (TGCTs). It consists of neoplastic gonocytes with latent totipotent (naïve) developmental potential, located as strings of beads in the spermatogonial niches of seminiferous tubules.

## ICD-O coding
9064/2 Intratubular germ cell neoplasia (male gonadal)

## ICD-11 coding
2C80.2 & XH8AD3 Germ cell tumour of testis & Intratubular malignant germ cells

## Related terminology
*Not recommended:* carcinoma in situ of the testis; intratubular germ cell neoplasia, unclassified; testicular intraepithelial neoplasia.

## Subtype(s)
None

## Localization
GCNIS occurs in the postpubertal testis. In patients with disorders of sex development it may be found in the prepubertal testis.

## Clinical features
Adults with isolated GCNIS are usually symptomless or present with mild testicular pain and relatively small testes (6–12 mL) {647,2717,1952,6040}. GCNIS is bilateral in 4–5% of cases {7330,1746}. About 80% show a heterogeneous ultrasound pattern, sometimes due to microlithiasis {2956,1617,1952}. GCNIS diagnosis requires a testicular biopsy in suspected cases. It may be detected in ejaculate by immunocytology {4581,2931, 7190,198}.

## Epidemiology
GCNIS and the invasive type II germ cell tumours originating from it share epidemiological associations and risk factors. The risk of GCNIS is increased in developmental reproductive disorders, in which gonocytes, failing to differentiate into spermatogonia, become the source of GCNIS cells {5738,6511}. The highest risk is seen in disorders of sex development, in which the GBY region, containing *TSPY1*, is involved; in those conditions the prevalence of GCNIS can reach 70% {1429,6528, 7204,3435,7322}. The risk is also increased (with a prevalence as high as 5%) in the testicular dysgenesis syndrome {6512, 6513,5738}, which groups overlapping anomalies such as cryptorchidism {3722}, hypospadias, and some forms of infertility {5048,5158,5973}, and in the contralateral testis of patients with unilateral type II TGCT {7330,1746}.

## Etiology
The etiology of GCNIS can be inferred from studies on gonadal dysgenesis and type II TGCT {5199}. In brief, GCNIS and derived germ cell tumours have a developmental origin, in which mutations play a minor role; these mutations most often affect *KIT*, its negative regulator *CBL*, and downstream KRAS and NRAS signalling pathways {6399}. These mutations may be initiating, but more often they drive progression {5198,1800}. Type II TGCTs have a strong familial component due to dozens of low-penetrance recessive gene variants (discovered in

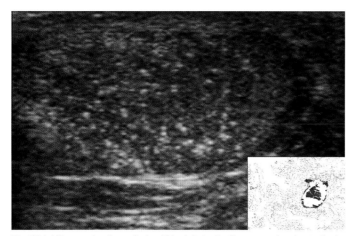

**Fig. 7.01** Ultrasound pattern of microlithiasis in testis. Sonogram showing testicular microlithiasis with numerous intratesticular echogenic foci, 1–2 mm in diameter. This speckled appearance is characteristic of testicular microlithiasis. **Inset:** Microscopy of microlith.

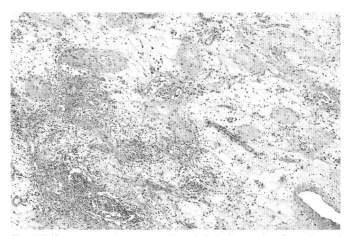

**Fig. 7.02** Host response clears germ cell neoplasia in situ over time. Parenchyma of seminoma in an elderly patient. The host response has almost completely wiped out the seminoma. It has also virtually cleared germ cell neoplasia in situ from the tubules, which have become entirely fibrotic in the process.

Chapter 7

genome-wide association studies), in particular in *KITLG* {5780, 3403}, involved in germ cell development, sex determination {3759}, DNA repair, apoptosis, and centrosome function, among other processes {7433}. A high dose of these variants leads to familial clustering of cases {7433}. In concert with internal and environmental hormone disruptors {5737,5741} they cause disturbances in testicular development and in the maturation of gonocytes to spermatogonia.

## Pathogenesis

Disturbed maturation of gonocytes is characterized by the aberrant expression of embryonic markers (in particular the pluripotency protein OCT4 {4206,7322}) and early differentiation markers (in particular TSPY {3958,3957}) in gonocytes relocating from the centre of the developing tubules to the spermatogonial niches {2966}. Persistent OCT4 expression in centrally located gonocytes beyond 6 months of age signifies delayed maturation. Failure to downregulate OCT4 expression, which leads to its coexpression with TSPY in gonocytes relocated to the niches in a heterogeneous pattern, is consistent with pre-GCNIS. KITLG then usually shows focal, patchy expression in the testis {5200, 3435,1427}. (Notably, in androgen insensitivity syndromes, the development of pre-GCNIS is associated with a *KITLG* variant {1432}.) Expansion of gonocytes homogeneously expressing OCT4, not always in combination with TSPY {7322}, in multiple pre-spermatogonial niches, as the beginning of a string of beads, characterizes the earliest manifestation of GCNIS {3435}. The nuclei of these cells may be enlarged and angular due to tetraploidization {5193,2382}. KITLG is diffusely expressed in a testis containing GCNIS {6719}. Delayed maturation and pre-GCNIS may be diagnosed in biopsies from cryptorchid testes at infancy {5200}. GCNIS is variably detected in prepubertal individuals with disorders of sex development {3435,7322} but is otherwise highly unlikely to occur prepubertally {4208}.

By the acquisition of specific chromosome copy-number variations, in particular overrepresentation of 12p {4205,5984,5252, 196} and the increased expression (and sometimes amplification) of *KIT* {4521}, GCNIS cells become independent from the spermatogonial niches. This enables them to float within the tubules and form intratubular and ultimately invasive seminoma, which is the default developmental outcome of GCNIS. Reprogramming of a GCNIS or intratubular seminoma cell {5196, 5195} results in an embryonal carcinoma cell, the stem cell of non-seminoma, which is the neoplastic counterpart of a naïve, totipotent human embryonic stem cell {5199}, thus giving rise to intratubular non-seminoma.

The phenomenon of reprogramming has been demonstrated in the TCam-2 seminoma cell line {1621} in vivo {4969} and in vitro {4968,4967}, whereby OCT4 switches partner from SOX17 to SOX2 as demonstrated in human tumour specimens {1620}. Reprogramming is initiated by the inhibition of BMP {4968} and requires the expression of SOX2 {4967}. Thus, it is in fact the reversal of germline specification that induces primordial germ cells in the early embryo upon BMP signalling, whereby OCT4 switches partner from SOX2 to SOX17 {3138,3706}.

## Macroscopic appearance

There is no specific macroscopic pattern.

## Histopathology

GCNIS consists of atypical cells resembling gonocytes with ample clear cytoplasm and large (10–11 μm) angulated nuclei with (usually) one nucleolus and coarse chromatin, typically located in the niche of spermatogonia, in one layer resembling a string of beads. This pattern can be recognized at low power; however, reliable diagnosis of GCNIS requires immunohistochemistry {7189}. GCNIS is usually a disperse, patchy process, in which the number of affected tubules may vary from few to all {647,1746,7188}. It is virtually always present in the testicular parenchyma surrounding a type II TGCT {3187,5194,3955}. Isolated GCNIS may be found in the workup of male infertility {6510} and in contralateral biopsies in cases of a clinically unilateral type II TGCT {1746}. It can be the only neoplastic manifestation in the testis of a patient with a burnt-out type II TGCT who presents with metastases (most often retroperitoneal) {5195, 2194,4524,6646}.

Often the GCNIS cells are stacked in layers and float in the lumen of the seminiferous tubules. Seminiferous tubules with

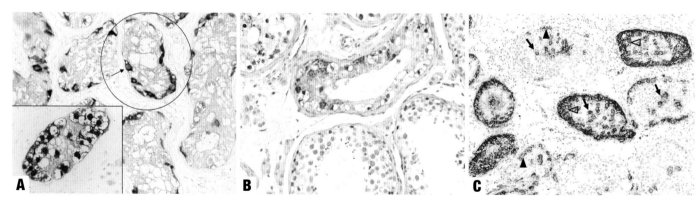

**Fig. 7.03** Intratubular germ cell neoplasia (male gonadal). **A** Early germ cell neoplasia in situ. The encircled tubule shows within the spermatogonial niches a clonal expansion of germ cells with enlarged nuclei (arrow), coexpressing OCT4 (nuclear, brown) and TSPY (membranous, blue), arranged as the beginning of a string of beads, characterizing this lesion as early germ cell neoplasia in situ. The other tubules show germ cells in the niches expressing TSPY with and without OCT4. The morphology in these tubules is still compatible with pre–germ cell neoplasia in situ. **Inset:** For comparison, full-blown germ cell neoplasia in situ is shown, in which all tumour cells express OCT4 (and in this case also TSPY, but this is not essential). **B** Testicular germ cell neoplasia in situ. KITLG is diffusely expressed, mostly (but not exclusively) in a granular pattern in the Sertoli cells of tubules containing germ cell neoplasia in situ. **C** Floating germ cell neoplasia in situ cells. Progression to independence from Sertoli cells allows germ cell neoplasia in situ cells to leave the spermatogonial niches, get stacked in multiple layers (open arrowheads), float within the tubules (arrows), and colonize adjacent normal tubules (solid arrowheads) by reoccupying spermatogonial niches,

GCNIS may contain trophoblastic giant cells in as many as 20% of cases, virtually always in combination with seminoma with trophoblastic giant cells {633}. Via the spermatogonial niches, GCNIS cells can spread in a pagetoid manner into neighbouring normal tubules, entrapping and replacing spermatogonia, whereby spermatogenesis is disturbed. Pagetoid spread of GCNIS cells into the rete testis is common. It follows the plane between rete epithelium and basement membrane, and it can be so extensive that clusters of GCNIS cells cause polypoid bulging of the rete epithelium. The tumour cells in the rete are in situ and do not worsen the prognosis {7288}. Floating GCNIS cells can colonize remote tubules and be released in seminal fluid. Testicular parenchyma surrounding GCNIS may show normal morphology or changes of testicular dysgenesis: clusters of maldeveloped tubules with undifferentiated Sertoli cells, a Sertoli cell–only pattern, intratubular microliths, and occasionally branching tubules {2932,6901}. In parenchyma adjacent to seminoma, infiltrates of lymphocytes are invariably present, particularly around and in GCNIS tubules. They cause tubular atrophy and fibrosis {5194,3085} comparable to the fibrosis of burnt-out seminoma.

Ongoing accumulation of GCNIS cells in the lumina of seminiferous tubules results in intratubular seminoma. It typically expands the tubules, and ultimately breaches their walls. Like invasive seminoma it contains lymphocytes. The tubules are often also surrounded by lymphocytic infiltrates. Intratubular seminoma is found in about 30% of seminoma specimens and 15% of non-seminoma specimens {5194,3955}. Intratubular non-seminoma is virtually always composed of pure embryonal carcinoma, which is usually largely necrotic and calcified. Differentiation into other components only starts upon invasion {5195,6229}. Intratubular non-seminoma is confined to parenchyma surrounding non-seminomas, occurring in about 15% of testicular germ cell tumours {5194,3955}. It is most frequently associated with small tumours, suggesting that larger tumours overgrow and obscure their intratubular precursor {5194}.

The amount of GCNIS decreases with age – particularly in parenchyma adjacent to a seminoma or a seminoma component, where it may completely disappear, probably owing to the host response towards seminoma that also targets GCNIS.

*Immunohistochemistry*
The immunoprofiles of gonocytes, GCNIS, and seminoma are similar {5735,5892}. The protein markers absent in normal spermatogonia include PLAP {940}, OCT4 {4206,5736, 3325,1619}, SOX17 {1620}, AP-2γ {2934}, NANOG {2930,2731, 4966}, LIN28A {7508,2425}, and podoplanin {6587}. KIT {5740}, although expressed in spermatogonia {767,690}, is useful because it is overexpressed in GCNIS and seminoma {4521}. Enzyme reactivity of alkaline phosphatase is utilized to diagnose GCNIS on frozen sections {6720} during operation, to assist in testis-sparing surgery. Immunoreactions may vary depending on the fixatives used and the origin of the antibodies. However, heterogeneity of expression may also be due to genuine maturation-dependent variations {5739,3334,4715}. The overall DNA epigenetic profile of GCNIS is hypomethylation {7503,4970, 3793,3792} also at the histone level {200}. The genome-wide transcriptomes of GCNIS and gonocytes are nearly identical and in addition to the markers listed above include numerous other embryonic and germ cell–specific genes {197,6586}.

*Differential diagnosis*
In the infantile and prepubertal testis, GCNIS should be distinguished from normal and delayed-matured gonocytes and from pre-GCNIS; in the postpubertal testis, it should be distinguished from arrested spermatogonia, intratubular seminoma, and intratubular non-seminoma. The morphological criteria are described above. Crucially, a reliable diagnosis of GCNIS requires immunohistochemistry {7189}.

Extensive pagetoid involvement of the rete testis may lead to the erroneous diagnosis of a non-seminoma combining teratoma (simulated by rete epithelium) and seminoma.

Absence of GCNIS in a postpubertal testis with teratoma must raise suspicion of a type I teratoma, a benign tumour {7827, 1583}.

## Cytology
The cytology of GCNIS is similar to that of seminoma.

## Diagnostic molecular pathology
Not relevant

## Essential and desirable diagnostic criteria
*Essential:* neoplastic gonocytes located as strings of beads in the spermatogonial niches of seminiferous tubules; positive immunohistochemistry for SOX17, AP-2γ, NANOG, LIN28A, and podoplanin; the gonocytes must stain for OCT4 and PLAP.

## Staging
By definition, GCNIS is staged as pTis {7288}.

## Prognosis and prediction
Approximately 90% of GCNIS cases will progress to an overt TGCT within 7 years {7330}. In some cases the interval may be as long as 15–20 years {1745}.

# Gonadoblastoma

Reyes-Múgica M
González-Peramato P
Stoneham SJ
Ulbright TM

## Definition
Gonadoblastoma is an in situ form of malignant germ cell tumour consisting of germ cell neoplasia in situ (GCNIS) / seminoma / dysgerminoma cells and incompletely differentiated sex cord cells reminiscent of Sertoli/granulosa cells.

## ICD-O coding
9073/1 Gonadoblastoma

## ICD-11 coding
2C73.Y & XH0K61 Other specified malignant neoplasms of the ovary & Gonadoblastoma

2F76 & XH0K61 Neoplasms of uncertain behaviour of female genital organs & Gonadoblastoma

2F77 & XH0K61 Neoplasms of uncertain behaviour of male genital organs & Gonadoblastoma

## Related terminology
*Not recommended:* dysgenetic gonadoma.

## Subtype(s)
None

## Localization
Gonads

## Clinical features
Most patients present as neonates with ambiguous genitalia in the setting of a disorder of sex development (DSD) {1428, 3000,7139}, although occasional patients do not present until their fourth decade of life {6309}. Approximately 50% of cases appear in virilized female patients, 30% in non-virilized female patients, and 20% in male patients with hypospadias and an empty scrotum {6309,7287}. A common initial presentation in young women is primary amenorrhoea {7139}. Advanced presentations usually feature an abdominal mass.

## Epidemiology
Although gonadoblastomas are almost always associated with DSDs {5050,5051,6011}, a subset occur in patients with no apparent DSD and normal peripheral blood karyotypes {6012}. As many as 60% of dysgenetic gonads develop gonadoblastoma {6309,3000,1428,7139}. Frequent entities associated with gonadoblastoma include 46,XY pure gonadal dysgenesis (bilateral streak gonads), mixed gonadal dysgenesis, ovotesticular DSD, Turner syndrome (see below), and androgen insensitivity syndrome {5050,5051}. Gonadoblastoma is bilateral in about 33–40% of cases {6309,7139,628}.

## Etiology
Mutations (many hereditary) leading to DSDs cause gonadoblastoma {3158,4335,6366}. DSDs are caused by abnormalities in genes implicated in the 46,XY developmental pathway, including *SRY, SOX9, WT1*, and *NR5A1* {1426,1428,4203}. Multiple genes may be affected in a single patient {2872}. An essential element is the presence of the GBY region of the Y chromosome, including the candidate gene encoding TSPY {7092,3958}. Abnormalities in this pathway result in immature sex cord cells instead of normal Sertoli cells. This undervirilized environment causes the delayed development of the embryonic germ cells, allowing coexpression of embryonal and early differentiation genes, particularly *POU5F1* (which encodes OCT3/4) and *TSPY1* {1431,3534}. This, combined with enhanced KIT/

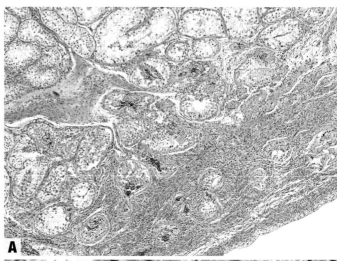

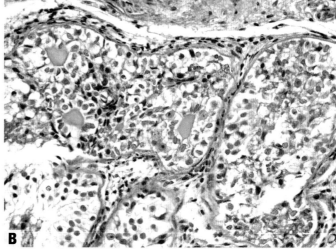

**Fig. 7.04** Gonadoblastoma in a dysgenetic gonad. **A** Dysgenetic testis from a 4-year-old girl with a disorder of sex development and 45,X/46,XY mosaicism in whom a gonadoblastoma is starting to develop. Note the dysplastic testicular cords/tubules and an early focus of gonadoblastoma in the centre left. **B** A closer view of the developing gonadoblastoma in the same case. Note the basement membrane hyaline deposits and nests of two cellular populations (germ cells and sex cord cells).

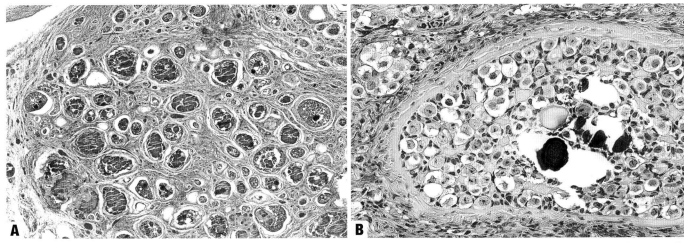

**Fig. 7.05** Gonadoblastoma. **A** Low-power view of a gonadoblastoma in a streak gonad shows the characteristic small nests in a cellular stroma. This case shows extensive calcifications, some with a mulberry-like configuration. **B** High-power view of a gonadoblastoma shows the three components: germ cells (most resembling those of germ cell neoplasia in situ), sex cord cells, and round deposits of basement membrane matrix. A dissecting pattern is at the top, mimicking a focus of invasive germinoma.

KITLG signalling {6719}, promotes the neoplastic transformation of germ cells into GCNIS-like cells. Concurrent GCNIS and gonadoblastoma have been reported within a single gonad, indicating an underlying DSD {2871,4094}. Patients with germline or somatic mutations in *WT1* (Denys–Drash and Frasier syndromes) or *SRY* (Swyer syndrome) feature dysgenetic gonads and gonadoblastomas {2640}. As many as 35% of patients with Turner syndrome with Y-chromosomal material (which may be cryptic) develop gonadoblastomas {7819,1467}, as do about 5% of those with androgen insensitivity syndrome {3026,3267}.

## Pathogenesis

Most patients with gonadoblastoma feature a female phenotype. However, their gonads carry Y chromosome material and show either a dysgenetic/dysplastic testicular histology (20%) or streak gonad appearance (20%) {6309}. Because the genetic male developmental pathway is faulty, or androgen effects are deficient, SOX9 expression is insufficient to support the normal

formation of seminiferous cords and Sertoli cells, leading to a predominance of FOXL2 {2869,925} and causing a delay in germ cell maturation, with the expression of OCT3/4 and TSPY, which together with KIT/KITLG signalling seems to promote neoplastic transformation.

## Macroscopic appearance

Gonadoblastomas range from soft to firm; they are brown, yellow, or grey in appearance, and they measure as large as 80 mm. They often show multifocal calcification. If they progress to invasive germ cell tumours, they show soft, grey nodules {7139,6011}.

## Histopathology

Like all blastomas, gonadoblastoma recapitulates the developmental process of its organ of origin. Gonadoblastomas feature round nests and cords composed of germ cells, small sex cord cells, and globoid deposits of hyaline basement membrane material in variable proportions. The germ cells have large nuclei, one or more prominent nucleoli, and pale/clear cytoplasm. Many resemble GCNIS or seminoma/dysgerminoma cells; others appear as spermatogonia. Mitotic figures can be seen. The sex cord cells show angulated, sometimes grooved nuclei; they are similar to Sertoli cells and may also show Charcot–Böttcher crystals {3149,6013}. The germ cells are scattered between the sex cord cells, which may form palisades at the periphery of nests, rosettes around the basement membrane deposits, or circular arrays around the germ cells. The basement membrane material frequently develops laminated calcifications, resembling psammoma bodies, with occasional coalescence to form mulberry-like structures. Rarely, calcifications can be so extensive as to obliterate the cellular detail (burnt-out gonadoblastoma). Scattered Leydig-like cells may be present in adjacent gonadal stroma. The immunophenotype includes PLAP, KIT (CD117), and podoplanin staining in the germ cells; inhibin, nuclear SOX9 (weak), and FOXL2 (strong) in the sex cord cells; and inhibin plus calretinin in Leydig-like cells. Gonadoblastoma is a precursor of invasive germ cell tumours. Depending on the degree of development in the dysgenetic gonad, the lesion may develop into a GCNIS or gonadoblastoma. Infiltration by the neoplastic germ cells into the surrounding stroma may result in any of the usual types of germ

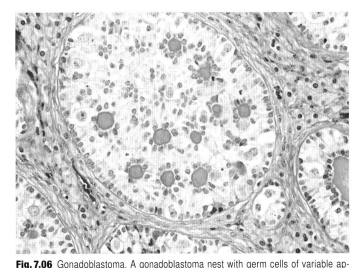

**Fig. 7.06** Gonadoblastoma. A gonadoblastoma nest with germ cells of variable appearance, ranging from spermatogonia-like cells to cells resembling those of germinoma/dysgerminoma/seminoma, incompletely differentiated sex cord cells, and round hyaline material. The surrounding spindle cell gonadal stroma contains Leydig-like or lutein-like cells.

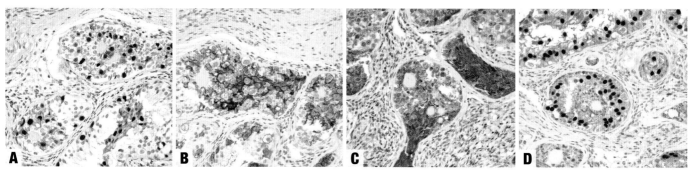

**Fig. 7.07** Gonadoblastoma. **A** Germ cells of gonadoblastoma showing nuclei positive for OCT3/4. **B** Germ cells of gonadoblastoma showing membranous staining for PLAP. **C** Sex cord cells of gonadoblastoma showing positive staining for inhibin. **D** Sex cord cells of gonadoblastoma showing positive nuclear staining for SOX9.

cell tumour, most frequently seminoma/dysgerminoma. The differential diagnosis in fetuses and neonates includes the lesion known as fetal gonadoblastoid testicular dysplasia {6610,3059, 5052}, and in postpubertal patients, Sertoli cell nodules colonized by GCNIS. Immunohistochemistry facilitates their distinction, because Sertoli cell nodules are negative for FOXL2 and strongly positive for SOX9 {3417}. Gonadoblastoma seems to originate from surviving OCT3/4-positive germ cells within undifferentiated gonadal tissue {1430} present in dysgenetic gonads, which may precede the development of fully recognizable gonadoblastoma. The morphological features of undifferentiated gonadal tissue overlap with what Scully called "dissecting gonadoblastoma", which is present in approximately 75% of cases. In these areas the neoplastic cells adopt a cord-like pattern {3415}.

## Cytology
Not relevant

## Diagnostic molecular pathology
FISH analysis may be useful to demonstrate the Y chromosome in tissues or other materials (urine) of phenotypically female patients {628} (see also *Pathogenesis* and *Etiology*, above).

## Essential and desirable diagnostic criteria
*Essential:* a nested to corded arrangement of germ cells (similar to that seen in germinoma/dysgerminoma/seminoma) and small sex cord cells with deposits of basement membrane material; immunopositivity for OCT3/4 and PLAP.
*Desirable:* background of a DSD; germ cells positive for podoplanin; sex cord cells coexpressing SOX9 (weak) and FOXL2 (strong), inhibin, calretinin and SF1.

## Staging
Gonadoblastoma is an in situ malignancy and is staged as pTis according to the eighth-edition American Joint Committee on Cancer (AJCC) and Union for International Cancer Control (UICC) system.

## Prognosis and prediction
Given the potential of gonadoblastoma to transform into an invasive germ cell tumour, gonadectomy is recommended in all cases. Surgical excision and bilateral gonadectomy result in cure of the tumour and prevention of contralateral gonadoblastoma. In cases that have progressed to an invasive tumour, staging and prognosis vary accordingly.

# Germinoma/dysgerminoma/seminoma

Bode PK
Looijenga LHJ
Stoneham SJ
Wong TT

## Definition

Germinomas, dysgerminomas, and seminomas are malignant germ cell tumours whose cells are considered the neoplastic counterparts of primordial germ cells. Despite different clinical manifestations and anatomical localization, they share the same morphology, immunophenotype, and molecular phenotype.

## ICD-O coding

9061/3 Seminoma
9061/3 Seminoma with syncytiotrophoblast cells
9060/3 Dysgerminoma
9060/3 Dysgerminoma with syncytiotrophoblast cells
9064/3 Germinoma
9064/3 Germinoma with syncytiotrophoblast cells

## ICD-11 coding

2A00.1Y & XH1E13 Other specified embryonal tumours of brain & Germinoma
2C73.1 Dysgerminoma of ovary
2C80.27 & XH9FM4 Germ cell tumour of testis & Seminoma, NOS
2C80.25 Mixed seminoma and non-seminomatous germ cell tumour of testis

## Related terminology

*Acceptable:* testicular germinoma; ovarian germinoma; gonadal germinoma; mediastinal germinoma; intracranial germinoma.

## Subtype(s)

Germinoma/dysgerminoma/seminoma with syncytiotrophoblast cells

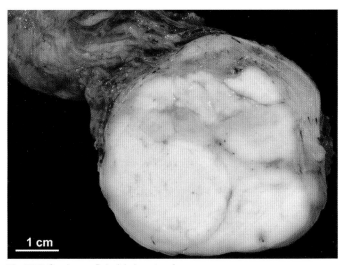

**Fig. 7.09** Seminoma. Pale, lobular cut surface.

## Localization

The nomenclature for germinoma/dysgerminoma/seminoma (GDS) varies with site. In gonads, the same tumour type is known as "dysgerminoma" in the ovary and "seminoma" in the testis. At extragonadal sites, the term "germinoma" is preferred.

Like all human germ cell tumours, GDSs occur not only in the gonads but also in extragonadal sites along the migratory pathway of primordial germ cells {5198}, especially in the retroperitoneal and mediastinal regions and in the midline of the brain {353,6255}. GDSs never develop in the sacrococcygeal region {6255}.

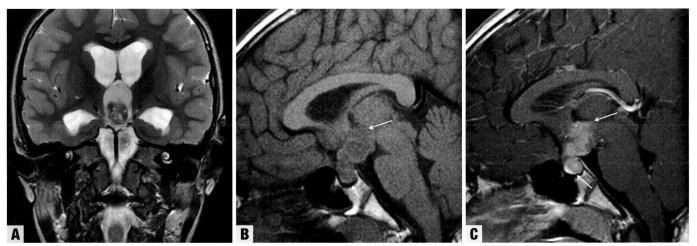

**Fig. 7.08** Germinoma. **A** MRI showing a sellar germ cell tumour. **B** T1-weighted sagittal MRI shows a poorly defined heterogeneous isointense to hypointense mass (extent marked by the two arrows) at the sellar and suprasellar region. Note the loss of the normal T1 bright spot of the posterior pituitary gland. **C** Contrast-enhanced T1-weighted sagittal MRI shows moderate enhancement of the tumour, the extent of which is shown by the two arrows.

In the CNS, typical sites include the pineal region (most commonly), followed by the suprasellar compartment (in the neuro-hypophysial/infundibular stalk) and the basal ganglia / thalamus {6841,6843}. Sites less frequently affected are the cerebrum, posterior fossa structures, spinal cord, and sella. The tumours can be bifocal or multifocal. Bifocal/multifocal examples are nearly all pure germinomas {6841}. Germinomas can grow as diffuse periventricular lesions {3799}.

## Clinical features

Clinical manifestations usually result from mass effect and depend on the anatomical location. Uncommon paraneoplastic syndromes may be seen in patients with GDS {7763} and

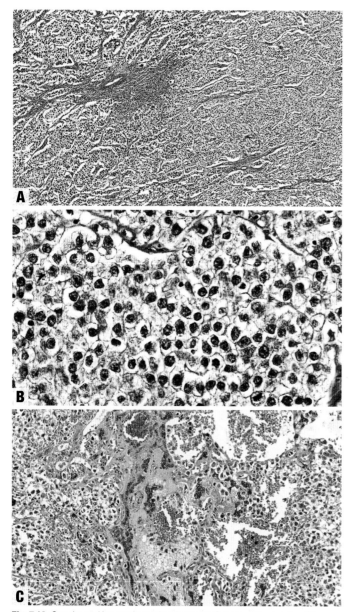

**Fig. 7.10** Germinoma/dysgerminoma/seminoma. **A** Overview showing the diffuse arrangement of pale cells interrupted by fibrovascular septa containing lymphocytes. **B** High-power view showing tumour cells with clear cytoplasm, crisp cytoplasmic membranes, and polygonal nuclei. **C** This example shows admixed multinucleated syncytiotrophoblast cells.

include hypercalcaemia {1516,4117}, polycythaemia {3371, 5837}, autoimmune haemolytic anaemia {4265}, exophthalmos {4378,6925}, limbic or brainstem encephalopathy {607,953, 7571}, and membranous glomerulonephritis {6254}.

*Brain:* Tumours in the pineal region compress the cerebral aqueduct, causing hypertensive hydrocephalus, and can produce paralysis of vertical and convergent eye movement (Parinaud syndrome) by compressing or invading the tectal plate. Posterior pituitary / suprasellar lesions produce visual disturbances by impinging on the optic chiasm, and they often cause diabetes insipidus, delayed growth, and delayed sexual maturation by disrupting the hypothalamic–pituitary axis. Germ cell tumours that produce β-hCG can cause precocious puberty in boys and also (rarely) in girls {5178,6650}.

*Testis:* Generally, patients are postpubertal and present with a testicular mass, sometimes associated with localized pain. About 3% of patients present with symptoms secondary to metastatic disease – usually lower back pain attributable to the involvement of retroperitoneal lymph nodes. Patients who present with metastatic disease typically have smaller testicular tumours, and there may be a large disparity between the size of the testicular tumour and the metastatic tumour. Usually, seminoma metastasizes initially to retroperitoneal lymph nodes, with subsequent involvement of the mediastinal and cervical (particularly left supraclavicular) lymph nodes. Visceral involvement (liver and lungs) typically develops only later in the disease course. Surprisingly, despite its marked tendency to spread by the lymphatic route, seminoma is the most common testicular germ cell tumour to metastasize to bone {851}.

*Ovary:* Dysgerminomas are usually rapidly growing tumours, which may come to clinical attention as a huge abdominal mass, occasionally with abdominal pain. Bilateral involvement is seen in 10–15% of cases {2499}. Some tumours may be clinically misdiagnosed as pregnancy, owing to their size and the clinical signs of a space-occupying lesion (loss of appetite, nausea, heartburn, constipation, etc.) {2370}. More than 50% are confined to the ovary {960,1643}. However, because of the high rate of undetected micrometastases in the retroperitoneal lymph nodes, recurrence may occur {960}, indicating that some dysgerminomas might initially be under-staged {4368}.

*Mediastinum:* GDSs usually occur in the anterior mediastinum and are typically associated with the thymus {7481}. The majority (75%) are very large and symptomatic at diagnosis. They can manifest with chest pain, dyspnoea, cough, weight loss, and/or superior vena cava syndrome {768}.

### Serum markers

Serum AFP levels are not markedly elevated in patients with pure GDS {2423}. Elevated AFP levels indicate the presence of a non-GDS component (yolk sac tumour [YST]) {3233}. Serum β-hCG is slightly increased in 10–20% of tumours with admixed syncytiotrophoblast cells {5907,6066,5127,768}; it may even reach 200 mIU/mL {5127}. Serum LDH is increased in about 80% of patients with advanced-stage disease {2193}, although it is less sensitive and specific than AFP and β-hCG {2423}.

### Epidemiology

In general, GDS is extremely rare in children aged < 5 years {6255}. Exceptions may be seen in patients with disorders of sex

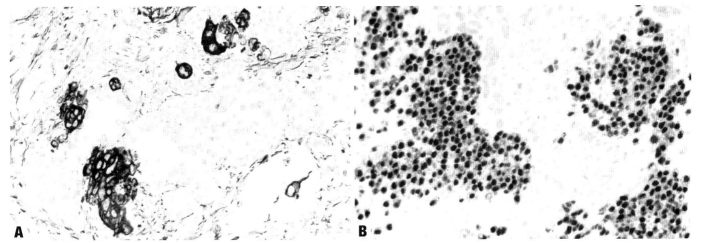

**Fig. 7.11** Germinoma/dysgerminoma/seminoma with syncytiotrophoblast cells. **A** β-hCG staining highlights clusters of syncytiotrophoblast cells. The germinoma/dysgerminoma/seminoma tumour cells are negative. **B** OCT3/4 staining highlights the germinoma/dysgerminoma/seminoma tumour cells. The syncytiotrophoblast cells are negative.

development {7287,1426,4387,6198} and Down syndrome {1427}, who may develop seminoma or dysgerminoma. Overall, the age spectrum varies depending on the anatomical localization.

The majority (as many as two thirds) of CNS germ cell tumours are germinomas. The M:F ratio is 3–4:1. The incidence of CNS germinoma peaks at 11–15 years (median patient age: 18.1 years) {6841,2432}. CNS germ cell tumours are more prevalent in eastern Asia than in Europe and the USA. Age-adjusted annual incidence rates of 0.45 cases per 100 000 population aged < 15 years and 0.49 cases per 100 000 population aged < 19 years have been reported from Japan {4338} and the Republic of Korea {3407}, respectively. These rates (the highest recorded) are more than three times as high as those reported in Germany {3358} and the USA {5240}.

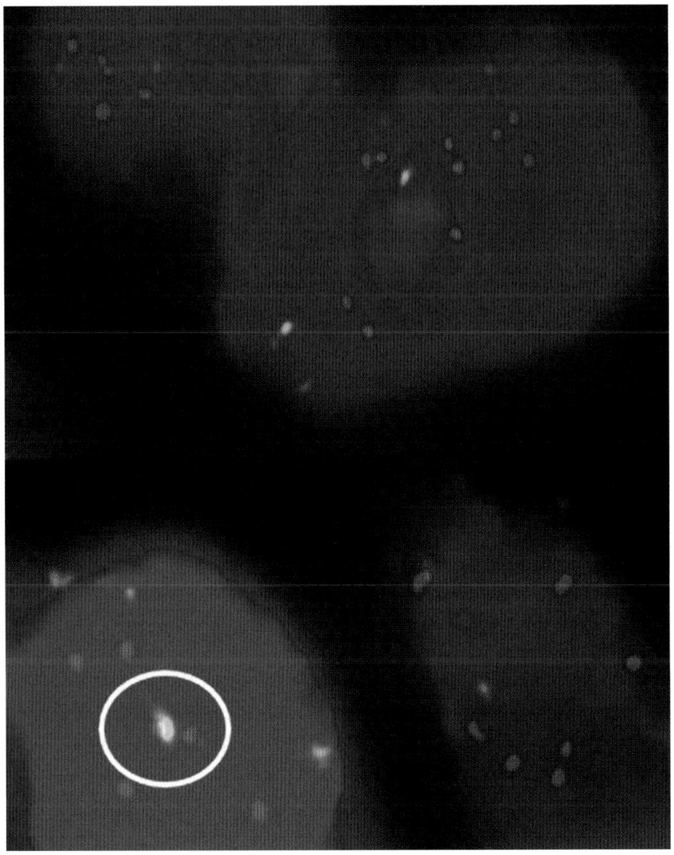

In contrast to their counterparts in the brain, pure GDSs at other sites usually occur after puberty {353}.

Seminoma accounts for about 50% of testicular germ cell tumours and occurs at a mean age of 37–41 years {3772,7334} and not before puberty {353,6255}, except in children with a disorder of sex development {635,963}. Seminoma generally has the same epidemiological and etiological factors as all germ cell tumours derived from germ cell neoplasia in situ. However, higher proportions of seminomas have been noted in patients with non-corrected cryptorchidism {2676,2081,7425} or immunodeficiency disorders {4032} than in the general population.

In the ovary, the equivalent of seminoma is called dysgerminoma. It accounts for one third of malignant germ cell tumours {6538} and predominantly arises in adolescents and young adults (peak incidence between the ages of 15 and 20 years) {353,3969}. Because of the predominance of dysgerminomas in the fertile age range, they are frequently discovered during pregnancy {6260,2383}. Dysgerminoma can develop from gonadoblastoma and is typically associated with a disorder of sex development {6310,7139,6309,2873}.

Pure GDSs are the second most common germ cell tumours in the mediastinum after teratomas {4784,6845}. Typically, patients are male and aged 11–79 years, but most patients are diagnosed in their third or fourth decade of life {353,4784, 6845}. Although Klinefelter syndrome was identified in as many as 20% of male patients with primary mediastinal germ cell tumour {5003,1724}, it is almost always associated with a non-GDS germ cell tumour {7327}.

### Etiology

See *Germ cell tumours: Introduction* (p. 648) and *Intratubular germ cell neoplasia (male gonadal)* (p. 649).

### Pathogenesis

See *Germ cell tumours: Introduction* (p. 648) and *Intratubular germ cell neoplasia (male gonadal)* (p. 649).

**Fig. 7.12** Postpubertal germ cell tumour. FISH showing 12p gain and isochromosome 12p (circle).

**Table 7.01** Usual patterns of immunoreactivity in testicular germ cell tumours and metastatic carcinoma, with markers listed alphabetically and the reported proportions of positive tumours shown in parentheses

| Marker | GCNIS | Seminoma | Embryonal carcinoma | Yolk sac tumour | Chorio-carcinoma | Teratoma | Spermatocytic tumour | Metastatic carcinoma | Other positive tumours |
|---|---|---|---|---|---|---|---|---|---|
| AE1/AE3 | – | ± (20–36%) | + (95%) | + | + | + | – | + | Many |
| AFP | – | – | ± (8–33%) | + (74–100%) | – | ± | – | ± | Hepatocellular neoplasms, hepatoid carcinomas, occasional other non–germ cell tumours |
| AP-2γ (TFAP2C) | + | + | ± (67%) | – | + | – | – | ± | Many carcinomas |
| CD30 (Ki-1, BerH2) | – | – | + (84–93%) | – | – | – | – | ± | Lymphoma, nasopharyngeal carcinoma, benign and malignant mesenchymal tumours, melanoma, (rarely) carcinomas |
| CK7 | ± | ± | + | – | + | + | ND | ± | Many carcinomas (not usually of colon or prostate), some sarcomas (e.g. synovial sarcoma, epithelioid angiosarcoma) |
| DMRT1 | – (< 2%) | ± (8%) | – | ND | ND | – | + (90%) | ± | Prostate carcinoma |
| EMA | – | – | – (2%) | – (5%) | ± (46%) | + | – | + | Many carcinomas, synovial sarcoma |
| GPC3 | – | – | – (5%) | + (100%) | + (80%)ᵃ | ± (17%) | ND | ± | Syncytiotrophoblasts, hepatocellular and gastric cancers |
| KIT (CD117) | +ᵇ | + (100%) | – | ± (59%) | – | – | ± (41–100%) | ± | Various tumours of epithelial and mesenchymal differentiation |
| MAGEA4 | + (87%) | + (74%) | – | ± (47%) | (rare) | – | + (100%) | ± | Many carcinomas, melanoma, CNS tumours, gastrointestinal stromal tumours |
| NANOG | + (100%) | + (100%) | + (100%) | – | – | – | – | – | Gliomas, some carcinomas |
| OCT3/4 (POU5F1, OCT3, OCT4) | + (100%) | + (100%) | + (100%) | – | – | – | – | – | Rare non-small cell lung cancer, clear cell renal carcinoma, large cell lymphomas |
| PLAP | + | + (90–100%) | + (79–86%) | ± (1–85%) | + | – | – | ± | Numerous adenocarcinomas (of colon, ovary, endometrium, etc.) |
| Podoplanin (D2-40, M2A) | + | + | – (29%)ᶜ | – | – | ± | – | ± | Gliomas, meningiomas, mesothelial tumours, lymphatic tumours, some adenocarcinomas |
| SALL4 | + | + (100%) | + (100%) | + (100%) | ± (69%)ᵈ | ± (52%) | + | ± | Haematological malignancies, rhabdoid tumour, nephroblastoma (also called Wilms tumour), gastrointestinal adenocarcinoma, other high-grade carcinomas |
| SOX17 | + | + (95%) | – | ± (50%) | – | ± | ND | ND | ND |
| SOX2 | – | – (< 1%) | + (96%) | – | – | ± | ND | ND | Neuroectodermal elements in teratoma, melanoma, rhabdoid tumour |
| β-hCG | – | – | – | – | + (100%)ᵃ | – | – | ± | Other trophoblastic tumours, syncytiotrophoblasts in germ cell tumours, some non–germ cell tumours |

–, usually negative; +, usually positive; ±, variable staining; GCNIS, germ cell neoplasia in situ; GPC3, glypican-3; ND, no data.
ᵃSyncytiotrophoblasts > mononucleated trophoblasts. ᵇNormal spermatogonia may be positive. ᶜCell apices only. ᵈMononucleated trophoblasts only.

## Macroscopic appearance

Most GDSs are solid, relatively homogeneous, often lobulated, pale-grey to tan or pale-yellow nodules that on cut surface bulge above the surrounding parenchyma. Foci of necrosis and haemorrhage may be present but are usually not extensive. They have a soft texture.

## Histopathology

Most commonly, there is a diffuse arrangement of pale cells interrupted by fibrovascular septa containing lymphocytes. The tumour cells characteristically have pale to clear cytoplasm, crisp cytoplasmic membranes, and polygonal nuclei with finely granular chromatin and frequently flattened edges. One or more large, centrally located nucleoli are present. The abundant cytoplasm results in relatively evenly spaced, non-overlapping nuclei in most cases. The cytoplasmic clarity is attributable to abundant glycogen particles that are demonstrable with the PAS stain. Less commonly, the cytoplasm is denser and the nuclei more crowded. This may result in a plasmacytoid appearance. Several morphological patterns may occur, including corded growth, microcystic, and tubular-like patterns {7135}, plus signet-ring cell change {7140}. Mitotic activity and necrosis are variable. A variably prominent lymphocytic infiltrate occurs in almost every case {1749,6688}. A granulomatous reaction, present in more than half of the cases, most commonly appears as small clusters of epithelioid cells, but occasional multinucleated giant cells may be seen. In rare cases, the granulomatous reaction may be so pronounced that the underlying tumour is largely effaced {3725}.

In seminoma, intertubular growth, particularly at the periphery of the tumour, is common and infrequently predominant {2840}. Intratubular growth with tubular expansion is designated intratubular seminoma. Germ cell neoplasia in situ is found in the residual seminiferous tubules in > 85% of cases {1370,5194}.

GDSs express antigens characteristic of immature, fetal-type germ cells (gonocytes) (see Table 7.01), including KIT (CD117) (in 90–100% of cases; cytoplasmic/membranous staining) {3177,4047,3107,2314}, OCT3/4 (100%; nuclear) {3324, 4206,5894,2425,2773,1245}, SALL4 (100%; nuclear) {3107, 1019,5065,1018}, and SOX17 (95%; nuclear) {753,1620,5073}. Podoplanin is also positive (100%; cytoplasmic/membranous) {3107,1159,3956}. Cytokeratin AE1/AE3 immunoreactivity varies (20–36%) {1263,5012,4694} but is frequently negative or stains the cytoplasm of only a minority of tumour cells, often in a paranuclear dot-like pattern. CD30 is characteristically negative, as is EMA (2%). Stains for AFP are always negative {7138}. Although PLAP is positive in seminoma (86–95%; cytoplasmic/membranous) {941,3188}, it is also expressed by other germ cell tumour components, such as embryonal carcinoma and YST {3756,4371,719,2920}.

GDS with syncytiotrophoblast cells is a subset of tumours containing admixed syncytiotrophoblast cells that vary from widely scattered individual cells to prominent aggregates {4814, 7331}. The cells are characteristically multinucleated, with the nuclei sometimes producing mulberry-like clusters, often associated with small foci of haemorrhage. These cells can be highlighted by β-hCG or broad cytokeratin immunostaining, which correlates with β-hCG serum levels.

GDS may be a component in a mixed germ cell tumour.

Syncytiotrophoblastic elements expressing hPL and β-hCG may be found and should not prompt the diagnosis of choriocarcinoma. Tumours with such components must be reported as GDS with syncytiotrophoblast cells.

### Differential diagnosis

Seminoma may be mistaken for solid-pattern embryonal carcinoma. The well-defined cytoplasmic membranes, more regular and less crowded nuclei, fibrous septa, and more frequent and prominent lymphocytic infiltrate of seminoma contrast with the findings in most embryonal carcinomas. Staining for KIT (CD117), podoplanin, and SOX17, as well as an absence of CD30, SOX2, and cytokeratin AE1/AE3 expression, also support a diagnosis of seminoma versus embryonal carcinoma. Solid YST may resemble seminoma but is usually differentiated by its admixture with other YST patterns, less prominent lymphocytic infiltrate, and absence of fibrous septa. Its negative staining with OCT3/4, expression of AFP and glypican-3 (GPC3), and strong immunoreactivity for cytokeratin AE1/AE3 contrast with the immunoprofile of seminoma. Lymphoma may be distinguished from GDS by its more irregular nuclear contours and expression of lymphoid markers. Testicular lymphoma features a more prominent intertubular growth and lacks germ cell neoplasia in situ.

## Cytology

In smear and squash preparations, large tumour cells with delicate, vacuolated cytoplasm and prominent nucleoli are admixed with small lymphocytes {4990,3280}. A tigroid extracellular background may be appreciated in material examined with Giemsa staining or related methods {4990}. This is particularly useful for excluding lymphoma, which lacks the tigroid extracellular background. A pseudopapillary arrangement of tumour cells can be encountered in squash preparations {389}.

## Diagnostic molecular pathology

Molecular analyses are virtually never necessary. The diagnosis is usually established by morphology. Immunohistochemistry may help in difficult cases. Nevertheless, GDSs harbour 12p alterations (isochromosome 12p, 12p gains), which are typical for all type II germ cell tumours {5152,6762,6947,1450,394,1087, 6780,4207}. Mutations of oncogenes do occur in germinomas, but their percentage depends on the anatomical localization. KIT is most frequently mutated, followed by KRAS and NRAS. The percentage of mutations is low in testicular seminoma (20%) {1511,6399,4150,6932}, whereas it is about 50% in ovarian dysgerminomas {2870,2933,7220} and in mediastinal GDSs {5660}, and as high as 80% in CNS germinomas {2260,7408, 6282}. Because KIT mutations in GDSs are mostly detected in exon 17, unlike in gastrointestinal stromal tumours where they occur in exons 11 and 9, GDSs do not respond to targeted therapy with imatinib {1902}.

## Essential and desirable diagnostic criteria

*Essential:* identification of large tumour cells with typical cytological characteristics.

*Desirable (in selected cases):* confirmation by immunohistochemistry (positive for OCT3/4, KIT, D2-40; negative for CD30 or AFP; no diffuse staining for cytokeratins).

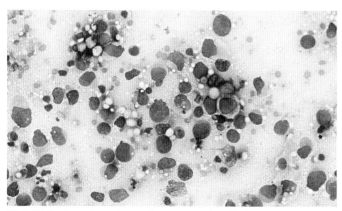

**Fig. 7.13** Cytology of germinoma. Smear preparation with large tumour cells in a homogeneous and tigroid background.

## Staging

Different classification systems exist depending on the anatomical location, although a poor concordance between paediatric and adult classification systems has been reported {2221}.

*Testis:* Staging follows the Union for International Cancer Control (UICC) TNM classification of germ cell tumours of the testis and the Children's Oncology Group (COG) staging system for germ cell tumours.

*Ovary:* Staging follows the UICC TNM system and the FIGO classification of tumours of the ovary.

*Brain:* A combination of radiological and cytological staging workup is recommended in the Delphi consensus for the management of intracranial germ cell tumours {4871}.

*Mediastinum:* For metastatic and mediastinal germ cell tumours, risk stratification is done according to the International Germ Cell Consensus Classification (IGCCC) {668,3130}.

## Prognosis and prediction

### Testis

The overall prognosis is excellent but stage-dependent. Clinical stage I disease cases, managed by surveillance protocols, adjuvant radiation, or single-agent chemotherapy, achieve a 95–98% overall 5-year survival rate {3320,5164}. Approximately 80% of patients with clinical stage I disease under surveillance do not require additional treatment after orchiectomy {4424}, a growing treatment trend in this group {2965}.

Indicated predictors of relapse on surveillance are primary tumour size (> 40 mm, but a definitive cut-off is controversial) and rete testis stromal (but not pagetoid) infiltration {2965}. For patients with advanced-stage disease (TNM stages IIC–IIIC), the disease-specific survival with cisplatin-based chemotherapy is 83% {2387}. An adverse prognostic finding in the advanced-stage group is the occurrence of non-pulmonary visceral metastases {2195}.

### Ovary

The prognosis for dysgerminoma is excellent. The overall survival rate reaches almost 100% with surgery only in localized tumours, and adjuvant platinum-based chemotherapy is recommended for advanced tumours {1842,6360}.

### Mediastinum

Long-term disease-free survival is achieved in about 90% of cases treated with cisplatin-based chemotherapy. Although most patients treated with primary radiotherapy are cured, the distant recurrence rate is high, and the 5-year disease-free survival rate is only 60–67% {768}.

### Brain

Pure CNS germinomas (curable by irradiation or chemoradiotherapy) show 10-year survival rates of about 90% {6841,4480, 982}. Comparable rates of control have been achieved with appropriate radiation dosing {5127,6415} and combined radiochemotherapy {6841} of germinomas harbouring syncytiotrophoblastic elements or associated with elevated β-hCG levels in the serum or cerebrospinal fluid. Some series have shown that atypical locations (e.g. basal nuclei / thalamus), evidence of chromosomal instability {6841}, and high intratumoural levels of macrophage-derived NOS2 are negative prognostic indicators {6842}, whereas conspicuous immune cell infiltration and high levels of CD4 expression may carry positive implications {6842}.

# Non-germinomatous germ cell tumours: Introduction

Looijenga LHJ

Within the germ cell tumours (see *Germ cell tumours: Introduction*, p. 648), the teratoma family represents a special group. Unlike the other non-seminomatous tumours, teratomas have variable clinical characteristics, although they all are composed of one or multiple histological elements of the embryonic germ layers: ectoderm, mesoderm, and endoderm. Their classification is predominantly determined by their anatomical localization, including various extragonadal sites, as well as the ovary and testis (see Table 7.02). Overarching patterns can be recognized, related to the specific maturation stage of the cell of origin. Because of the different stages and timing of the development of female and male (embryonic) germ cells, the repertoires of teratoma types diagnosed in the ovary and in the testis differ in their behaviours, with those in the testis having an overall benign behaviour, and those in the ovary having a dual pattern (related to prepubertal vs postpubertal diagnosis). Most of the extragonadal teratomas represent the (overall benign) prepubertal type.

**Table 7.02** Classification and occurrence of paediatric germ cell tumours: organizational framework (continued on next page)

| Morphological category | Pathogenetic category | Usual anatomical sites |
|---|---|---|
| **Intratubular germ cell neoplasia family** | II | T |
| GCNIS | | |
| Intratubular seminoma | | |
| Intratubular embryonal carcinoma | | |
| Other rare intratubular patterns | | |
| **Germinoma family** | II | |
| Germinoma | | C |
| Dysgerminoma | | O |
| Seminoma | | T, M |
| **Non-germinoma family** | | |
| Embryonal carcinoma subfamily | II | T, O, C, M |
| Teratoma subfamily | | |
| • GCNIS-independent (prepubertal) teratoma | I | T |
| • GCNIS-associated (postpubertal) teratoma | II | T |
| • Ovarian mature teratoma | IV, I | O |
| • Ovarian immature teratoma | IV, I | O |
| • Non-gonadal teratoma | I | C, M, other |
| • Monodermal teratoma | | T, O |
| • Teratoma with somatic malignancy | I, II, IV | T, O, C, M |
| Trophoblastic subfamily | | |
| • Choriocarcinoma | II | T, O, C, M |
| • Non-choriocarcinomatous trophoblastic tumour | II | T |
| ° Placental site trophoblastic tumour | | |
| ° Epithelioid trophoblastic tumour | | |
| ° Cystic trophoblastic tumour | | |

C, CNS; GCNIS, germ cell neoplasia in situ; M, multiple; n/a, not applicable; O, ovary; T, testis.

**Table 7.02** Classification and occurrence of paediatric germ cell tumours: organizational framework (continued)

| Morphological category | Pathogenetic category | Usual anatomical sites |
|---|---|---|
| Yolk sac subfamily | | |
| • Prepubertal-type yolk sac tumour | I | T, O, C, M |
| • Postpubertal-type yolk sac tumour | II | T, O, C, M |
| **Mixed germ cell tumour family** | | |
| Mixed germinoma and non-germinoma subfamily | II | T, O, C, M |
| Mixed non-germinoma subfamily | | |
| • Mixed teratoma and yolk sac tumour (prepubertal type; GCNIS-independent) | I | T, O, C, M |
| • Mixed non-germinomatous germ cell tumour (postpubertal type; GCNIS-associated) | II | T, O, C, M |
| ° Special patterns (polyembryoma, diffuse embryoma) | | |
| **Mixed germ cell and sex cord stromal tumour family** | n/a | |
| Gonadoblastoma | | |
| Mixed germ cell / sex cord stromal tumour NOS | n/a | |

C, CNS; GCNIS, germ cell neoplasia in situ; M, multiple; n/a, not applicable; O, ovary; T, testis.

# Mature cystic teratoma

Vang R
Stoneham SJ
Ulbright TM

## Definition
Mature cystic teratoma is a tumour composed exclusively of mature tissue derived from two or three germ layers (ectoderm, mesoderm, and/or endoderm). In the testis, mature cystic teratoma is a subtype of prepubertal-type teratoma.

## ICD-O coding
9080/0 Teratoma, benign

## ICD-11 coding
2F32.Y & XH3GV5 Other specified benign neoplasm of ovary & Teratoma, benign
2F34 & XH52Q4 Benign neoplasm of male genital organs & Teratoma, prepubertal type

## Related terminology
*Not recommended:* dermoid cyst; mature solid teratoma.

## Subtype(s)
None

## Localization
Mature cystic teratomas occur in extragonadal sites (including the sacrococcygeal region, mediastinum, head and neck, retroperitoneum, CNS, and various sites within the abdominal cavity), as well as in the ovary and testis.

## Clinical features
In the testis, mature cystic teratoma is a type I germ cell tumour.
Teratomas occur from birth through the third decade of life, but they can also occur after this period. Presentation with

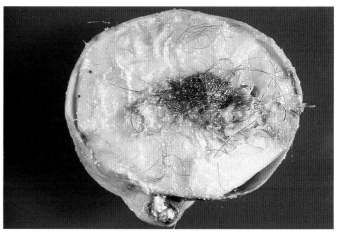

**Fig. 7.15** Mature cystic teratoma. Gross specimen showing cut surface with abundant sebaceous material and hair.

abdominal pain or a mass is common; some are incidentally detected. Congenital anomalies may be associated with sacrococcygeal teratomas {1672}. Rarely, patients with ovarian teratomas may present with anti-NMDAR encephalitis {1517,1345, 5070}. About 10% of ovarian tumours are bilateral {5485,6016, 6313}.

The average age of paediatric patients with mature cystic teratoma of the testis is 1.5–2.5 years, but older children and adults may also be affected {117,1335,4594,7827}. Virtually all cases come to clinical attention as testicular masses discovered by parents/patients or on physical examination. Ultrasound typically shows cystic and solid components with internal calcifications and heterogeneous echogenicity {1162,1970}.

## Epidemiology
Sacrococcygeal teratoma is the most common germ cell tumour in children, and the ovary is the second most common site in this age group {1672}. The majority of paediatric germ cell tumours are mature cystic teratomas {2719,1672,4156,7764, 113}. A small subset of cases may have metachronous disease or a familial association.

Unlike the postpubertal-type teratoma of the testis, mature cystic teratoma has no distinct epidemiological associations, although there are suggestive reports of a link to Klinefelter syndrome and a familial predisposition, supporting a genetic role {6904,2632,6448}. These tumours did not have the marked rise in incidence during the 20th and early-21st centuries seen in testicular postpubertal-type (type II) germ cell tumours {5737, 5026}; rather, their incidence was stable and much lower {3058, 7375,7661}.

## Etiology
Unknown

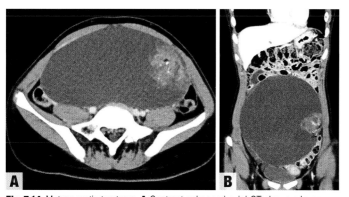

**Fig. 7.14** Mature cystic teratoma. **A** Contrast-enhanced axial CT shows a large cystic mass with a focal enhancing soft tissue protuberance, known as the Rokitansky nodule. Within the nodule, there are multiple foci of calcification and a focus of very low density suggestive of fat. **B** Contrast-enhanced coronal reformatted CT shows a large cystic mass in the central abdomen displacing the bowel loops. There is a focal Rokitansky nodule containing multiple internal foci of calcifications. Additional foci of very low density suggestive of a fat component are also evident within the mass.

Chapter 7

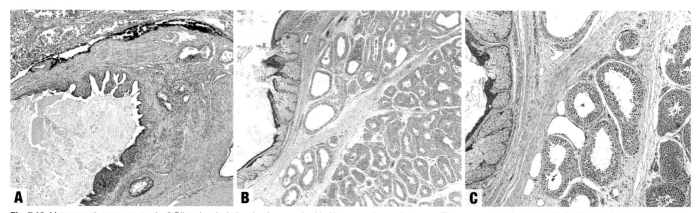

**Fig. 7.16** Mature cystic teratoma, testis. **A** Dilated and tubular glands are embedded in a smooth muscle stroma. There was no cytological atypia in this prepubertal-type teratoma from a teenage boy. **B** A stratified squamous epithelial lining with associated pilosebaceous units lines a cyst. The adjacent testis of this teenage boy shows normal seminiferous tubules. **C** Higher-magnification view of the same case.

## Pathogenesis

The favoured explanation is the parthenogenetic theory, which suggests an origin from primordial germ cells {4131,4132,5782, 5362,6557}. For the majority of ovarian cases, studies support a derivation from post-meiotic I or pre-meiotic II germ cells {7335, 4130,4131}.

In testicular sites, there is an absence of the genetic abnormalities seen in germ cell neoplasia in situ (GCNIS)-derived teratomas, including isochromosome 12p {7827,963,4812}. High-throughput DNA methylation analyses support the notion that the originating germ cell has a partially erased pattern of genomic imprinting {6480,5893}.

## Macroscopic appearance

Most teratomas are cystic (mature cystic teratoma) but some can be solid. Their size is variable, ranging from < 50 to 300 mm. The cysts may contain sebaceous and keratinous material, hair, and sometimes teeth or cartilage. A solid nodule lined by hair-bearing skin (Rokitansky protuberance) is typically present along the cyst lining in ovarian teratomas. Mature cystic teratomas may be solid with interspersed cysts {7573,5484}. Those resembling a malformed human fetus have been termed "fetiform teratoma" {11}. Solid areas should be liberally sampled (ideally, 1 section per 10 mm of solid area).

## Histopathology

Ectodermal derivatives include squamous epithelium and cutaneous adnexal structures, as well as neuroectoderm (glia, ependyma, and cerebellum). Mesodermal derivatives include adipose tissue, bone, cartilage, and smooth muscle. Endodermal derivatives include gastrointestinal and respiratory/bronchial epithelium, thyroid, and salivary glands. Rarely, prostate {2667}, pituitary, adrenal, and parathyroid tissue can be seen. Rare microscopic foci of immature neuroectodermal tissue may be present {7694}. Fat necrosis and foreign body reaction to keratin are common. In patients with anti-NMDAR encephalitis, neuroglial tissues are surrounded by lymphoid aggregates with germinal centres {5070,1517}.

All elements in testicular sites lack marked atypia, and the surrounding parenchyma lacks GCNIS as well as the dysgenetic features {7827,5049} seen in GCNIS-derived / postpubertal-type teratoma.

## Cytology

Not clinically relevant

## Diagnostic molecular pathology

Not clinically relevant

## Essential and desirable diagnostic criteria

*Essential:* mature tissue representing ≥ 2 germ layers.

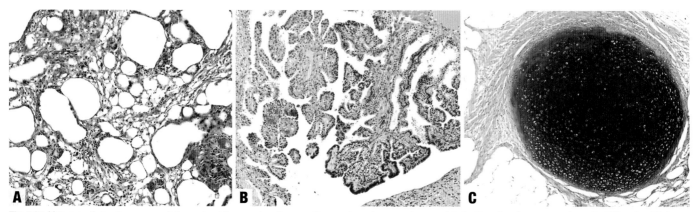

**Fig. 7.17** Mature cystic teratoma, ovary. **A** A prominent lipogranulomatous reaction, as shown here, can be associated with ruptured squamous elements. **B** The choroid plexus, as in this example, may be associated with glial components. **C** A nodule of cartilage is noted adjacent to smooth muscle and adipose tissue.

*Desirable:* in the testis, all elements lack atypia, GCNIS, and the dysgenetic tubules seen in GCNIS-derived / postpubertal-type teratoma.

## Staging

Not clinically relevant

## Prognosis and prediction

These are typically benign except in rare instances of concurrent malignant transformation and rare cases of development of immature teratoma in residual ovary after partial excision of a mature cystic teratoma (associated with cyst rupture) {7694}. Furthermore, paediatric teratomas in critical anatomical sites, such as the CNS, pericardium, or mediastinum, can cause death by local effects {1672}. The presence of rare microscopic foci of immature neuroectodermal tissue in a mature teratoma is associated with an excellent outcome and does not merit overall classification as immature teratoma {7694}. Gliomatosis peritonei can occur in patients with mature cystic teratoma but does not adversely affect prognosis {5913}. Of note, testicular mature cystic teratoma is benign, in contrast to postpubertal-type teratomas {7827}.

# Extragonadal teratoma

Bode PK
Jacques TS
Srigley JR
Stoneham SJ

## Definition

Pure extragonadal teratomas consist of tissue components of the three germ cell layers and occur predominantly in neonates and infants. They arise along the migratory path of primordial germ cells.

## ICD-O coding

None

## ICD-11 coding

2A00.1Y & XH83G5 Other specified embryonal tumours of brain & Teratoma, NOS

2F36.3 & XH83G5 Teratoma of orbit & Teratoma, NOS

2F71.3 & XH5MG2 Immature teratoma of the lung & Neoplasms of uncertain behaviour of trachea, bronchus, or lung

2F71.0 & XH2KP9 Immature teratoma of the thymus & Neoplasms of uncertain behaviour of thymus

2F7A.Y & XH5PC3 Immature teratoma of thyroid & Other specified neoplasms of uncertain behaviour of endocrine glands

## Related terminology

*Acceptable:* teratoma, prepubertal type; germ cell tumour type I; congenital teratoma.

## Subtype(s)

Sacrococcygeal teratoma

## Localization

The sacrococcygeal area is the most common site, followed by the head and neck, CNS, and mediastinum {2808,2721}.

## Clinical features

Congenital teratoma manifests in utero, usually during the second trimester. Sonography reveals a solid or mixed cystic and solid mass {7565}. Large lesions (> 100 mm) are associated with an increased risk of fetal demise and a high perinatal mortality {596}. Rapidly growing tumours can cause a vascular steal phenomenon with consecutive fetal hydrops, especially when the tumour is detected before the thirtieth week of gestation {776,834,2805}.

Depending on their anatomical extension, sacrococcygeal teratomas (SCTs) can be classified into different types (see Table 7.03). Type IV teratomas are diagnosed later in infancy than teratomas with external components and are frequently associated with yolk sac tumour (YST) foci {5850, 5851}.

In neonates, serum levels of AFP are physiologically elevated at least for the first 6–8 months of life {7637,735} and do not necessarily correlate with the presence of YST components {2808}. After tumour resection, AFP levels usually decrease slowly but continuously {509}.

## Epidemiology

Extragonadal teratoma typically affects prepubertal patients {2808,2721}. SCT constitutes 40–50% of extragonadal type I germ cell tumours and is one of the most common congenital tumours, with a reported incidence of 3.7–7.1 cases per 100 000 live births and an M:F ratio of 1:3–4 {6646,6805,5851, 6275,5405,2678}. Beyond the age of 6 months, the incidence of pure teratoma decreases, whereas the frequency of YST rises {6255}. In postpubertal patients, pure teratoma is rare; in this age group teratomas are typically components of mixed germ cell tumours {6255}.

## Etiology

SCTs are normally sporadic but can also be part of the autosomal dominant inherited Currarino triad (anorectal malformation, sacral agenesis, presacral mass) {1508}.

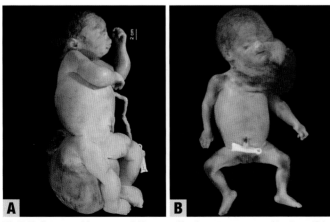

**Fig. 7.18** Extragonadal teratoma. **A** Neonate with a large sacrococcygeal teratoma. **B** Induced abortion of a fetus with a rapidly growing cervical teratoma (22nd gestational week).

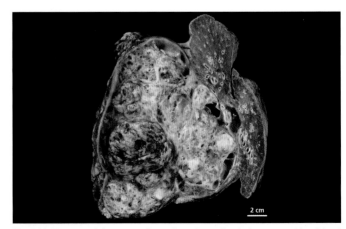

**Fig. 7.19** Extragonadal teratoma. Cut surface of a mediastinal teratoma with solid and cystic areas.

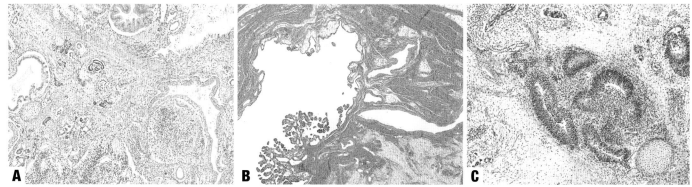

**Fig. 7.20** Extragonadal teratoma. **A** Histology from a mediastinal teratoma in a premature newborn (29th gestational week) showing various tissue types (respiratory and intestinal epithelium, acinic proliferations, a small cartilage island, and a few predominantly immature neuroepithelial elements). **B** Histology from a resected sacrococcygeal teratoma in a newborn showing mature elements (brain tissue, a cyst with papillary epithelial proliferation, and fat tissue islands, in a dense collagenous stroma). **C** Histology from a sacrococcygeal teratoma in a fetus (25th gestational week) showing a focus of immature neuroepithelial tissue.

## Pathogenesis

The postulated cell of origin is a mismigrated primordial germ cell that escaped apoptosis {4360,5201} and failed to maintain the primordial germ cell phenotype {5198}. Extragonadal teratomas are diploid and do not harbour driver mutations {5198,2722}. Whereas 12p alterations are a common feature of postpubertal type II germ cell tumour {4207,6928}, extragonadal type I teratomas, especially SCT, lack chromosome 12p abnormalities {2627,4890}.

## Macroscopic appearance

Extragonadal teratomas vary in size but can reach > 15 mm {496, 2808}. They are well demarcated, with a heterogeneous cut surface showing solid or cystic components containing fluid, debris, or hairy material. Congenital teratomas do not have a (pseudo) capsule, which can make complete resection difficult {2722}.

## Histopathology

Teratomas contain tissue of all three germ cell layers: ectoderm, mesoderm, and endoderm. Immature tissue components like primitive neuroectodermal rosettes are a common feature of congenital SCT {2808,2722}. Two grading systems for estimating the degree of immaturity have been proposed (see Table 7.04), although the presence or degree of immaturity does not predict malignant behaviour in SCT {2818,4403}. However, the frequency of admixed YST foci in teratoma rises with increasing grades of immaturity {2818,2808}.

## Cytology

Insufficient data

## Diagnostic molecular pathology

Not clinically relevant

## Essential and desirable diagnostic criteria

*Essential:* teratoma without other germ cell tumour components and without evidence of a gonadal primary.
*Desirable:* prepubertal age.

## Staging

Pure extragonadal teratomas are benign and are not staged.

## Prognosis and prediction

Pure extragonadal teratomas do not metastasize. In congenital teratomas, prognosis is dependent on size, structure (cystic better than solid), and the presence of hydrops fetalis {426}. In order to avoid local recurrence, complete resection (including coccygectomy in SCT) is mandatory {3048,4403}. The degree of immaturity is not associated with malignant behaviour, which means that patients with immature teratoma do not benefit from adjuvant chemotherapy {4379,2453,4403}. In SCT with malignant elements (e.g. YST), adjuvant platinum-based chemotherapy is recommended, especially at a metastasized stage or after incomplete resection {2453,4402,4380}.

**Table 7.03** Sacrococcygeal teratoma types according to anatomical location (Altman classification {210})

| Type | Anatomical location |
|------|---------------------|
| I | Posterior extension (externalized) with no presacral involvement |
| II | Externalized with pelvic extension |
| III | Externalized with intra-abdominal extension |
| IV | Entirely presacral (no externalization) |

**Table 7.04** Grading systems for immature teratoma

| Grade | Amount of incompletely differentiated (embryonal) tissues | |
|-------|----------------------|-----------------------------|
| | **Gonzalez-Crussi {2486}** | **Norris[a] {5082}** |
| 1 | < 10% | < 1 low-power field in any slide |
| 2 | 10–50% | 1–3 low-power fields in any slide |
| 3 | > 50% | > 3 low-power fields in any slide |

[a]The grading of immature teratoma according to Norris {5082} is based on the number of low-power microscopic fields (4.5 mm in diameter and 15.9 mm[2] in area, 40× total magnification) containing aggregated amounts of immature neuroepithelium in any one slide.

# Monodermal teratomas (female gonadal)

Vang R
Stoneham SJ
Ulbright TM

## Definition
Monodermal teratomas are teratomas composed exclusively or predominantly of a single type of tissue derived from one embryonic layer and include struma ovarii, carcinoid, neuroectodermal-type tumours, and monodermal cystic teratoma. Also included in this section are somatic-type tumours derived from teratomas.

## ICD-O coding
9090/0 Struma ovarii, NOS
9090/3 Struma ovarii, malignant
9091/1 Strumal carcinoid
9080/0 Monodermal cystic teratoma
9084/3 Teratoma with malignant transformation

## ICD-11 coding
2F76 & XH22M4 Neoplasms of uncertain behaviour of female genital organs & Struma ovarii, NOS
2F76 & XH2XW3 Neoplasms of uncertain behaviour of female genital organs & Strumal carcinoid
2F76 & XH7K24 Neoplasms of uncertain behaviour of female genital organs & Neuroectodermal tumour, NOS
2F32.0 Cystic teratoma
2C73.3 & XH33E8 Malignant teratoma of ovary & Teratoma with malignant transformation

## Related terminology
*Acceptable:* strumal carcinoid; struma ovarii; neuroectodermal-type tumours; monodermal cystic teratoma; somatic-type tumours derived from teratomas.
*Not recommended:* grade 1 neuroendocrine tumour; well-differentiated neuroendocrine tumour.

## Subtype(s)
None

## Localization
Ovary

## Clinical features
Patients may present with signs and symptoms related to a pelvic mass {2016, 7735, 6823, 6853, 5915, 3643, 3499, 5245, 1273, 4097, 4864, 1221, 1801, 2651, 5483, 2906}. Ascites (with or without pleural effusion) is seen in about one third of patients with struma ovarii, and hyperthyroidism in < 10% {5916,6853, 5915}. Carcinoid syndrome (including cardiac manifestations) is seen in 30% of insular carcinoid cases {5912,1598}.

## Epidemiology
Monodermal teratomas typically occur in adults. When diagnosed in young women, they are more frequently found in the third decade of life, and tumours occurring in the first and second decades are rare {7764}. Struma ovarii was the most common type of monodermal teratoma (~3%) in a pathological case series {6822}. The most common type of ovarian carcinoid is the insular type (~50%) {5912} followed by strumal carcinoid (~40%) {5914}, whereas trabecular carcinoid {5915, 6854} and mucinous carcinoid {456} are rare. The setting of somatic-type tumours arising from teratomas is more common in older women but has been described in paediatric patients {708,6948}.

## Etiology
Unknown

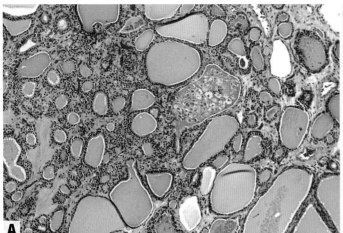 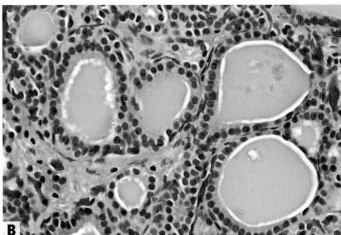

**Fig. 7.21** Struma ovarii. **A** The tumour is composed of thyroid follicles filled with colloid. **B** Higher-power magnification of the same case. The follicles are lined by low cuboidal cells with round and small nuclei without atypia. Colloid is evident within the follicles.

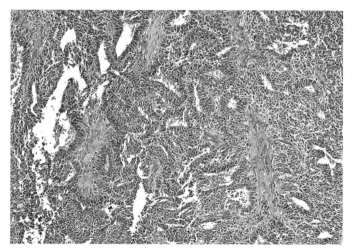

**Fig. 7.22** Medulloepithelioma. The tumour predominantly consists of distinct primitive tubules in this field. Other areas (not shown here) demonstrated papillary architecture. Note that the histological appearance can mimic that of immature teratoma.

## Pathogenesis

*Struma ovarii:* Mutations in *BRAF*, *KRAS*, and *HRAS*, as well as *RET*/PTC rearrangements have been found in papillary carcinomas (including the follicular form), and *PAX8::PPARG* rearrangement in follicular carcinoma arising in struma ovarii {817,6247,6860,7098,1468}.

*Carcinoid:* These tumours are thought to arise from neuroendocrine cells within intestinal-type epithelium of mature cystic teratoma.

*Neuroectodermal-type tumours, monodermal cystic teratoma, and somatic-type tumours derived from teratomas:* The pathogenesis of these tumours is unknown.

## Macroscopic appearance

The macroscopic features vary according to histological type. Tumours are typically unilateral, and their size is variable. The gross appearance may be solid, cystic, or solid-cystic, although struma ovarii usually is solid, whereas monodermal cystic teratomas have simple thin-walled cysts. Struma ovarii has a solid (sometimes nodular) beefy-red to brown cut surface resembling normal thyroid or goitre. Carcinoid has a homogeneous yellow to tan cut surface, which can be glistening if mucinous {456}. The cut surface of neuroectodermal-type tumours in the solid component is white, tan, or pink; haemorrhage and necrosis can be prominent. Extraovarian spread is common with somatic-type tumours derived from teratomas.

## Histopathology

In struma ovarii, thyroid tissue is the predominant or sole component. It usually resembles normal thyroid tissue, with variably sized follicles (most frequently macrofollicles) lined by cuboidal to flat cells and filled with colloid. Other patterns include solid, trabecular, pseudopapillary, pseudotubular {6823}, and predominantly cystic {6822}. Hyperplastic changes (proliferative struma) and adenomatous changes may be seen {1720}. Papillary, follicular (including highly differentiated) {5916,2327,6015,817,6247,6355,6014,1720, 7479}, or anaplastic carcinoma may rarely develop {2256}. Tumour cells express thyroglobulin, thyroid transcription factor 1 (TTF1), and PAX8 {3929,4509}.

Carcinoids are well-differentiated neuroendocrine tumours (NETs) resembling those arising in the gastrointestinal tract. Insular, trabecular, strumal (intimately admixed or juxtaposed with thyroid follicles {5914}), and mucinous (goblet cell) types occur. Teratomatous elements in the ipsilateral or contralateral ovary {6853,5915,5914} and fibromatous stroma may be present. Carcinoids are variably positive for neuroendocrine markers.

Neuroectodermal-type tumours are malignant tumours resembling those of the CNS or Ewing sarcoma. They are characterized either by a variable degree of neuronal or glial differentiation or by a small round cell proliferation. Most resemble ependymoma, astrocytoma, oligodendroglioma, neurocytoma, medulloblastoma, ependymoblastoma, medulloepithelioma, or glioblastoma {5208,2914,4864,3642,4102,7730}, although one study failed to find mutations characteristic of the CNS counterparts {4102}. A component of mature teratoma may be present. Tumours may show membranous CD99 and nuclear FLI1 expression, and they are often positive for CD56, NSE, and synaptophysin {1273,4864}.

Monodermal cystic teratoma includes neuroectodermal cysts lined by ependymal cells with choroid plexus–like epithelium along the cyst lining {2165,6609,7551} and epidermoid cysts lined by mature, often keratinizing, stratified squamous epithelium. Keratinaceous debris fills the cyst lumen {2032,5068,3547,7768}.

Somatic-type neoplasms arising from teratomas are composed of benign or malignant tumours derived from any of the elements within a teratoma. These can consist of squamous cell carcinoma, melanoma, melanocytic naevi, basal cell carcinomas, sebaceous lesions (including sebaceous hyperplasia, adenoma, sebaceoma, and carcinoma), adenocarcinoma, benign and low-grade appendiceal-type mucinous epithelial neoplasms, and sarcomas of various types {4502,2251,827, 1361,5483,5767,7238,4526,5970,6201,7709,1420,427,3511, 1316,1592,2613,3831,248,4472,5018}.

## Cytology

Not clinically relevant

## Diagnostic molecular pathology

Not clinically relevant

## Essential and desirable diagnostic criteria

*Struma ovarii*
*Essential:* benign thyroid tissue alone or constituting > 50% of a dermoid cyst.

*Carcinoid*
*Essential:* insular, trabecular, strumal, or mucinous (goblet cell) architectural types; salt-and-pepper chromatin pattern of the nuclei, with or without cytoplasmic granules.
*Desirable:* immunohistochemical expression of neuroendocrine markers.

*Neuroectodermal-type tumours*
*Essential:* a primitive tumour with a variable degree of neuroectodermal differentiation, as seen in brain tumours.

*Monodermal cystic teratoma*
*Essential:* a cyst lined by benign keratinizing squamous epithelium or by neuroectodermal tissues.

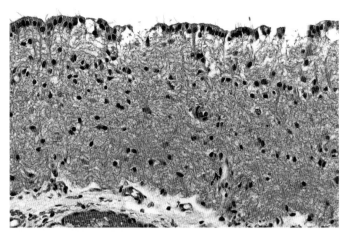

**Fig. 7.23** Monodermal cystic teratoma. This neuroectodermal cyst is lined by low cuboidal ependymal-type cells with cilia, and the stroma is composed of a glial matrix.

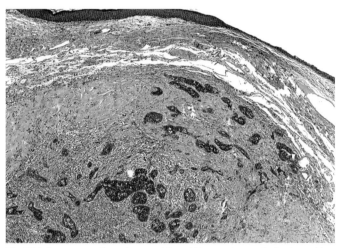

**Fig. 7.24** Squamous cell carcinoma arising within a mature cystic teratoma. Haphazardly arranged nests of squamous cell carcinoma with variable size and shape infiltrate the underlying stroma. The lining of the mature cystic teratoma is present at the top of the photograph.

*Somatic-type tumours derived from teratomas*

The essential and desirable diagnostic criteria are based on the histological type of the somatic neoplasm (see *Histopathology*, above).

## Staging

For struma ovarii, carcinoid, and monodermal cystic teratoma, staging is not clinically relevant.

Neuroectodermal-type tumours and malignant somatic-type tumours derived from teratomas are staged according to the Union for International Cancer Control (UICC) TNM classification {870} and the FIGO staging system.

## Prognosis and prediction

Struma ovarii (without thyroid-type carcinoma) is clinically benign. The presence of peritoneal implants of well-differentiated thyroid tissue in a patient with a histologically benign struma ovarii, known as strumosis, is now thought to represent metastasis from a highly differentiated follicular carcinoma arising in struma ovarii {6355,6014}.

The prognosis of carcinoid is generally excellent, with rare exceptions.

Limited clinical data for neuroectodermal-type tumours suggest that stage is the most important prognostic factor for these neoplasms {3643,1273}. Differentiated tumours are associated with a better prognosis {3643,1273,4864}.

Monodermal cystic teratomas are benign.

For malignant somatic-type tumours derived from teratomas, prognosis is highly dependent on stage, and most data are derived from squamous cell carcinoma in adults. Overall, patients with tumours limited to the ovary have a favourable outcome. The 5-year overall survival rate is 15–52% for all stages combined {2906} and 76% for stage I tumours {1221,1267,1801, 2651}. The prognosis of advanced disease is worse than that of more common ovarian cancers {1221,1801,2651,3074,2278}. Patients should not be treated with germ cell tumour chemotherapy regimens but rather by the most effective treatment for the specific type of malignancy.

# Immature teratoma (female gonadal)

Vang R
Stoneham SJ
Ulbright TM

### Definition
Immature teratoma is a teratoma containing immature and variable amounts of mature tissue.

### ICD-O coding
9080/3 Immature teratoma, NOS

### ICD-11 coding
2C73.3 & XH0N49 Malignant teratoma of ovary & Immature teratoma, malignant

### Related terminology
None

### Subtype(s)
None

### Localization
Ovary

### Clinical features
Immature teratoma usually manifests as a pelvic mass {5066}. Elevated serum AFP should prompt more extensive sampling of the tumour to rule out a component of yolk sac tumour (YST), but immature teratomas with hepatoid components may have elevated AFP {4182}.

### Epidemiology
This is the second most common malignant ovarian germ cell tumour in the USA {6538}, usually arising within the first three decades of life {5066}. Immature teratoma is much less common than its mature counterpart {2719,4156,113}.

### Etiology
Unknown

### Pathogenesis
Immature teratoma may develop, like mature cystic teratoma, via a common origin involving germ cells at the same developmental stage {7866,6557}. They usually do not exhibit 12p gain or isochromosome 12p unless they are part of a mixed germ cell tumour (MGCT) {5899,3773,5608}.

### Macroscopic appearance
Immature teratoma is usually unilateral, large, fleshy, grey-tan, and solid-cystic, with haemorrhage and necrosis {5082}.

### Histopathology
Variable amounts of immature tissues, mostly neuroectodermal tubules and rosettes, are admixed with ectodermal and endodermal tissues of varying maturation. The tubules and rosettes are composed of mitotically active hyperchromatic cells. Cellular, mitotically active glia may also be present. Immature mesodermal and, less commonly, endodermal tissues can be seen. A trabecular or nested proliferation of thin-walled blood vessels may be present, mimicking a vascular neoplasm {457,5064}.

It is unclear whether an immature teratoma with microscopic foci of YST should be classified as MGCT {5368A}. Quantitative criteria, however, have not been established for the minimal amount of a second component to qualify as clinically significant. Nonetheless, immature teratomas containing a focus of YST measuring > 3 mm were classified as MGCTs in one study {5116}. To facilitate clinical management, any foci of YST should be quantified (size and/or percentage) in the pathology report. An apparently pure immature teratoma associated with elevated serum levels of AFP requires additional sampling to locate a YST component and then be classified as MGCT.

Grading (see Table 7.05) is based on the number of low-power microscopic fields (diameter: 4.5 mm) containing aggregated amounts of immature neuroectoderm in any one slide {5082,5116}. Metastatic sites of immature teratoma are graded using the same criteria; pure gliomatosis peritonei is considered mature (grade 0).

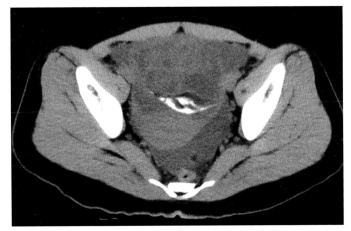

**Fig. 7.25** Immature teratoma, ovarian. Contrast-enhanced axial CT shows a heterogeneous mixed solid-cystic pelvic mass containing calcifications (dense material) and punctate foci of fat (very low density material).

**Table 7.05** Grading of immature teratoma

| Number of fields[a] | Grade (3-tier system) {5082} | Grade (2-tier system) {5116} |
|---|---|---|
| ≤ 1 | Grade 1 | Low-grade |
| > 1 to ≤ 3 | Grade 2 | High-grade |
| > 3 | Grade 3 | High-grade |

[a]The grading of immature teratoma is based on the number of low-power microscopic fields (4.5 mm in diameter, ×40 total magnification) containing aggregated amounts of immature neuroectoderm in any one slide.

Chapter 7

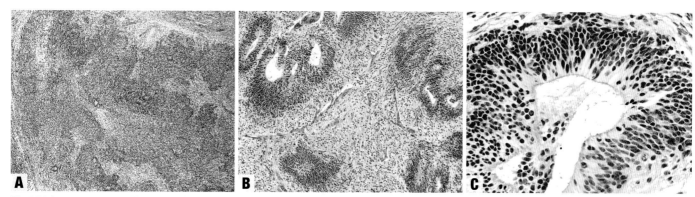

**Fig. 7.26** Immature teratoma. The extent of immature neuroectodermal tissue in these cases is consistent with grade 3 (**A**) and grade 1 (**B**). **C** The immature neuroectodermal tissue forms primitive neural tubules lined by cells with increased N:C ratios. The nuclei are enlarged and hyperchromatic. Mitotic figures and apoptotic bodies are present.

SALL4 can be positive in immature neuroectoderm and intestinal elements {1018,5708}. SOX2 and glypican-3 (GPC3) may be expressed in neuroectoderm. AFP may stain immature gastrointestinal-type glands.

## Cytology
Not clinically relevant

## Diagnostic molecular pathology
Not clinically relevant

## Essential and desirable diagnostic criteria
*Essential:* a germ cell tumour with immature neuroectodermal tissue.

## Staging
Immature teratoma is staged according to the Union for International Cancer Control (UICC) TNM classification and the FIGO staging system. Although gliomatosis peritonei represents stage III disease, its behaviour is generally regarded as benign, and overtreatment should be avoided.

## Prognosis and prediction
The stage and grade of the primary tumour and the grade of the metastatic tumour (if present) are the main prognostic factors.

The 5-year overall survival rate is > 90%. For stage I tumours, the 5-year survival rate approaches 100% {1142,7295,3333,775}. Of note, opinions differ between paediatric and gynaecological oncologists regarding the role of chemotherapy for immature teratoma. Furthermore, microscopic foci of YST (see *Histopathology*, above) do not necessarily warrant chemotherapy.

There is also controversy about the best way to stage immature teratoma and gliomatosis. Gliomatosis is currently considered benign and not requiring chemotherapy {5913,4103, 7736}. Some cases occur in patients with or even without benign ovarian tumours {2891}. Therefore, implants must be adequately sampled by surgeons and carefully evaluated by pathologists. The current UICC recommendation is that gliomatosis should be staged when associated with an ovarian immature teratoma {7584}, but no outcome-based evidence exists to support this advice. Therefore, many clinicians and pathologists discount the presence of pure gliomatosis and upstage ovarian tumours only if the implants contain immature elements (i.e. grade 1 or higher). Whichever approach is taken, the nature of the implants must be carefully documented and the prognostic significance clearly communicated to the treating clinicians.

After chemotherapy treatment, rare patients may develop enlarging extraovarian deposits of pure mature teratomatous tissue (growing teratoma syndrome) {7219,4596,1767}.

# Prepubertal-type testicular teratoma

Kao CS
Stoneham SJ
Williamson SR

## Definition

Prepubertal-type teratoma is a germ cell tumour usually seen in the prepubertal testis, although rarely it occurs in postpubertal patients (benign postpubertal teratoma). It is composed of elements resembling somatic tissue derived from one or more of the germinal layers.

## ICD-O coding

9084/0 Prepubertal-type testicular teratoma
9084/0 Dermoid cyst
9084/0 Epidermoid cyst
9084/3 Well-differentiated neuroendocrine tumour (monodermal teratoma)

## ICD-11 coding

2C80.4 & XH52Q4 Malignant teratoma of testis & Teratoma, prepubertal type

## Related terminology

Acceptable: type I germ cell tumour of the testis; benign postpubertal testicular teratoma.

## Subtype(s)

Dermoid cyst; epidermoid cyst; well-differentiated neuroendocrine tumour (monodermal teratoma)

## Localization

Testis

## Clinical features

Most prepubertal-type teratomas manifest as lumps discovered by patients or parents, or during physical examination or

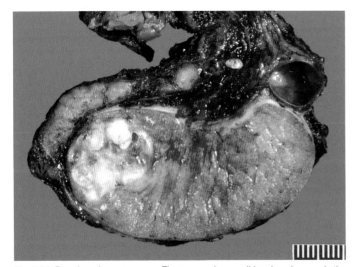

**Fig. 7.27** Prepubertal-type teratoma. The tumour shows solid and cystic areas in the testis of a 17-year-old boy. FISH hybridization for isochromosome 12p was negative.

imaging. Most are at least partially cystic on ultrasound examination, but they may also be solid {1970}.

## Epidemiology

Prepubertal-type teratoma typically occurs before the age of 6 years {6646}. It is thought that prepubertal-type teratoma in an adult represents a persistent lesion from a young age. No ethnicities, geographical locales, or exposures to certain substances have been linked to its development. No genetic susceptibility is known.

## Etiology

The cause is unknown. There is no established cell of origin for prepubertal-type teratoma, but an early embryonic germ or stem cell has been proposed as a possible candidate {5198}.

## Pathogenesis

It has been postulated that gonocytes or non-transformed primordial germ cells undergo reprogramming by a lack of maintenance of phenotype and reversal of germline specification {5198}.

## Macroscopic appearance

The tumours may be solid or have a variably prominent cystic component filled with keratinaceous or mucoid material; they may also show calcification or bone formation. Grossly identifiable hair may be present in the dermoid subtype, which is a finding never reported in postpubertal-type testicular teratomas.

## Histopathology

The prepubertal-type testicular teratomas exhibit distinct differences from the postpubertal-type ones. The various elements are often arranged in an organoid pattern and all lack marked cytological atypia. No germ cell neoplasia in situ (GCNIS) is present; therefore, the background testicular parenchyma should be closely examined, especially in the postpubertal setting, to exclude the possibility of a GCNIS-derived tumour. No tubular atrophy, parenchymal scars, tubular microlithiasis, necrosis, or impaired spermatogenesis (dysgenetic features) should be observed. In difficult cases, molecular investigation for 12p gain should be considered.

### Dermoid cyst

Dermoid cyst is a specialized subtype of prepubertal-type teratoma that is morphologically identical to its much more common ovarian counterpart. This tumour is cured by complete excision {952,2611,7827}.

### Epidermoid cyst

Grossly a unilocular cyst that contains keratinaceous material; microscopy shows a stratified squamous epithelium lining without skin appendages or other elements. This tumour is also cured by complete excision.

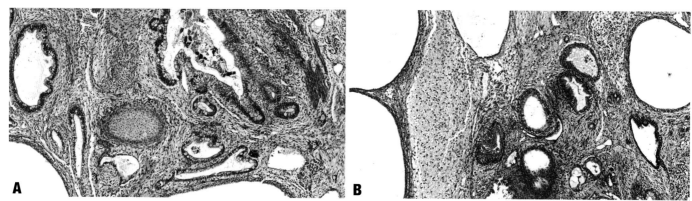

**Fig. 7.28** Prepubertal-type teratoma. **A** This prepubertal-type teratoma occurring in a child includes glandular epithelium, cartilage, spindle cell stroma, and focal smooth muscle. **B** This prepubertal-type teratoma includes cysts with glandular epithelium, glial tissue (left), and focal pigmented epithelium (right).

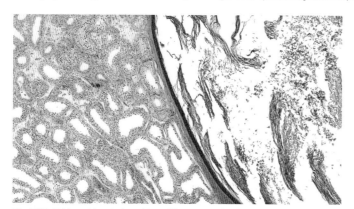

**Fig. 7.29** Epidermoid cyst. An epidermoid cyst occurring in the postpubertal testis is considered a form of prepubertal-type teratoma. This example includes a single cyst lined by keratinizing squamous epithelium, associated with normal seminiferous tubules.

### Well-differentiated neuroendocrine tumour (monodermal teratoma)

This subtype accounts for < 1% of all testicular tumours and is found in children and adults. The morphology is usually typical of midgut well-differentiated neuroendocrine tumours, with well-defined cords or solid nests of cells arranged in trabecular, follicular, pseudoglandular, or spindled patterns. This tumour occurs in several forms: pure primary neoplasms, primary neoplasm with teratoma, primary neoplasms with epidermoid or dermoid cysts, and metastatic neoplasms from an extratesticular primary {615, 5856,7424,6735}. Most reported cases associated with teratoma have occurred in postpubertal male patients. Of the 15 cases with mature teratoma, 2 metastasized. From a total of 6 primary and teratoma-associated neoplasms analysed for isochromosome 12p, 2 were negative and 4 positive {9,3477,7424}.

### Cytology
Not relevant

### Diagnostic molecular pathology
Prepubertal-type teratomas are diploid and lack the usual genetic abnormalities seen in the postpubertal-type teratomas or other GCNIS-associated tumours, including chromosome 12p gain. No recurrent somatic mutations have been identified {1440,4812,5197}.

### Essential and desirable diagnostic criteria
*Essential:* no association with GCNIS, dysgenetic parenchymal changes, scarring, or chromosome 12p amplification.
*Desirable:* prepubertal age.

### Staging
Staging follows the system outlined in the TNM classification of germ cell tumours of the testis and the staging of germ cell tumours by the Pediatric Oncology Group (POG).

### Prognosis and prediction
There have been no documented cases of prepubertal-type teratomas exhibiting malignant behaviour {7827}. Well-differentiated neuroendocrine tumour (monodermal teratoma) is a low-grade malignant neoplasm with a metastatic rate of approximately 15% {6735}; atypical morphology (necrosis and mitotic activity) correlates with a greater risk of metastasis {7424}.

# Postpubertal-type teratoma

Looijenga LHJ
Bode PK
Stoneham SJ
Wong TT

## Definition
Teratomas are composed of somatic-type tissues that recapitulate the differentiating potential of the ectoderm, endoderm, and mesoderm.

## ICD-O coding
9080/3 Teratoma, postpubertal-type

## ICD-11 coding
2C80.4 Malignant teratoma of testis

## Related terminology
*Not recommended:* malignant teratoma.

## Subtype(s)
None

## Localization
Postpubertal-type teratomas occur in the gonad, mediastinum, sacrococcygeal region, and the head and neck. Within the CNS, pure infantile immature teratomas are most frequent in cerebral ventricles {6465}. After early childhood, both pure mature teratomas and immature teratomas arise most commonly in the pineal region, followed by the suprasellar compartment, and rarely in the basal ganglia / thalamic region, spine, and other locations {6465,3808,4026,90}. Teratomas with somatic-type malignancy are rare {4480,2225,1219,4364,5273}.

## Clinical features
Infantile teratomas usually manifest as large congenital lesions, particularly immature teratoma {3142}. For tumours arising beyond early childhood, representing postpubertal (type II) teratomas, the treatment and prognosis vary with tumour subtype, tumour marker (AFP, indicative of yolk sac tumour progression), and staging {4480,982,981}. Pineal region tumours can cause hydrocephalus, intracranial hypertension, and ocular paralysis (Parinaud syndrome). Posterior pituitary / suprasellar lesions can result in visual disturbances, diabetes insipidus, and delayed growth and sexual maturation. hCG production can result in precocious puberty, predominantly in boys {5178,6650}. Spinal tumours may induce back pain, paraparesis, and loss of excretory function. Imaging shows heterogeneous appearances with variable attenuations and signal intensities, whereas CT reveals a tumour with different degrees of calcification, fat, and cystic components {4101}. MRI shows usually hypointense to isointense T1-weighted images and hyperintense T2-weighted images, and the solid part is well enhanced. In mature teratomas, a well-marginated mass with associated fat is helpful for radiological diagnosis. Immature teratomas have less calcification and cystic components than mature teratomas. Malignant tumours are poorly marginated, with irregular contours, homogeneous enhancement, and sometimes perifocal oedema in surrounding brain tissues {3855}. Unlike in their benign counterparts, fat and calcified components are not seen. Leptomeningeal dissemination of immature teratomas and of teratomas with somatic-type malignancy is rare {7315, 1698}. When it occurs, treatment follows the regimens of specific histological risk subgroups with and without metastasis, and staging follows the management of intracranial germ cell tumours {4871}.

## Epidemiology
In one study, CNS teratoma, mature teratoma, immature teratoma, and teratoma with somatic-type malignancy accounted for 19.6%, 12.4%, 4.6%, and 2.6%, respectively, of 153 intracranial germ cell tumours {4480}. The mean patient ages for mature teratoma, immature teratoma, and teratoma with somatic-type malignancy are 11.6 ± 8.5, 16.1 ± 11.7, and 31 ± 14.6 years, respectively {4480}.

## Etiology
See *Germ cell tumours: Introduction* (p. 648).

## Pathogenesis
See *Germ cell tumours: Introduction* (p. 648).

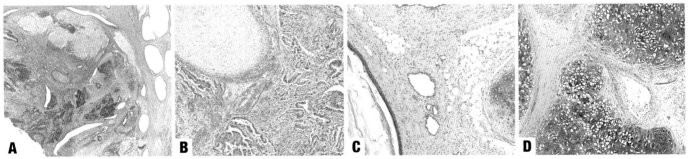

**Fig. 7.30** Teratoma, postpubertal-type. **A** Mixed teratomatous elements with embryonic-type neuroectodermal components. **B** This example shows mature cartilage and an embryonal-type neuroectodermal component. **C** This example shows several mature tissue types, including squamous epithelium, mature cartilage, glandular epithelium, adipose tissue, and myofibroblastic stroma. **D** Cartilage and glandular tissue are seen in this teratoma. The cartilage appears hypercellular and shows prominent cellular atypia.

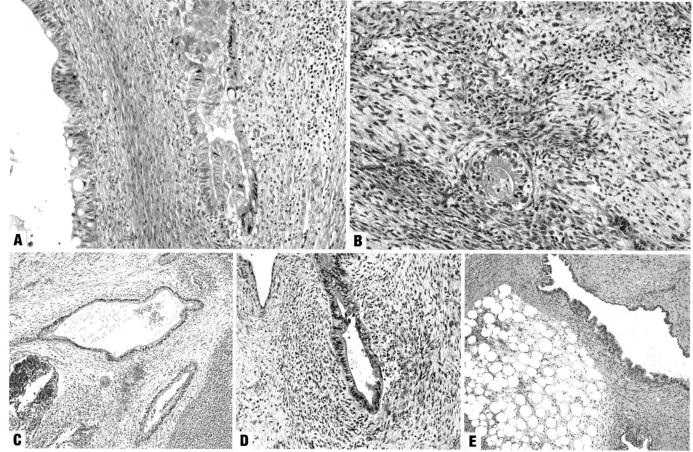

**Fig. 7.31** Teratoma, postpubertal-type. **A** Glandular epithelium showing goblet cells. The surrounding spindle cell stroma is predominantly aggregating around the glands. **B** A single gland is surrounded by highly cellular spindle cell stroma in a myxoid matrix. **C** Mature glandular elements with mild nuclear atypia and pleomorphism. Note the syncytio-trophoblast with intracytoplasmic red blood cells and the spindle cell stroma displaying variable cellularity. **D** Periglandular stromal cuffing. Both mesenchymal and epithelial components show nuclear atypia. **E** Glandular tissue, fibrous stroma, and adipose tissue (high-power view).

## Macroscopic appearance

Postpubertal teratomas are nodular and firm, with heterogeneous cut surfaces showing solid and cystic areas, possibly including cartilage, bone, and pigmented areas. Mature teratomas typically have both solid components and cysts possibly containing mucinous material. Areas of calcification and chondroid nodules may be appreciable, whereas haemorrhage and necrosis are typically absent. Immature teratomas may contain cysts, regions of calcification, and chondroid nodules, but generally have soft, fleshy components. Teratomas with somatic-type malignancy may resemble mature or immature teratomas but frequently exhibit regional necrosis. Overgrowth by sarcomatous components may lend a fleshy appearance, and mucoid/gelatinous regions may reflect the presence of mucin-producing adenocarcinoma.

## Histopathology

Virtually any epithelial, mesenchymal, and neural tissue type can be seen. Organoid arrangements characteristic of the skin, respiratory tract, gastrointestinal tract, and genitourinary tract may also be seen, but they occur in a much smaller proportion of postpubertal-type teratomas than prepubertal-type teratomas. Cytological atypia can be present (e.g. mature glandular tissue with features of high-grade dysplasia or carcinoma in situ, and cartilage resembling chondrosarcoma). Fetal or embryonic-type

tissue may also be seen (ectodermal, endodermal, and/or mesodermal/mesenchymal tissues). Immature neuroectodermal structures are particularly common. In contrast to epidermoid cysts and many dermoid cysts, which are considered to be prepubertal-type teratomas, postpubertal-type teratomas often contain multiple cysts lined by glandular or squamous epithelium, neuroectodermal tissue, non-cystic glands, and mesenchymal elements such as adipose tissue and cartilage. Within the testis, teratoma can show invasion of paratesticular tissue, as well as intratesticular and extratesticular vascular invasion. Like other malignant germ cell tumours, the typical postpubertal-type teratoma shows testicular atrophy with impaired spermatogenesis in the surrounding testis. The uninvolved testis may also harbour microlithiasis and germ cell neoplasia in situ. The differentiated elements express the immunophenotype expected for that specific cell type. The glandular elements of a teratoma are positive for EMA {3107}. hCG can be seen in syncytiotrophoblastic cells. PLAP is also demonstrable in glandular structures {4816}. It is important to differentiate postpubertal-type teratomas from prepubertal-type teratomas because the latter may also occur in postpubertal patients {7827,5202}.

### Mature teratoma

Mature teratomas harbour only fully differentiated, adult-type tissue elements that exhibit little if any mitotic activity. Ectodermal

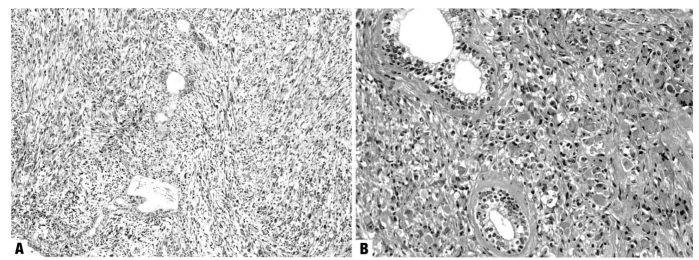

**Fig. 7.32** Teratoma, postpubertal-type. **A** Glandular and mesenchymal component with prominent rhabdomyomatous differentiation. **B** Rhabdomyomatous differentiation.

components commonly include epidermis and skin adnexa, central nervous tissue, choroid plexus, and salivary gland acini. Smooth and striated muscle, as well as cartilage, bone, and adipose tissue, are typical mesodermal representatives. Glands that are lined by respiratory or enteric-type epithelia and are often cystically dilated are the usual endodermal participants, but hepatic and pancreatic tissue may be encountered. Gut-like structures replete with mucosa and muscular coats, and bronchus-like structures with cartilaginous rings, can be formed. Exceptional intracranial teratomas contain remarkably organized, fetus-like bodies {4947}. Re-resection specimens deriving from germ cell tumours displaying progressive enlargement in the course of adjuvant therapy or recurrence after an initially complete response to treatment may be composed solely of mature teratomatous elements, a seemingly paradoxical scenario termed "growing teratoma syndrome" {5259, 7101}. Although the simple expansion of cystic components can play a role in this phenomenon, Ki-67 immunohistochemistry may reveal surprisingly elevated labelling within their ostensibly differentiated tissues {5259}.

The identification of even minor tissue components with incompletely differentiated, fetal-like appearances mandates the classification of a teratoma as immature. Commonly represented are hypercellular and mitotically active stromal elements resembling embryonic mesenchyme, glands lined by crowded columnar cells with clear subnuclear and apical cytoplasm (reminiscent of fetal gut and respiratory mucosa), and primitive central neuroepithelial elements that may feature multilayered rosettes or canalicular arrays of neural tube–like appearance. Abortive retinal differentiation is represented by clefts lined by melanotic neuroepithelium. Immature teratomas exhibit the immunophenotype expected of their somatic tissue counterparts. Retained expression of SMARCB1 (INI1), a general feature of CNS germ cell tumours {2648}, may assist in distinguishing teratomas with multilayered neuroepithelial rosettes from atypical teratoid/rhabdoid tumours containing similar structures {7400}.

*Teratoma with somatic-type malignancy*
Somatic-type cancers most commonly encountered in this setting are rhabdomyosarcomas and undifferentiated sarcomas {719,4480,6049}, enteric-type adenocarcinomas {2225, 3575}, and squamous carcinomas {4480}. The possibility of a

teratomatous derivation must also be considered when evaluating primitive-appearing neuroepithelial neoplasms in age groups and locations favoured by CNS germ cell tumours {7137}. Erythroleukaemia {2822}, leiomyosarcoma {6522}, and neuroendocrine tumour associated with an intradural spinal teratoma {3139} have been described. The pathogenesis of a composite intrasellar tumour containing elements of Burkitt-like B-cell lymphoma and germinoma is unclear {7169}. Yolk sac tumour components have been the speculated progenitors of enteric-type adenocarcinomas encountered in selected cases {2225}. Cytological atypia alone may be seen, especially after adjuvant chemotherapy, and should not be interpreted as somatic-type malignant transformation, even when pronounced.

## Cytology
In each subtype (mature teratoma, immature teratoma, and teratoma with somatic-type malignancy), the cytological appearances reflect the tissue type components.

## Diagnostic molecular pathology
See *Intratubular germ cell neoplasia (male gonadal)* (p. 649) for postpubertal-type teratoma. Prepubertal (type I) teratomas are diploid without chromosomal anomalies or genetic mutations.

## Essential and desirable diagnostic criteria
Differentiation between prepubertal (type I) and postpubertal (type II) teratoma.
*Mature teratoma:* components exhibiting differentiation along at least two of the three somatic tissue lines (ectoderm, endoderm, mesoderm); fully differentiated, adult-type histology (absence of fetal-type elements); absence of other germ cell tumour components.
*Immature teratoma:* incompletely differentiated elements of at least two of the three blastodermal layers, or the presence of any such elements within a tumour otherwise qualifying as a mature teratoma; absence of non-teratomatous germ cell tumour components.
*Teratoma with somatic-type malignancy:* identification of a distinct histological component having the cytological features, architecture, mitotic activity, and disorderly growth pattern expected of a sarcoma, carcinoma, or other defined type of somatic cancer.

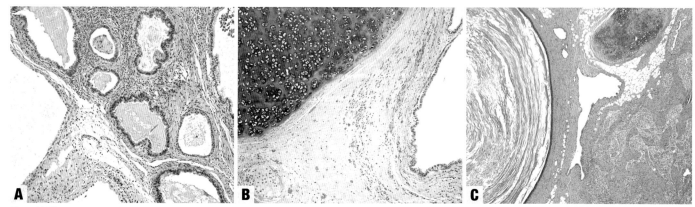

**Fig. 7.33** Teratoma, postpubertal-type. **A** Glandular tissue, fibrous stroma, and adipose tissue (low-power view). **B** Cartilage tissue showing hypercellularity and chondrocyte atypia. **C** Squamous epithelial and glandular tissue, fibrous stroma, adipose tissue, and glial proliferation (lower right).

## Staging

Not relevant

## Prognosis and prediction

In the postpubertal testis, teratoma occurs with metastases in 22–37% of cases {4033}. Excepting somatic-type malignancy, the presence of epithelium or mesenchymal elements with cytological atypia or immaturity has no prognostic impact. In patients with clinical stage I teratoma, the risk of metastasis in retroperitoneal lymphadenectomies is 16.7% {1244}. Nearly 37% of referred patients with pure teratoma present with advanced disease. Teratoma is the most common component in treated germ cell tumours; when it is the only component present in metastases, the prognosis is generally favourable, in contrast to the prognosis for persistent, postchemotherapy, non-teratomatous germ cell tumours {6900}. Teratoma metastases are typically synchronous; they are metachronous in only about 13% of cases. Late recurrences (≥ 2 years after an initial complete response to chemotherapy) are most commonly teratomas, and these have a better prognosis than late recurrences of other germ cell tumours {4641}. In postchemotherapy lymph nodes, the finding of mature rhabdomyocytes with abundant eosinophilic cytoplasm (lacking mitotic activity and a primitive cellular component) is associated with a favourable prognosis and must be differentiated from metastatic rhabdomyosarcoma as a component of a somatic malignancy arising in teratoma {1356}.

A literature survey of 90 fetal intracranial teratomas identified only 7 survivors after resection {3142}. In teratoma arising beyond early childhood, the best outcomes are seen in pure and fully mature teratomas (curable by surgical means alone). In a series of 153 patients treated in 1963–1994, immature teratomas and teratomas with somatic malignancy were associated with 3-year survival rates of 70% {4480}, increased to overall 5- and 10-year survival rates of patients with aggressive lesions to 75–80% more recently {981,6841}. An important scenario occurs when a persistent or enlarging posttherapy tumour consists of mature teratoma only (growing teratoma syndrome); in such cases, radical resection effects disease control {3573}.

# Embryonal carcinoma

Looijenga LHJ
Kao CS
Stoneham SJ
Wong TT

## Definition

Embryonal carcinoma is composed of cells resembling embryonic stem cells, with ovoid to columnar profiles, clear to granular or amphophilic cytoplasm, and markedly pleomorphic nuclei, with diverse morphological patterns.

## ICD-O coding

9070/3 Embryonal carcinoma

## ICD-11 coding

2C73.Y & XH8MB9 Other specified malignant neoplasms of the ovary & Embryonal carcinoma, NOS

2C80.2 & XH8MB9 Germ cell tumour of testis & Embryonal carcinoma, NOS

2A00.1Y & XH8MB9 Other specified embryonal tumours of brain & Embryonal carcinoma, NOS

2C28.0 & XH8MB9 Malignant germ cell neoplasms of heart, mediastinum, or non-mesothelioma of pleura & Embryonal carcinoma, NOS

## Related terminology

*Not recommended:* undifferentiated malignant teratoma.

## Subtype(s)

None

## Localization

Embryonal carcinoma arises in the gonads, mediastinum, and CNS (in which most cases occur in the pineal region or suprasellar compartment, and fewer occur in the basal ganglia / thalamus and other locations) {3270}.

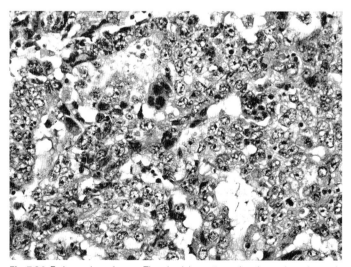

**Fig. 7.34** Embryonal carcinoma. The glandular pattern of embryonal carcinoma is composed of pleomorphic tumour cells and syncytiotrophoblastic giant cells.

## Clinical features

After seminoma, embryonal carcinoma is the most prevalent testicular germ cell tumour (pure embryonal carcinomas account for 2.3–16% of testicular germ cell tumours) {3418,4815,7334}); it is present in 87% of non-seminomatous tumours {3772,4815}. It is rare in childhood, except in patients with disorders of sex development {2785,3772}. Most testicular examples come to clinical attention as a mass, with 10% showing metastatic disease {5945}. Retroperitoneal lymph node involvement relates to the proportion of embryonal carcinoma in mixed germ cell tumour (MGCT) {5945}. Serum β-hCG is generally not elevated {3234}, although LDH and PLAP can be {801,7100}. Imaging does not distinguish embryonal carcinoma from MGCT. Embryonal carcinoma in the CNS manifests with symptoms depending on location, β-hCG level, and associated hydrocephalus {3270}. Spinal leptomeningeal metastases rarely occur {3250, 7183}. Levels of AFP and β-hCG can be elevated {6841}.

## Epidemiology

See *Intratubular germ cell neoplasia (male gonadal)* (p. 649). CNS embryonal carcinoma accounts for 3.3–5% of all germ cell tumours {4480,3250} and in 5.6% of non-germinomatous tumours {4480}, with a male predominance and a peak in incidence at 16–18 years (mean age: 11.8 ± 7.1 years) {4480, 3250}.

## Etiology

See *Intratubular germ cell neoplasia (male gonadal)* (p. 649) {6259,6947,2260,7408,6282}. Fewer CNS germ cell tumours exhibit gains of 12p than do testicular and mediastinal examples {5152,6762,6947,2260}. Gains of *CCND2* and *PRDM14* (primordial germ cell specification regulator) and losses of *RB1* imply involvement of the cyclin/CDK/RB1/E2F pathway {6947}. Activating mutations involving the MAPK pathway (KIT, RAS family members) and (less frequently) the PI3K/AKT/mTOR pathway have been identified in germ cell tumours beyond infancy / early childhood {2260,7408,3106,6282}. More CNS germ cell tumours appear to occur in Down syndrome {4726} and Klinefelter syndrome (47,XXY) {3370,7553,5270} than in the general population.

## Pathogenesis

See *Intratubular germ cell neoplasia (male gonadal)* (p. 649). Clinical and epigenetic studies of CNS germ cell tumours arising after infancy / early childhood {3106,6282,2261} suggest a primordial germ cell origin, although alternative origins have also been suggested {5201,6861}.

## Macroscopic appearance

The cut section has a variegated, granular, solid, grey-white to tan appearance and may exhibit haemorrhage, necrosis, and cysts.

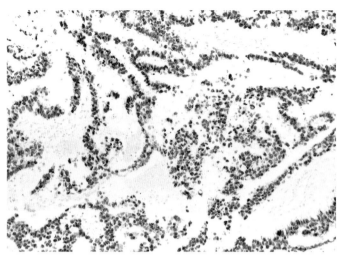

**Fig. 7.35** Embryonal carcinoma. SOX2 stains embryonal carcinoma in a nuclear pattern.

## Histopathology

Embryonal carcinoma cells are epithelioid, with vesicular nuclei, dense amphophilic cytoplasm, and poorly defined cytoplasmic membranes, and they show prominent mitoses (atypical) and apoptosis. Nuclear crowding, overlapping, and marked pleomorphism can be characteristic; necrotic foci are common. The most frequent patterns are solid, glandular, papillary, and combined {3418}. Embryonal carcinoma cells can mimic germinoma-like cells {3418} and may show syncytiotrophoblast cells and lymphocytic infiltrates, although a granulomatous reaction is rare {3418}. Immunohistochemically, embryonal carcinomas express CD30 (possibly lost after chemotherapy) {634}, OCT3/4 and SOX2 {6168}, LIN28A {1020}, cytokeratin AE1/AE3 {3107}, and SALL4.

## Cytology

Squash and smear preparations show cohesive clusters of large epithelioid cells with prominent nucleoli and abundant cytoplasm.

## Diagnostic molecular pathology

Isochromosome 12p and increased gains of 12p in most embryonal carcinomas are helpful diagnostic findings to differentiate from non–germ cell, poorly differentiated malignancies {4204, 7207}. Embryonal carcinoma has a lower DNA index than seminoma {1942,5193}.

## Essential and desirable diagnostic criteria

*Essential:* large epithelioid cells with a defined immunohistochemical pattern (OCT3/4, SOX2, LIN28A, AE1/AE3, and SALL4).

## Staging

See *Intratubular germ cell neoplasia (male gonadal)* (p. 649). CNS embryonal carcinomas rarely show leptomeningeal metastasis at diagnosis {3250}; if present, treatment follows the regimen for poor prognostic groups with metastasis {4479}. Staging is according to the Delphi consensus {4871}.

## Prognosis and prediction

Prognosis correlates with stage and the proportion of embryonal carcinoma in testicular MGCT {145,4823,6807,7572}. Pure embryonal carcinoma behaves more aggressively than MGCT {3189,7572}, with frequent lymphovascular invasion and an increased risk of metastasis. Haematogenous spread to the lungs and other sites may occur. Post-orchiectomy combination chemotherapy plus retroperitoneal lymph node dissection is necessary in many cases {144,2212,6569}. For CNS embryonal carcinoma, pure or mixed, outcomes are dismal {4480, 6203,4479}, but combined irradiation and chemotherapy increase 5- and 10-year survival rates to 75–80% {981,6841}. Logarithmic decreases of AFP and hCG augur favourably {3490}, whereas AFP levels of > 1000 ng/mL and residual disease after treatment have negative implications {981}. Long-term survivors are at risk of premature death due to subsequent treatment-associated malignant neoplasms, stroke, and other iatrogenic effects {38}.

# Yolk sac tumour

Looijenga LHJ
Kao CS
Stoneham SJ
Tan GC
Wong TT

## Definition

Yolk sac tumour (YST) is a malignant neoplasm resembling extraembryonic structures, including the yolk sac, allantois, and extraembryonic mesenchyme.

## ICD-O coding

9071/3 Yolk sac tumour
9071/3 Prepubertal (type I) yolk sac tumour
9071/3 Postpubertal (type II) yolk sac tumour

## ICD-11 coding

2C73.Y & XH09W7 Other specified malignant neoplasms of the ovary & Yolk sac tumour
2C80.Y & XH09W7 Other specified malignant neoplasms of testis & Yolk sac tumour
2A00.1Y & XH09W7 Other specified embryonal tumours of brain & Yolk sac tumour

## Related terminology

*Not recommended:* endodermal sinus tumour; yolk sac carcinoma; orchioblastoma; infantile embryonal carcinoma.

## Subtype(s)

Prepubertal (type I) yolk sac tumour; postpubertal (type II) yolk sac tumour (germ cell neoplasia in situ–related)

## Localization

Prepubertal YST arises in the gonads, mediastinum, and many other sites. Prepubertal and postpubertal YSTs occur within the CNS, most frequently in the pineal and suprasellar compartment, followed by the basal ganglia / thalamus, spinal cord, and other locations {4480,7386,3829,7095}. During the first 2 years of life the most common germ cell tumour in the vagina is a YST.

## Clinical features

Prepubertal YST develops at a median age of 16–20 months (range: 3 months to 8 years); it rarely arises beyond 6 years of age {1441,4019,5998,6646}. Postpubertal YST is rarely pure (only in 0.6% of tumours containing YST). Although AFP is positive in most cases (95%) {4019}, neonates have high AFP normally (≥ 100 ng/mL at ≤ 6 months {735}), limiting its significance. About 80% of paediatric cases are clinical stage I {4019, 5998}, and only 6% recur during surveillance (retroperitoneal and pulmonary {4019}). In contrast, 33% of postpubertal YSTs show occult retroperitoneal metastases {2198}. The risk for haematogenous spread is higher in prepubertal YST than in postpubertal YST. CNS YST occurs at 2.6–14.5 years of age (peak incidence: 11–15 years {6841}; mean age: ~13 years {4480,7616}). Although systemic dissemination is rare {3250}, intra-abdominal metastasis via ventriculoperitoneal shunt can occur {440}. Clinical symptoms and signs correlate with tumour location and associated hydrocephalus.

## Epidemiology

For postpubertal YST, see *Intratubular germ cell neoplasia (male gonadal)* (p. 649).

Prepubertal YST has a stable incidence in the first 6 years of life of (2–3 cases per 1 million person-years) {6646}, with no racial or geographical predilection {7661}. Testicular prepubertal YSTs have no association with cryptorchidism or germ cell neoplasia in situ {2594,2784,3335,4373}, are pure in most cases, and represent the most common neoplasm (accounting for 48–62% of all neoplasms) at this age {4019,5998}. There are

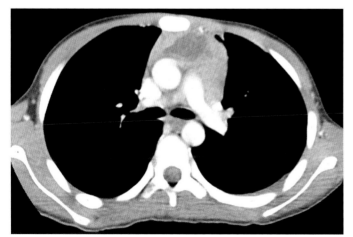

**Fig. 7.36** Yolk sac tumour. Contrast-enhanced axial CT shows a heterogeneous anterior mediastinal mass abutting the ascending aorta and pulmonary trunk. A cystic component is noted within the mass and there is no calcification.

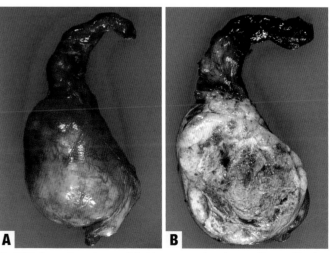

**Fig. 7.37** Pure yolk sac tumour. **A** Orchiectomy specimen from an 18-year-old patient with Down syndrome. **B** Cut surface of the same specimen.

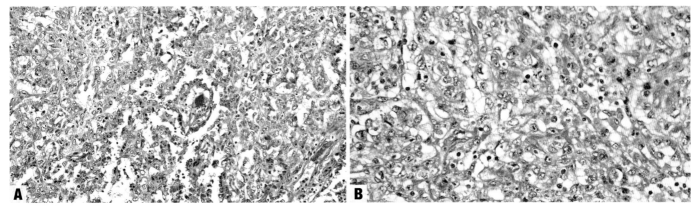

**Fig. 7.38** Yolk sac tumour. **A** Classic Schiller–Duval body surrounded by cells with intracytoplasmic eosinophilic globules. **B** At higher magnification, the intracellular globular globules and band-like intercellular deposits of basement membrane (parietal differentiation) are clearly seen.

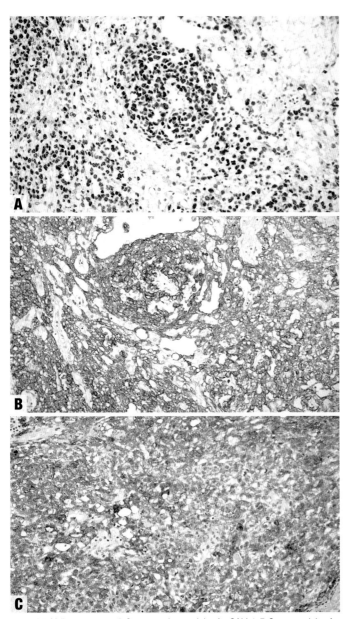

**Fig. 7.39** Yolk sac tumour. **A** Strong nuclear staining for SALL4. **B** Strong staining for AE1/AE3. **C** Positive immunohistochemistry for glypican-3 (GPC3).

no established epidemiological associations. Within the CNS, YSTs constitute 2–7.2% of intracranial germ cell tumours and 3.3–19.1% of the non-germinomas {4480,7616,3250}. There is an equal sex distribution {6465}.

### Etiology

For postpubertal YST see *Intratubular germ cell neoplasia (male gonadal)* (p. 649); for CNS YST see *Embryonal carcinoma* (p. 679).

### Pathogenesis

See *Intratubular germ cell neoplasia (male gonadal)* (p. 649). Clinical and epigenetic studies of germ cell tumours arising after infancy / early childhood {3106,6282,2261} suggest a primordial germ cell origin, although alternative origins have also been suggested {5201,6861}. Prepubertal-type YST is a type I germ cell tumour {5195}, which probably progressed from a pure (type I) teratoma, showing recurrent gains of 1q, 12p13, 20q, and 22, and losses of 1p, 4, and 6q {4812,5367, 6258,7267}. Association with a SNP variant of *BAK1* has been reported {5612}, suggesting that primitive germ cell apoptosis plays a pathogenetic role.

### Macroscopic appearance

YSTs are predominantly solid, relatively homogeneous nodular masses, yellow to tan in colour and possibly friable or gelatinous (owing to myxoid changes). Focal cysts may be present. Necrosis and haemorrhage are uncommon.

### Histopathology

Similar morphological patterns (possibly in combination) and immunophenotypes are seen in prepubertal and postpubertal YST. Both show intracytoplasmic and extracellular hyaline globules with a refractile eosinophilic quality and irregular, often band-like intercellular deposits of basement membrane, called parietal differentiation. Schiller–Duval bodies are commonly present. In testicular postpubertal-type YST, germ cell neoplasia in situ and regressive changes in the surrounding parenchyma are absent. The prepubertal type may be mixed with teratoma, whereas the other elements can also be found in the postpubertal type (all associated with 12p gain). The prepubertal type rarely arises after puberty {5202}. Immunoreactivity for AFP (which is potentially also found in the glandular components of teratomas) characterizes YST {719,2920,2314}, in addition to cytokeratins, SALL4 {1019}, glypican-3 (GPC3) {5249,7898}, LIN28A {1020}, possibly KIT (CD117) {3416}, and PLAP {4557}.

## Cytology

Smear and squash preparations show cohesive clusters of epithelioid cells with distinct nucleoli and feature spindle mesenchymal elements and myxoid material.

## Diagnostic molecular pathology

Not clinically relevant

## Essential and desirable diagnostic criteria

*Essential:* epithelioid cells in various patterns, with or without mesenchymal constituents.
*Desirable:* AFP expression by immunohistochemistry.

## Staging

See *Intratubular germ cell neoplasia (male gonadal)* (p. 649). For CNS pure YST with leptomeningeal metastasis, treatment follows the regimens for poor prognostic groups with metastasis {4479}. Staging of these tumours follows the Delphi consensus {4871}.

## Prognosis and prediction

Limited prognostic information is available for YST, owing to its rarity. Patients aged > 2 years may be more likely to have advanced-stage disease at diagnosis {5611}, but effective chemotherapy results in survival rates approaching 100% {4019,5952,6949}. Specific microRNA elevation after orchiectomy may predict metastasis {2424,4872,199}. Surgical excision of residual masses after chemotherapy may be performed but is usually not necessary. Postpubertal patients with stage III germ cell tumours containing YST elements have a poorer outcome than patients with tumours lacking such elements, probably indicating relative chemoresistance. This also correlates with an increased prevalence of YST in late recurrences {4641} and in autopsy assessments of patients who died of progressive germ cell tumours in the current treatment era {5100}. Therefore, it may be that the histological patterns of YST disproportionately found in chemoresistant cases and late recurrences (glandular predominant, hepatoid, parietal, and sarcomatoid) are adverse findings in the primary tumour, but this remains to be proved. Within the CNS, combined irradiation and chemotherapy resulted in 5- and 10-year survival rates of 75–80% {981,6841}, in which logarithmic decreases of AFP and hCG predict favourable outcomes {3490}. AFP levels of > 1000 ng/mL and residual disease after treatment have negative implications {981}. Long-term survivors are at risk of premature death due to subsequent treatment-associated malignant neoplasms {38}.

# Fetus in fetu

Reyes-Múgica M
Stoneham SJ

## Definition
Fetus in fetu (FIF) is an exceptional developmental anomaly in which a parasitic fetus is contained within the body of its twin.

## ICD-O coding
None

## ICD-11 coding
None

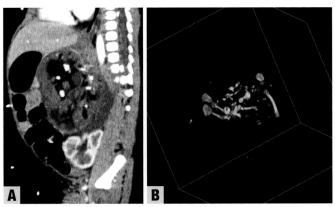

**Fig. 7.40** Fetus in fetu. **A** Contrast-enhanced sagittal reformatted CT showing a large heterogeneous abdominal mass between the liver and the left kidney, with multiple calcified components favouring fetal parts. **B** 3D CT with volume-rendering display in bone algorithm showing multiple calcified components within the abdominal mass, resembling the long bones, scapula, and pelvis of a fetus.

## Related terminology
*Acceptable:* internal parasitic twin; external parasitic twin; epignathus; fetiform teratoma.

## Subtype(s)
None

## Localization
FIF is most commonly intra-abdominal (70–80% of cases) {6187, 487}, although it may occur in many different locations, including the gonads {3916}, sacrum, oropharynx, orbit, intracranial structures, and thorax {7781,7043,3583,1339,5198}.

## Clinical features
FIF most commonly manifests as an asymptomatic abdominal mass and is usually discovered by prenatal ultrasound {3312}. The original term is attributed to Johann Friedrich Meckel, circa 1800 {4068}. It is currently considered a type 0 germ cell tumour {5198}.

## Epidemiology
The estimated incidence is of FIF is 1 case per 500 000 live births {6187}. Most occur in neonates or young children, but rare cases in adults have been reported {3814}.

## Etiology
Genetic data point towards an abnormality in the development of monozygotic/diamniotic twins.

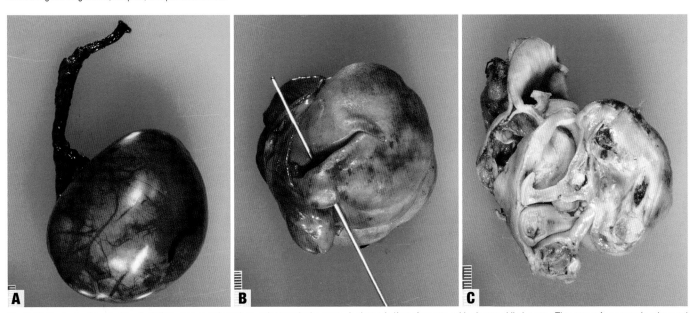

**Fig. 7.41** Testicular fetus in fetu. **A–C** This case manifested as an intratesticular mass. It shows fetiform features, with abnormal limb parts. The cut surface reveals advanced organic development.

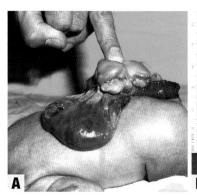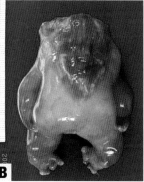

**Fig. 7.42** Fetus in fetu. **A** This example was located in the lumbosacral region of a newborn immediately before excision. The lesion showed a well-developed half of a face, which was able to move the lips and eyebrow. **B** Fetus in fetu from the back aspect, showing a combination of anencephaly and craniorachischisis. Note the well-formed limbs and trunk.

## Pathogenesis
More than 15% of FIF cases have a family history of twinning. It is currently thought that blastomeres in the two-cell (2C) stage, which are defined as omnipotent, are prone to escaping the organizing influence of the developing embryo or their developmental potential, leading to FIF {5198}.

## Macroscopic appearance
By definition, FIF appears as a tumour mass with variable fetiform features. Some reach a strikingly fetus-like stage of development, including mobility of the limbs {3312} and the development of other recognizable portions of a fetal body. FIF should be distinguished from mature/fetiform teratoma by the presence of metameric segmentation, demonstrated radiologically by evidence of vertebral organization.

## Histopathology
The histopathology of FIF is similar to that of mature teratomas but with a higher degree of organization. Full bowel and multiple organs are commonly recognized.

## Cytology
Not relevant

## Diagnostic molecular pathology
Most analyses reveal genotypic identity between the host and the FIF {3583}.

## Essential and desirable diagnostic criteria
*Essential:* advanced organoid development; evidence of axialization and metameric segmentation (vertebral organization).
*Desirable:* enclosure by a distinct sac; partial or complete normal skin coverage; grossly recognizable anatomical parts; attachment to the host by only a few relatively large blood vessels; immediate adjacency to one of the sites of attachment of conjoined twins, or association with the neural tube or gastrointestinal system.

## Staging
Not relevant

## Prognosis and prediction
Most are cured with simple surgical resection. There are reports of recurrences with a malignant component, especially yolk sac tumour {2974}.

# Choriocarcinoma (non-gestational)

Looijenga LHJ
Kao CS
Stoneham SJ
Wong TT

### Definition
Choriocarcinoma is composed of cells of the extraembryonic chorion, including cytotrophoblast, intermediate trophoblast, and syncytiotrophoblast cells.

### ICD-O coding
9100/3 Choriocarcinoma (non-gestational)

### ICD-11 coding
2C73.Y & XH8PK7 Other specified malignant neoplasms of the ovary & Choriocarcinoma, NOS

2C80.02 & XH8PK7 Germ cell tumour of testis & Choriocarcinoma, NOS

2A00.1Y & XH8PK7 Other specified embryonal tumours of brain & Choriocarcinoma, NOS

### Related terminology
*Not recommended:* trophoblastic malignant teratoma; chorionepithelioma.

### Subtype(s)
None

### Localization
Choriocarcinoma occurs in the gonads, mediastinum, and CNS (mostly in the pineal region, followed by the suprasellar compartment, basal ganglia / thalamus, spine, and other locations) {6447,3269,3830}.

### Clinical features
Choriocarcinoma occurs in 6.4–17.8% of mixed testicular germ cell tumours and is pure in 0.3% {3772,4804,4813,211}. It is rare in childhood, except in patients with disorders of sex development {2785,3772}. Detection often follows signs or symptoms attributed to a distant metastasis, such as haemoptysis, an abdominal mass, neurological dysfunction, anaemia, or hypotension. β-hCG is invariably elevated (often > 50 000 IU/L {211}), possibly related to gynaecomastia (10%) and thyrotoxicosis (rare). Clinical features of CNS primary pure choriocarcinomas correlate with tumour location, high β-hCG, associated hydrocephalus, and tumoural haemorrhage {6447,3269,5677}. Metastatic choriocarcinomas in the brain and spinal cord occur and are frequently associated with tumoural haemorrhage. The symptoms and signs vary from headache to acute change of consciousness. In cases of spinal tumour haemorrhage, patients may present with back pain.

### Epidemiology
See *Intratubular germ cell neoplasia (male gonadal)* (p. 649). CNS choriocarcinoma occurs in 3.3–5% of all germ cell tumours {4480,3250} and in 5.6% of non-germinomatous tumours {4480}. It is more frequent in male patients (M:F ratio: 3.4:1). The mean patient age is 13 years (range: 5–22 years), with two peaks in incidence, at 6–11 years and at 13–18 years {3269}.

### Etiology
See *Intratubular germ cell neoplasia (male gonadal)* (p. 649) {6259,6947,2260,7408,6282}. Fewer CNS germ cell tumours

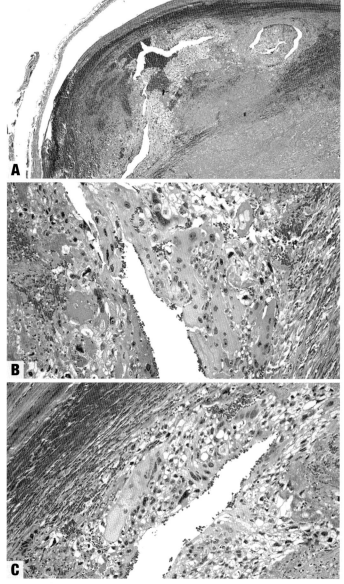

**Fig. 7.43** Choriocarcinoma. **A** Panoramic view of an area of haemorrhage and necrosis with foci of choriocarcinoma from a 17-year-old patient. **B** Cytotrophoblastic and syncytiotrophoblastic cells in a haemorrhagic background, characteristic of choriocarcinoma. **C** Cytotrophoblast with multiple mitoses in a focus of choriocarcinoma.

exhibit gains of 12p than do testicular and mediastinal examples {5152,6762,6947,2260}. Gains of *CCND2* and *PRDM14* (primordial germ cell specification regulator) and losses of *RB1* imply involvement of the cyclin/CDK/RB1/E2F pathway {6947}. Activating mutations involving the MAPK pathway (KIT, RAS family members) and (less frequently) the PI3K/AKT/mTOR pathway have been identified in germ cell tumours beyond infancy / early childhood {2260,7408,3106,6282}. More CNS germ cell tumours appear to occur in Down syndrome {4726} and Klinefelter syndrome (47,XXY) {3370,7553,5270} than in the general population.

## Pathogenesis

See *Intratubular germ cell neoplasia (male gonadal)* (p. 649). Clinical and epigenetic studies of germ cell tumours arising after infancy / early childhood {3106,6282,2261} suggest a primordial germ cell origin, although alternative origins have also been suggested {5201,6861}.

## Macroscopic appearance

Choriocarcinoma appears as mostly solid, haemorrhagic and necrotic nodules containing foci (sometimes as a peripheral rim) of solid, greyish-tan tumour.

## Histopathology

Choriocarcinoma classically consists of mononucleated trophoblasts (cytotrophoblasts and intermediate trophoblasts) and multinucleated syncytiotrophoblasts, mostly in a haemorrhagic background. Mononucleated trophoblasts (small cytotrophoblasts with some medium-sized and fewer large intermediate trophoblasts) are capped by syncytiotrophoblasts forming plexiform aggregates and protrusions. Cytotrophoblasts have clear to lightly eosinophilic cytoplasm, distinct cell boundaries, slightly irregular nuclei, and one or multiple prominent nucleoli displaying frequent mitotic figures. Syncytiotrophoblasts are large, with deeply eosinophilic cytoplasm (often containing internalized erythrocytes) and one or multiple nuclei (often dark and smudgy). They may have spindly configurations. Monophasic choriocarcinoma, i.e. sheets of cytotrophoblasts with syncytiotrophoblasts, may occur {7142}. Vascular invasion is common. β-hCG and hPL are expressed, as well as keratin and sometimes PLAP {3107, 719,2920,2314}. Syncytiotrophoblasts express inhibin and glypican-3 (GPC3) {4501,7898}, and cytotrophoblasts express SALL4, GDF3, p63, and GATA3 {482,1019,2498,211}.

## Cytology

Diagnosis requires examination of tissue sections and immunohistochemical evaluation, but the presence of syncytiotrophoblastic giant cells in squash or smear preparations raises concern for choriocarcinoma, particularly in a haemorrhagic/necrotic background.

## Diagnostic molecular pathology

Isochromosome 12p and increased copy numbers of 12p in the majority of choriocarcinomas are helpful diagnostic findings to

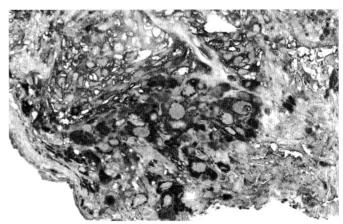

**Fig. 7.44** Choriocarcinoma. Immunohistochemistry is strongly positive for β-hCG in choriocarcinoma.

differentiate from non–germ cell, poorly differentiated malignancies {4204,7207}.

## Essential and desirable diagnostic criteria

*Essential:* identification of both syncytiotrophoblastic and cytotrophoblastic elements; β-hCG expression; absence of KIT, D2-40, AFP, and OCT3/4.

## Staging

See *Intratubular germ cell neoplasia (male gonadal)* (p. 649). In CNS choriocarcinoma, extraneural metastasis is more frequent than leptomeningeal metastasis at diagnosis {3250,6544,3269}. Staging without extraneural metastasis follows the Delphi consensus {4871}.

## Prognosis and prediction

Choriocarcinoma is highly aggressive, with early haematogenous spread, high stage, and haemorrhagic complications {535, 2845,3252,211}. Choriocarcinoma commonly metastasizes to the lungs, liver, gastrointestinal tract, brain, spleen, and adrenals {4813,5321,211}. Elevated serum β-hCG (> 50 000 IU/L) after treatment indicates a poor response {4189}. Pure/predominant choriocarcinomas have similar outcomes {211}. After combination chemotherapy, a 3-year survival rate of 21% is reported {211}. Outcome may not be uniformly fatal with standard chemotherapy for metastases confined to the lungs, or after complete resection of residual mass with high-dose chemotherapy and stem cell support {4018,5321,211}.

CNS pure choriocarcinoma (intracranial-predominant) has a median survival time of 22 months, and survival rates of 58.8% and 45.8% at 36 and 60 months, respectively {1337}. Haematogenous metastases occur in 26.8%, predominantly in the lung {3269}. Negative prognostic factors are extraneural metastasis {3269} and a pineal or suprasellar location {1167,3269}; positive indicators include gross total resection {3269}, postresectional chemotherapy {1167,3269}, and postresectional radiotherapy {1167}. A high β-hCG level has no prognostic significance {1167}.

# Malignant mixed germ cell tumours

Looijenga LHJ
Kao CS
Stoneham SJ
Wong TT

## Definition

Malignant mixed germ cell tumours (MMGCTs) are composed of more than one histological element. They are regarded as non-seminoma, despite the presence of a seminoma-like component.

## ICD-O coding

9085/3 Malignant mixed germ cell tumours

9085/3 Mixed germinoma and teratoma

9085/3 Mixed germ cell tumour consisting of germinoma or teratoma with a small portion of malignant element

9085/3 Mixed tumour consisting mainly of choriocarcinoma, embryonal carcinoma, or yolk sac tumour

## ICD-11 coding

2C80.26 & XH2PS1 Germ cell tumour of testis & Mixed germ cell tumour

2A00.1Y & XH2PS1 Other specified embryonal tumours of brain & Mixed germ cell tumour

2D4Y & XH2PS1 Other specified malignant neoplasms of ill-defined or unspecified primary sites & Mixed germ cell tumour

## Related terminology

*Not recommended:* combined tumour; intermediate malignant teratoma.

## Subtype(s)

Mixed germinoma and teratoma (MGT); mixed germ cell tumour consisting of germinoma or teratoma with a small portion of malignant element (MXB); mixed tumour consisting mainly of choriocarcinoma, embryonal carcinoma, or yolk sac tumour (MXM)

## Localization

MMGCTs occur in the gonads, mediastinum, and CNS (in which most occur in the pineal region or suprasellar compartment and

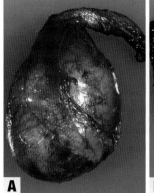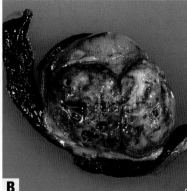

**Fig. 7.46** Malignant mixed germ cell tumour. **A** Orchiectomy specimen from a 17-year-old boy. **B** Cut surface shows a multicystic and fleshy tumour with multifocal haemorrhage replacing most of the testicular parenchyma in this example from a 17-year-old boy.

fewer arise in the basal ganglia / thalamus and other locations) {4480,7616,5053}.

## Clinical features

MMGCTs represent the majority of non-seminomatous tumours. Although embryonal carcinomas with teratoma, seminoma, or yolk sac tumour (YST) are frequent, any combination, often with more than two components, can be seen. MMGCTs in prepubertal patients are extremely rare. Tumour markers are often elevated, but their absence is associated with an increased incidence of metastases {559,6066}. Different components and their proportions, particularly in clinical stage I testicular germ cell tumour, may have clinical implications {1575}; therefore, determination of their percentages is required, for which immunohistochemistry is usually helpful. In CNS MMGCTs, the classified subgroups have clinical and therapeutic implications {4480,4479}. The presence of more than two components is common. The mean ages at diagnosis of CNS MMGCT in two studies were 10.1 years (range:

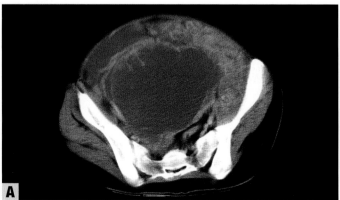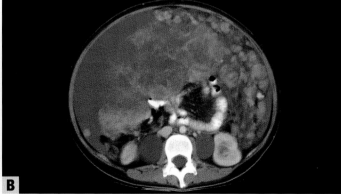

**Fig. 7.45** Malignant mixed germ cell tumour. Contrast-enhanced axial CT shows a mixed solid and cystic mass with irregular enhancing fibrovascular septa (**A**) and extensive metastatic peritoneal deposits and ascites (**B**).

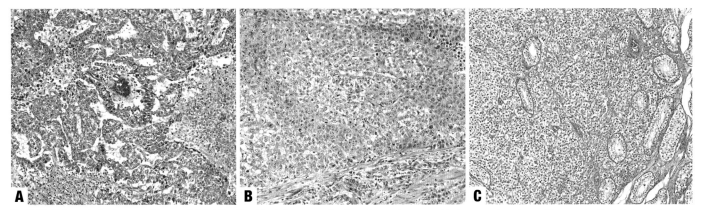

**Fig. 7.47** Malignant mixed germ cell tumour. **A** A Schiller–Duval body in an area of yolk sac tumour from an orchiectomy specimen from a 17-year-old patient. Cytogenetic analysis revealed two copies of the short arm of chromosome 12 (isochromosome 12p), along with four copies of chromosome 12, resulting in five or six copies of 12p and other chromosomal abnormalities. **B** An area of embryonal carcinoma from the same tumour. **C** A focus of seminoma at the borderline with the testicular parenchyma showing seminiferous tubules with germ cell neoplasia in situ. This example is from an 18-year-old male patient.

1.6–15.4 years) and 15 ± 6.6 years, respectively {4480,7616}. The level of AFP elevation is low (< 200 ng/mL) in the MGT subtype and in the MXB subtype with an embryonal carcinoma component; it may be high in MXBs containing a YST component (90–1810 ng/mL); and it is invariably high in MXMs consisting mainly of a YST component (3380–6700 ng/mL) {4480}. The level of hCG elevation may be low in MGT (61 mIU/mL, 1 case), in MXB containing YST (770 mIU/mL, 1 case), or in MXM consisting mainly of YST (167 mIU/mL, 1 case), and it is high in MXM consisting mainly of choriocarcinoma {4480}. Systemic dissemination rarely occurs {368}. The clinical symptoms and signs of CNS mixed germ cell tumours correlate with tumour location and associated hydrocephalus.

## Epidemiology

See *Intratubular germ cell neoplasia (male gonadal)* (p. 649). CNS MMGCTs principally affect children and are more prevalent in eastern Asia than in Europe and the USA. Age-adjusted annual incidence rates of 0.45 cases per 100 000 population aged < 15 years and of 0.49 cases per 100 000 population aged < 19 years have been reported, respectively, from Japan {4338} and the Republic of Korea {3407}. These (the highest recorded) are more than three times as high as the rates in Germany {3358} and the USA {5240}. The incidence of CNS germ cell tumours in Canadian children aged < 18 years is 0.29 ± 0.18 cases per 1 million person-years {3505}. Pure germinomas outnumber other types, followed by mixed lesions and teratomas; embryonal carcinomas, YSTs, and choriocarcinomas occur uncommonly in pure form {2920,719,4480, 6843}. CNS MMGCTs (intracranial-predominant) accounted for 13.8–32.0% of all germ cell tumours and 30.2–54.4% of non-germinoma germ cell tumours in two reported series {4480, 7616}. The M:F: ratio is 3.9:1. In mixed tumours arising in the suprasellar compartment (posterior pituitary), a reversal of the M:F ratio is observed (0.8:1) {4480}.

## Etiology

See *Intratubular germ cell neoplasia (male gonadal)* (p. 649) and *Embryonal carcinoma* (p. 679). Germline variants of *JMJD1C*, which encodes a jumonji domain–containing histone demethylase, have been associated with a heightened risk of CNS germ cell tumours in Japanese people {3834}.

## Pathogenesis

See *Intratubular germ cell neoplasia (male gonadal)* (p. 649) and *Embryonal carcinoma* (p. 679).

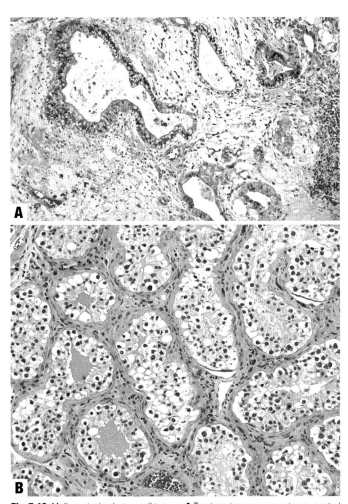

**Fig. 7.48** Malignant mixed germ cell tumour. **A** Teratomatous component represented by intestinal glandular structures in an 18-year-old male patient. **B** Peritumoural testicular parenchyma showing seminiferous tubules with the classic appearance of germ cell neoplasia in situ. This is from the 17-year-old boy with multiple copies of isochromosome 12p (see Fig. 7.47A).

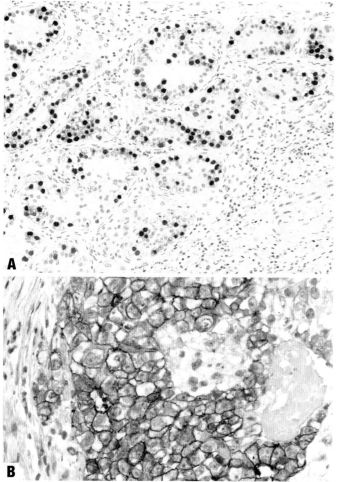

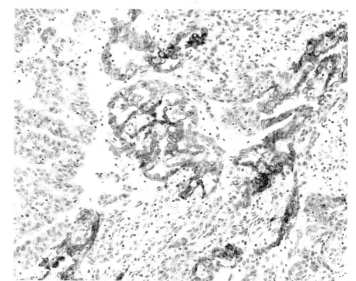

**Fig. 7.50** Malignant mixed germ cell tumour. A yolk sac tumour area is highlighted by glypican-3 (GPC3) immunohistochemistry in this example from a 17-year-old boy.

**Fig. 7.49** Malignant mixed germ cell tumour. **A** OCT4 immunohistochemistry shows strong nuclear staining in tubules with germ cell neoplasia in situ in this specimen from a 17-year-old boy. **B** An area of embryonal carcinoma showing a characteristic membranous staining pattern with CD30.

## Macroscopic appearance

MMGCTs appear variegated according to the presence of different components; solid white to grey areas may reflect a seminoma-like component, whereas non-seminomatous elements are more often associated with areas of necrosis, haemorrhage, and cystic change.

## Histopathology

The histopathological features of the individual components are identical to those seen in pure forms. Closely associated components of embryonal carcinoma and YST are particularly common, and the YST component is often missed. The distinction of foci of choriocarcinoma from syncytiotrophoblastic giant cells in association with seminoma is important. Two patterns of mixed germ cell tumour are sufficiently distinct to be separately subcategorized: polyembryoma {2006} and diffuse embryoma {1039,1645}.

## Cytology

See the various pure elements.

## Diagnostic molecular pathology

See *Intratubular germ cell neoplasia (male gonadal)* (p. 649) and the sections on non-germinomatous germ cell tumours.

## Essential and desirable diagnostic criteria

See *Intratubular germ cell neoplasia (male gonadal)* (p. 649) and the sections on non-germinomatous germ cell tumours.

## Staging

See *Intratubular germ cell neoplasia (male gonadal)* (p. 649) and the other pure elements.

## Prognosis and prediction

See *Intratubular germ cell neoplasia (male gonadal)* (p. 649), *Embryonal carcinoma* (p. 679), and *Yolk sac tumour* (p. 681). A teratomatous component in the testis is associated with a higher probability of teratoma in postchemotherapy retroperitoneal lymph nodes in higher-stage tumours {1072}. Like in pure tumours, the predominance of a choriocarcinomatous component in mixed germ cell tumour is associated with high stage at presentation and aggressive behaviour {211}.

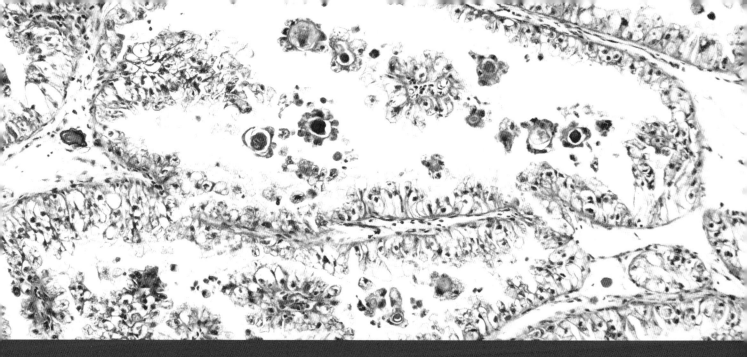

# 8

# Renal and male genital tumours

Edited by: Hill DA, Moch H, Pritchard-Jones K, Srigley JR, Tsuzuki T

Renal tumours
  Nephroblastic and related tumours
    Paediatric cystic nephroma
    Nephroblastoma
  Molecularly defined renal tumours
    Renal cell carcinoma with MiT translocations
    *ALK*-rearranged renal cell carcinoma
    Eosinophilic solid and cystic renal cell carcinoma
    SMARCB1-deficient renal medullary carcinoma
  Metanephric tumours
    Metanephric adenoma
    Metanephric adenofibroma
    Metanephric stromal tumour
  Mesenchymal renal tumours
    Ossifying renal tumour of infancy
    Mesoblastic nephroma
    Clear cell sarcoma of the kidney
    Malignant rhabdoid tumour of the kidney
    Anaplastic sarcoma of the kidney
    Renal Ewing sarcoma
Testicular tumours
    Juvenile granulosa cell tumour of the testis

# Renal and male genital tumours: Introduction

Pritchard-Jones K
Bode PK

This chapter includes major sections on nephroblastoma and renal carcinomas, whereas germ cell tumours of the testis are dealt with in another chapter, alongside germ cell tumours of the female genital tract and non-gonadal tumours (Table 8.01). Metanephric tumours are dealt with in this chapter, as are epithelial or biphasic renal tumours unique to the kidney.

## Nephroblastoma

Nephroblastoma, also known by the eponym "Wilms tumour", is the commonest primary kidney tumour in childhood. It accounts for > 90% of malignant kidney tumours diagnosed in children aged ≤ 7 years, with other entities in the differential diagnosis accounting for 2–3% individually {4918}. On this basis, chemotherapy may be started empirically without histological diagnosis if the clinical and imaging features are typical. This approach, recommended by International Society of Paediatric Oncology (SIOP) protocols in common use around the world, aims to provide a more favourable tumour stage distribution when assessed at nephrectomy, including reducing the risk of tumour rupture during surgery. In infancy, the relative likelihood of rhabdoid tumour increases, as does that of mesoblastic nephroma, particularly in the first 3 months of life. For these reasons, immediate nephrectomy without preceding chemotherapy is recommended by both SIOP and the Children's Oncology Group (COG) protocols in younger children. The incidence of renal cell carcinoma (RCC) starts to increase in older children, but nephroblastoma is still the more common tumour type up to the age of 13 years and constitutes 23% of all renal cancers diagnosed in patients aged 15–19 years {4918}.

Histological diagnosis of nephroblastoma can be straightforward when all three elements of the classic triphasic tumour are identified. However, when the tumour has only a monophasic or biphasic appearance, the differential diagnosis expands and it is important to take account of the full clinical context (age, associated syndromes, presence and pattern of metastasis) as well as immunohistochemistry and molecular testing. The latter may be necessary to exclude rarer entities that can show morphological overlap with some components of nephroblastoma.

Needle biopsy, when indicated, should be performed using a percutaneous cutting needle approach. It is recommended to use a coaxial technique under image guidance to avoid areas of necrosis and so that multiple cores sufficient for histological diagnosis can be obtained. FNAB is not recommended for diagnosis of nephroblastoma. Needle biopsy is not reliable for the diagnosis of diffuse anaplasia, missing 90% of cases where this was found in the subsequent nephrectomy specimen {3185}.

Treatment context is critical for assigning both histological risk and tumour stage. Both SIOP and COG systems recognize diffuse anaplasia as a high-risk category of nephroblastoma, but only the SIOP classification takes account of histological response to pre-nephrectomy chemotherapy. The high-risk blastemal-type nephroblastoma can only be defined in the setting of prior chemotherapy. It constitutes < 10% of all nephroblastomas, in contrast to chemotherapy-naïve tumours that can be described as "blastemal predominant", which constitute approximately one third of all nephroblastomas {7343}. Owing to the range of histological appearances of nephroblastoma and its relative rarity, a system of pathology review is offered through the clinical study groups {7348,5457}. This should be welcomed, because historically, 38% of cases with diffuse anaplasia were not classified as such by the institutional pathologist {1781}.

Molecular correlates of histological subtypes and of prognosis are not as well established in nephroblastoma as in some other childhood cancers, but they continue to emerge {2277, 7344}. Somatic gain of chromosome 1q is on the point of being introduced as a clinical risk-stratification factor by COG and is under investigation by SIOP for its relative prognostic impact in relation to residual blastemal volume after chemotherapy {1783, 7344}. One challenge is intratumoural heterogeneity of somatic genetic changes {1485}. This may be overcome by the analysis of circulating tumour DNA {3274}. Molecular analysis of specific histological subtypes may also reveal mutations in genes that may reflect genetic predisposition – for example, WT1 in stromal-type/predominant tumours.

## Paediatric renal cell carcinomas

For this first classification of paediatric tumours, a chapter called *Carcinomas usually occurring in adults* was originally planned. However, it became apparent that such a chapter can hardly cover all aspects of paediatric RCC. On the one hand, paediatric

**Table 8.01** Tumours that may occur in childhood but are not covered further in this chapter

| Name of tumour | Features specific to childhood occurrence | | | |
| --- | --- | --- | --- | --- |
| | Approximate occurrence (prevalence/incidence, if known) | Clinical features | Pathological features | Genes involved |
| Clear cell renal cancer | < 5% | None | Occurs in VHL syndrome | VHL |
| Papillary renal cell carcinoma | < 5% | None | Occurs in HLRCC or PRCC syndrome | MET and FH |
| Chromophobe renal cell carcinoma | < 5% | None | None (BHD syndrome) | |

BHD, Birt–Hogg–Dubé; HLRCC, hereditary leiomyomatosis and renal cell carcinoma; PRCC, papillary renal cell carcinoma; VHL, von Hippel–Lindau.

RCC does not represent only one entity but includes numerous subtypes. On the other hand, several adjustments were made in the fifth edition of the WHO classification of renal cell tumours. Roughly summarized, RCC is now divided into morphologically and molecularly defined tumours. The molecularly defined RCC group involves tumours with a very broad range of morphological patterns but with a specific gene alteration. Some of these molecularly defined RCCs are relatively common in children,

for example *TFE3*-rearranged RCC, *TFEB*-rearranged RCC, SMARCB1-deficient medullary RCC, and *ALK*-rearranged RCC. Other molecularly defined RCCs may occur in a hereditary tumour syndrome, for example fumarate hydratase–deficient RCC (hereditary leiomyomatosis and RCC–associated RCC) or succinate dehydrogenase–deficient RCC. Whereas most of these molecularly defined RCCs require a molecular test to make a definite diagnosis, most morphologically defined RCCs can be

**Table 8.02** Relative proportions of kidney cancer types[a] recorded by population-based cancer registries by age and geographical region, cases diagnosed in 2001–2010[b,c]

| Renal cancer type | Age group (years) | | | | |
|---|---|---|---|---|---|
| | 0[d] | 1–4 | 5–9 | 10–14 | 15–19 |
| **Total number of cases in each age group, all world regions combined** | | | | | |
| Wilms tumour (VIa1) | 1812 | 8751 | 2813 | 462 | 181 |
| Rhabdoid renal tumour (VIa2) | 197 | 109 | 15 | 6 | 4 |
| Kidney sarcomas (VIa3) | 57 | 286 | 55 | 33 | 7 |
| Renal cell carcinomas (VIb) | 13 | 69 | 155 | 306 | 564 |
| Unspecified (VIc) | 33 | 87 | 38 | 23 | 44 |
| All malignant renal tumours | 2112 | 9302 | 3076 | 830 | 800 |
| **Cases as a percentage of all malignant renal tumours** | | | | | |
| Wilms tumour | 85.8% | 94.1% | 91.4% | 55.7% | 22.6% |
| Rhabdoid renal tumour | 9.3% | 1.2% | 0.5% | 0.7% | 0.5% |
| Kidney sarcomas | 2.7% | 3.1% | 1.8% | 4.0% | 0.9% |
| Renal cell carcinomas | 0.6% | 0.7% | 5.0% | 36.9% | 70.5% |
| Unspecified | 1.6% | 0.9% | 1.2% | 2.8% | 5.5% |
| **Relative proportions of Wilms tumour and renal cell carcinomas (*n* = total number of renal cancer cases registered per region)** | | | | | |
| **North America (*n* = 5943)** | | | | | |
| Wilms tumour | 82.9% | 93.8% | 90.8% | 48.6% | 18.4% |
| Renal cell carcinomas | 0.8% | 0.6% | 6.1% | 46.5% | 78.4% |
| **Europe (*n* = 5682)** | | | | | |
| Wilms tumour | 87.4% | 95.1% | 92.5% | 60.7% | 26.0% |
| Renal cell carcinomas | 0.4% | 0.5% | 4.3% | 34.0% | 64.4% |
| **Latin America and the Caribbean (*n* = 1174)** | | | | | |
| Wilms tumour | 90.2% | 93.4% | 90.6% | 58.7% | 40.0% |
| Renal cell carcinomas | 0.6% | 0.9% | 2.1% | 24.0% | 48.6% |
| **Asia (*n* = 1734)** | | | | | |
| Wilms tumour | 84.2% | 91.0% | 89.6% | 57.5% | 33.3% |
| Renal cell carcinomas | 1.2% | 2.1% | 5.5% | 23.8% | 52.4% |
| **Africa (*n* = 1157)** | | | | | |
| Wilms tumour | 90.7% | 95.7% | 95.8% | 83.9% | 21.7% |
| Renal cell carcinomas | 0.0% | 0.1% | 2.5% | 9.7% | 60.9% |
| **Oceania (*n* = 403)** | | | | | |
| Wilms tumour | 86.3% | 94.7% | 96.1% | 33.3% | 36.4% |
| Renal cell carcinomas | 0.0% | 1.3% | 1.3% | 63.0% | 54.5% |

[a]Tumours classified in group VI (renal tumours) according to the International Classification of Childhood Cancer (ICCC), third edition, 2017 update (ICCC-3-2017) {6785}. [b]Numbers derived from population-based cancer registry data submitted by International Incidence of Childhood Cancer 3 (IICC-3) contributors {6669}. [c]Data extracted from supplementary Table S3 of Nakata et al. (2020) {4918}. [d]Numbers do not include the benign entity mesoblastic nephroma; this entity is reported by a collaborative effort of international childhood renal tumour study groups to account for 54% of all renal tumours diagnosed in the first month, 33% in the second, 16% in the third, and < 10% of all tumours diagnosed in the fourth and subsequent months of life {7197}.

**Table 8.03** Reported relative frequencies of renal cell carcinoma (RCC) subtypes in children and young adults {976}

| RCC subtype | Relative frequency (%) |
|---|---|
| MiT RCC | 41.5 |
| Papillary RCC | 16.5 |
| Renal medullary RCC | 12.3 |
| Unclassified RCC | 7.5 |
| Chromophobe RCC | 6.6 |
| Tuberous sclerosis–associated RCC | 4.2 |
| ALK-rearranged RCC | 3.8 |
| Clear cell RCC | 3.3 |
| Fumarate hydratase–deficient RCC | 1.4 |
| Succinate dehydrogenase–deficient RCC | 0.5 |
| Others | 2.4 |

**Table 8.04** Hereditary renal cell carcinoma (RCC) syndromes in children and adolescents {1472}

| Tumour type | Hereditary tumour syndrome | Gene | Gene locus |
|---|---|---|---|
| Clear cell RCC | Von Hippel–Lindau syndrome | VHL | 3p25.3 |
| | Succinate dehydrogenase–deficient RCC syndrome | SDHB SDHD | 1p36.13 11q23.1 |
| Papillary RCC | Hereditary papillary RCC | MET | 7q31 |
| | Hereditary leiomyomatosis RCC | FH | 1q43 |
| Chromophobe RCC | Birt–Hogg–Dubé syndrome | FLCN | 17p11.2 |

diagnosed by morphology and immunohistochemistry alone. The p.V600E mutations of *BRAF* are present in approximately 90% of metanephric adenomas. Most, but not all, can be detected by immunohistochemistry for BRAF using the VE1 clone. Therefore, these tumours remained in the group of morphologically defined renal tumours.

Taking all this into account, we have decided to replace the originally planned chapter with this introduction, which aims to highlight important differences between RCC in children and in adults. The morphological and molecular details of the individual subtypes are included in the fifth edition of the WHO classification of renal cell tumours.

### Epidemiology

Overall, paediatric RCC is rare and accounts for 2–4% of all renal neoplasms in childhood and adolescence {5379,2349, 6338,910,5794} (see Table 8.02, p. 693). Whereas nephroblastoma dominates in the first decade of life, RCC accounts for about half of all renal tumours after the age of 12–14 years (median ages at presentation: 11–17 years) {6814,2349,4918}. There is an equal sex distribution {6814,114,7760}, which contrasts with the male predominance of adult RCC. Although most translocation RCCs occur in children and young adults, they are not infrequent in adults. Among all RCCs in children and young adults, about one third are accounted for by papillary, chromophobe, clear cell, and unclassified RCCs together (see Table 8.03). A slowly increasing incidence of paediatric RCC has been observed over the past few decades {4918}. A possible link to obesity {7880,3914}, dietary habits {4570}, and better imaging techniques {3992} has been discussed.

### Clinical features

Children and adolescents with RCC present with more advanced disease and a higher stage than adults. Therefore, > 80% of patients are symptomatic at the time of diagnosis. The most common manifestations include abdominal pain, haematuria, palpable mass, or fever. Furthermore, as many as one third of paediatric patients have metastases, including lymph node metastases, which are rarely seen in adults {114, 6195,6338}.

### Etiology

RCC can be associated with different familial syndromes (see Table 8.04). In a hereditary context, it frequently manifests at a younger age {1472}.

### Staging, prognosis, and prediction

Unlike for Wilms tumour, TNM classification is used for RCC. Despite the advanced stage at the time of diagnosis, the prognosis is more favourable in children than in adults with RCC. This is because the survival rate of paediatric patients with regional lymph node involvement still reaches 70% {2348}. Distant metastasis (stage IV) predicts a poor outcome, with survival rates of < 15% {2348,4356}.

## Metanephric neoplasms

Metanephric neoplasms are bland renal neoplasms that microscopically resemble differentiated components of nephroblastoma {313}. These lesions are benign, although they may (rarely) coexist with nephroblastoma or papillary RCC. The pathological spectrum includes pure epithelial neoplasms, termed "metanephric adenoma"; pure stromal neoplasms, termed "metanephric stromal tumour"; and composite stromal-epithelial lesions, termed "metanephric adenofibroma". Metanephric neoplasms are united by the common occurrence of *BRAF* p.V600E mutations in all three entities.

# Paediatric cystic nephroma

Vujanic GM
Chang KTE
de Krijger RR
Tanaka Y
Tsuzuki T

## Definition
Paediatric cystic nephroma is a benign, multilocular, cystic neoplasm of the kidney associated with *DICER1* syndrome.

## ICD-O coding
8959/0 Paediatric cystic nephroma

## ICD-11 coding
2F35 & XH7TJ0 Benign neoplasm of urinary organs & Paediatric cystic nephroma

## Related terminology
None

## Subtype(s)
None

## Localization
Paediatric cystic nephroma is localized in the kidney.

## Clinical features
Paediatric cystic nephroma may manifest as a palpable abdominal mass or be detected on screening in a child with a germline *DICER1* mutation and/or pleuropulmonary blastoma. About 25% of cases are bilateral {1799}. Cystic nephromas are typically treated by complete nephrectomy.

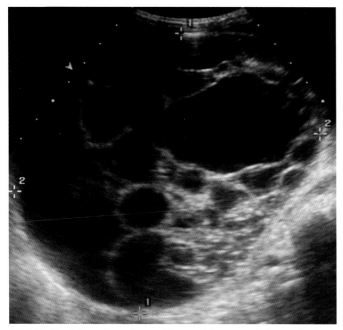

**Fig. 8.01** Paediatric cystic nephroma. Ultrasound shows a well-circumscribed multiseptated cystic mass. The cysts are anechoic with no nodular solid components.

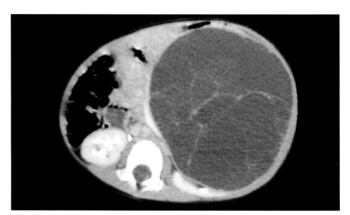

**Fig. 8.02** Paediatric cystic nephroma. Contrast-enhanced axial CT shows an encapsulated multiseptated cystic mass. The cysts are isoattenuating or slightly hyperattenuating relative to water. The capsule and septa are mildly enhancing. Herniation of the tumour into the collecting system is a characteristic feature.

## Epidemiology
Paediatric cystic nephroma occurs slightly more often in boys than in girls. Most patients are aged < 2 years (median: 16 months). Cases are rare in patients aged > 4 years {978}. Familial cases of cystic nephroma and an association with pleuropulmonary blastoma were recognized in the early 1990s {1681}. Cystic nephroma is now considered a pathognomonic neoplasm in *DICER1* syndrome {6524}.

## Etiology
Paediatric cystic nephroma is associated with *DICER1* mutations in about 90% of cases {1799}.

## Pathogenesis
Mouse models with conditional ablation of *DICER1* in ureteric bud epithelium during development show cystic masses of the kidney resembling cystic nephroma {4900}.

## Macroscopic appearance
Paediatric cystic nephromas are generally large tumours, with a median diameter of about 100 mm and a median weight of 540 g. They are usually well circumscribed and consist entirely of cysts of variable size and shape, and they have no macroscopically noticeable expansive, solid nodules. In many cases, there is a direct continuity between the tumour and the pelvicalyceal structures {978}.

## Histopathology
Paediatric cystic nephromas are sharply demarcated from the renal parenchyma in about 55% of cases, and poorly demarcated in the rest. They are composed entirely of cysts separated by septa of different thicknesses. The septa are lined by flattened, cuboidal, or hobnailing epithelium. The septa are usually thin and hypocellular, and they contain fibrous tissue with focal

Chapter 8

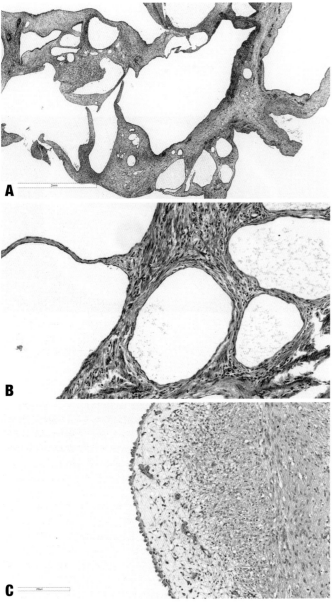

cellular condensations and well-differentiated tubules, but no blastema – its presence is a diagnostic criterion for cystic partially differentiated nephroblastoma {978}. ER and PR staining may be absent, unlike in adult cystic nephroma {4839}.

## Cytology
Not relevant

## Diagnostic molecular pathology
Germline analysis of tumour-specific *DICER1* mutations may be helpful in the diagnosis.

## Essential and desirable diagnostic criteria
*Essential:* a circumscribed neoplasm composed of epithelial-lined cysts separated by fibrous septa, which typically contain bland mesenchymal cells and chronic inflammation.
*Desirable:* DICER1 mutations may be detected.

## Staging
Not applicable

## Prognosis and prediction
Paediatric cystic nephroma is treated with surgery only, usually by complete nephrectomy, or in selected cases by partial nephrectomy {7199}. Its prognosis is excellent, with event-free and overall survival rates of 100% {4258}. Very rare cases of cystic nephroma transformation into *DICER1* sarcoma have been described, but the risk is regarded as very low {1799}.

**Fig. 8.03** Paediatric cystic nephroma. **A** There are mature tubules within the septa, but no blastema. **B** The cysts are lined with a flat epithelium. **C** The cysts are lined with a hobnail epithelium.

# Nephroblastoma

Vujanic GM
Chang KTE
Tanaka Y
Tsuzuki T

## Definition
Nephroblastoma is a malignant renal tumour that originates from the nephrogenic blastema and resembles the histology of developing kidney.

## ICD-O coding
8960/3 Nephroblastoma

## ICD-11 coding
2C90.Y & XH5QN3 Other specified malignant neoplasms of kidney, except renal pelvis & Nephroblastoma, NOS

## Related terminology
*Acceptable:* Wilms tumour.
*Not recommended:* fetal rhabdomyomatous nephroblastoma; botryoid nephroblastoma; teratoid nephroblastoma.

## Subtype(s)
See Table 8.05 (p. 698).

## Localization
Nephroblastoma develops in the kidney, and in about 5–10% of cases it is bilateral {1181}. In rare cases it may develop outside of the kidney {5957}.

## Clinical features
Patients with nephroblastoma usually present with an abdominal mass incidentally noticed by parents. In some 20–30% of cases there are signs and symptoms including abdominal pain, haematuria, hypertension (due to increased renin production), and/or anaemia.

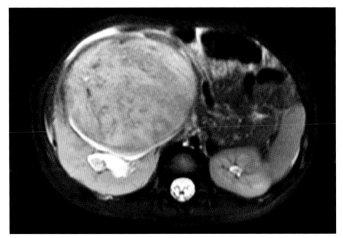

**Fig. 8.04** Nephroblastoma. T2-weighted axial MRI. The tumour is isointense to the renal cortex. The tumour is typically lobulated with heterogeneous signal due to foci of necrosis and old haemorrhage.

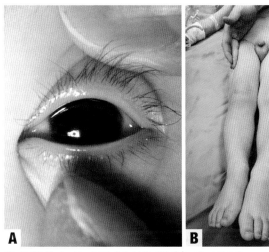

**Fig. 8.05** Nephroblastoma. **A** Aniridia. **B** Left hemihypertrophy.

In 10–15% of patients, nephroblastoma is associated with a predisposition syndrome. Some of these syndromes are associated with a high risk (> 20%) of developing nephroblastoma, including WAGR syndrome (Wilms tumour, aniridia, genitourinary anomalies, and a range of developmental delays) and Denys–Drash syndrome; some with a moderate risk (5–20%), including Beckwith–Wiedemann syndrome, Simpson–Golabi–Behmel syndrome, and Frasier syndrome; and some with a low risk (< 5%), including Bloom syndrome, *DICER1* syndrome, Li-Fraumeni syndrome, and isolated hemihypertrophy {7054}.

There are two main treatment approaches in nephroblastoma. The International Society of Paediatric Oncology (SIOP) approach, followed in most countries around the world, includes preoperative chemotherapy followed by surgery, with further chemotherapy and radiotherapy if necessary. The Children's Oncology Group (COG) approach, followed mainly in the USA and Canada, is based on primary surgery, followed by chemotherapy and radiotherapy if necessary {1783}. Pretreatment biopsy is not recommended in either approach, except in indicated cases (unusual clinical presentation, age > 10 years) {3185}.

## Epidemiology
Nephroblastoma most commonly occurs at 3–4 years of age, with a slight female predominance {862}. The European and North American prevalence rates are very similar (1 in 10 000 children), but nephroblastoma is more common in African and African-American populations, and least common in eastern Asian populations. The incidence in Europe is between 0.17 and 0.27 cases per million, and it very rarely occurs in adults {4718}. The majority of nephroblastoma cases are non-syndromic, but in 10–15% of children it is associated with

Chapter 8

**Table 8.05** Histological risk classifications for nephroblastoma; in the Children's Oncology Group (COG) classification there are two subtypes: non-anaplastic nephroblastoma (favourable histology) and anaplastic (focal and diffuse) nephroblastoma (unfavourable histology); the International Society of Paediatric Oncology (SIOP) classification distinguishes the following types of nephroblastoma: completely necrotic, epithelial, stromal, mixed, regressive, focal anaplasia, diffuse anaplasia, and blastemal {1783}

| Risk category | SIOP | COG |
|---|---|---|
| Low risk | Cystic partially differentiated nephroblastoma[a] | Cystic partially differentiated nephroblastoma[a] |
| | Completely necrotic nephroblastoma | |
| Intermediate risk | Epithelial, stromal, mixed, regressive types | Favourable histology |
| | Focal anaplasia | No evidence of anaplasia |
| High risk | Diffuse anaplasia | Diffuse anaplasia |
| | Blastemal type | Focal anaplasia |

[a]Treated with surgery only.

syndromes and congenital anomalies {6308}, and in 1–2% it is familial {6068}.

## Etiology

Nephroblastoma is thought to develop from its precursor lesions – nephrogenic rests. A number of genes are implicated in its development, including *WT1* at chromosome 11p13 and other, unidentified genes {7054}.

Nephrogenic rests are precursor lesions of nephroblastoma {564}, and they are found in 40% of unilateral tumours and > 90% of bilateral tumours {7342}. It is still not clear how nephrogenic rests progress to tumour. There are two main types of nephrogenic rests: perilobar and intralobar. They are further subclassified into incipient or dormant, sclerosing or regressive, or hyperplastic. They can be single, multiple, or diffuse. "Nephroblastomatosis" is the term used to describe two or more nephrogenic rests of any type, and it is not automatically associated with an increased risk of developing nephroblastoma in a contralateral kidney. Only the finding of perilobar nephrogenic rests in a unilateral nephroblastoma in children aged < 1 year is associated with a markedly increased risk of developing a contralateral nephroblastoma {1436}. Hyperplastic perilobar nephroblastomatosis is a condition in which the cortical layers of the kidney are replaced with hyperplastic nephrogenic tissue resulting in massive enlargement of the affected kidney(s), and it requires prolonged chemotherapy because of an increased risk of developing nephroblastoma {5459,2271}.

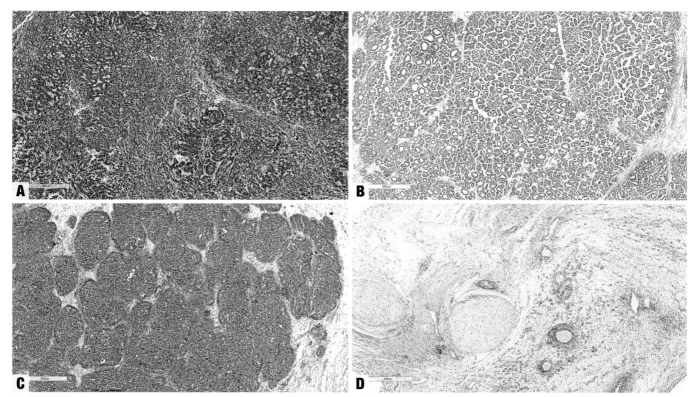

**Fig. 8.06** Nephroblastoma. **A** This example is composed of closely mixed blastemal and epithelial components. **B** This nephroblastoma is composed of the epithelial component only (monophasic). **C** This nephroblastoma is composed of the blastemal component only (nodular appearance). **D** The stromal component with heterologous elements, including cartilage and skeletal muscle.

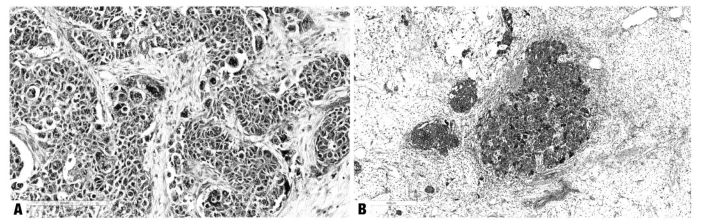

**Fig. 8.07** Anaplastic nephroblastoma. **A** Diffuse anaplasia with markedly enlarged and hyperchromatic nuclei and enlarged multipolar, atypical mitoses. **B** Focal anaplasia surrounded by chemotherapy-induced changes.

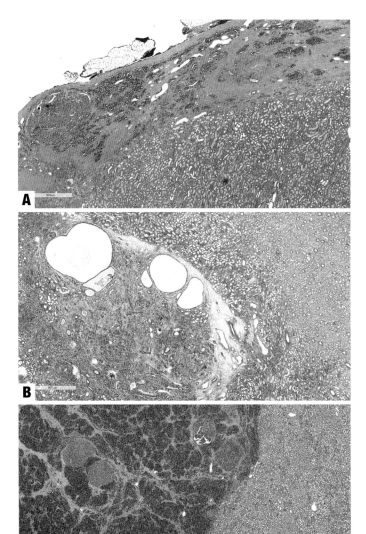

**Fig. 8.08** Nephrogenic rests. **A** A perilobar nephrogenic rest showing sclerosing and a hyperplastic rest. **B** An intralobar nephrogenic rest mingling with the normal renal parenchyma. **C** Perilobar hyperplastic nephroblastomatosis.

## Pathogenesis

The pathogenesis of nephroblastoma is incompletely understood. It seems that several signalling pathways, microRNA processing, and epigenetics play important roles. Nephroblastoma represents a genetically mixed group, demonstrating a low incidence of known somatic alterations and a high degree of intratumoural heterogeneity.

## Macroscopic appearance

Nephroblastomas are usually large, solitary, spherical masses, sharply demarcated from the renal parenchyma and distorting kidney contours. In about 10% of cases they are multifocal. In cases that have undergone primary surgery, the tumour is grey-white or pink-grey in colour, lobulated, soft, and friable. In nephroblastomas treated with preoperative chemotherapy, necrosis and haemorrhage are usually extensive. Some tumours may have a prominent cystic appearance.

## Histopathology

Nephroblastoma typically consists of three components – blastemal, epithelial, and stromal – but tumours comprising two components, or only one, are not rare. Because of the different lines and degrees of differentiation of its components, nephroblastoma manifests with innumerable patterns. Preoperative chemotherapy given in SIOP studies results in chemotherapy-induced changes that may involve 0–100% of the tumour and that alter its histological features {7343}.

Blastema is the least differentiated component, consisting of small to medium-sized undifferentiated cells with relatively small, regular nuclei and small nucleoli. It may show different patterns (diffuse, serpentine, nodular, and basaloid), which are of no prognostic significance. Mitotic figures are frequent.

The epithelial component includes poorly differentiated elements (rosette-like structures), moderately differentiated elements (tubules and papillary structures), and well-differentiated elements (glomerular-like structures and small mature tubules). It may also contain heterologous elements (squamous and mucinous epithelium, glial tissue).

The stromal component may show a variable appearance, ranging from hypocellular or hypercellular undifferentiated areas to well-differentiated areas that often contain heterologous elements (rhabdomyoblasts, adipose tissue, cartilage) {7349}.

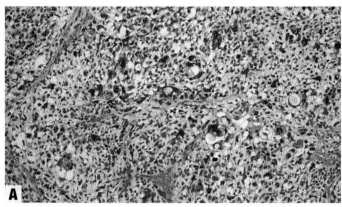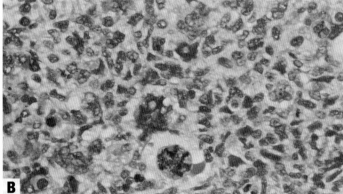

**Fig. 8.09** Anaplastic nephroblastoma. **A** H&E staining. **B** Anaplasia cell.

Descriptive terms such as "fetal rhabdomyomatous nephroblastoma", "botryoid nephroblastoma", and "teratoid nephroblastoma" should not be used, because they are not separate entities, do not exist in any classification, and have no prognostic significance {7349,1733}.

Anaplasia is a histological feature found in 7–10% of nephroblastomas. It is defined as the presence of enlarged, atypical, tripolar or multipolar mitotic figures; marked nuclear enlargement; and hyperchromasia. The presence of all three features is required for the diagnosis, and it may occur in any of the components. Anaplasia is subclassified into focal and diffuse anaplasia. Focal anaplasia is defined as a clearly delineated focus within a primary intrarenal tumour, but in rare cases more than one focus is allowed for its diagnosis: in the COG definition it is as many as 4 foci, and in the SIOP definition it is as many as 2 foci of ≤ 15 mm {2055,7344}. Diffuse anaplasia is defined as follows: non-localized anaplasia; focal anaplasia with marked nuclear unrest in the remaining tumour; anaplasia beyond the tumour capsule; anaplastic cells in intrarenal or extrarenal vessels, renal sinus, extracapsular sites, and/or metastatic deposits; or anaplasia in a biopsy. Nephroblastomas with diffuse anaplasia show a different age distribution from that of non-anaplastic nephroblastomas: the former are extremely rare in the first year of life, and rare in the second year, but then more than half of the patients are aged > 4 years at presentation. The stage distribution for nephroblastoma with diffuse anaplasia is also markedly different, with fewer stage I cases and more stage IV and V cases than in non-anaplastic nephroblastoma. Nephroblastoma with focal anaplasia has a similar age and stage distribution to non-anaplastic nephroblastoma, except that it is also very rare in the first 2 years of life {1781}. The prognosis for nephroblastoma with diffuse anaplasia is significantly worse than that for non-anaplastic nephroblastoma, whereas focal anaplasia has a similar prognosis to non-anaplastic nephroblastoma in SIOP studies {7345}.

Monophasic nephroblastoma may be difficult to distinguish from other tumours, and in such cases immunohistochemistry may be helpful. WT1 is the most sensitive and specific marker (positive in ~90% of cases) and shows nuclear staining with antibodies directed to the C-terminal and N-terminal portions of the WT1 protein. The blastemal component shows diffuse expression of WT1, PAX8, and vimentin, and variable staining for CD56, CD57, cytokeratins, EMA, and desmin. The epithelial component shows expression of cytokeratin, EMA, CD56, and it stains variably for PAX8 and WT1. The stromal component is positive for vimentin and variable for BCL2 and CD34, whereas WT1 is weak or absent {5192}.

There are two histological classification systems of nephroblastoma: the SIOP histological classification (see Table 8.06) is based on the assessment of percentage of chemotherapy-induced changes and viable tumour components, and it includes eight types of nephroblastoma {7344}. The COG histological

**Table 8.06** Histological criteria for nephroblastoma types in International Society of Paediatric Oncology (SIOP) pretreated cases

| Tumour type | Histological features | | | |
| --- | --- | --- | --- | --- |
| | Chemotherapy-induced changes | Viable components[a] | | |
| | | Blastema | Epithelium | Stroma |
| Completely necrotic | 100% | 0% | 0% | 0% |
| Regressive | > 66% | 0–100% | 0–100% | 0–100% |
| Mixed | < 66% | 0–65% | 0–65% | 0–65% |
| | < 66% | 11–65% | 0–89% | 0–89% |
| Epithelial | < 66% | 0–10% | 66–100% | 0–33% |
| Stromal | < 66% | 0–10% | 0–33% | 66–100% |
| Blastemal | < 66% | 66–100% | 0–33% | 0–33% |

[a]The percentages of the components of the viable tumour should add up to 100%. The presence of diffuse anaplasia in any of the above types supersedes the underlying types. Focal anaplasia must also be specifically mentioned in the diagnosis (e.g. "focal anaplasia in mixed type").

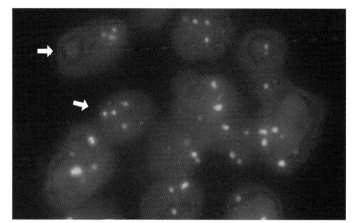

**Fig. 8.10** Nephroblastoma. FISH showing chromosome 1q gain.

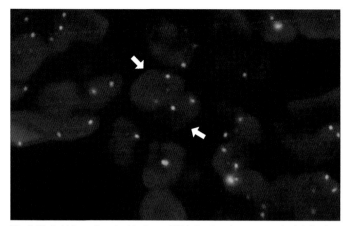

**Fig. 8.11** Aniridia and nephroblastoma. FISH showing chromosome 1p deletion in a 3-year-old girl with aniridia and a right Wilms tumour.

classification includes only anaplastic (unfavourable-histology) and non-anaplastic (favourable-histology) nephroblastoma {1783}.

## Cytology
Not relevant

## Diagnostic molecular pathology
Nephroblastoma demonstrates a number of genetic changes with variable prevalence, including *WT1* on chromosome 11p13 (prevalence: 10–20%; regarded as an early event, associated with stromal histology), *CTNNB1* on chromosome 3p22 (prevalence: ~15%; regarded as a late event, not associated with nephrogenic rests), *IGF2* on chromosome 11p15 (prevalence: ~70%; regarded as an early event, associated with perilobar nephrogenic rests and with epithelial and blastemal histology), *TP53* on chromosome 17p13 (prevalence: ~70%; associated with anaplasia), *MYCN* on chromosome 2p24 (prevalence: ~15%; associated with anaplasia), and 1q gain (prevalence: ~30–40%; associated with reduced event-free and overall survival) {7054}.

## Essential and desirable diagnostic criteria
*Essential:* presence of ≥ 2 of the following components: blastemal, epithelial, and/or stromal.
*Desirable:* for monophasic nephroblastoma: immunohistochemistry or molecular testing to distinguish it from other tumours with similar histological features.

## Staging
The SIOP and COG staging systems are used, and they are similar, but they still have some differences related to the initial treatment of nephroblastoma {1783}. SIOP staging is done on the basis of findings recognized at the time of nephrectomy {7344}. The important difference is that a pretreatment fine-needle or Tru-Cut biopsy is not a criterion for upstaging a tumour according to SIOP, whereas in the COG system any biopsy results in a stage III assignment.

## Prognosis and prediction
The overall survival for nephroblastoma is approximately 90%. Relapses occur in about 15% of children, the majority within 2 years of diagnosis. There are a number of prognostic factors in nephroblastoma that differ between the two main approaches to its treatment {1783}. In both the COG and the SIOP approaches, tumour histology and stage are important prognostic factors. However, in the COG studies, prognostic factors also include age, tumour weight, rapidity of lung metastasis response, and molecular markers (loss of heterogeneity at chromosomes 1p and 16q; and 1q gain, identified very recently). In the SIOP studies, prognostic factors include histological risk stratification into three treatment groups, tumour volume before and after preoperative chemotherapy in defined cases, and responsiveness of lung metastases to initial chemotherapy in some groups. Molecular markers are still not used as prognostic factors according to SIOP. The main difference in histological risk stratification is that nephroblastoma with focal anaplasia is regarded by SIOP as an intermediate-risk tumour, and the blastemal type (in addition to diffuse anaplasia) is regarded as a high-risk nephroblastoma {7347}.

# Renal cell carcinoma with MiT translocations

Argani P
Bode PK
Geller J
He LJ
Matoso A

## Definition

Renal cell carcinoma (RCC) with MiT translocations harbours gene fusions involving members of the MiT subfamily of transcription factors, *TFE3* and *TFEB*.

## ICD-O coding

8311/3 Renal cell carcinoma with MiT translocations
8311/3 *TFE3*-rearranged renal cell carcinoma (Xp11 translocation renal cell carcinoma)
8311/3 *TFEB*-rearranged renal cell carcinoma (t(6;11) renal cell carcinoma)

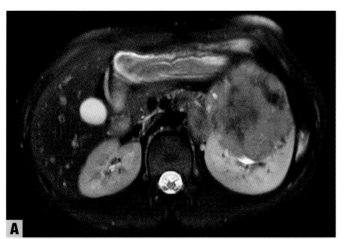

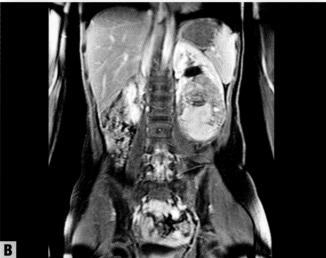

**Fig. 8.12** Renal cell carcinoma. **A** T2-weighted axial MRI. The tumour is lobulated and hypointense compared with the kidney. It is heterogeneous in signal, related to internal haemorrhage, necrosis, cystic change, and calcification. There is evidence of tumour invasion and left renal vein thrombosis. **B** Postcontrast T1-weighted coronal MRI. After intravenous administration of gadolinium contrast material, the tumour enhances moderately and less intensely than the adjacent cortex.

## ICD-11 coding

2C90.0 Renal cell carcinoma of kidney, except renal pelvis

## Related terminology

None

## Subtype(s)

*TFE3*-rearranged renal cell carcinoma (Xp11 translocation renal cell carcinoma); *TFEB*-rearranged renal cell carcinoma (t(6;11) renal cell carcinoma)

## Localization

Kidney

## Clinical features

The clinical features of RCC with MiT translocations are the same as those of other RCCs.

## Epidemiology

Although MiT translocation RCCs occur both in children and in adults, they have a greater tendency than other RCCs to affect young people. Overall, the median age of patients with MiT translocation RCC is approximately 30 years {2306, 6551}.

## Etiology

*TFE3*-rearranged RCCs account for approximately 40% of paediatric RCCs but only 1.6–4% of adult RCCs {3713}. *TFEB*-rearranged RCCs are less common than *TFE3*-rearranged RCCs; only about 100 cases have been reported in the world literature. Prior exposure to cytotoxic chemotherapy is a risk factor for MiT-family translocation RCC {324}.

## Pathogenesis

*TFE3*-rearranged RCCs harbour fusions of the transcription factor gene *TFE3* (which maps to Xp11) with one of multiple reported genes including *ASPSCR1* (*ASPL*), *PRCC*, *NONO* (*P54NRB*), *SFPQ* (*PSF*), *RBM10*, *MED15*, *CLTC*, and many others {315,314,5774,1344,337}. The three most common *TFE3*-rearranged RCCs are those bearing t(X;1)(p11.2;q21), which fuses *PRCC* and *TFE3*; those bearing t(X;17)(p11.2;q25), which fuses *ASPSCR1* and *TFE3* (the same gene fusion found in alveolar soft part sarcoma) {329}; and those bearing t(X;1)(p11.2;p34), which fuses *SFPQ* and *TFE3*. The *SFPQ::TFE3* fusion is also commonly found in the Xp11 translocation perivascular epithelioid cell tumours (PEComas) and melanotic Xp11 translocation renal cancers {5775,337}. The t(6;11) translocation fuses *TFEB* with *MALAT1* (*Alpha*), an untranslated gene of unknown function, resulting in overexpression of native TFEB {3871,1593}. Rare alternative *TFEB* fusion partners have been reported {1009}. *TFEB* amplification in RCC represents an alternative means of overexpressing native TFEB; however,

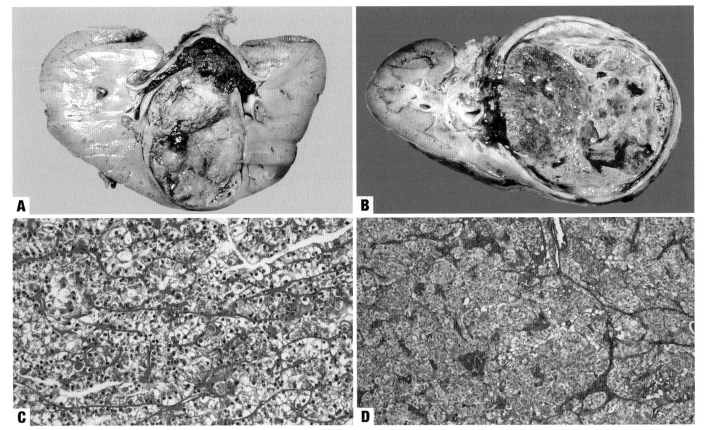

**Fig. 8.13** Renal cell carcinoma with MiT translocations. **A** *TFE3*-rearranged renal cell carcinoma. The gross appearance is a well-circumscribed tumour with a tan-yellow cut surface, focal haemorrhage, and necrosis. **B** *TFE3*-rearranged renal cell carcinoma. Macroscopic appearance with focal haemorrhage. **C** *TFEB* renal cell carcinoma. This example shows a focal papillary architecture with nests. **D** *TFE3*-rearranged renal cell carcinoma. This example has a solid histological pattern.

such neoplasms typically affect adults {333,6515,2622,7557}. Overexpressed TFE3 fusion proteins and native TFEB act as aberrant transcription factors that activate the expression of multiple downstream targets, including those normally activated by the related MiT-family transcription factor MITF (such as melanocytic markers and cathepsin K) {3809,7093,3677, 2621}.

## Macroscopic appearance
MiT-family translocation RCCs do not have a distinctive gross appearance.

## Histopathology
The most distinctive histological pattern of *TFE3*-rearranged RCCs is that of a papillary neoplasm composed of epithelioid

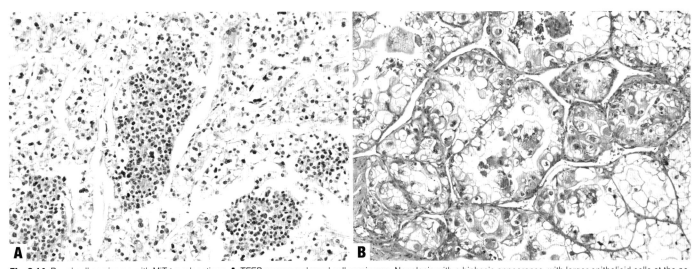

**Fig. 8.14** Renal cell carcinoma with MiT translocations. **A** *TFEB*-rearranged renal cell carcinoma. Neoplasia with a biphasic appearance, with larger epithelioid cells at the periphery of the nests and smaller cells clustered in the centre. **B** *TFE3*-rearranged renal cell carcinoma. This example exhibits an alveolar component.

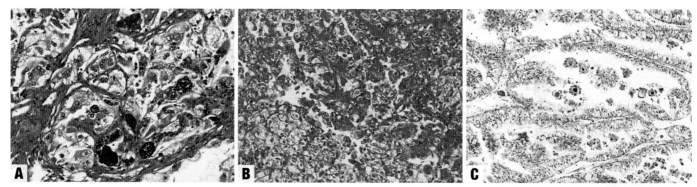

**Fig. 8.15** *TFE3*-rearranged renal cell carcinoma. **A** At higher power, there is patchy, fine to slightly coarse cytoplasmic melanin pigmentation. **B** Eosinophilic and clear cell components are present. **C** Papillary pattern with many psammoma bodies.

clear cells with abundant psammoma bodies {315,314}. *TFE3*-rearranged RCCs can also mimic other renal neoplasms, including clear cell RCC, papillary RCC, clear cell papillary RCC, multilocular cystic RCC, oncocytoma, and epithelioid angiomyolipoma {330,2542}. Occasional *TFE3*-rearranged RCCs contain melanin pigment, creating an overlap with Xp11 translocation pigmented PEComas {317,316}. Xp11 translocation PEComas typically affect young patients but are not associated with tuberous sclerosis. They almost always have an exclusively epithelioid clear cell morphology, have minimal to no immunoreactivity for muscle markers, and do not demonstrate inactivation of *TSC1* or *TSC2*. A similar malignant epithelioid cell renal neoplasm with *TFE3* gene fusions and melanin pigment was originally described as melanocytic Xp11 translocation cancer but most likely represents pigmented Xp11 translocation PEComa. Unlike *TFE3*-rearranged RCCs, Xp11 translocation PEComas do not label for the renal tubular marker PAX8 and lack overtly epithelial architectures such as tubules and well-formed papillae.

The most distinctive pattern of *TFEB*-rearranged RCC is that of a biphasic neoplasm, comprising nests of larger epithelioid cells and smaller cells clustered around basement membrane material {321,334,325}. *TFEB*-rearranged RCC characteristically entraps single native renal tubules at their periphery. *TFEB*-rearranged RCC can overlap morphologically with *TFE3*-rearranged RCC, and vice versa. When the population of smaller cells is small or absent, the differential diagnosis of *TFEB*-rearranged RCC is broader and includes clear cell RCC and oncocytic renal neoplasms.

In contrast to most RCCs, MiT translocation RCCs underexpress epithelial markers such as cytokeratins and EMA but consistently express PAX8 and other renal tubular markers {6551, 322}. *TFEB*-rearranged RCCs consistently express the melanoma markers melan-A and HMB45 and the cysteine protease cathepsin K, whereas only occasional *TFE3*-rearranged RCCs express melanocytic markers and approximately 60% label for cathepsin K {4418,4417}. Strong nuclear TFE3 immunoreactivity using an antibody to the C-terminal portion of TFE3 is highly sensitive and specific for *TFE3*-rearranged RCC {326}, but *TFE3* break-apart FISH assays have generally proved to be more useful because they suffer less from fixation issues {2542,7852}. The key exceptions are the *TFE3*-rearranged RCCs resulting from paracentric inversions involving Xp11 that are often impossible to detect by conventional *TFE3* break-apart FISH, giving a false negative result. These resulting fusions include *RBM10::TFE3*, *GRIPAP1::TFE3*, *RBMX::TFE3*, and *NONO::TFE3*. The diagnosis can be suspected when a neoplasm demonstrates other typical features of *TFE3*-rearranged RCC (such as cathepsin K immunoreactivity and characteristic morphology) along with strong diffuse TFE3 nuclear labelling by immunohistochemistry. The diagnosis can then be confirmed by RNA sequencing or RT-PCR, or by FISH using specialized fosmid break-apart probes {335,5417,336,1350}.

Similarly, nuclear immunoreactivity for TFEB is highly specific for *TFEB*-rearranged RCC {325}, but a *TFEB* break-apart FISH assay is less affected by variable fixation and thus represents the preferred diagnostic test for establishing the diagnosis in formalin-fixed, paraffin-embedded material {334,4805}.

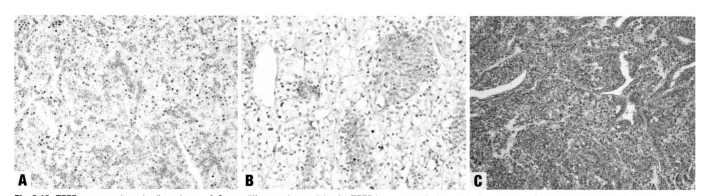

**Fig. 8.16** *TFEB*-rearranged renal cell carcinoma. **A** Strong diffuse nuclear staining for TFEB in tumour cells, but not in the stroma. **B** Characteristic focal HMB45 immunohistochemical staining. **C** The tumour cells show nuclear and cytoplasmic labelling for TFEB.

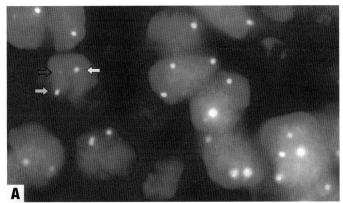

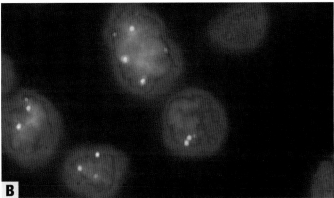

**Fig. 8.17** Renal cell carcinoma with MiT translocations. **A** *TFE3*-rearranged renal cell carcinoma. Typical FISH image of a dual-colour break-apart *TFE3* (Xp11.2) locus from a female patient. **B** *TFEB*-rearranged renal cell carcinoma. Typical image of dual-colour break-apart FISH for the *TFEB* (6p21) locus.

## Cytology

Not relevant

## Diagnostic molecular pathology

*TFE3*-rearranged RCCs harbour gene fusions involving the TFE3 transcription factor–encoding gene, which maps to chromosome Xp11. *TFEB*-rearranged RCCs harbour gene fusions involving the TFEB transcription factor–encoding gene, which maps to chromosome 6p21; the typical fusion is *MALAT1* (*Alpha*)::*TFEB*, resulting from a t(6:11)(p21;q12) translocation.

## Essential and desirable diagnostic criteria

*Essential:* RCC with strong nuclear labelling for TFE3 or TFEB in a clean background OR *TFE3* or *TFEB* gene fusion identified by molecular techniques such as RNA sequencing.

*Desirable:* clear cells with papillary architecture, psammoma bodies, or biphasic large cell / small cell morphology (typical morphology but not seen in all cases); cathepsin K immunoreactivity (not seen in all cases); aberrant immunoreactivity for melanocytic markers (e.g. HMB45 or melan-A) (not seen in all cases).

## Staging

Union for International Cancer Control (UICC) TNM RCC tumour staging is used.

## Prognosis and prediction

Survival of patients with *TFE3*-rearranged RCC is similar to that of patients with clear cell RCC, and significantly worse than that of patients with papillary RCC {5503}. In a multivariate analysis, only distant metastasis and older age at diagnosis independently predicted death {6765}. Paediatric patients have a lower burden of genomic events than do adults, which may explain their better prognosis {4394}.

Fusion subtype impacts presentation; *ASPSCR1*::*TFE3* RCCs are more likely to manifest with regional lymph node metastasis (24 of 32 evaluable cases, 75%) than are *PRCC*::*TFE3* RCCs (5 of 14 cases, 36%); however, most of the former patients remained disease-free without adjuvant therapy {6765,1922}. Hence, locally advanced stage may not predict adverse outcomes. *TFEB*-rearranged RCCs have generally been more indolent neoplasms than *TFE3*-rearranged RCCs. Of the evaluable cases (~50) in the published literature, only 4 developed metastases, which led to patient death in 3 cases. Most patients presented with low-stage disease (pT1 or pT2) and had benign follow-up. Probably reflecting their usually low proliferative indices, MiT-family translocation RCCs have the potential to metastasize late – as many as 20 or 30 years after diagnosis.

# *ALK*-rearranged renal cell carcinoma

Argani P
Bode PK

## Definition

*ALK*-rearranged renal cell carcinomas (RCCs) harbour gene fusions resulting from chromosome translocations involving the chromosome 2p23 breakpoint.

## ICD-O coding

8311/3 *ALK*-rearranged renal cell carcinoma

## ICD-11 coding

2C90.0 Renal cell carcinoma of kidney, except renal pelvis

## Related terminology

None

## Subtype(s)

None

## Localization

Kidney

## Clinical features

These RCCs have no specific clinical features, aside from the association of *VCL::ALK* RCC with young patients who have sickle cell trait (see below).

## Epidemiology

There have been approximately 40 reported cases, with a nearly equal sex distribution, in both children and adults (patient age range: 3–85 years).

## Etiology

Unknown

## Pathogenesis

Unknown

## Macroscopic appearance

Most of the tumours have been small and organ-confined (pT1) at presentation.

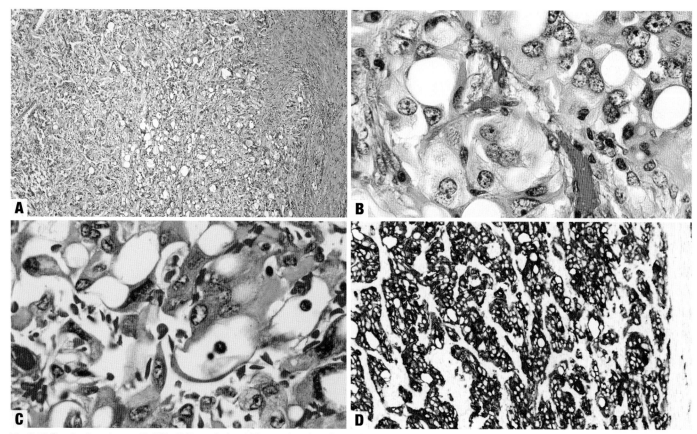

**Fig. 8.18** Renal cell carcinoma with *VCL::ALK* gene fusion. **A** The neoplasm is well delineated from the native kidney by the fibrous capsule to the right. **B** The neoplastic cells demonstrate striking cytoplasmic vacuolization. **C** There are numerous sickled erythrocytes scattered among the vacuolated neoplastic cells. **D** The neoplastic cells demonstrate diffuse cytoplasmic immunoreactivity for ALK protein by immunohistochemistry.

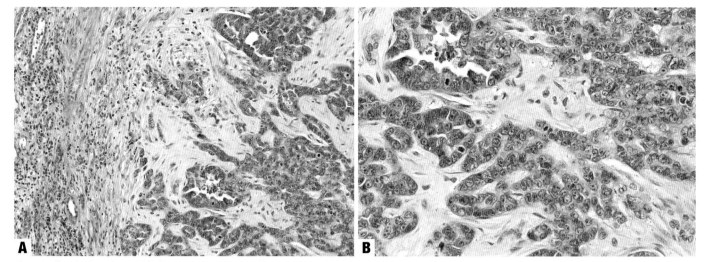

**Fig. 8.19** Renal cell carcinoma with *EML4::ALK* gene fusion. **A** The neoplastic cells form glands and cribriform structures within an oedematous, desmoplastic stroma. The native kidney is to the left. **B** The morphology is that of a nondescript high-grade adenocarcinoma with desmoplastic stroma.

## Histopathology

The 4 known cases with a *VCL::ALK* gene fusion (3 reported) are distinctive in that they affected young patients with sickle cell trait and have a distinctive morphology. These neoplasms are typically well circumscribed and may have chronic inflammation at their periphery. They are composed of polygonal neoplastic cells with abundant eosinophilic cytoplasm and striking vacuolization {1659,4406,6550}. Sickle-shaped erythrocytes are more readily seen in extravasated blood than in the blood vessels. These neoplasms have been proposed to be the eighth sickle cell nephropathy {6550}. *ALK*-rearranged RCCs with fusion partners other than *VCL* – such as *TPM3*, *EML4*, *STRN*, and *HOOK1* – are more heterogeneous {6755,6764, 3845,977,3832}. They may show cytoplasmic vacuolization but often have a papillary or cribriform architecture and mucinous stroma. Other morphologies resembling metanephric adenoma or mucinous tubular and spindle cell carcinoma have also been reported {3832}. By immunohistochemistry, ALK labelling is a useful screening tool for these neoplasms. SMARCB1 protein (also known as INI1, SNF5, or BAF47), which is typically lost in the renal medullary carcinomas that affect patients with sickle cell trait, is retained. TFE3 immunoreactivity is frequently seen using automated staining techniques, but it is usually negative in more standard overnight incubation procedures, and *TFE3* gene rearrangements are not present.

## Cytology

Not relevant

## Diagnostic molecular pathology

Demonstration of *ALK* rearrangement with various partners is required for the diagnosis.

## Essential and desirable diagnostic criteria

*Essential:* RCC with documentation of *ALK* rearrangement by break-apart FISH or demonstration of an *ALK* fusion using sequencing methods.
*Desirable:* ALK immunoreactivity.

## Staging

Union for International Cancer Control (UICC) TNM RCC tumour staging is used.

## Prognosis and prediction

Follow-up is limited in the reported cases. Ten patients had no evidence of disease in limited follow-up. Two adults died of disease, and three other patients had lymph node metastases or local recurrence. Three patients with metastatic disease had dramatic responses to a targeted ALK inhibitor, indicating that ALK inhibition is a non-toxic and potentially highly effective treatment in these patients {5289}.

# Eosinophilic solid and cystic renal cell carcinoma

Argani P
Bode PK

## Definition

Eosinophilic solid and cystic renal cell carcinoma (ESC-RCC) is characterized by a solid and cystic architecture, polygonal neoplastic cells with voluminous eosinophilic cytoplasm and basophilic cytoplasmic stippling, and frequent patchy immunoreactivity for CK20.

## ICD-O coding

8311/3 Eosinophilic solid and cystic renal cell carcinoma

## ICD-11 coding

2C90.0 Renal cell carcinoma of kidney, except renal pelvis

## Related terminology

None

## Subtype(s)

None

## Localization

Kidney

## Clinical features

ESC-RCC was originally described exclusively in women {7077}. More recently, cases in children and men have been reported {4092}, as have multifocal cases and rare cases with lymph node or haematogenous metastasis {5294,4525,7057}.

## Epidemiology

The reported age range is 14–75 years.

## Etiology

ESC-RCC closely resembles the granular eosinophilic-macrocystic subtype of RCC that has been associated with tuberous sclerosis {2604,7699} and is now considered its somatic counterpart. Other RCC subtypes reported in tuberous sclerosis include papillary carcinomas with clear cells and prominent smooth muscle, and chromophobe-like tumours. Sporadic forms of all of these RCCs associated with somatic TSC gene mutations have now been described {5340,6514}. Some cases previously reported as oncocytoid RCC after neuroblastoma have also proved to be ESC-RCC {4551}.

## Pathogenesis

Recently, biallelic somatic mutations in *TSC1* or *TSC2* have been identified in a majority of ESC-RCCs {5294,5341,4556}.

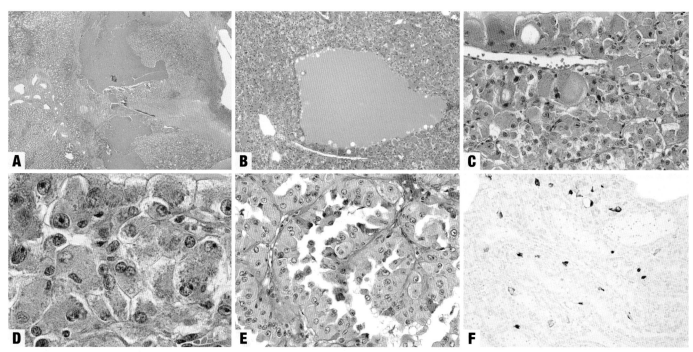

**Fig. 8.20** Eosinophilic solid and cystic renal cell carcinoma. **A** At low power, this well-delineated neoplasm demonstrates both cystic and solid architecture. **B** The neoplasm has a predominantly solid architecture and cysts containing pale-pink proteinaceous fluid. **C** The cells lining the cysts are frequently multinucleated and have particularly voluminous eosinophilic cytoplasm. **D** The neoplastic cells characteristically demonstrate basophilic cytoplasmic stippling. **E** The neoplasms occasionally demonstrate a papillary architecture. **F** The neoplasms typically demonstrate patchy but intense single-cell immunoreactivity for CK20.

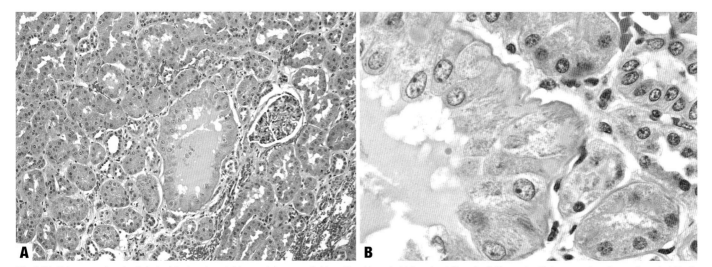

**Fig. 8.21** Tuberous sclerosis. **A** An incipient cyst containing proteinaceous fluid and lined by cuboidal eosinophilic cells. **B** The cysts of tuberous sclerosis are characteristically lined by cells with voluminous eosinophilic cytoplasm. Note the basophilic stippling, similar to that of eosinophilic solid and cystic renal cell carcinoma.

This results in upregulation of the mTOR pathway, which regulates cellular metabolism, proliferation, and survival.

## Macroscopic appearance
ESC-RCCs are typically well circumscribed, tan, and solid and cystic, with reported sizes ranging from < 10 to 135 mm. Most are organ-confined and small (pT1), although some are multifocal.

## Histopathology
ESC-RCCs are typically unencapsulated. Although a solid and cystic architecture is typical, some are extensively papillary. The neoplastic cells are polygonal and have voluminous eosinophilic cytoplasm with basophilic cytoplasmic stippling. The stippling may include eosinophilic to purple cytoplasmic granules surrounded by a clear rim, reminiscent of leishmaniasis. The cysts are typically lined by a single layer of hobnail cells that are often multinucleated. Prominent cytoplasmic vacuolization (consisting of either large or small vacuoles) may produce a clear cell appearance. The nuclei are round to oval, with minimal pleomorphism and variably prominent nucleoli. Scattered binucleated cells are common. Psammoma bodies are often present. Ultrastructural examination shows that the stippling corresponds to aggregated rough endoplasmic reticulum.

By immunohistochemistry, the carcinoma cells typically label for PAX8. CK20 characteristically yields patchy immunoreactivity ranging from isolated positive cells to more extensive immunoreactivity in 30–40% of the carcinoma cells. Similarly, cathepsin K is usually positive in a patchy fashion, although occasional tumours are negative and some are diffusely positive. CK7 and KIT (CD117) are usually negative. Occasional tumours are immunoreactive for melan-A {5294,7057}.

When extensively papillary, ESC-RCC can resemble type 2 papillary RCC {5294}. The cytoplasmic stippling, psammoma bodies, frequent cathepsin K immunoreactivity, and occasional immunoreactivity for melan-A raise the differential diagnosis of MiT-family translocation RCC. The binucleation and solid areas of these neoplasms, as well as cytoplasmic vacuolization, can closely resemble chromophobe RCC. More recently, a subset of

RCCs characterized by eosinophilic and vacuolated cytoplasm, prominent nucleoli, and stromal oedema have been reported to be associated with *TSC2* or *MTOR* somatic mutations, with associated upregulation of the mTOR pathway {1232}. Although these neoplasms were negative for CK20 in the initial report of 7 cases and have a distinctive appearance, they may be pathogenetically related to ESC-RCC. Another cohort of similar cases, termed "high-grade oncocytic renal tumour" (despite their benign outcome so far) labelled for CK20 in 5 of 14 cases {2796}.

In addition to angiomyolipomas, the kidneys of children with tuberous sclerosis frequently have renal cysts characteristically lined by hypertrophic renal tubular cells with prominent eosinophilic cytoplasm, not unlike the cells of ESC-RCC {638}.

## Cytology
Not relevant

## Diagnostic molecular pathology
Identification of biallelic somatic mutations in *TSC1* or *TSC2* with the morphological features described above is diagnostic {5294,5341,4556}.

## Essential and desirable diagnostic criteria
*Essential:* an eosinophilic solid-cystic RCC; focal or diffuse CK20 positivity.
*Desirable:* TSC gene mutation.

## Staging
Staging follows the Union for International Cancer Control (UICC) TNM system.

## Prognosis and prediction
Albeit with limited follow-up data, the majority of ESC-RCCs appear to have been cured by resection. A few patients with lymph node or haematogenous metastases have been reported. One patient with haematogenous liver metastases at diagnosis had a complete response to mTOR pathway inhibitors, and the patient remains disease-free 10 years after diagnosis {5294}.

# SMARCB1-deficient renal medullary carcinoma

Argani P
Bode PK

## Definition

SMARCB1-deficient renal medullary carcinoma is a high-grade adenocarcinoma typically centred in the renal medulla, which occurs mainly in patients with sickle cell trait.

## ICD-O coding

8510/3 SMARCB1-deficient renal medullary carcinoma

## ICD-11 coding

2C90.Y & XH2YP5 Other specified malignant neoplasms of kidney, except renal pelvis & Medullary carcinoma, NOS

## Related terminology

None

## Subtype(s)

None

## Localization

Kidney

## Clinical features

Age at diagnosis ranges from childhood to the seventh decade of life (median: 21 years) {1591,3098}. There is a male predominance (M:F ratio: 2:1). Virtually all patients are symptomatic at diagnosis, with haematuria and flank or abdominal pain being the most common symptoms. Other common presenting symptoms are an abdominal mass, dysuria, and weight loss.

## Epidemiology

Several hundred cases of renal medullary carcinoma have been reported. The vast majority of cases have been in patients of African ancestry in the USA and Brazil {7458}. Almost all patients have had sickle cell trait or haemoglobin SC disease, but a few have had sickle cell disease. A few patients without a haemoglobinopathy have been reported to have tumours identical to renal medullary carcinoma {5122}.

## Etiology

Sickle cell trait is far more common than sickle cell disease and it appears that patients with sickle cell trait and sickle cell disease have similar risks (~1 case per 40 000 patients over a 10-year period) of developing renal medullary carcinoma {4828,254}.

## Pathogenesis

The hypoxic and hypertonic environment of the renal medulla, exacerbated by microvascular occlusion by sickle-shaped erythrocytes, may promote the DNA double-strand breaks that are prerequisites for the translocations and deletions that inactivate SMARCB1 and drive tumorigenesis {4828}. About three quarters of the tumours occur in the right kidney. This may be accounted for by the relative hypoxia in the right kidney due to the lesser blood flow caused by the greater length of the right renal artery.

## Macroscopic appearance

Renal medullary carcinomas are usually large and poorly circumscribed, ranging in size from 40 to 120 mm (mean: 70 mm). Smaller tumours are often centred in the renal medulla, which experiences hypoxia and sometimes undergoes papillary necrosis in patients with sickling haemoglobinopathies. The cut surface of the tumour is frequently tan or grey-white and often shows extensive necrosis and haemorrhage.

## Histopathology

Renal medullary carcinoma cells typically grow as infiltrating cords, nests, microcysts, sheets, and tubules. Round empty spaces from individual cell necrosis are common and when numerous can impart a cribriform, adenoid cystic carcinoma–like appearance. There is usually a pronounced myxoid desmoplastic reaction with a chronic inflammatory cell infiltrate. The carcinoma cells may show marked nuclear pleomorphism, but many have vesicular chromatin, prominent nucleoli, and eosinophilic cytoplasm, imparting a rhabdoid appearance. Mitotic figures are numerous. Sickle-shaped erythrocytes are a frequent finding within the vasculature of the tumour and kidney but are most commonly seen among extravasated red blood cells.

By immunohistochemistry, medullary carcinomas {1243} demonstrate loss of SMARCB1 (also known as INI1, SNF5, or BAF47). Renal medullary carcinomas typically label diffusely for PAX8, broad-spectrum cytokeratins, EMA, and vimentin {4162, 2620}. There is variable labelling for CK7, high-molecular-weight cytokeratin, CEA, and p53. OCT3/4 is strongly positive in about 50% of cases {5773}, creating a potential diagnostic pitfall with metastatic germ cell tumour when these young patients present with extensive retroperitoneal nodal involvement.

Ultrastructurally, the carcinoma cells contain vesicles lined by long microvilli, prominent desmosomes, and condensed fibrillary electron-dense deposits. Intracytoplasmic glycogen or lipids are not prominent {7452}.

The main differential diagnostic considerations for renal medullary carcinoma in children are rhabdoid tumour and VCL::ALK fusion renal cell carcinomas, which also occur in patients with sickle cell trait. Rhabdoid tumours typically affect younger children, and SMARCB1 is intact in VCL::ALK carcinomas. In adults, the differential diagnosis is mainly high-grade invasive urothelial carcinoma. Clinical evidence of sickle cell trait and young age at presentation are typical of renal medullary carcinoma, whereas the presence of in situ urothelial carcinoma or CK20 positivity favour urothelial carcinoma.

## Cytology

Not relevant

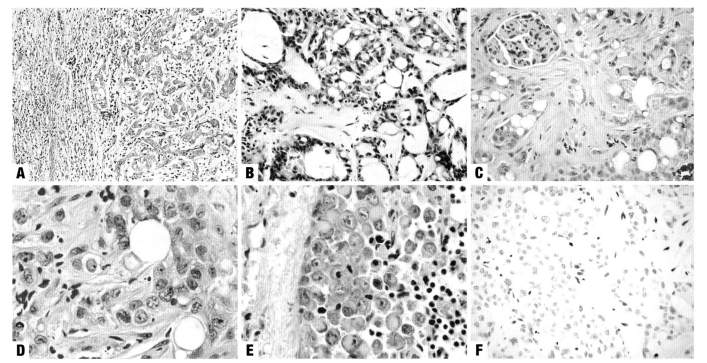

**Fig. 8.22** Renal medullary carcinoma. **A** The neoplastic cells form cords and tubules within an oedematous desmoplastic stroma. Native kidney is present to the left. **B** The neoplasm has a cribriform architecture, reminiscent of adenoid cystic carcinoma. **C** The neoplastic cells are vacuolated and form cords in a desmoplastic stroma. They permeate the kidney, surrounding a native glomerulus at the upper left. **D** Extravasated red blood cells within the neoplasm demonstrate sickling. **E** The renal medullary carcinoma cells in this lymph node metastasis have a rhabdoid phenotype. They demonstrate vesicular chromatin, prominent nucleoli, and hyaline intracytoplasmic inclusions. **F** The neoplastic cells demonstrate a loss of SMARCB1 (INI1). The surrounding non-neoplastic stromal cells demonstrate appropriate nuclear immunoreactivity.

## Diagnostic molecular pathology

The most common genetic abnormality is the inactivation of *SMARCB1* by chromosomal translocations or deletions {1046}. *SMARCB1* is located in a fragile region at 22q11.2 and is commonly lost by mutation and deletion in rhabdoid tumour of the kidney. In medullary carcinoma, loss of SMARCB1 protein expression arises through mechanisms of concurrent hemizygous loss and translocation, or by homozygous loss {3265}.

## Essential and desirable diagnostic criteria

*Essential:* a high-grade SMARCB1-deficient infiltrating renal adenocarcinoma.
*Desirable:* clinical/laboratory evidence of a haemoglobinopathy.

## Staging

Renal medullary carcinomas are staged using conventional renal cell carcinoma staging protocols (Union for International Cancer Control [UICC]).

## Prognosis and prediction

Renal medullary carcinoma has a poor prognosis, with > 90% of patients presenting with metastases to lymph nodes or other sites (most frequently lung and liver) at the time of diagnosis {3098}. Patients with localized disease at presentation have only slightly better survival. Overall, the median survival time is 8 months {2014}. Preoperative chemotherapy has been suggested, but there is little evidence that this will make a notable difference in outcome {4827,6358}.

# Metanephric adenoma

Argani P
Bode PK

## Definition
Metanephric adenoma is a highly cellular epithelial neoplasm composed of small, uniform, embryonic-appearing cells that are generally mitotically inactive.

## ICD-O coding
8325/0 Metanephric adenoma

## ICD-11 coding
2F35 & XH0JC7 Benign neoplasm of urinary organs & Metanephric adenoma

## Related terminology
None

## Subtype(s)
None

## Localization
Kidney

## Clinical features
Approximately 50% of cases are identified incidentally. Abdominal pain and haematuria are the most common presenting symptoms. Approximately 10% of patients have polycythaemia at presentation, due to erythropoietin production by the neoplasm {3318,1590}.

## Epidemiology
More than 100 cases of metanephric adenoma have been reported. Patients with metanephric adenoma have ranged in age from 5 to 83 years, but most are in their fifth or sixth decade of life. There is a distinct female predominance (M:F ratio: 1:2) {2555}.

## Etiology
Unknown

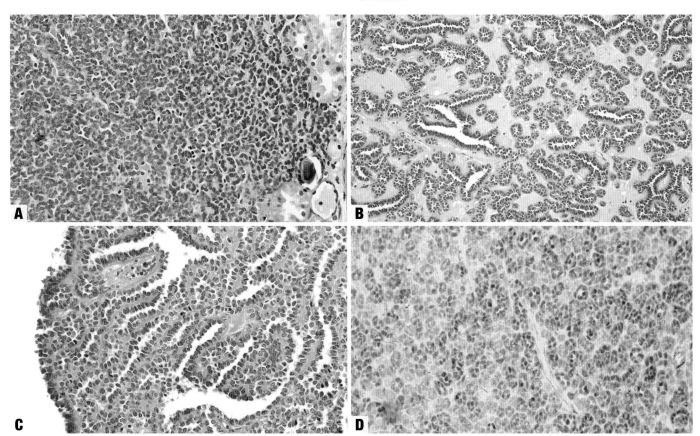

**Fig. 8.23** Metanephric adenoma. **A** The neoplasm is unencapsulated and directly abuts the native kidney to the right. The neoplasm is composed of cuboidal cells with primitive basophilic nuclei and minimal cytoplasm, forming small tubules. Mitotic activity is not evident. A psammoma body is noted at the lower right. **B** The stroma is oedematous and contains branching tubules and tubulopapillary structures, creating a fingerprint-like appearance. **C** Tumours with more prominent papillary areas can be confused with low-grade papillary renal cell carcinoma. The more hyperchromatic nuclei and absence of stromal foam cells are clues to the diagnosis of metanephric adenoma. **D** Metanephric adenomas typically demonstrate diffuse nuclear immunoreactivity for WT1 protein.

## Pathogenesis

*BRAF* mutation or (more rarely) *KANK1::NTRK3* gene fusion is often present.

## Macroscopic appearance

Metanephric adenomas are typically unicentric, sizeable lesions; the mean diameter is 50–60 mm but tumours can reach 150 mm. On sectioning, metanephric adenomas are solid and tan to grey, and they may be soft or firm. Most metanephric adenomas are solid, but degenerative cyst formation, haemorrhage, and necrosis are not uncommon in larger tumours.

## Histopathology

Metanephric adenomas usually lack pseudocapsules but are well-circumscribed neoplasms composed of embryonal epithelial cells with small round nuclei (only slightly larger than those of lymphocytes), even chromatin without prominent nucleoli, and minimal cytoplasm. These monotonous primitive blue cells typically form small, crowded acini in a hyalinized, oedematous, paucicellular stroma. Long, curved, branching tubules commonly impart a fingerprint-like appearance. Stubby papillae that project into small cysts resemble glomeruli. Very tightly packed acini with overlapping nuclei create a solid appearance. Oedematous polypoid structures with microacini within their stroma and microcysts are occasionally found. Psammoma bodies are common and often abundant. Mitotic figures are usually absent or rare. Vascular invasion is not seen.

By immunohistochemistry, metanephric adenomas usually demonstrate diffuse nuclear labelling for WT1 and cytoplasmic/membranous labelling for CD57. CK7 is either negative or patchy, labelling more intensely in areas of elongated tubule formation. EMA and AMACR (racemase) are typically negative {4832,3608,4386,5159}. Most cases show positivity for BRAF p.V600E immunohistochemistry.

The differential diagnosis of metanephric adenoma is essentially the solid subtype of low-grade papillary renal cell carcinoma (RCC) and epithelial-predominant nephroblastoma. Papillary RCC has slightly more vesicular chromatin and more abundant cytoplasm than metanephric adenoma. Unlike metanephric adenoma, solid papillary RCC usually labels diffusely for CK7 and EMA. WT1 is characteristically negative in papillary RCC (glomerular podocytes provide an excellent internal control for WT1 labelling) {3608,4386,5159}. Papillary RCC almost always demonstrates trisomy of chromosomes 7 and 17, which is not present in metanephric adenoma {915}. Epithelial-predominant nephroblastoma is typically distinguished from metanephric adenoma by the younger age of the patient, the presence of a pseudocapsule, elongate nuclei with small nucleoli, and abundant mitotic activity {313,1590}. Occasional cases span the morphological spectrum of metanephric adenoma and nephroblastoma {5845}, but most epithelial-predominant nephroblastomas do not harbour *BRAF* mutations {986}, making a direct relationship to metanephric adenoma unlikely. However, a subset of epithelial-predominant nephroblastomas that have areas that overlap with metanephric adenoma do have *BRAF* mutations, supporting a relationship between this subset of nephroblastoma and metanephric adenoma {7592}.

## Cytology

Not relevant

## Diagnostic molecular pathology

Mutations of *BRAF* (p.V600E) are present in approximately 90% of metanephric adenomas {986,1304,7128}. Most, but not all, can be detected by immunohistochemistry for BRAF using the VE1 clone {5554}. Rare cases have *BRAF* p.V600D or *BRAF* p.K601L mutations. *BRAF* mutations are associated with older age at diagnosis. Two cases lacking *BRAF* mutations have demonstrated a t(9;15)(p24;q24) translocation resulting in a *KANK1::NTRK3* gene fusion {1101,5744}.

## Essential and desirable diagnostic criteria

*Essential:* a cellular renal epithelial neoplasm composed of small uniform embryonal cells that are mitotically inactive.
*Desirable: BRAF* mutation; WT1 immunoreactivity.

## Staging

Not relevant

## Prognosis and prediction

Metanephric adenomas have a benign outcome. Polycythaemia associated with the tumour disappears after complete resection.

# Metanephric adenofibroma

Argani P
Bode PK

## Definition

Metanephric adenofibroma is a rare biphasic neoplasm that combines a spindle cell component that is morphologically identical to metanephric stromal tumour with an epithelial component that is morphologically identical to metanephric adenoma.

## ICD-O coding

9013/0 Metanephric adenofibroma

## ICD-11 coding

2F35 & XH7ZU2 Benign neoplasm of urinary organs & Metanephric adenofibroma

## Related terminology

*Not recommended:* nephrogenic adenofibroma.

## Subtype(s)

None

## Localization

Kidney

## Clinical features

Patients with metanephric adenofibroma presented with polycythaemia in 4 of 14 cases and with haematuria in 3 of 14 cases {356,2842,7117,5561}.

## Epidemiology

Fewer than 30 cases have been reported. Patients with metanephric adenofibroma have ranged in age from 13 months to 36 years (median: 81 months) {356,2842}.

## Etiology

Unknown

## Pathogenesis

All tumours have so far contained *BRAF* p.V600E mutations.

## Macroscopic appearance

Metanephric adenofibromas are typically solitary, tan, partially cystic masses with indistinct borders. The mean diameter is 40 mm. Many of these lesions have been centred on the renal pelvis, accounting for the presentation with haematuria.

## Histopathology

The relative amounts of the spindle cell and epithelial components vary. The border of the tumour with the kidney is typically irregular and the spindle cell component entraps tubules and glomeruli. Like that of metanephric stromal tumour, the stroma of metanephric adenofibroma frequently labels for CD34. The epithelial elements label similarly to metanephric adenoma.

Composite cases in which epithelial mitotic activity, nephroblastoma, or papillary renal cell carcinoma are associated with metanephric adenofibroma have been reported {356,2293}.

## Cytology

Not relevant

## Diagnostic molecular pathology

All metanephric adenofibromas tested to date have harboured the *BRAF* p.V600E mutations that are characteristic of the other metanephric neoplasms, metanephric stromal tumour and

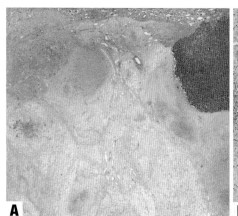 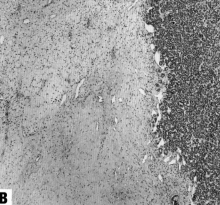 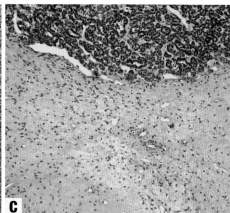

**Fig. 8.24** Metanephric adenofibroma. **A** The majority of this biphasic neoplasm is a stromal neoplasm identical to metanephric stromal tumour, and an epithelial nodule that is identical to metanephric adenoma is present at the upper right. Note the unencapsulated border with the native kidney at the top of the image. **B** The metanephric stromal tumour component on the left is composed of bland spindle cells, and the metanephric adenoma component composed of primitive but mitotically inactive tubules is to the right. **C** The bland spindle cell stromal component is at the bottom, and the primitive but mitotically inactive epithelial component is at the top.

metanephric adenoma {327,4369}. One composite metanephric adenofibroma–papillary renal cell carcinoma had the same *BRAF* p.V600E mutation in both the adenoma and carcinoma components {1131}.

## Essential and desirable diagnostic criteria

*Essential:* a biphasic stromal-epithelial renal neoplasm with areas identical to metanephric stromal tumour and metanephric adenoma.

*Desirable: BRAF* p.V600E mutations.

## Staging

Not relevant

## Prognosis and prediction

All reported metanephric adenofibromas have had a benign course, with no reports of metastases. One local recurrence has been reported {1644}. Excision is adequate therapy. Rare patients have experienced morbidity or died from the manifestations of extrarenal angiodysplasia, apparently induced by metanephric stromal tumour.

# Metanephric stromal tumour

Argani P
Bode PK

## Definition
Metanephric stromal tumour is a rare benign renal stromal neoplasm of uncertain histogenesis that is identical to the stromal component of metanephric adenofibroma.

## ICD-O coding
8935/1 Metanephric stromal tumour

## ICD-11 coding
2F35 & XH4N88 Benign neoplasm of urinary organs & Metanephric stromal tumour

## Related terminology
None

## Subtype(s)
None

## Localization
Kidney

## Clinical features
Metanephric stromal tumour is approximately one-tenth as common as congenital mesoblastic nephroma. Patients typically present with an abdominal mass, although haematuria is not rare and a few patients have presented with manifestations of extrarenal vasculopathy such as hypertension or haemorrhage. The mean age at diagnosis is 24 months. Rare adult cases have been described {737,1190}, as has a case in a patient with neurofibromatosis type 1 {4516}.

## Epidemiology
Unknown

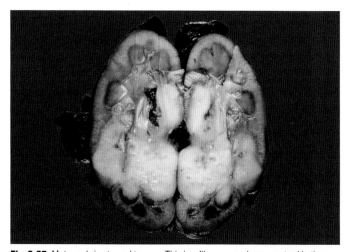

**Fig. 8.25** Metanephric stromal tumour. This is a fibrous neoplasm, centred in the medulla of this bivalved kidney. Note the scalloped border with the native kidney.

## Etiology
Unknown

## Pathogenesis
Most tumours have *BRAF* p.V600E mutations.

## Macroscopic appearance
Metanephric stromal tumour is typically a tan, lobulated, fibrous mass centred in the renal medulla. The mean diameter is 50 mm. Approximately half of the cases are grossly cystic, and one sixth are multifocal.

## Histopathology
Metanephric stromal tumour lacks a pseudocapsule and is a subtly infiltrative neoplasm composed of spindle-shaped to stellate cells with thin, hyperchromatic nuclei and thin, indistinct cytoplasmic extensions. Epithelioid stromal cells are not rare but typically are focal. Many of the characteristic features of metanephric stromal tumour result from its interaction with entrapped native renal elements. Metanephric stromal tumour characteristically surrounds and entraps renal tubules and blood vessels to form concentric, onion skin–like rings or collarettes around these structures in a myxoid background. More cellular, less myxoid spindle cell areas at the periphery of these collarettes yield nodular variations in cellularity. Most neoplasms induce angiodysplasia of entrapped arterioles, consisting of epithelioid transformation of medial smooth muscle and myxoid change, similar to that commonly seen in neurofibromatosis type 1. Rarely, such angiodysplasia results in intratumoural aneurysms. One quarter of metanephric stromal tumours induce juxtaglomerular cell hyperplasia within entrapped glomeruli, which may occasionally lead to hypertension associated with hyperreninism. One fifth of metanephric stromal tumours demonstrate heterologous differentiation in the form of glia or cartilage. Glial elements are commonly associated with metaplastic embryonal epithelium, forming glial–epithelial complexes.

Necrosis is unusual in metanephric stromal tumour. Most metanephric stromal tumours are mitotically inactive, but cellular foci may have multiple mitotic figures in a given high-power field. Whereas metanephric stromal tumour may involve the renal sinus and nerves and undermine the renal pelvic urothelium (suburothelial pads), vascular invasion is absent. Metanephric stromal tumours are typically immunoreactive for CD34, but labelling may be patchy. CD34 labelling is typically most prominent in the collarettes surrounding native tubules and blood vessels. Desmin, cytokeratins, PAX8, and S100 are negative, although heterologous glial areas label for GFAP and S100. Unlike clear cell sarcoma of the kidney, metanephric stromal tumour is typically negative for BCOR {331}. Unlike cellular congenital mesoblastic nephroma, metanephric stromal tumour lacks the *ETV6::NTRK3* gene fusion {318}.

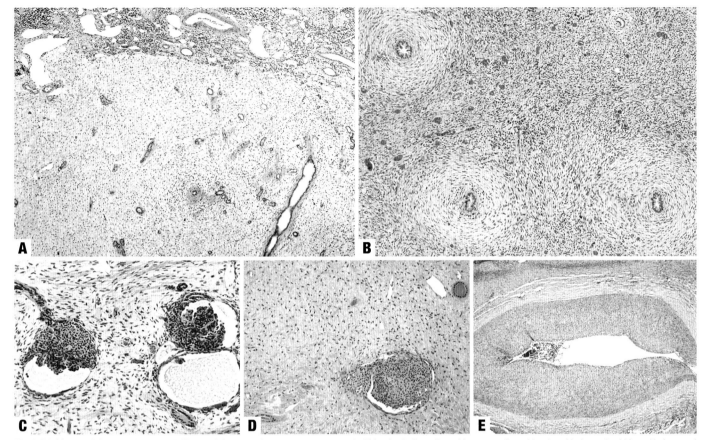

**Fig. 8.26** Metanephric stromal tumour. **A** Metanephric stromal tumours are composed of bland spindle cells and have a scalloped border with the native kidney. Native renal tubules are present within the lesion. **B** Neoplastic spindle cells encircle entrapped native tubules in a concentric fashion, yielding an onion-skin pattern. **C** Glomeruli entrapped within a metanephric stromal tumour frequently demonstrate florid juxtaglomerular cell hyperplasia. This may result in hyperreninism. **D** The neoplastic cells are bland and have indistinct cytoplasmic processes within a fibromyxoid stroma. Note the striking juxtaglomerular cell hyperplasia in the entrapped glomerulus at the lower right. **E** Arterioles within and occasionally outside of a metanephric stromal tumour frequently demonstrate angiodysplasia. Compared to the normal arterial wall (lower right), the majority of this arterial wall is markedly thickened and has undergone myxoid degeneration. The normally spindle-shaped smooth muscle cells have become epithelioid. These vessels can rupture, leading to haemorrhage.

## Cytology
Not relevant

## Diagnostic molecular pathology
The majority of metanephric stromal tumours harbour *BRAF* p.V600E mutations {327}. Because these are not found in clear cell sarcoma of the kidney, congenital mesoblastic nephroma, or ossifying renal tumour of infancy, the presence of these mutations may support the diagnosis in difficult cases.

## Essential and desirable diagnostic criteria
*Essential:* a bland, predominantly spindle cell neoplasm of the kidney, which encircles entrapped native renal tubules in a concentric growth pattern, yielding a nodular growth pattern.

*Desirable:* angiodysplasia of entrapped arterioles; juxtaglomerular cell hyperplasia of entrapped glomeruli; *BRAF* p.V600E mutations.

## Staging
Not relevant

## Prognosis and prediction
All reported metanephric stromal tumours have had a benign course, with no reports of metastases. One local recurrence has been reported {1644}. Excision is adequate therapy. Rare patients have experienced morbidity or died from the manifestations of extrarenal angiodysplasia, apparently induced by metanephric stromal tumour.

# Ossifying renal tumour of infancy

de Krijger RR
Chang KTE
Okita H
Tanaka Y
Tsuzuki T
Vujanic GM

## Definition
Ossifying renal tumour of infancy (ORTI) is an intracalyceal neoplasm composed of a combination of osteoid, osteoblastic cells, and spindle cells.

## ICD-O coding
8967/0 Ossifying renal tumour of infancy

## ICD-11 coding
2F35 & XH3SR2 Benign neoplasm of urinary organs & Ossifying renal tumour

## Related terminology
None

## Subtype(s)
None

## Localization
Renal pelvis

## Clinical features
ORTI has no specific clinical presentation, but most patients present with gross haematuria and a calcified mass protruding into the renal pelvis on imaging. No association with any other renal tumour type or syndrome has been published.

## Epidemiology
These tumours are extremely rare, with only about 25 cases published in the literature. There is a clear male predominance (M:F ratio: 7:1), and patients are between 6 days and 2.5 years old {2574,2665}.

## Etiology
Unknown

## Pathogenesis
Unknown

## Macroscopic appearance
The tumours are well circumscribed and measure 10–60 mm in diameter. Almost all tumours show signs of calcification on imaging studies and this is also reflected in the gross appearance.

## Histopathology
ORTIs are composed of two types of cells: osteoblast-like cells that are located between and around areas of osteoid, and a spindle cell (blastema-like) component found mostly at the periphery of the tumour. Both osteoblast-like cells and spindle cells are bland, without features of malignancy. The osteoblast-like cells are almost always immunopositive for EMA and vimentin.

## Cytology
Not relevant

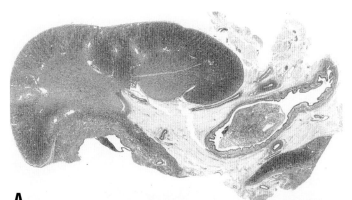

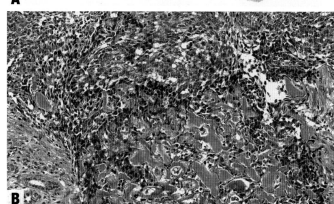

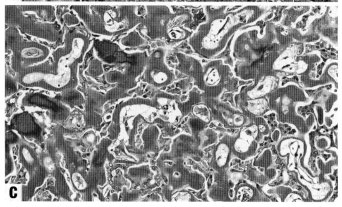

**Fig. 8.27** Ossifying renal tumour of infancy. **A** Low-power view showing the relationship of the tumour to the kidney and calyces. **B** High-power view showing the spindle cell component. **C** High-power view of the calcified part with osteoblastic cells.

## Diagnostic molecular pathology

Two different papers have now described 5 cases of ORTI with clonal trisomy 4, so this seems to be a relevant and recurrent molecular abnormality {4157,2574}.

## Essential and desirable diagnostic criteria

*Essential:* the typical histological combination of osteoid, osteoblastic cells, and spindle cells is required to make the diagnosis.

## Staging

All tumours are limited to the kidney and are regarded as benign lesions. No particular staging protocol applies.

## Prognosis and prediction

This is a benign tumour for which conservative surgical management is sufficient. Outcome has been uniformly favourable.

# Mesoblastic nephroma

Vujanic GM
Chang KTE
de Krijger RR
Tanaka Y
Tsuzuki T

## Definition
Mesoblastic nephroma (MN) is a spindle cell renal tumour of infancy, with classic and cellular forms.

## ICD-O coding
8960/1 Mesoblastic nephroma
8960/1 Classic mesoblastic nephroma
8960/1 Cellular mesoblastic nephroma
8960/1 Mixed mesoblastic nephroma

## ICD-11 coding
2C90.Y & XH10F1 Other specified malignant neoplasms of kidney, except renal pelvis & Mesoblastic nephroma

## Related terminology
None

## Subtype(s)
Classic mesoblastic nephroma; cellular mesoblastic nephroma; mixed mesoblastic nephroma

## Localization
MN is localized in the kidney. It is never multifocal or bilateral.

## Clinical features
MN accounts for 2–4% of renal tumours of childhood {5379}. Patients usually present with an abdominal mass (in ~75% of cases), hypertension (in ~20%), or haematuria (in ~10%). It may be diagnosed by prenatal ultrasound.

## Epidemiology
MN is the most common renal tumour in the first 3 months of life. In 90% of cases it occurs in the first year of life, and it virtually never arises after the age of 3 years; in 63% of patients, the median age at diagnosis is < 1 month. In ~15% of patients, MN is detected prenatally, usually associated with polyhydramnios {2495}.

## Etiology
There are no recognized risk factors, and no familial cases have been reported.

## Pathogenesis
A specific chromosomal translocation, t(12;15)(p13;q25), which results in the fusion of *ETV6* and *NTRK3*, has been found in about 70% of cases of cellular MN {7323,1908}. *EGFR* internal tandem duplication (ITD) is a consistent and recurrent genetic event in classic MN, whereas mixed MN may have either *EGFR* ITD or *ETV6::NTRK3* gene fusion {7848}. A recurrent *EGFR* ITD is found in classic MN {7475,7848}.

## Macroscopic appearance
MN is always solitary, and most cases arise in the medial renal sinus. The classic type has a firm, whorled, myomatous consistency and is poorly demarcated from the normal renal parenchyma. The cellular type is usually soft; it sometimes has cysts, haemorrhage, and necrosis; and the tumour–kidney junction is better demarcated than in the classic type.

## Histopathology
Classic MN, representing about 25% of cases, is characterized by intermingling fascicles of spindle cells; collagen deposition; low mitotic activity; and often prominent, dilated, thin-walled vascular spaces. There is no capsule, and the tumour–kidney border is irregular, with many finger-like protrusions of the tumour into the renal parenchyma, resulting in numerous islands of entrapped renal elements, which may undergo metaplastic changes. Islands of hyaline cartilage may be found at the tumour–kidney interface. Foci of extramedullary haematopoiesis are common. Because of their infiltrative growth into the renal sinus or perirenal fat, the vast majority of tumours are stage II. Cellular MN (~65% of cases) is characterized by increased cellularity of plump cells with vesicular nuclei and a moderate amount of cytoplasm, growing in a sheet-like pattern. There is a high mitotic activity (which is of no prognostic significance). Despite a relatively clear border between the tumour and the renal parenchyma, there is no capsule, and the tumour subtly infiltrates the kidney. Mixed-type MN (~10% of cases) shows features of both types. SMA and cyclin D1 immunostains are positive in MN {4705}. Desmin is usually negative. Nuclear staining with a pan-TRK antibody is supportive of a diagnosis of cellular MN with *ETV6::NTRK3* gene fusion {7848}.

## Cytology
Not relevant

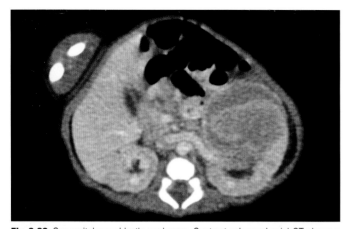

**Fig. 8.28** Congenital mesoblastic nephroma. Contrast-enhanced axial CT shows a fairly homogeneous mass with predominantly peripheral enhancement at the anterior region of the left kidney extending to the renal hilum but without invasion of the renal vessels.

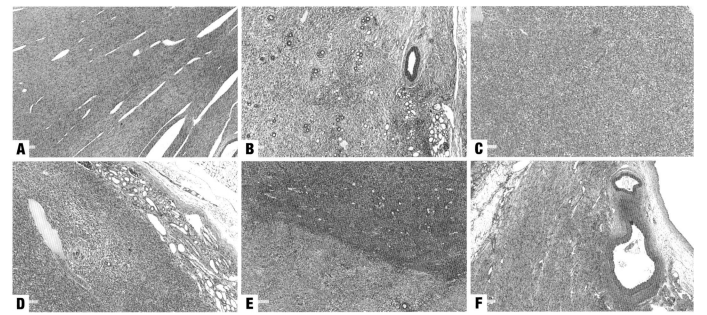

**Fig. 8.29** Mesoblastic nephroma. **A** Classic-type mesoblastic nephroma composed of interlacing fascicles of spindled cells and thin-walled vascular spaces. **B** The tumour–kidney interface is irregular, with many islands of entrapped normal renal parenchyma. **C** Cellular type, composed of densely packed plump cells growing in a sheet-like pattern. **D** The tumour–kidney border in the cellular type is sharp, despite the absence of the capsule. **E** Mixed type, composed of cellular areas (upper part of the figure) that are sharply demarcated from the classic type. **F** Renal sinus infiltration by tumour, which is very common because no capsule is present.

## Diagnostic molecular pathology

Cellular MN shows a t(12;15)(p13;q25) translocation in about 70% of cases, resulting in the expression of the fusion protein ETV6::NTRK3 {7323}. The same translocation is found in infantile fibrosarcoma, indicating that they are pathogenetically related neoplasms {3664}.

## Essential and desirable diagnostic criteria

*Essential:* patient age < 3 years; characteristic histological features.
*Desirable:* for cellular MN: presence of *ETV6::NTRK3* fusion.

## Staging

MN is staged according to the same staging criteria as nephroblastoma {7344}.

## Prognosis and prediction

MN has an excellent prognosis, even in stage II or III disease {2495}. It is treated with nephrectomy with wide margins, and chemotherapy is not routinely given, even for stage III cases. Local relapse and/or metastasis has been reported in 38 children in the literature, all with the cellular type; all cases of relapse and metastasis occurred within 12 months after surgery. Local recurrences are related to incomplete surgical removal and are still best cured by complete resection. The most common site of metastasis is the lung (~40%), followed by the liver (28%) and brain (22%). Fifty per cent of children with recurrence and/or metastasis died {3241}.

# Clear cell sarcoma of the kidney

Chang KTE
Okita H
Tanaka Y
Tsuzuki T
Vujanic GM

## Definition

Clear cell sarcoma of the kidney (CCSK) is a rare malignant renal tumour of childhood, characterized histologically by variably clear tumour cells and distinctive arborizing fibrovascular septa, and molecularly by *BCOR* mutations or *YWHAE*::NUTM2 gene fusion.

## ICD-O coding

8964/3 Clear cell sarcoma of the kidney

## ICD-11 coding

2C90.Y & XH0765 Other specified malignant neoplasms of kidney, except renal pelvis & Clear cell sarcoma of kidney

## Related terminology

*Not recommended:* bone-metastasizing renal tumour of childhood.

## Subtype(s)

None

## Localization

CCSK arises in the kidney and is often centred in the renal medulla. Bilateral CCSK has not been reported.

## Clinical features

The affected child may have nonspecific features of abdominal distension, pain, a palpable abdominal mass, or gross haematuria.

## Epidemiology

CCSK constitutes 3–5% of malignant renal tumours in childhood, ranking a distant second after nephroblastoma. The M:F ratio is 2:1. The mean age at diagnosis is 3 years {6598}.

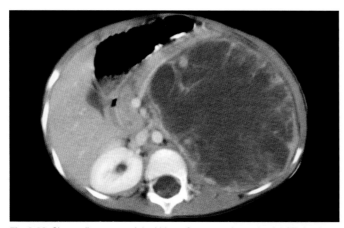

**Fig. 8.30** Clear cell sarcoma of the kidney. Contrast-enhanced axial CT showing a large heterogeneous enhancing mass (predominantly a central large fluid space with enhancing septa). The tumour crosses the midline and markedly displaces the pancreas and its adjacent splenic vein.

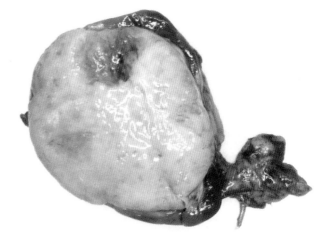

**Fig. 8.31** Clear cell sarcoma of the kidney. Gross examination shows a well-circumscribed fleshy mass.

## Etiology

There are no known risk factors. CCSK is a sporadic tumour. There are no reports of familial CCSK.

## Pathogenesis

CCSK is characterized by mutations affecting *BCOR* (either an in-frame internal tandem duplication [ITD] affecting exon 15 {7129} or a *BCOR::CCNB3* gene fusion {7613}) or by *YWHAE*::NUTM2 gene fusion {5180}. These mutations result in oncogenic upregulation of BCOR, which is a component of non-canonical PRC1.1 {2345}. The specific mechanism of molecular pathogenesis is currently unknown.

## Macroscopic appearance

CCSK often manifests as a solitary large renal tumour with its epicentre at the renal medulla. The cut surface is pale tan-grey and fleshy; mucoid to cystic areas may be present.

## Histopathology

CCSK has varied histological patterns {332}. The classic pattern is most common and is usually present at least focally {332, 415}. The features include plump ovoid tumour cells demarcated into broad trabeculae or nests by distinctive arborizing fibrovascular septa. Tumour cells have barely perceptible cytoplasm and monomorphic nuclei with dispersed chromatin and indistinct nucleoli. The nuclei and cytoplasm often have a clear appearance, from which this tumour derives its name. The cellular pattern has similar tumour cells that are more closely packed, with frequent nuclear overlapping {332}. The myxoid pattern features increased mucopolysaccharide matrix, which may form mucoid pools and cysts {332}. The sclerosing pattern features hyalinized collagen, which may resemble osteoid {332}. The epithelioid pattern has tumour cells aligned in acini

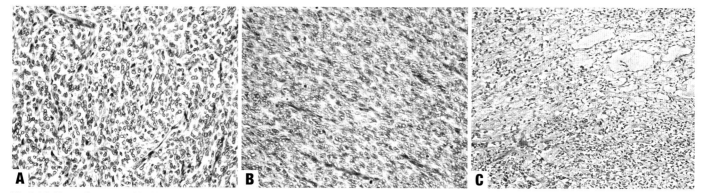

**Fig. 8.32** Clear cell sarcoma of the kidney. **A** Classic areas feature ovoid tumour cells with variably clear nuclei and cytoplasm; note the delicate branching vasculature. **B** Cellular areas feature overlapping of the nuclei. **C** Myxoid areas show increased extracellular matrix. Cyst formation is possible.

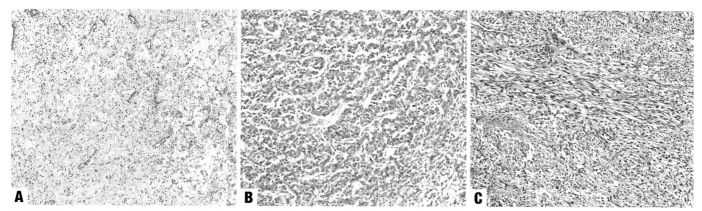

**Fig. 8.33** Clear cell sarcoma of the kidney. **A** Sclerosing areas show deposits of eosinophilic hyalinized material that may resemble osteoid. **B** Epithelioid areas feature tumour cells arranged as tubules or trabeculae. **C** Spindled areas feature fascicular groups of elongated tumour cells, resembling a spindle cell sarcoma.

or elongated trabeculae mimicking the epithelial structures that may be seen in nephroblastoma {332}. The palisading pattern features nuclear palisading that resembles Verocay bodies of schwannomas {332}. The spindled pattern has elongated tumour cells resembling those of spindle cell sarcomas {332}. Rare tumours have anaplasia, defined in the same way as for nephroblastomas {332}. Posttreatment relapses may resemble myxoma or fibromatosis histologically.

*Immunohistochemistry*
Immunoreactivity for both cyclin D1 and BCOR in a diffuse nuclear staining pattern provides robust support for the diagnosis of CCSK {7613,3259,4705}. However, although sensitive, cyclin D1 is not perfectly specific; and BCOR is neither perfectly sensitive nor specific. Other positive markers include vimentin, p75-NGFR, BCL2, TLE1, and SATB2 {3523,359}. CCSK is negative for CD34, S100, desmin, cytokeratins, and EMA {4202}. CCSK with *BCOR::CCNB3* gene fusion expresses cyclin B3 {4482}.

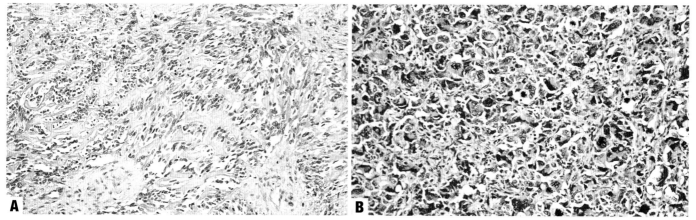

**Fig. 8.34** Clear cell sarcoma of the kidney. **A** Palisading areas resemble Verocay bodies of schwannomas. **B** Anaplasia may rarely occur in clear cell sarcoma of the kidney and is defined as for nephroblastoma.

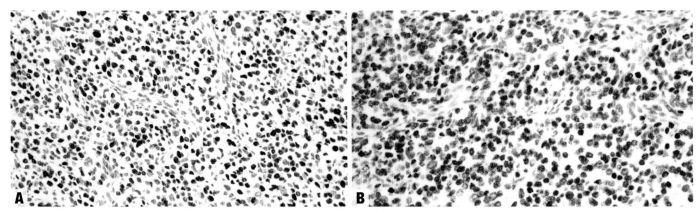

**Fig. 8.35** Clear cell sarcoma of the kidney. Tumour cell nuclei stain for cyclin D1 (**A**) and BCOR (**B**) in a strong and diffuse pattern. Note that vascular endothelial cells are negative.

## Cytology

Not relevant

## Diagnostic molecular pathology

The three characteristic mutations of CCSK are (in decreasing order of frequency) *BCOR* exon 15 ITD, *YWHAE*::NUTM2 fusion, and *BCOR*::*CCNB3* fusion. These three sequence alterations are mutually exclusive.

## Essential and desirable diagnostic criteria

*Essential:* characteristic histomorphology (ovoid tumour cells with nuclear and/or cytoplasmic clearing at least focally, distinctive arborizing fibrovascular septa, and immunoreactivity for cyclin D1 and BCOR).

*Desirable:* in cases with atypical histomorphology or immunophenotype: molecular identification of *BCOR* exon 15 ITD or *YWHAE*::NUTM2 fusion or *BCOR*::*CCNB3* fusion.

## Staging

Staging follows the same International Society of Paediatric Oncology (SIOP) or Children's Oncology Group (COG) staging systems as used for nephroblastomas.

## Prognosis and prediction

CCSK has 5-year event-free and overall survival rates of 65–85% and 75–90%, respectively, with intensive multiagent chemotherapy and radiation therapy {2494}. Approximately 16% of patients relapse {2493}. Relapse may be late {332}. CCSK may metastasize to unusual sites such as bone, orbit, and brain. The clinical course is not predicted by histological pattern or mutation findings.

# Malignant rhabdoid tumour of the kidney

de Krijger RR
Okita H
Tanaka Y
Tsuzuki T
Vujanic GM

## Definition

Malignant rhabdoid tumour of the kidney (MRTK) is a highly malignant tumour, typically composed of sheets of cells that have eccentric pleomorphic nuclei with prominent nucleoli and characteristic intracytoplasmic inclusions, complemented by loss a of SMARCB1 (INI1) immunostaining and frequent *SMARCB1* genetic abnormalities.

## ICD-O coding

8963/3 Malignant rhabdoid tumour of the kidney

## ICD-11 coding

2C90.Y & XH3RF3 Other specified malignant neoplasms of kidney, except renal pelvis & Rhabdoid tumour, NOS
2B5F.2 & XH3RF3 Sarcoma, not elsewhere classified, of other specified sites & Malignant rhabdoid tumour
2A00.1Y & XH3RF3 Other specified embryonal tumours of brain & Malignant rhabdoid tumour

## Related terminology

*Acceptable:* rhabdoid tumour (of soft tissues); rhabdoid tumour predisposition syndrome.

## Subtype(s)

None

## Localization

Kidney parenchyma

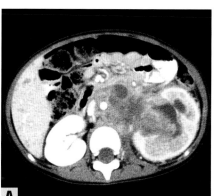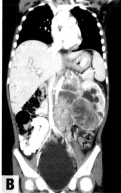

**Fig. 8.36** Malignant rhabdoid tumour of the kidney. **A** Contrast-enhanced axial CT showing a heterogeneous mass with an indistinct margin in the central portion of the left kidney, with invasion to the renal pelvis and extracapsular spread with encasement of the renal vessels, aorta, and inferior vena cava. There is an associated enlargement of retroperitoneal lymph nodes. **B** Contrast-enhanced coronal reformatted CT showing a heterogeneous mass arising from the lower pole of the left kidney, with extracapsular spread and encasement of the renal vessels, aorta, and inferior vena cava. There is obstructive dilatation of the upper pole calyces.

## Clinical features

There are no specific clinical features, but patients generally present with haematuria and/or an abdominal mass.

## Epidemiology

MRTKs account for approximately 2% of paediatric renal tumours, which makes them extremely rare tumours. They occur in infants and young children, with a mean/median patient age of 1 year and with 80% of patients diagnosed before the age of 2 years. Although congenital cases have been described, it is rare to find MRTK in children aged > 3 years {7472}. In as many as 15% of cases there is a synchronous or metachronous occurrence of atypical teratoid/rhabdoid tumours in the brain.

## Etiology

Biallelic inactivation of *SMARCB1* (also known as *BAF47*, *SNF5*, or *INI1*), located on chromosome 22q11.23, is the almost universal hallmark of renal and extrarenal rhabdoid tumours, including atypical teratoid/rhabdoid tumour of the brain. Inactivation may occur through mutation, segmental chromosomal deletion, or whole-chromosome loss (loss of heterozygosity). *SMARCB1* mutations may occur in the germ line in as many as one third of patients; if so, they are affected by the familial rhabdoid tumour predisposition syndrome type 1. A small proportion (≤ 5%) of patients with MRTK have biallelic inactivation of *SMARCA4*, another component of the SWI/SNF complex, instead of *SMARCB1* inactivation {5409}.

## Pathogenesis

Because MRTK and other rhabdoid tumours are genetically silent tumours, almost exclusively characterized by *SMARCB1* inactivation, it is thought that deregulation of the SWI/SNF chromatin-remodelling complex leads to carcinogenesis by its epigenetic effect on the promoter and enhancer regions of other genes.

## Macroscopic appearance

These are large, highly infiltrative tumours with a haemorrhagic and necrotic appearance.

## Histopathology

MRTK is composed of disorganized sheets of poorly cohesive large cells that grow in a diffuse infiltrative pattern with abundant necrosis. The tumour cells have large vesicular nuclei with one or two prominent eosinophilic nucleoli, and moderate amounts of pink cytoplasm. Rounded pink cytoplasmic inclusions, ultrastructurally composed of balls of intermediate filaments, give the tumour its descriptive "rhabdoid" name. MRTK, like other rhabdoid tumours, may have different architectural growth patterns, including solid, sclerosing, epithelioid, spindled, cystic, vascular, or myxoid. Tumour cells with classic rhabdoid inclusions may be only focally present. Apart from the typical morphology,

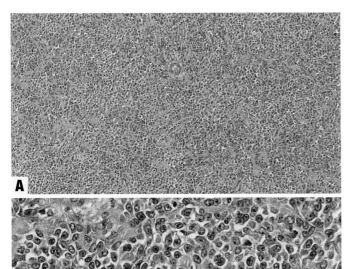

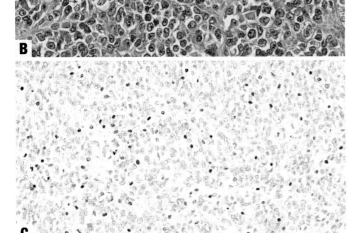

**Fig. 8.37** Malignant rhabdoid tumour of the kidney. **A** Diffuse growth pattern of tumour cells. **B** High-power view showing the typical cellular aspect with prominent nucleoli and cytoplasmic inclusions in some cells. **C** Absence of SMARCB1 (INI1) immunostaining in tumour cells, with retention in normal cells (which serve as an internal positive control).

MRTKs are characterized by a loss of nuclear SMARCB1 (INI1) staining, which is otherwise universally present in all cells (staining of normal cells is an internal positive control) {3345}. It should be noted that a limited spectrum of other tumours may also show a loss of SMARCB1 (INI1) staining, including renal medullary carcinoma. For MRTK with *SMARCA4* inactivation, SMARCA4 (BRG1) immunohistochemistry may be used; these tumours show a loss of nuclear staining in tumour cells and normal expression in all other cells {5409}.

### Cytology
Not relevant

### Diagnostic molecular pathology
Mutation analysis by next-generation sequencing techniques will show *SMARCB1* or *SMARCA4* mutations. This should be complemented by other techniques aiming to demonstrate the loss of the other allele (e.g. SNP arrays). Patients with mutations should be referred to clinical genetics for germline analysis and counselling.

### Essential and desirable diagnostic criteria
*Essential:* typical morphology with absence of SMARCB1 (INI1) immunostaining.
*Desirable: SMARCB1* mutation and/or loss of 22q11.

### Staging
No separate staging system exists for renal MRTK, but the staging systems from the International Society of Paediatric Oncology (SIOP) 2016 UMBRELLA protocol or from the Children's Oncology Group (COG) may be used. Most patients present with advanced-stage tumours; only 6–21% present with stage I disease {7011,7198}.

### Prognosis and prediction
MRTKs have a uniformly dismal prognosis, with reported 5-year overall survival rates ranging from < 15% to 25%. Younger age and presence of metastases at diagnosis are adverse prognostic factors for survival {7011,7198}.

# Anaplastic sarcoma of the kidney

Vujanic GM
Chang KTE
de Krijger RR
Tanaka Y
Tsuzuki T

## Definition
Anaplastic sarcoma of the kidney (ASK) is a multipatterned cystic and solid sarcoma with anaplasia. It is regarded as part of the *DICER1* spectrum of tumours.

## ICD-O coding
8802/3 Anaplastic sarcoma of the kidney

## ICD-11 coding
2C90.Y & XH4UM7 Other specified malignant neoplasms of kidney, except renal pelvis & Sarcoma, NOS

## Related terminology
*Acceptable: DICER1* sarcoma of the kidney.

## Subtype(s)
None

## Localization
ASK is localized in the kidney, but tumours with similar features have been described in other organs (pleuropulmonary blastoma {1678}).

## Clinical features
ASK usually manifests as a large renal mass. Some patients present with flank pain and haematuria.

## Epidemiology
ASK is extremely rare, with < 30 cases published in the English-language literature. Patient age at presentation ranges from 10 months to 41 years (median: 9.4 years), and about 70% of patients are aged < 15 years {7346,3419}.

## Etiology
ASK is associated with *DICER1* pathogenic variants.

## Pathogenesis
Similarly to how purely cystic (type I) pleuropulmonary blastoma in the lung shows potential to progress to cystic and solid (type II) pleuropulmonary blastoma, cystic nephroma of the kidney can progress to anaplastic sarcoma {7638,7639,1799}. Like in pleuropulmonary blastoma, in some cases of ASK there are biallelic loss-of-function and missense RNase IIIb mutations in *DICER1*. This combination of mutations is expected to alter

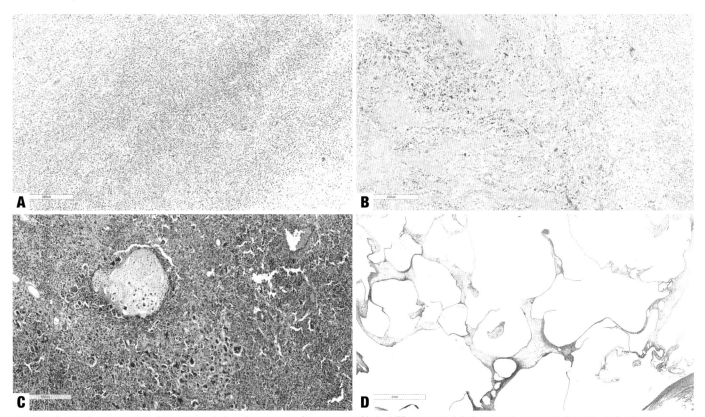

**Fig. 8.38** Anaplastic sarcoma of the kidney. **A** A spindle cell component of the tumour. **B** Marked diffuse anaplasia in the stromal component. **C** An island of malignant cartilage is one of the key features. **D** A cystic component of the tumour, closely resembling cystic nephroma.

Chapter 8

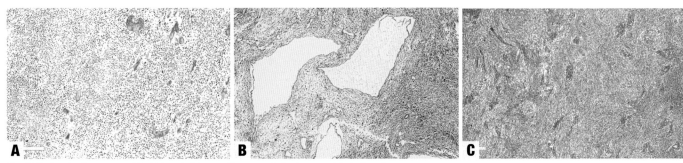

**Fig. 8.39** Anaplastic sarcoma of the kidney. **A** Blastema-like areas. **B** Cystic areas. **C** Spindle cell area.

expression of microRNAs important in regulating the cell cycle and limiting differentiation {5661}.

## Macroscopic appearance

ASK is typically large (median diameter: 150 mm) and located centrally in the kidney. Many tumours have a distinct cystic component {7346,3419}.

## Histopathology

ASK is a multipatterned sarcoma with cystic and solid sarcomatous components. The predominant pattern is spindle cell sarcoma with scattered large cells that have large hyperchromatic and irregular nuclei and enlarged multipolar anaplastic figures. Malignant cartilage nodules and embryonal rhabdomyosarcomatous areas can also be seen. Residual cystic nephroma can be seen at the periphery of the tumours {7346,1799}.

## Cytology

Not relevant

## Diagnostic molecular pathology

ASK has biallelic *DICER1* loss-of-function and missense RNase IIIb pathogenic variants {1799,7640}.

## Essential and desirable diagnostic criteria

*Essential:* a multipatterned sarcoma containing spindle cell sarcoma, cartilage, and diffuse anaplasia, with or without a residual cystic nephroma.

*Desirable:* biallelic *DICER1* pathogenic sequence variants in tumour tissue.

## Staging

No separate staging system exists for ASK, but the International Society of Paediatric Oncology (SIOP) or Children's Oncology Group (COG) staging systems may be used {1782,7344}.

## Prognosis and prediction

Follow-up is limited in these cases. In reported cases, the overall survival rate is 75% {7346,3419}.

# Renal Ewing sarcoma

de Krijger RR
Chang KTE
Okita H
Tanaka Y
Tsuzuki T
Vujanic GM

## Definition

Renal Ewing sarcoma, like other extraosseous Ewing sarcomas, is a sarcoma composed of small round cells, characterized by a fusion of a FET gene family member (most frequently *EWSR1*) and an ETS gene family member (most frequently *FLI1*).

## ICD-O coding

9364/3 Renal Ewing sarcoma

## ICD-11 coding

2B52.3 Ewing sarcoma of soft tissue

## Related terminology

*Acceptable:* peripheral neuroectodermal tumour; Ewing sarcoma family of tumours.

## Subtype(s)

None

## Localization

Renal parenchyma

## Clinical features

There are no specific symptoms or imaging characteristics that may distinguish Ewing sarcoma from other primary renal tumours, but a classic triad of haematuria, pain, and palpable tumour has been reported.

## Epidemiology

Ewing sarcoma is the second most common sarcoma of bone and soft tissues in children and adolescents, representing 2–3% of cancers in these age groups. Primary Ewing sarcoma of the kidney is extremely rare, representing 1.5% of all cases of Ewing sarcoma in one study. The median patient age is 27 years, and there is a slight male preponderance {7881}.

## Etiology

See *Ewing sarcoma* (p. 579).

## Pathogenesis

See *Ewing sarcoma* (p. 579).

## Macroscopic appearance

There are no specific gross features, but tumours are usually large (110–120 mm on average).

## Histopathology

The morphology of renal Ewing sarcoma is identical to that of Ewing sarcoma in other bone or soft tissue locations. Because most cases occur in adolescents, diagnosis will frequently be biopsy-based. The aspect of a highly cellular tumour composed of small cells with little cytoplasm, organized in sheets and possibly rosettes, should stimulate the use of ancillary techniques. Diffuse strong membranous CD99 expression is a hallmark, although molecular confirmation is recommended {1927}. In addition, nuclear NKX2-2 staining in ≥ 5% of tumour cells shows high sensitivity but imperfect specificity for Ewing sarcoma {7740}. A panel of markers, including WT1, SMARCB1 (INI1), keratins, neuroendocrine markers, desmin, PAX8, PHOX2B, and NB84, may be used to exclude other entities, such as blastemal Wilms tumour, neuroblastoma, malignant rhabdoid tumour, and desmoplastic round cell tumour. It should be noted that as many as 30% of Ewing sarcomas may show keratin expression, which should not lead to an erroneous diagnosis of undifferentiated carcinoma.

## Cytology

Not relevant

## Diagnostic molecular pathology

The majority (90%) of Ewing sarcomas, including renal Ewing sarcoma, show a characteristic t(11;22)(q24;q12) translocation with fusion between various exons of the genes *EWSR1*

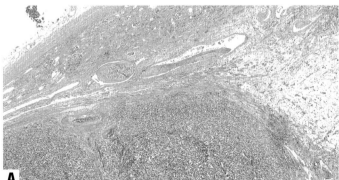 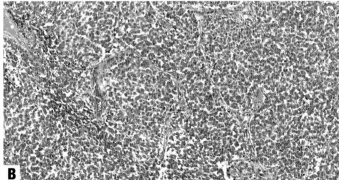

**Fig. 8.40** Renal Ewing sarcoma. **A** Low-power view showing the tumour in relation to the kidney. **B** High-power view showing the typical appearance of Ewing sarcoma with uniform small round cells with little cytoplasm and slightly nodular growth.

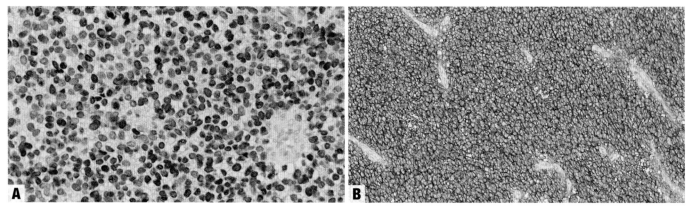

**Fig. 8.41** Renal Ewing sarcoma. Tumour cells show strong diffuse immunostaining for NKX2-2 (nuclear) (**A**) and CD99 (membranous) (**B**).

and *FLI1*. In addition, translocations of *EWSR1* with a number of other ETS genes (including *ERG*, *ETV1*, and *FEV*), or between another gene (*FUS*) and ETS-family genes, have been described {6163}. Together, these translocations are found in almost 100% of cases.

### Essential and desirable diagnostic criteria
*Essential:* typical (small blue round cell) morphology with diffuse strong membranous CD99 staining.

### Staging
No separate staging system exists for renal Ewing sarcoma, but the staging system for renal cell carcinoma from the International Society of Paediatric Oncology (SIOP) 2016 UMBRELLA protocol or from the Children's Oncology Group (COG) may be used.

### Prognosis and prediction
The current overall survival rate for patients with localized renal Ewing sarcoma is about 70%, but it drops to 10–40% for those with metastases at diagnosis {7881}. No other predictive factors are currently known. The presence of vascular thrombus and the exact nature of the molecular genetic translocation do not seem to affect the prognosis.

# Non–germ cell testicular tumours: Introduction

Bode PK
Schneider DT
Tsuzuki T

At first glance, the present chapter on testicular tumours in children may seem incomplete, because it provides only one short section about juvenile granulosa cell tumour. However, germ cell tumours, which represent 80–90% of all testicular neoplasms in children and adolescents {7141,5998,3005,5050}, are addressed with other germ cell tumours in their own chapter (see Chapter 7: *Germ cell tumours*). For the very first WHO classification of paediatric tumours, it was decided that all germ cell tumours would be grouped into one chapter to highlight the common features of this tumour class regardless of anatomical location. However, this also presented several challenges. In the WHO classification of urinary and male genital tumours, testicular germ cell tumours were subdivided into those derived from germ cell neoplasia in situ (GCNIS) (postpubertal-type germ cell tumours) and those unrelated to GCNIS (prepubertal-type germ cell tumours). Of course, this quite reasonable subdivision could not be adopted for a cross-organ classification, because GCNIS occurs exclusively in the testis. In the present classification of paediatric tumours, this resulted in the following: postpubertal-type germ cell tumours of the testis are discussed in the sections on germinoma-family tumours (seminoma) and non-germinomatous germ cell tumours; for prepubertal-type germ cell tumours, which include two main entities, the benign prepubertal-type teratoma is addressed in a separate section (*Prepubertal-type testicular teratoma*), although there is some overlap with extragonadal teratomas, and prepubertal-type yolk sac tumour is discussed in the *Yolk sac tumour* section together with its postpubertal counterpart (this section explicitly discusses the differences in tumour biology between the two subtypes). Finally, GCNIS has its own section in the sections on non-invasive germ cell neoplasia.

Sex cord stromal tumours are the second most common primary tumours of the testis, although in terms of absolute numbers they are very rare in the paediatric population {1114, 2943}. Proportionally, they are more frequent in the first decade of life (10–15% of primary tumours of the testis) than thereafter (5%) {5998,895}. This is due to the fact that before puberty germ cell tumours are less represented than in adolescents and adults. Because it occurs almost exclusively in children, juvenile granulosa cell tumour is the only sex cord stromal tumour discussed in this chapter. Leydig cell tumours {4256} and Sertoli cell tumours {791} have also been reported in children, although cases in adults far outweigh those in the paediatric population {2048,2564}. However, one important difference should be explicitly emphasized: sex cord stromal tumours occurring in the first decade of life are almost always benign {6026,2048, 2564}. From the paediatric pathological perspective, two more peculiar entities should be mentioned: large cell calcifying Sertoli cell tumour, which may be associated with the Carney complex (cardiac myxoma, spotty skin pigmentation, and endocrine overactivity), and intratubular large cell hyalinizing Sertoli cell neoplasia, which represents a possible testicular manifestation of Peutz–Jeghers syndrome. Both are extraordinarily rare, so for reasons of space, a detailed presentation has been omitted. Therefore, we refer here to the WHO classification of urinary and male genital tumours.

# Juvenile granulosa cell tumour of the testis

Bode PK
Schneider DT
Tsuzuki T

## Definition
Juvenile granulosa cell tumour (JGCT) is a sex cord tumour composed of primitive-appearing granulosa cells, which is similar in appearance to its ovarian counterpart.

## ICD-O coding
8622/0 Juvenile granulosa cell tumour of the testis

## ICD-11 coding
2F34 & XH2U25 Benign neoplasm of male genital organs & Granulosa cell tumour of the testis, juvenile

## Related terminology
*Not recommended:* interstitial tumour; stromal tumour.

## Subtype(s)
None

## Localization
JGCT is exclusively intratesticular and does not occur in paratesticular sites.

## Clinical features
Almost all patients present with a testicular mass or testicular enlargement. Unlike in its ovarian counterpart, hormonal changes like gynaecomastia or premature puberty are extremely rare in JGCT {2565}. There are no well-established risk factors, although a few cases are associated with karyotypic abnormalities {5050,7141} or cryptorchidism {2565}.

## Epidemiology
Unlike its ovarian counterpart, JGCT manifests predominantly in the first 6 months of life or even congenitally. Beyond the first year of life only anecdotal cases have been described. It accounts for 6–7% of all prepubertal testicular tumours {3972, 2720,7888,1114,2565}.

## Etiology
Unknown

## Pathogenesis
Unknown

## Macroscopic appearance
The reported average tumour size is 20 mm (range: 5–50 mm). The cut surface usually shows cystic parts, which contain watery or mucous fluid. The colour ranges from grey to tan-white or yellow {2565,3414,3972}.

## Histopathology
Although the histomorphological spectrum is broad in JGCT, a lobulated pattern with macrocystic and microcystic areas is characteristic in the overview. At higher power, the cysts correspond to ovarian-like follicles filled with eosinophilic or basophilic fluid. In addition to the cystic pattern, a solid component is usually present. Rarely, unusual morphology (e.g. papillary, basaloid, or spindle cell pattern) may occur. The tumour cells are polygonal with sometimes vacuolated or eosinophilic cytoplasm. The nuclei are ovoid with small nucleoli and no nuclear grooves. The tumour cells are embedded in a fibrous or fibromyxoid stroma. Mitotic activity can be very high (> 5 mitoses/mm2), and apoptosis with regressive changes is often prominent {3414,3972}.

JGCT shares a common immunophenotype with other sex cord stromal tumours, expressing SF1, calretinin, inhibin, SOX9, WT1, and FOXL2 {3414,3376}. Low-molecular-weight cytokeratins may be focally positive.

The differential diagnosis includes yolk sac tumour (YST) and other sex cord stromal tumours. Unlike JGCTs, the majority of YSTs arise in children beyond the first year of life; only one fifth of YSTs affect children aged < 1 year {1441}. In this context, it must be emphasized that serum AFP levels in neonates and infants have to be interpreted carefully, because physiological elevation is seen in the first few months of life. Microscopically, follicular elements are not a feature of YST, but solid growth patterns can cause potential confusion. In difficult cases, immunohistochemistry is usually straightforward. YSTs are negative for SF1, inhibin, calretinin, and the other already mentioned sex cord stromal tumour markers, whereas JGCTs do not express SALL4, AFP, or glypican-3 (GPC3) {3414}.

The differential diagnosis with other sex cord stromal tumours (Sertoli cell tumour NOS and mixed sex cord stromal tumours)

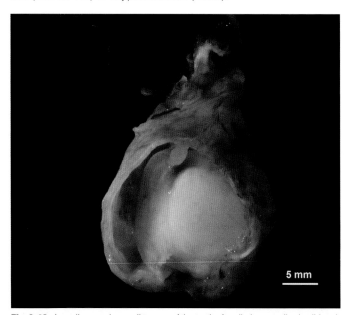

**Fig. 8.42** Juvenile granulosa cell tumour of the testis. A well-circumscribed solid nodule with a yellow cut surface.

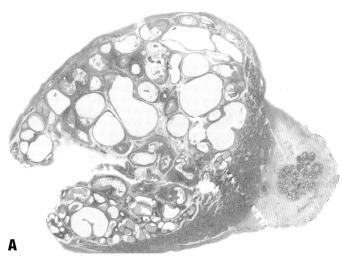
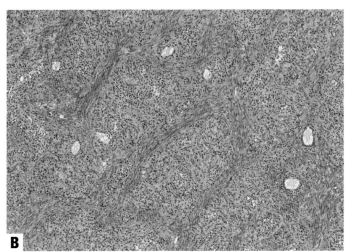

**Fig. 8.43** Juvenile granulosa cell tumour of the testis. **A** Overview of the multicystic appearance. **B** Solid area with a lobular growth pattern and microcysts containing basophilic fluid.

may be difficult and is sometimes impossible. However, the presence of follicles and a young age should favour the diagnosis of JGCT. Unlike JGCTs, the majority of Sertoli cell tumours NOS harbour *CTNNB1* mutations resulting in nuclear expression of β-catenin {5466,7830}.

### Cytology
Not relevant

### Diagnostic molecular pathology
*FOXL2* mutations, recently described in ovarian and some testicular adult granulosa cell tumours, have not yet been systematically investigated in JGCT. The only case investigated to date was *FOXL2*-wildtype {4123,6362}.

### Essential and desirable diagnostic criteria
*Essential:* a partially macrocystic or microcystic tumour of the testis composed of primitive granulosa cells with diffuse or lobular growth punctuated by variably sized and shaped follicles.
*Desirable:* manifestation in neonates and infants aged < 1 year; sex cord stromal tumour immunophenotype (SF1, calretinin, inhibin).

### Staging
Not relevant

### Prognosis and prediction
All of the reported cases showed a benign behaviour without evidence of metastatic potential {2565}.

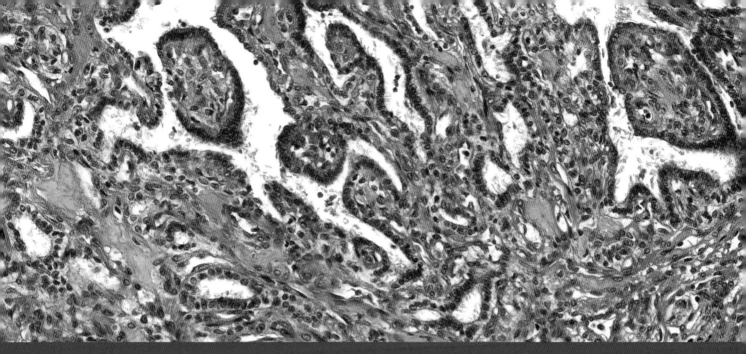

# 9

# Female genital tumours

Edited by: Cheung AN, Lax SF, Reyes-Múgica M

Ovarian tumours
   Sex cord stromal tumours
      Ovarian fibroma
      Sclerosing stromal tumour
      Juvenile granulosa cell tumour of the ovary
      Sex cord tumour with annular tubules
      Papillary cystadenoma
      Sertoli–Leydig cell tumour
      Gynandroblastoma
   Other ovarian tumours
      Small cell carcinoma of the ovary, hypercalcaemic type
Lower female genital tract tumours
   Epithelial tumours
      Mesonephric remnants and hyperplasia
      Müllerian papilloma
      Condyloma acuminatum
Peritoneal tumours
   Mesothelial tumours
      Peritoneal inclusion cysts

# Non–germ cell tumours of the female genital tract: Introduction

Reyes-Múgica M
Cheung AN
Lax SF

In childhood and adolescence, tumours of the female reproductive organs are generally rare, and only a subset of the tumours occurring in adults are observed. In particular, neither tumours of the uterine corpus nor epithelial ovarian tumours (which are both important in adults) play a role in the paediatric age group, so they have not been included here. Epithelial ovarian tumours are very unusual in the paediatric age group and are mostly benign cystadenomas. Borderline tumours (e.g. serous, mucinous) and carcinomas (e.g. mucinous) occur very rarely {4797,2532}. In the setting of Lynch syndrome, ovarian and endometrial carcinomas are also exceptional in patients aged < 18 years, although colorectal carcinoma may occur {3037}. Germline mutations of BRCA1 or BRCA2 are not associated with an increased risk for ovarian or tubal carcinoma in childhood; these entities are unusual in this age group {1916,891}. A variety of sex cord stromal tumours reported in the paediatric age group, some quite rare, are listed and discussed in this chapter.

Ovarian germ cell tumours, which are covered together with their male counterparts in Chapter 7: Germ cell tumours, affect adolescents and young adults more frequently than older age groups, with the exception of mature teratoma. Another rare but aggressive tumour almost exclusively occurring in adolescents and young adults is small cell carcinoma of the hypercalcaemic type, characterized by SMARCA4 and (rarely) SMARCB1 deficiency as distinctive molecular alterations. In childhood it is frequently associated with germline mutations.

Metastases to the ovaries are also very rare in children and adolescents, but they can be seen with neuroblastoma, rhabdomyosarcoma, and other childhood tumours {7766}. Only a few (mostly benign) tumours of the lower female genital tract affect paediatric patients. However, HPV infection – the most important tumorigenic factor for cervical, vaginal, and vulvar neoplasms – may affect adolescent girls and lead to mostly squamous or, less frequently, glandular precursor lesions requiring surveillance or treatment. Nevertheless, invasive carcinomas, particularly of the cervix, are unusual before the age of 18 years. HPV-associated tumours are broadly covered in the fifth-edition WHO classification of female genital tumours.

A typical tumour of childhood, embryonal rhabdomyosarcoma of the vagina is discussed in Chapter 6: Soft tissue and bone tumours, with other tumours of the rhabdomyosarcoma family. Finally, it needs to be mentioned that mesothelial tumours, particularly mesothelioma, are very rare in the paediatric age group. Mesothelioma seems to be distinct from its counterpart in adulthood, the paediatric form occurring more frequently in the peritoneum, being less frequently associated with asbestos exposure, and having a better prognosis {5209}.

# Ovarian fibroma

Irving JA
Dale AE

## Definition
Ovarian fibroma is a benign fibroblastic stromal tumour with a variably collagenous stroma.

## ICD-O coding
8810/0 Fibroma, NOS
8810/1 Cellular fibroma

## ICD-11 coding
2F32.1 Ovarian fibroma

## Related terminology
None

## Subtype(s)
Cellular fibroma

## Localization
Ovary

## Clinical features
Most cases are unilateral, but bilateral cases occur occasionally, especially in young patients with naevoid basal cell carcinoma syndrome (NBCCS, also known as Gorlin syndrome) {2503}. Symptoms referable to an ovarian mass are most common. Less frequently, hormonal manifestations or Meigs syndrome (ascites and pleural effusion) may occur.

## Epidemiology
Fibroma is the most common ovarian stromal tumour in adults and may occur in any decade of life, most often arising in patients aged > 30 years {5624}. It is rare in children, accounting for < 2% of paediatric ovarian tumours, and when encountered at a young age, should prompt consideration of NBCCS {2503,475}. However, even among patients with NBCCS, this tumour is usually discovered in adulthood. Ovarian fibromas may be more common among NBCCS patients with underlying *SUFU* mutations than in those with underlying *PTCH1* mutations, but they are common in both populations {2000,3595}. Mulibrey nanism, an autosomal recessive condition caused by *TRIM37* mutations, has a very high frequency of benign ovarian tumours including fibromas {3478,4877}. Ovarian fibromas have been reported rarely in other genetic syndromes but are not seen more frequently than expected by chance alone.

## Etiology
NBCCS (Gorlin syndrome, MIM number: 109400) is responsible for many cases of ovarian fibroma, but approximately 40% of cases occur as a de novo mutation.

## Pathogenesis
Cytogenetic studies often show trisomy and/or tetrasomy of chromosome 12 as well as imbalances (both gain and loss) of chromosomes 4 and 9 {6731}. The drivers of these cytogenetic alterations are not clear, although a loss of chromosome 9 may reflect a loss of one copy of *PTCH1*, the tumour suppressor gene underlying most cases of NBCCS. Loss of heterozygosity at the *PTCH1* locus and at the *STK11* (Peutz–Jeghers syndrome) locus are seen frequently in hereditary and sporadic cases. Mutations in these genes have rarely been demonstrated in sporadic tumours, and a loss of heterozygosity may reflect contributions from other drivers at these locations. Alternatively, the remaining allele may, in some cases, be silenced epigenetically {3478, 4877}. Point mutations have been reported in *IDH1* {3525}, and epigenetic silencing of *TRIM37* is frequent in sporadic tumours {3448}. Activation of oncogenes and mutations of DNA repair genes have not been demonstrated in ovarian fibromas, but the somatic mutation landscape of these tumours remains to be comprehensively evaluated.

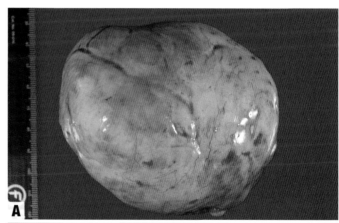
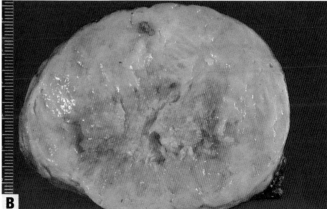

**Fig. 9.01** Ovarian fibroma in Gorlin syndrome. External appearance (**A**) and cut surface (**B**) of an ovarian fibroma from a 15-year-old girl.

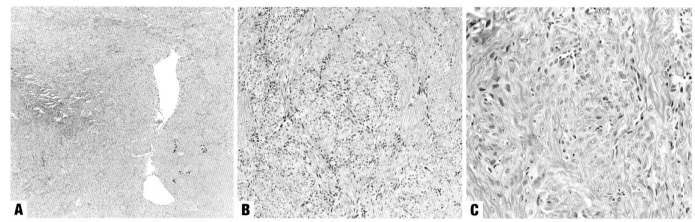

**Fig. 9.02** Ovarian fibroma in Gorlin syndrome. **A** Intersecting fascicles of spindle cells and focal calcifications. **B** This example (the same case as shown in Fig. 9.01) shows densely packed spindle cells without marked atypia or mitotic figures. **C** Spindle and ovoid cells are surrounded by collagen bundles.

## Macroscopic appearance

The ovarian capsule is usually smooth or nodular, with a hard, chalky, white-yellowish cut surface; calcifications are common in female patients with NBCCS. Cellular tumours may be soft and tan. Areas of cystic degeneration may be present, and occasional tumours may show haemorrhage or necrosis, especially with torsion.

## Histopathology

Fibromas are characterized by intersecting fascicles of spindle to ovoid cells with bland nuclei and scant cytoplasm, within a variably collagenous, hyalinized stroma; in most cases, mitoses are negligible {5624}. Calcifications may be present, and tumours may rarely contain eosinophilic hyaline globules {4644} or melanin pigment {6924}. Approximately 10% of fibromas are densely cellular (cellular fibroma) and may exhibit higher mitotic activity (mitotically active cellular fibroma) {3140}. Haemorrhage and infarct-type necrosis may occur and should not be misinterpreted as coagulative tumour cell necrosis. On rare occasions, luteinized cells or a minor component (< 10%) of sex cord elements can be seen. Fibromas typically exhibit immunoreactivity for WT1, FOXL2, CD56, SF1, and hormone receptors; inhibin and calretinin may show positive staining, but it is usually focal and/or weak {3716,1656}.

## Cytology

Not clinically relevant

## Diagnostic molecular pathology

Not clinically relevant

## Essential and desirable diagnostic criteria

*Essential:* fascicles of bland fibromatous spindle cells; minor sex cord elements are permissible but must constitute < 10% of the tumour.

## Staging

Not clinically relevant

## Prognosis and prediction

The vast majority of tumours are benign, but they may rarely recur in patients with NBCCS {5724}. A small proportion are associated with ovarian surface rupture and extraovarian adhesions, and such tumours are at risk of local recurrence, often after a long interval {5624,3140}.

# Sclerosing stromal tumour

Bennett JA
Gwin K
Weigelt B

## Definition

Sclerosing stromal tumour is a benign stromal neoplasm characterized by a pseudolobular architecture with a prominent vasculature and epithelioid and spindled cells, separated by oedematous or densely collagenous stroma.

## ICD-O coding

8602/0 Sclerosing stromal tumour

## ICD-11 coding

2F32.Y & XH6NZ8 Other specified benign neoplasm of ovary & Sclerosing stromal tumour

## Related terminology

None

## Subtype(s)

None

## Localization

Sclerosing stromal tumour occurs in the ovary; rarely, it is paraovarian {7720}.

## Clinical features

Patients present with menstrual abnormalities, abnormal uterine bleeding, or abdominal pain. Precocious puberty {4876,2799, 1194,6634}, virilization {5352,6634}, and an association with ascites (Meigs syndrome) {693,247} have occasionally been reported. Most tumours are unilateral, but bilateral cases have been described {1165,4904}.

## Epidemiology

Sclerosing stromal tumours account for 7–28% of all sex cord stromal tumours in childhood and adolescence {6256, 2724}. They typically occur in adolescents and young women (median age: 29 years) {2641,3589} but can also arise in premenarchal girls as well as in infants as young as 7 months {2669,1844,7718}.

## Etiology

Unknown

## Pathogenesis

*GLI2* rearrangements have been detected in > 80% of sclerosing stromal tumours, with the *FHL2::GLI2* fusion being present in > 60% of cases {3589}. No recurrent mutations have been identified.

## Macroscopic appearance

Tumours range in size from 15 to 190 mm (mean: 110 mm) {1128, 7818,2462,5344}. They are well circumscribed, often with a yellow to white cut surface that may show central oedema and cyst formation.

## Histopathology

Sclerosing stromal tumour has a pseudolobular appearance and a prominent vasculature, typically composed of thin-walled dilated vessels with a haemangiopericytoma-like appearance. Pseudolobules are separated by a hypocellular oedematous, collagenous, or (occasionally) myxoid stroma. Cellular nodules are composed of an admixture of bland epithelioid and spindled cells. The former have clear to eosinophilic vacuolated cytoplasm, sometimes resulting in a signet ring–like appearance {1128}, and may show prominent luteinization, especially during pregnancy {606}. Mitotic activity is often low, but large numbers of mitoses are seen in a small subset of cases {2462}. Tumours are usually positive for sex

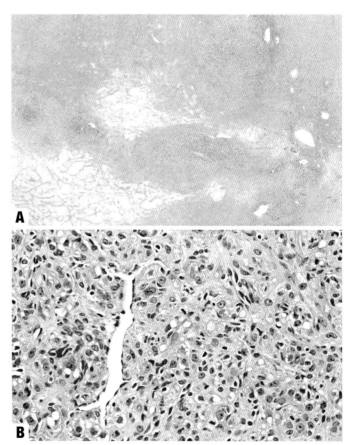

**Fig. 9.03** Sclerosing stromal tumour. **A** Cellular pseudolobules separated by densely collagenous to focally oedematous stroma. Note the conspicuous haemangiopericytoma-like vessels. **B** A nodule composed of an admixture of epithelioid and spindled cells.

cord markers, such as inhibin, calretinin, and FOXL2, but are negative for cytokeratins and EMA.

## Cytology
Not clinically relevant

## Diagnostic molecular pathology
Not clinically relevant

## Essential and desirable diagnostic criteria
*Essential:* pseudolobules composed of epithelioid and spindled cells separated by hypocellular stroma; thin-walled haemangiopericytoma-like vessels.

## Staging
Not clinically relevant

## Prognosis and prediction
One recurrence has been reported. The primary tumour had capsular disruption, necrosis, and marked mitotic activity {2462}.

# Juvenile granulosa cell tumour of the ovary

Stewart CJR
Galmiche L
Hicks MJ

## Definition
Juvenile granulosa cell tumour (JGCT) is a sex cord tumour composed of primitive-appearing granulosa cells arranged in intermixed solid and follicular patterns.

## ICD-O coding
8622/1 Juvenile granulosa cell tumour of the ovary

## ICD-11 coding
2F76 & XH2KH2 Neoplasms of uncertain behaviour of female genital organs & Granulosa cell tumour, juvenile

## Related terminology
None

## Subtype(s)
None

## Localization
Ovary

## Clinical features
Patients may show manifestations of a pelvic mass, as well as estrogenic effects in 80% of cases, including precocious pseudopuberty, menstrual disturbances, or virilization {7765}. JGCTs are predominantly unilateral (> 95% of cases) and rarely spread beyond the ovary. However, haemoperitoneum secondary to tumour rupture is an occasional presentation. Rare patients have *DICER1* syndrome, Maffucci syndrome, or Ollier disease {6283,6877,6856}.

## Epidemiology
JGCTs usually occur within the first three decades of life (mean age: 13 years), and 50% occur in prepubertal patients. They represent approximately 5% of all ovarian granulosa cell tumours {7765}.

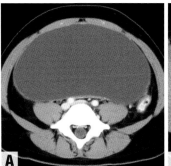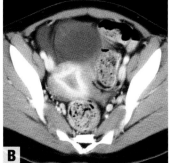

**Fig. 9.04** Juvenile granulosa cell tumour of the ovary. **A** Contrast axial CT showing a large, almost completely cystic mass arising from the pelvis of a prepubertal girl. **B** Contrast axial CT showing a poorly enhancing solid component at the uppermost aspect of the cystic mass. Note there is endometrial thickening within the uterus as a result of the estrogenic effect.

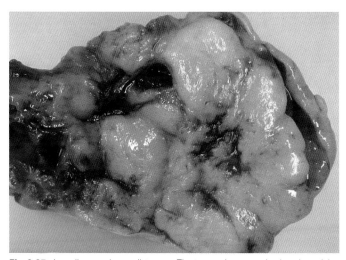

**Fig. 9.05** Juvenile granulosa cell tumour. The tumour has a predominantly nodular, solid, yellow cut surface with focal cystic and haemorrhagic areas.

## Etiology
Unknown

## Pathogenesis
Activating alterations in *AKT1* and *GNAS* have been detected in 60% and 30% of tumours, respectively {661,3375}. Somatic mosaic *IDH1* and *IDH2* mutations have been reported in tumours associated with Ollier disease or Maffucci syndrome {5580}. Rare reports describe an association with tuberous sclerosis and germline *TP53* and *PTEN* mutations {2603,5582}. Somatic *DICER1* mutations are rare {2849,2511,4118}. FISH analysis may identify monosomy 22 or trisomy 12 {4488A}.

## Macroscopic appearance
The mean tumour size is 120 mm (range: 30–320 mm). JGCTs are typically solid or solid and cystic, and rarely predominantly cystic, with a tan to yellow to grey cut surface, commonly with areas of necrosis and haemorrhage (especially if ruptured) {7765}.

## Histopathology
Tumours show a nodular or diffuse architecture and scattered interspersed follicles of varying size with irregular contours, frequently containing basophilic secretions lined by cell layers of variable thickness. The stroma is typically inconspicuous but sometimes prominently sclerotic or myxoid. Tumour cells have round, vesicular, non-grooved nuclei, and (usually) abundant pale or eosinophilic cytoplasm. There is minimal to marked nuclear atypia with variable mitotic activity {7765}. Variably luteinized and sometimes spindled theca cells may be seen. Occasional pseudopapillae may develop due to cystic degeneration {3141}. Tumours usually express SF1, inhibin, calretinin, WT1, CD99, and CD56; some express EMA and FOXL2 (without associated mutation).

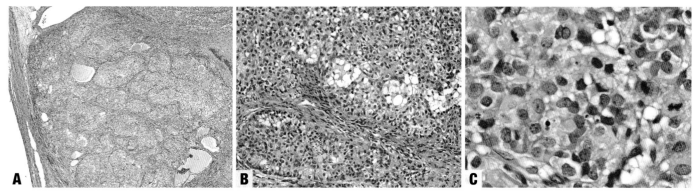

**Fig. 9.06** Juvenile granulosa cell tumour. **A** Low-magnification view showing nodular tumour architecture with variably sized follicle-like spaces. **B** Predominantly solid growth pattern with small follicle-like spaces (upper part of image). The cells have eosinophilic or focally vacuolated cytoplasm. **C** High-magnification view showing mitotic activity and apoptosis.

## Cytology

See *Prognosis and prediction*, below.

## Diagnostic molecular pathology

Not relevant

## Essential and desirable diagnostic criteria

*Essential:* primitive granulosa cells with diffuse or nodular growth punctuated by irregularly shaped follicles.
*Desirable:* positive staining for sex cord markers.

## Staging

Not relevant

## Prognosis and prediction

Patients with tumours confined to the ovary have an excellent prognosis with simple oophorectomy. Rupture, positive cytology, and extraovarian spread increase the risk of recurrence (most often within the first 3 years) {7765}.

# Sex cord tumour with annular tubules

Stewart CJR
Chen L
Nucci MR

## Definition
Sex cord tumour with annular tubules (SCTAT) is a sex cord tumour with sharply circumscribed nests composed of ring-like tubules that encircle basement membrane–like material.

## ICD-O coding
8623/1 Sex cord tumour with annular tubules

## ICD-11 coding
2F76 & XH5BV8 Neoplasms of uncertain behaviour of female genital organs & Sex cord tumour with annular tubules

## Related terminology
None

## Subtype(s)
None

## Localization
Ovary

## Clinical features
SCTAT can be seen at any age and may represent an incidental finding in Peutz–Jeghers syndrome (PJS). Non-syndromic cases may be associated with nonspecific symptoms, but estrogenic effects, seen in approximately 50% of patients, may cause isosexual pseudoprecocity or menstrual disturbance. Less commonly, there may be signs related to progesterone production {6312,6311,7772,5680}.

## Epidemiology
SCTAT is rare overall, accounting for 1–2% of all sex cord tumours {7772,5680}. In one large series, 36% of patients with sex cord tumours had PJS {7772}.

## Etiology
Approximately one third of SCTATs occur in patients with PJS, and about 75% of these patients have a germline mutation in *STK11*. The mechanism by which patients with PJS develop SCTAT is unclear {4611}.

## Pathogenesis
Syndromic cases have germline *STK11* mutations on chromosome 19p13.3 {6863}. SCTAT is not associated with *DICER1* mutations {5185}.

## Macroscopic appearance
Lesions in PJS are often small (microscopic to 30 mm), bilateral, and multifocal. Non-syndromic tumours are typically unilateral tan to yellow masses as large as 200 mm; they are usually solid, but cysts may be seen and occasionally predominate {6311, 7772}.

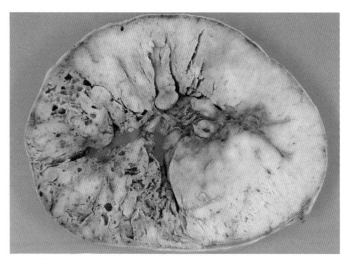

**Fig. 9.07** Sex cord tumour with annular tubules. Non-syndromic tumour with a predominantly solid, yellow, and focally nodular cut surface.

## Histopathology
Syndromic and non-syndromic tumours are both characterized by variably sized, usually rounded nests composed of simple or complex tubules that encircle hyaline basement membrane–like material, which may also be present around the tubules. Cells are tall, with pale cytoplasm and basally located round nuclei that often display an antipodal distribution within the tubules. In PJS lesions, calcification within the tubules may be present and there may be a solid proliferation of indifferent sex cord cells, whereas in non-syndromic cases classic morphology may focally transition to granulosa or Sertoli cell morphology. Cytological atypia and mitotic activity may be seen, rarely, in the non-syndromic setting {6311,7772}. The tumour cells are typically positive for calretinin, WT1, inhibin, SF1, FOXL2, and CD56 {7705,4505,136,1656}. They are typically negative for EMA and CD10 {5160}.

## Cytology
Not clinically relevant

## Diagnostic molecular pathology
Not clinically relevant

## Essential and desirable diagnostic criteria
*Essential:* simple or complex tubules that encircle basement membrane–like material; tall cells with pale cytoplasm and round nuclei with an antipodal distribution.
*Desirable:* sex cord marker positivity.

## Staging
Not relevant

Chapter 9

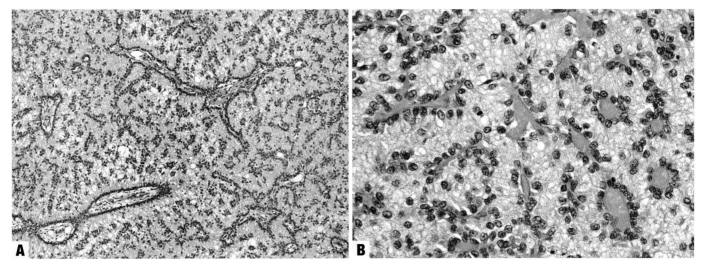

**Fig. 9.08** Sex cord tumour with annular tubules. **A** Complex interconnecting tubules are separated by relatively scant fibrovascular stroma. **B** The tubules are lined by cells with uniform, radially arranged nuclei and abundant pale cytoplasm encircling basement membrane–like material.

### Prognosis and prediction

Syndrome-associated tumours are typically benign, whereas as many as 20% of non-syndromic cases exhibit extraovarian spread {6311,7772}.

# Papillary cystadenoma

Usubutun A
Lax SF

## Definition
Papillary cystadenoma is a benign papillary-cystic tumour of probable mesonephric origin, usually seen in patients with von Hippel–Lindau syndrome.

## ICD-O coding
8450/0 Papillary cystadenoma

## ICD-11 coding
2F33.Y & XH0FM6 Benign neoplasm of other specified female genital organs & Papillary cystadenoma, NOS

## Related terminology
None

## Subtype(s)
None

## Localization
Uterine ligaments

## Clinical features
Patients may present with abdominal pain, although in children papillary cystadenoma is likely to be an incidental finding {5067, 2283}.

## Epidemiology
Most patients have von Hippel–Lindau syndrome {5067,836, 2369,3741}. As yet this tumour has only been described in adults aged > 20 years.

## Etiology
The anatomical location and immunophenotype suggest a mesonephric origin {5067}. Allelic loss of VHL has been reported {6401}.

## Pathogenesis
Unknown

## Macroscopic appearance
The tumours are about 50 mm (reported sizes range from < 10 to 80 mm), have a thick fibrotic capsule, and are traversed by fibrous bands creating a solid-cystic lobulated appearance {5067,7504}.

## Histopathology
There is complex tubulopapillary growth with varying broad-based and delicate branching and stromal hyalinization. Focal tubular or solid growth may be present. The cells are non-ciliated and cuboidal, with minimal clear to eosinophilic cytoplasm. Prominent subepithelial blood vessels are common. The cells are positive for CK7, PAX8, PAX2, and CD10. WT1 and calretinin are variably positive; ER and PR are negative {5067,836,1462,425}.

## Cytology
Not clinically relevant

## Diagnostic molecular pathology
Demonstration of germline VHL mutation may be helpful.

## Essential and desirable diagnostic criteria
Essential: a cystic/lobulated mass; complex tubulopapillary growth of non-ciliated and cuboidal cells.
Desirable: VHL mutation.

## Staging
Not clinically relevant

## Prognosis and prediction
These are benign, except for a single report of peritoneal metastases in a patient without von Hippel–Lindau syndrome {5067}.

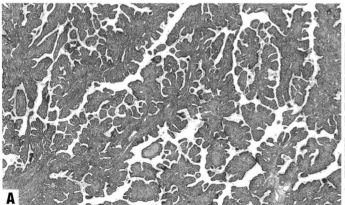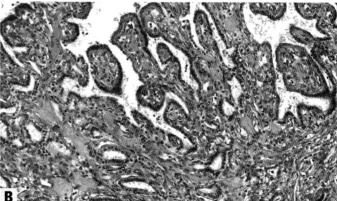

**Fig. 9.09** Papillary cystadenoma. **A** Complex papillary structures with hyalinized stromal cores. **B** Tubulopapillary architecture with cuboidal cells that have clear to eosinophilic cytoplasm and stromal hyalinization.

# Sertoli–Leydig cell tumour

Buza N
Hill DA

## Definition

Sertoli–Leydig cell tumours (SLCTs) are composed of varying proportions of Sertoli and Leydig cells. Most paediatric cases occur in the context of *DICER1* syndrome.

## ICD-O coding

8631/1 Sertoli–Leydig cell tumour
8631/0 Sertoli–Leydig cell tumour, well differentiated
8631/1 Sertoli–Leydig cell tumour, moderately differentiated
8631/3 Sertoli–Leydig cell tumour, poorly differentiated
8633/1 Sertoli–Leydig cell tumour, retiform

## ICD-11 coding

2F32.Y Other specified benign neoplasm of ovary &
XH6FQ9 Sertoli–Leydig cell tumour, NOS
XH0UP7 Sertoli–Leydig cell tumour, intermediate differentiation
XH8U56 Sertoli–Leydig cell tumour, intermediate differentiation, with heterologous elements
XH6XB6 Sertoli–Leydig cell tumour, retiform
XH7E53 Sertoli–Leydig cell tumour, well differentiated
XH29E0 Sertoli–Leydig cell tumour, poorly differentiated
XH3PN1 Sertoli–Leydig cell tumour, retiform, with heterologous elements
XH3BT2 Sertoli–Leydig cell tumour, poorly differentiated, with heterologous elements

## Related terminology

None

## Subtype(s)

Sertoli–Leydig cell tumour, well differentiated; Sertoli–Leydig cell tumour, moderately differentiated; Sertoli–Leydig cell tumour, poorly differentiated; Sertoli–Leydig cell tumour, retiform

## Localization

Ovary

## Clinical features

Patients may present with pelvic pain or a pelvic mass, or rarely with ascites and tumour rupture. Androgenic manifestations including hirsutism, clitoromegaly, breast atrophy, menstrual irregularity, or secondary amenorrhoea are common (seen in approximately 50% of patients) {2583,7798}. Estrogenic effects are rare and include isosexual pseudoprecocity and menometrorrhagia.

## Epidemiology

SLCTs account for < 0.5% of ovarian neoplasms and 1–2% of paediatric ovarian tumours {5595}. The patient age range is 1–84 years (mean: 25 years) {7771,2583,7798,2549}; the median age of paediatric patients is 14 years {6257}. Tumours with a retiform pattern or germline *DICER1* mutation occur at a

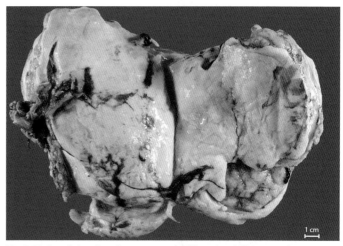

**Fig. 9.10** Sertoli–Leydig cell tumour, poorly differentiated. The cut surface shows a predominantly solid, fleshy, tan-yellow cut surface with focal haemorrhage.

younger age {6285}. Nearly all paediatric SLCTs are moderately or poorly differentiated, and they often show a retiform pattern or heterologous elements.

## Etiology

In the paediatric age group, most SLCTs occur in patients with *DICER1* syndrome {2892,5898,6283,6524,2199}, but paediatric SLCTs may also be sporadic, without detectable germline *DICER1* mutation {6285,1630}.

## Pathogenesis

SLCT has three molecular subtypes: *DICER1*-mutant (younger age, moderately/poorly differentiated, retiform or heterologous elements), *FOXL2* c.402C>G (p.C134W)–mutant (postmenopausal patients, moderately/poorly differentiated, no retiform or heterologous elements), and *DICER1/FOXL2*-wildtype (intermediate age, no retiform or heterologous elements, including all well-differentiated tumours) {3451}.

Patients with *DICER1* syndrome harbour a germline mutation in *DICER1*, encoding RNase IIIb in the microRNA maturation pathway {2849,7577}. The second-hit somatic mutation is a hotspot missense mutation affecting the RNase IIIb domain of *DICER1* {7578}. *DICER1* mutations may alter global gene expression, differentiate an ovarian cell into a sertoliform phenotype, and induce androgenic symptoms {7428,272}.

Sporadic tumours may have two somatic hotspot *DICER1* mutations without a germline mutation. Somatic hotspot *DICER1* mutations are present in approximately half (range: 15–97%) of all cases and in nearly all paediatric SLCTs {1630,2849,1415, 2511,3588,6285,7883,7577}. Most paediatric patients with SLCT also harbour germline *DICER1* mutations {2892,5898, 6283,6524,2199}.

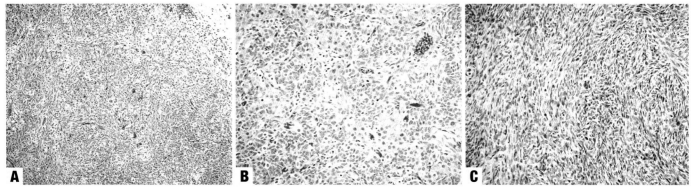

**Fig. 9.11** Sertoli–Leydig cell tumour. **A** A moderately differentiated tumour in a young patient with *DICER1* syndrome. The tumour is composed of compressed basophilic Sertoli cell tubules and scattered small clusters of eosinophilic Leydig cells. **B** A moderately differentiated tumour in a young patient with *DICER1* syndrome. **C** A poorly differentiated example, composed of diffuse sheets of immature, sarcomatoid Sertoli cells resembling primitive gonadal stroma.

## Macroscopic appearance

Almost all SLCTs (97%) are unilateral. Bilaterality may be associated with *DICER1* syndrome {4503}. Tumour size ranges from 10 to 350 mm (mean: ~130 mm). The cut surface is solid, cystic, or solid and cystic; fleshy; tan-yellow; and occasionally has focal haemorrhage and necrosis.

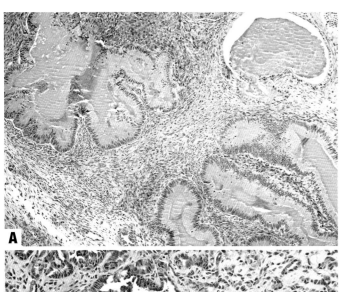

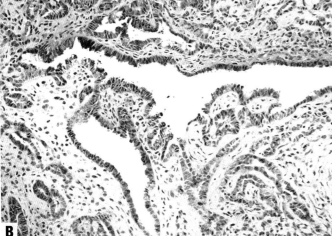

**Fig. 9.12** Sertoli–Leydig cell tumour. **A** The tumour contains heterologous mucinous epithelium surrounded by immature Sertoli cells and rare Leydig cell clusters. **B** Retiform subtype, in which the tumour cells form anastomosing, slit-like, irregular spaces resembling the rete testis.

## Histopathology

SLCTs are subdivided into three forms – well-differentiated, moderately differentiated, and poorly differentiated – based on the degree of tubular differentiation of the Sertoli cell component.

Well-differentiated SLCTs are composed of open or compressed Sertoli cell tubules without marked nuclear atypia or mitotic activity. Leydig cells are present in clusters, cords, and singly, and they contain cytoplasmic lipofuscin and Reinke crystals.

Moderately differentiated SLCTs have a diffuse or lobulated pattern, with Sertoli cells arranged in compressed tubules, cords, or diffuse sheets, and they have hyperchromatic oval or spindled nuclei with mild to moderate atypia and occasional mitotic figures. Rare small clusters of Leydig cells are admixed with the Sertoli cells.

Poorly differentiated SLCTs consist of diffuse sheets of immature, sarcomatoid Sertoli cells resembling primitive gonadal stroma. The nuclear atypia is moderate to marked, and mitotic figures are conspicuous. Leydig cells are sparse and are typically located at the periphery of tumour.

Approximately 15% of SLCTs demonstrate a focal or diffuse retiform pattern, forming either anastomosing, slit-like, irregular spaces or a multicystic, sieve-like, or papillary architecture {7771,2583,7798,5626,7769,7770}.

Heterologous elements may be seen in approximately 20% of moderately or poorly differentiated SLCTs and in retiform SLCT {7771,2583,7798,5626,7769,7770}. The most common form is mucinous (intestinal or gastric type) epithelium, which may be benign, borderline, or malignant {7769}. Neuroendocrine tumour and focal hepatocyte differentiation have also been described {7769,4775}. Heterologous mesenchymal (cartilage or skeletal muscle) elements are less common {7769}.

### *Immunohistochemistry*

Sertoli cells are typically positive for vimentin and pancytokeratin, as well as for sex cord markers (α-inhibin, calretinin, SF1, WT1, and FOXL2) {136,1100,1656,2890,3716,4825,7846}. Retiform and poorly differentiated tumours are more likely to be negative. CK7 and EMA immunostains are negative and are helpful in distinguishing SLCTs from epithelial ovarian tumours. Leydig cells typically show no or only minimal staining for FOXL2 and WT1, but they usually express α-inhibin and melan-A. Heterologous elements exhibit the immunoprofile of their constituent tissues.

## Cytology

Not clinically relevant

## Diagnostic molecular pathology

*DICER1* mutation analysis of tumour tissue shows pathogenic RNase IIIb missense mutations in moderately and poorly differentiated SLCT {6285,1630}.

## Essential and desirable diagnostic criteria

*Essential:* a sex cord stromal tumour consisting of an admixture of Sertoli cell and Leydig cell components.
*Desirable:* positive immunohistochemical staining for sex cord markers; *DICER1* RNase IIIb missense (hotspot) mutation.

## Staging

Malignant tumours are staged according to the Union for International Cancer Control (UICC) TNM classification and the FIGO staging system.

## Prognosis and prediction

Behaviour correlates with tumour grade and histological subtype: well-differentiated tumours are essentially benign; approximately 10% of moderately differentiated tumours and 13–59% of poorly differentiated tumours have malignant behaviour {7771,6482,2583,671}. Heterologous mesenchymal elements, a retiform pattern, tumour rupture, and spread outside the ovary (stage II or higher) are adverse prognostic factors {6482,671, 7771,7770}. Germline *DICER1* mutations have been shown to confer a favourable prognosis compared with somatic *DICER1* mutations alone {6285}. Genetic counselling and testing for *DICER1* syndrome is recommended for paediatric patients with SLCT {6286}.

# Gynandroblastoma

Hill DA

## Definition
Gynandroblastoma is a composite sex cord stromal tumour with elements of Sertoli–Leydig cell tumour and juvenile granulosa cell tumour.

## ICD-O coding
8632/1 Gynandroblastoma

## ICD-11 coding
2F76 & XH0Q64 Neoplasms of uncertain behaviour of female genital organs & Gynandroblastoma

2C73.Y & XH0Q64 Other specified malignant neoplasms of the ovary & Gynandroblastoma

## Related terminology
*Acceptable:* mixed sex cord stromal tumour.

## Subtype(s)
None

## Localization
Ovary

## Clinical features
Patients can present with abdominal pain or distension and androgenic symptoms {7430,6844,7675,5217}.

## Epidemiology
The reported patients with gynandroblastoma have ranged in age from 13 to 80 years (median: 24.5–28 years) {7430,5217}.

## Etiology
Unknown

## Pathogenesis
In the largest study to date, heterozygous hotspot mutations in the RNase IIIb domain of *DICER1* were discovered in both tumour components in 3 of 16 cases, all of which showed an admixture of juvenile granulosa cell tumour (JGCT) and Sertoli–Leydig cell tumour (SLCT). All tumours were *FOXL2*-wildtype, including 7 cases with an adult granulosa cell tumour component, and none showed a mutation within the pleckstrin homology domain of *AKT1* {7430}. Several additional *DICER1*-mutant (but only very few *FOXL2*-mutant) gynandroblastomas have been reported {1415,5203,6285}. Because SLCT is also strongly associated with mutations in *DICER1* {2849,6285}, and because SLCT has a wide range of heterologous differentiation, there is consideration that gynandroblastoma may represent an alternative morphology of SLCT {5217}. Gynandroblastoma containing a component of adult granulosa cell tumour seems

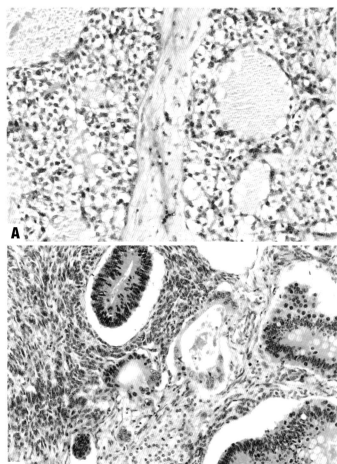

**Fig. 9.14** Gynandroblastoma. Gynandroblastoma composed of juvenile granulosa cell tumour (**A**) and moderately differentiated Sertoli–Leydig cell tumour with heterologous intestinal mucinous differentiation (**B**).

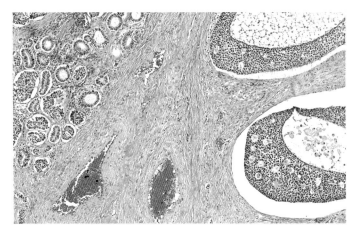

**Fig. 9.13** Gynandroblastoma. Gynandroblastoma composed of Sertoli–Leydig cell tumour (left) and adult granulosa cell tumour (right).

Chapter 9

to be different from pure adult granulosa cell tumour, almost all cases of which harbour a hotspot mutation in *FOXL2* (c.402C>G p.C134W) {6362,4510}.

## Macroscopic appearance
Tumours are usually unilateral and large. The average tumour size is 110 mm (range: 55–200 mm). The cut surface is solid or cystic and pale-yellow or white {4972}.

## Histopathology
Typical tumours are composed of (1) deep purple solid lobules of Sertoli cells, or Sertoli cells growing in nests and cords; (2) small clusters of Leydig cells with abundant pink cytoplasm; and (3) pale nodules containing small clusters of cells and variably sized follicles containing pink flocculent material similar to that seen in JGCT {7430,5217}.

## Cytology
Not clinically relevant

## Diagnostic molecular pathology
Gynandroblastomas composed of SLCT and JGCT elements show biallelic *DICER1* loss-of-function and missense RNase IIIb mutations.

## Essential and desirable diagnostic criteria
*Essential:* a sex cord stromal tumour showing an admixture of Sertoli–Leydig cell tumour and JGCT elements.
*Desirable: DICER1* missense RNase IIIb mutation may be present in tumour tissue.

## Staging
Tumours are staged according to the Union for International Cancer Control (UICC) TNM classification {870} and the FIGO staging system.

## Prognosis and prediction
Most tumours are low-stage at diagnosis. Only rare recurrences have been reported {1285}.

# Small cell carcinoma of the ovary, hypercalcaemic type

Karnezis AN
Bush JW
Huntsman DG

## Definition
Hypercalcaemic-type small cell carcinoma of the ovary is an aggressive undifferentiated tumour composed of small cells, with or without a large-cell component, usually with hypercalcaemia.

## ICD-O coding
8044/3 Small cell carcinoma of the ovary, hypercalcaemic type
8044/3 Small cell carcinoma of the ovary, hypercalcaemic type, large cell subtype

## ICD-11 coding
2C73.0Y & XH8ZR8 Other specified carcinomas of ovary & Small cell carcinoma, hypercalcaemic type

## Related terminology
*Acceptable:* SMARCA4-deficient carcinoma of ovary.

## Subtype(s)
Small cell carcinoma of the ovary, hypercalcaemic type, large cell subtype

## Localization
Ovary

## Clinical features
Symptoms are usually related to pelvic/abdominal disease. Two thirds of patients have paraneoplastic hypercalcaemia. Familial cases due to germline mutation in *SMARCA4* (rhabdoid tumour predisposition syndrome type 2) are usually bilateral {7767,7575}.

## Epidemiology
This rare tumour accounts for < 1% of ovarian carcinomas. It occurs almost exclusively in young women and children

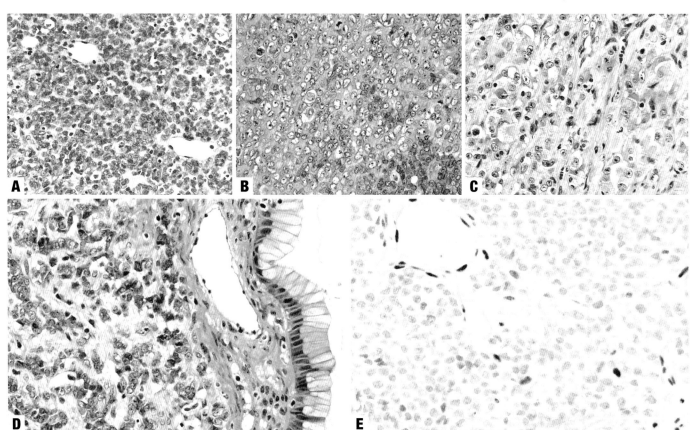

**Fig. 9.15** Small cell carcinoma of the ovary, hypercalcaemic type. **A** Small nests of tumour cells separated by minimal fibrous stroma. The tumour cells are round to oval, with occasional prominent nucleoli and chromocentres and with scant cytoplasm. **B** Comparison between the small cell (lower right) and large cell (remaining area) morphology. The large cells often show larger, open nuclei with vesicular chromatin and prominent nucleoli. Abundant eosinophilic cytoplasm is present, and cellular borders can occasionally be delineated. **C** The large-cell regions occasionally contain rhabdoid cells with eccentric nuclei, prominent nucleoli, and dense to glassy eosinophilic cytoplasmic inclusions that displace the nucleus. **D** A focus of benign mucinous epithelium (right) within the small-cell component. **E** SMARCA4 (BRG1) immunohistochemistry showing a loss of expression in the tumour cells and retained expression in endothelial and stromal cells. Dual loss of SMARCA4 and SMARCA2 (BRM) is highly sensitive and specific for this tumour.

(median age: 25 years) {1740,7767,7575}. Familial cases occur at a younger age; germline mutations have been identified in all cases diagnosed in patients aged < 15 years {7575}.

## Etiology

Almost all tumours harbour somatic or germline inactivating mutations in *SMARCA4*, encoding SMARCA4 (BRG1), an ATPase in the SWI/SNF chromatin-remodelling complex. Rare *SMARCA4*-wildtype tumours have mutations in *SMARCB1* (*INI1*, *BAF47*) {4508,3245,5763,5764,7574,65,4739}. A germ cell tumour relationship is suggested by foci of mature/immature teratoma or yolk sac tumour, or by the expression of SALL4 in some tumours {3826,4508}. A possible origin from a neuronal lineage is suggested by the upregulation of neural markers upon the reintroduction of SMARCA4 into tumour cells, and by morphological and genetic similarities with malignant rhabdoid tumour {7429}.

## Pathogenesis

SWI/SNF complex mutations and a diploid karyotype indicate the importance of epigenetic perturbations impacting the expression of genes involved in differentiation and growth arrest {2830}. Genetic similarities with malignant rhabdoid tumours and dedifferentiated carcinomas in multiple organs indicate that SWI/SNF defects induce a common aggressive, undifferentiated clinicopathological phenotype.

## Macroscopic appearance

Tumours are usually large (mean size: 150 mm, range: 60–260 mm), solid, fleshy, and tan to white to grey, with haemorrhage, necrosis, and cystic degeneration.

## Histopathology

Tumour cells are loosely cohesive and grow in sheets, nests, cords, and trabeculae with minimal intervening stroma. Follicle-like spaces with eosinophilic or basophilic secretions are often present. The small-cell component has monomorphic round, ovoid, or occasionally spindled nuclei with vesicular chromatin, small nucleoli, scant cytoplasm, and brisk mitotic activity. The large-cell component, which is present in half of the tumours,

has eccentric nuclei, prominent nucleoli, and abundant eosinophilic cytoplasm, sometimes imparting a rhabdoid appearance. When large cells predominate, this is designated as the large cell subtype (rare). Approximately 15% of tumours have a focal mucinous component. Rare tumours have foci of mature/immature teratoma or yolk sac tumour {7767,3826,4508}.

Immunohistochemistry reveals loss of SMARCA4 (by mutation) and SMARCA2 (by silencing) in almost all tumours; diffuse WT1 expression; and variable expression of epithelial markers (especially in the large-cell component), CD10, and calretinin. SALL4 can be positive, but OCT3/4, inhibin, and thyroid transcription factor 1 (TTF1) are negative {3826,4508,3245,5763, 7574,65,1347,1416,3246,3444,3452,4507}.

## Cytology

Not relevant

## Diagnostic molecular pathology

Inactivating mutations in *SMARCA4* are present in almost all tumours.

## Essential and desirable diagnostic criteria

*Essential:* an undifferentiated tumour composed mostly of monomorphic small cells with follicle-like spaces, sometimes with a large-cell component.
*Desirable:* SMARCA4 or SMARCA2 deficiency.

## Staging

This entity is staged according to the Union for International Cancer Control (UICC) TNM classification and the FIGO staging system.

## Prognosis and prediction

The prognosis is poor, even with combined surgery and aggressive chemoradiation. Stage is the most important prognostic factor; only one third of patients with stage IA tumours are alive without disease after surgery. Favourable prognostic factors include age > 30 years, normal calcium levels, tumour size < 100 mm, and an absence of large cells {7767,7575}.

# Mesonephric remnants and hyperplasia

Howitt BE
Ganesan R
Kong CS
Mirkovic J
Moritani S

## Definition
Mesonephric remnants are embryonic remnants of mesonephric duct, and mesonephric hyperplasia is their benign proliferation.

## ICD-O coding
None

## ICD-11 coding
GA15.Y Other specified acquired abnormalities of cervix uteri

## Related terminology
None

## Subtype(s)
None

## Localization
Mesonephric remnants and hyperplasia are typically localized in the lateral uterine cervical wall, but they may be found anywhere along the lateral aspects of the urogenital tract.

## Clinical features
Mesonephric remnants and hyperplasia are usually an incidental finding. Hyperplasia may rarely manifest with abnormal cervical cytology or as a mass or expansion of the cervical wall.

## Epidemiology
Mesonephric remnants and hyperplasia are detected in as many as 20% of cervixes.

## Etiology
Unknown

## Pathogenesis
Mesonephric remnants and hyperplasia are thought to arise from residual (non-regressed) cells of the mesonephric (Wolffian) duct.

## Macroscopic appearance
Mesonephric remnants are generally an incidental microscopic finding. Rarely, mesonephric hyperplasia may form a mass.

## Histopathology
Remnants are composed of clusters or linear arrays of small to medium-sized tubules lined by cuboidal cells with scant eosinophilic cytoplasm and round to ovoid nuclei with fine chromatin. Dense eosinophilic PAS-positive intraluminal secretions are usually present. Mitoses are inconspicuous. Hyperplasia is a more robust proliferation of mesonephric tubules with histological features similar to those of remnants. It may be of lobular (most common), diffuse, ductal, or mixed type {2110,3008}. Diffuse hyperplasia lacks lobular growth and has tubules that are architecturally simple and separated by stroma. Ductal hyperplasia shows proliferation of ductal structures, which often have clefts; it may be associated with peripheral tubules. Although not necessary for diagnosis, CD10 (luminal/apical), calretinin, GATA3, thyroid transcription factor 1 (TTF1), and PAX8 are frequently positive {3006,5959,3524}, and ER, PR, and p16 are negative {2513}.

## Cytology
Mesonephric remnants rarely extend to the cervical canal, showing cuboidal, hyperchromatic cells without pseudostratification or mitoses in cervical cytology sampling {2827}.

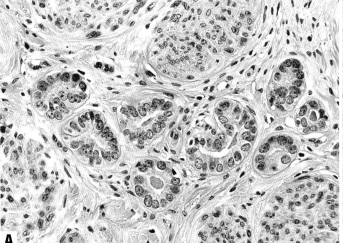 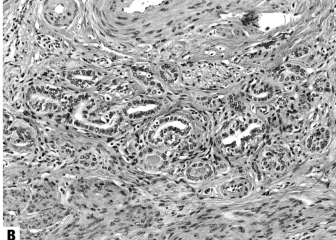

**Fig. 9.16** Mesonephric remnants. **A** Mesonephric remnants are composed of bland cuboidal cells with pale eosinophilic cytoplasm and nuclei with fine chromatin. **B** Mesonephric remnants in the lateral cervical wall are composed of simple tubules lined by bland cuboidal epithelium with characteristic eosinophilic luminal secretions.

## Diagnostic molecular pathology
Not clinically relevant

## Essential and desirable diagnostic criteria
*Essential:* small to medium-sized tubules lined by cuboidal cells with scant eosinophilic cytoplasm and round to ovoid bland nuclei; location in the lateral walls of the cervix, vagina, or uterus.

## Staging
Not applicable

## Prognosis and prediction
Mesonephric remnants and hyperplasia are benign. Occasionally, renal abnormalities, including ipsilateral renal dysgenesis or ureterocoele, occur in association with mesonephric remnants or tubulocystic anomalies of the mesonephric duct {1396}.

# Müllerian papilloma

Pantanowitz L
Gang DL
Wong RW

## Definition
Müllerian papilloma is a benign papillary tumour composed of Müllerian-type epithelium.

## ICD-O coding
None

## ICD-11 coding
GA15.0 Polyp of cervix uteri
GA14.0 Polyp of vagina

## Related terminology
*Acceptable:* Müllerian papilloma of infancy.
*Not recommended:* mesonephric papilloma.

## Subtype(s)
None

## Localization
Müllerian papillomas may arise in the cervix or vagina, and in some cases both sites may be involved {4540}. The tumours are usually mucosal, but some vaginal examples are intramural. Their anatomical location in the cervix/vagina is variable {4540}.

## Clinical features
Most patients present with vaginal bleeding {4540}.

## Epidemiology
These are rare cervical/vaginal neoplasms that mostly occur in prepubertal girls, typically aged 2–5 years, with a few cases reported in adolescents or young adults (age range: 15 months to 24 years) {4540,2953,7669,7105,1386,4506}.

## Etiology
The etiology is unknown, but it is likely to be developmental.

## Pathogenesis
The pathogenesis of Müllerian papillomas is uncertain, but they are believed to arise from Müllerian epithelium {4506, 7136}. There have been reports of isolated cases with a history of another tumour/disorder, including renal cysts and Wilms tumour {3919}, osteosarcoma {4540}, and Proteus syndrome {6556}, but there is insufficient evidence for a specific association. They are unrelated to either acquired or maternal HPV infection.

## Macroscopic appearance
Mucosal-based papillomas manifest as a friable polypoid lesion in the cervix and/or vagina {4540,2953,7669}, whereas intramural tumours manifest as a solid-cystic mass in the vaginal wall {4506,7136}.

## Histopathology
Müllerian papillomas have a papillary architecture with branching fibrovascular stromal cores lined by cuboidal or columnar epithelium with no hobnail appearance or cytological atypia {2953,1386,4506,5800}. Nuclei are bland with fine chromatin. Mitoses are normally absent. Squamous metaplasia may be seen. A rare case associated with melanin pigmentation has been reported {1386}. There should be no stromal cell atypia or cambium layer; if present, these should raise the suspicion of rhabdomyosarcoma.

## Cytology
There is little published information. The presence of glandular and papillary fragments with epithelial cells with hyperchromatic

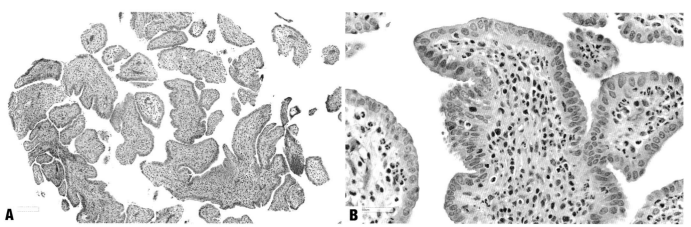

**Fig. 9.17** Müllerian papilloma. **A** Papillary structures with branching fibrovascular cores are covered by cuboidal to columnar epithelium. **B** The columnar epithelial lining over the papillae displays bland nuclear features.

nuclei and a high N:C ratio was reported in 1 case of cervical Müllerian papilloma {2953}.

## Diagnostic molecular pathology
Not clinically relevant

## Essential and desirable diagnostic criteria
*Essential:* papillary architecture; cuboidal or columnar epithelium without cytological atypia.

## Staging
Not clinically relevant

## Prognosis and prediction
The clinical outcome is favourable {4540,5800}, although recurrence has been noted in a few cases {6553,1837,4267,1769}. Malignant transformation to clear cell carcinoma was reported in 1 case with multiple recurrences {37}.

# Condyloma acuminatum

Oligny LL
Lieberman RW

## Definition

Condyloma acuminatum is a benign verrucous papillary lesion caused by HPV.

## ICD-O coding

None

## ICD-11 coding

1A95.1 & XA2GU7 Genital warts & Female genital organs

## Related terminology

*Acceptable:* anogenital wart; low-grade squamous intraepithelial lesion, condylomatous type; CIN 1, condylomatous type; Buschke–Löwenstein tumour; genital seborrhoeic keratosis.

## Subtype(s)

None

## Localization

Anogenital skin and mucosa; lower female genital tract (including the cervix)

## Clinical features

Condylomas are asymptomatic lesions identified in anogenital skin and mucosa, including the cervix. They are macroscopically indistinguishable from warts in the paediatric population {4396,177}. The majority (75%) of anogenital warts are acquired through a non-sexual route, for example by vertical transmission from the mother, inoculation by a carer, autoinoculation from warts in other sites, or infection from shared personal items. In a small percentage of cases, sexual abuse is confirmed; this percentage increases with age {4396}.

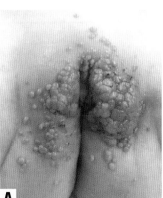
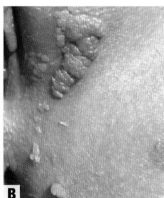

**Fig. 9.18** Paediatric genital condyloma. **A** Preoperative photograph of a 2-year-old girl with congenitally acquired condyloma of the vulva, grossly and microscopically a genital seborrhoeic keratosis subtype. PCR was positive for HPV6. **B** This 5-year-old girl was subjected to repeated sexual assault by her mother's boyfriend and presented with persistent "scratching of her private parts". The clinical photo shows multiple exophytic papillomatous lesions of the labia majora.

## Epidemiology

HPV infections affect as many as 80% of women in their early twenties {177}; 70% of young women infected with any HPV type and 90% of those infected with low-risk types will spontaneously revert to an HPV-negative status within 24 months {4802}. Low-grade squamous intraepithelial lesions (LSILs) architecturally resembling condylomata acuminata are much more common in external genital sites than in the cervix.

## Etiology

Condylomas are associated predominantly with low-risk venereal HPV types, particularly types 6 and 11.

Anogenital warts can result from non-sexual or sexual transmission, and venereal-type HPV infections can be acquired non-sexually. A meticulous familial/social history and physical examination are required in paediatric cases {4396,7524}.

## Pathogenesis

HPV infection induces squamous cell proliferation. In condylomas, the HPV genome (both low- and high-risk types) replicates but remains as an episome not integrated within the host's genome; it is integrated in cancer.

## Macroscopic appearance

Condyloma acuminatum is an exophytic, benign keratosis-like lesion that may be single or multiple on anogenital skin and mucosa. White cervical lesions are observed on colposcopy, but they are usually invisible to the naked eye {4396}.

## Histopathology

The squamous epithelium exhibits acanthosis, papillomatosis, and koilocytosis. LSIL features proliferation of basal/parabasal-like cells that may be minimal and extends no further than the lower third of the epithelium. Mitotic activity is confined to this zone. In the upper three quarters to two thirds of the epithelium, the cells differentiate and gain cytoplasm; nuclear enlargement persists, with an increased N:C ratio. Nuclear hyperchromasia and nuclear membrane irregularities are usually present, and often a well-defined halo-like vacuole develops around the nucleus (koilocytosis). A less mature pattern with a metaplastic appearance (immature papillary squamous metaplasia) has been described. Marked atypia of single cells in the basal third of the epithelium, or abnormal mitotic figures, exclude LSIL. Block positive staining for p16 (p16INK4a) (nucleus and cytoplasm involving contiguous epithelium from the base (≥ 70%) indicates a high-grade squamous intraepithelial lesion {5799,7865}.

Histology does not distinguish between venereal papillomas (caused by HPV types 6, 11, 16, 18, etc.) and common warts (caused by HPV types 1, 2A, 3, 7, etc.). Venereal lesions may be hyperkeratotic or parakeratotic with keratohyalin granules, and they may lack koilocytes. Non-venereal papillomas may show epidermal hyperplasia, hypergranulosis, koilocytosis, and

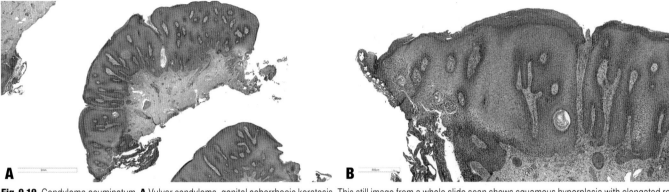

**Fig. 9.19** Condyloma acuminatum. **A** Vulvar condyloma, genital seborrhoeic keratosis. This still image from a whole slide scan shows squamous hyperplasia with elongated rete pegs and keratin horn cysts. **B** Vulvar condyloma, seborrhoeic keratosis–like. High-magnification view demonstrates parakeratosis atop squamous hyperplasia. An embedded keratin horn cyst is seen in the mid-lower epidermis. Scattered koilocytes are also noted (nuclear chromatin irregularities with perinuclear clearing). PCR was positive for HPV6.

diffuse hyperkeratosis. Attempts to distinguish venereal from non-venereal lesions using histological criteria in children fail in 62% of cases {2080}.

## Cytology
Cervical Pap smears show nuclear enlargement with chromatin clumping, with or without perinuclear clearing (koilocytosis).

## Diagnostic molecular pathology
Typing of HPV by sequencing may be helpful.

## Essential and desirable diagnostic criteria
*Essential:* acanthosis and papillomatosis, with formation of papillary structures and thickened rete ridges; parakeratosis, hyperkeratosis, and variable degrees of koilocytic atypia.

## Staging
Not applicable

## Prognosis and prediction
Spontaneous regression is expected in most cases of HPV infection through a combination of innate and adaptive immunity {5927}, including a role for HLA antigens {5272}.

Vaccination allows neutralizing antibodies (nAbs) to destroy the virus before its uptake into epithelial cells. nAbs from vaccination are protective but cannot eliminate virus-infected cells {5927}. Lesions acquired at an early age are more likely to persist or progress, possibly through virus-induced immunomodulation – more so in children – enhancing the likelihood of persistence or progression to cancer {5927}. Vaccination remains a major public health issue around the world, despite its proven efficacy and cost-effectiveness. The 9-valent HPV vaccine prevents persistent infections related to HPV types 31, 33, 45, 52, and 58 with an efficacy of 90.4–100% {2328}. Immunosuppression increases the likelihood of aggressive disease. Immunosuppressed patients, including those with systemic lupus and HIV, should be vaccinated against HPVs.

The cervicovaginal microbiome correlates with high-risk HPV progression {7157,3854,4717}. HIV infection alters the gut biome and promotes immune dysfunction; specific faecal and mucosal bacteria predict the existence of precancerous anal lesions, possibly providing diagnostic tools or therapeutic targets {6345}.

# Peritoneal inclusion cysts

Malpica A

## Definition
Peritoneal inclusion cysts are benign cysts lined by mesothelium.

## ICD-O coding
9055/0 Peritoneal inclusion cysts

## ICD-11 coding
DC51.Y & XH8U12 Other specified disorders of peritoneum or retroperitoneum & Peritoneal inclusion cysts

## Related terminology
*Acceptable:* multilocular peritoneal inclusion cysts.
*Not recommended:* benign cystic mesothelioma.

## Subtype(s)
None

## Localization
Peritoneum, spleen, liver, and testis {6021,7893}

## Clinical features
Peritoneal inclusion cysts can be detected incidentally or manifest with abdominal or pelvic pain, abdominal distension, or as an inguinal hernia {5778,3}. One patient who presented with pelvic pain passed the lesion in the form of string-like material through her cervix {6684}. A rare case has been associated with ascites {4514}. Occasionally, this lesion is seen in patients with renal developmental anomalies {6709}.

## Epidemiology
Peritoneal inclusion cysts are uncommon. They have a slight female predilection and are seen from the gestational period to the age of 19 years {6021,3717,5778}.

## Etiology
Although some lesions are congenital and others are reactive (i.e. secondary to abdominal/pelvic surgery, inflammation, or bleeding) {6021,3717,2472}, in many cases no etiological factor is identified {235,1861}.

## Pathogenesis
FISH shows no *CDKN2A* (*P16*) deletion {1332}.

## Macroscopic appearance
There are single or multiple cysts, which can be unilocular or multilocular and range in size from a few millimetres to 400 mm {7185,5778,5707}. Their inner and outer surfaces are usually smooth, and some cases can have a pedicle {235}.

## Histopathology
Peritoneal inclusion cysts are lined by a single layer of bland, flat or cuboidal mesothelial cells. Metaplastic or reactive changes,

hobnail cells, and adenomatoid areas can be seen. The septa are composed of fibroconnective tissue without smooth muscle bundles. There is no invasion into the adjacent tissue. Calretinin and CK5/6 are expressed, and PAX8, ER, and PR are variably positive {5778,1171,7653,6204}. BAP1 expression is retained.

## Cytology
Cytology shows bland or reactive mesothelial cells.

## Diagnostic molecular pathology
Not clinically relevant

## Essential and desirable diagnostic criteria
*Essential:* cyst(s) lined by bland mesothelial cells, with no invasion into adjacent tissue.
*Desirable:* positive staining for mesothelial markers.

## Staging
Not clinically relevant

## Prognosis and prediction
Peritoneal inclusion cysts are benign. Recurrences are seen infrequently {235,6709}.

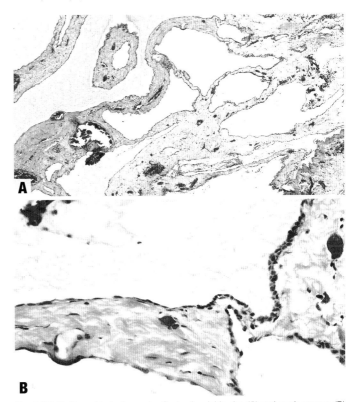

**Fig. 9.20** Peritoneal inclusion cysts. Cysts of variable size (**A**) and cystic spaces (**B**) lined by bland, flat and cuboidal mesothelial cells.

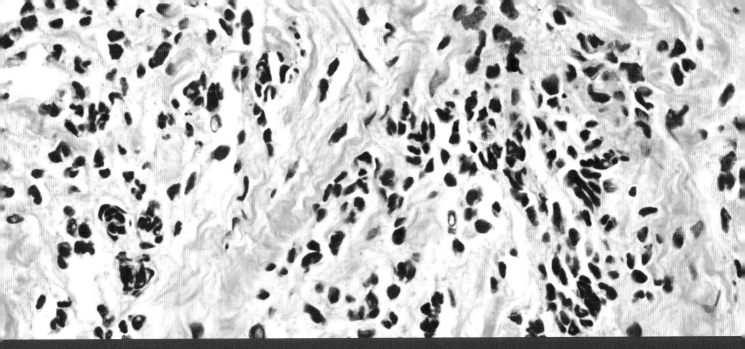

# 10

# Breast tumours

Edited by: Hill DA, Lakhani SR, Tan PH

Breast tumours
    Fibroepithelial tumours
    Juvenile fibroadenoma
    Juvenile papillomatosis

# Breast tumours: Introduction

Tan PH

Breast tumours in the paediatric age group are uncommon, and the vast majority are benign lesions {3400,3521,2315}. Breast tumours are overwhelmingly represented by fibroadenomas, which account for 91% of all solid breast masses {6148}.

When a paediatric patient presents clinically with a breast mass, it is important to consider non-neoplastic processes, including developmental changes such as premature thelarche and asymmetrical breast growth, for which surgical intervention is contraindicated because it may lead to damage to the breast, resulting in hypoplasia or aplasia. Neonatal breast enlargement can occur as a result of transient estrogen elevations from transplacental passage, whereas pubertal gynaecomastia in boys may be related to hormonal changes, although the exact etiology is largely unknown {3400}. Less commonly, pathological gynaecomastia from testicular tumours and adrenocortical neoplasms has to be ruled out.

Inflammatory conditions like mastitis and abscesses may lead to breast masses mimicking tumours. Juvenile papillomatosis is a benign proliferative epithelial lesion that can become clinically palpable, manifesting as a breast mass.

Apart from fibroadenomas, other neoplasms that can occur within the paediatric breast are intraductal papilloma and phyllodes tumour, the latter being mostly benign, although borderline and malignant phyllodes tumours can also (rarely) be seen.

Primary breast carcinomas are extremely uncommon, accounting for < 1% of childhood cancers and < 0.1% of all breast cancers {3447}. Secretory carcinoma is the most frequent tumour type described in the paediatric age group, although it can be diagnosed at all ages and is in fact more commonly found in adult patients {7519}. Secretory carcinoma is histologically characterized by microcystic, solid, tubular,

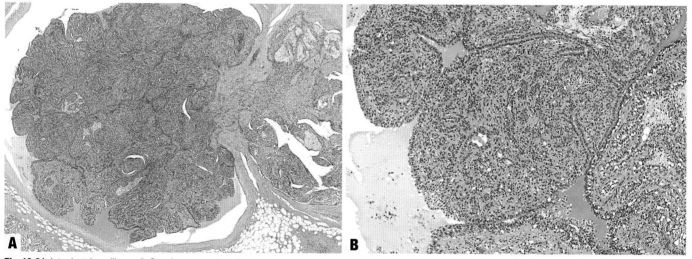

**Fig. 10.01** Intraductal papilloma. **A** On microscopy, there is a papillary tumour with fronds covered by bilayered epithelium, projecting into a cystically dilated duct space. **B** Higher magnification shows fibrovascular stromal cores covered by luminal epithelium and myoepithelium. Several foamy histiocytes are noted.

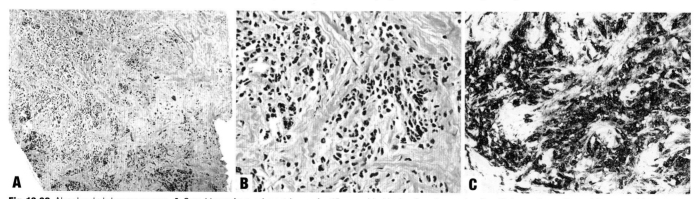

**Fig. 10.02** Alveolar rhabdomyosarcoma. **A** Core biopsy from a breast lump of a 15-year-old girl, showing abnormal cells with hyperchromatic nuclei, arranged in loose aggregates and cords within the breast parenchyma. **B** Higher magnification shows tumour cells with high N:C ratios and occasional pink cytoplasm. **C** Immunohistochemistry for desmin shows cytoplasmic reactivity of tumour cells, indicating muscle differentiation.

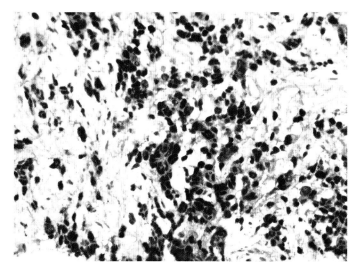

**Fig. 10.03** Alveolar rhabdomyosarcoma. Immunohistochemistry for myogenin shows nuclear reactivity of tumour cells, indicating muscle differentiation.

and papillary patterns formed by polygonal cells with pink granular and vacuolated cytoplasm with intracytoplasmic and luminal eosinophilic colloid-like secretions. Usually histological grade 1 or 2, these tumours possess pathognomonic *ETV6*::*NTRK3* gene fusions and have an indolent clinical course, especially in children and young adults {7519}. Anecdotal reports of breast carcinomas with inflammatory and medullary features have been reported {3521}. When breast cancer is diagnosed in a young patient, the possibility of a familial association ought to be considered.

Before concluding that a malignant neoplasm in the paediatric breast is of primary origin, it is necessary to exclude extramammary metastases to the breast, which are more common than primary breast malignancies in children {2315}. These include rhabdomyosarcoma, neuroblastoma, lymphoma, Ewing sarcoma, and melanoma {1328}. Some of these may arise in the chest wall and directly involve the overlying breast through contiguous extension {2315}.

Evaluation of breast masses in the paediatric patient requires close clinicoradiological correlation, with ultrasonography being the radiological modality usually applied {2315}. Because these paediatric breast lesions are predominantly benign, a conservative approach is recommended. For worrisome breast masses, FNAB or core biopsy can offer a preoperative diagnosis, although there may be a basis for excisional biopsy to avoid repeated traumatic procedures {3521}.

# Fibroepithelial tumours

Tay TKY
Gudi M
Shin SJ

## Definition

Fibroadenoma is a biphasic neoplasm of the terminal duct lobular unit composed of a proliferation of epithelial and stromal elements.

Phyllodes tumour is generally a circumscribed fibroepithelial neoplasm showing a prominent intracanalicular architectural pattern with leaf-like stromal fronds, capped by luminal epithelial and myoepithelial cell layers, accompanied by stromal hypercellularity.

## ICD-O coding

9010/0 Fibroadenoma
9020/1 Phyllodes tumour

## ICD-11 coding

2F30.5 & XH9HE2 Fibroadenoma of breast & Fibroadenoma, NOS
2F30.3 & XH50P7 Benign phyllodes tumour of breast & Phyllodes tumour, benign
2F75 & XH5NK4 Neoplasms of uncertain behaviour of breast & Phyllodes tumour, borderline
2C63 & XH8HJ7 Malignant phyllodes tumour of breast & Phyllodes tumour, malignant

## Related terminology

*Not recommended:* adenofibroma; cystosarcoma phyllodes.

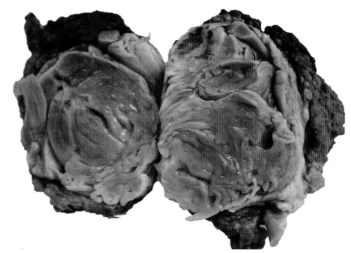

**Fig. 10.05** Benign phyllodes tumour. A large tumour from a 19-year-old female patient, with a tan-coloured and fleshy cut surface, cleft-like spaces, and focal haemorrhage.

## Subtype(s)

None

## Localization

Fibroepithelial tumours may occur in any part of the breast.

## Clinical features

Fibroepithelial tumour of the breast often manifests as a palpable mass, with some patients also experiencing pain {1859, 908}. Fibroadenomas can occur synchronously as multiple masses in the same breast or bilaterally {6922,1389,5996}. In contrast, phyllodes tumours tend to be unifocal {5733}. Both can grow to large sizes (> 100 mm) {7650,6774,908}, resulting in breast distortion and asymmetry. There may be thinning of the overlying skin with dilatation and prominence of the superficial veins {371}. The breast may feel warm as a result of the increased blood supply, and ischaemia and erosion of the overlying skin may occur in extremely large tumours. Infarction can occur in both tumours and lead to nipple discharge {7879}.

When assessing breast tumours in the paediatric population, ultrasonography is generally performed because it can detect lesions in dense breast tissue and does not expose paediatric patients to ionizing radiation {4002}. On ultrasound, both fibroadenomas and phyllodes tumours appear as hypoechoic, oval, solid masses with well-circumscribed margins and posterior acoustic enhancement {6148,4108}. There is considerable overlap of ultrasonographic features, and distinguishing the two on imaging is not always possible {7726}. Anechoic cysts or clefts may be seen in phyllodes tumour and correspond to the gross appearance of the tumour, but they

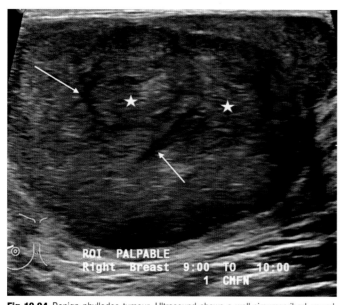

**Fig. 10.04** Benign phyllodes tumour. Ultrasound shows a well-circumscribed, round, solid mass with bulging, lobulated borders and posterior enhancement. This tumour in a 14-year-old girl shows apparent nodular compartments (stars) surrounded by slit-like cystic spaces (arrows), probably corresponding to leaf-like fronds seen microscopically.

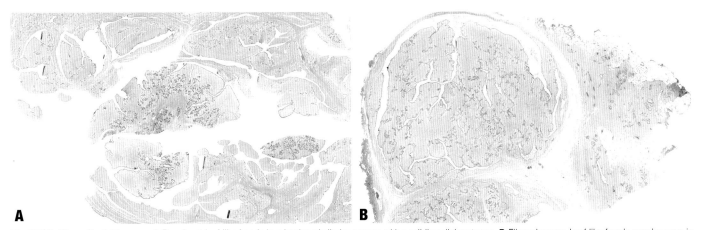

**Fig. 10.06** Fibroepithelial tumours. **A** Prominent leaf-like fronds in a benign phyllodes tumour with a mildly cellular stroma. **B** Fibroadenoma. Leaf-like fronds may be seen in fibroadenomas, but they are usually not as well-developed, prominent, or diffuse as those in phyllodes tumours.

are not entirely specific because they may also be seen in juvenile fibroadenomas.

### Epidemiology

Fibroadenoma is the most common breast tumour in adolescent girls {6713,2823} and can occur in children as young as 8–9 years old {5177,4043}. In the USA, phyllodes tumours in the paediatric population are reported to be more common in Black children than in White children {7650,4043,7509}. Malignant phyllodes tumours are the second most common malignant breast tumours in adolescent girls, after carcinomas {7650,5874,7509}.

### Etiology

The exact etiology of fibroadenoma and phyllodes tumour is unclear, because most cases occur sporadically. However, a relationship with estrogenic stimulation has been postulated for fibroadenomas {7047}. Myxoid fibroadenomas have also been described in women with Carney complex {1053}. More recently, ciclosporin immunosuppression has been implicated in the development of fibroadenomas in both liver and renal transplant recipients {6871,700,453}, with resolution of the fibroadenomas observed in some patients upon cessation of ciclosporin immunosuppression {3101}.

### Pathogenesis

Like adult fibroadenomas, paediatric fibroadenomas also contain *MED12* exon 2 mutations in a subset of cases, as seen in two studies {5334,6922}. In addition, in one of the studies, 8 benign phyllodes tumours were sequenced and *MED12* mutations were found in 7 tumours {5334}. A majority of the *MED12* exon 2 mutations in benign fibroepithelial tumours were found to be in-frame deletions. *MED12* mutations were also associated with the intracanalicular type of growth pattern {5334}. However, this was not reproduced in the other study, which found *MED12* missense mutations in a majority of paediatric fibroepithelial tumours but no correlation between *MED12* mutations and type of growth pattern; instead, a correlation was found between *MED12* and stromal mitotic counts {6922}. In both studies, none of the fibroadenomas or benign phyllodes tumours had *TERT* promoter mutations.

### Macroscopic appearance

Fibroadenomas are solid, ovoid tumours with a firm, greyish-white cut surface with slit-like spaces. Phyllodes tumours are often larger and show a bulging cut surface with or without cystic spaces. The cut surface can also show a variety of appearances, ranging from firm to soft and fleshy, tan to yellow or greyish, and with gelatinous mucoid areas or papillary

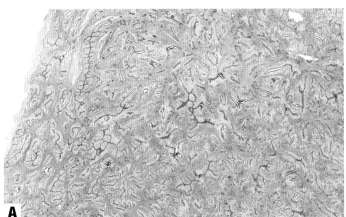
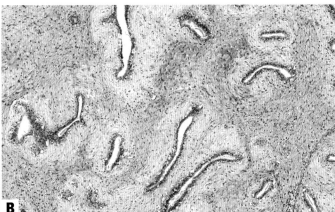

**Fig. 10.07** Fibroadenoma. **A** Intracanalicular growth pattern. **B** A more cellular stroma is often seen in paediatric fibroadenomas than in adult fibroadenomas.

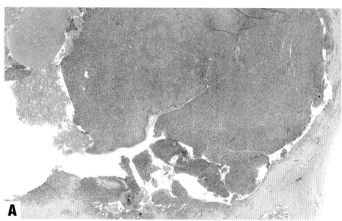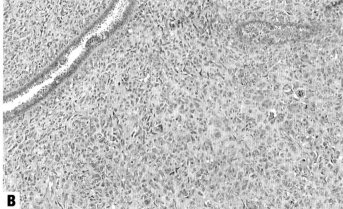

**Fig. 10.08** Malignant phyllodes tumour from a 15-year-old girl. **A** A leaf-like frond is vaguely discernible with an epithelial lining capping a markedly cellular stroma. **B** Markedly atypical stromal cells with brisk mitotic activity including atypical mitotic figures. Benign epithelial components are admixed within.

excrescences. Haemorrhage and necrosis may be seen in malignant phyllodes tumours {5733}.

## Histopathology

Fibroepithelial tumours show a biphasic proliferation of stromal and epithelial elements. Fibroadenomas classically display a mildly cellular stroma, but in the paediatric population, increased stromal cellularity is not uncommon {6921} and stromal mitotic counts may even reach 2.5–5 mitoses/mm$^2$ (equating to 5–10 mitoses/10 HPF of 0.5 mm in diameter and 0.2 mm$^2$ in area) in rare cases {5996}. Small leaf-like fronds may also be present. These features do not necessarily warrant a diagnosis of phyllodes tumour {6774,6921}. Phyllodes tumours in the paediatric age group show similar morphological features to those seen in adults {5733}. They are characterized by a prominent leaf-like architecture secondary to an exaggerated intracanalicular growth pattern and are associated with a hypercellular stroma. Periductal stromal tumour is regarded as a subtype of phyllodes tumour with a pericanalicular growth pattern. Phyllodes tumour can be divided into benign, borderline, and malignant categories based on the criteria used for adults.

## Cytology

The cytological features of fibroepithelial tumours are similar to those seen in adults. Because paediatric fibroadenomas may have increased stromal cellularity, it may be challenging to distinguish them from phyllodes tumours on cytology.

## Diagnostic molecular pathology

Not clinically relevant

## Essential and desirable diagnostic criteria

*Fibroadenoma*

*Essential:* a circumscribed biphasic tumour; an intracanalicular and/or pericanalicular growth pattern; no stromal overgrowth; absence of well-developed fronds; no stromal atypia; low mitotic activity in the stromal component.

*Phyllodes tumour*

*Essential:* stromal fronds and hypercellularity; a dominant intracanalicular growth pattern with stromal fronds capped by luminal/myoepithelial cell layers.

## Staging

Not clinically relevant

## Prognosis and prediction

The majority of fibroadenomas do not recur after excision, even with positive margins {6921,5996}. Phyllodes tumours may recur locally, and malignant phyllodes tumours have the potential to metastasize. Infiltrative tumour borders and positive surgical margins may increase the risk of local recurrence {5733}. However, a lack of local recurrence has also been reported in some case series of benign phyllodes tumours with positive surgical margins, with clinical follow-up being recommended for phyllodes tumours in the benign category instead of further excision {6945,2657}. Paediatric patients with malignant phyllodes tumours have been found to have better overall survival than older patients {7650}.

# Juvenile fibroadenoma

Tay TKY
Gudi M
Shin SJ

## Definition

Juvenile fibroadenoma is a biphasic proliferation of stromal and epithelial elements with a cellular stroma, gynaecomastoid usual-type ductal hyperplasia, and (often) a pericanalicular growth pattern.

## ICD-O coding

9030/0 Juvenile fibroadenoma
9030/0 Giant juvenile fibroadenoma

## ICD-11 coding

2F30.5 & XH70H4 Fibroadenoma of breast & Juvenile fibroadenoma

## Related terminology

*Not recommended:* juvenile adenofibroma; cellular fibroadenoma; giant fibroadenoma.

## Subtype(s)

Giant juvenile fibroadenoma

## Localization

Juvenile fibroadenoma may occur in any part of the breast and may be multifocal or bilateral.

## Clinical features

Juvenile fibroadenoma may manifest as solitary or multiple unilateral or bilateral masses in the breast, often in adolescent girls {5534}. It can grow rapidly and reach a large size (> 50 mm), resulting in breast distortion and asymmetry {5534,5996,6921}. Juvenile fibroadenomas > 50 mm in size have been termed "giant juvenile fibroadenomas". Most juvenile fibroadenomas

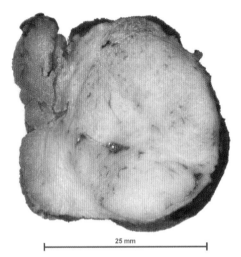

**Fig. 10.10** Juvenile fibroadenoma. A well-circumscribed tumour from a 17-year-old girl, with a greyish-white cut surface and slit-like spaces.

occur in postmenarchal women, but they can occur in prepubertal patients {5534,6921}. They also tend to occur at a younger age and grow to larger sizes than conventional adult-type fibroadenomas {6921}. Although juvenile fibroadenoma occurs more commonly in adolescent girls than in adults, conventional adult-type fibroadenomas are still more common in adolescents {371}.

On ultrasound, juvenile fibroadenomas most commonly appear as well-circumscribed, round to oval, solid, isoechoic or hypoechoic masses with hypervascularity on colour Doppler sonography. Posterior acoustic enhancement is common {3591}. Thin fluid-filled clefts may also be seen.

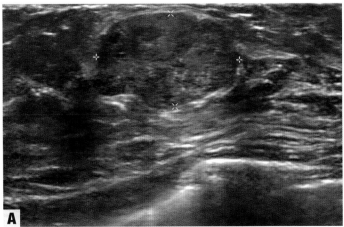

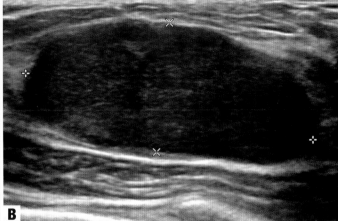

**Fig. 10.09** Juvenile fibroadenoma. **A** Transverse ultrasound shows a macrolobulated, circumscribed, wider-than-tall hypoechoic mass within the fibroglandular breast tissue. **B** Ultrasound of this tumour from an 18-year-old female patient shows a well-defined, wider-than-tall, oval solid mass. The internal echoes are fairly homogeneous and there is posterior enhancement. No internal cystic spaces are present.

## Epidemiology

Juvenile fibroadenoma has been reported to be seen more commonly in Black patients {5534}.

## Etiology

The exact etiology of fibroadenoma and phyllodes tumour is unclear because most occur sporadically. However, like for conventional fibroadenomas, a relationship with estrogenic stimulation has been postulated.

## Pathogenesis

The pathogenetic mechanisms of juvenile fibroadenoma are not completely understood. There are scant data on the molecular genetics of juvenile fibroadenomas. In one study, where targeted DNA sequencing of 50 genes was performed on 17 juvenile fibroadenomas, *MED12* mutations were found in a subset of cases, similarly to conventional adult fibroadenomas {6922}. Juvenile fibroadenomas had a higher rate of mutations in *FLNA*, *DYNC2H1*, *SMAD4*, *CHD8*, *FSIP2*, *MAP3K1*, *MAP4K5*, *NCOR1*, *STAT3*, and *TBX3*, whereas conventional fibroadenomas had a higher rate of mutations in *DNAH11*, *KMT2D*, *FOXA1*, *NOTCH2*, *PIK3CA*, *ROS1*, and *KMT2C*. *TERT* promoter mutations were absent in both. Juvenile fibroadenomas with *MED12* mutations were more likely to have a higher stromal mitotic count (1–1.5 mitoses/mm$^2$, equating to 2–3 mitoses/10 HPF of 0.5 mm in diameter and 0.2 mm$^2$ in area) than those without (< 0.5 mitoses/mm$^2$, equating to < 1 mitosis/10 HPF). Among

the 17 juvenile fibroadenomas sequenced, 7 were giant juvenile fibroadenomas (> 50 mm); 3 cases had no mutations detected in the panel of 50 genes, and the remaining 4 cases disclosed various mutations in *MED12*, *KMT2C*, *KMT2D*, *SMAD4*, *FLNA*, *OPA1*, and *FSIP2*. More studies are required to further elucidate the molecular genetic mechanisms of juvenile fibroadenoma.

## Macroscopic appearance

The macroscopic appearance of juvenile fibroadenoma is not well documented, with isolated case reports describing a circumscribed, solid, greyish-white tumour. The external surface may be bosselated or multilobulated and the cut surface may have a myxoid appearance with slit-like spaces and tiny cysts {5036,7667,1115}.

## Histopathology

Juvenile fibroadenoma is a neoplasm with circumscribed borders and a predominant pericanalicular growth pattern, although a mixture of pericanalicular and intracanalicular growth patterns may also be seen {5534,5996,6921}. The stroma is cellular, and usual ductal hyperplasia in the form of gynaecomastia-like micropapillary tufting is often present {5996,5534,6921}. There may be stromal multinucleated giant cells in rare cases. Mitotic activity in the stromal component is usually low: < 1 mitosis/mm$^2$ (< 2 mitoses/10 HPF of 0.5 mm in diameter and 0.2 mm$^2$ in area) and should not exceed 5 mitoses/mm$^2$ {5996,2058}. Some tumours may have intratumoural heterogeneity, with focal areas

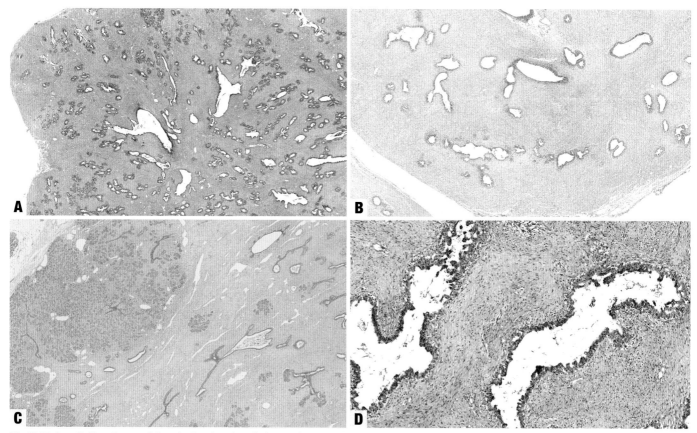

**Fig. 10.11** Juvenile fibroadenoma. **A** A predominantly pericanalicular growth pattern with a cellular stroma. **B** Mixed pericanalicular and intracanalicular growth patterns. **C** Some juvenile fibroadenomas can have intratumoural heterogeneity, with areas featuring an increased number of glands and with a tubular arrangement resembling a tubular adenoma. **D** Cellular stroma and usual-type ductal hyperplasia in the form of gynaecomastoid epithelial tufting.

featuring an increased number of glands and with a tubular arrangement resembling a tubular adenoma {5996}. Patients with multiple juvenile fibroadenomas may also have synchronous or recurrent tumours resembling conventional adult-type fibroadenomas {5534}. Although some studies have used the terms "giant fibroadenoma" or "cellular fibroadenoma" interchangeably with "juvenile fibroadenoma", it is recommended that the term "giant" be reserved for tumours > 50 mm in size, and this term can be applied to both conventional fibroadenomas (i.e. giant fibroadenoma) and juvenile fibroadenomas (e.g. giant juvenile fibroadenoma). The term "cellular fibroadenoma" may be reserved for tumours that show increased stromal cellularity without the gynaecomastia-like epithelial hyperplasia, or for those with a predominant intracanalicular growth pattern. Although juvenile fibroadenoma shows increased stromal cellularity similar to that of a benign phyllodes tumour, it lacks the well-developed leaf-like fronds seen in phyllodes tumour.

## Cytology

Because juvenile fibroadenomas have increased stromal cellularity, it may be challenging to distinguish them from phyllodes tumours on cytology.

## Diagnostic molecular pathology

Not clinically relevant

## Essential and desirable diagnostic criteria

*Essential:* a circumscribed biphasic neoplasm with stromal and epithelial elements; predominant pericanalicular growth patterns, cellular stroma, and usual-type epithelial hyperplasia with gynaecomastia-like micropapillary tufting; an absence of prominent leaf-like fronds, stromal atypia, stromal overgrowth, and malignant heterologous elements.

## Staging

Not clinically relevant

## Prognosis and prediction

A majority of solitary juvenile fibroadenomas do not recur after excision, even with positive margins {5996,5534}. Patients with multiple juvenile fibroadenomas may have a higher risk of recurrence {5534}. In patients with large tumours occupying most parts of the breast, preservation of apparently minimal amounts of normal breast tissue can result in normal breast development subsequently {5534}.

# Juvenile papillomatosis

Gudi M
Shin SJ
Tay TKY

## Definition
Juvenile papillomatosis (JP) is a benign proliferative lesion seen commonly in adolescent girls and characterized by duct papillomatosis, apocrine and non-apocrine cysts, papillary apocrine hyperplasia, sclerosing adenosis, and duct stasis.

## ICD-O coding
None

## ICD-11 coding
2F30.2 & XH4LZ4 Intraductal papilloma of breast & Intraductal papilloma

## Related terminology
*Not recommended:* Swiss cheese disease.

## Subtype(s)
None

## Localization
JP may occur in various parts of the breast but is most commonly located in the upper lateral quadrant {1237,5980}.

## Clinical features
The most common presenting symptom is a palpable lump {5982}. Examination usually reveals a localized, firm, mobile nodule. Pain and nipple discharge are rare {7420,5980}. The clinical presentation resembles that of a fibroadenoma, for which it is often mistaken. However, JP tends to be larger and firmer than a fibroadenoma {2587}. It is usual for patients to have had one or more biopsies of the ipsilateral or contralateral breast for fibroadenomas or other proliferative breast diseases before obtaining a diagnosis of JP {2929}.

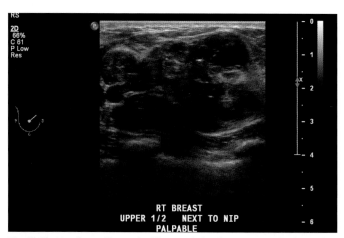

**Fig. 10.12** Juvenile papillomatosis. Ultrasound showing a retroareolar hypoechoic mass with an indistinct margin and multiple cystic areas especially at the periphery, findings that reflect the macroscopic features.

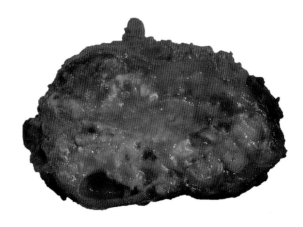

**Fig. 10.13** Juvenile papillomatosis. The gross appearance of juvenile papillomatosis comprises a discrete mass with cysts and intervening fibrous areas with interspersed yellowish and whitish appearances.

### Imaging
Ultrasonography is the preferred imaging technique for JP because of the young age of these patients. Characteristically, JP is seen as a poorly defined hypoechoic mass usually associated with multiple cysts, frequently located at the periphery of the lesion on ultrasound. On MRI these lesions are lobulated in shape, are hypointense on T1-weighted images, contain internal cystic areas that are bright on T2-weighted images, and show a benign enhancement pattern {5142,7727}.

## Epidemiology
As the name implies, JP tends to occur in young women, usually aged < 30 years, although the age range is 10–48 years in the largest series (median: 21 years) {5980}. Since that series, approximately 400 cases have been described, with the majority occurring in White patients and only rare cases seen in patients of Asian origin {7420}. Male patients are extremely rare {7314}.

## Etiology
There are no specific etiological factors found to be linked to JP. No association with abnormal menstrual history or with the use of exogenous hormones has been found. More research is required to assess the genetic cause of JP.

## Pathogenesis
Hotspot mutations in *PIK3CA* and *AKT1* have been demonstrated in cases of JP where there is a positive family history of breast cancer. However, these mutations are not specific for JP. The genetic link between JP, a positive family history, and the subsequent risk of breast cancer needs to be analysed in further studies {2587}.

## Macroscopic appearance

Macroscopic examination reveals a well-defined, firm, discrete, usually unencapsulated mass measuring 10–80 mm (average size: ~40 mm). Cut sections have an appearance resembling Swiss cheese, with multiple cysts varying in size from 1 to 20 mm and with greyish-white intervening stroma often showing yellowish white spots or flecks {5980,5982}.

## Histopathology

JP is characterized by multiple cysts or ectatic ducts, many of which contain inspissated secretions or intraluminal foamy macrophages. Papillary epithelial hyperplasia or papillomatosis of the ducts is very often present. The epithelium of the cysts frequently shows flat or papillary apocrine metaplasia. Ducts stasis is manifested by intraluminal lipid-laden macrophages/histiocytes or secretions that may correspond to the yellowish and whitish spots or flecks seen grossly. In most cases, the proliferative changes within the ducts consist of usual-type ductal hyperplasia, which may be quite florid and occasionally may exhibit a cribriform or micropapillary growth pattern with or without necrosis. There is histological merging of apocrine metaplasia/hyperplasia with usual ductal hyperplasia within the lesional cysts. There may be accompanying sclerosis producing a radial scar–like appearance. Atypical ductal hyperplasia is sometimes present. The stroma in combination with the epithelial alterations tends to be dense and fibrous, which in combination with the multiple cysts gives rise to the classic Swiss-cheese appearance grossly. Foci of sclerosing adenosis and fibroadenomatoid change can also be seen {2929}.

The florid epithelial hyperplasia shows mosaic-type staining for basal cytokeratins (CK5/6), a heterogeneous staining pattern of ER, and preservation of the myoepithelial cells (p63) around the ducts with usual ductal hyperplasia and within the papillary proliferations. Epithelial atypia can be found in JP; however, the grade of the atypia was not shown to be associated with the subsequent development of breast cancer {5982,5979,3867}.

The types of breast carcinoma associated with JP include ductal carcinoma in situ, lobular carcinoma in situ, infiltrating duct carcinoma, infiltrating lobular carcinoma, and secretory carcinoma, and the prevalence is 4–15% {5981}.

### *Differential diagnosis*

"Sclerosing papillary duct hyperplasia" is a term reserved for papillomas that are distorted and disrupted by a desmoplastic proliferation of myoepithelial and stromal cells, giving a radial scar–like appearance, but differing from a radial scar by being well circumscribed.

"Papillomatosis" is a term used to describe papillary hyperplasia of the usual type involving multiple ducts.

Fibroadenomas in children with multiple cysts have multiple cysts within the fibroadenoma, as the name suggests, but without the proliferative ductal component.

None of the above entities shows the constellation of prominent cyst formation, extensive apocrine metaplasia, stasis, and other benign proliferative changes that characterize JP.

## Cytology

The smears are cellular, with large, antler horn–like sheets of ductal epithelial cells with some nuclear overlapping and bare nuclei, as well as cyst macrophages and clusters of apocrine cells. It is difficult to establish a confident diagnosis of JP just on cytology. However, in the appropriate clinical context of a firm circumscribed mass in a young adolescent patient, which yields cyst fluid, demonstrates a residual mass after aspiration, and exhibits the above cytological features, a diagnosis of JP can be rendered {5244}.

## Diagnostic molecular pathology

Not clinically relevant

## Essential and desirable diagnostic criteria

*Essential:* duct papillomatosis; apocrine and non-apocrine cysts; papillary apocrine hyperplasia; sclerosing adenosis; duct stasis.

## Staging

Not applicable

## Prognosis and prediction

In Rosen's original series of 180 cases of JP, a family history of breast carcinoma was observed in 28% {5980}. In subsequent studies, a positive family history in first- or second-degree relatives was reported in 26–58% of patients with JP, with cases in

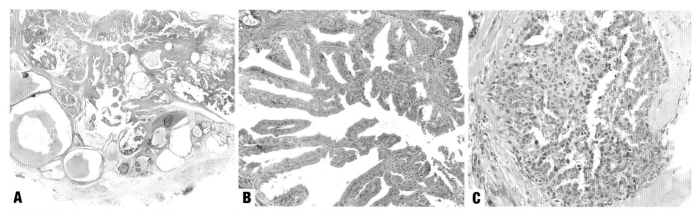

**Fig. 10.14** Juvenile papillomatosis. **A** A low-power scanning view of juvenile papillomatosis shows cysts, intraductal papillomas, and apocrine metaplasia within dense stroma. **B** Papillary apocrine hyperplasia in a cyst of juvenile papillomatosis. **C** A distended duct shows florid usual-type ductal hyperplasia.

mothers and maternal aunts being associated with the highest risk {5980,3867,2587}. A positive family history together with recurrent bilateral JP has therefore been suggested as a risk factor for developing invasive breast cancer {5981}. Treatment of JP is usually achieved by complete excision followed by histological confirmation. No additional treatments are necessary if no coexisting carcinomatous lesions are seen. Recurrence is inevitable if incompletely excised. Re-excision is prudent if the lesion has not been completely excised and/or has atypical ductal hyperplasia and is a recurrence with involved margins. Patients with a positive family history together with recurrent bilateral JP lesions have the highest risk of developing breast carcinoma {3867}. Follow-up including a physical examination and ultrasonography is recommended on a yearly basis. JP may be a marker of breast cancer in a family of patients with JP, so a thorough medical follow-up is recommended for patients and their families {7420}.

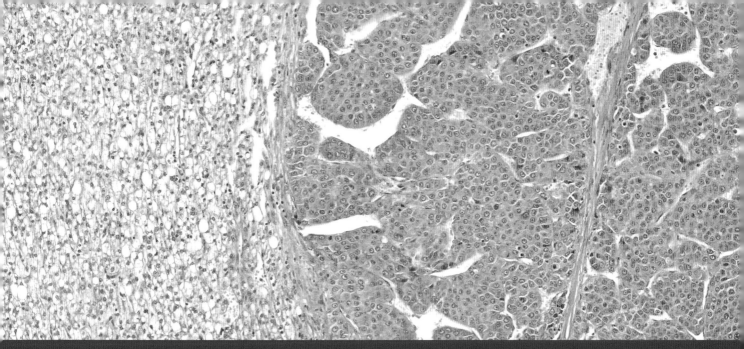

# 11

# Digestive system tumours

Edited by: Carneiro F, López-Terrada DH, Reyes-Múgica M, Washington MK

Liver tumours
    Epithelial tumours
        Hepatoblastoma
        Fibrolamellar variant of hepatocellular carcinoma
        Paediatric hepatocellular carcinoma
    Mesenchymal tumours unique to the liver
        Mesenchymal hamartoma
        Calcifying nested stromal-epithelial tumour
        Embryonal sarcoma of the liver
        Hepatic congenital haemangioma
        Hepatic infantile haemangioma
        Hepatic angiosarcoma
Pancreatic tumours
    Epithelial tumours
        Pancreatoblastoma
        Pancreatic acinar cell carcinoma
        Solid pseudopapillary neoplasm
Gastrointestinal tumours
    Epithelial tumours
        Gastroblastoma
        Appendiceal neuroendocrine tumours

# Digestive system tumours: Introduction

López-Terrada DH
Carneiro F
Reyes-Múgica M

Primary tumours of the liver, pancreas, and gastrointestinal tract are rare in children and, similarly to other paediatric cancers, their histology, pathogenesis, and clinical presentation often differ from those of corresponding cancers in adults. This chapter will focus on tumour types that are either exclusively or most commonly diagnosed in children and adolescents, including embryonal neoplasms arising early in life (such as hepatoblastoma [HBL]), as well as malignancies seen often in older children and adolescents, such as pancreatoblastoma (an embryonal neoplasm that recapitulates pancreatic development) and gastroblastoma (a rare gastric tumour whose pathogenesis has been recently characterized). Other gastrointestinal neoplasms seen in children, such as gastrointestinal lymphomas, gastrointestinal stromal tumours, and neoplasms associated with polyposis syndromes, are discussed in the *Digestive system tumours* volume of this series {7521}. Clear cell sarcoma–like tumour of the gastrointestinal tract (malignant gastrointestinal neuroectodermal tumour) is also covered in that volume and will not be discussed here.

Primary digestive neoplasms in children represent < 1% of paediatric tumours, with the most common being gastrointestinal lymphomas, colorectal carcinomas, neuroendocrine tumours, and gastrointestinal stromal tumours (discussed in Chapter 5: *Soft tissue and bone tumours*) {378}. Primary malignant liver tumours are similarly rare during childhood, representing approximately 1% of all paediatric cancers, but their incidence appears to be rising. The most common type is HBL, usually diagnosed during the first few years of life, followed by hepatocellular carcinoma (HCC), which is more common in older children {1559}. These tumours are generally sporadic, but they can be seen in association with familial cancer and genetic syndromes, as well as metabolic disorders and underlying liver disease in patients with HCC {3500}. Primary liver tumours of mesenchymal origin are less common in children, with the exception of vascular tumours (haemangiomas). Primary sarcomas of the liver are very rare, with embryonal sarcoma, sometimes associated with mesenchymal hamartoma, being the most common {3483}.

Recent cooperative international clinical trials and scientific partnerships have facilitated diagnostic and therapeutic improvements, in particular for children with HBL {1513}. The recently proposed International Pediatric Liver Tumors Consensus Classification was based on histological data collected by central reviewers and other pathologists participating in the systematic histopathological examination of tumours diagnosed in children enrolled in these trials. Experts participating in this effort attempted to create a standardized, clinically meaningful classification to be used in international trials that may serve as a template to integrate newly recognized biological parameters, and to improve diagnosis and patient outcomes {4219}.

Molecular characterization of a subset of these tumours has recently contributed valuable information that has been incorporated into the WHO classification. One of the important updates was the recognition that the previously designated "small cell undifferentiated HBL" (also termed "anaplastic variant of HBL"), believed to be an aggressive HBL subtype with low AFP expression, really represents primary malignant rhabdoid tumour of the liver characterized by *SMARCB1* abnormalities and loss of SMARCB1 (INI1) nuclear expression {7070}. Another important addition was the creation of a new provisional category, hepatocellular neoplasm NOS, to recognize a subset of difficult-to-classify paediatric hepatocellular tumours showing either intermediate or hybrid features between HBL and HCC, and to reflect the need to identify and molecularly characterize this group of tumours, proposed to represent progressed HBLs with histological and biological features of both HBL and HCC (HBL with HCC features) {6772,1899}.

Hepatocellular carcinomas (HCC) are more often seen in older children, with two thirds being diagnosed in patients aged > 10 years {3872}. The fibrolamellar variant represents almost one third of all HCCs diagnosed in patients aged < 20 years without underlying liver disease, and it constitutes a distinct histological and biological entity characterized by the activation of PKA, either through a *DNAJB1::PRKACA* fusion gene or (rarely) through *PRKAR1A* mutations {2967,1958}. Other HCCs in children represent a wide disease spectrum, with tumours that can arise either de novo or in the context of congenital or chronic liver disease {3482,2664}. HBV and HCV infections still represent important associated factors, mostly in Asian populations with high infection rates.

Ongoing molecular characterization and genomic profiling studies promise to dramatically improve our understanding of the pathogenesis and oncogenic mechanisms underlying liver, pancreatic, and gastrointestinal neoplasms in children. These advances, some currently underway through international clinical trials and collaborative scientific and precision medicine initiatives, should facilitate the identification of biomarkers and the development of new therapies for some of these young patients.

# Hepatoblastoma

Ranganathan S
Alaggio R
Czauderna P
de Krijger RR
Tanaka Y

## Definition

Hepatoblastoma (HBL) is a primary malignant embryonal tumour that recapitulates the developmental stages of the liver and consists of either epithelial or epithelial and mesenchymal components.

## ICD-O coding

8970/3 Hepatoblastoma, NOS
8970/3 Pure fetal hepatoblastoma with low mitotic activity (well-differentiated fetal hepatoblastoma)
8970/3 Fetal hepatoblastoma, mitotically active (crowded fetal hepatoblastoma)
8970/3 Pleomorphic hepatoblastoma, poorly differentiated
8970/3 Embryonal hepatoblastoma
8970/3 Small cell undifferentiated hepatoblastoma, SMARCB1 (INI1) retained (positive)
8970/3 Small cell undifferentiated hepatoblastoma, SMARCB1 (INI1) lost (negative)
8970/3 Cholangioblastic hepatoblastoma
8970/3 Epithelial mixed hepatoblastoma
8970/3 Epithelial macrotrabecular pattern of hepatoblastoma
8970/3 Mixed epithelial and mesenchymal hepatoblastoma without teratoid features
8970/3 Mixed epithelial and mesenchymal hepatoblastoma with teratoid features
8000/3 Hepatoblastoma, hepatocellular neoplasm NOS subtype

## ICD-11 coding

2C12.01 Hepatoblastoma

## Related terminology

None

## Subtype(s)

Epithelial and mixed epithelial and mesenchymal hepatoblastoma subtypes (see Box 11.01); hepatocellular neoplasm NOS

**Box 11.01** International Pediatric Liver Tumors Consensus Classification (modified) for hepatoblastoma {4219}

**Hepatoblastoma**
  Epithelial subtypes
    Pure fetal hepatoblastoma with low mitotic activity (well-differentiated fetal hepatoblastoma)
    Fetal hepatoblastoma, mitotically active (crowded fetal hepatoblastoma)
    Pleomorphic hepatoblastoma, poorly differentiated
    Embryonal hepatoblastoma
    Small cell undifferentiated hepatoblastoma
      SMARCB1 (INI1) retained (positive)
      SMARCB1 (INI1) lost (negative)
    Cholangioblastic hepatoblastoma
    Epithelial mixed hepatoblastoma
    Epithelial macrotrabecular pattern of hepatoblastoma
  Mixed epithelial and mesenchymal subtypes
    Mixed epithelial and mesenchymal hepatoblastoma without teratoid features
    Mixed epithelial and mesenchymal hepatoblastoma with teratoid features

## Localization

HBL usually arises as a solitary mass affecting the right lobe (in 55–60% of cases), the left lobe (in 15–20%), or both lobes of the liver. Multifocal lesions at presentation do occur. Metastases at diagnosis, usually to the lungs, are present in 5% of cases.

## Clinical features

The majority (80–90%) of HBLs occur in children aged 6 months to 5 years (median age: 18 months). They can be congenital. This tumour can also occur in older children, and it has (rarely) been reported in adults. The most common presentation is of an abdominal mass incidentally discovered by family members or the paediatrician. Other constitutional symptoms may be seen, including weight loss, anorexia, nausea, vomiting, and abdominal pain. Liver enzyme levels are generally normal, and serum AFP is frequently highly elevated (to thousands or even millions

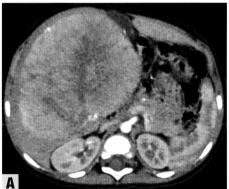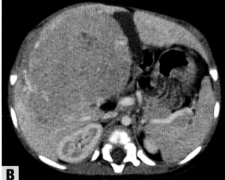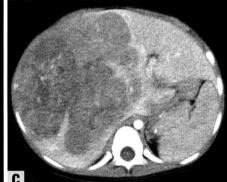

**Fig. 11.01** Hepatoblastoma. **A** Axial CT image obtained in the arterial phase of enhancement, showing a circumscribed, heterogeneously enhanced mass in the right lobe of the liver, displacing the gallbladder. **B** Axial CT image obtained in the portal phase of enhancement, showing that the tumour is hypoattenuating relative to adjacent liver. **C** Contrast-enhanced axial CT shows a large lobular mass with slight heterogeneous enhancement but with less attenuation than the adjacent liver parenchyma. There are speckled calcifications within the mass.

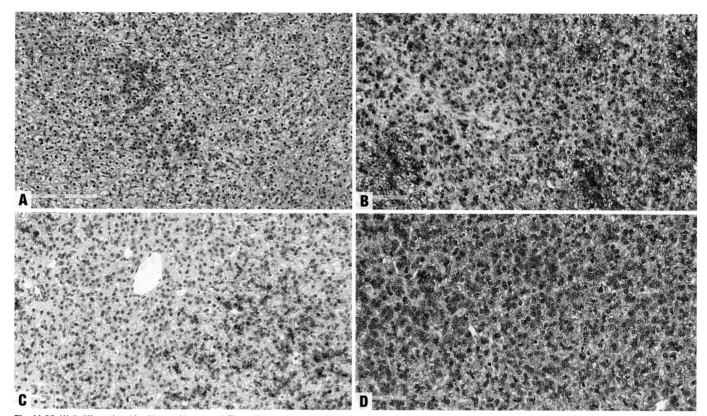

**Fig. 11.02** Well-differentiated fetal hepatoblastoma. **A** The uniform polygonal cells show a light and dark cell pattern and no mitotic activity. **B** Strong nuclear β-catenin staining is present. **C** Fine granular glypican-3 (GPC3) immunostaining staining is seen in the cells of well-differentiated fetal hepatoblastoma. **D** Glutamine synthetase (GS) staining in the same case, showing strong cytoplasmic staining.

of nanograms per millilitre) and is only rarely < 100 ng/mL, without any clear association with specific histological subtypes. Thrombocytosis with platelet counts > 450 000/μL is frequent. On ultrasound, HBLs usually appear as well-defined, lobulated, heterogeneous, and mildly echogenic masses that may show calcifications and areas of haemorrhage. Imaging studies serve as the modality for pretreatment extent of disease (PRETEXT) staging of these tumours (see Box 11.02) {6269,7042}. On

CT, HBLs appear as well-defined hypodense or occasionally isodense masses. Intratumoural cystic changes, haemorrhage, and necrotic foci may be observed. On MRI, most tumours are heterogeneous, hypoenhancing, T2-hyperintense, and T1-hypointense lesions, and they are hypointense with gadolinium in the hepatobiliary phase.

### Epidemiology

The overall incidence of HBL is increasing worldwide {3045}. A recent SEER database analysis showed an increase from 1.89 cases per 1 million population in the year 2000 to 2.16 cases per 1 million in 2015 {2076}. There was a significant rise in incidence in boys, with an overall M:F ratio of 2:1. The incidence was highest in children aged 0–1 years (11.19 cases per 1 million), followed by children aged 2–4 years (5.66 cases per 1 million) and those aged 5–18 years (0.18 cases per 1 million) {2076}. An association with prematurity and very low birth weight (< 1500 g) is well documented {6614,4528}. Other associations have been reported including maternal smoking, use of infertility treatment, and younger maternal age {4528,6615, 6613,4883}.

### Etiology

Several congenital abnormalities and constitutional genetic syndromes have been associated with HBL {6274,3483} (see Box 11.03). An increased incidence, warranting surveillance, is seen in patients with Beckwith–Wiedemann syndrome and other syndromes {4879,6613}. However, the majority of HBLs appear to be sporadic.

**Box 11.02** The 2017 pretreatment extent of disease (PRETEXT) staging system for liver tumours {7042}

**PRETEXT group**
PRETEXT I: One section is involved and three adjoining sections are free.
PRETEXT II: One or two sections are involved and two adjoining sections are free.
PRETEXT III: Two or three sections are involved and no two adjoining sections are free.
PRETEXT IV: All four sections are involved.

**Annotation factors**
V: Hepatic venous / inferior vena cava involvement
P: Portal venous involvement
E: Extrahepatic spread of disease
F: Multifocal tumour
R: Tumour rupture
C: Tumour involving caudate lobe
N: Lymph node metastases
M: Distant metastases

Note: PRETEXT groups the liver into four sections (previously referred to as sectors): the left lateral section (segments 2 and 3), the left medial section (segments 4a and 4b), the right anterior section (segments 5 and 8), and the right posterior section (segments 6 and 7).

## Pathogenesis

HBLs are thought to arise from progenitor cells (hepatoblasts) with the propensity to differentiate along different lineages, giving rise to the histological spectrum of this tumour.

In general, HBLs are tumours that have relatively stable genomes with a very low rate of somatic mutations {2558}. The WNT/β-catenin pathway appears to be central to HBL development, with as many as 90% of cases harbouring *CTNNB1* mutations, resulting in upregulation of downstream WNT targets {589,4266}. *NFE2L2* is the second most commonly mutated gene documented in HBL (5–10%), followed by mutations in the *TERT* promoter; both are associated with a poor prognosis. The presence of *TERT* promoter mutations is characteristic of the provisional subtype hepatocellular neoplasm NOS (HCN-NOS). Other pathways reported to be involved in HBL pathogenesis and potentially implicated in its clinical behaviour include the NOTCH, sonic hedgehog, PI3K/AKT, EGFR (HER1) and Hippo/YAP1 pathways, among others {4266,4220,1899,5770,6772, 6891}.

Gene expression profiling initially demonstrated two distinct genotype–phenotype HBL subtypes, C1 and C2, the C1 subtype with a more mature phenotype corresponding to fetal histology, and the C2 subtype recapitulating early fetal liver (embryonal histology) {974}. Further genomic studies demonstrated three distinct molecular HBL risk–associated subtypes, with high-risk tumours being characterized by high NFE2L2 activity; high expression of LIN28B, HMGA2, SALL4, and AFP; low let-7 expression; and low HNF1α activity {6772}. Recently, HBL epigenomic profiling demonstrated genome-wide dysregulation of RNA editing in HBL and identified additional epigenomic clusters, including an aggressive subgroup recognized by characteristic methylation features, strong expression of the 14q32 locus, mutations in *CTNNB1* and *NFE2L2*, and a progenitor-like phenotype {1058}.

## Macroscopic appearance

HBLs are usually single, well-circumscribed, lobulated, tan masses arising in normal liver. They may be grossly heterogeneous and are often surrounded by a pseudocapsule. After therapy, the tumours usually show cystic changes, with areas of haemorrhage and necrosis, as well as a more accentuated pseudocapsule. Large-vessel invasion can be seen. Areas of calcification or osteoid formation may be present.

## Histopathology

HBLs are classified according to the different components present (see Box 11.01, p. 775) as either epithelial HBL or mixed HBL (the latter when both epithelial and mesenchymal components are present).

Well-differentiated fetal HBL (pure fetal with low mitotic activity) is characterized by uniform polygonal cells with a low N:C ratio and few mitoses {4355,7487}, arranged in trabeculae that are 2 or 3 cells thick. This diagnosis can only be made on a primary tumour resection when the entire lesion can be evaluated, and not on a biopsy or after therapy. The cytoplasm is variably clear to eosinophilic and finely granular, and frequently a light and dark cell pattern is seen. These are generally low-stage tumours without necrosis or haemorrhage {3484}.

Crowded fetal HBL (fetal HBL with mitoses) is characterized by fetal areas showing polygonal cells with dense eosinophilic to amphophilic cytoplasm and round, centrally placed nuclei with inconspicuous to prominent nucleoli; there is no pleomorphism, and the cells are arranged in trabeculae. These areas frequently merge imperceptibly into embryonal areas. Extramedullary haematopoiesis is frequently present.

Embryonal HBL is characterized by smaller cells with a high N:C ratio, arranged in sheets or nests, that may merge with fetal cells. The nuclei are angulated rather than round. Nucleoli and mitoses are frequent. The tumour cells are frequently arranged

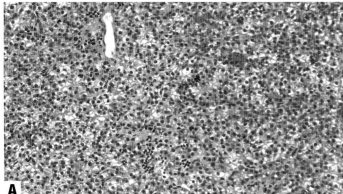
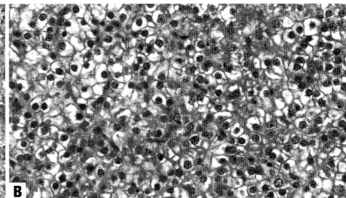

**Fig. 11.03** Hepatoblastoma. **A** Crowded fetal pattern. An area with monotonous polygonal cells with increased N:C ratios and round nuclei. Note the extramedullary haematopoiesis. **B** Crowded fetal pattern showing fetal cells with larger nuclei and mitoses.

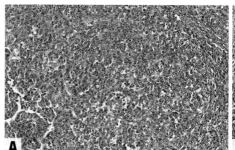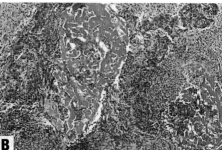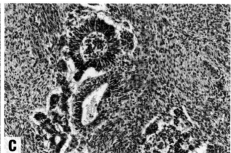

**Fig. 11.04** Hepatoblastoma. **A** Embryonal hepatoblastoma with a small cell undifferentiated component, cells with scant cytoplasm and oval to angulated nuclei, and a focus of small cells in the upper quadrant. **B** Mixed hepatoblastoma showing the epithelial fetal pattern, osteoid, and blastema. **C** Primitive neuroepithelial rosettes in a teratoid hepatoblastoma.

in rosettes and tubular forms. Extramedullary haematopoiesis may be seen.

The macrotrabecular pattern of HBL is characterized by trabeculae > 5 cells thick, mimicking the pattern seen in hepatocellular carcinoma. These cells can have either a fetal or an embryonal phenotype. The macrotrabecular pattern of HBL should not be mistaken for hepatocellular carcinoma, especially on a biopsy.

The pleomorphic epithelial (poorly differentiated) pattern is characterized by fetal or embryonal cells showing nuclear pleomorphism (including giant cells or frank anaplasia with large prominent nucleoli). These areas are noted occasionally in posttherapy resections and have been reported to be associated with chemoresistance and poor outcome, but they can also be seen in biopsies.

The category of pure small cell undifferentiated HBL is no longer accepted, because tumours showing loss of SMARCB1 (INI1) nuclear staining should be classified as malignant rhabdoid tumours. The more frequent occurrence is the presence of the small cell undifferentiated pattern as scattered small nests within other areas of the tumour. Cells have scant cytoplasm and stippled chromatin with variable mitoses and are arranged in different patterns, sometimes forming sheets and nests of small round to ovoid cells {7068}.

Another epithelial element that can be encountered is biliary differentiation (cholangioblastic HBL), which is usually seen at the periphery or intermixed with other epithelial areas. This is to be differentiated from the reactive biliary proliferation seen after therapy. Tumour cholangioblastic areas are positive for nuclear

β-catenin, unlike reactive ducts. A squamous component with keratin production may also be seen occasionally.

Mixed HBL is characterized by any of the epithelial elements associated with stromal derivates, including osteoid and other mesenchymal elements (e.g. spindle cells [blastemas], cartilage, and rhabdomyoblastic and fat components). Some of the mesenchymal elements are detected on imaging, so the presence of calcifications is suggestive of mixed HBL at diagnosis. Posttherapy specimens tend to show cells differentiating into bone, still considered neoplastic. The presence of a mixture of heterologous components – including endoderm, neural elements (e.g. glial tissue), and neuroectodermal derivates (e.g. neuromelanin or primitive neuroepithelial rosettes) – warrants the diagnosis of a teratoid HBL. Rare examples of neuroendocrine differentiation and yolk sac–like glands in teratoid areas, all demonstrating nuclear expression of β-catenin, have been documented.

Posttherapy resections may show areas of differentiation and chemotherapy effects including necrosis, haemorrhage, peliosis-like spaces, and extensive bone formation. Large areas of fibrous reaction, histiocytic infiltrate, and haemosiderin pigment may be seen. It is important not to mistake haemosiderin-laden cells for melanin pigment.

Immunohistochemistry may be useful to identify different components, as shown in Table 11.01. Other immunohistochemical stains that can be used include AFP, which highlights tumour cells. Arginase and HepPar-1 do not help distinguish from nonneoplastic liver but are generally positive.

HCN-NOS is a new provisional category that includes tumours previously designated as transitional cell liver tumours

**Table 11.01** Immunohistochemistry (IHC) in the diagnosis of hepatoblastoma

| IHC stain | Histology | | | | | | | |
|---|---|---|---|---|---|---|---|---|
| | WDF | CF | E | SCUD | Blastema | Osteoid | Cholangio | HCN-NOS |
| β-catenin nuclear | +/++ | ++ | +++ | +++ | Neg/++ | ++ | ++ | +/+++ |
| GPC3 | + | ++/+++ | +++/Neg | Neg | Neg | Neg | Neg | +/++ |
| GS | +++ | +++ | +/+++ | Neg | Neg/+ | Neg | Neg/+ | + |
| MOC31 | + | +++ | +++ | Neg | Neg | Neg | +++ | ++ |
| SALL4 | Neg | Neg | ++/+++ | Neg | Neg | Neg | Neg | +/++ |
| SMARCB1 (INI1) | + | + | + | + | + | + | + | + |
| CK19 | Neg | Neg/+ | +/++ | ++ | ++ | Neg | +++ | Neg/+ |

CF, crowded fetal; Cholangio, cholangioblastic; E, embryonal; GPC3, glypican-3; GS, glutamine synthetase; HCN-NOS, hepatocellular neoplasm NOS; Neg, negative; SCUD, small cell undifferentiated; WDF, well-differentiated fetal.

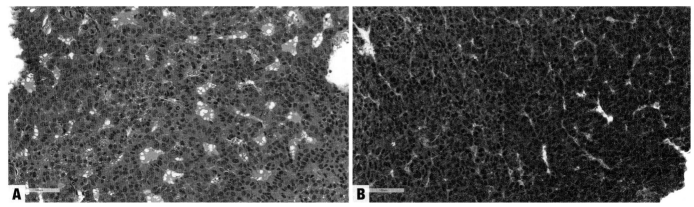

**Fig. 11.05** Hepatocellular neoplasm NOS. **A** Biopsy of a lesion composed of primitive cells, some with angulated nuclei, but with an acinar arrangement, mimicking hepatocellular carcinoma. **B** There is nuclear β-catenin staining in almost every tumour cell.

{5656} and thought to represent lesions with intermediate or combined biology and histological features of both HBL and hepatocellular carcinoma, sometimes in distinct areas of the tumour. The tumour cells may also be monotonous and resemble crowded fetal cells. There may be a macrotrabecular arrangement. Hepatocellular carcinoma features are often seen in posttherapy specimens. HCN-NOS carries mutations in *CTNNB1* (encoding β-catenin), as well as other mutations seen in hepatocellular carcinoma, such as *TERT* promoter mutations, which are associated with a poor prognosis {6772,1899}. HCN-NOS can occur at any age but is more frequent in children aged > 8 years without underlying liver disease. These tumours are usually aggressive, and those recorded in the literature appear to be associated with a poor outcome. They are treated as group D (high-risk HBL) in the current Paediatric Hepatic International Tumour Trial (PHITT) {1359}.

For the differential diagnosis of HBL, see Table 11.02.

## Cytology

Cytological diagnosis is not recommended, because it limits the evaluation of histological components, tumour architecture, and the amount of tissue for sometimes-needed ancillary studies. Neoplastic cells in the fetal component can be difficult to distinguish from normal hepatocytes in such specimens.

**Table 11.02** Differential diagnosis of hepatoblastoma (HBL), malignant hepatocellular neoplasm NOS (HCN-NOS), and hepatocellular carcinoma (HCC)

| Characteristic | HBL | HCN-NOS | HCC |
|---|---|---|---|
| Cytology | Uniform: WDF<br><br>Mixed pattern: fetal cells (polygonal, uniform, clear to eosinophilic cytoplasm, round nuclei ± nucleoli)<br><br>Embryonal: scant cytoplasm, high N:C ratio, oval nuclei, nucleoli+, mitoses++<br><br>SCUD: small cells, monotonous<br><br>Blastema: ovoid to spindle to round in sheets<br><br>Mixed: with osteoid, fat, muscle | Monotonous population of cells with high N:C ratios; sheet-like arrangement rather than trabecular (some macrotrabecular); 5–10 cells thick; no clear embryonal/fetal distinction; variable pleomorphism, difficult diagnosis on biopsy without immunohistochemistry; in rare cases, hepatoblastoma and HCC occur in different nodules | Well-differentiated tumours; monotonous; large nuclei with magenta nucleoli and intranuclear inclusions; cytoplasmic globules; higher grades with pleomorphism; trabeculae 15–20 cells thick; sheet-like arrangement possible; necrosis+; mitosis++; hyaline globules++; fat present; sclerosis in fibrolamellar HCC |
| Background liver | Normal | Normal | Either cirrhotic or normal |
| Age | Most 0–4 years, some > 4 years | Usually ≥ 8 years; can be < 8 years | Usually second decade of life; can be 2–10 years; fibrolamellar HCC second decade |
| AFP | Elevated (> 100 ng/dL) | Variable usually elevated | Elevated or normal |
| PHITT group | Groups A–D | Group D | Groups E and F |
| **Immunohistochemistry** | | | |
| β-catenin nuclear | Fetal focal+; crowded fetal / embryonal +++ | +/++ | Often negative but can be positive |
| GS cytoplasmic | +++ fetal; + to +++ embryonal | + to +++ patchy | Variable; weak to positive |
| GPC3 cytoplasmic | + to +++ | +/++ patchy, weak | +/++ patchy |
| MOC31 membranous | + | + | + |
| PROX1 nuclear | + | + | – |
| SALL4 nuclear | + | Often + | Occasionally + |
| Molecular | *CTNNB1* mutation in 90% | *CTNNB1* + *TERT* / other HCC mutations | Occasionally *CTNNB1*; *TERT*+; *TP53*+ other HCC mutations |

GPC3, glypican-3; GS, glutamine synthetase; PHITT, Paediatric Hepatic International Tumour Trial; SCUD, small cell undifferentiated; WDF, well-differentiated fetal.

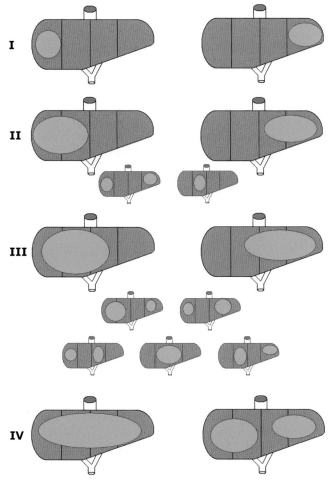

**Fig. 11.06** PRETEXT staging. An illustration of pretreatment extent of disease (PRE-TEXT) staging as determined by the involvement of contiguous segments of liver.

## Diagnostic molecular pathology

About 90% of HBLs carry *CTNNB1* mutations, and the remainder may be associated with germline *APC* mutations or with mutations in other WNT pathway genes. Mutation testing of the *TERT* promoter and of *NFE2L2* and other prognostically relevant genes may be useful in aggressive tumours {974A}, particularly for the diagnosis of HCN-NOS and tumours demonstrating chemoresistance.

## Essential and desirable diagnostic criteria

*Essential:* sheets of neoplastic cells – either solely epithelial cells resembling fetal/embryonal liver cells, and/or undifferentiated cells alone or in various combinations, or malignant epithelial and stromal derivates (including spindle cells, osteoid, or other components in addition to the epithelial component[s]); for the teratoid subtype: heterologous elements including endoderm, neuroectodermal derivates, melanin-containing cells, and/or other elements.

*Desirable:* *CTNNB1* mutation or nuclear β-catenin expression by immunohistochemistry; for HCN-NOS: *TERT* promoter mutation and/or other hepatocellular carcinoma–associated mutations.

## Staging

The pretreatment extent of disease (PRETEXT) system is used for the staging of HBL and has been adopted for risk stratification in the current PHITT {1359,7042,5950}. It describes the extent of tumour involvement of surgical liver segments and is reflective of the extent of involvement of the liver. Annotation factors include venous and extrahepatic tumour, as well as metastasis.

## Prognosis and prediction

The salient known prognostic factors are listed in Table 11.03. The 5-year survival rate for the combined stages of HBL is 60–70%. The survival rate is > 80% for patients with surgically resectable tumours after chemotherapy, but it is worse for children with higher-stage, chemoresistant, or metastatic tumours.

**Table 11.03** Prognostic markers in hepatoblastoma

| Factor | Prognosis | |
|---|---|---|
| | **Good/unaffected** | **Poor/worse** |
| **Age** | 0–7 years (provisional) | > 8 years; 6 years by CHIC data |
| **AFP** | > 1000 ng/dL | < 100 ng/dL |
| **PRETEXT stage** | I, II | III, IV, positive annotation<br>Metastasis |
| **Surgical** | Complete resection | Positive margins<br>Tumour rupture |
| **Vascular invasion** | Absent | Present |
| **Histological** | WDF pattern | Pleomorphic, HCN-NOS, macrotrabecular |
| **Chemotherapy response** | > 50% | < 50% |
| **Molecular** | *CTNNB1*<br>C1 genotype/phenotype[a] | C2 genotype/phenotype[a]<br>*NFE2L2* mutations<br>*TERT* promoter mutations<br>High expression of oncofetal proteins and stem cell markers |

CHIC, Children's Hepatic Tumors International Collaboration; HCN-NOS, hepatocellular neoplasm NOS; PRETEXT, pretreatment extent of disease; WDF, well-differentiated fetal.
[a]C1 and C2 are expression profile clusters as described by Cairo et al. {974}.

# Fibrolamellar variant of hepatocellular carcinoma

Cho SJ
Makhlouf HR
Ranganathan S

## Definition

The fibrolamellar variant of hepatocellular carcinoma (FLHCC) is a primary malignancy of the liver composed of epithelial cells showing hepatocellular differentiation with characteristic morphological features and recurrent genomic abnormalities typically involving the *PRKACA* gene.

## ICD-O coding

8171/3 Hepatocellular carcinoma, fibrolamellar

## ICD-11 coding

2C12.02 & XH9Q35 Hepatocellular carcinoma of liver & Hepatocellular carcinoma, fibrolamellar

## Related terminology

*Acceptable:* fibrolamellar carcinoma; hepatocellular carcinoma, fibrolamellar.

## Subtype(s)

None

## Localization

FLHCC can occur in any portion of the liver but is most common in the left lobe {1471}, and it has a propensity to involve the hilum.

## Clinical features

Patients present with an abdominal mass or hepatomegaly, and/or with otherwise nonspecific symptoms including nausea, vomiting, abdominal pain, malaise, and weight loss {7018}. Less common are mass effects due to the tumour, including biliary or vena caval obstruction. Rarely, FLHCC may occur with gynaecomastia, recurrent deep vein thrombosis, Budd–Chiari syndrome, non-bacterial thrombotic endocarditis, fulminant liver failure, or encephalopathy {3907,4500,6346}. Other uncommon clinical features include increased serum neurotensin or increased serum transcobalamin 1 (TCN1, also called haptocorrin) {2525}.

Patients with FLHCC typically do not have underlying liver disease, and almost all cases (95%) arise in non-cirrhotic livers. No elevation in serum AFP is seen. Lymphatic spread is common, as are peritoneal spread and lymphovascular invasion {3105,6700, 5550,1971,6687}. Ovarian metastasis has been reported {603}.

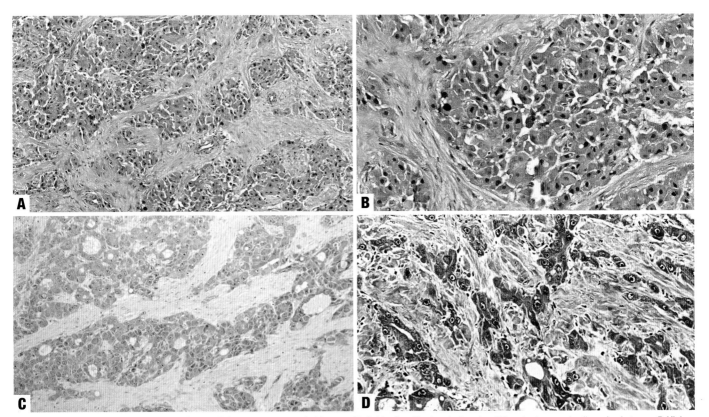

**Fig. 11.07** Fibrolamellar hepatocellular carcinoma. **A** A tumour composed of large epithelioid cells with abundant eosinophilic cytoplasm and collagenized stroma. **B** Higher-magnification view showing pleomorphic nuclei with variable nucleoli and eosinophilic cytoplasm. **C** A tumour showing areas with glandular architecture. **D** Trichrome stain highlighting fibrous stroma.

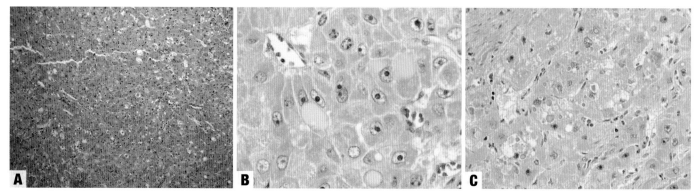

**Fig. 11.08** Fibrolamellar hepatocellular carcinoma. **A** A tumour showing a solid pattern of growth. **B** Higher-magnification view showing tumour cells with pleomorphic nuclei, variable nucleoli, and granular eosinophilic cytoplasm, focally containing pale bodies (centre). **C** Tumour cells may also contain cytoplasmic hyaline bodies (centre).

## Imaging

On CT, FLHCC is usually a large, heterogeneous, well-defined mass that is predominantly hypoattenuating on unenhanced images {3104,2234}. Calcification is seen in 50% of cases {3104, 2234}. Although a central stellate scar is seen in two thirds of FLHCCs {3104,720}, it is not pathognomonic. On MRI, FLHCC is usually hypointense on T1-weighted images and hyperintense on T2-weighted images {3104}. The central scar is typically hypointense on both T1- and T2-weighted images, a feature that can help distinguish FLHCC from focal nodular hyperplasia (in which the scar is predominantly T2-hyperintense) {2307}. With gadolinium contrast, FLHCC shows arterial hyperenhancement and early venous washout {2307,1789}.

## Epidemiology

FLHCC accounts for 15–25% of paediatric hepatocellular carcinomas (HCCs) and is exclusive to children aged > 5 years {175}. Children with FLHCC are older than those with HCC (88% vs 29% aged > 12 years, respectively), and unlike in HCC there is no male predominance {7470}.

## Etiology

Unknown

## Pathogenesis

Activation of PKA (a tetramer composed of two regulatory and two catalytic subunits) via the increased activity of *PRKACA* appears to be a central mechanism in FLHCC tumorigenesis. In nearly all sporadic cases, this activation occurs through a *DNAJB1::PRKACA* fusion, which results from a 400 kb deletion of chromosome 19 {2967}. The fusion transcript leads to increased PKA Cα subunit expression and PKA activity. Studies in mice have shown that the fusion transcript is sufficient to induce hepatic tumours that are morphologically similar to FLHCC {1958}.

The *DNAJB1::PRKACA* fusion is present in the vast majority of cases of FLHCC, but rare cases have been reported that lack

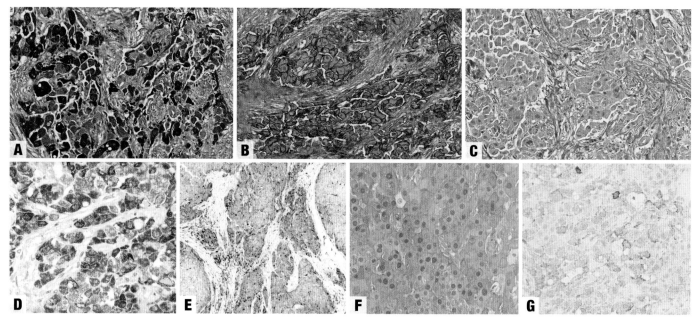

**Fig. 11.09** Fibrolamellar hepatocellular carcinoma. **A** There is strong diffuse cytoplasmic staining of tumour cells for CK7. **B** There is a predominantly membranous pattern of staining for β-catenin. **C** A glypican-3 (GPC3) stain shows focal positivity in tumour cells. **D** Tumour cells demonstrate positivity for immunohistochemical markers of hepatocellular differentiation, including HepPar-1. **E** Positive CD68 cytoplasmic staining in tumour cells. **F** An arginase-1 (ARG1) stain showing diffuse positivity in tumour cells. **G** In situ hybridization for albumin is positive in the cytoplasm of tumour cells.

the fusion and instead demonstrate mutations in *PRKAR1A*. The majority of these cases occur in patients with Carney complex, 60–70% of whom have a germline mutation in *PRKAR1A* {2522}. PRKAR1A is the regulatory subunit of PKA {2967}, the loss of which results in a gain of *PRKACA* function {3618}.

Although cytogenetic changes have been reported in FLHCC, no recurrent structural abnormalities other than the deletion in chromosome 19 have been identified {1561}. FLHCC lacks the common gene alterations seen in conventional HCC, including in *TP53* and *CTNNB1*.

## Macroscopic appearance
Most tumours are solitary and large (range: 90–140 mm) at the time of resection {5550}. Tumours consist of well-circumscribed, multinodular, yellow to tan to green masses that may range from soft to firm to hard in consistency. Cut sections reveal a central scar in approximately 70% of cases {3104}. Gross vascular invasion may be seen (25% of cases) {5550}. The background liver is non-cirrhotic.

## Histopathology
FLHCC consists of large polygonal cells with vesicular nuclear chromatin, prominent single nucleoli, and abundant granular and eosinophilic cytoplasm due to abundant mitochondria {2054}, lysosomes {2054}, and/or endosomal cytoplasmic accumulations {5997}. Binucleated and multinucleated tumour cells can be seen. The tumour cells are arranged in trabeculae, cords, and nests in a dense fibrous stroma classically arranged in parallel lamellae.

Other classic (but nonspecific) features of FLHCC include pale eosinophilic cytoplasmic bodies, thought to be composed at least partly of fibrinogen, and hyaline bodies, which may be seen in approximately 50% of cases.

Other features include calcifications, bile production, and pseudoglandular structures with mucin production, as well as solid and peliotic patterns.

Immunohistochemically, tumour cells express markers of hepatocellular differentiation, including HepPar-1 and arginase-1 (ARG1); albumin mRNA can be detected by in situ hybridization. FLHCC may show a canalicular staining pattern for polyclonal CEA. Glypican-3 (GPC3) positivity is also reported (in 17–64% of cases) {19,6356,7438}. AFP is usually negative. Characteristically, almost all cases (85–90%) of FLHCC demonstrate strong diffuse expression of CK7 and CD68 due to abundant lysosomes {2526,5997}; these findings are also seen in conventional HCC (CK7 in 20–30% of cases {19,7438}; CD68 in 10–25% {5997}). The expression of CK7 and CD68 may be patchy, and rare cases may be negative. FLHCC also stains for α1-antitrypsin and copper. It shows strong expression of AGR2 {7317}. Rarely, expression of neuroendocrine markers is seen {7402}. Other markers that may be positive in FLHCC but are not in routine diagnostic use include EpCAM, CD56 (NCAM), CD113, and CD44 {7438}; liver fatty acid–binding protein expression may be absent {2524}.

## Cytology
FLHCC is characterized by aggregates of loosely cohesive polygonal cells with large nuclei, prominent nucleoli, and abundant oncocytic granular cytoplasm, which may contain pale bodies and hyaline bodies. Characteristic lamellar fibrosis may be seen within tumour fragments. A background of proliferating capillaries may be present {1582,3822,5450,6751}.

## Diagnostic molecular pathology
The *DNAJB1::PRKACA* fusion can be detected by RT-PCR, or by FISH {2520,2526}, which has a sensitivity of 97% and specificity of 100% for FLHCC in the context of a primary liver neoplasm {2526}. The fusion is not specific to FLHCC and has been reported in pancreatobiliary malignancies {7352}.

In the rare cases with mutations in *PRKAR1A* rather than the *DNAJB1::PRKACA* fusion, loss of PRKAR1A expression can be confirmed by immunohistochemistry {2522}.

## Essential and desirable diagnostic criteria
*Essential:* large polygonal cells with eosinophilic cytoplasm and macronucleoli; dense fibrosis; CK7 expression.
*Desirable:* demonstration of *DNAJB1::PRKACA* fusion.

## Staging
The current staging system is the eighth-edition American Joint Committee on Cancer (AJCC) or Union for International Cancer Control (UICC) system {238}. However, studies have shown limitations in the predictive value of this system in FLHCC {7689, 6700,3462}. Other proposed staging systems include the pre-treatment extent of disease (PRETEXT) system currently in use for hepatoblastoma {7042}, including in the ongoing Paediatric Hepatic International Tumour Trial (PHITT).

## Prognosis and prediction
In early studies of FLHCC, some showed that the survival of patients with FLHCC was better than that of patients with other HCC {1471,1971,2053,4903}, whereas others did not {3481, 7470}. Subsequent larger case series and meta-analyses have shown that overall survival is similar between patients with FLHCC and those with conventional HCC {5057,7689}. Likewise, studies of FLHCC in children have shown no differences in outcomes between FLHCC and other HCCs {3481,7470}, with a reported 5-year event-free survival rate of 30% in US trials {3481} and 3-year event-free and overall survival rates of 22% and 42%, respectively, in the SIOPEL studies {7470}; cases in younger patients (aged < 12 years) and with no multifocality show a trend towards better outcomes {4485}.

Cases of FLHCC with increased mitochondrial DNA levels {7316} and those with a greater number of chromosomal imbalances {3372} show aggressive behaviour.

Lymph node metastasis in FLHCC is common and does not affect prognosis {6700,7689}. Adverse prognostic features include vascular invasion, multifocality, and incomplete surgical resectability, including resectability of regional lymph node metastases {3462}. In children, FLHCC, like conventional HCC, has shown a poor response to chemotherapy, and the prognosis is determined by surgical resectability {3481,7470}.

# Paediatric hepatocellular carcinoma

Cho SJ
Guettier C
Hiyama E
Makhlouf HR
Ranganathan S
Rangaswami A

## Definition

Paediatric hepatocellular carcinoma (HCC) is a primary malignancy of the liver composed of epithelial cells showing hepatocellular differentiation, occurring before the age of 18 years.

## ICD-O coding

8170/3 Hepatocellular carcinoma, NOS
8170/3 Conventional hepatocellular carcinoma
8174/3 Clear cell hepatocellular carcinoma

## ICD-11 coding

2C12.02 & XH4W48 Hepatocellular carcinoma of liver & Hepatocellular carcinoma, NOS
2C12.02 & XH4T58 Hepatocellular carcinoma of liver & Hepatocellular carcinoma, clear cell type

## Related terminology

None

## Subtype(s)

Conventional hepatocellular carcinoma; clear cell hepatocellular carcinoma

## Localization

HCC can occur anywhere within the liver as a single nodule or multiple nodules.

## Clinical features

Common symptoms include abdominal pain, distension, a mass, fatigue, and weight loss, as well as cachexia and jaundice in advanced disease. In the setting of chronic liver disease, children may present with signs of end-stage liver disease. As many as one third of cases are asymptomatic and detected on

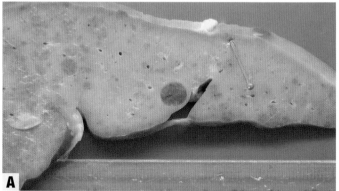

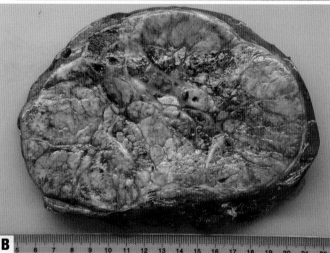

**Fig. 11.11** Hepatocellular carcinoma. **A** An encapsulated small hepatocellular carcinoma of 8 mm in a 9-month-old child, occurring in cirrhotic liver due to progressive familial intrahepatic cholestasis type 2. **B** Hepatocellular carcinoma of the conventional type. A well-limited and partially encapsulated large tumour of 160 mm within normal liver parenchyma. Tumoural tissue is polychromatic with some necrotic changes.

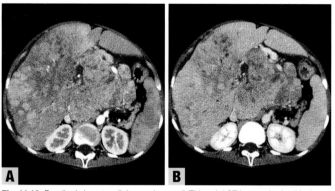

**Fig. 11.10** Paediatric hepatocellular carcinoma. **A** This axial CT image obtained in the arterial phase of enhancement shows multiple nodular enhancement, giving rise to a mosaic appearance within a large tumour. **B** This axial CT image obtained in the portal phase of enhancement shows washout of the previously enhanced area, with areas of non-enhancement suggestive of necrosis. There is also associated portal vein thrombosis.

imaging during systematic follow-up of chronic liver disease or incidentally diagnosed at pathological examination of the explanted liver {3544,4740}.

Serum AFP level is elevated in 67–92% of cases and can be as high as $1.4 \times 10^6$ ng/mL {3544,5961,7824}. Children with tyrosinaemia, however, can present with very high AFP values due to liver regeneration alone, without HCC.

Ultrasound is useful for detecting tumours in the setting of chronic liver disease, but multiphase contrast-enhanced CT or MRI is necessary to confirm the diagnosis. In children, CT is preferred for the evaluation of tumour extent, vascular invasion, and resectability, because of the technical complexity, limited availability, and intubation requirements of MRI in young patients. Contrast-enhanced ultrasound is promising because it avoids exposure to ionizing radiation {3544}.

The European, US, and Asia-Pacific {1987,2821,5179} recommendations for the diagnosis of HCC in adults have not been validated in children; however, it is suggested that diagnosis of paediatric HCC in non-cirrhotic livers needs histological confirmation, whereas in cirrhotic livers, diagnosis may be based on suggestive imaging and high AFP levels {3512}.

## Epidemiology

Malignant primary liver tumours account for 1–2% of paediatric solid tumours, with hepatoblastoma (HBL) accounting for the majority of cases (70–80%) and HCC being the second most common (20–30%). In patients aged < 5 years, 91% of primary liver tumours are HBLs, whereas HCCs account for 87% of primary liver tumours among patients aged 15–19 years {1559}. The overall age-adjusted incidence rate of HCC is 0.41 cases per 1 million person-years, with a slight male predominance (0.45 vs 0.37 cases per 1 million person-years for male and female populations, respectively) {1559}.

The epidemiology of non-fibrolamellar paediatric HCC varies substantially depending on the level of endemic HBV infection (see Table 11.04). HBV vaccination programmes have resulted

**Table 11.04** Conditions associated with the development of paediatric hepatocellular carcinoma (HCC)

| Condition | Characteristic features and epidemiology |
|---|---|
| **HBV infection** | In Asian countries:<br>• Most commonly due to perinatally acquired infection<br>• Sharp decrease in incidence with HBV vaccination programmes {1161,3057}<br><br>In African countries:<br>• HBV transmission mostly horizontal in early childhood {1160}<br><br>In North America<br>• Minority of paediatric HCC {4740}<br><br>HCCs occur at 12–15 years of age<br><br>Marked male predominance (M:F ratio: 1.2–13.1:1)<br><br>Can arise in cirrhotic (> 50% of cases) and non-cirrhotic liver<br><br>HCC is associated with HBV genotypes B and F {5001} |
| **Tyrosinaemia** {4488,7826} | Prevalence of HCC: 14–75%<br><br>Prevalence increases with age<br><br>Dietary restriction and nitisinone treatment lead to decreased incidence, but nitisinone must be started early |
| **GSD type 1 and type 3** | HCC rare in childhood<br><br>GSD type 1<br>• Develops through adenoma–carcinoma sequence<br><br>GSD type 3<br>• Occurs in background of cirrhosis |
| **Progressive familial intrahepatic cholestasis**<br>• BSEP deficiency<br>• MDR3 deficiency {7299}<br>• TJP2 deficiency {7855,7300} | BSEP deficiency:<br>• HCC occurs early, at 13–52 months of age {3665}<br>• Risk of HCC at 2 years of age is 5–10% {4959} |
| **Biliary atresia** | Prevalence of HCC: ~1%<br>Most tumours diagnosed before 5 years of age {2656}<br>Some HCCs incidental in explanted liver |
| **Alagille syndrome** {3570,669} | |
| **Vascular liver disease**<br>• Congenital portosystemic shunt (Abernethy malformation)<br>• Hepatic venous outflow obstruction / Budd–Chiari syndrome<br>• Congenital heart disease +/− Fontan procedure {3714} | Congenital portosystemic shunt<br>• 20–50% of patients develop hepatocellular nodules (median age: 8 years), including FNH-like (60%), HCA (30%), regenerative, HBL, and HCC (2.5%) {3544}<br>• HCC may occur de novo or via malignant transformation of benign nodules {631,5669,6146} |
| **α1-antitrypsin deficiency** | HCC mostly in adults; rarely in children {2655} |
| **Mitochondrial respiratory chain disorders** {6219} | |
| **Genetic syndromes**<br>• Fanconi–Bickel syndrome {5584}<br>• Ataxia telangiectasia<br>• Fanconi anaemia<br>• Familial adenomatous polyposis<br>• Neurofibromatosis | |

BSEP, bile salt export pump; FNH, focal nodular hyperplasia; GSD, glycogen storage disease; HBL, hepatoblastoma; HCA, hepatocellular adenoma; MDR3, multidrug resistance protein 3; TJP2, tight junction protein 2.

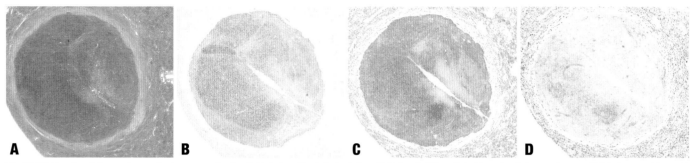

**Fig. 11.12** Hepatocellular carcinoma due to progressive familial intrahepatic cholestasis type 2. **A** A well-differentiated hepatocellular carcinoma with intratumoural haematopoiesis. **B** Diffuse positivity of tumour cells for glypican-3 (GPC3). **C** Diffuse positivity of tumour cells for EpCAM. **D** Heterogeneous positivity of tumour cells for CK19.

in a sharp decrease in the incidence of paediatric HCCs {1161, 3057}, but chronic HBV infection still accounts for the majority of cases worldwide.

Two distinct subsets of paediatric HCC are observed in Europe and North America, the first occurring in the setting of inherited liver disease, biliary atresia, or vascular malformations, and occurring most often in cirrhotic livers; the second is sporadic / de novo HCC, which occurs in normal liver {3544,3950, 5186}. The proportion of each subset is unclear. In the USA, the first subset represents one third of paediatric HCC cases {1827, 2664}, whereas in European countries, it seems predominant {545,7824}. In some inherited liver diseases, HCC develops within the first few years of life, whereas sporadic HCC usually occurs in children aged > 10 years {2656}. Patients with sporadic HCC typically present at an advanced stage, with unresectable or metastatic disease {5186}. The incidence of HCC can be reduced by universal HBV vaccination, improvement in medical therapies (e.g. treatment for tyrosinaemia), and early transplantation for inherited liver disease {2656}.

## Etiology

Chronic HBV infection is the most common etiology of paediatric HCC. The main underlying inherited conditions that predispose to paediatric HCC are tyrosinaemia type 1 and bile salt export pump (BSEP) deficiency. Other conditions include biliary atresia, mitochondrial respiratory chain disorders, Fanconi–Bickel syndrome (*SLC2A2* [*GLUT2*] mutation), and glycogen storage disease type 1. HCC also occurs in children with vascular liver diseases, including congenital portosystemic shunts, venous outflow obstruction / Budd–Chiari syndrome, and liver disease related to congenital heart disease with or without the Fontan procedure. These and other less common etiologies are summarized in Table 11.04 (p. 785).

## Pathogenesis

The pathogenesis of paediatric HCC is still largely unknown compared with adult HCC, because of its rarity and etiological diversity. The genetic alterations and pathogenesis have largely been inferred from studies of adult HCCs. However, unlike adult HCCs, HCCs in children often arise de novo, without underlying cirrhosis, so the mechanisms of transformation appear to be different.

For HBV-associated HCC, carcinogenesis may follow the classic pattern as described in adults (chronic hepatitis – cirrhosis – premalignant lesions – HCC), but approximately 50% of paediatric HCCs develop without cirrhosis {3544}.

A recent study evaluating 15 cases using various molecular methods found that alterations seen in adult HCCs were also seen in paediatric HCCs, including multiple molecular alterations in WNT pathway genes (most commonly intragenic deletions of *CTNNB1*; also *APC* inversion and *AMER1* somatic mutation) and telomerase pathway genes (*TERT* activation or *ATRX* mutation), but *TP53* mutations, although detected, were much less frequent {2664}. Potentially therapeutically targetable mutations in the MAPK/ERK signalling pathway (*MAPK1* and *BRAF*) were seen in 20% of cases {2664}. Tumours arising in children with underlying liver disease were found to be molecularly distinct and lacked obvious oncogenic drivers compared with those arising de novo. Molecular alterations in paediatric HCC are summarized in Table 11.05.

Massive gene amplification has been observed in paediatric HCC occurring in the setting of BSEP deficiency {3099}, along with somatic mutations in *CTNNB1* and *NFE2L2* {7301}. In children with congenital portosystemic shunts, *CTNNB1* mutations seem to be a major event in the malignant transformation of benign hepatocellular nodules {6146,6593}.

Germline mutations in *CDKN2A* (*P16INK4A*), *APC*, and *BRCA2* have been reported to be associated with the development of de novo HCC {5269}.

Additional information on the biology of paediatric HCC and potential therapeutic targets may become available in the future,

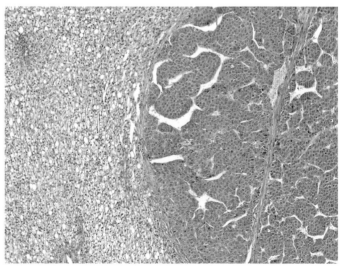

**Fig. 11.13** Hepatocellular carcinoma in a 9-year-old child with tyrosinaemia type 1. Macrotrabecular and steatotic subtypes in the same tumour.

**Table 11.05** Summary of molecular alterations in paediatric non-fibrolamellar hepatocellular carcinoma {2664,3931,5354,7685,7301}

| Pathway | Molecular alterations | No underlying liver disease | Underlying liver disease |
|---|---|---|---|
| WNT pathway | CTNNB1 deletion | ++ | – |
| | CTNNB1 mutation | – | + (BSEP) |
| | AMER1 mutation | + | – |
| | APC germline inversion | + | – |
| | WNT expression cluster | ++ | + |
| Telomeres | TERT promoter deletion | + | – |
| | TERT focal gain | + | – |
| | TERT promoter mutation | – | – |
| | ATRX mutation | – | + |
| MAPK/ERK signalling pathway | MAPK1 mutation | + | – |
| | BRAF mutation | + | – |
| | RPS6KA3 mutation | + | – |
| DNA repair and surveillance | CDKN2A copy-number loss | ++ | – |
| | CDKN2A mutation | + | – |
| | RB1 copy-number loss | ++ | + |
| | TP53 mutation | – | + |
| Hippo pathway | YAP1 nuclear localization | ++ | n/a |
| | YAP1 target increases | + | |
| Oxidative stress | NFE2L2 mutation | – | + (BSEP) |
| c-Met | MET mutation | n/a | ++ (HBV) |

BSEP, bile salt export pump; n/a, not applicable.

given the inclusion of HCC in the current Paediatric Hepatic International Tumour Trial (PHITT).

## Macroscopic appearance

Like HCCs reported in adults, HCCs in children are variably light-tan to yellow to green, depending on the amount of bile production or fat content. HCCs occurring in the setting of underlying liver disease tend to be multifocal and small, with > 90% of tumours measuring < 3 mm and 100% measuring < 10 mm {7824,3665}. A pseudocapsule may be present, particularly when occurring in a background of cirrhosis. Tumours occurring in normal liver are usually unifocal and larger (50–120 mm) {7305}, and they may be associated with satellite nodules and macrovascular invasion.

## Histopathology

The histopathological findings in paediatric HCC are overall similar to those seen in adult HCC, and the histological classification and grading of paediatric HCC follow the WHO classification of digestive system tumours. Tumours are graded as well, moderately, or poorly differentiated {7521}. Features more specific to paediatric HCC are discussed below. Microscopic vascular invasion is seen in 25–33% of cases {7824,2664}.

Subtypes in children reported in the SEER registry from 1973 to 2009 include conventional (73%), fibrolamellar (25%, see

*Fibrolamellar variant of hepatocellular carcinoma*, p. 781), and clear cell (2%) HCC {175}.

HCC in the setting of tyrosinaemia is notable for diffuse clear cell change and solid architecture, as well as nodules of different grades {2664}.

### Immunohistochemistry

See Table 11.06. Hepatocellular differentiation can be demonstrated by immunohistochemistry, including positivity for Hep-Par-1 and arginase-1 (ARG1). Paediatric HCC more frequently expresses glypican-3 (GPC3), EpCAM (usually diffuse), and CK19 than does adult HCC. Nuclear β-catenin is less frequent in HCC than in HBL {7824}.

### Premalignant lesions

Premalignant lesions, including dysplastic foci and dysplastic nodules (low-grade and high-grade), are found almost exclusively in cirrhotic livers and are overall rare in paediatric HCC, but they have been reported in the setting of tyrosinaemia {2664} and TJP2 deficiency {7855,7300}.

### Differential diagnosis

The distinction between HCC and HBL is critical for appropriate patient care. Differentiating HCC from pleomorphic and/or macrotrabecular epithelial HBL may be difficult; the patient's age (< 5 years) and the presence of more typical HBL areas or a mesenchymal component favour HBL. In older children, tumours with features of both HBL and HCC have been recognized and given a provisional diagnosis of malignant hepatocellular neoplasm NOS (see *Hepatoblastoma*, p. 775) {4219,7856, 5656}.

Hepatocellular adenomas are benign liver tumours in children, and they follow the recent molecular classification of adult hepatocellular adenomas {4948}. Differentiating between well-differentiated HCC and hepatocellular adenoma can be difficult; GPC3 expression, if present, favours HCC. A reticulin stain may be helpful in identifying areas of decrease or loss of the reticulin framework in HCC. Like those in adults, hepatocellular adenomas with mutations in *CTNNB1* (encoding β-catenin) occurring in children are at risk of malignant transformation.

**Table 11.06** Immunohistochemical staining patterns of paediatric and adult conventional hepatocellular carcinoma (HCC) and the fibrolamellar variant of hepatocellular carcinoma (FLHCC) {7824,7439,2664,5997,2526,4119}

| Marker | Staining pattern | Non-FLHCC paediatric HCC | Non-FLHCC adult HCC | FLHCC |
|---|---|---|---|---|
| GPC3 | M/Cy | 90% | 40–50% | 0–60% |
| β-catenin | N | 8% | 35% | 0% |
| EpCAM | M | 75–100% | 15% | 15–25% |
| CK19 | Cy | 33–50% | 5–10% | 20–25% |
| CK7 | Cy | 17% | 30% | 90–100% |
| CD68 | Cy | n/a | 20% | 95% |

Cy, cytoplasmic; GPC3, glypican-3; M, membranous; N, nuclear; n/a, not applicable.

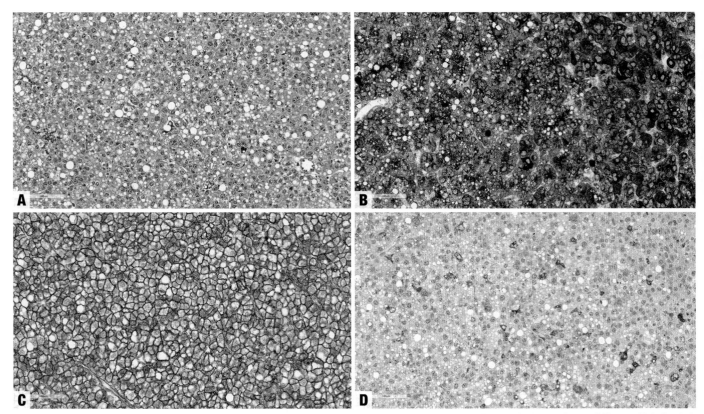

**Fig. 11.14** Well-differentiated hepatocellular carcinoma. **A** A higher-magnification image showing large nuclei with nucleoli and fat in the cytoplasm. **B** Diffuse positivity for glypican-3 (GPC3). **C** β-catenin immunohistochemistry showing mainly membranous staining and minimal cytoplasmic staining. **D** Glutamine synthetase (GS) immunohistochemistry showing weak and patchy staining of tumour cells.

Cholangiocarcinomas in children have been reported in the setting of biliary cysts, biliary atresia, and other biliary tract anomalies {4986}, including primary sclerosing cholangitis {1702,3330} and BSEP deficiency {6221}. Paediatric cholangiocarcinomas are histologically identical to adult cholangiocarcinomas {7521} and should be distinguished by histological (ductal/ductular/tubular morphology with or without mucin secretion) and immunophenotypic features (CK7 and CK19 expression without hepatocellular differentiation).

Neuroendocrine neoplasms (NENs) are rarely seen in the liver in the paediatric population; when they occur, they are predominantly metastases from extrahepatic primaries. Rare primary hepatic NENs have been reported {878}. Characteristic morphology and immunophenotype (e.g. synaptophysin, chromogranin) are necessary to confirm the diagnosis and to exclude primary hepatic neoplasms that may rarely or focally express neuroendocrine markers.

## Cytology
FNAB is not recommended in the evaluation of paediatric liver tumours.

## Diagnostic molecular pathology
Like that of adult HCC {7521}, the diagnosis of paediatric HCC primarily relies on imaging and histopathology, and diagnostic molecular tests are not available.

## Essential and desirable diagnostic criteria
*Essential:* hepatocellular differentiation as demonstrated by histology and immunohistochemical markers; proven malignancy, based on histological criteria and immunohistochemical markers; absence of other tumour components.

## Staging
There is no universally accepted staging system for paediatric HCC. The current TNM staging system is the same as that used for adult HCC, published by the American Joint Committee on Cancer (AJCC) and the Union for International Cancer Control (UICC) {238}. However, most international groups, including those participating in the ongoing PHITT, use the pretreatment extent of disease (PRETEXT) system currently used for HBL {7042}. The different staging systems for stratifying patients for liver transplantation have not been tested in children, but several studies have shown that children with non-metastatic HCC who fall beyond the Milan criteria may still benefit from transplantation {4490,1827,557}.

## Prognosis and prediction
Overall, the prognosis of paediatric HCC is poor (5-year survival rate: 17–28%) {1512,4862,175}. Two thirds of patients with paediatric HCC present with unresectable disease and there is limited benefit from chemotherapy {4862,3482}, although data from prior paediatric trials in North America and Europe suggest that de novo HCC in children may be more responsive to chemotherapy than that in adults {3482,4862}.

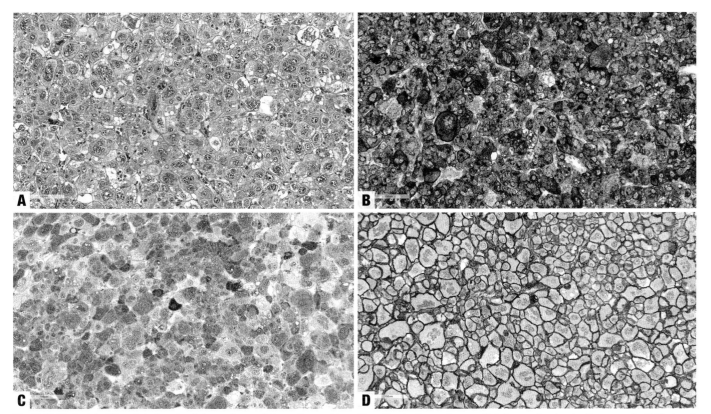

**Fig. 11.15** Moderately differentiated hepatocellular carcinoma. **A** Some pleomorphism with multinucleation can be seen. Note the prominent nucleoli in many cells. **B** Glypican-3 (GPC3) immunohistochemistry showing strong diffuse staining of cells. **C** Glutamine synthetase (GS) immunohistochemistry showing positive staining of tumour cells. **D** Membranous staining for β-catenin is seen in this example.

The most important prognostic factor appears to be tumour resectability, given that lymphovascular invasion, extrahepatic tumour, and metastatic disease precluding complete resection are poor prognostic factors {1514}. The subset of children with complete surgical resection or a liver transplant for a localized unresectable tumour have a much better prognosis, with 5-year overall survival rates ranging from 53% to 80%, even reaching 100% in the most recent series {4495,545,2015,4862, 7876}. The best results are achieved after liver transplantation, even outside the Milan criteria {3161,1827}, and in children with underlying inherited liver disease {4495,5291,545}. In these patients, vascular invasion is the most important prognostic factor {7305}.

# Mesenchymal hamartoma

Tsui WMS
Ranganathan S
Saxena R

## Definition
Mesenchymal hamartoma (MH) of the liver is a benign tumour characterized by a multicystic, loose connective tissue mass accompanied by a ductal component with ductal plate malformation.

## ICD-O coding
None

## ICD-11 coding
2E92.7 Benign neoplasm of liver or intrahepatic bile ducts

## Related terminology
None

## Subtype(s)
None

## Localization
MHs occur in the right lobe of the liver in 75% of cases, the left lobe in 22%, and both lobes in 3%.

## Clinical features
Patients with MH typically present with abdominal distension and an upper abdominal mass, although some cases are found incidentally. Pain is rarely a dominant feature, and only a few patients show anorexia, vomiting, or failure to thrive {1690}. Abdominal distention may progress rapidly and cause respiratory distress {6639}. Large MHs in neonates and infants may compromise blood circulation and evolve into life-threatening lesions. MH may be associated with mesenchymal stem villous hyperplasia of the placenta and Beckwith–Wiedemann syndrome {1062,979}. A subset of MHs are detectable prenatally (fetal MH), usually in the last trimester of pregnancy. Liver function is usually normal, but serum levels of AFP may be slightly elevated {773}; in exceptional cases, MH is associated with high levels of serum AFP {2599}. Rare association with neonatal

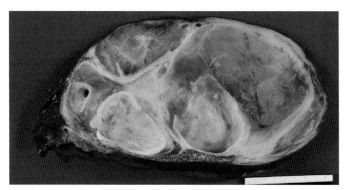

**Fig. 11.16** Mesenchymal hamartoma. A well-circumscribed tumour with solid and cystic areas.

hyperbilirubinaemia is reported {6702}. CT features are a well-circumscribed multilocular or multicystic mass that contains low-density cysts separated by a solid septum and stroma.

## Epidemiology
MH is the third most common hepatic tumour in childhood after hepatoblastoma and infantile haemangioma {6702,6733}. It accounts for 12% of all liver tumours occurring during the first 2 years of life and 8% of those occurring from birth to the age of 21 years. It occurs almost exclusively in young children (average age: 15 months). About 85% of affected children present before the age of 3 years, and < 5% of MHs are diagnosed after the age of 5 years {1690}. About 15% of cases have been observed in the neonatal period {4852}. MH is slightly more common in boys than in girls. In contrast, the rare MHs occurring in adults are more frequent in women than in men {7721}.

## Etiology
MH is primarily mesenchymal in origin and is believed to arise from a developmental abnormality in the formation of ductal plates during late embryogenesis, resulting in disordered arrangement of the mesenchyme, bile ducts, and hepatic parenchyma.

## Pathogenesis
There is cytogenetic and molecular genetic evidence that MH is neoplastic and not only a developmental process {6855}. This is supported by the documented evolution of MH to undifferentiated embryonal sarcoma {3968}.

Recurrent genetic alterations found in MH include either chromosomal rearrangements involving chromosome 19q13.4 (in sporadic cases) {5745,6382} or androgenetic-biparental mosaicism (in cases associated with placental mesenchymal dysplasia and Beckwith–Wiedemann syndrome) {5808,979}. The chromosomal breakpoint (19q13.4) is in the vicinity of the microRNA cluster C19MC, which is activated in both scenarios {3436}. Cytogenetic analyses of some cases of undifferentiated embryonal sarcomas have also revealed chromosomal rearrangements involving 19q13.4, similar to those in MH {5734, 4470}.

## Macroscopic appearance
Most MHs manifest as expanding, well-delineated masses without a capsule. They are frequently multiloculated and cystic, with solid components. Multiple cystic spaces lacking a communication with bile ducts are noted on cut surfaces in 85% of cases. Very young patients show fewer cysts and more solid masses, suggesting that cysts develop in parallel with progressive tumour growth. In one series, 41% of tumours were solid and 59% were cystic {1157}. The cysts, ranging in size from a few millimetres to 150 mm, contain yellow fluid or gelatinous material.

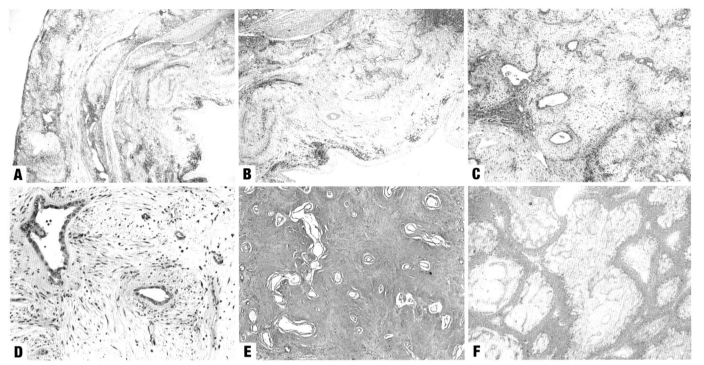

**Fig. 11.17** Mesenchymal hamartoma. **A** The cyst wall of this tumour is composed of a composite mixture of loose connective tissue, malformed bile ducts, hepatocyte islands, and dilated vessels. **B** Higher-magnification image of the cyst wall showing a mixture of stromal and epithelial components and the inner surface of the cyst devoid of any lining cells. **C** Dilated and branched ductal structures in a loose mesenchymal stroma containing bland spindle-shaped cells. **D** Dilated bile ducts surrounded by a concentric cuff of collagenous tissue. **E** Dense collagenized stroma arranged concentrically around bile ducts. **F** Solid tumour area featuring lobulated islands of haphazardly arranged loose connective tissue and bile ducts separated by hepatocytic parenchyma.

## Histopathology

Microscopically, the lesion is composed of loose connective tissue and epithelial bile ducts in varying proportions, arranged in lobulated islands. The mesenchyme is typically loose, myxoid, and rich in glycosaminoglycans, and it contains bland-looking spindled fibroblasts, dilated vessels, and fluid-filled spaces. It may be collagenous and arranged concentrically around the ducts. The biliary structures are often tortuous, branched, and occasionally dilated, reminiscent of a ductal plate malformation pattern. Islets of hepatocytes without acinar architecture may be present. Non–epithelial-lined cysts develop within the mesenchyme because of an accumulation of fluid. Foci of extramedullary haematopoiesis are observed in > 85% of cases. In older children, atypical features such as scarcity of the ductal component and stromal calcification may occur {7311,6667}.

By immunohistochemistry, the spindle cells are positive for vimentin, actin, and desmin (focal), and the ducts stain positively for CK7 and CK19 but not CK20. The vessels are highlighted by CD31, CD34, and D2-40. Nuclear β-catenin is not expressed in any of the components. The intervening hepatocytes as well as the tumour components may express glypican-3 (GPC3), causing confusion with hepatoblastoma {4063}.

Principal differential diagnoses include mixed epithelial-mesenchymal hepatoblastoma, infantile haemangioma, and

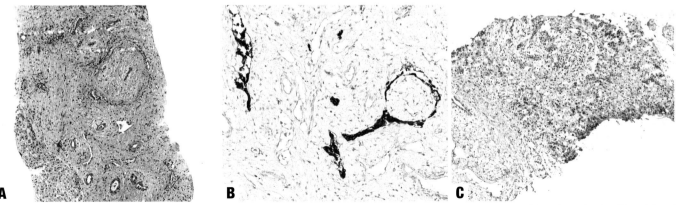

**Fig. 11.18** Mesenchymal hamartoma. **A** Liver biopsy showing an abnormal mixture of mesenchymal tissue and epithelial components. **B** Liver biopsy showing CK7 staining of the abnormal ductal structures, which are partly in a ductal plate arrangement. **C** Liver biopsy with glypican-3 (GPC3) expression of the intervening non-lesional hepatocytes, causing confusion with hepatoblastoma.

Chapter 11

embryonal sarcoma. The cystic form of MH is often confused with other hepatic cystic lesions, especially in adults {1422, 7721}. The two cases of MH reported with *DICER1* syndrome probably represent hepatic lesions analogous to other *DICER1*-related cystic tumours instead of bona fide MH {298,978}.

## Cytology
Not clinically relevant

## Diagnostic molecular pathology
MH demonstrates a characteristic molecular signature with chromosomal rearrangements involving the breakpoint 19q13.4, termed "mesenchymal hamartoma of the liver breakpoint 1" (MHLB1).

## Essential and desirable diagnostic criteria
*Essential:* a hypocellular fibromyxoid stroma with bland spindle cells, accompanied by malformed bile ducts in a ductal plate configuration.
*Desirable:* rearrangements involving chromosome 19q13.4.

## Staging
Not clinically relevant

## Prognosis and prediction
MH generally has a benign course in the absence of complications, with an excellent prognosis if the mass is resected {7719}. Exceptions are cases with severe cardiopulmonary complications and rare instances of evolution to undifferentiated embryonal sarcoma {5750,3455}.

# Calcifying nested stromal-epithelial tumour

Hornick JL
Makhlouf HR
Ranganathan S

## Definition
Calcifying nested stromal-epithelial tumour (CNSET) of the liver is a rare, low-grade hepatic neoplasm of uncertain lineage characterized by a distinctive nested architecture surrounded by a cellular myofibroblastic stroma and psammomatous calcifications.

## ICD-O coding
8975/1 Calcifying nested stromal-epithelial tumour

## ICD-11 coding
2F70.5 & XH8X78 Neoplasms of uncertain behaviour of liver, gallbladder, or bile ducts & Calcifying nested epithelial stromal tumour

## Related terminology
*Acceptable:* nested stromal-epithelial tumour; ossifying stromal-epithelial tumour; desmoplastic nested spindle cell tumour; ossifying malignant mixed epithelial and stromal tumour.

## Subtype(s)
None

## Localization
CNSET most often arises in the right hepatic lobe (65% of cases) {2809,2895,4337}.

## Clinical features
CNSET is often discovered incidentally, sometimes in patients with a history of a calcified hepatic nodule. Occasional patients present with abdominal pain, a palpable mass, or nausea. Around 20% of patients present with Cushing syndrome {2809,4337}.

## Epidemiology
CNSET is rare, with about 40 reported cases. There is a female predominance and a predilection for children and adolescents (80% of cases) {2809,2895,4337,2361A}.

## Etiology
Most CNSETs are sporadic. Several cases have been associated with Beckwith–Wiedemann syndrome {4357,3549}.

## Pathogenesis
*CTNNB1* deletions have been identified in several cases {379}.

## Macroscopic appearance
CNSET is well circumscribed but unencapsulated, with a multinodular, sharp interface with adjacent liver. Tumours range in size from 20 to 300 mm (median: 125 mm). The cut surface is yellow or white and granular {4337}.

## Histopathology
The tumours are composed of ovoid to irregular nests of variably spindled to epithelioid cells, cuffed by a cellular stroma. A focally trabecular architecture is sometimes observed. Occasional nests contain central necrosis. The tumour cells are bland and uniform, with vesicular chromatin, indistinct nucleoli, eosinophilic cytoplasm, and low mitotic activity. The nests often harbour psammomatous calcifications, and sometimes ossification. The stroma may contain a bile ductular proliferation.

By immunohistochemistry, the tumour cells are positive for broad-spectrum keratins and WT1 (usually nuclear but sometimes cytoplasmic or paranuclear dot-like), with aberrant nuclear and cytoplasmic β-catenin staining {2809,2895,4337, 379}. Expression of CD56, EMA, PR, NSE, and KIT (CD117) is variable. Desmin, chromogranin, synaptophysin, HepPar-1 (CPS1), and polyclonal CEA are negative. The spindle cells in the stroma are positive for SMA.

## Cytology
Not relevant

## Diagnostic molecular pathology
Not relevant

## Essential and desirable diagnostic criteria
*Essential:* a nested architecture surrounded by cellular myofibroblastic stroma; bland and uniform epithelioid and spindle cells; expression of keratins, WT1, and nuclear β-catenin.

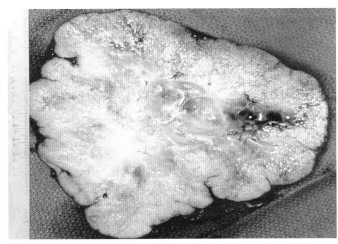

**Fig. 11.19** Calcifying nested stromal-epithelial tumour. Cross-section of the tumour showing a pale yellowish-tan cut surface with focal cystic change and calcifications at the periphery.

Chapter 11

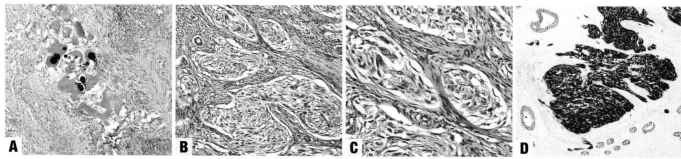

**Fig. 11.20** Calcifying nested stromal-epithelial tumour. **A** Psammomatous calcifications are often seen, sometimes with osseous metaplasia. **B** The tumour is composed of nests of epithelioid and spindle cells surrounded by cellular stroma. **C** The tumour cells contain irregular nuclei with fine chromatin, variably prominent small nucleoli, and abundant pale eosinophilic cytoplasm. **D** Immunohistochemistry for β-catenin shows aberrant cytoplasmic and nuclear staining. Note the normal membranous staining in the surrounding bile ducts.

## Staging
Not relevant

## Prognosis and prediction
Many patients with CNSET are cured by surgical excision, although several reported patients have developed local recurrence requiring liver transplantation {2809,2895,4337, 884}. Lymph node or lung metastases are rare; several reported patients have died of the disease {2963,4569}.

# Embryonal sarcoma of the liver

Vokuhl C
Ranganathan S
Saxena R

## Definition

Embryonal sarcoma of the liver (ESL) is a malignant mesenchymal tumour with a heterogeneous morphology and no specific differentiation pattern.

## ICD-O coding

8991/3 Embryonal sarcoma

## ICD-11 coding

XH42Q2 Embryonal sarcoma (of liver)

## Related terminology

*Acceptable:* undifferentiated (embryonal) sarcoma of the liver.

## Subtype(s)

None

## Localization

ESL usually affects the right lobe of the liver, but it may occur in either lobe or involve both lobes.

## Clinical features

Patients with ESL present with a rapidly growing, palpable abdominal mass; abdominal pain and swelling; and nonspecific symptoms such as fever and weight loss. Serum AFP levels are not elevated.

## Epidemiology

ESL is the third most common malignant liver tumour, constituting 6–13% of all malignant childhood liver tumours. ESL shows no sex predilection and occurs mostly in children aged 6–10 years {7487,6703,6411,3863}; however, it may occur in patients of any age, including very young children and older adults {1022,5045}.

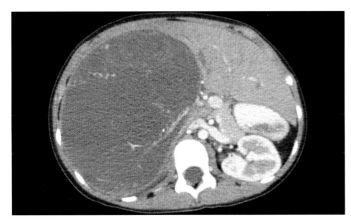

**Fig. 11.21** Embryonal sarcoma of the liver. Contrast-enhanced axial CT shows a large hepatic mass showing predominantly water attenuation, consistent with the myxoid stroma. Enhancement is limited to the septa and periphery.

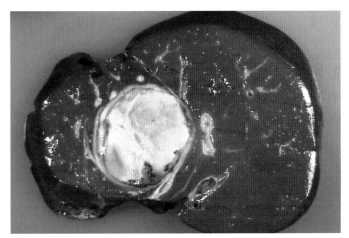

**Fig. 11.22** Embryonal sarcoma of the liver. Gross image of a posttherapy explant showing a predominantly necrotic tumour abutting the large vessels in the medial aspect of the liver.

## Etiology

There are no known environmental or biological etiological agents. Most cases are sporadic, although cases progressing from and/or sharing molecular signatures with mesenchymal hamartoma have been identified {5246,5734,3968,6395,1613}.

## Pathogenesis

Pathogenesis appears to involve C19MC, a potential oncomir that exhibits a negative correlation with *TP53* and *KRAS* regulatory microRNAs, with potential effects on cell differentiation and autophagy. It appears that t(11;19)(q13;q13.4) and other 19q13 abnormalities shared with mesenchymal hamartoma represent the first hit, with *TP53* abnormalities being the second hit leading to malignant transformation {6349}. WNT and telomerase pathways do not appear to play a role in the pathogenesis of ESL {4042}.

The t(11;19)(q13;q13.4) translocation has been reported in ESL arising from mesenchymal hamartoma, supporting the proposed link between the two neoplasms. This translocation affects a non-coding region with linkage to *MALAT1*. Recent genomic profiling of ESL demonstrated that this and other chromosomal structural events result in a combination of C19MC hyperexpression and *TP53* mutation or loss, which are highly recurrent genomic events of ESL {6349,4042,4470,6604,5734}.

## Macroscopic appearance

ESLs are generally large tumours (100–300 mm), sharply demarcated by a pseudocapsule formed by compression of the adjacent liver. The cut surface is heterogeneous, with solid, myxoid, and variably sized cystic areas. Degenerative changes such as necrosis and haemorrhage are often present, especially after therapy.

## Histopathology

ESL is composed of medium-sized to large spindle and stellate cells embedded in a myxoid stroma. Cellularity is variable. The

Chapter 11

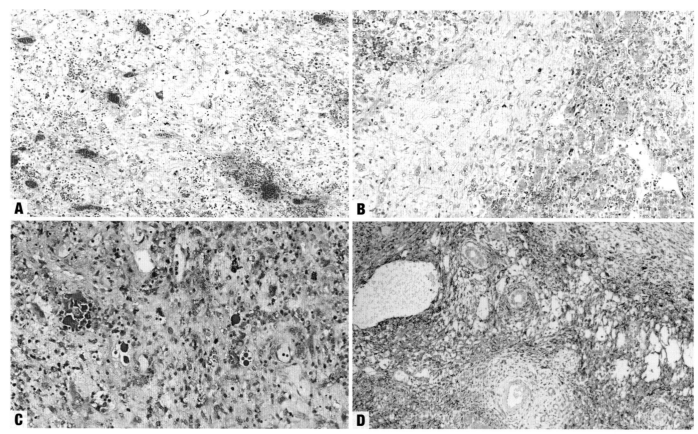

**Fig. 11.23** Embryonal sarcoma of the liver. **A** The tumour is composed of medium to large spindle and stellate cells embedded in a myxoid stroma. The nuclei are pleomorphic and hyperchromatic and the cytoplasm is often eosinophilic. Mitotic figures are numerous. **B** Entrapped liver tissue can be seen at the periphery of the tumour. **C** PASD staining highlights the intracytoplasmic globules. **D** The tumour cells are strongly positive for desmin.

nuclei are pleomorphic and hyperchromatic, containing stippled chromatin and inconspicuous nuclei. The cytoplasm is often eosinophilic and may be vacuolated. Giant, bizarre cells and numerous, often atypical, mitoses are usually present. PAS-positive, diastase-resistant intracytoplasmic globules are characteristic. Extramedullary haematopoiesis and entrapped hepatocytes and bile ducts are often noted; the latter may be cystically dilated {6703,7487}. Loose myxoid areas that are hypocellular and associated with dilated bile ducts suggestive of mesenchymal hamartoma may be seen. Immunohistochemically, ESL shows diffuse vimentin and α1-antitrypsin, especially in the intracytoplasmic globules, and variable positivity for desmin, cytokeratin, SMA, BCL2, glypican-3 (GPC3), and CD56. Most tumours show nuclear p53 positivity. AFP and HepPar-1 are negative {3553, 6395,5005,5449,4659,3863}. Negative myogenin and MYOD1 help to distinguish ESL from biliary rhabdomyosarcoma {5005}. Electron microscopy shows undifferentiated, fibroblastic, or fibrohistiocytic cells with characteristically dilated rough endoplasmic reticulum and electron-dense lysosomal material, which correspond to the eosinophilic globules seen on light microscopy. Intracytoplasmic fat, glycogen, intermediate filaments, and cell junctions have been noted {4659,3504,68,297,5045,3863}.

## Cytology

FNAB of ESL shows variable cellularity with loose clusters of pleomorphic, spindle-shaped, or stellate cells in a metachromatic matrix containing arborizing vascular channels. Numerous dissociated tumour cells, giant bizarre forms, and intracytoplasmic globules are often seen {5528,2612,462}.

## Diagnostic molecular pathology

FISH for the t(11;19)(q13;q13.4) translocation may be done in cases where tissue is limited, to help confirm the diagnosis of ESL arising from mesenchymal hamartoma.

## Essential and desirable diagnostic criteria

*Essential:* spindle to stellate cells with marked pleomorphism embedded in a myxoid background.

*Desirable:* giant cells with intracytoplasmic eosinophilic, PAS-positive, diastase-resistant globules; no specific pattern of differentiation; *TP53* mutation or loss.

## Staging

Not clinically relevant

## Prognosis and prediction

Metastases occur in about 5–13% of patients. Multimodal therapy comprising surgical resection and chemotherapy, with radiotherapy if needed, constitutes the current standard of care, ensuring a median survival time of 4–5 years. Total hepatectomy with transplantation is a viable option for unresectable, refractory, and locally recurrent tumours {5576,1022,4471,6411,6936}. Negative surgical margins are not associated with improved outcomes {6411}.

# Hepatic congenital haemangioma

Gupta A
Kozakewich HP

## Definition

Hepatic congenital haemangioma (HCH) is a benign, GLUT1-immunonegative, vascular neoplasm that is fully developed at birth, with most cases involuting in infancy.

## ICD-O coding

9131/0 Congenital haemangioma
9131/0 Rapidly involuting congenital haemangioma
9131/0 Partially involuting congenital haemangioma
9131/0 Non-involuting congenital haemangioma

## ICD-11 coding

2E81.2Y & XH27G6 Other specified benign vascular lesions of infancy and childhood & Congenital haemangioma, NOS

## Related terminology

*Not recommended:* haemangioendothelioma, type 1; cavernous haemangioma; congenital arteriovenous malformation.

## Subtype(s)

Rapidly involuting congenital haemangioma (RICH); partially involuting congenital haemangioma (PICH); non-involuting congenital haemangioma (NICH)

## Localization

HCH occurs most commonly in the right lobe of the liver.

## Clinical features

HCHs are primarily asymptomatic and incidentally found on imaging in infancy or on prenatal ultrasound {1741,1311,5863}. Some newborns may present with hepatomegaly, thrombocytopenia, and mild hypofibrinogenaemia, and rarely with cardiac failure from arteriovenous or portohepatic venous shunting {784, 1741,7493}, which may also result in hydrops fetalis {2481}.

RICHs, PICHs, and NICHs are high-flow lesions, with NICHs demonstrating only minimal enlargement of the dysplastic veins compared to RICHs and PICHs. HCHs are fully developed at birth. HCH may become larger between prenatal ultrasound and postpartum imaging, secondary to the sudden shift from fetal to postnatal circulation, resulting in peripartum intratumoural bleeding and thrombus formation. On morphology, the capillary component of most HCHs spontaneously recedes partially or entirely postpartum. The clinical recommendation is to monitor HCH for at least 1 year, until two consecutive hepatic ultrasounds show stable size and vascularity {3092}.

## Epidemiology

The true incidence of HCH is unknown. HCH and infantile haemangioma combined account for 12% of all paediatric liver

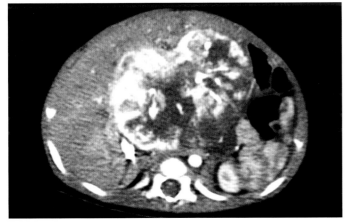

**Fig. 11.24** Hepatic congenital haemangioma. Contrast-enhanced axial CT showing a large hepatic tumour with an intense centripetal pattern of enhancement; the centre is not completely enhanced due to central necrosis.

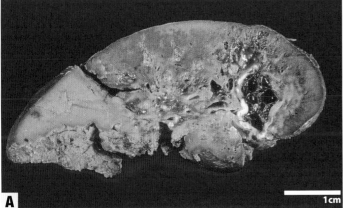 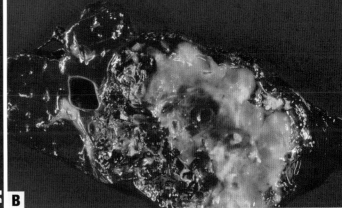

**Fig. 11.25** Hepatic rapidly involuting congenital haemangioma. **A** Liver resection showing a vascular lesion with dilated central vascular channels surrounded by a rim of calcification. **B** Liver resection of an ovoid mass with large areas of central necrosis, haemorrhage, and fibrosis.

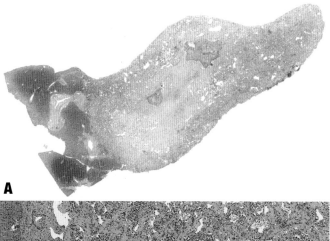

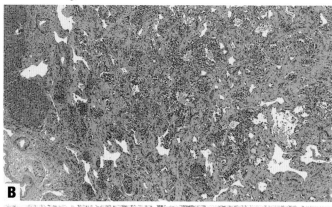

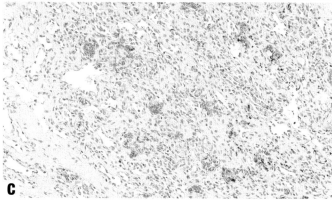

**Fig. 11.26** Hepatic rapidly involuting congenital haemangioma. **A** A scanned slide demonstrating central less-cellular areas with calcification and fibrosis, and more-cellular peripheral areas. **B** High-power view of the periphery demonstrates aggregates or lobules of capillary-type channels lined by plump to hobnailed endothelial cells and pericytes. **C** GLUT1 is negative within the endothelial cells. Red blood cells serve as the internal control.

tumours. HCH is more common in girls and may be associated with cutaneous infantile haemangioma or cavernous haemangioma {1741,5863}.

## Etiology
Unknown

## Pathogenesis
Most RICHs are secondary to missense mutations that alter the glutamine at amino acid position 209 (Q209), resulting in hyperactivation of *GNAQ* and *GNA11* {428} at variant allele

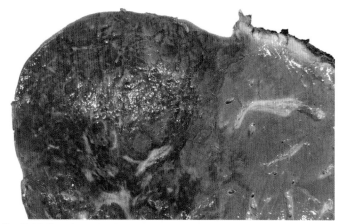

**Fig. 11.27** Hepatic non-involuting congenital haemangioma. A solitary, diffusely red-brown mottled vascular lesion within the left lobe of the liver in a 17-month-old.

frequencies of 3–33%. Similar mutations have been identified in both cutaneous RICH and NICH, suggesting that additional factors influence the phenotype. A subset also have *PIK3CA* mutation {7059}.

## Macroscopic appearance
HCHs are usually solitary {1311}, and only rarely are there several foci. They range from a few millimetres to > 100 mm in size. HCH is circumscribed, firm to soft, tan-white, and often has calcification and fibrosis. Central haemorrhage and necrosis may be present in the early stages, attributed to the cessation of umbilical blood flow at the time of delivery. Large central or peripheral veins are often present.

## Histopathology
HCH is composed of variably sized aggregates or lobules of capillary-type channels lined by plump to hobnailed endothelial cells and pericytes. As HCH involutes, the aggregates or lobules are replaced by fibrous stroma. The intervascular stroma is fibrotic with entrapped hepatocytes that are occasionally immunoreactive for glypican-3 (GPC3), dispersed bile ducts, foci of extramedullary haematopoiesis, and occasional dilated sinusoids. Central necrosis, macrophages (occasionally haemosiderin-laden), dystrophic calcification, chronic inflammatory cells, and dysplastic veins with thrombi are frequently observed. Lesions with one or more arteriovenous or portohepatic venous fistulae may mimic a vascular malformation. The hepatic sinusoids adjacent to the lesion tend to be dilated. Lesional endothelial cells are immunoreactive for CD31, CD34, and WT1, and immunonegative for GLUT1 {617}. There is minimal information on the histopathology of PICH, but presumably it shares many features with RICH. NICH lacks involutional changes such as necrosis, haemorrhage, fibrosis, and haemosiderin.

## Cytology
Cytological features are not specific; red blood cells, blood vessels with bland endothelium, extramedullary haematopoiesis, calcification, and necrosis are often present.

## Diagnostic molecular pathology
Not clinically relevant

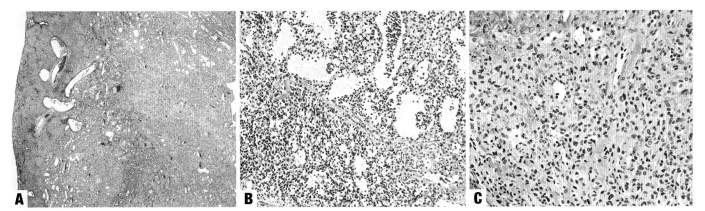

**Fig. 11.28** Hepatic non-involuting congenital haemangioma. This example is from a 2-year-old child with two hepatic lesions measuring 42 mm and 5 mm, the larger of which was identified on antenatal Doppler ultrasound. **A** Left lateral segmentectomy demonstrates an unencapsulated hepatic lesion composed of vascular channels tracking along hepatic sinusoids. **B** Higher magnification highlights lobules of capillary-type channels lined by plump to hobnailed endothelial cells and pericytes. Endothelial cells lack pleomorphism and endothelial redundancy. Solid areas are absent. GLUT1 (not shown here) was negative. **C** Lip lesion in the same patient, showing similar histology.

## Essential and desirable diagnostic criteria

*Essential:* capillary-type aggregates and lobules; stromal fibrosis; enlarged sinusoids and veins; GLUT1-immunonegative endothelium.

## Staging

Not relevant

## Prognosis and prediction

RICHs undergo spontaneous involution (90% reduction in size in 13 months), leaving only a small calcified remnant. Most lesions do not require any treatment {1741}, but a small subset of large lesions may result in morbidity and even mortality due to intratumoural haemorrhage, hypofibrinogenaemia and thrombocytopenia, or high-output cardiac failure from arteriovenous or portohepatic venous shunting. PICHs undergo only partial involution, and NICHs show no involution {3092}.

# Hepatic infantile haemangioma

Gupta A
Kozakewich HP

## Definition
Hepatic infantile haemangioma (HIH) is a benign, proliferative, vascular neoplasm with GLUT1 endothelial immunopositivity.

## ICD-O coding
9131/0 Infantile haemangioma
9131/0 Single infantile haemangioma
9131/0 Multifocal infantile haemangioma
9131/0 Diffuse infantile haemangioma

## ICD-11 coding
2E81.2Y Other Specified benign vascular lesions of infancy and childhood

## Related terminology
*Acceptable:* infantile hepatic haemangioma.
*Not recommended:* haemangioendothelioma, type 1, type 2, or type 3; infantile haemangioendothelioma; juvenile haemangiomas; hepatic small vessel neoplasm.

## Subtype(s)
Single infantile haemangioma; multifocal infantile haemangioma; diffuse infantile haemangioma

## Localization
One or both lobes of the liver

## Clinical features
The natural history of HIH remains unclear. Some HIHs may manifest as early as the first day of life {784,1741} and show progressive growth followed by gradual involutional changes. Generally, HIHs are not visualized ultrasonographically beyond 18–24 months of age {3092}.

Most HIHs are asymptomatic and found incidentally on imaging. However, some patients present with hepatomegaly, abdominal enlargement, abdominal compartment syndrome, failure to thrive, and cardiac failure {784,1311,1741,3833}. HIH produces type 3 iodothyronine deiodinase (D3), which inactivates thyroid hormone and can result in clinical hypothyroidism {3034}. Because HIH proliferates weeks to months after birth, hypothyroidism may not be detected on newborn screening.

Approximately 70% of infants with HIH have one or more cutaneous lesions {1741}. Screening for HIH should be performed when ≥ 5 cutaneous infantile haemangiomas (CIHs) are present. Imaging demonstrates multifocal, diffuse, or (rarely) solitary hepatic lesions with mixed echogenicity {1311}. MRI findings of HIH often overlap with those of hepatic congenital haemangioma, with a typical dynamic pattern of early peripheral enhancement (with HIH showing more confluency than

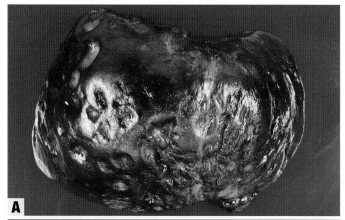

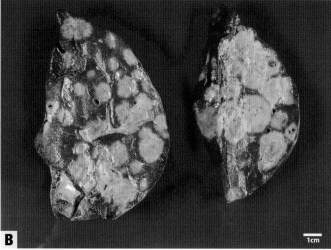

**Fig. 11.30** Hepatic infantile haemangioma. **A** Liver explant from a 3-month-old with abdominal compartment syndrome, showing multiple lesions. **B** The cut section shows a cholestatic liver with diffuse tan-white, occasionally coalescing masses.

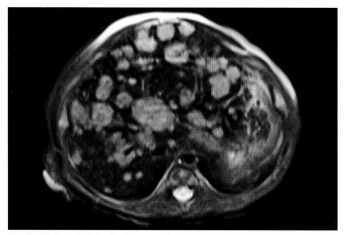

**Fig. 11.29** Hepatic infantile haemangioma. Fat-saturated T2-weighted axial MRI showing numerous well-defined hyperintense nodules in the liver.

hepatic congenital haemangioma, which is discontinuous), followed by gradual central enhancement {3711,4605}. Continued surveillance with serial ultrasounds is recommended until involution is complete. Growth beyond 2 years and/or new lesions after 1 year are concerning for a possible transition into an angiosarcoma {3092}. HIH may occur in association with hepatoblastoma, mesenchymal hamartoma {583,579,646,4291}, and Beckwith–Wiedemann syndrome. Mesenchymal hamartoma can, on occasion, have a prominent vascular component {6733, 646}, mimicking HIH.

## Epidemiology

HIH is the most common hepatic mesenchymal tumour in children {3015}, and the liver is the most common extracutaneous site for infantile haemangioma {5079}. HIH is associated with the female sex, multigestational pregnancy, low birth weight, and prematurity {784,1821,1278,2831,6351,3559,4853}.

## Etiology

The exact mechanism is unclear, but uterine, placental, or local hypoxia is thought to play a key role in the development of these lesions; this notion is supported by endothelial expression of GLUT1, IGF2, VEGF-A, and HIF1α in HIHs {5902, 1822,1625}.

## Pathogenesis

HIH undergoes the same proliferative and involutive phases as its cutaneous counterpart. CIH studies based on the X-linked human *AR* (*HUMARA*) assay {828,7376} and methylation- and transcription-based PCR clonality assays {7376} have shown an allelic loss within HIH endothelial cells as compared with normal skin, thus a non-random X-inactivation pattern supporting a monoclonal origin. This is postulated to result in an imbalance of vasculogenic factors including endothelial markers, stem cell markers (e.g. CD133 and LYVE1), IGF2, FGF, VEGF, VEGFR {7376,7779,3543,3281}, and other markers, thereby promoting proliferation. During involution, in both CIH and HIH, there is an increase in tissue metalloproteinases, which inhibit new vessel formation {6839,7434}. Aggressive forms of HIH have shown overexpression of the hedgehog signalling components

sonic hedgehog and GLI2 and their target gene *FOXA2* {7499}. Genomic imprinting of *IGF2* {7780} in Beckwith–Wiedemann syndrome may relate to its association with HIH.

## Macroscopic appearance

HIH is usually multifocal or diffuse, and rarely single; the diffuse pattern is usually seen as innumerable, often coalescent nodules that virtually replace the hepatic parenchyma {1311}. Individual nodules can range from a few millimetres to > 100 mm and are well demarcated, tan-white, oval to round, and spongy. Areas of haemorrhage and necrosis may occur, although this may also herald transformation to an angiosarcoma.

## Histopathology

HIH, especially in the central portions of the nodules, is characterized by anastomosing, sinusoid-like channels lined by flattened or minimally plump endothelial cells with small, bland, hyperchromatic nuclei without marked atypia and with infrequent mitoses. Occasionally, there are foci of endothelial redundancy with pseudopapillary formation that can mimic Masson papillary endothelial hyperplasia. Solid epithelioid to spindled areas, necrosis, and marked endothelial atypia are absent. The intervening stroma is fibrotic, and entrapped bile ducts and hepatocytes can also be present; the hepatocytes may be immunopositive for glypican-3 (GPC3). The masses are not encapsulated and their margins are irregular and composed of capillary-like channels extending along sinusoids. Individual masses are separated by normal hepatic parenchyma. Lesional endothelial cells are immunopositive for GLUT1, CD31, and CD34. The endothelial proliferation is greatest in the centre of the nodules {2139}.

Moderate to marked endothelial atypia, solid spindled or epithelioid foci, necrosis, and variability in GLUT1 endothelial immunoexpression suggest transition into angiosarcoma.

## Cytology
Not relevant

## Diagnostic molecular pathology
Not relevant

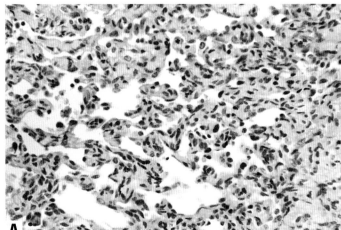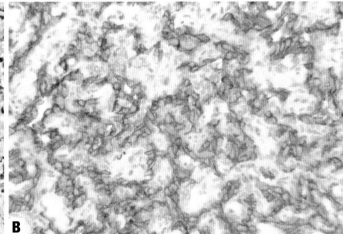

**Fig. 11.31** Hepatic infantile haemangioma. **A** Histology shows complex anastomosing vascular/sinusoidal channels and pseudopapillae with foci of endothelial redundancy and rare mitotic figures. Solid areas, endothelial atypia, necrosis, and atypical mitoses are absent. **B** Tumour cells are immunoreactive for GLUT1.

## Essential and desirable diagnostic criteria

*Essential:* wide, anastomosing, sinusoid-like channels with mostly small and bland GLUT1-immunopositive endothelial cells with absent or only minor atypia.

## Staging

Not relevant

## Prognosis and prediction

Screening for HIH in infants with ≥ 5 CIHs has led to the earlier detection and treatment of HIH {5864}. Oral propranolol {3015} or corticosteroids have been used to hasten involution of HIH, and interferon has also been used in cases of steroid resistance. Thyroid replacement therapy has been effective in cases of diffuse or multifocal HIH–acquired hypothyroidism. Because some infants with diffuse HIH deteriorate quickly, transplant evaluation should be considered early in the treatment {1311}. HIH has a mortality rate as high as 16%. Most of these children have diffuse HIH, abdominal compartment syndrome, and cardiac failure {5864}. If the proliferative phase continues beyond 2 years of age, there is a greater risk of transition into angiosarcoma {3247,2534}.

# Hepatic angiosarcoma

Gupta A
Kozakewich HP

## Definition
Hepatic angiosarcoma (HA) is a rare, malignant endothelial cell neoplasm with potential for distant metastases.

## ICD-O coding
9120/3 Angiosarcoma

## ICD-11 coding
2B56.3 Liver angiosarcoma

## Related terminology
*Not recommended:* haemangioendothelioma, type 1 or type 2; malignant haemangioendothelioma.

## Subtype(s)
None

## Localization
Right lobe, left lobe, or both lobes of the liver

## Clinical features
HA manifests in early childhood, is locally aggressive, and has the potential to metastasize. HA presentations may include abdominal pain or distension, jaundice, constipation, vomiting, fever, and difficulty in breathing due to a large abdominal volume {5872,6336}. The average length of time from symptoms to a diagnosis of HA is 1 year {2534}. Often, a history of cutaneous infantile haemangioma and/or hepatic infantile haemangioma (HIH) with involutional changes is obtained {6336,7487,51, 3247}. AFP is typically normal or only minimally elevated, and children may present with anaemia and/or thrombocytopenia. Fulminant hepatic failure is rare. MRI findings are nonspecific

and depict a single or multifocal lesion with intense diffusion restriction and heterogeneous enhancement throughout, suggesting intense vascularity. Intralesional haemorrhage and necrosis are common.

## Epidemiology
HA accounts for 1–2% of all paediatric hepatic tumours {2534}, and most commonly occurs between 1 and 7 years of age {6336}; however, the youngest patient reported with metastasis was a 6-week-old infant {4529}. More girls are affected than boys {416,6336}. It is most often found in association with HIH {25,2534}. Growth of HIH beyond 2 years of age, or a new lesion that appears on imaging after a year, warrants a biopsy to exclude HA {2534}.

## Etiology
Although adult HA seems to arise spontaneously {1674,7773}, most paediatric HA cases arise within pre-existing HIH {416, 1756,7645,5692,7435}. Risk factors in adults and children include exogenous exposure to chemical carcinogens (including vinyl chloride {4408,7487,1921}, androgens {2030}, cyclophosphamide {5987}, diethylstilbestrol, and arsenic {1189}), as well as exposure to Thorotrast {5659}, radium, and radiation.

## Pathogenesis
The exact pathogenesis of HA remains uncertain; however, molecular diagnostic findings have provided some insight. HA associated with vinyl chloride exposure has been shown to carry activating mutations in RAS genes {5659,7484,3247}. Gain-of-function mutations promote angiogenesis through the constitutive activation of the MAPK/ERK signalling pathway, which promotes transcription of proangiogenic factors {7871, 3163,5350,5692}.

*ROS1* rearrangements {4411,3351} and activating RAS mutations {3247,5659} have been found in HA, and cumulative HA studies have also shown mutations in *HRAS*, *KRAS* (*KRAS2*), *AKT1*, *PTEN* {6905}, *TP53* (p53) {2955}, and *PIK3CA* {2534, 5692}. Some vascular-specific receptor tyrosine kinases like VEGFR2 (KDR), TEK, VEGFR1 (FLT1), and TIE1 are reportedly upregulated in cutaneous and visceral angiosarcomas {291}. *MYC* amplification has been associated with postirradiation angiosarcoma.

## Macroscopic appearance
Macroscopically, there is nodular involvement of either or both lobes, which is usually multicentric and (in rare cases) can virtually replace the entire liver. Central regions may demonstrate haemorrhage, fibrosis, and necrosis {7435}.

## Histopathology
In HIH, there is abnormal proliferation of endothelial cells and minimal to no atypia; however, moderate endothelial atypia

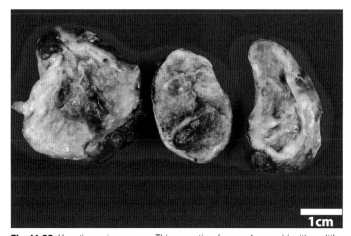

**Fig. 11.32** Hepatic angiosarcoma. This resection from a 4-year-old with multifocal hepatic infantile haemangiomas, a rapidly enlarging liver mass, and a new lung mass shows a large, tan, ovoid to round mass with central areas of haemorrhage and necrosis.

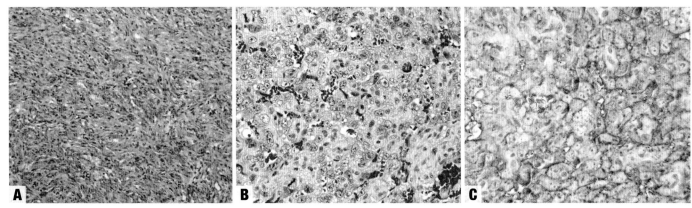

**Fig. 11.33** Hepatic angiosarcoma. This example is from a 4-year-old with multifocal hepatic infantile haemangiomas, a rapidly enlarging liver mass, and a new lung mass. **A** Scattered foci of solid areas show sheets of spindled endothelial cells with several mitotic figures. **B** Lung metastasis showing a solid, cellular mass composed of pleomorphic epithelioid to focally spindled endothelial cells with numerous mitoses. **C** Tumour cells are immunoreactive for GLUT1.

with nuclear enlargement, irregular cytoplasmic and nuclear contours, and occasional prominent nucleoli are worrisome features that may herald the transition to HA. More convincing features to support HA are solid foci with markedly atypical, pleomorphic, spindled to epithelioid endothelial cells and readily identified mitoses. Like HIH, HA has infiltrative margins that extend into existing sinusoids. The Ki-67 proliferation index, especially within the solid areas, is > 10% {7435, 2422}. The endothelial cells of HA show variable immunopositivity for GLUT1, rather than the diffuse and intense immunopositivity seen in HIH. In addition, HA is immunopositive for CD34, CD31, ERG {7436}, and von Willebrand factor, and 10% of cases show focal immunoreactivity for pancytokeratin. PAS-positive, diastase-resistant, eosinophilic cytoplasmic globules can occasionally be present {6336}. Entrapped bile ducts and hepatocytes can also be present, like in HIH and hepatic congenital haemangioma. Intrahepatic lymphovascular invasion is common. Sinusoidal growth occurs in HA as well as in HIH and hepatic congenital haemangioma, and by itself should not be interpreted as a sign of malignancy {7707,44}. Because HA can coexist with HIH and (rarely) with hepatic congenital haemangioma, sampling bias may be an issue {5079,44}, so image-guided biopsy and correlation are essential.

## Cytology
Not clinically relevant

## Diagnostic molecular pathology
Not relevant

## Essential and desirable diagnostic criteria
*Essential:* moderate to marked endothelial atypia; solid spindled or epithelioid foci; necrosis; conspicuous mitotic activity; variable endothelial GLUT1 immunoexpression.

## Staging
Because of the rarity of paediatric HA and its association mostly with HIH, it is difficult to obtain reliable data from a cohort of cases. Clinical staging of adult HA is currently based on the Union for International Cancer Control (UICC) and American Joint Committee on Cancer (AJCC) system for soft tissue sarcomas, which is based on tumour size, regional lymph nodes, and distant metastasis. All HAs per the adult classification for soft tissue angiosarcomas are considered deep lesions, with the majority of cases being stage I or IV {3027}.

## Prognosis and prediction
The overall outcome of HA in children is poor {1741}. HA is highly metastatic, most commonly to the lung {3247}. A few children have successfully undergone hepatic transplantation {44}; however, complete cure is rare. Complete surgical resection should be attempted and systemic chemotherapy initiated. Biological angiogenic inhibiting agents (VEGF) have shown some reduction in tumour size {3247,5692,51,1677}; however, the overall 5-year survival rate is < 35% {1677,51,1726,6336}.

# Pancreatoblastoma

Singhi AD
Klimstra DS
Ohike N
Singhi AD
Tanaka Y

## Definition
Pancreatoblastoma is a malignant epithelial neoplasm of the pancreas showing predominantly acinar differentiation with squamoid nests.

## ICD-O coding
8971/3 Pancreatoblastoma

## ICD-11 coding
2C10.Y & XH27L5 Other specified malignant neoplasms of pancreas & Pancreatoblastoma

## Related terminology
*Not recommended:* pancreaticoblastoma; infantile pancreatic carcinoma; pancreatic carcinoma of childhood.

## Subtype(s)
None

## Localization
Pancreatoblastomas can occur throughout the pancreas, with no predilection for anatomical location {3703,1732}. However, an extrapancreatic pancreatoblastoma has been reported, originating within the mesentery {7702}.

## Clinical features
Pancreatoblastomas are slow-growing and are often clinically occult until they are quite large. Therefore, symptoms are typically the result of mass effect in the upper abdomen and include a palpable abdominal mass, abdominal distention, upper abdominal pain, weight loss, nausea, diarrhoea, and failure to thrive {4889,1732,2446}. These neoplasms can produce considerable amounts of AFP, and 50–75% of patients have elevated serum AFP levels {686,1668,1148,4796}. When

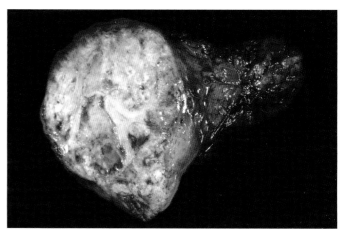

**Fig. 11.35** Pancreatoblastoma. On cross-section, the tumours are soft, solid, and well demarcated, and they may be haemorrhagic and necrotic.

elevated, serum AFP levels can be used to monitor the patient's response to therapy. Cushing syndrome secondary to ectopic secretion of ACTH from the pancreatoblastoma has also been described in rare cases {3650,5373,5704}. The radiographic images of pancreatoblastoma are reported to be distinct {6407,1329}. CT demonstrates a well-marginated and lobulated mass with heterogeneous and septal enhancement {2855}. Calcifications are frequently observed and correspond to small, punctate, clustered or rim-like hyperdense foci. Neonatal cases of pancreatoblastoma are also often cystic. Similarly, MRI shows a well-circumscribed mass. Pancreatoblastomas typically have low to intermediate signal intensity on T1-weighted images and heterogeneously high signal intensity on T2-weighted images. The heterogeneous signal intensity reflects the presence of haemorrhage and necrosis within a pancreatoblastoma {6681}.

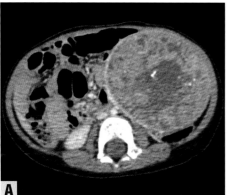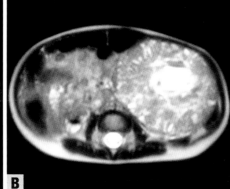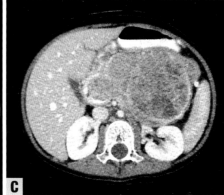

**Fig. 11.34** Pancreatoblastoma. **A** Contrast-enhanced axial CT shows a large, well-circumscribed, heterogeneous mass growing exophytically from the body and tail of the pancreas. Non-enhancing cystic areas and foci of intense enhancement are noted within the mass. **B** T2-weighted axial MRI shows a well-marginated mass with heterogeneous high signal arising from the body and tail of the pancreas. The tumour typically compresses rather than invades the surrounding structures. **C** Transaxial abdominal CT reveals a well-marginated and lobulated mass with heterogeneous and septal enhancement.

Chapter 11

## Epidemiology

Although pancreatoblastomas account for < 1% of all pancreatic exocrine neoplasms, it is the most common malignant pancreatic neoplasm in children aged < 10 years {6460,4889, 5514}. Affected patients range in age from 2 months to 17 years (mean age: 5 years) {1732,4889}. Some cases are congenital, particularly in patients with Beckwith–Wiedemann syndrome {1824,3696,5428}. There is also a slight preponderance of male patients (M:F ratio: 1.14:1) and patients of Asian descent {3654, 1732,2977,3044}.

## Etiology

The majority of cases are sporadic; however, neonatal cases of pancreatoblastoma can be associated with Beckwith–Wiedemann syndrome {1824,3696,5428}.

## Pathogenesis

The pathogenesis of pancreatoblastomas is unknown, but transcriptome studies suggest that these neoplasms arise from a primitive cell origin, similarly to hepatoblastomas {3162}. In fact, there are several clinical and pathological parallels between pancreatoblastoma and hepatoblastoma. Both neoplasms occur in similar age groups, both are associated with the Beckwith–Wiedemann syndrome and familial adenomatous polyposis (in adult patients with pancreatoblastoma), and both often

express high levels of AFP. Additionally, pancreatoblastomas and hepatoblastomas share genomic similarities that include somatic alterations in *CTNNB1* and *APC*, loss of heterozygosity of chromosome 11p15.5, dysregulation of *IGF2*, and upregulation of the R-spondin/LGR5/RNF43 module {3162}. These findings suggest, in principle, a similar pathogenesis for these tumours.

## Macroscopic appearance

Pancreatoblastomas are solitary and well circumscribed, and they tend to be large at clinical presentation (mean: 117 mm, range: 20–200 mm) {4889}. On cross-section, tumours are usually well circumscribed, lobulated, soft, and fleshy. Some cases are firm and fibrous, depending on the proportion of stroma to epithelium. Haemorrhage and necrosis can also be identified. As noted earlier, pancreatoblastomas in neonates are often cystic {6753}.

## Histopathology

Pancreatoblastomas are characterized by variably sized epithelial lobules that are separated by broad bands of fibrous stroma {3652}. The lobules consist of highly cellular sheets of neoplastic cells that exhibit a geographical or lymphoid follicular appearance. These growth patterns reflect the different cell types of a pancreatoblastoma. The acinar component

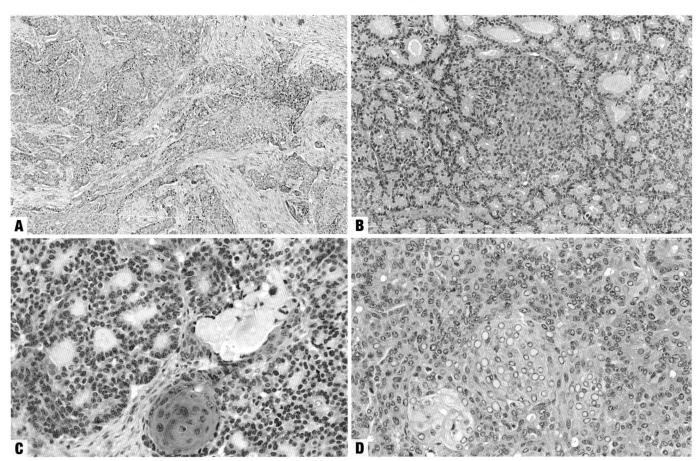

**Fig. 11.36** Pancreatoblastoma. **A** Neoplastic lobules and nests are separated by a fibrous stroma. **B** Acinar differentiation akin to acinar cell carcinoma predominates, with neoplastic cells polarized around small lumina. **C** Squamoid nests are, by definition, present at least focally in every case and composed of whorled, plump cells with eosinophilic cytoplasm that is more abundant than that of the surrounding cells. **D** Although most squamoid nests are uniform, there can be a gradient of differentiation and the nuclei are often large and clear with intranuclear biotin accumulation.

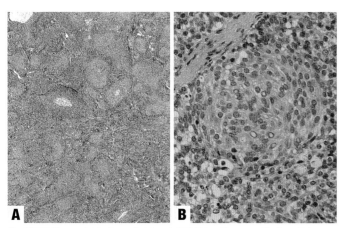

**Fig. 11.37** Pancreatoblastoma. **A** A lymphoid follicle at low magnification. **B** A squamoid nest of epithelioid cells. Note the nuclear clearing in some cells.

usually predominates, consisting of sheets and nests of uniform polygonal epithelial cells with distinct borders, pale basophilic cytoplasm, central nuclei, and prominent nucleoli, often with the formation of small lumina. Acinar differentiation is supported by the detection of PASD-positive cytoplasmic granules and immunolabelling for trypsin, chymotrypsin, lipase, and BCL10 {3857}. In addition, these cells often label for AFP. Half to two thirds of pancreatoblastomas also show evidence of neuroendocrine differentiation by immunolabelling. The cells showing neuroendocrine differentiation are usually diffusely scattered among the acinar cells, but in some cases they form trabeculae or solid nests. As expected, the neuroendocrine cells stain for neuroendocrine markers, such as chromogranin A and synaptophysin. Ductal (mucin-containing) and primitive round cell components can be found in a minority of cases; when identified, they are typically focal.

The defining feature of pancreatoblastoma is the presence of squamoid nests {3654,562,2978}. Squamoid nests are usually located in the centre of the lobule and may adopt a distinctive whorled appearance. The cells within these nests often have an epithelioid to spindled shape and abundant eosinophilic cytoplasm, and their nuclei are large, ovoid, and frequently optically clear with intranuclear biotin accumulation {6873}. The nuclei lack cellular atypia, prominent nucleoli, and mitoses. Rarely, keratinization is found as well. It is important to note that the density and distribution of squamoid nests can vary within a pancreatoblastoma, and they may be

difficult to detect in small samples. Unlike the aforementioned components of a pancreatoblastoma, squamoid nests do not demonstrate a consistent direction of differentiation by immunohistochemistry. However, squamoid nests and a subset of other neoplastic cells often show abnormal cytoplasmic and nuclear expression for β-catenin {6875}. This pattern of labelling is due to alterations in *CTNNB1* or *APC* that result in the impaired degradation of β-catenin. The nuclear accumulation of β-catenin coincides with WNT pathway signal transduction and the transcription of downstream target genes (e.g. *LEF1* and *CCND1*). Thus, LEF1 and cyclin D1 also exhibit nuclear expression within squamoid nests {6875,6497}. In comparison to adult cases, the fibrous stroma of paediatric pancreatoblastomas is often hypercellular. In addition, in rare cases, it appears to be neoplastic, with heterologous osseous and cartilaginous formation. A high-grade spindle cell component is also rare but has been reported {3654}.

## Cytology

FNAB smears are highly cellular and composed of clusters and single cells {2839,5569,6488}. Consistent with the histopathological findings, most of the cells are acinar in differentiation and characterized by a polygonal shape, round to ovoid nuclei, fine or vesicular chromatin, and distinct nucleoli. Pleomorphism and mitotic activity have only rarely been described. A second population of larger squamoid cells are more frequently found in cell blocks than on smears. They may contain biotin-rich, optically clear nuclei. Other reported cytological findings in pancreatoblastoma include spindle cells, immature mesenchyme, and stromal fragments.

## Diagnostic molecular pathology

Sequencing studies have shown that pancreatoblastomas, like other tumour types occurring in childhood, harbour a low tumour mutation burden. However, recurrent mutations affecting the genes in the WNT/β-catenin signalling pathway (including *CTNNB1* and *APC*) have been identified {27,3273, 3162}. Additionally, loss of heterozygosity of chromosome 11p15.5 is a frequent finding and results in the dysregulation of *IGF2* {30,3532,3162}. The importance of these genomic alterations is underscored by reports of pancreatoblastomas occurring in patients with familial adenomatous polyposis and Beckwith–Wiedemann syndrome {3696,30,3998,3883, 6596,3533}. Familial adenomatous polyposis and Beckwith–Wiedemann syndrome are due to germline mutations and/

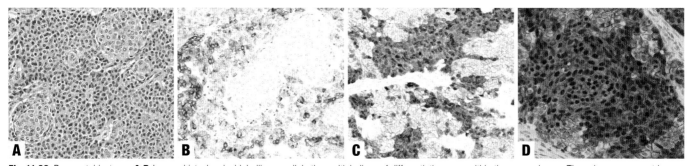

**Fig. 11.38** Pancreatoblastoma. **A,B** Immunohistochemical labelling parallels the multiple lines of differentiation seen within these neoplasms. The acinar component is supported by trypsin expression. **C** In most cases, an abnormal nuclear and cytoplasmic pattern of β-catenin staining is seen within the squamoid nests and surrounding neoplastic cells. **D** Abnormal cytoplasmic and nuclear expression of β-catenin in the squamoid nest.

or deletions in *APC* and chromosome 11p15.5, respectively. Among other driver genes associated with pancreatic neoplasms, *SMAD4* mutations have been reported in 2 cases {3273,3162}. At the transcriptome level, pancreatoblastomas exhibit upregulation of the R-spondin/LGR5/RNF43 module {3162}.

## Essential and desirable diagnostic criteria

*Essential:* a neoplasm exhibiting multiple lines of pancreatic epithelial differentiation; squamoid nests.

## Staging

The TNM classification of pancreatoblastomas follows the criteria for classifying exocrine pancreatic neoplasms.

## Prognosis and prediction

At diagnosis, the majority of patients with pancreatoblastoma have tumours that locally extend beyond the pancreas or have metastatic disease. These neoplasms often invade into adjacent structures, such as the duodenum, spleen, colon, and portal vein. The liver is the most common site of distant metastases, followed by the lymph nodes, lung, and peritoneum {3654,1320, 1732}. Although no standard of treatment has been established, the most important prognostic factor is complete resection. Therefore, in the absence of metastatic disease, surgical resection is the mainstay of treatment. In addition, neoadjuvant therapy may improve margin-negative resection rates {5514}. Recurrence after surgical resection with curative intent is 15% at a mean follow-up time of 24 months {4889}. Despite aggressive therapy, patients with pancreatoblastomas have a 5-year overall survival rate of 54% {1732}. Stage and response to treatment are predictors of patient outcome.

# Pancreatic acinar cell carcinoma

La Rosa S
Cho SJ
Singhi AD

## Definition
Pancreatic acinar cell carcinoma is a malignant epithelial neoplasm showing acinar cell differentiation.

## ICD-O coding
8550/3 Acinar cell carcinoma
8551/3 Acinar cell cystadenocarcinoma

## ICD-11 coding
2C10.0 & XH3PG9 Adenocarcinoma of pancreas & Acinar cell carcinoma

## Related terminology
None

## Subtype(s)
Acinar cell cystadenocarcinoma

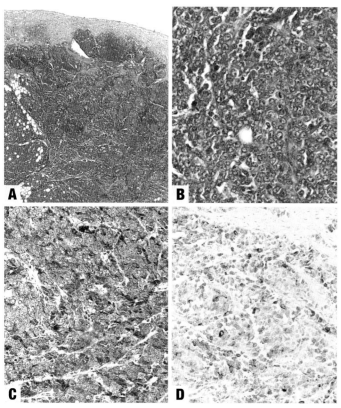

**Fig. 11.39** Pancreatic acinar cell carcinoma. **A** At low magnification, pancreatic acinar cell carcinoma shows solid and lobular growth and appears highly cellular, with scant fibrous stroma. **B** This case shows a solid pattern of growth characterized by large sheets of cells that have large nuclei with dispersed chromatin and prominent nucleoli. Only rare lumina are observed. Tumour cells are diffusely and strongly positive for BCL10 (**C**) and more focally positive for AFP (**D**), which was also elevated in the serum in this 10-year-old patient.

## Localization
Acinar cell carcinoma diagnosed in the paediatric population can involve any portion of the pancreas; it is most common in the tail (41% of cases), followed by the head (32%), the body (13.5%), the body-tail (9%), and the head-body (4.5%) {3934}.

## Clinical features
In most cases, patients present with vague and nonspecific symptoms, including abdominal pain or discomfort, abdominal swelling or mass, nausea, vomiting, mild fever, and anaemia. Jaundice is unusual. Unlike in adults, polyarthralgia, panniculitis, and subcutaneous fat necrosis, which are symptoms related to lipase release by tumour cells, have not been reported in children {3934}.

Serum AFP levels were found to be elevated in all paediatric patients with acinar cell carcinoma in whom AFP was measured {1340,4389,1920}. The capacity of neoplastic cells to produce and secrete AFP has important diagnostic and clinical implications and may be useful for posttherapy monitoring.

Patients presenting with Cushing syndrome due to the ectopic production of ACTH by tumour cells have been described, and it is important to recognize this clinical manifestation because it may lead to the erroneous diagnosis of pancreatic neuroendocrine neoplasm (PanNEN) {4389,3119,4465}.

## Epidemiology
Pancreatic neoplasms are rare in children and adolescents. Their annual incidence in individuals aged 0–19 years is 0.018 cases per 100 000 (adjusted to the 2000 US standard population) in the SEER database, 0.20 cases per 100 000 in the Italian cooperative TREP project report, and 0.018 cases per 100 000 in a German study {5448,1542,1920}. The reported annual incidence of acinar cell carcinoma in individuals aged 0–19 years (age-adjusted to the 2000 US standard population for tumour histology) was 0.003 cases per 100 000 population {5448}.

Acinar cell carcinomas account for approximately 7% of paediatric pancreatic neoplasms, with a slight male predilection and an average age at diagnosis of 9.57 years (range: 3–16 years).

## Etiology
The etiology of paediatric acinar cell carcinomas is unknown and they probably appear as sporadic tumours, although a detailed family history has not been reported in published cases. It is worth noting that acinar cell carcinomas diagnosed in the context of Lynch syndrome, Carney complex, and familial adenomatous polyposis have been documented in adults {2342,3857,3439,4166,6328}.

## Pathogenesis
Mechanisms involved in the pathogenesis of paediatric acinar cell carcinomas are unknown, and the limited available data mainly pertain to acinar cell carcinomas diagnosed in adults {7521}.

Although the molecular landscape of adult acinar cell carcinomas has been widely investigated over the past few years, molecular data concerning paediatric acinar cell carcinomas are scant. In the 2 paediatric cases investigated, allelic loss of chromosome 11p was found in 1 case, and no mutations in the APC/β-catenin pathway were detected {29}. The genetic alterations in paediatric acinar cell carcinomas would have to be extrapolated from the work that has previously been done on adult acinar cell carcinomas, which showed chromosome instability characterized by high degrees of allelic losses and gains. The more frequently involved chromosomal regions of loss included 1p, 3p, 5q, 6q, 8p, 9p, 11, 17p, and 18q, whereas the main chromosomal regions gained were 1q, 7, 8q, 12, 17q, and 20q {3273,2972,6902,623}. MYC amplification and/or chromosome 8 polysomy have been described in a subset of acinar cell carcinomas as well {623,3859}. Alterations in the APC/β-catenin pathway are well documented and include mutations of both APC and CTNNB1, although the most frequent alterations of APC are gene loss and/or promoter hypermethylation {2269}. TP53 mutations as well as TP53 gene loss have been identified in 12–24% of cases {1287,3273,3858, 1722}. BRAF mutations are very rare {3273}, but approximately 23% of acinar cell carcinomas harbour rearrangements involving BRAF and RAF1, and the most prevalent fusions are SND1::BRAF and HERPUD1::BRAF {1287,7405}. RET rearrangement has also been identified in a subset of pancreatic acinar cell carcinomas {1301}.

### Macroscopic appearance

Paediatric acinar cell carcinomas are usually large at the time of diagnosis, with an average diameter of 118 mm (range: 32–200 mm). They are well circumscribed, fleshy, and pink to tan, and they generally contain areas of necrosis and/or haemorrhage. Cystic patterns have rarely been described {3043}.

### Histopathology

Acinar cell carcinomas in children show the same histological features and immunohistochemical phenotype as those observed in adults. Acinar cell carcinomas are highly cellular, with scant fibrous stroma, a lobular pattern of growth, and frequent and abundant necrosis. Cells have moderate amounts of granular eosinophilic cytoplasm containing zymogen granules, which are PAS-positive and diastase-resistant. Nuclei are generally uniform with a single prominent nucleolus. The mitotic count is variable but generally high. The most frequent architectural patterns observed in paediatric acinar cell carcinomas are acinar and solid patterns, frequently present in the same tumour. The acinar pattern is characterized by structures resembling normal acini, sometimes with minute lumina. Cells are distributed in a monolayer with basally located nuclei. The solid pattern is characterized by large sheets of cells without lumina, making the differential diagnosis with PanNENs sometimes difficult. The trabecular pattern has rarely been observed. Other uncommon patterns described in adults, including oncocytic, spindled, clear, pleomorphic, and follicular-like thyroid cell types {3857,3934, 6105}, have not been described in paediatric acinar cell carcinomas. Extremely rare cases of acinar cell cystadenocarcinoma have been described.

### Immunohistochemistry

Immunohistochemistry plays a key diagnostic role in demonstrating acinar cell differentiation. However, commercially available antibodies commonly used in routine diagnostic practice (against trypsin, chymotrypsin, lipase, amylase, and carboxyl ester lipase) show different sensitivities {3857,3860}. The monoclonal antibody directed against the C-terminal portion of the BCL10 protein (clone 331.3), which recognizes the C-terminal portion of pancreatic carboxyl ester lipase, is highly specific and sensitive in detecting acinar cell differentiation {3860}. Amylase is rarely expressed, and lipase antibodies show low sensitivity. Trypsin, chymotrypsin, and BCL10 antibodies are the most sensitive. The simultaneous use of two of these three antibodies allows the detection of nearly 100% of cases {3860,3857}. Acinar cell carcinomas may also express CK7 and CK19, and they are positive for PDX1. Scattered chromogranin A–positive and/or synaptophysin-positive neuroendocrine cells are frequently observed. Acinar cell carcinomas associated with Cushing syndrome surprisingly show a scant immunohistochemically detectable neuroendocrine component that is weakly and focally immunoreactive for ACTH {4389}. AFP immunoreactivity can be demonstrated in acinar cell carcinomas, although it is focal {374}.

### Cytology

The cytological features are the same as those of tumours observed in adults, and smears are moderately cellular with a clean background, although cytoplasmic granules and naked nuclei can be observed. Neoplastic cells are polygonal with

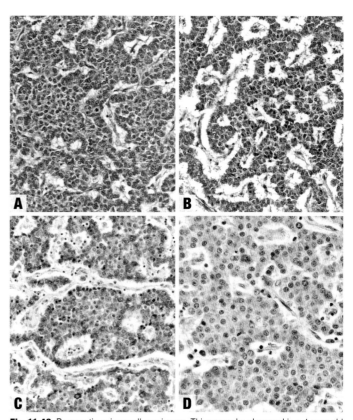

**Fig. 11.40** Pancreatic acinar cell carcinoma. This example, observed in a 1-year-old boy presenting with Cushing syndrome, shows a mixed architectural pattern including solid and acinar/glandular features in some areas (**A**) and trabeculae in others (**B**). Tumour cells are immunoreactive for trypsin (**C**) and focally immunoreactive for ACTH (**D**).

abundant finely granular cytoplasm and uniform nuclei with one or two evident nucleoli; the cells are generally arranged in irregularly shaped groups, small glandular structures, or large sheets.

## Diagnostic molecular pathology
Not clinically relevant

## Essential and desirable diagnostic criteria
*Essential:* a lobular pattern of growth; scant to absent fibrous stroma; moderate to abundant necrosis; high cellularity; cells with moderate amounts of granular eosinophilic cytoplasm with uniform nuclei showing single prominent nucleoli; demonstration of acinar cell differentiation.

*Desirable:* immunohistochemistry with specific antibodies, including against trypsin, chymotrypsin, and BCL10.

## Staging
The staging system is the same as that used for pancreatic carcinoma, published by the American Joint Committee on Cancer (AJCC) or the Union for International Cancer Control (UICC).

## Prognosis and prediction
Metastases have been reported in approximately 40% of paediatric acinar cell carcinomas; they are locoregional in 26% of cases and distant in 22%. In the reported cases, 43% of patients were only treated with surgical resection, 36% were treated with surgical resection combined with chemotherapy and/or radiotherapy, and 21% received palliative chemotherapy. Although aggressive, paediatric acinar cell carcinomas seem to have a better prognosis than adult acinar cell carcinomas {3653}. After chemotherapy, 45% of patients were alive with no evidence of disease at an average follow-up time of 25.5 months (range: 3–132 months); 13.7% were alive with disease at an average follow-up time of 14.7 months; and 27.5% died of disease, with an average survival time of 34.4 months. No specific studies on prognostic markers in paediatric acinar cell carcinomas have been performed. By analogy with adult acinar cell carcinomas, stage may play a major prognostic role {3857}.

# Solid pseudopapillary neoplasm

Singhi AD
Tanaka Y

## Definition

Solid pseudopapillary neoplasm of the pancreas is a low-grade malignant tumour composed of poorly cohesive polygonal cells that surround delicate blood vessels, form solid masses with frequent cystic degeneration and intracystic haemorrhage, and lack a specific line of cell differentiation.

## ICD-O coding

8452/3 Solid pseudopapillary neoplasm of the pancreas
8452/3 Solid pseudopapillary neoplasm with high-grade carcinoma

## ICD-11 coding

2C10.Y & XH3FD4 Other specified malignant neoplasms of pancreas & Solid pseudopapillary tumour

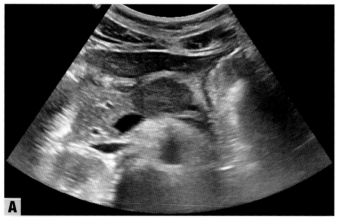

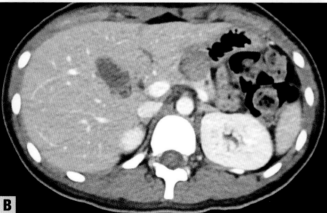

**Fig. 11.41** Solid pseudopapillary neoplasm. **A** Ultrasound shows a well-defined hypoechoic cystic mass at the body of the pancreas. The echogenicity of the mass is higher than the fluid in the gallbladder, probably owing to the presence of blood products and debris. **B** Contrast-enhanced axial CT shows a well-defined, fairly homogeneous, cystic mass arising in the body of the pancreas. The mass enhances less than the adjacent normal pancreatic tissue.

## Related terminology

*Acceptable:* solid pseudopapillary tumour.
*Not recommended:* solid-cystic tumour; papillary-cystic tumour; solid and papillary epithelial neoplasm; Frantz tumour.

## Subtype(s)

Solid pseudopapillary neoplasm with high-grade carcinoma

## Localization

Solid pseudopapillary neoplasms can occur throughout the pancreas, but in children there is a slight predilection for the pancreatic body and tail {598,1494,4889,1983,4020,3088}. Rare cases of extrapancreatic solid pseudopapillary neoplasms have been reported to arise in the ovary and in an ectopic pancreas in the mesocolon {1717,3715,3155}.

## Clinical features

Unlike adults, most children with solid pseudopapillary neoplasm of the pancreas present with nonspecific symptoms related to an intra-abdominal mass, including abdominal pain, dyspepsia, early satiety, and nausea and vomiting {4889,1494}. A palpable mass or fullness can often be appreciated on abdominal examination. In rare instances, a solid pseudopapillary neoplasm can rupture after trauma and patients may present acutely with haemoperitoneum {6836,4704}. Serum pancreatic enzymes and known tumour markers (e.g. AFP, CEA, and β-hCG) are typically negative {4889}.

The radiographic findings of a solid pseudopapillary neoplasm reflect the variable macroscopic features of these tumours. CT tends to demonstrate a large, well-defined, isodense lesion that is heterogeneously hypoenhancing on postcontrast images, with predominantly mixed solid-cystic morphology. A pseudocapsule can be identified in nearly half of all cases, as can internal calcification {927}. MRI may also be useful. Solid portions are isodense to hypointense to the pancreas on T1-weighted images and slightly hyperintense to the pancreas on T2-weighted images {1016,1395}. A surrounding hypointense pseudocapsule and internal haemorrhagic necrosis or debris, seen as high signal intensity on T1-weighted images, are distinguishing features of solid pseudopapillary neoplasms. In the appropriate clinical context these imaging findings are reasonably suggestive of the diagnosis.

## Epidemiology

Solid pseudopapillary neoplasms account for 60–70% of paediatric pancreatic tumours {4889}. The majority of patients are adolescent girls (mean age: 14 years, range: 5–18 years) {4889, 598}. Although earlier reports suggested these neoplasms are more common in Asian and African-American populations, subsequent studies have not identified an ethnic predilection {7460}.

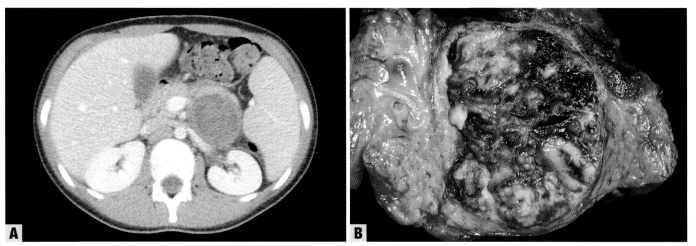

**Fig. 11.42** Solid pseudopapillary neoplasm. **A** Axial CT reveals a solid pseudopapillary neoplasm involving the pancreatic body and tail and characterized by a variable solid and pseudocystic mass. **B** Gross image showing a large, well-demarcated neoplasm that is partially haemorrhagic and necrotic.

## Etiology

Rare cases have been reported in patients with familial adenomatous polyposis syndrome and Lynch syndrome {6052,3127, 1501}.

## Pathogenesis

Despite numerous morphological, immunohistochemical, ultrastructural, and multiomic studies, the cell of origin and pathogenesis of solid pseudopapillary neoplasms remain unknown {5495,4110,3757,1106,5349,6337,995}. However, several hypotheses have been proposed for the histogenesis of these tumours. Given the high prevalence of solid pseudopapillary neoplasms in the female population, as well as the expression of PR and AR and the lack of expression of transcription factors associated with pancreatic glandular development (PDX1, SOX9, PTF1A, and NKX2-2), it has been postulated that solid pseudopapillary neoplasms are derived from a pluripotent stem cell within the genital ridges {3757,3715,995,1717}. In support of this hypothesis, the genital ridges are in close proximity to the pancreatic anlage during embryogenesis. Furthermore, solid pseudopapillary neoplasms reported to occur in the ovary are morphologically identical to those in the pancreas. Considering that somatic mutations in *CTNNB1*, which encodes the cell adhesion protein β-catenin, are essentially ubiquitous in solid pseudopapillary neoplasms, it is possible that loss of adhesion within a pluripotent stem cell from the genital ridge may

translocate to the pancreatic parenchyma during embryogenesis {27,6874}.

Missense activating mutations in exon 3 of *CTNNB1* or inactivating alterations in *APC* have been consistently identified in solid pseudopapillary neoplasms {27,7636,229,6337}. Unlike in other pancreatic neoplasms, alterations in *KRAS*, *GNAS*, *CDKN2A*, *SMAD4*, and *VHL* are distinctly absent in solid pseudopapillary neoplasms. However, alterations in *CTNNB1* and *APC* have been seen in as many as 80% of pancreatoblastomas and 50% of acinar cell carcinomas {2269,1287,3273}. Of note, in the setting of a cystic lesion, preoperative testing of pancreatic cyst fluid for *CTNNB1* mutations and *APC* deletions can be highly sensitive and specific for solid pseudopapillary neoplasms {6498}.

## Macroscopic appearance

Solid pseudopapillary neoplasms are typically solitary, but rare cases of multicentric tumours have been described {3676,5219}. Tumours are round, well-demarcated, and generally large (average diameter: 82 mm, range: 12–200 mm). On cross-section, solid pseudopapillary neoplasms appear grossly encapsulated and exhibit a variable amount of solid, cystic, haemorrhagic, and necrotic components. Small tumours tend to be solid, whereas larger neoplasms can be almost entirely cystic with prominent haemorrhage, necrosis, and a thin peripheral rim of remaining neoplastic tissue {1759,4388}. Calcifications may be present

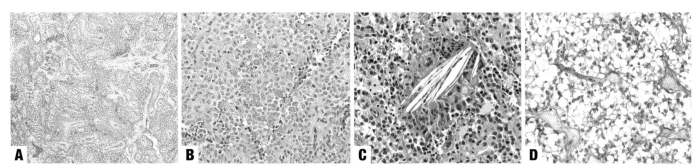

**Fig. 11.43** Solid pseudopapillary neoplasm. **A** Prominent pseudopapillary growth pattern with fibrovascular cores surrounded by loosely cohesive neoplastic cells. **B** Many of the neoplastic cells contain intracytoplasmic, eosinophilic hyaline globules that are variable in size and shape. **C** Other findings include degenerative changes, such as the presence of foamy macrophages, cholesterol crystals, and haemorrhage. **D** Although the neoplastic cells are frequently eosinophilic, cytoplasmic vacuolization is a common occurrence.

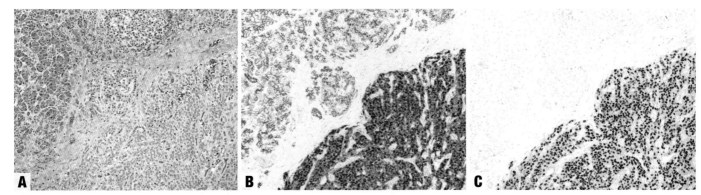

**Fig. 11.44** Solid pseudopapillary neoplasm. **A,B** Genomic alterations in exon 3 of *CTNNB1* or *APC* are consistently identified within these tumours. These mutations result in strong nuclear and cytoplasmic expression of β-catenin, while the adjacent non-neoplastic pancreatic parenchyma shows a normal membranous labelling. **C** LEF1 is diffusely positive within tumour nuclei but absent in the non-neoplastic pancreatic parenchyma.

within the wall of the neoplasm. Rarely, tumours will extend into adjacent structures, such as the duodenal wall {6242}.

## Histopathology

The microscopic findings of a solid pseudopapillary neoplasm are heterogeneous and include variable proportions of solid and pseudopapillary structures. The solid areas contain sheets of relatively uniform polygonal cells with an admixture of numerous delicate, capillary-sized blood vessels {5495,6711,4110}. Other areas of the neoplasm show dramatic degenerative changes that include the formation of pseudopapillae, foamy macrophages, cholesterol crystals, and haemorrhage. Pseudopapillae are the result of neoplastic cells detaching from one another and are characterized by loosely cohesive cells that cling to the blood vessels. The cytoplasm of these neoplastic cells is usually eosinophilic, but it can also be clear, foamy, and/or vacuolated {147}. The cytoplasm often contains aggregates of small hyaline PAS-positive globules, although this is a nonspecific feature {4603}. The globules are not uniformly distributed and may be absent in much of the neoplasm but innumerable in isolated clusters of neoplastic cells. The nuclei are round to ovoid, with uniform and finely stippled chromatin and frequent longitudinal nuclear grooves. Mitoses are rare, and bizarre nuclear pleomorphism may be observed {4080}. Of note, solid pseudopapillary neoplasms with foci of high-grade malignant transformation including undifferentiated and sarcomatoid features constitute a recognized histological subtype {6881}. These neoplasms are characterized by diffuse sheets of cells with increased nuclear atypia and abundant mitotic figures.

Abnormal cytoplasmic and nuclear immunohistochemical expression of β-catenin is a characteristic finding in solid pseudopapillary neoplasms {27,6874,6876}. This pattern of labelling is secondary to *CTNNB1* or *APC* mutations that result in the impaired degradation of β-catenin. The nuclear accumulation of β-catenin coincides with WNT pathway signal transduction and transcription of downstream target genes (e.g. *LEF1*). Thus, LEF1 is also diffusely expressed within the nuclei of tumour cells {6497}. There is also loss or abnormal cytoplasmic expression of E-cadherin {1252}. Other diagnostic markers include cyclin D1, CD10, CD99 (dot-like), PR, AR, glutamine synthetase (GS), TFE3, and SOX11 {4847,6994,5096,2607,3757,2730}. Immunoreactivity for cytokeratins, synaptophysin, and CD56 has been observed in 30–70% of cases. However, solid pseudopapillary neoplasms are negative for chromogranin A, PDX1, and acinar cell markers such as trypsin and BCL10 {3860,4999}. Considering that the differential diagnosis for a solid pseudopapillary neoplasm includes pancreatoblastoma, acinar cell carcinoma, and pancreatic neuroendocrine tumour (PanNET), a panel of immunohistochemical stains is often warranted.

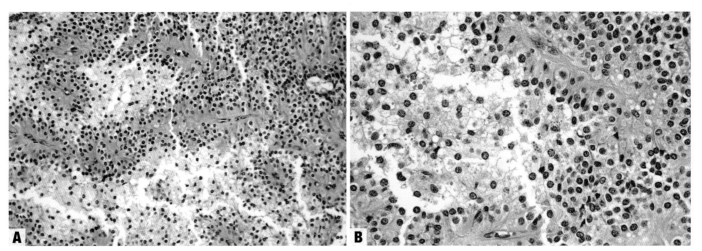

**Fig. 11.45** Solid pseudopapillary neoplasm. **A** Pseudopapillae with fibrovascular stalks surrounded by loosely cohesive tumour cells. **B** Pseudopapillae and loosely cohesive tumour cells, some containing aggregates of hyaline globules.

## Cytology

FNAB smears are highly cellular and predominantly composed of tissue fragments {493,5495,5492}. The neoplastic cells in these fragments are aggregated around slender branching capillary vessels. In addition, the neoplastic cells can be present singly or in small, loosely cohesive aggregates, or they may form acini or rosettes. The cytoplasm of the neoplastic cells is often eosinophilic and finely vacuolated, and it may contain hyaline globules. Some of the single cells can exhibit cytoplasmic tails (cercariform cells) {6142}. The nuclei are uniform, round to ovoid, stippled, and located eccentrically. Few cells have well-formed nuclear grooves, so the differential diagnosis often includes a pancreatic NET.

## Diagnostic molecular pathology

Not clinically relevant

## Essential and desirable diagnostic criteria

*Essential:* a neoplasm occurring in a patient of the characteristic age and sex; solid, papillary, and cystic structures; positive nuclear and cytoplasmic immunolabelling for β-catenin.

*Desirable:* PAS-positive granules; cholesterol crystals; foamy macrophages.

## Staging

The TNM classification of solid pseudopapillary neoplasms follows the criteria for classifying exocrine pancreatic neoplasms. However, rarely do these neoplasms extend beyond the pancreas {6242}.

## Prognosis and prediction

The prognosis for patients with solid pseudopapillary neoplasms is excellent {598,1494,4889,1983}. For the majority of patients, pancreatectomy with negative margins is curative. As many as 7% of paediatric patients develop recurrence or distant metastases to the liver, omentum, mesentery, or peritoneum. Most of these lesions are also surgically resectable, and long-term survival can be achieved in many patients with metastatic disease.

All solid pseudopapillary neoplasms are classified as low-grade malignant neoplasms. There are no proven morphological predictors of outcome, although vascular invasion, pleomorphism, and necrosis have been associated with recurrence and poor survival. Furthermore, it has been suggested that the outcome for adult patients is worse than that for paediatric patients, and patients with aneuploid neoplasms do worse than those with diploid neoplasms {3356,4020,3390}. Solid pseudopapillary neoplasms with foci of high-grade malignant transformation are also noted to be particularly aggressive, with death due to disease reported within 16 months of initial diagnosis {6881}.

# Gastroblastoma

Pawel BR
Graham RP

## Definition
Gastroblastoma is a rare, low-grade gastric biphasic epitheli-omesenchymal neoplasm with metastatic potential that is composed of epithelial and spindle cells. The tumour arises in the stomach in children and young adults.

## ICD-O coding
8976/1 Gastroblastoma

## ICD-11 coding
2F70.1 & XH4VQ1 Neoplasms of uncertain behaviour of stomach & Gastroblastoma

## Related terminology
None

## Subtype(s)
None

## Localization
Gastroblastoma is an intramural gastric tumour, most commonly arising in the antrum, but it may also arise from the gastric body {1116,4655}.

## Clinical features
Patients usually present with nonspecific abdominal pain or discomfort, in some cases accompanied by a palpable abdominal mass. Patients may also present with gastrointestinal bleeding and anaemia {1116,4655}. Depending on tumour size and localization, endoscopy may reveal a mass with endoluminal growth with or without ulceration {1116}. Imaging modalities such as CT and MRI will commonly reveal a mixed solid-cystic mass involving the stomach, with variable compression of adjacent structures {6442}.

## Epidemiology
The ages of the reported patients with gastroblastoma from North America, Europe, Asia, and northern Africa have ranged from 9 to 56 years (mean: 24 years, median: 27 years). There appears to be a male predominance, with cases reported in 8 male patients and 4 female patients to date {4655,6442,7511, 4285,2085,2523,7039}.

## Etiology
Unknown

## Pathogenesis
Gastroblastoma is characterized by a *MALAT1::GLI1* fusion, and it has been proposed that this fusion gene probably drives *GLI1* oncogenic properties and hedgehog activation. Further evidence in support of the oncogenic properties of the *MALAT1::GLI1* fusion gene is its presence in a subset of another gastric tumour, plexiform fibromyxoma {6606}.

## Macroscopic appearance
Gastroblastoma manifests as a solid or solid-cystic mass involving gastric wall structures with variable degrees of haemorrhage and mucosal ulceration. It is well demarcated from surrounding

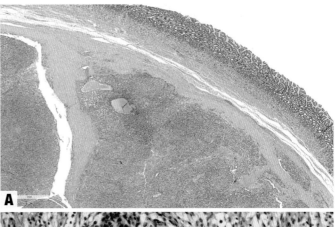

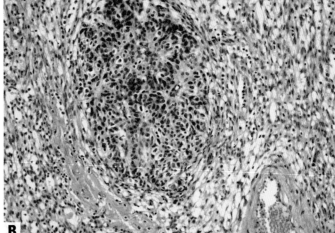

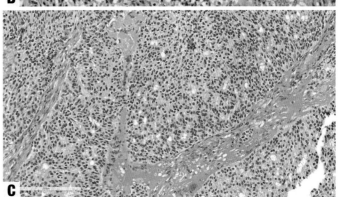

**Fig. 11.46** Gastroblastoma. **A** A vaguely biphasic tumour arising in the wall of the gastric antrum. **B** An epithelial cell nodule surrounded by bland spindle cells. **C** Epithelial cells forming small rosettes.

tissues and may project intraluminally to form a polypoid mass. The tumour can be as large as 150 mm in maximum dimension {4655}.

## Histopathology

Gastroblastoma has a multinodular growth pattern, with mesenchymal and epithelial components present in variable proportions. Neither component is histologically malignant. The mesenchymal component is composed of bland, uniform, ovoid to spindle cells with pale, clear, or eosinophilic cytoplasm, and it often shows a reticular pattern. The epithelial component may consist of rosettes with eosinophilic secretions, epithelial cords, or solid epithelioid nests, which may be either admixed with mesenchymal elements or well demarcated from them. Mitoses are rare in most cases (with exceptions {4655,6442}), and mitotic counts seem to be unrelated to outcome. Neither the epithelial nor the mesenchymal components display marked atypia or pleomorphism {4655}.

### Immunohistochemistry

The mesenchymal component of gastroblastoma expresses CD10, CD56, and vimentin. The epithelial component expresses cytokeratin (AE1/AE3 and CAM5.2) {1116}. KIT may rarely be expressed {6442,7511}. Both components show strong and diffuse staining for GLI1 {2523}. SMA, calretinin, CD34, desmin, and S100 are negative {1116,4655}.

## Cytology

Not clinically relevant

## Diagnostic molecular pathology

Gastroblastoma is characterized by a recurrent in-frame, oncogenic *MALAT1::GLI1* fusion gene, which can be identified with both clinical molecular studies and FISH. This genomic event occurs in both the epithelial and mesenchymal component of the tumour {2523}. The transcriptome of gastroblastoma is

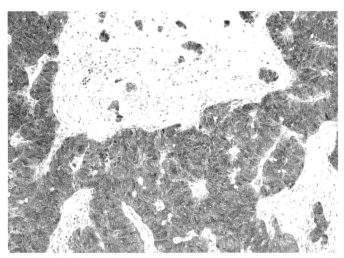

**Fig. 11.47** Gastroblastoma. Strong diffuse nuclear and cytoplasmic staining for GLI1.

characterized by upregulation of GLI1, a key effector of the hedgehog pathway {3054,2523}.

## Essential and desirable diagnostic criteria

*Essential:* gastric origin; biphasic epithelial and spindle cell histopathology; expression of cytokeratin in the epithelial component.
*Desirable:* demonstration of *MALAT1::GLI1* fusion.

## Staging

Not clinically relevant

## Prognosis and prediction

Gastroblastoma rarely recurs after partial or subtotal gastrectomy {1116}. Regional and distant lymph node metastases may occur, as well as distant organ metastases. Deaths attributable to gastroblastoma have not been documented {1116}.

# Appendiceal neuroendocrine tumours

Klimstra DS

## Definition

Neuroendocrine neoplasms (NENs) arising in the appendix in children are well-differentiated neuroendocrine tumours (NETs), which show an organoid, nested architecture; cytological features typical of neuroendocrine neoplasms; low proliferation; and immunolabelling for chromogranin and/or synaptophysin.

## ICD-O coding

8240/3 Neuroendocrine tumour, NOS
8240/3 Neuroendocrine tumour, grade 1
8249/3 Neuroendocrine tumour, grade 2

## ICD-11 coding

2B81.2 & XH9LV8 Neuroendocrine neoplasms of appendix & Neuroendocrine tumour, grade 1
2B81.2 Neuroendocrine neoplasms of appendix

## Related terminology

Not recommended: carcinoid tumour; well-differentiated endocrine tumour/carcinoma.

## Subtype(s)

None

## Localization

Appendiceal NETs in children mainly occur in the tip of the appendix (54–73%) {2835,5058,5787}, with involvement of the body in 21% of cases; the base is uncommonly involved.

## Clinical features

Girls are more commonly affected than boys (M:F ratio: 1:1.65), and the mean age at presentation is 11.65 years {4181,5058}.

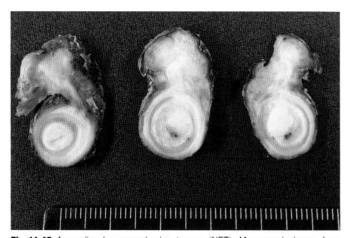

**Fig. 11.48** Appendiceal neuroendocrine tumour (NET). Macroscopic image from a 10-year-old. Most of the tumour is intraluminal. The tumour replaces most of the mucosa and penetrates through the wall layers, focally reaching the mesoappendix.

Most patients (85%) present with acute appendicitis, with the neoplasm incidentally detected during pathological evaluation of the appendectomy specimen {6306,4181,5058}; chronic abdominal pain or an appendiceal mass are uncommon. In some patients the neoplasm is incidentally detected after appendectomy performed during abdominal surgery for other indications {5058}. The carcinoid syndrome of flushing and diarrhoea is very uncommon {3592}, and there are no elevated serotonin metabolites in the urine {2774}.

## Epidemiology

Appendiceal NETs are very rare in childhood. According to the SEER database, the incidence in children is 2.9 cases per 1 million person-years. However, the appendix is the most common gastrointestinal location for NETs in children, and appendiceal NET is the most common gastrointestinal epithelial neoplasm in this age group {6633}. Among appendectomy specimens largely performed for acute appendicitis, 0.2–0.4% contain a NET {1772}, which contrasts with 1.9% in adult patients {7521}.

## Etiology

Unknown

## Pathogenesis

Appendiceal NETs may arise from neuroendocrine cells within the mucosal crypts, but some evidence also suggests an origin from subepithelial neuroendocrine cells, particularly for enterochromaffin (EC)-cell NETs, which commonly display S100-positive sustentacular-like cells surrounding the nests of neoplastic cells {2457}.

## Macroscopic appearance

Macroscopically, appendiceal NETs appear as well-demarcated yellow to tan nodules, most commonly at the tip of the appendix and centred within the wall. In cases with coexisting acute appendicitis and in appendices removed incidentally, the NET may not be identifiable grossly, indicating that the tip of the organ should always be examined microscopically. The majority (71%) of appendiceal NETs in children are < 10 mm in diameter; 22% are 10–20 mm, and only 6% exceed 20 mm {5058}.

## Histopathology

Microscopically, paediatric appendiceal NETs are essentially always EC-cell NETs {2774}. They consist of uniform polygonal tumour cells that are frequently arranged in large nests, often with peripheral nuclear palisading and luminal formations. Nuclei are uniform, with coarsely stippled chromatin and indistinct nucleoli. Mitoses are infrequent to absent and necrosis is very uncommon {1118,5058}. In areas involved by acute appendicitis, the cytological features may be more

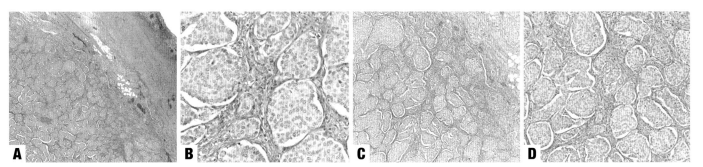

**Fig. 11.49** Appendiceal neuroendocrine tumour (NET) in the appendix of a 10-year-old child. **A** Low-power view. The tumour features the classic Zellballen pattern of neuroendocrine neoplasia. **B** High-power view. The chromatin pattern is classically stippled, without prominent nucleoli. **C** Typical nested pattern of NET. **D** Higher-magnification view.

atypical and the nested architecture may be disrupted. The tumours are associated with a fibrotic stromal response in most cases. Even when small, the bulk of the tumour often lies in the deep muscular wall and subserosa, with minimal mucosal involvement {6699}. Within the muscularis propria, the nests can be compressed into ribbons. About one third of appendiceal NETs infiltrate the mesoappendix, including 50–82% that are < 3 mm in thickness {5787,7326}. Production of serotonin can be demonstrated by immunohistochemistry, along with staining for chromogranin A and synaptophysin. The vast majority of paediatric appendiceal NETs are WHO grade 1 {5787,7326}.

## Cytology
Not relevant

## Diagnostic molecular pathology
Not clinically relevant

## Essential and desirable diagnostic criteria
*Essential:* a uniform population of cells with round nuclei and finely stippled chromatin; architectural patterns include trabeculae, acini, nests, and ribbons; expression of synaptophysin and chromogranin A or chromogranin B.

## Staging
The staging of appendiceal NETs has been greatly modified in the eighth (2017) editions of the Union for International Cancer Control (UICC) TNM classification {870} and the American Joint Committee on Cancer (AJCC) cancer staging manual {238}. It is based mainly on tumour size and infiltration of the serosa and/or mesoappendix. In this classification, many NETs are staged as pT3 because of invasion of the subserosa or mesoappendix.

## Prognosis and prediction
The prognosis of appendiceal NETs in children is excellent. In a meta-analysis of 958 cases, there were no recurrences after surgery and no tumour-related deaths after a mean follow-up of 4.8 years {5058}. Regional lymph node metastases are rare but are found in 1.4% of cases, and the risk of nodal metastases is significantly increased in tumours measuring > 20 mm {5058}. Traditionally, indications for right hemicolectomy after appendectomy include tumour size > 20 mm, involvement of the mesoappendix, vascular invasion, a positive margin, or an elevated mitotic count. However, given the outstanding prognosis in this age group, some authorities question whether right colectomy is indicated {3592,4181,5058}, and among the patients with indications for surgery who instead underwent observation, there still have been no deaths or recurrences {5058}.

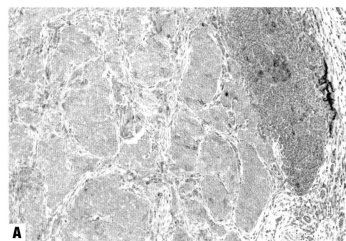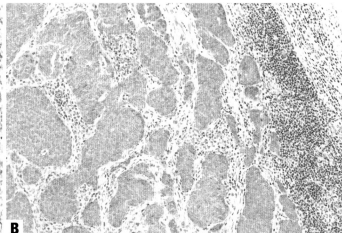

**Fig. 11.50** Appendiceal neuroendocrine tumour (NET). **A** Immunohistochemical staining for chromogranin is a reliable marker in NETs of the appendix. **B** Synaptophysin staining is also consistently positive in these tumours.

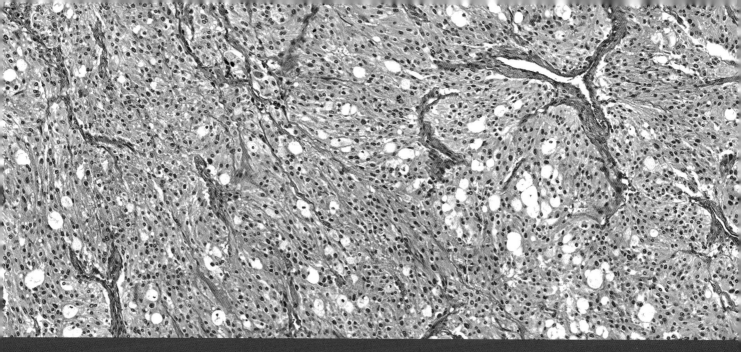

# 12

# Endocrine tumours

Edited by: Jarzembowski JA, Thompson LDR

Thyroid tumours
    Thyroid epithelial tumours
        Follicular adenoma of the thyroid
        Papillary thyroid carcinoma
        Cribriform morular thyroid carcinoma
        Medullary thyroid carcinoma
        Spindle epithelial tumour with thymus-like elements
Parathyroid tumours
    Parathyroid endocrine tumours
        Parathyroid adenoma
Adrenal tumours
    Adrenal cortical tumours
        Adrenal cortical tumours
Tumours of the adrenal medulla and extra-adrenal paraganglia
    Sympathetic paraganglioma
    Parasympathetic paraganglioma (head and neck paraganglioma)
    Phaeochromocytoma
    Composite phaeochromocytoma/paraganglioma
Neuroendocrine neoplasms
    Neuroendocrine tumours
        Other neuroendocrine tumours

# Endocrine tumours: Introduction

Jarzembowski JA
Thompson LDR

Paediatric endocrine tumours are rare and rarely fatal. Cases in children account for just 0.7% of deaths in the USA and about 9% of all paediatric deaths related to cancer {6474}. The top five leading causes of cancer death in both male and female patients do not include tumours from endocrine organs but are instead related to CNS tumours, leukaemia, bone and soft tissue neoplasms, and lymphomas {6474}. With many endocrine tumours, children have much more favourable outcomes than adults, for reasons known (genetics) and unknown {5771,3231}. Nonetheless, prompt and accurate diagnosis of endocrine organ tumours in children is essential because of their frequent association with syndromes and heritable disease risk.

Peripheral neuroblastic tumours are the third most common childhood neoplasm, and the most common neoplasm during the first year of life. Because a large proportion develop within the adrenal gland and abdominal cavity, this neoplastic category has been separated into its own chapter, rather than being included with the rest of the endocrine organ tumours. Within the endocrine organs (pituitary gland, thyroid gland, parathyroid glands, endocrine pancreas, adrenal cortex, adrenal medulla/paraganglia), the majority of neoplasms occur in the thyroid gland, and in children there are disproportionately more carcinomas than benign neoplasms as compared with adults. Therefore, papillary thyroid carcinoma and medullary thyroid carcinoma are much more likely to be identified in paediatric patients than are follicular carcinomas. Follicular carcinoma in paediatric patients (diagnosed with the same criteria as are used for adult cases) is extremely rare, and it should be recognized that the presence of a follicular carcinoma may be a sentinel event in syndrome presentation or familial disease detection.

One of the most important considerations in all endocrine organ neoplasms, whether benign or malignant, is syndromic or familial association. Pituitary neuroendocrine tumours (PitNETs; see Chapter 3: CNS tumours), when present in paediatric patients, are frequently part of a genetic association, such as X-linked acrogigantism, McCune–Albright syndrome, Carney complex, or multiple endocrine neoplasia (MEN) type 1 (MEN1) {6697,7067,3097,5905,2848}. Furthermore, pancreatic neuroendocrine tumours (PanNETs) are recognized in MEN, along with tuberous sclerosis and von Hippel–Lindau syndrome, among others. Specifically, the gastroenteropancreatic NETs (GEP-NETs) are covered in *Other neuroendocrine tumours* (p. 867) rather than in the gastrointestinal tract sections, but appendiceal NETs are presented within the gastrointestinal sections (see *Appendiceal neuroendocrine tumours*, p. 818). Parathyroid carcinoma is extremely rare and therefore not presented here, but parathyroid adenoma is included. Parathyroid adenoma is known to have a strong association with syndromes, including MEN1, MEN2A, and MEN4, along with the hyperparathyroidism–jaw tumour syndrome {7109,1684, 125}. Medullary thyroid carcinoma is identified as the presenting tumour in paediatric patients with MEN2B or MEN2A, or in those with related familial medullary thyroid carcinoma {1093, 6649}. Papillary thyroid carcinoma, recognized as the most common thyroid gland malignancy in paediatric patients {2609, 2668}, develops in paediatric patients with early exposure to radiation, autoimmune disorders, or nutritional deficiency, and as part of various genetic predisposition syndromes, such as APC-associated polyposis, DICER1 syndrome, Carney complex, PTEN hamartoma tumour syndrome / Cowden syndrome, Werner syndrome, Beckwith–Wiedemann syndrome, familial phaeochromocytoma–paraganglioma syndrome, Li–Fraumeni syndrome, and McCune–Albright syndrome {6578,3386,6343, 6540,4994,5536,3962,3930,5319,4444,1402,7061}. Many of these syndromes, in addition to the familial phaeochromocytoma–paraganglioma syndromes caused by SDHB, SDHC, and SDHD mutations, as well as von Hippel–Lindau syndrome and Lynch syndrome, have additional manifestations of tumours in the adrenal cortex (adrenal cortical adenoma and carcinoma) and the adrenal medulla or paraganglia in paediatric patients. Of note, congenital adrenal hyperplasia is not a tumour per se, but it has been included in the forthcoming *Endocrine and neuroendocrine tumours* volume {7522} as part of the differential consideration with neoplasms..

Therefore, to ensure appropriate workup and treatment, a good understanding of genetic predisposition syndromes and family history is required whenever a diagnosis of an endocrine organ tumour is made in a paediatric patient. Practitioners in the discipline of paediatric pathology always take great pride in recognizing the extraordinary achievement in overall outcome for the single most common endocrine organ malignancy: a 5-year survival rate of > 99% for paediatric papillary thyroid carcinoma {6474}.

# Follicular adenoma of the thyroid

Seethala R
Volante M

## Definition

Follicular adenoma (FA) is a benign encapsulated and non-invasive epithelial neoplasm showing thyroid follicular cell differentiation, without the nuclear features of papillary thyroid carcinoma.

## ICD-O coding

8330/0 Follicular thyroid adenoma
8330/0 Follicular thyroid adenoma with papillary architecture
8330/0 Hyperfunctioning (toxic) follicular adenoma
8290/0 Oncocytic adenoma of the thyroid

## ICD-11 coding

2F37.Y & XH0LM0 Other specified benign neoplasm of endocrine glands & Follicular adenoma

## Related terminology

None

## Subtype(s)

Follicular adenoma with papillary hyperplasia; hyperfunctioning (toxic) follicular adenoma; oncocytic (Hürthle cell) adenoma

## Localization

FA can occur in any part of the thyroid gland in association with thyroglossal duct cysts and lingual thyroid tissue, but it is not recognized in ovarian teratoma (struma ovarii).

## Clinical features

The majority (75–85%) of cases manifest as solitary or dominant palpable masses. About 15% of patients demonstrate compressive symptoms. Palpable lymph nodes are fairly common (occurring in as many as 25% of patients) but are reactive

{1445}. The majority of patients (except for those with the hyperfunctioning or papillary architecture subtype) are euthyroid at presentation {2111,3063,987}.

### Imaging

Ultrasonographically, FAs have a variable appearance (ranging from anechoic to hyperechoic compared to surrounding thyroid tissue) and a smooth, well-defined border. Non-chaotic low blood flow suggests adenoma, but ultrasound features are not specific. Calcification and abnormal lymph nodes are seldom seen {1445}. By radionucleotide scintigraphy, the majority of FAs are cold {3063}, except for those hyperfunctioning clinically.

## Epidemiology

The prevalence of FA is obfuscated by the clinical and histological overlap with benign hyperplastic nodules, as well as verification bias (i.e. patients with benign nodules that do not go to surgery), so the reported rates vary from 12% to 60% of solitary thyroid nodules {7729,3877,1445,3063}. There is a female predilection (M:F ratio: 1:3–4), and the mean age at presentation is about 11–12 years {1445,3063}. Hyperfunctioning (toxic) adenomas are rare (~1–5% of solitary thyroid nodules) {381,94,3063}.

## Etiology

Radiation exposure and iodine deficiency are among the most common risk factors for sporadic FA. Risk from radiation is dose-dependent and may persist for > 40 years after exposure {6458,6253,39}. An important patient subgroup comprises childhood cancer survivors treated with radiation for leukaemia, lymphoma, or a CNS tumour {2208}. Although the link between iodine deficiency and autonomous thyroid nodules including FA and toxic adenomas has been established {586},

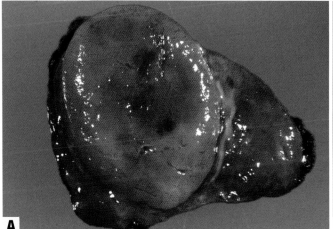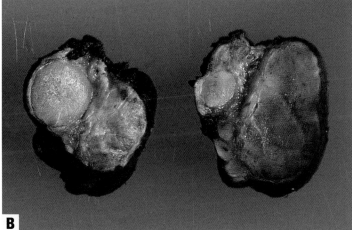

**Fig. 12.01** Follicular adenoma. **A** This example is encapsulated and well delineated from the adjacent thyroid parenchyma and shows a homogeneous light-pink to tan cut surface. **B** Multiple follicular adenomas in *PTEN* hamartoma tumour syndrome. There are multiple encapsulated tan-white follicular adenomas in a multinodular background in this patient with *PTEN* hamartoma tumour syndrome.

the mechanism is not clear. The presumption is that the iodine deficiency results in secondary chronic growth stimulation of the gland, leading to an increased risk of mutation. Family and personal histories of goitre are also risk factors, with syndrome association reported (see Table 12.01) {5536,4025}.

## Pathogenesis

Thyroid nodules occur in as many as 25% of patients with Carney complex {648}, and about 25% of patients with Carney complex have FA; about 20% are aged < 20 years at presentation {1052}. The presence of FA and multiple hyperplastic nodules qualifies as a minor criterion to support the diagnosis of *PTEN* hamartoma tumour syndrome. Although the prevalence of FA in patients with *PTEN* hamartoma tumour syndrome is about 25% overall {3967,5095}, when restricting the population to paediatric patients, the aggregate prevalence of benign tumours (including FA) is lower, at 2–14% {5536}. FAs are rarely reported in *DICER1* syndrome, although hyperplastic nodules and differentiated thyroid carcinomas are more frequently reported {4025}. Hyperfunctioning FAs are known to have activating mutations of *TSHR* or *GNAS* and mutations in *EZH1*, often coexistent {7079, 5359,985}. No molecular markers reliably distinguish FA from follicular carcinoma, the follicular variant of papillary thyroid carcinoma, or non-invasive follicular thyroid neoplasm with papillary-like nuclear features {4817,94,4759,2208}.

## Macroscopic appearance

FAs are characteristically well circumscribed and encapsulated. The cut surface may vary from light tan to a dark brown, generally distinct from the background thyroid parenchyma. Cystic change may be noted, particularly after FNAB. FA in the setting of *PTEN* hamartoma tumour syndrome may manifest as dominant encapsulated nodules in a multinodular background {3967}.

## Histopathology

By definition, FAs lack invasion and typically demonstrate a thin, easily recognizable fibrous connective tissue capsule containing smooth muscle–walled vessels. A follicular architecture predominates, varying from microfollicular to macrofollicular, usually with mixed patterns. Solid and trabecular patterns are

**Table 12.01** Hereditary tumour syndromes associated with follicular adenoma (FA)

| Syndrome | Gene | Thyroid findings |
| --- | --- | --- |
| Carney complex | *PRKAR1A* (17q24.2) | Multinodular goitre, FA, differentiated thyroid carcinomas |
| *PTEN* hamartoma tumour syndromes (including Cowden syndrome, Bannayan–Riley–Ruvalcaba syndrome) | *PTEN* (10q23.31) | Multinodular goitre, FA, differentiated thyroid carcinomas |
| *DICER1* syndrome | *DICER1* (14q32.13) | Multinodular goitre, FA, differentiated thyroid carcinomas |

usually a minor component. Tumour stroma is scant with a delicate vascular network, although prior FNAB or core needle biopsy may induce a stromal reaction. Neoplastic cells recapitulate the appearance of normal follicular cells and are cuboidal with pale to eosinophilic cytoplasm and small, round, dark, regular nuclei. Mitotic figures are rare (except around a needle tract) and do not change the diagnosis when present. The background thyroid varies from normal to multinodular, sometimes with chronic lymphocytic thyroiditis {7607}.

A histological subtype seen in adolescents is FA with papillary hyperplasia. This subtype is characterized by projections of microfollicles into dilated follicle spaces, imparting what can be designated a pseudopapillary architecture {4334}. Cells show cuboidal to columnar cytoplasm but still retain evenly spaced, round, dark, regular nuclei polarized to the basement membrane with little overlap or stratification. Hyperfunctioning (i.e. toxic, hot) adenomas overlap with FA with papillary hyperplasia and show slightly more variation in nuclear size, more prominent columnar and eosinophilic to vacuolated cytoplasm, and scalloped colloid resorption (histologically similar to the diffuse hyperplasia seen in Graves disease). There are rare reports of oncocytic adenomas {3680}. Histological patterns (clear cell, signet-ring cell, spindle cell, lipoadenoma, and FA with bizarre nuclei) are not well characterized in paediatric patients. Pigmented (or black) adenomas are rare in paediatric patients because they require chronic exposure to

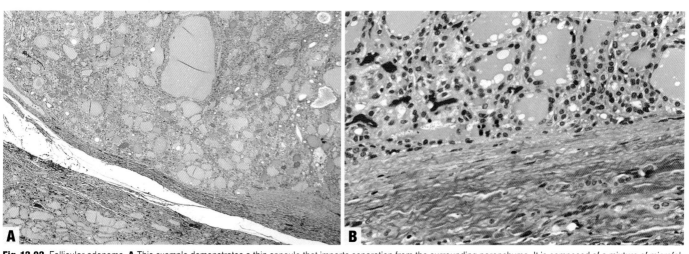

**Fig. 12.02** Follicular adenoma. **A** This example demonstrates a thin capsule that imparts separation from the surrounding parenchyma. It is composed of a mixture of microfollicles and macrofollicles, and it is overall more cellular and distinct from the surrounding thyroid. **B** The nuclei are bland and monomorphic and have round to ovoid nucleoli with condensed chromatin. The nuclei should not deviate much from those in the adjacent normal tissue, seen here as a compressed follicle.

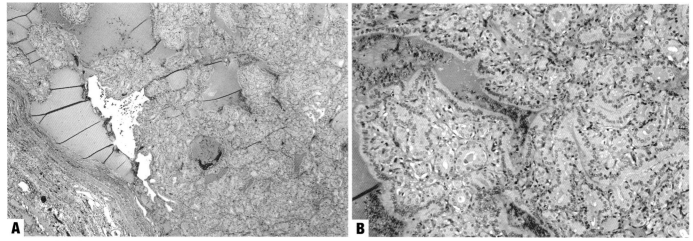

**Fig. 12.03** Follicular adenoma (FA) with papillary architecture. **A** Like conventional FAs, those with papillary architecture are demarcated from the surrounding thyroid by a capsule but often show cystic change and a pseudopapillary architecture, reminiscent of a hyperplastic nodule. These are fairly common in adolescents. **B** The pseudopapillae seen in FA with papillary architecture show cuboidal to columnar cells with bland ovoid nuclei, similar to those seen in typical FA, and are polarized towards the basement membrane without much stratification or overlap. In contrast to the fibrovascular cores of true papillae seen in conventional papillary thyroid carcinoma, these papillae often show follicles within. The cytoplasm is often somewhat oncocytic. Hyperfunctioning adenomas may show some overlap with FA with papillary architecture but often show more vacuolated cytoplasm and scalloped colloid.

tetracyclines {3738}. FAs in Carney complex do not have any distinctive features. FAs in *PTEN* hamartoma tumour syndrome are multiple (there may be as many as 100) and tend to be more solid or hypercellular. Although they are well demarcated, tumoural capsules may not be readily apparent, making their distinction from hyperplastic nodules difficult. Oncocytic change, background lymphocytic thyroiditis, inflammation, and physiological C-cell hyperplasia are common.

### Immunohistochemistry

The neoplastic cells in FA are reactive for thyroglobulin, thyroid transcription factor 1 (TTF1), and PAX8, but negative for calcitonin and PTH. Malignancy-related markers are scarcely investigated in paediatric FAs. Galectin-3 has been found to be expressed in as many as 30% of benign follicular lesions in children, whereas HBME1 and CD56 are more specific, potentially aiding in the diagnosis {6519}. Loss of nuclear PTEN protein by immunohistochemistry has been suggested as a screening tool to detect *PTEN* hamartoma tumour syndrome–associated cases {497}.

### Differential diagnosis

FA is difficult and occasionally impossible to distinguish from hyperplastic nodules, although this distinction is usually academic (see Table 12.02). The presence of clear demarcation from the adjacent parenchyma and a well-formed tumour capsule support the diagnosis of FA. The presence of a clonal genetic alteration also favours FA. To ensure accurate diagnosis, the entire tumour capsule/periphery should be evaluated microscopically. Follicular carcinoma is delineated from FA by the presence of tumour capsular and/or lymphovascular invasion. Follicular carcinoma in the paediatric population is usually minimally invasive, requiring microscopic evaluation of the entire tumour capsule–parenchyma junction to exclude this. FA is distinguished from non-invasive follicular thyroid neoplasm with papillary-like nuclear features by the absence of papillary thyroid carcinoma nuclear features; the latter entity appears to be less common in the paediatric population {6002}. Intrathyroidal or perithyroidal parathyroid adenomas are rare in children but may mimic FA {1784} with a follicular architecture, but they have more prominent cell borders, smaller nuclei, no colloid,

**Table 12.02** Key differential diagnostic considerations for follicular adenoma

| Feature | Hyperplastic nodule | Follicular adenoma | NIFTP | Follicular carcinoma |
|---|---|---|---|---|
| Border | Unencapsulated | Encapsulated | Encapsulated | Encapsulated with capsular or lymphovascular invasion |
| Growth pattern | Variable follicle size; overlaps with follicular variation of background thyroid | Variable follicle size; typically more cellular, microfollicular, and distinct from surrounding thyroid | Variable follicle size; typically more cellular, microfollicular, and distinct from surrounding thyroid; distinctive accentuation of cellularity at periphery | Variable follicle size; typically more cellular, microfollicular, and distinct from surrounding thyroid |
| Stroma | Scant to fibrotic if degenerative | Scant to fibrotic if traumatized or degenerative | Often delicate to abundant sclerosis | Scant to fibrotic if traumatized or degenerative; capsule thickened at areas of invasion |
| Cytonuclear features | Round, dark, regular nuclei | Round, dark, regular nuclei | Subtle papillary thyroid carcinoma nuclei | Round, dark, regular nuclei |

NIFTP, non-invasive follicular thyroid neoplasm with papillary-like nuclear features.

Chapter 12

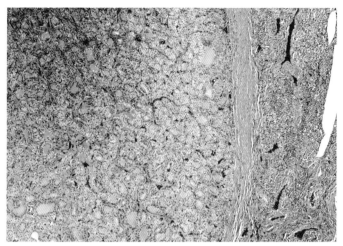

**Fig. 12.04** Follicular adenoma in a background of thyroiditis. This example shows a prominent microfollicular pattern and is notably spared by the lymphocytic infiltrates, which is typically the case for neoplasms in a thyroiditis background.

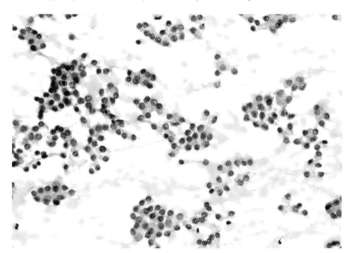

**Fig. 12.05** Thyroid follicular adenoma. The Pap-stained smear is cellular, with limited colloid. The follicular cells are arranged in tight follicles and have round nuclei.

and more typical nested trabecular areas. In some cases, PTH immunohistochemistry may be useful.

## Cytology

The Bethesda System for Reporting Thyroid Cytopathology (BSRTC) is used for paediatric patients. The relative malignancy rates for each category are affected by the overall higher prevalence of malignant neoplasms in the paediatric population {2817}. FAs more frequently fall in the benign categories of atypia of undetermined significance / follicular lesion of undetermined significance (AUS/FLUS) or follicular neoplasm / suspicious for a follicular neoplasm (FN/SFN) {7396}. Cytological samples of FA are usually hypercellular, with follicular cells either arranged in microfollicles or dispersed in a background containing scant colloid. Because of the heterogeneity of follicle size, some cases may display more abundant colloid content. Nuclei are small, round, and regular, with finely dispersed chromatin.

## Diagnostic molecular pathology

Molecular findings aid in categorizing neoplasia but are not validated in children for defining a specific tumour entity (i.e. not diagnostically useful).

## Essential and desirable diagnostic criteria

*Essential:* an encapsulated tumour distinct from surrounding thyroid; no capsular or lymphovascular invasion; no nuclear features of papillary thyroid carcinoma.
*Desirable:* thyroglobulin confirmation of follicular derivation (in selected cases).

## Staging

Not applicable

## Prognosis and prediction

FAs are benign, cured by conservative surgery. Mutation-positive FAs, particularly RAS-mutated tumours, have the potential to progress to carcinoma if not resected.

# Papillary thyroid carcinoma

Faquin WC
Dauer AJ
Nga ME
Rossi ED

## Definition

Papillary thyroid carcinoma (PTC) is a malignant epithelial neoplasm derived from thyroid follicular cells showing characteristic nuclear features identified in diverse growth patterns.

## ICD-O coding

8260/3 Papillary thyroid carcinoma
8340/3 Follicular variant of papillary thyroid carcinoma
8350/3 Diffuse sclerosing papillary thyroid carcinoma
8260/3 Solid/trabecular papillary thyroid carcinoma
8344/3 Tall cell papillary thyroid carcinoma
8342/3 Oncocytic papillary thyroid carcinoma
8341/3 Papillary thyroid microcarcinoma

## ICD-11 coding

2D10.1 Papillary carcinoma of thyroid gland

## Related terminology

*Not recommended:* papillary thyroid adenocarcinoma.

## Subtype(s)

Follicular variant of papillary thyroid carcinoma; diffuse sclerosing papillary thyroid carcinoma; solid/trabecular papillary thyroid carcinoma; tall cell papillary thyroid carcinoma; oncocytic papillary thyroid carcinoma

## Localization

PTC can arise anywhere in the thyroid gland. Rare cases develop in association with ectopic thyroid tissue (such as struma ovarii or lingual tissue) or within thyroglossal duct cysts {4259,6247,7479,6984,7878}.

## Clinical features

PTC typically manifests as an asymptomatic nodule in the thyroid gland or as cervical lymphadenopathy detected by palpation of an enlarged lymph node {2208,7494}. In some cases, PTCs are first detected as incidental nodules after imaging or surgery {7494}. In rare cases, there may be tracheal compression by a large tumour or extrathyroidal invasion with involvement of the recurrent laryngeal nerve, leading to hoarseness and dysphagia.

### Imaging

Ultrasound examination is the standard imaging protocol for the evaluation of a paediatric thyroid nodule, with ultrasonographic features such as composition, echogenicity, shape, margin, and echogenic foci (standardized into a number of reporting systems, such as the Thyroid Imaging Reporting and Data System [TI-RADS]) {6956,7662,2531} and the presence of abnormal lymph nodes in the central or lateral neck determining which nodules warrant an ultrasound-guided FNAB {7066}.

## Epidemiology

Thyroid nodules are uncommon in children, but approximately 25% are malignant {5396,1135}. Most paediatric thyroid cancers occur in the second decade of life, accounting for > 6% of all paediatric cancers {5076,5396}. PTC is the leading type of thyroid cancer, accounting for 90% of cases {2609,2668}. Its incidence has been increasing over the past four decades {7281}. There is a female predominance in adolescents (M:F ratio: 1:5), unlike in younger children {2946,7643,2208}.

## Etiology

In the past 60 years, the incidence of PTC in children has shown two specific peaks {5965,4248,4332,4863,5337,7550}. The first

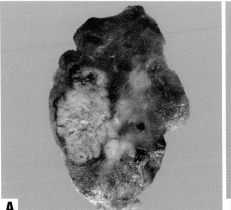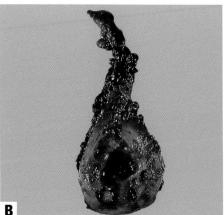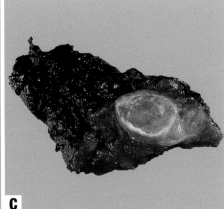

**Fig. 12.06** Papillary thyroid carcinoma. **A** Gross appearance shows an irregular, infiltrative, off-white tumour. The coarse granular appearance reflects the presence of papillary structures. **B** Gross appearance of a papillary thyroid carcinoma of a predominantly cystic nature, with intraluminal papillary protrusions. **C** Encapsulated papillary thyroid carcinoma. Gross appearance shows a relatively circumscribed encapsulated nodule with a fleshy, solid cut surface. This pattern is more common in the follicular variant of papillary thyroid carcinoma. Note the area of capsular invasion at the 3 to 6 o'clock position, with new secondary capsule formation.

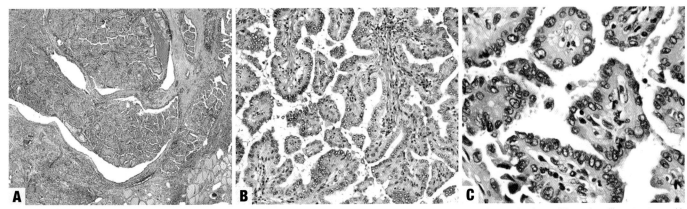

**Fig. 12.07** Classic papillary thyroid carcinoma. **A** Low-magnification view of an unencapsulated classic papillary thyroid carcinoma showing well-formed papillary structures with fibrovascular cores, and infiltration of the tumour into the adjacent non-neoplastic thyroid parenchyma (lower-right corner). **B** Papillary structures with fibrovascular cores lined by cells with oval, pale, overlapping nuclei. **C** Nuclei exhibit open, ground-glass chromatin, with frequent intranuclear cytoplasmic inclusions.

occurred in about 1950 and was mostly due to the use of external radiation for treating *Tinea capitis*, acne, chronic tonsillitis, and thymus hyperplasia, with an average of 10–20 years between the radiation therapy and the development of PTC {5965,4248}. The second peak occurred in the mid-1990s in Eastern Europe, due mostly to the Chernobyl nuclear power plant meltdown on 26 April 1986 {4332,4863,5337,7550}. The first cases of PTC were diagnosed approximately 4–5 years after the nuclear event in children who had been < 5 years of age at the time of the incident. The Chernobyl accident demonstrated the higher sensitivity of the paediatric population to radiation effects as compared to the adult population.

Several reported risk factors are associated with the development of PTC in children, including thyroid disease (e.g.

autoimmune thyroid disorders), nutritional (iodine) deficiency, prior radiation exposure, and familial tumour predisposition syndromes {6670,6089,7277,2208,1923,1964}. One group at risk for developing PTC are childhood cancer survivors who had been treated with radiation therapy for Hodgkin lymphoma, leukaemia, and CNS tumours {871,4629,6521,4546}. In children with Hashimoto thyroiditis, the prevalence of PTC ranges from 0.67% to about 3%, well above the background risk of about 0.02% in the general paediatric population {1444, 4530}. Rarely, genetic predisposition syndromes including *APC*-associated polyposis, *DICER1* syndrome, Carney complex, *PTEN* hamartoma tumour syndrome / Cowden syndrome, and Werner syndrome are associated with PTC and follicular thyroid carcinoma, accounting for approximately 5% of cases

**Table 12.03** Common familial thyroid cancer predisposition syndromes with clinical features

| Predisposition syndrome | Gene (locus) with GeneReviews link | Thyroid phenotype | Other features |
|---|---|---|---|
| ***PTEN* hamartoma tumour syndrome** (Cowden syndrome, Bannayan–Riley–Ruvalcaba syndrome) | *PTEN* (10q23) https://www.ncbi.nlm.nih.gov/books/NBK1488/ | • Thyroid adenomas and multinodular goitre<br>• Thyroid carcinoma (PTC and FTC) | • Macrocephaly (≥ 95%)<br>• Mucocutaneous lesions, papillomatous papules, trichilemmomas, acral keratoses, pigmented macules of the glans penis<br>• Breast cancer (women only)<br>• Endometrial carcinoma / uterine fibroids<br>• Genitourinary tumours<br>• Autism |
| ***DICER1* syndrome** (*DICER1* pleuropulmonary blastoma familial tumour predisposition syndrome) | *DICER1* (14q32.13) https://www.ncbi.nlm.nih.gov/books/NBK196157/ | • Multinodular goitre (thyroid follicular nodular disease)<br>• Thyroid carcinoma (PTC, FTC, and poorly differentiated thyroid carcinoma [rare]) | • Pleuropulmonary blastoma<br>• Sertoli–Leydig cell ovarian tumour<br>• Cystic nephroma<br>• Wilms tumour<br>• Botryoid embryonal rhabdomyosarcoma<br>• Eye and nose tumours<br>• Pituitary blastoma |
| ***APC*-associated polyposis** (familial adenomatous polyposis) | *APC* (5q22.2) https://www.ncbi.nlm.nih.gov/books/NBK1345/ | • Cribriform morular thyroid carcinoma | • Adrenocortical tumours<br>• Colorectal polyps/carcinoma<br>• Osteomas<br>• Desmoid tumours<br>• Pancreatic adenocarcinomas<br>• Medulloblastoma<br>• Hepatoblastoma |

FTC, follicular thyroid carcinoma; PTC, papillary thyroid carcinoma.

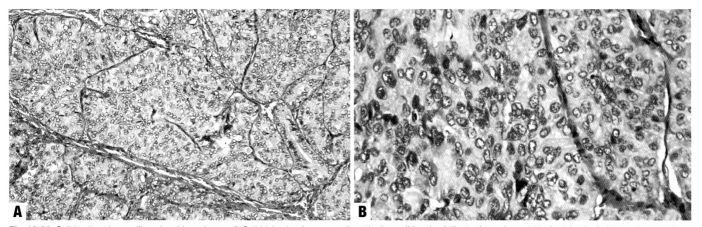

**Fig. 12.08** Solid/trabecular papillary thyroid carcinoma. **A** Solid islands of tumour cells with discernible microfollicular formations within the islands. A delicate but prominent vascular network is seen. **B** Nuclear features of papillary thyroid carcinoma are preserved, with well-formed nuclear pseudoinclusions.

(see Table 12.03) {6578,3386,6343,6540,4994,5536,3962}. In addition, PTC has also been reported in children with the following syndromes: Beckwith–Wiedemann, succinate dehydrogenase (SDH)-deficient tumour syndrome, Li–Fraumeni, McCune–Albright, and Peutz–Jeghers {3930,5319,4444,1402,7061}.

## Pathogenesis
The molecular mechanisms of PTC development involve activation of the RAS/RAF/MEK/ERK (MAPK) pathway and other intracellular signalling pathways via point mutations, gene fusions, and somatic copy-number alterations {1007,538, 6566,7625,7688,7654}. The oncogenic driver alterations in paediatric PTC are the same as those found in adults. However, gene fusions occur more frequently in thyroid cancers in children (60–70%) than those in adults (~15%) {5396,538}. Thus, point mutations of RAS and *BRAF* genes account for as many as 70% of genetic abnormalities in adult PTCs {5032, 538,4719,6095,5396} but are seen in about 30% of paediatric patients (*BRAF* p.V600E mutations are the most common) {5396,538,5440} and are virtually absent in the youngest patients {5440}. *RET* proto-oncogene fusions are the most commonly observed alteration, reported in approximately 25–30% of sporadic paediatric PTC cases, with an increase to 35–50% in paediatric patients with a history of radiation exposure {2079,5396,538}. *RET::CCDC6* and *RET::NCOA4* (paracentric intrachromosomal inversions) are the most commonly observed *RET* fusions. These rearrangements are not linked with genomic instability, possibly influencing the improved response to radioiodine therapy in children with PTC and the rare progression to less differentiated tumours {2079,5382}. Additional oncogenic fusions involve *NTRK1* or *NTRK3, BRAF, ALK*, the transcription factor gene *PAX8*, and the receptor tyrosine kinase gene *MET* {5396,538,5426}; less frequently there are mutations in *PTEN, RAS, DICER1*, and *PIK3CA* {5396,538}. These alterations are seen in 10–15% of PTCs in children and adolescents exposed to ionizing radiation {1895,5396}, as well as in sporadic PTC {5426}. The mechanism involved in the association between Hashimoto thyroiditis and PTC seems to be based on the overproduction of TSH or chronic inflammation leading to proliferation, angiogenesis, and/or reduced apoptosis {5443}.

In children and adolescents, the presence of thyroid oncogene mutations (*BRAF* p.V600E) or rearrangements (e.g. *RET*, NTRK, *BRAF, ALK*, or other fusions) in a nodule with indeterminate cytology is associated with a very high likelihood of PTC {539,5396,538}. In contrast, mutations in *PTEN*, RAS genes, and *DICER1* have a lower specificity for PTC and may be found in both benign and malignant thyroid nodules. There are few to no data on the presence and role of alterations in *TERT, EIF1AX, CHEK2, GNAS*, or *TSHR*, or of several other oncogenic alterations that have been previously detected in adults with PTC {1007}. Until additional molecular markers are available, diagnostic lobectomy for unilateral nodules with indeterminate oncogenes is still the best approach to assessing malignant potential.

## Macroscopic appearance
Grossly, PTCs may be solitary, multifocal (same lobe or isthmus), or multicentric (different lobes or isthmus). They form firm, off-white to tan, irregular masses that may feel gritty on sectioning because of the presence of microcalcifications. The median tumour size is 12–30 mm (range: 1–110 mm) {1399,3892,6756, 2232,2786}. Cystic change and multifocality/multicentricity are not uncommon. Close examination may reveal a somewhat granular cut surface, reflecting the presence of microscopic papillary structures. Some PTCs may appear grossly encapsulated, with thorough sampling of the capsule necessary to assess for the presence of capsular and/or lymphovascular invasion. Extrathyroidal extension, when grossly present, may be recognized as tumour infiltrating into adherent skeletal muscle. Lymph node metastases may be solid or cystic, sometimes with extranodal extension.

## Histopathology
### Classic PTC
Classic PTC is among the three most frequent forms of paediatric PTC, both among sporadic and radiation-associated cohorts {1399,2707,1713,4173,2233}. It is characterized by the presence of well-formed papillary structures composed of a central fibrovascular stalk covered by cuboidal to low columnar epithelial cells. Papillary structures are often seen in cystic areas, sometimes with background histiocytes. Follicular structures may be intermingled with the papillary areas. Psammoma

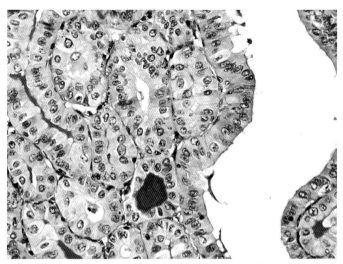

**Fig. 12.09** Tall cell papillary thyroid carcinoma. Tall columnar cells, two to three times taller than wide, showing abundant eosinophilic cytoplasm.

bodies may be present. Sclerotic fibrosis, correlating with the off-white gross appearance, may be seen. Lymphatic invasion is frequently present, reflecting the most common route of metastatic spread by PTC {1399,2232,2786}.

Tumour cells exhibit the classic nuclear features of PTC, which include nuclear enlargement and elongation; pale, open, ground-glass chromatin; small, marginated nucleoli; longitudinal nuclear grooves; and variable numbers of intranuclear cytoplasmic inclusions. The nuclei are often crowded and overlapping. Multinucleated histiocytic giant cells with small nuclei and abundant eosinophilic cytoplasm may be seen between papillary structures and within neoplastic follicular lumina.

The diagnosis of PTC is typically made based upon histomorphology alone. Nevertheless, some cases may benefit from the application of immunohistochemical markers, either to support the diagnosis or to confirm the follicular cell origin of primary or metastatic thyroid tumours {1255,4155,1760,4759, 6001}. PTCs are positive for thyroglobulin, thyroid transcription factor 1 (TTF1), PAX8, and cytokeratins (pancytokeratin, CK7, CAM5.2, and AE1/AE3) {582,3954,5075,5263}. Galectin-3 and HBME1 are expressed in the majority of classic PTCs {519,1081, 523,6003,6098,6005} and at a lower frequency in the follicular variant of PTC (FVPTC) {6003}; their expression is sometimes used to support a diagnosis of PTC over one of benign papillary hyperplasia {6003}. Pertinent negative immunohistochemical stains include calcitonin, CEA, neuroendocrine markers, and CK20 {997}. CK19 is usually not helpful in differentiating between benign and malignant thyroid lesions {1081,523,6227, 6111,3552}. Loss of CD56 expression is noted in almost 100% of classic PTC cases and in two thirds of FVPTC cases {1909,1848, 714,790}. Nuclear and cytoplasmic overexpression of CITED1 is seen in two thirds of classic PTCs and in 50% of cases of FVPTC {6304,5622}. The BRAF p.V600E mutation–specific antibody VE1 in thyroid tumours shows 90–100% sensitivity and nearly 100% specificity for *BRAF* p.V600E mutation–positive PTC {5034,5032,2392,3732,6000,5999}. The diagnostic utility of other markers (thyroperoxidase, fibronectin, S100A4, cyclin D1, p27) has not been defined.

### Follicular variant of PTC

FVPTC is relatively common in the paediatric population, making up 10–33% of non–radiation-induced PTCs {1399,2707, 1713,2233}. Grossly, FVPTC, particularly when encapsulated, may have a more homogeneous, pale tan, fleshy appearance, reminiscent of follicular neoplasms. These tumours may be infiltrative or encapsulated and are composed exclusively of follicular structures, without well-formed papillary structures, while exhibiting many of the classic nuclear features of PTC. The follicles may be round or elongated, and they contain small amounts of brightly hypereosinophilic colloid. Multifocality has been reported in 28–39% of FVPTC cases {4044,6145}.

Infiltrative forms of FVPTC can be associated with nodal and sometimes distant metastases, as well as with extrathyroidal extension {4173,2233}. Encapsulation has been documented in 50–67% of paediatric FVPTCs {6145,4400}. Like in adults, encapsulated tumours with capsular or lymphovascular invasion in children have been shown to be associated with nodal metastases {4400}. In the absence of capsular or angioinvasion (after completely examining the tumour periphery), metastasis or recurrence is rare to absent {6145,4400,6002,5975,7394}, so

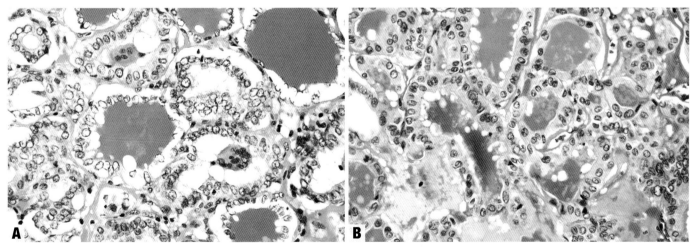

**Fig. 12.10** Follicular variant of papillary thyroid carcinoma. **A** Follicular structures lined by cells with glassy, round to oval nuclei with pale chromatin. Scattered multinucleated giant cells are noted within some of the lumina. The luminal colloid appears bright pink. **B** Follicular structures (some of which are elongated) lined by cells with oval grooved nuclei, pale chromatin, and an occasional nuclear pseudoinclusion.

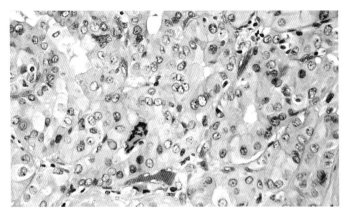

**Fig. 12.11** Oncocytic papillary thyroid carcinoma. Polygonal oncocytic cells with abundant dense eosinophilic cytoplasm, displaying classic nuclear features of papillary thyroid carcinoma. A pseudoinclusion is evident here, close to a multinucleated giant cell.

the same nomenclature as in adults can be applied, i.e. non-invasive follicular thyroid neoplasm with papillary-like nuclear features (NIFTP).

*Diffuse sclerosing PTC*

Diffuse sclerosing PTC (DSPTC) most commonly occurs in adolescents and young adults, in both sporadic and radiation-associated settings {1399,2232,2707,4173,2233,463}. It has a striking female predominance, with female patients making up > 80% of patient cohorts {4341,3891,6982,5814}. Grossly, there may not be a discernible dominant mass, and microscopic tumour foci may not be grossly appreciated. It is characterized by the diffuse involvement of one or both thyroid lobes by numerous foci of PTC including papillary structures with psammoma bodies. The psammoma bodies are characterized by a concentrically lamellated pattern of calcification, often associated with the fibrovascular papillary cores of the tumour. There is associated stromal fibrosis and a prominent chronic lymphocytic thyroiditis {6982,3891,5814}. Another characteristic feature is the presence of squamous morules, which appear as solid whorls or nests of cells with dense eosinophilic cytoplasm. Lymphatic invasion is extensively present, and DSPTC has a greater

predilection than classic PTC for extrathyroidal extension, nodal and distant metastases, and persistent or residual disease, with > 50% of cases showing documented nodal metastases at presentation {4341,3891,6982}.

*Solid/trabecular PTC*

Solid/trabecular PTC accounts for 10–35% of paediatric PTCs {7254} in both radiation-associated and sporadic cases {1399, 2707,4173,2233,5031}. An association with younger age (≤ 10 years) has been suggested but not universally confirmed {1399,2707,2233}. Histologically, there is a predominant solid, nested, insular, or trabecular pattern with a prominent fine vascular network. The defining amount of solid/trabecular areas can vary from about 50% to virtually 100% {5140,5033}. However, even solid areas constituting < 50% have been associated with disease recurrence or higher stage {5140, 1037}. Within the nests, the cells may be arranged in sheets or in follicular structures with minimal colloid, or they may form compressed papillary structures. Classic nuclear features of PTC are present. The main differential diagnosis is poorly differentiated thyroid carcinoma, which lacks classic PTC nuclei and shows necrosis and elevated mitotic activity (unlike solid/trabecular PTC) {7325}.

By immunohistochemistry, solid areas exhibit diminished reactivity with CK19 and HBME1, as well as a somewhat elevated Ki-67 nuclear labelling index (although it is still lower than that seen in poorly differentiated thyroid carcinoma) {5141,5139}. Nuclear reactivity with TTF1 and PAX8 is usually retained. Molecular alterations include the presence of *RET/PTC* and *NTRK1* and/or *NTRK3* gene fusions, but this subtype has a relative rarity of *BRAF* mutations compared with classic PTC {5033,7351}.

*Tall cell PTC*

Tall cell PTC (TCPTC) may be diagnosed when ≥ 30% of the tumour is composed of cells whose height is at least two to three times their width {4180,999}. TCPTCs are composed of prominent papillary fronds with delicate thin fibrovascular cores, or of elongated, compressed follicular structures. The elongate cells contain abundant eosinophilic cytoplasm and

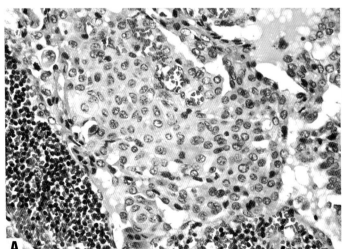
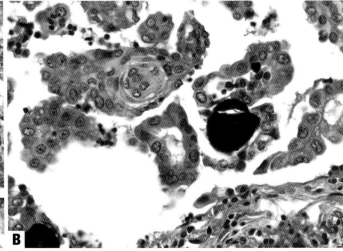

**Fig. 12.12** Diffuse sclerosing papillary thyroid carcinoma. **A** Squamous morule with cells arranged in a swirling manner. Note the prominent lymphoid infiltrate. **B** Papillary structures with a small squamous morule and psammoma bodies within the stromal cores.

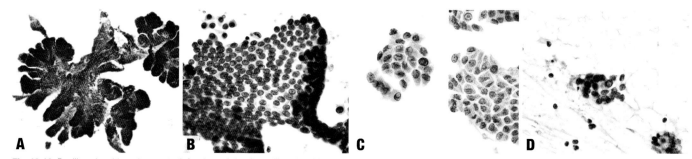

**Fig. 12.13** Papillary thyroid carcinoma. **A–C** Cytology of classic papillary thyroid carcinoma. **A** Well-formed papillary structure with central fibrovascular core and finger-like papillary projections (Pap stain). **B** Flat, monolayered syncytial sheet of follicular cells with enlarged, oval, overlapping, grooved nuclei; powdery chromatin; and small nucleoli (Pap stain). **C** Enlarged, oval, overlapping nuclei with pale chromatin, longitudinal grooves, and intranuclear pseudoinclusions (Pap stain). **D** Cytology of the follicular variant of papillary thyroid carcinoma. A small, crowded group of follicular cells with oval nuclei; fine, delicate chromatin; and a nuclear pseudoinclusion. In the absence of papillary structures and psammoma bodies, this can be categorized as a follicular neoplasm or as suspicious for papillary thyroid carcinoma (Pap stain).

usually intranuclear cytoplasmic inclusions. Mitoses and apoptotic cells can be seen. TCPTC should be distinguished from Warthin-like PTC, which features broad papillae expanded by lymphoplasmacytic cells, which are in turn lined by oncocytic cells. Another differential diagnosis is the oncocytic subtype of PTC, in which the cells are not as tall. *BRAF* mutations (particularly *BRAF* p.V600E) are found in as many as 80% of TCPTCs {7304,4171,4172}.

### Oncocytic PTC
Pure oncocytic PTC is very rare in paediatric patients {2232, 2707}. The cells may form follicular or papillary structures and are polygonal with abundant granular to dense eosinophilic cytoplasm surrounding nuclei, with classic nuclear features of PTC. The main differential diagnoses include oncocytic cell neoplasms, which lack the characteristic nuclear features of PTC and TCPTC as described previously.

### Papillary microcarcinoma
See the forthcoming *Endocrine and neuroendocrine tumours* volume {7522}.

## Cytology
FNAB is the key first-line diagnostic tool for the evaluation of clinically significant thyroid nodules in the paediatric age group. All FNAs in children should be performed under ultrasound guidance, with the six-category Bethesda System for Reporting Thyroid Cytopathology (BSRTC) applied {2208,163}. Within the paediatric population, there is a wide variation in the risk of malignancy in nodules with indeterminate cytology (BSRTC categories 3, 4, and 5), and, in general, the risk in each category appears to be higher than in adults {540,1555}. Classic PTC and most PTC subtypes (with the exception of FVPTC and NIFTP) can be accurately diagnosed by FNAB, although subclassification into a particular subtype of PTC may not be possible from cytological samples. FNAB samples of classic PTC are cellular and show syncytial and branching sheets of neoplastic cells as well as intact papillary structures with fibrovascular cores. Nuclei are enlarged, oval to elongated, and often overlapping. The chromatin is fine and evenly distributed, and most nuclei exhibit longitudinal nuclear grooves. Small eccentric nucleoli are present, as well as occasional intranuclear cytoplasmic pseudoinclusions. The amount of colloid is variable, and it often has a thickened, hypereosinophilic appearance in air-dried

preparations. Multinucleated giant cells are also encountered. A definitive cytological diagnosis of PTC requires, in addition to classic nuclear features, architectural features such as papillary structures or flat syncytial monolayered sheets and psammoma bodies {163,3776}. Strict cytological criteria should be applied to avoid overdiagnosis of indolent follicular-patterned lesions, such as NIFTP.

The cytological diagnosis of FVPTC is more challenging, because of its substantial cytomorphological overlap with NIFTP {6732,4327}. Cytological features of both entities include a predominantly follicular microarchitecture, with variable nuclear enlargement, pallor, and grooves {163,3776,6732, 4327}. Notably, papillary structures and psammoma bodies are absent, and intranuclear pseudoinclusions are uncommon. In these instances, cytological classification in the BSRTC usually falls into categories 3, 4, or 5 {163,2050}.

The specific cytological diagnosis of PTC subtypes is not required, because a diagnosis of PTC is usually sufficient to direct appropriate management. However, there are some cytological clues that may suggest the presence of non-classic PTC. DSPTC, in addition to classic nuclear features, has rounded groups of cells with outer scalloped borders, distinct cytoplasmic vacuoles, frequent psammoma bodies, squamoid-appearing cells, and background lymphocytes {6837}. TCPTC smears exhibit typical PTC nuclear features, with the additional findings of nuclear palisading with basally located nuclei, tall columnar-shaped cells with tapering cytoplasm, and (occasionally) spindle-shaped tumour cells {6867}. Mitoses, apoptosis, and necrosis are sometimes seen. The cytological distinction between oncocytic PTC and oncocytic cell neoplasms is important, albeit very challenging. Nuclear features are the key discriminators: chromatin pallor, grooves, and pseudoinclusions favour oncocytic PTC, whereas large round hyperchromatic nuclei with prominent central nucleoli favour oncocytic cell neoplasm {4787}.

## Diagnostic molecular pathology
Oncogene panels, gene expression classifier panels, and microRNA panels have been incorporated into clinical practice (see Table 12.04) within the adult population to improve the accuracy and reliability of pathological diagnosis {5777}; however, data in the paediatric population are primarily limited to somatic oncogenic alterations {2213,5396,538}, which are used to predict an increased risk of malignancy in a patient aged

**Table 12.04** Thyroid oncogene, risk of invasive disease, and anticipated surgical approach in paediatric papillary thyroid carcinoma (modified from Bauer 2019 {540})

| Point mutation or oncogene fusion | Increased risk of DTC with invasive disease? | Surgical approach |
|---|---|---|
| BRAF p.V600E | Yes | Total thyroidectomy with central neck lymph node dissection; lateral neck lymph node dissection based on clinical findings and FNAB confirmation of metastasis |
| RET/PTC | Yes | |
| NTRK fusion | Yes | |
| BRAF fusion | Yes (limited data) | |
| ALK fusion | Yes (limited data) | |
| TERT + additional mutation | No data in paediatrics | |
| RAS, PTEN, DICER1, PAX8::PPARG | No (lower risk of invasive disease) | Lobectomy<br>Consider completion thyroidectomy if invasive features on histology |
| TSHR | No/minimal | |
| THADA | No | Surveillance or definitive treatment if associated with autonomous function and no evidence of invasive behaviour |
| GNAS | No | |
| AKT1, CTNNB1, EIF1AX, and others | Unknown | No specific recommendation |

DTC, differentiated thyroid cancer.

< 19 years with a nodule with indeterminate cytology on FNAB {540}. In addition, there are no data in children to support using the results of oncogenic profiling to identify the likelihood of a benign lesion.

### Essential and desirable diagnostic criteria
*Essential:* PTC nuclear features (including nuclear enlargement and elongation; crowding and overlap; pale, open, ground-glass chromatin; small marginated nucleoli; longitudinal nuclear grooves; and variable numbers of intranuclear pseudoinclusions); papillary or follicular-patterned growth.
*Desirable:* demonstration of a molecular alteration with a high specificity for PTC (in selected cases).

### Staging
PTCs are staged using the TNM system as published by the Union for International Cancer Control (UICC), although it is not specific for paediatric patients {5682}.

### Prognosis and prediction
PTC in paediatric patients is associated with an excellent prognosis, with > 98% of patients surviving for ≥ 30 years after initial treatment. Some PTC subtypes (including classic PTC, DSPTC, solid PTC, and widely invasive FVPTC), as well as the presence of extrathyroidal extension and lymphatic invasion, are associated with an increased risk of regional and distant metastasis, most commonly to the lungs {3658, 6145,540}. Encapsulated FVPTC and PTC associated with *PTEN* hamartoma tumour syndrome and *DICER1* syndrome appear to have a more indolent course, with a reduced risk of regional and distant metastasis. Pathological classification to predict tumour behaviour includes cytological, histological, biochemical, and oncogenic driver data {1007}. Preliminary paediatric data suggest that a similar approach, i.e. identification of the oncogenic driver mutation, may provide improved diagnostic accuracy as well as an opportunity to stratify surgery and optimize medical care.

# Cribriform morular thyroid carcinoma

Erickson LA
Mete O

## Definition
Cribriform morular thyroid carcinoma (CMTC) is a malignant thyroid tumour with a particular growth pattern secondary to constitutive activation of the WNT/β-catenin pathway that can occur with familial adenomatous polyposis (FAP) or sporadically.

## ICD-O coding
8201/3 Cribriform carcinoma, NOS

## ICD-11 coding
2D10.Y & XH1YZ3 Other specified malignant neoplasms of thyroid gland & Cribriform carcinoma, NOS

## Related terminology
*Not recommended:* cribriform morular variant of papillary thyroid carcinoma; papillary thyroid carcinoma, cribriform morular variant.

## Subtype(s)
None

## Localization
CMTC is usually multifocal and/or bilateral in FAP, whereas sporadic cases occur as a solitary nodule {999,5093A,5094,2593A}.

## Clinical features
Almost all CMTCs (97%) occur in young women, with 89% of cases occurring in individuals aged < 40 years (mean: 28 years, range: 8–69 years) {3890}, including paediatric patients. The M:F ratio is 1:31–61 {3890,999B}. As many as 53% of CMTC cases are associated with FAP {3890}. Tumours may present as a painless mass, hoarseness, or dysphagia, or they may be incidentally discovered on ultrasound.

## Epidemiology
In review of 129 CMTCs in the English-language literature, 63% of reported cases were from Asia, 26% from America, and 11% from Europe {3890}. The frequency of thyroid carcinoma in FAP has increased with screening ultrasound and FNAB {999B}.

## Etiology
In patients with FAP, CMTC is secondary to germline *APC* pathogenic variants. Somatic mutation resulting in permanent activation of the WNT/β-catenin signalling pathway is responsible for sporadic tumours {999B}. Female sex is a risk factor {1122C,999B}.

## Pathogenesis
Most germline *APC* pathogenic sequence variants in FAP with thyroid tumours occur in exon 15 (codons 463–1387), and codon 1061

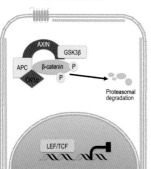

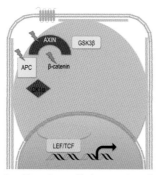

**Fig. 12.14** Pathogenesis of cribriform morular thyroid carcinoma. Under normal conditions, in the absence of WNT binding to frizzled (FZD) receptors, β-catenin interacts with the destruction complex (CK1, GSK3B, APC, and AXIN1), resulting in its phosphorylation by CK1 and GSK3B and its subsequent degradation by the proteasome. In sporadic cribriform morular thyroid carcinoma, somatic mutations in the *APC, CTNNB1,* and/or *AXIN1* genes alter the destruction complex, impairing β-catenin phosphorylation and degradation. β-catenin accumulates in the cytoplasm and subsequently translocates to the nucleus, where it acts as an activator of LEF/TCF proteins that lead to constitutive expression of WNT target genes. In cribriform morular thyroid carcinomas associated with familial adenomatous polyposis, there are germline *APC* mutations.

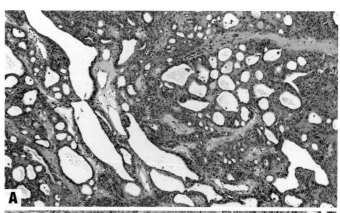
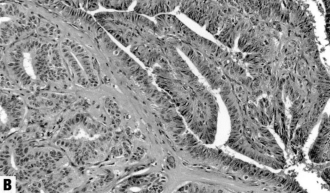

**Fig. 12.15** Cribriform morular thyroid carcinoma. **A** The cribriform structures lack intervening fibrous stroma and merge with tubular follicles that lack colloid. **B** Papillae and pseudopapillae are lined by tall, cuboidal, or pseudostratified columnar cells. Tubular follicles lacking colloid are seen.

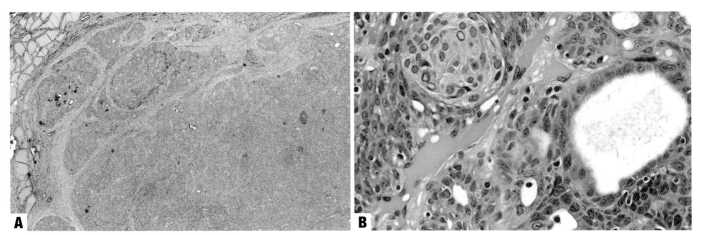

**Fig. 12.16** Cribriform morular thyroid carcinoma. **A** These tumours are usually circumscribed or encapsulated, but they can have fibrous bands imparting a multilobulated appearance. **B** There is a morule in the upper left and cribriform tubular growth in the lower right.

is a hotspot for hepatoblastoma and CMTC {1122B}. *APC* mutation leads to a truncated APC protein, which is unable to contribute to β-catenin proteasomal degradation. Stabilized β-catenin is translocated into the nucleus and binds LEF/TCF proteins, leading to constitutive expression of WNT target genes involved in proliferation and loss of differentiation {999B}. In FAP with multiple CMTCs, each tumour has a different somatic *APC* variant (second hit) {4726A}. Second-hit somatic variants in *KMT2C* and *KMT2D* have been described in some familial CMTCs {5024A}.

Somatic alterations involving *RET* (in the form of rearrangements) {6589A,1122A}, *PIK3CA* {3853A}, and *KRAS* {2401A}, as well as *TERT* promoter variants {5153A}, may be additional effectors of the WNT/β-catenin pathway in familial and sporadic CMTC {999B}.

## Macroscopic appearance

CMTCs in FAP are often multifocal (4–13 foci), bilateral, and small; sporadic tumours are larger (mean: 30 mm), single nodules {830A,2707A,999,5094,999B,5344A}. CMTCs are well circumscribed or encapsulated, solid (but may be cystic), and white-tan {999B}.

## Histopathology

CMTCs are circumscribed or encapsulated and may appear lobulated due to fibrous septa {5093A,999B,2707A}. Angioinvasion occurs in 30% of cases and capsular invasion in 40% {999B}.

CMTCs have an admixture of growth patterns not seen in other thyroid carcinomas {5093A,2707A}. As originally described, CMTCs display "an intricate blending of cribriform, follicular, papillary, trabecular, and solid patterns of growth, with squamoid morulae" {999}. The cribriform structures are composed of anastomosing bars and arches, without intervening fibrous stroma, that merge with tubular follicles that lack colloid {999, 999B}. Papillae and pseudopapillae are lined by tall, cuboidal or pseudostratified cells, and trabecular areas show spindle cells reminiscent of hyalinizing trabecular tumour {999,5094,999B}. Squamoid morulae are whorls of spindle to ovoid cells that lack keratinization and show nuclear clearing due to biotin accumulation {999,2593A,999B}. Psammoma bodies are rare {3890, 999B}. With these distinctive features, the tumour was initially called the cribriform-morular subtype of papillary thyroid carcinoma {999}. But correlation between the tumour's morphological features and recently understood molecular alterations brought about a name change to CMTC {5095A,5094,999B,999C,830A}.

### *Immunohistochemistry*

Aberrant strong nuclear and cytoplasmic β-catenin staining is the hallmark of this thyroid tumour {5094,2593A,999B}. CMTC is positive for thyroid transcription factor 1 (TTF1, clones SPT24 and 8G3G7/1), various keratins, EMA, ER, and PR, and negative for CK20, calcitonin, and WT1 {998A,998B,2401A,3853A,

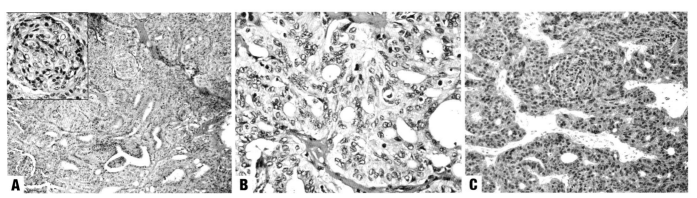

**Fig. 12.17** Cribriform morular thyroid carcinoma. **A** Cribriform architecture, with irregularly shaped follicular structures devoid of colloid, interspersed with morular areas. **Inset:** Scattered optically clear nuclei within morules, caused by the accumulation of biotin. **B** Non-morular area showing oval, overlapping grooved nuclei. **C** β-catenin immunohistochemistry, showing strong nuclear and moderate cytoplasmic reactivity in both follicular and morular cells.

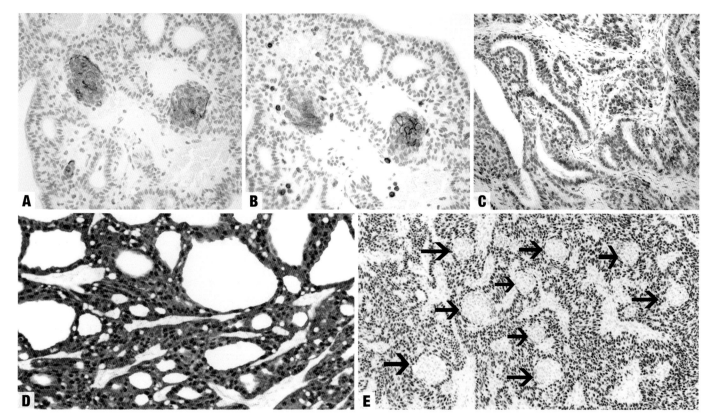

**Fig. 12.18** Cribriform morular thyroid carcinoma. **A** The morular component is positive for CK5. **B** Immunostaining for CD5 highlights the morular component of these tumours, as well as scattered CD5-positive T lymphocytes. **C** This tumour is diffusely positive for ER. **D** β-catenin immunostaining shows characteristic aberrant immunopositivity in the nuclei and in the cytoplasm of the tumour cells. **E** The tumour is positive for thyroid transcription factor 1 (TTF1) by immunostaining, except for the morules (arrows).

2593A,999B}. Thyroglobulin expression is typically negative; however, focal nonspecific diffusion-type staining can occur due to entrapped non-tumorous thyroid follicles {830A}. PAX8 immunohistochemistry using either the monoclonal BC12 antibody or polyclonal antisera shows no or only focal weak staining in these tumours {830A}. Morulae are negative for keratin 34βE12, thyroglobulin, TTF1, PAX8, ER, PR, and E-cadherin, but they stain for CDX2, CD10, CD5, and CK5 {998A,998B, 2401A,3853A,999B,830A}. The Ki-67 proliferation index is usually < 5%. High-grade CMTCs have increased mitotic activity, necrosis, and a Ki-67 index of 15–60%; they may have neuroendocrine differentiation, and they can occur in both sporadic and familial settings {999A,4921A,1439A,7095A}. In a study of 33 CMTCs, high-grade features were present in 2 sporadic CMTCs and in none of the FAP-associated CMTCs {830A}.

## Cytology
Findings in paediatric patients have been reported but are not unique {3349A,2908}.

## Diagnostic molecular pathology
Evaluation for germline *APC* pathogenic sequence variants is desirable in patients with CMTC. About 85% of germline *APC* variants are in exon 15, usually outside the mutation cluster region {1122B,999B}. In familial and sporadic cases, constitutive WNT/β-catenin pathway activation is evidenced by strong nuclear β-catenin immunostaining – a hallmark of CMTC and an important diagnostic criterion. *BRAF* variants are absent.

## Essential and desirable diagnostic criteria
*Essential:*
- A well-circumscribed or locally invasive TTF1-positive thyroid neoplasm
- Diffuse nuclear β-catenin expression
- Predominant complex architecture including cribriform areas and squamoid morulae, with no colloid formation

*Desirable:*
- Cribriform areas: positive for pancytokeratin, ER, and PR; negative (or focal weak) reactivity for PAX8; negative for thyroglobulin
- Morulae: positive for CD10, CDX2, CD5, and CK5; negative for TTF1, PAX8, thyroglobulin, ER, and PR

## Staging
These tumours are staged according to the Union for International Cancer Control (UICC) eighth-edition TNM system.

## Prognosis and prediction
At presentation, CMTC is associated with lymph node metastases in 12% of cases and distant metastases in 3%, with an overall cancer mortality rate of 2% {3890}. High-grade CMTCs behave aggressively {4921A,5153A,7095A}.

# Medullary thyroid carcinoma

Collini P
Cipriani NA

## Definition

Medullary thyroid carcinoma (MTC) is a malignant tumour derived from the calcitonin-producing parafollicular C cells of the thyroid gland.

## ICD-O coding

8345/3 Medullary thyroid carcinoma
8345/3 Medullary thyroid microcarcinoma

## ICD-11 coding

2D10.4 Medullary carcinoma of thyroid gland

## Related terminology

*Acceptable:* C-cell carcinoma.
*Not recommended:* parafollicular cell carcinoma; C-cell adenoma; solid carcinoma with amyloid stroma.

## Subtype(s)

Medullary thyroid microcarcinoma

## Localization

Sporadic MTC is usually a single nodule in the thyroid gland. Syndrome-associated tumours (i.e. those occurring in patients

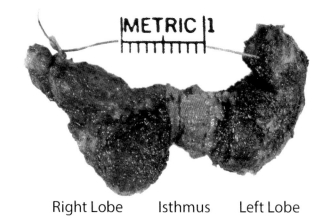

Right Lobe    Isthmus    Left Lobe

**Fig. 12.20** Outer surface of a prophylactic thyroidectomy. Prophylactic total thyroidectomy in a 3-year-old girl with multiple endocrine neoplasia type 2. The total weight of the gland was 1.53 g. The greatest dimension (longitudinal) of the right lobe was 21 mm and that of the left lobe was 17 mm. Microscopically, C-cell hyperplasia was identified.

with multiple endocrine neoplasia type 2 [MEN2]) tend to be bilateral and multicentric, typically in the upper outer parts of the lobes, and associated with C-cell hyperplasia.

## Clinical features

*Sporadic MTC:* In 70% of cases, patients present with a painless thyroid nodule, or with cervical lymphadenopathy. Metastases are noted in 10% of cases at presentation. There can be upper airway obstruction and dysphagia. Patients with metastatic disease can have severe diarrhoea, flushing, or Cushing syndrome related to circulating high levels of calcitonin, CRH, ACTH, and other tumour-related products. Serum levels of calcitonin correlate with the tumour burden. In < 1% of cases the tumours are non-secretory; in these cases, CEA levels can be monitored {6649}.

*Hereditary MTC:* Most MTCs are associated with multiple endocrine neoplasia type 2A (MEN2A), although this association is much less common in paediatric patients than in adult patients. In fully developed MTC, usually discovered in the second decade of life, the signs and symptoms are comparable to those of sporadic MTC. However, MTC in patients with MEN2B is characterized by an early onset, usually within the first year of life – earlier than other MEN2B-associated tumours such as phaeochromocytoma {1093,6649,2421}. In prophylactic thyroidectomies, there can be medullary thyroid microcarcinoma (MTmC) associated with primary C-cell hyperplasia, without palpable nodules. Patients with MEN2B may present with gastrointestinal symptoms (constipation and/or diarrhoea, feeding intolerance), alacrima (tearless crying), mucosal neuromas, marfanoid body habitus along with other skeletal disorders, and other tumours. In a European multicentre study (EUROMEN) of 207 asymptomatic patients with multiple endocrine neoplasia (MEN) who underwent prophylactic thyroidectomy, the mean ages at diagnosis of C-cell hyperplasia and node-negative

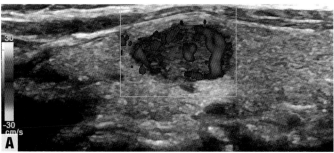
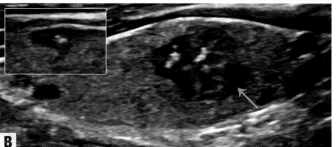

**Fig. 12.19** Medullary thyroid carcinoma. **A** Longitudinal colour Doppler sonography of the thyroid of a syndromic patient. In a patient with a *RET* p.V804M germline pathogenic sequence variant, longitudinal colour Doppler sonography shows flow within a hypoechoic 13 mm nodule, confirming its solid composition. **B** Ultrasound image of the thyroid of a syndromic patient. Bilateral sonographically abnormal thyroid nodules are present in this patient with a *RET* p.G533C germline variant: longitudinal greyscale sonography reveals a dominant left-lobe hypoechoic solid 12 mm nodule (yellow arrow) and a similar subcentimetre right-lobe nodule (**inset**), both containing dystrophic calcifications (red arrows).

MTmC were, respectively, 8.3 and 10.2 years among patients with extracellular domain mutations, and 11.2 and 16.6 years among those with intracellular domain mutations {4301}.

### Imaging

Ultrasound, the preferred imaging modality for thyroid nodules, shows certain high-suspicion findings that include hypoechogenicity, hypervascularity, microcalcifications, taller-than-wide orientation, or spiculated margins {2208,2777,2528}. Coarse, irregularly shaped calcifications indicative of tissue necrosis are most commonly encountered in MTC {2922}, but round calcifications and smooth borders may also be seen {6975}. In paediatric patients, ultrasound-guided FNAB is indicated for clinically and/or ultrasonographically suspicious nodules, even if they measure < 10 mm {2208}.

### Tumour markers

The most frequently evaluated serum marker in MTC is calcitonin, which is directly proportional to C-cell mass {7496}. Although most children with a known MEN syndrome undergo prophylactic total thyroidectomy before the development of MTC, basal and stimulated calcitonin is often performed in order to preoperatively screen for MTC and to establish the baseline in case of disease development/recurrence {837}. Immunochemiluminometric calcitonin assays are considered highly sensitive and specific for monomeric calcitonin {7496}. In the first 2 years of life, serum calcitonin levels are relatively increased (mean: 5–10 pg/mL), with the highest levels occurring in the first 6 months (mean: 11 pg/mL) {1085}. Some studies demonstrate slightly higher levels in male than female patients {1888}. Calcitonin levels decrease as early as the third year of life, approaching adult levels (mean: 0.5–1.5 pg/mL) {1085,1888,1212}. Reference ranges for paediatric patients have not been systematized, and interpretative caution should be exercised. Serum levels of CEA correspond to tumour dedifferentiation, especially when out of proportion to calcitonin {6975,1212}.

### Epidemiology

Approximately 4–8% of paediatric thyroid carcinomas are MTC, with the highest incidence occurring between birth and 4 years of age {1713}. The incidence of MTC in children is 0.03 cases per 100 000 person-years, with a fairly equal sex distribution {6649}. In contrast to adult cases, most paediatric MTCs are

hereditary, related to autosomal dominant germline pathogenic sequence variants in the *RET* proto-oncogene. MEN2A (including familial MTC) affects 95% of syndromic patients; MEN2B affects the remainder {5396,7496,6649}.

### Etiology

Approximately 75% of MEN2B cases occur in patients with de novo germline *RET* pathogenic sequence variants; only 25% have a known family history {7496}. To date, 199 *RET* gene anomalies have been catalogued, including mutations, duplications, insertions, deletions, and rearrangements {4399}.

### Pathogenesis

The *RET* gene on chromosome 10q11.21 contains 21 exons and encodes a receptor tyrosine kinase that is expressed in neural crest–derived cells, including C cells {6649}. It is activated by the glial cell line–derived neurotrophic factor (GDNF) family of ligands, and it regulates cell proliferation and survival via the intracellular PI3K and MAPK signalling pathways {6649}. Extracellular ligand-binding induces dimerization, autophosphorylation of the intracellular kinase domain, and subsequent cell signalling. In MEN2A, gain-of-function mutations occur in the extracellular domain (most often at codon 634 on exon 11 but also at codons 609, 611, 618, 620, and 630 on exon 10), promoting constitutive ligand-independent dimerization. In MEN2B, mutations occur in the tyrosine kinase domain (TKD), most often at codon 918 on exon 16 but also at codon 883 on exon 15, conferring ligand-independent activity to monomeric proteins {1713,6649,7496}. Some patients with atypical MEN2B have double *RET* germline pathogenic sequence variants (one of which involves codon 804 plus a second hit on the same allele) and develop MTC at a slightly older age (20–30 years) {7496}. The risk of aggressive behaviour varies depending on the codon mutated. The American Thyroid Association (ATA) stratified mutations into three relative risk groups: moderate, high, and highest {7496}, corresponding loosely to the North American Neuroendocrine Tumor Society (NANETS) groups: level 1 (high), level 2 (higher), and level 3 (highest) {1212}. Aggressive behaviour is defined by the development of MTC at an early age as well as the development of metastatic disease. The majority (95%) of patients with MEN2B are in the highest risk group, because they have a *RET* p.M918T mutation. Fewer than 5% have a p.A883F mutation

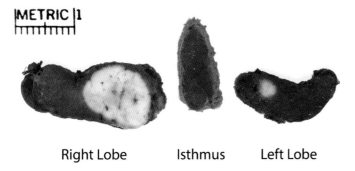

**Fig. 12.21** Cut surface of a total thyroidectomy in a syndromic patient. Total thyroidectomy in an 11-year-old boy with known multiple endocrine neoplasia type 2 and clinically suspected medullary thyroid carcinoma. The total weight of the gland was 10.3 g. The greatest dimension (longitudinal) of the right lobe was 35 mm and that of the left lobe was 22 mm. A 19 mm tumour was present in the right upper-mid lobe and a 3 mm tumour was in the left upper lobe.

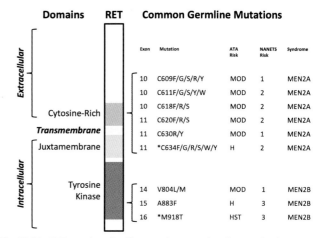

**Fig. 12.22** *RET* gene/protein. Diagram demonstrating the protein domains, most common germline pathogenic sequence variants in multiple endocrine neoplasia syndromes, and relative risks for aggressive carcinomas.

{1713,7496}. Given that as many as 50% of sporadic MTCs harbour *RET* mutation, the definitive diagnosis of a syndrome hinges on germline testing {7496}, because presumed sporadic MTC may carry *RET* germline pathogenic sequence variants {7119,837, 7496}. Patients with a known or suspected family history of a MEN syndrome should undergo genetic counselling and germline testing for a mutant *RET* allele as early as the neonatal period {5988, 5989}, as regionally available.

## Macroscopic appearance

Prophylactic/therapeutic thyroidectomies for a known MEN syndrome or MTC should be weighed and measured fresh, differentially inked, and fixed overnight for ease of sectioning. The lobes should be serially sectioned transversely and thinly (~3 mm) from superior to inferior and entirely submitted. The isthmus can be sectioned transversely or sagittally. Because C cells reside at the upper-mid to outer portions of each lobe, C-cell hyperplasia or MTC should be expected to arise in this location. Tumours tend to be unencapsulated but well demarcated, with a white-yellow, firm, gritty cross-sectional appearance. Sporadic MTC is usually unilateral and solitary, whereas familial tumours are often smaller, bilateral, and multicentric {5094,1212}.

## Histopathology

*Sporadic MTC*: MTC characteristically demonstrates a variety of patterns, ranging from the more classic solid, trabecular, and insular growth patterns to a series of infrequent morphological patterns resembling follicular cell–derived carcinomas and other epithelial and mesenchymal histotypes. The histological patterns do not impact the prognosis, but they may cause confusion with diagnosis. At present, quantitative criteria are not defined, with the following patterns or cell types recognized: papillary, pseudopapillary, follicular (tubular/glandular), spindle cell, giant cell, clear cell, oncocytic, melanotic, squamous, amphicrine, paraganglioma-like, angiosarcoma-like, encapsulated, and small cell (this last cell type may be calcitonin-negative). Neoplastic cells can be round, spindled, plasmacytoid, or small, frequently admixed in the same tumour. Overt anaplasia is usually absent, but variability in nuclear shape and size (random endocrine atypia) can be present. Proliferation is usually low. The cytoplasm ranges from eosinophilic to clear to amphophilic and is usually finely granular. There may be mucin vacuoles and psammoma bodies. In about 90% of cases, amyloid stroma is present, formed by full-length calcitonin.

*Hereditary MTC:* MTCs in patients with MEN2B are usually smaller, multicentric, and bilateral, and associated with primary (neoplastic) C-cell hyperplasia.

*Immunohistochemistry*
Tumour cells are immunoreactive for calcitonin, CGRP, synaptophysin, chromogranins, and CEA, in addition to keratins, thyroid transcription factor 1 (TTF1), and PAX8. MTC can be reactive for peptide products, such as ACTH, somatostatin, GRP, and neurotensin.

*Primary C-cell hyperplasia and MTC:* The progression from primary C-cell hyperplasia to MTC is characteristic of MTC in MEN2B. Primary C-cell hyperplasia is defined as > 6–8 cells per cluster in several foci with > 50 C cells per 2 mm$^2$ (approximately). Primary C-cell hyperplasia is usually recognizable on H&E-stained slides as a growth of intrafollicular C cells (with varying degrees of dysplasia) lining the follicles and filling them. MTC occurs when C cells

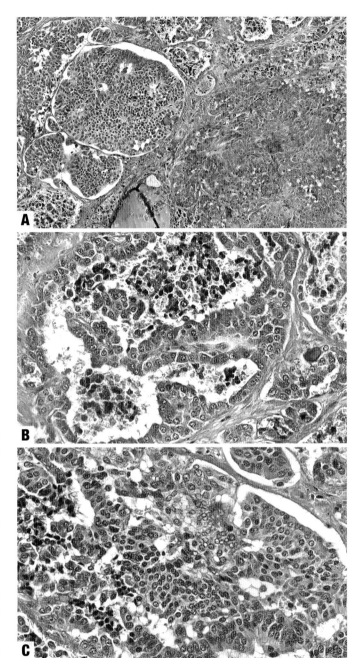

**Fig. 12.23** Medullary thyroid carcinoma. **A** Medullary thyroid carcinoma showing an admixture of round and spindle cells with minimal atypia, in a solid, cribriform, and follicular growth pattern. **B** A pseudopapillary architecture can be seen in some tumours, showing areas of necrosis. **C** Many different patterns of growth can be seen in a medullary thyroid carcinoma, including a cribriform pattern, showing apoptosis in the centre.

infiltrate through the basal membrane and beyond, with induction of a sclerotic stroma or amyloid deposition. Collagen IV or Congo red staining can be of help. MTmC measures < 10 mm in diameter. In prophylactic thyroidectomies performed before 1 year of age, there is usually primary C-cell hyperplasia, potentially with MTmC in the upper third of the lobes. Primary C-cell hyperplasia can be associated with sporadic MTCs. Physiological C-cell hyperplasia is not aggregated to > 50 cells per 2 mm$^2$ (approximately), is not atypical, usually needs calcitonin immunohistochemistry to highlight the cells, and is not considered a precursor to MTC {372}.

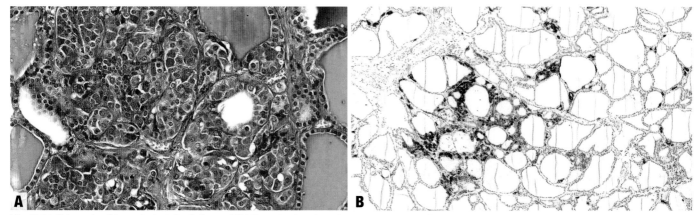

**Fig. 12.24** Primary C-cell hyperplasia. **A** C cells line and fill follicles, but there is no destructive invasion. **B** Calcitonin staining highlights primary C-cell hyperplasia in a prophylactic thyroidectomy in a syndromic child.

## Cytology

Smears from MTCs are highly cellular, with dispersed or loosely cohesive cells. Individual cell morphology may range from epithelioid to spindled to plasmacytoid with eccentrically placed nuclei. Binucleated cells may be frequent. Anisonucleosis (representing random endocrine atypia) and occasional intranuclear cytoplasmic pseudoinclusions (mimicking papillary thyroid carcinoma) can be seen. Chromatin tends to be coarsely granular. Amyloid may be present in the background, manifesting as homogeneously staining translucent fragments that can be orange-pink (Pap stain) or pale blue (Giemsa stain) {5673,7062}.

## Diagnostic molecular pathology

Although molecular testing is not required for the diagnosis, germline testing and genetic counselling is recommended for any paediatric patient with MTC.

## Essential and desirable diagnostic criteria

*Essential:* an invasive proliferation of neoplastic cells with parafollicular C-cell differentiation.

*Desirable:* associated primary C-cell hyperplasia in familial cases.

## Staging

MTCs are staged using the TNM system as published by the Union for International Cancer Control (UICC), according to International Collaboration on Cancer Reporting (ICCR) guidelines and/or other expert-initiated reporting guidelines {2391}.

## Prognosis and prediction

Prophylactic total thyroidectomy is indicated for all patients with known MEN2B {7361}, with timing determined partly by the specific germline pathogenic sequence variant identified {7496,1212,7119}. Lymph node dissection is usually reserved for patients with high serum calcitonin levels or clinically and/ or radiographically abnormal lymph nodes {837}. In a large, multicentre cohort of asymptomatic patients with MEN {4301}, the risk for nodal metastasis began at the age of 14 years and steadily increased. Only patients with mutations in codon 634 or 918 developed MTC before the age of 1 year {4301}. Overall, patients with germline *RET* p.M918T mutations are at the highest risk of aggressive tumours, with lymph node metastases identified as early as the first year of life {7496,7361}. When uncontrolled, MTC is the most common cause of cancer death in patients with MEN2B {7361}. Syndromic mortality occurs earlier in MEN2B than in MEN2A.

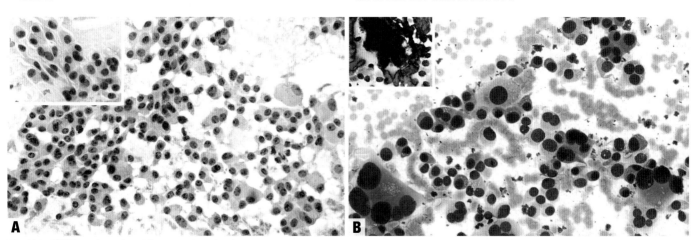

**Fig. 12.25** FNAB cytology of medullary thyroid carcinoma. **A** Pap-stained alcohol-fixed smear showing vaguely cohesive cells with round to oval nuclei with finely stippled chromatin and small nucleoli. **Inset:** Spindled cells. **B** Romanowsky-stained smear showing cellular dyscohesion, anisocytosis, binucleation/multinucleation, and small intracytoplasmic vacuoles. **Inset:** Coarse amyloid fragment.

# Spindle epithelial tumour with thymus-like elements

Chan JKC
Folpe AL

## Definition

Spindle epithelial tumour with thymus-like elements (SETTLE) is a malignant tumour of the thyroid or mediastinum, characterized by a lobulated architecture and a biphasic cellular composition, with spindle epithelial cells that merge into glandular structures.

## ICD-O coding

8588/3 Spindle epithelial tumour with thymus-like elements

## ICD-11 coding

2D10.Y & XH6ZG8 Other specified malignant neoplasms of thyroid gland & Spindle epithelial tumour with thymus-like element

## Related terminology

*Acceptable:* spindle epithelial tumour with thymus-like differentiation.

## Subtype(s)

None

## Localization

SETTLE occurs primarily in the thyroid and rarely in the lateral neck or superior mediastinum {6686}.

## Clinical features

The usual presentation is a painless thyroid mass of variable duration. Less common presentations include a rapidly enlarging neck mass, local tenderness, and diffuse thyroid enlargement. The tumour appears cold on thyroid scan and displays heterogeneous solid and cystic density on CT. Approximately 10% of patients have cervical lymph node metastasis at presentation {5801,3134,4925}. SETTLE has a propensity for late metastasis, most commonly to the lung, lymph node, kidney, and liver {2175,1144,5801,3134}.

## Epidemiology

SETTLE is very rare. It predominantly affects children and young adults (median age: 19 years, range: 2–73 years), with a slight male predilection (M:F ratio: 1.5:1) {5801,3134}.

## Etiology

Unknown

## Pathogenesis

Single cases have been reported to show *KRAS*, *NRAS*, *SMYD1* (*KMT3D*), or *KMT2C* mutation {7657,6686}.

## Macroscopic appearance

The tumour is grossly encapsulated, partially circumscribed, or infiltrative, with a mean size of 42 mm (range: 11–120 mm) {3134}. The cut surface is firm, greyish-white to tan, and vaguely lobulated.

## Histopathology

SETTLE is a highly cellular tumour with a vaguely lobulated pattern delineated by fibrous septa {1144}. The growth pattern is biphasic, although rare cases may be almost exclusively composed of spindled cells or glandular structures (monophasic pattern) {1251}. Compact interlacing to reticulated long fascicles of spindled cells merge imperceptibly with tubulopapillary and gland-like structures, with areas of stromal hyalinization. Cleft-like spaces containing grey-blue mucosubstances are often seen. The spindled cells have elongated nuclei with fine chromatin and inconspicuous nucleoli, and scant cytoplasm (ultrastructurally shown to be epithelial with tonofilaments), desmosomes, and basal lamina {1144}. Mitotic figures are rare, although high mitotic activity and necrosis may be present in rare cases {3614}. The glandular component usually takes the form of tubules, papillae, glomeruloid formations, cords, small pale-staining islands, and epithelium-lined cystic spaces. The

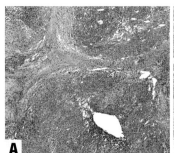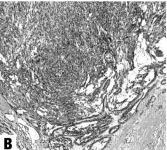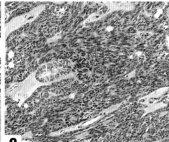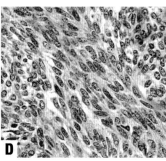

**Fig. 12.26** Thyroid spindle epithelial tumour with thymus-like elements. **A** A highly cellular tumour with a lobulated growth pattern. Even at this low magnification it is evident that there are interspersed reticulated spaces, some apparently empty and some containing basophilic mucosubstance. **B** The biphasic tumour comprises long, sweeping fascicles of spindle cells merging into complex glandular structures. Basophilic mucosubstance is present in the reticulated spaces among the spindle cells as well as the glandular lumina. **C** Fascicles of spindle cells merge into elongated glandular structures, some with a glomeruloid appearance. The glandular structures are lined by uniform cuboidal to low columnar cells. **D** The spindle cells appear uniform and have elongated, bland-looking nuclei.

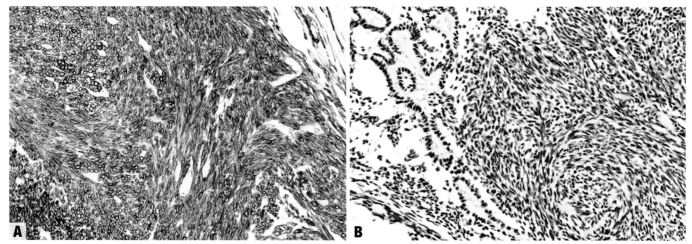

**Fig. 12.27** Thyroid spindle epithelial tumour with thymus-like elements. **A** All the spindle cells and the cuboidal epithelial cells are immunopositive for pancytokeratin. **B** Both the spindle cells (right) and the cuboidal epithelial cells (left) are extensively immunopositive for p40.

epithelial cells are cuboidal to columnar and are sometimes mucinous or ciliated. In exceptional cases, there is focal squamous differentiation. Lymphocytes are usually scant. Vascular invasion may be present {6686}.

### Immunohistochemistry

Both the spindled and glandular cells are diffusely positive with pancytokeratin antibodies. Expression of high-molecular-weight cytokeratins is more extensive than that of low-molecular-weight cytokeratins {2175}. p63 and/or p40 are commonly positive. Rarely, the spindled cells may express markers suggestive of myoepithelial differentiation, such as actins {7657,6744}. The tumour cells are negative for thyroglobulin, calcitonin, CEA, thyroid transcription factor 1 (TTF1), S100, and CD5.

### Differential diagnosis

SETTLE can be distinguished from synovial sarcoma by the lobulated growth pattern, lower overall nuclear grade, diffuse keratin and p63/p40 expression, and lack of *SS18* or *SS18L1* gene

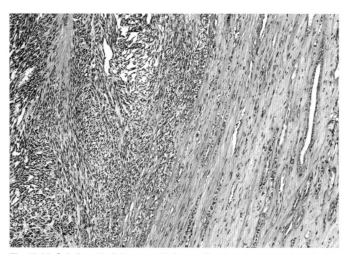

**Fig. 12.28** Spindle epithelial tumour with thymus-like elements, metastatic to the kidney. Residual renal parenchyma is seen (right). The metastatic tumour (left) comprises spindle cells in fascicles, interspersed with reticulated spaces.

rearrangement {2175}. Ectopic type A thymoma can greatly mimic SETTLE, but it differs by showing jigsaw puzzle–like lobulation, more haphazard orientation of the spindle cell fascicles, infrequent presence of reticulated or microcystic spaces among spindled cells, a frequent pericytomatous vascular pattern, and less complex glandular elements.

### Cytology

Aspirates are highly or moderately cellular, including cohesive and single dissociated spindle cells with bland oval nuclei. Occasional groups of epithelioid and columnar cells can be seen. Mitotic figures are rare or absent. Extracellular metachromatic material should not be misinterpreted as amyloid {528A}.

### Diagnostic molecular pathology

SETTLE lacks the *SS18* or *SS18L1* gene rearrangements that characterize synovial sarcoma {2175,5801} and the *GTF2I* mutation characteristic of type A/AB thymoma {4925}.

### Essential and desirable diagnostic criteria

*Essential:* a biphasic tumour comprising fascicles of spindled cells merging into complex glandular elements; bland cytological features; a reticulated or sieve-like pattern in some areas; diffuse immunoreactivity for keratins (especially high-molecular-weight keratins)

*Desirable:* absence of *SS18* or *SS18L1* rearrangements (in selected cases).

### Staging

Not applicable

### Prognosis and prediction

SETTLE is a slow-growing tumour, with an overall survival rate of 86% (median follow-up: 6.3 years) {5801}. The metastatic rate is 26%, but this increases to 40% when follow-up exceeds 5 years {5801,1254}. Metastasis often occurs after a long latency (mean: 10 years) {5801}. The presence of cervical lymph node metastasis is associated with a high risk of subsequent development of distant metastasis {5801}. Metastatic disease can still be compatible with a long survival after treatment {1254}.

# Parathyroid adenoma

Gill AJ
Kruijff S
Larsson C
Mete O

## Definition
Parathyroid adenoma is a benign neoplasm of parathyroid epithelial cells.

## ICD-O coding
8140/0 Parathyroid adenoma

## ICD-11 coding
2F37.Y & XH3DV3 Other specified benign neoplasm of endocrine glands & Adenoma, NOS

5A51.0 & XH3DV3 Primary hyperparathyroidism & Adenoma, NOS

## Related terminology
None

## Subtype(s)
None

## Localization
Multigland disease and ectopic sites, including the thyroid, mediastinum, retro-oesophageal space, and thymus, are common in children {1054,1391,1890,5766,7109,1684,3710}.

## Clinical features
Children are more likely than adults to be symptomatic with marked hypercalcaemia and hypercalciuria {125,4838,4393, 7292,5830,7109,1684,5956,3710}.

## Epidemiology
The prevalence of childhood hyperparathyroidism is 2–5 cases per 100 000 individuals {3973,4351,125}, with an equal sex distribution and a bimodal age distribution {4838,4351}. CASR mutations dominate in infancy; true adenomas dominate in older adolescents {4113,1684,125}.

## Etiology
Hyperparathyroidism in childhood is commonly hereditary/syndromic (see Table 12.05) {7109,4113,1684,125}.

**Table 12.05** The most common hereditary syndromes occurring with hyperparathyroidism in childhood

| Disease | Inheritance | Gene (locus) | Morphology | Other syndromic features |
|---|---|---|---|---|
| Multiple endocrine neoplasia type 1 | Dominant | MEN1 (11q13) | Multigland disease common<br>Often nodular, mimicking hyperplasia | PitNETs, PanNETs, thymic NETs |
| Multiple endocrine neoplasia type 2A | Dominant | RET (10q11.2) | Multigland disease less common<br>Less nodular, appearance of conventional adenoma | Medullary thyroid carcinoma, phaeochromocytoma |
| Multiple endocrine neoplasia type 4 | Dominant | CDKN1B (12p13.1) | Multigland disease common<br>Often nodular, mimicking hyperplasia (similar to multiple endocrine neoplasia type 1) | PitNETs, PanNETs, thymic NETs, adrenocortical tumours, meningiomas, facial angiofibromas, lipomas |
| Hyperparathyroidism–jaw tumour syndrome | Dominant | CDC73 (1q31.2) | Sheet-like growth, cytological atypia, distinctive vasculature, microcystic change, often eosinophilic cytoplasm with perinuclear clearing, parafibromin loss by immunohistochemistry | Rare: Fibro-osseous jaw tumours<br>Extremely rare: renal cystic and uterine tumours |
| Familial hypocalciuric hypercalcaemia type 1 | Dominant | CASR (3q13.33-q21.1) | Glands normal size or very slightly hyperplastic | |
| Familial hypocalciuric hypercalcaemia type 2 | Dominant | GNA11 (19q13) | Glands normal size or very slightly hyperplastic | |
| Familial hypocalciuric hypercalcaemia type 3 | Dominant | AP2S1 (19q13) | Glands normal size or very slightly hyperplastic | |
| Neonatal severe hyperparathyroidism | Recessive | CASR (3q13.33-q21.1) | Increased size with diffuse chief cell hyperplasia | |
| Familial isolated hyperparathyroidism | Variable | Unknown | Nil distinctive | A diagnosis of exclusion |

NET, neuroendocrine tumour; PanNET, pancreatic neuroendocrine tumour; PitNET, pituitary neuroendocrine tumour.

Chapter 12

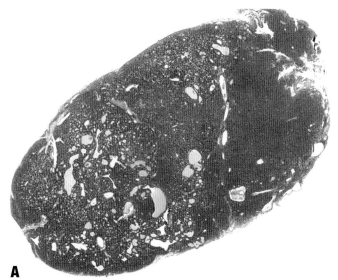

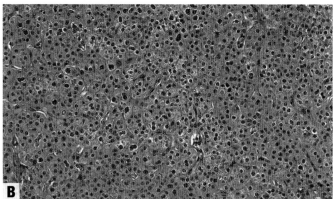

**Fig. 12.29** Parafibromin-deficient (hyperparathyroidism–jaw tumour type) parathyroid adenoma. **A** This tumour demonstrates the typical sheet-like architecture, eosinophilic cell type, prominent vasculature, and microcystic change of parathyroid tumours associated with hyperparathyroidism–jaw tumour syndrome. **B** There is eosinophilic cytoplasm with perinuclear cytoplasmic clearing, nuclear enlargement (often with preserved N:C ratios), and some multinucleation.

## Pathogenesis

In addition to germline pathogenic sequence variants, recurrent somatic mutations of *CCND1*, *MEN1*, and *CDC73* have been reported {2837}.

## Macroscopic appearance

Parathyroid adenomas range in size from < 10 mm (100 mg) to > 100 mm (1000 mg). They are usually oval to reniform in shape, with a pale-tan cut surface. Particularly if sectioned along the hilum, a rim of pale-tan to yellow normal parathyroid tissue may be identified.

## Histopathology

Most parathyroid adenomas are composed predominantly of chief cells, with a reduction or absence of stromal fat. Oxyphilic and water-clear cells may cause confusion in the differential diagnosis if they predominate. On examination of a single gland, the distinction between adenoma and hyperplasia may be difficult, although a rim of normal or suppressed (atrophic, compressed) parathyroid tissue is a clue to adenoma. Parathyroid

glands subjected to biopsy or trauma and hyperplastic glands arising secondary to chronic renal failure may show marked reactive cytological and architectural atypia (including heavy fibrosis) that can mimic invasion and should not be misinterpreted as evidence of malignancy {216,3580,7555}. Immunohistochemistry is rarely required for diagnosis, with expression of PTH and GATA3 supporting a parathyroid origin {5215,1975}.

Although morphology cannot be used to replace genetic testing, features associated with germline pathogenic *CDC73* variants and deletions (hyperparathyroidism–jaw tumour syndrome [HPT-JT]) include a sheet-like growth pattern, eosinophilic cell type, perinuclear cytoplasmic clearing, nuclear enlargement (occasionally with multinucleation), and a distinctive arborizing vasculature (often with staghorn vessels) {7109,2420}. Loss of immunohistochemical expression of parafibromin is usually seen in association with biallelic *CDC73* mutation/deletion {2416,2420,2419}. Although parafibromin immunohistochemistry is not completely sensitive or specific, and somatic-only mutations do occur, parafibromin-deficient parathyroid tumours in the paediatric population are almost always associated with HPT-JT {2420}. Multiple endocrine neoplasia type 1 tends to manifest with multiglandular disease with a multinodular appearance, whereas in multiple endocrine neoplasia type 2, single gland disease with the appearance of usual adenoma is more common {1975,1684,7109}.

### Differential diagnosis

Parathyroid carcinoma is virtually non-existent in childhood outside the setting of HPT-JT {2416,4038,7109}. The diagnosis of malignancy should be restricted to cases with unequivocal invasive growth and/or vascular space invasion {7555}.

## Cytology

Parathyroid adenoma is rarely intentionally biopsied, but the cytological findings may mimic a thyroid follicular neoplasm.

## Diagnostic molecular pathology

Although molecular pathology is not used diagnostically, a parathyroid adenoma or hyperplasia occurring in childhood is considered an indication for genetic evaluation.

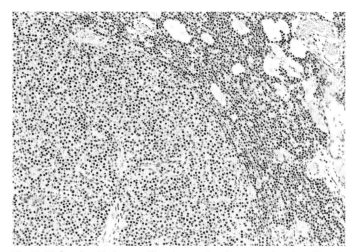

**Fig. 12.30** Parathyroid adenoma. There is normal nuclear expression of parafibromin in this tumour not associated with hyperparathyroidism–jaw tumour syndrome.

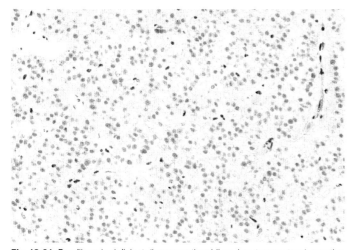

**Fig. 12.31** Parafibromin-deficient (hyperparathyroidism–jaw tumour type) parathyroid adenoma. Complete loss of nuclear expression of parafibromin in all neoplastic cells. The presence of the prerequisite internal positive control in non-neoplastic endothelial and stromal cells is emphasized.

## Essential and desirable diagnostic criteria

*Essential:* enlarged hypercellular (stromal fat–depleted) parathyroid tissue in the appropriate clinical context.

*Desirable:* a rim of non-neoplastic parathyroid or a marked drop in PTH after removal (> 50% reduction of PTH level).

## Staging

Not relevant

## Prognosis and prediction

Sporadic parathyroid adenomas rarely recur after simple excision. There is a high risk of recurrent hyperparathyroidism or other tumours in hereditary disease, depending on the underlying genetic abnormality. The lifetime risk of parathyroid carcinoma in the setting of HPT-JT may be as high as 15% {2420, 2416,1684}.

# Adrenal cortical tumours

Giordano TJ
Kletskaya IS

## Definition

Adrenal cortical adenoma is a benign epithelial tumour of adrenal cortical cells. Adrenal cortical carcinoma is a malignant epithelial tumour of adrenal cortical cells.

## ICD-O coding

8370/0 Adrenal cortical adenoma
8370/3 Adrenal cortical carcinoma

## ICD-11 coding

2F37.Y & XH3DV3 Other specified benign neoplasm of endocrine glands & Adenoma, NOS
2F37 & XH1YP0 Other specified benign neoplasm of endocrine glands & Adrenal cortical adenoma, clear cell
2F37.Y & XH2CT2 Other specified benign neoplasm of endocrine glands & Adrenal cortical adenoma, compact cell
2F37.Y & XH60N5 Other specified benign neoplasm of endocrine glands & Adrenal cortical adenoma, glomerulosa cell
2F37.Y & XH2VZ8 Other specified benign neoplasm of endocrine glands & Adrenal cortical adenoma, mixed cell
2F37.Y & XH2FJ6 Other specified benign neoplasm of endocrine glands & Adrenal cortical adenoma, pigmented
2D11.Y & XH0U20 Other specified malignant neoplasms of adrenal gland & Neuroendocrine carcinoma, NOS

## Related terminology

None

## Subtype(s)

Oncocytic adrenal cortical carcinoma; myxoid adrenal cortical carcinoma

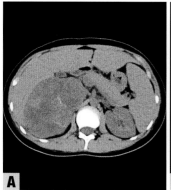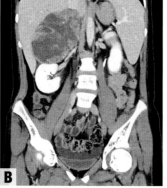

**Fig. 12.32** Adrenal cortical carcinoma. **A** Plain axial CT shows a large inhomogeneous but well-defined right suprasellar mass that displaces the adjacent structures. Low-attenuation areas consistent with necrosis are invariably present in large tumours (> 60 mm). Faint calcifications are also present within the tumour. **B** Contrast-enhanced reformatted coronal CT shows heterogeneous enhancement of the right suprarenal mass, with greater enhancement seen peripherally and relatively little enhancement centrally because of central necrosis. Note the tumour thrombus extending into the inferior vena cava.

## Localization

The large majority of adrenal cortical tumours are unilateral masses that arise in the adrenal gland. Tumours that arise in very young children are thought to arise in the fetal cortex {3888,7655}, but localization to a specific zone of the fetal or adult adrenal cortex is not feasible.

## Clinical features

Adrenal cortical tumours are most often associated with various endocrinopathies, which often leads to their early clinical identification {6155,4413}. Specific signs and symptoms reflect the underlying hormonal status. Excess androgen secretion (in as many as 80% of patients) results in signs and symptoms of virilization, including hirsutism, acne, and amenorrhoea {5946}. Excess cortisol secretion (in 15–40% of patients) results in Cushing syndrome with hypertension, obesity, and other typical signs and symptoms {5868}. Feminization and gynaecomastia (in 7% of patients) can result from excess estrogen secretion, and a small minority of patients (1–4%) have hypertension and hypokalaemia related to aldosterone secretion {5868}. Mixed endocrinopathies produce a mixture of signs and symptoms that reflect the specific endocrine milieu.

A minority of patients have non-functioning tumours; these tend to be more common in the adolescent population {5868}. Such non-functioning tumours are incidentally diagnosed during imaging for

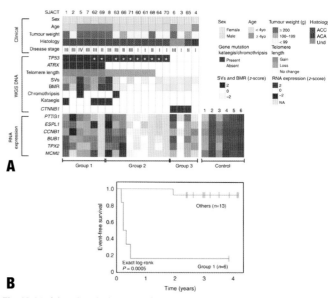

**Fig. 12.33** Adrenal cortical tumours. Overall genomic landscape of paediatric adrenal cortical tumours showing the association between clinical, pathological, and molecular attributes, with identification of three groups. **A** The upper panel details the clinico-pathological features of 19 patients. The middle panel details the genetic alterations, including essential molecular features. The lower panel displays the expression of selected cell-cycle genes. **B** Kaplan–Meier analysis of group 1 tumours as compared with the other groups combined.

other reasons (adrenal incidentaloma) or during evaluation for non-specific symptoms such as fatigue and abdominal pain {190}.

*Imaging*

The imaging characteristics of adrenal cortical adenoma and carcinoma are generally distinct, but imaging of paediatric tumours overall is not as diagnostically reliable as imaging of tumours in adults {2688}. Adenomas tend to be uniform and well circumscribed {2688}. Because carcinoma is difficult to absolutely exclude on imaging, evaluation for lung metastases by CT imaging is often indicated, especially for larger tumours. Carcinomas are generally larger (> 85 mm and > 212.5 mL tumour volume) and heterogeneous, with areas of necrosis, haemorrhage, and calcifications {95,2164}. Local invasion, such as soft tissue extension and/or vena cava involvement, can be present and supports a diagnosis of carcinoma {95,2164}. FDG PET-CT imaging can be useful for distinguishing adenomas from carcinomas and also has the benefit of identifying occult metastases {7612}.

## Epidemiology

The overall incidence of adrenal cortical tumours displays a bimodal distribution. Paediatric cases are concentrated during the first 5 years of life, with a smaller concentration of cases occurring during adolescence. In contrast, the incidence of adult cases peaks in the fourth decade of life. Adrenal cortical tumours in the paediatric population are extremely rare, especially in the USA and Europe. The incidence of adrenal cortical carcinoma in these regions is 0.2–0.3 patients per 1 million person-years {4496}, which is significantly lower than that observed in the adult population {1949}. Therefore, it is estimated that there are only 25 new paediatric cases of carcinoma per year in the USA {4496}. The incidence of adenomas is more difficult to establish, because given their benign diagnosis, such cases are not typically recorded by cancer registries. Interestingly, the incidence of adrenal cortical tumours in southern Brazil is strikingly (15–20 times) higher {5868}; this is related to a specific founder mutation of the tumour suppressor gene *TP53* (p.R337H) {2103,5556}. The prevalence of this mutation is very high in southern Brazil, where it is present in about 0.3% of the general population and in 90% of cases. Despite this germline genetic difference, the overall clinical and biological

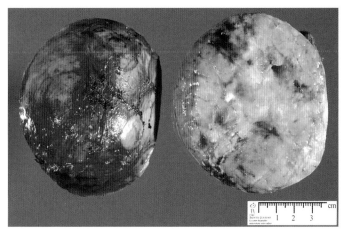

**Fig. 12.35** Adrenal cortical carcinoma. The mass is grossly well circumscribed. The cut surface shows areas of haemorrhage and necrosis.

characteristics of paediatric adrenal cortical tumours in southern Brazil are similar to those of cases around the world.

## Etiology

Adrenal cortical carcinoma is one of the most heritable cancers, especially in the paediatric population. Paediatric adrenal cortical tumours have a strong association with germline genetic defects, most often involving inactivating mutations of *TP53* {7358}. Thus, adrenal cortical tumours are a well-established component of Li–Fraumeni syndrome {7358,5165,1948,217}. The prevailing view is that loss of p53 function leads to genomic instability in the fetal adrenal cortex, which then predisposes to additional genetic alterations such as loss of heterozygosity at 11p15 with concomitant overexpression of IGF2. Overexpression of IGF2 leads to growth advantage, clonal expansion, and ultimately tumour formation. Additional genetic defects accumulate over time and increase the risk of malignant behaviour {1911}.

In addition, a large proportion of patients with adrenal cortical tumours (some of whom display clinical features of Beckwith–Wiedemann syndrome {1948}) harbour constitutional abnormalities of chromosome 11p15, resulting in constitutive overexpression of IGF2. In these patients, tumours tend to develop at a young age {1948}. Because of these strong genetic associations, genetic testing and counselling is recommended for all patients with these tumours {5487}. Beyond these genetic associations, little is known about additional etiological factors.

## Pathogenesis

The pathogenesis of paediatric adrenal cortical tumours has been investigated through genome-wide association studies of adenomas, carcinomas, and tumours of indeterminate malignant potential {1911,5555}. Gene expression profiles of adrenal cortical tumours are highly distinct from those of the normal cortex and can separate adenomas and carcinomas with reasonable accuracy {7507}. Integrated genomic analysis of a relatively large cohort of tumours revealed the genomic landscape of these tumours and confirmed the essential role of *TP53* germline deficiency combined with IGF2 overexpression as early events in pathogenesis, probably related to p53-mediated chromosomal instability {5555}. Somatic mutations of *ATRX* and *CTNNB1* were found to represent secondary events. Genomic classification

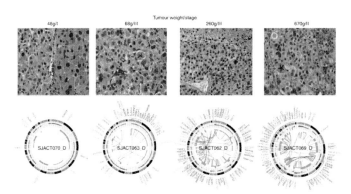

**Fig. 12.34** Adrenal cortical tumours. Circos plots demonstrating the overall association between pathological features and the degree of genetic alterations. Accumulation of genetic alterations is associated with increasing tumour weight and aggressive tumour phenotype.

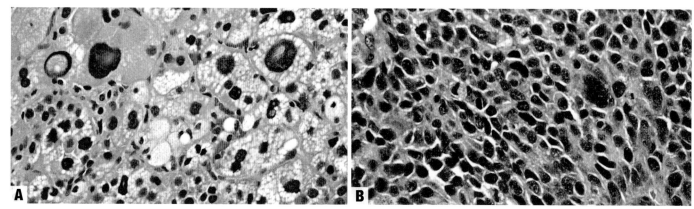

**Fig. 12.36** Adrenal cortical tumour. **A** This tumour shows a mixture of lipid-rich and lipid-poor cells with nuclear pleomorphism. **B** High-grade adrenal cortical carcinoma with small-cell features and mitotic figures.

identified three groups of tumours: group 1 was defined by *TP53* and *ATRX* mutations, group 2 had only *TP53* mutations, and group 3 were wildtype for *TP53* and *ATRX*. The combination of germline *TP53* and acquired *ATRX* mutations (group 1) was associated with a dismal clinical outcome compared to groups 2 and 3 {5555}. Most interestingly, a strong genotype–phenotype correlation was observed between overall histological features of malignancy and the accumulation of genomic alterations. These observations provide support for a model in which the progressive accumulation of genomic alterations drives histological progression and clinical behaviour {5555}.

## Macroscopic appearance

Adrenal cortical adenoma and carcinoma tend to have distinct macroscopic appearances. Adenomas are usually smaller than carcinomas, have a uniform cut surface without gross haemorrhage or necrosis, and are well circumscribed without invasion of extra-adrenal tissues. Conversely, carcinomas are larger, with marked heterogeneity (reflecting intratumoural evolution), and typically contain gross necrosis. The large majority of adrenal cortical tumours are localized to the gland. Direct invasion of adjacent structures (kidney, adipose, and large vessels) occurs in about 10% of cases.

## Histopathology

Adrenal cortical tumours, like their adult counterparts, consist predominantly of cortical cells with admixed vessels and capillaries, without substantial desmoplastic stroma or large numbers of intratumoural inflammatory cells. Adenomas are non-invasive tumours with a nested or trabecular architecture and often contain a mixture of lipid-rich and lipid-poor cells. The nuclei of the typical adenoma tend to be smaller with less variation. These tumours lack or have minimal mitotic activity and lack true tumour necrosis. Conversely, carcinomas display a loss of regular architecture, which can be demonstrated by highlighting the reticulin framework on special stains. The nuclei of carcinomas tend to be larger and can show significant hyperchromasia and marked pleomorphism. The mitotic count is elevated, and atypical mitoses are common. Necrosis is often present. Oncocytic cell changes may be seen. A myxoid stromal change may be prominent in selected cases. Immunohistochemical profiles of paediatric tumours are similar to those of adult tumours, i.e. the tumour cells express α-inhibin, synaptophysin, melan-A, and SF1, and they do not express chromogranin. Cytokeratin expression is variable in paediatric tumours.

Despite these differences between adenomas and carcinomas, their histopathological distinction has been and continues to be diagnostically challenging. This reflects, in part, their low incidence; however, these tumours sometimes defy histopathological classification, with some benign-appearing tumours behaving aggressively. Moreover, some frankly malignant tumours according to general pathological criteria never recur or metastasize after adequate surgical resection. Given these inconsistencies, classifying paediatric adrenal cortical tumours represents a diagnostic challenge beyond that of non-paediatric cases {1676}. Because of these considerations, paediatric tumours are best evaluated using different macroscopic and microscopic criteria

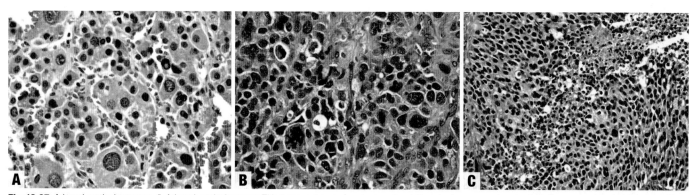

**Fig. 12.37** Adrenal cortical tumours. **A** Adrenal cortical tumour. This tumour shows abundant eosinophilic cytoplasm, occasional mitotic figures, and nuclear pleomorphism. **B** Adrenal cortical carcinoma. High-grade adrenal cortical carcinoma with an atypical mitotic figure and apoptotic body. **C** Adrenal cortical carcinoma. True tumour necrosis.

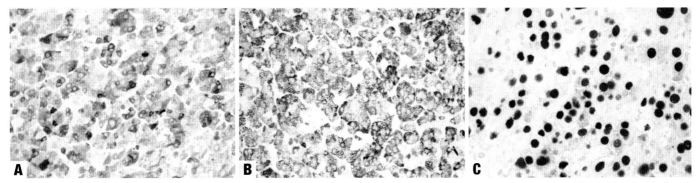

**Fig. 12.38** Adrenal cortical tumours. **A** Adrenal cortical tumour. Immunoreactivity for α-inhibin, which commonly shows a mosaic pattern of staining. **B** Adrenal cortical carcinoma. Immunoreactivity for melan-A. **C** Adrenal cortical carcinoma. Immunoreactivity for SF1.

from those used for adult tumours. The most reliable multifactorial scoring system, the Wieneke / US Armed Forces Institute of Pathology (AFIP) algorithm {7535}, consists of nine parameters focused on tumour size and weight, extra-adrenal extension, vena cava extension, capsular and venous invasion, tumour necrosis, mitotic count, and atypical mitotic figures. Tumours fulfilling two or fewer criteria are associated with a benign clinical course; tumours fulfilling three criteria are considered indeterminate for malignancy (uncertain malignant potential); and tumours fulfilling four or more criteria are associated with malignant behaviour and can be diagnosed as carcinoma. Of note, the size, weight, and mitotic count cut-off points are much higher for paediatric tumours than they are in most adult scoring systems. Importantly, paediatric oncocytic tumours are not included in these criteria. More recent studies have examined the role of Ki-67 immunohistochemistry; a Ki-67 proliferation index cut-off point of 15% was suggested as an additional criterion to be included with the Wieneke/AFIP algorithm {4437}.

## Cytology

FNAB is rarely performed for suspected paediatric adrenal cortical tumours. A few case reports highlight hypercellular specimens containing large cells with abundant eosinophilic granular cytoplasm and large vesicular nuclei with prominent nucleoli, marked pleomorphism, and variable mitotic activity {3410}.

## Diagnostic molecular pathology

The genomic investigation of paediatric tumours in general has advanced recently, with clear diagnostic and therapeutic

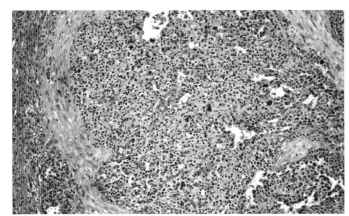

**Fig. 12.39** Adrenal cortical carcinoma. Liver metastasis.

implications {6809}. However, although much has been learned over the past two decades about the molecular and genomic basis of adult and paediatric adrenal cortical tumours, the routine use of diagnostic molecular pathology has not been clinically established. Some centres have deployed large next-generation sequencing–based genetic panels mostly for therapeutic purposes in an attempt to identify molecular targets, but the yield of this approach has been limited to date.

### Essential and desirable diagnostic criteria

*Adrenal cortical adenoma*
*Essential:*
- Tumour weight < 400 g
- Tumour size < 105 mm
- Absence of extra-adrenal tumour extension
- Absence of vena cava invasion
- Absence of venous invasion
- Absence of capsular invasion
- Absence of tumour necrosis
- Mitotic count ≤ 3 mitoses/mm² in 5 mm² (≤ 15 mitoses/20 HPF of 0.57 mm in diameter and 0.25 mm² in area)
- Absence of atypical mitoses
*Desirable:*
- p53 immunohistochemistry showing a wildtype pattern with weak nuclear staining
- Ki-67 proliferation index < 10% suggests a benign course

*Adrenal cortical carcinoma*
*Essential (but not all criteria are present in each case):*
- Tumour weight > 400 g
- Tumour size > 105 mm
- Presence of extra-adrenal tumour extension
- Presence of vena cava invasion
- Presence of venous invasion
- Presence of capsular invasion
- Presence of tumour necrosis
- Mitotic count > 3 mitoses/mm² in 5 mm² (> 15 mitoses/20 HPF of 0.57 mm in diameter and 0.25 mm² in area)
- Presence of atypical mitoses
*Desirable:*
- p53 immunohistochemistry showing either diffuse and strong staining or complete loss of staining correlates with *TP53* mutation
- Ki-67 proliferation index > 15% correlates with malignant behaviour

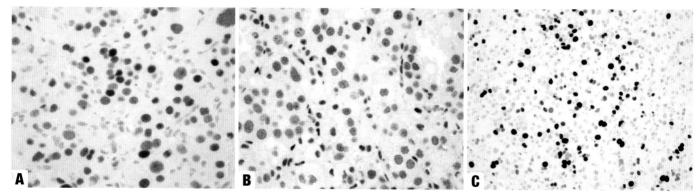

**Fig. 12.40** Adrenal cortical tumours. **A** Adrenal cortical carcinoma. Diffuse nuclear immunoreactivity for p53, suggesting the presence of a *TP53* mutation. **B** Adrenal cortical tumour. Retained nuclear immunoreactivity for ATRX, which is associated with a more indolent course. **C** Adrenal cortical carcinoma. Immunoreactivity for Ki-67. A Ki-67 proliferation index of < 10% predicts a benign course, whereas > 15% predicts a malignant course.

## Staging

Staging of paediatric adrenal cortical tumours divides tumours into three main groups. Disease localized to the adrenal gland represents the majority (75%) of cases and is subdivided into stage I (< 50 mm in greatest dimension, or < 200 g) and stage II (≥ 50 mm in greatest dimension, or ≥ 200 g). Stage III disease (10% of cases) is characterized by regional invasion, including lymph node metastases and invasion of the kidney or vena cava, or by residual disease postoperatively. Stage IV disease represents about 15% of cases and is characterized by distant haematogenous metastatic disease, most often involving the liver and lungs. A slightly different staging system, proposed by Sandrini et al. {6155} and endorsed by the Children's Oncology Group (COG), revised stage III disease to be cases with microscopic or gross residual tumour after resection or inoperable disease without distant metastases.

## Prognosis and prediction

Stage of disease represents the most meaningful predictor of outcome {4648,2597}. Accordingly, completely resected small tumours that are confined to the adrenal gland (stage I) have an excellent prognosis, even when the tumour displays malignant histopathological features. Tumours that are incompletely resected (stage III) or manifest with stage IV disease have a much worse prognosis {2597}.

Beyond disease stage, patients with excess glucocorticoids tend to have a worse prognosis than patients with virilization {4648}. Moreover, age has prognostic significance, with younger patients (aged < 5 years) doing better than older patients (≥ 5 years) {4648,2597}.

Development of additional prognostic and predictive tools is clearly needed, because some cases recur despite a good prognosis (completely resected small tumours) {2597}. Immunohistochemical assessment of p53 {1571}, β-catenin, and ATRX can be used to predict malignant behaviour {5555}, and Ki-67 immunohistochemistry is emerging as a strong predictive biomarker {1571,5515,4437}, like it is for other endocrine tumours; the emerging picture suggests that a Ki-67 proliferation index of < 10% predicts a benign clinical course and > 15% predicts malignant behaviour {4437}.

# Sympathetic paraganglioma

Tischler AS
de Krijger RR
Hicks MJ
Kimura N
Mete O

## Definition
Sympathetic paraganglioma is a neuroendocrine neoplasm (NEN) that develops from neural crest–derived progenitors in paraganglia associated with the perivertebral sympathetic chains, sympathetic nerve plexuses, and sympathetic nerves.

## ICD-O coding
8681/3 Sympathetic paraganglioma

## ICD-11 coding
2F7A.Y & XH4G21 Other specified neoplasms of uncertain behaviour of endocrine glands & Sympathetic paraganglioma

## Related terminology
Acceptable: extra-adrenal paraganglioma.
Not recommended: extra-adrenal phaeochromocytoma; phaeochromocytoma.

## Subtype(s)
None

## Localization
Sympathetic paragangliomas occur predominantly in the abdomen, retroperitoneum, pelvis, and thorax, as well as (occasionally) in or near the cervical sympathetic ganglia. Of patients aged < 18 years with a paraganglioma, about 50% have a phaeochromocytoma; others have abdominal (~25%), head and neck (20%), or thoracic (< 5%) paragangliomas; and the remainder have a pelvic paraganglioma {1653,7310}.

## Clinical features
See Phaeochromocytoma (p. 858).

## Epidemiology
Paragangliomas and phaeochromocytomas are developmentally and functionally related {2268,2928,3468}, and because of their commonalities they are often grouped together as paraganglioma and/or phaeochromocytoma in epidemiological studies. Sympathetic paragangliomas account for 10–18% of all paragangliomas and/or phaeochromocytomas in population-wide studies that consist mostly of adult patients {616}. Where national registries are reported, the incidence ranges from 0.18 to 0.5 cases per 100 000 person-years {616,3582}, with a prevalence of 2.13 cases per 100 000 population {3582}. Patients typically present in their fifth or sixth decade of life (age range: 0–88 years) {616}. An equal sex distribution or a slight female predominance is reported {616,3582}. About 10–20% of paragangliomas and/or phaeochromocytomas occur in paediatric patients {1653}; in this population, the reported median ages range from 11.6 to 13.3 years, and there is an equal sex distribution {1653,7310}.

## Etiology
There is an extremely high likelihood of a hereditary basis for paediatric paragangliomas. Pathogenic variants have been identified in as many as 78% of patients tested, with mutations in SDHB or VHL being the most common {1653,7310}.

## Pathogenesis
See Phaeochromocytoma (p. 858).

## Macroscopic appearance
Sympathetic paragangliomas may be identical to phaeochromocytomas and can be located close to the adrenal gland. Care should be taken during gross and microscopic examination to ascertain that their location is extra-adrenal, because a diagnosis of phaeochromocytoma would have different genetic implications {1904}.

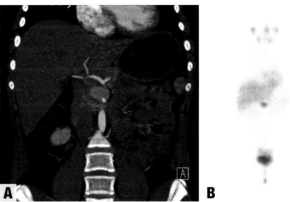

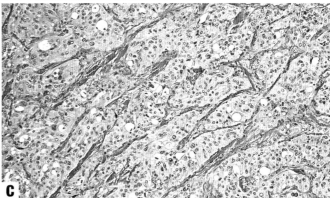

**Fig. 12.41** Anatomical and functional imaging in a patient with abdominal paraganglioma. The patient was a 13-year-old girl in a family with a known SDHB mutation; two older family members had already developed paragangliomas. Genetic testing confirmed that she also carried the mutation. Biochemical testing for metanephrines was negative. CT (**A**) and whole-body MIBG scan (**B**) showed a small midline paraganglioma, which had varied histological patterns including irregular nests and cords of cells with prominent intervening sclerosis (**C**). Intratumoural heterogeneity was also observed with respect to several immunohistochemical markers.

Chapter 12

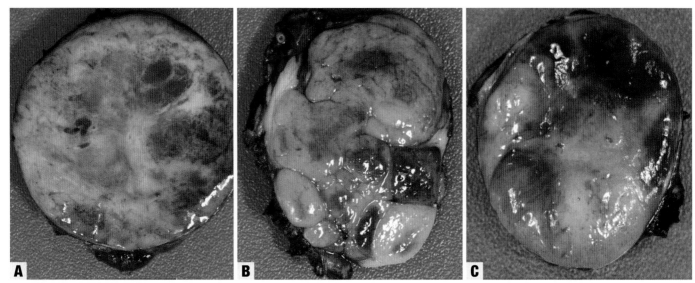

**Fig. 12.42** Multicentric paragangliomas. This patient with a hereditary *SDHB* mutation was screened for tumours in her early twenties. By that time, she had already developed three paragangliomas measuring 34–47 mm (**A–C**), adjacent to her lumbar vertebrae, each with a somewhat different gross appearance. Note the bulging nodule and cystic change (**A**) and large fleshy nodules with central necrosis (**C**), which are putative risk factors for metastasis. The tumour shown in **C** also had a diffuse growth pattern and high cellularity.

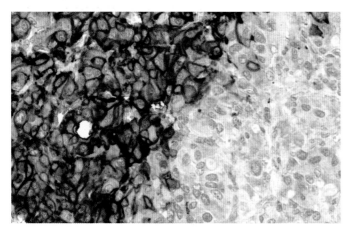

**Fig. 12.43** Abdominal paraganglioma. Staining of a resected paraganglioma for SSTR2A can be useful as a preliminary test to assess whether functional imaging or treatment with radiolabelled somatostatin analogues would be suitable to screen for or treat metastases. Most sympathetic paragangliomas express SSTR2A. However, intratumoural heterogeneity can be marked, like in this example.

## Histopathology

Paediatric paragangliomas are similar to phaeochromocytomas. Tumours are arranged in small nests (Zellballen) of neuroendocrine cells separated by a delicate fibrovascular stroma. The paraganglioma cells are intermediate, with basophilic, amphophilic, or clear cytoplasm surrounding nuclei with stippled to coarse nuclear chromatin. Isolated, extremely pleomorphic nuclei may be seen. Necrosis and increased mitoses are uncommon. Extension through a capsule and lymphovascular invasion may be present and are features used in risk stratification {6983}. When tumours have clear cytoplasm, they may mimic urinary bladder {7854}, prostate {7398}, or kidney {2832} carcinomas. Markers of differential diagnosis are the same as for phaeochromocytoma. Benign or malignant designations are not used, because all paragangliomas are considered to have metastatic potential {5897}.

## Cytology

Aspiration biopsy is generally not advised {7234,6983} but is occasionally performed either deliberately or inadvertently

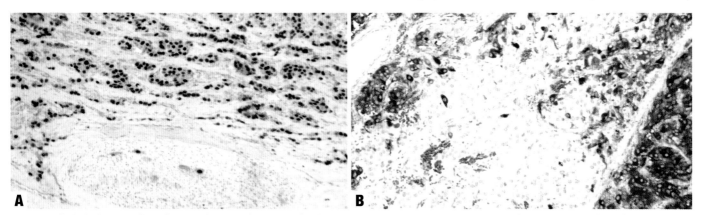

**Fig. 12.44** Abdominal paraganglioma. Sympathetic paragangliomas can show intratumoural heterogeneity with respect to biomarker expression, varying with both the type of marker and individual tumour. Transcription factors are often diffusely expressed, whereas expression of functional markers can be focal and weak. **A** Uniformly positive immunohistochemical stain for GATA3 showing characteristic nuclear staining in a paraganglioma and in two neurons in an adjacent normal ganglion at the bottom of the image. **B** Highly variable staining for tyrosine hydroxylase.

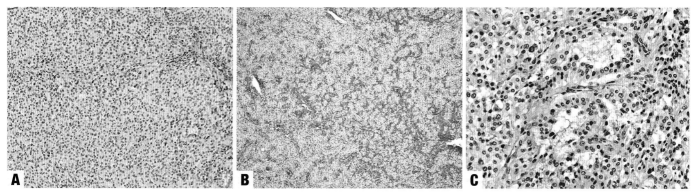

**Fig. 12.45** Histological findings in multicentric paragangliomas. Multiple histological patterns can be found in synchronous paragangliomas with the same genetic background. **A** This solid growth pattern with high cellularity was associated with tumour necrosis and coarse nodularity; all these features are putative risk factors for metastasis. Other morphological features included sharply defined tumour cell nests (Zellballen pattern) (**B**) and clear cells with patchy degenerative changes (**C**).

during workup for other tumours. Features are varied, but may help to exclude other tumours {2140}.

### Diagnostic molecular pathology
Molecular pathology is not required for diagnosis, but germline screening must be considered, guided by the clinical and pathological findings.

### Essential and desirable diagnostic criteria
*Essential:* Zellballen or a nested architecture; stippled nuclear chromatin; neuroendocrine histology.
*Desirable:* neuroendocrine immunohistochemistry and S100 sustentacular cells; biochemical testing for metanephrines; structural imaging; immunohistochemistry for SDHB and other relevant biomarkers (in selected cases).

### Staging
See *Phaeochromocytoma* (p. 858).

### Prognosis and prediction
Prognostic and risk factors are the same as for phaeochromocytoma, but location itself is a risk factor. Approximately 30% of abdominal paragangliomas may ultimately metastasize, versus about 8% for phaeochromocytoma {1496}. However, it is difficult to ascertain the contributions of genotype versus anatomical site. Extra-adrenal abdominal paragangliomas often harbour *SDHB* mutations, which may be the major cause of their aggressive behaviour {1496}.

# Parasympathetic paraganglioma (head and neck paraganglioma)

Tischler AS
de Krijger RR
Hicks MJ
Kimura N
Mete O

## Definition

Parasympathetic paraganglioma is a neuroendocrine neoplasm (NEN) that develops from neural crest–derived progenitors in paraganglia associated with the vagus and glossopharyngeal nerves in the head and neck.

## ICD-O coding

8682/3 Parasympathetic paraganglioma (head and neck paraganglioma)

## ICD-11 coding

2F7A.Y & XH5LK3 Other specified neoplasms of uncertain behaviour of endocrine & Parasympathetic paraganglioma

## Related terminology

*Not recommended:* glomus tumour; carotid body tumour; glomus caroticum tumour; glomus jugulare tumour; glomus tympanicum tumour; chemodectoma.

## Subtype(s)

None

## Localization

The designation "parasympathetic" is based on the anatomical association with parasympathetic nerves and does not imply a function. Although the terms "parasympathetic" and "head and neck" are used interchangeably, head and neck tumours may include tumours associated with cervical sympathetic chains or with mixed sympathetic and parasympathetic innervation {4765}.

These tumours are associated with the vagus and glossopharyngeal nerves within the head and neck, with topographic association used to designate the tumour, i.e. carotid body, jugulotympanic, vagal, and laryngeal paraganglioma.

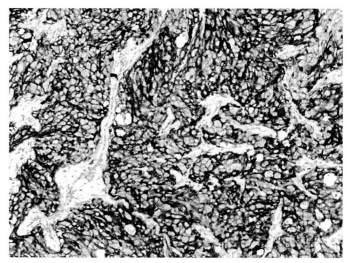

**Fig. 12.47** Carotid body paraganglioma. Diffuse strong expression of SSTR2A correlates with bright images in PET-CT using 68Ga-DOTATOC or other radiolabelled somatostatin analogues.

The most common tumour locations (identical in paediatric and adult patients) include the carotid body (~60%), the floor and wall of the middle ear (jugulotympanic, ~30%), and the trunk of the vagus nerve in or near the nodose ganglion (~10%) {6539}. Unusual head and neck locations include the larynx, thyroid, parathyroid, mandible, parotid gland, nasopharynx, paranasal sinuses, sella turcica, orbit, and clivus {362,6073,4064}.

## Clinical features

Only about 4% of head and neck paragangliomas are biochemically functional, producing predominantly dopamine and/or 3-methoxytyramine. Occasionally, norepinephrine or normetanephrine is elevated serologically or in urine. The

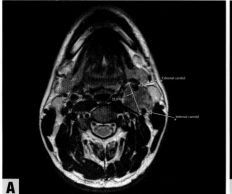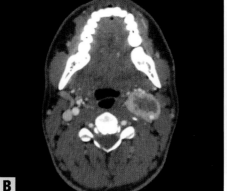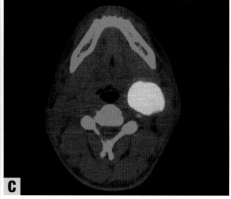

**Fig. 12.46** Carotid body paraganglioma. Classic anatomical and functional imaging characteristics in a 19-year-old patient. **A** T2-weighted MRI showed a hypervascular tumour in the bifurcation of the carotid artery. **B** To assess potential surgical options, CT angiography was performed, further demarcating the lesion, which was deemed unresectable because of the encasement of the internal and external carotid. **C** To exclude metastases, a 68Ga-DOTATOC PET-CT image was acquired, showing bright labelling consistent with intense expression of SSTR. Genetic testing showed a germline *SDHD* mutation.

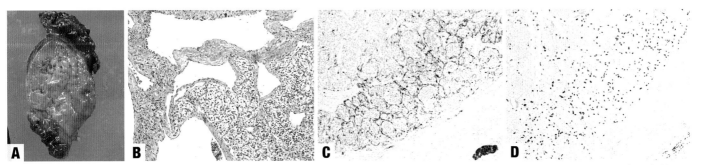

**Fig. 12.48** Carotid body paraganglioma. The spongy cut surface of this sporadic paraganglioma (**A**) corresponds to cavernous blood vessels (**B**) that communicated with vessels in the tumour capsule. Prominent, well-formed nests of clear tumour cells are highlighted by immunohistochemical stains for S100 (nuclear and cytoplasmic) (**C**) and SOX10 (nuclear) (**D**). Note the intratumoural variation in density of sustentacular cells, with a gradient in this case from periphery to centre. A small nerve outside the tumour is present in the lower-right corner.

presence of elevated metanephrine/epinephrine levels most likely points to a concurrent sympathetic paraganglioma or phaeochromocytoma {6539}. Most cases are discovered during evaluation after genetic testing in families with known histories, or as asymptomatic incidental mass lesions. Classically, carotid body paragangliomas manifest as masses at the angle of the mandible. Patients with jugulotympanic paragangliomas present with pulsatile tinnitus, hearing abnormalities, or a sensation of aural fullness. Large or infiltrative tumours, and most vagal paragangliomas, are associated with cranial nerve symptoms {7554}. Head and neck paragangliomas have a low metastatic potential, with a risk of metastasis of only 4–6% for those in the carotid body and 2% for those in the middle ear {7554}. Although few or no {1653} metastases have been reported in paediatric patients in the short term, they can occur after many years, especially in patients harbouring germline *SDHB* mutations {1925,4513}. Patients with SDH gene variants are also at risk of developing other tumours, including (but not limited to) gastrointestinal stromal tumours, pulmonary chondromas, renal cell carcinoma, thyroid carcinomas, pancreatic neuroendocrine tumours (PanNETs), and pituitary neuroendocrine tumours (PitNETs). Therefore, they require lifelong surveillance and treatment that may be tailored to their particular genotype {7556}.

## Epidemiology

The estimated incidence is 1.0–3.3 cases per 100 000 person-years {6539}, although this is without paediatric patient data

specifically. Unlike their sympathetic counterparts, parasympathetic paragangliomas show a female predominance, with an M:F ratio of about 1:1.7 {6539,1973,4381}. Paragangliomas represent < 0.5% of tumours in the head and neck. In a population-wide French series that included paediatric patients, the median patient age was 13.3 years (range: 4.6–18 years). Overall, 22.5% had head and neck tumours {1653}; this was higher than in a comparable Italian series, in which 9.1% of all patients with paragangliomas had head and neck tumours {7310}.

## Etiology
### Genetic factors
Parasympathetic paragangliomas have a hereditary predisposition in almost 85% of patients tested {6539}. Consequently, there is a high probability of synchronous or metachronous multicentric paragangliomas occurring, which may be confined to the head and neck or occasionally include sympathetic paragangliomas and phaeochromocytomas {6539, 1556}. The most common mutations are in *SDHD* (46.5%), followed by *SDHB* (30.2%) and *SDHC* (16.3%) {6539}. *SDHD* mutation is associated predominantly with single or multifocal tumours in the head and neck, with a lower probability of phaeochromocytomas and thoracoabdominal sympathoadrenal paragangliomas. The opposite is true for *SDHB*, which is more often associated with thoracoabdominal tumours {5123}. Regional differences in hereditary susceptibility genes may contribute to very different ratios of head and neck to thoracoabdominal paragangliomas. A rare, non-hereditary genetic

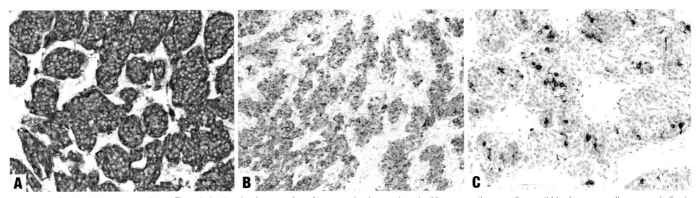

**Fig. 12.49** Carotid body paraganglioma. The relative levels of expression of neuroendocrine markers in this apparently sporadic carotid body paraganglioma are similar to those generally seen in other head and neck parasympathetic paragangliomas: synaptophysin (**A**) shows the strongest expression, followed by chromogranin A (**B**) and tyrosine hydroxylase (**C**). Chromogranin A can be expressed in a patchy pattern, and often in only a dot-like cytoplasmic distribution. Tyrosine hydroxylase is often absent or focal.

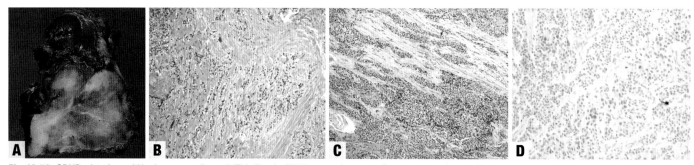

**Fig. 12.50** *SDHB*-related carotid body paraganglioma. **A** This fibrotic *SDHB*-mutated paraganglioma encases the carotid artery and extends to resection margins. **B,C** Areas with a nested Zellballen pattern are present focally at the periphery of the tumour, but the tumour mostly consists of small cells with solid and infiltrative growth. **D** S100 immunohistochemistry shows extremely rare sustentacular cells in these areas. The tumour was removed in an en bloc resection followed by a synthetic carotid artery graft. The patient, who was 22 years old when the tumour was discovered, had a germline *SDHB* mutation.

association is Carney triad, consisting of paraganglioma, gastrointestinal stromal tumour, and pulmonary chondroma {6348}.

### Risk factors

For carotid body paragangliomas in particular, tumour incidence is increased, and the M:F ratio is as high as 9:1 in some populations living at high altitudes, probably reflecting the effects of hypoxia as a phenotypic modifier in patients with *SDHD* {384, 1965} or *SDHB* {1117} mutations.

### Pathogenesis

See *Phaeochromocytoma* (p. 858).

### Macroscopic appearance

Parasympathetic paragangliomas are typically not well encapsulated tumours that are grey-pink to tan in colour. The surfaces may be somewhat firmer than those of sympathetic paragangliomas, and there may be areas of necrosis resulting from preoperative embolization.

### Histopathology

Carotid body paragangliomas show a particularly pronounced Zellballen architecture with clear cells and well-developed, sometimes cavernous, blood vessels {7003} that communicate with capsular and extratumoural vessels. The alveolar pattern ranges from a few to many chief cells. The cytoplasm ranges from amphophilic to pink and from epithelioid to spindled in appearance. The nuclei show hyperchromatic, salt-and-pepper chromatin clustering. Sustentacular supporting cells are inconspicuous with H&E stains. Isolated nuclear pleomorphism, tumour necrosis, bone invasion, and infiltration into adjacent tissues are occasionally seen and do not predict aggressive behaviour. Glands and/or mucin are not seen. Embolic material may be present after presurgical embolization.

### Immunohistochemistry

Head and neck paragangliomas are usually negative for keratins, distinguishing them from epithelial NENs. Still, neuroendocrine markers (chromogranin, synaptophysin) are variably expressed {7002}. Immunoreactivity for transcription factors may be helpful: INSM1 is detected in chromogranin-negative tumours {3789}, and GATA3 is useful to distinguish paragangliomas from most epithelial neuroendocrine tumours (NETs). GATA3 is also expressed in normal and neoplastic parathyroid and pituitary, so it must be interpreted with caution {362,1832,4664,4625,7111}. Immunoreactivity for tyrosine hydroxylase, a functional marker for paraganglioma, can be at least focally expressed in as many as 30% of head and

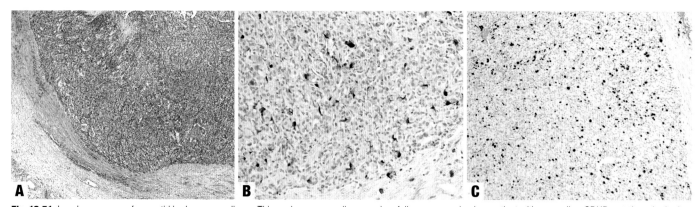

**Fig. 12.51** Local recurrence of a carotid body paraganglioma. This neck mass was discovered on follow-up scanning in a patient with a germline *SDHB* mutation who had an ipsilateral sclerotic infiltrating paraganglioma resected 4 years earlier. The lesion was 4–8 mm in diameter and protruded from the lumen of a vein (**A**). Unlike the initial tumour, which for the most part was highly cellular and consisted of small cells with infiltrative and solid growth patterns and extremely rare sustentacular cells, this tumour consisted of larger cells with relatively well-formed nests and readily identified sustentacular cells (immunohistochemical stain for S100) (**B**). The tumour was initially suspected of being a lymph node metastasis. Because no lymph node was present, it was considered to be a local recurrence, most likely from peripheral areas of the original neoplasm. The Ki-67 proliferation index (**C**) was comparable to that in solid areas of the initial tumour.

neck paragangliomas, even in patients with no biochemically detectable catecholamine hypersecretion {5234}. Furthermore, paragangliomas may show aberrant immunoreactivity for peptide hormones including calcitonin {4623,1832,477}. Although medullary thyroid carcinomas can also focally stain for tyrosine hydroxylase, they are typically negative for GATA3 and positive for CEA and thyroid transcription factor 1 (TTF1) {4623,477}. Sustentacular cells identified by staining for S100, SOX10, or (uncommonly) GFAP, can assist in the diagnosis of some tumours {7860} but are not specific for paraganglioma {1832,6602,42}. The proliferation index as determined by Ki-67 labelling may aid in risk stratification {3599}.

*Differential diagnosis*
In limited samples, metastatic disease to neck lymph nodes may represent another NET category (neuroendocrine carcinoma, Merkel cell carcinoma, medullary thyroid carcinoma), with epithelial markers generally aiding in the separation {4623}. NENs of the larynx should not be confused with paraganglioma {7556}. Heterotopic or adenomatous parathyroid may be found within the vagus nerve {7249}. Middle-ear NET (middle-ear adenoma) shows both epithelial and neuroendocrine features {6981}. In the sella turcica, pituitary paraganglioma is potentially misdiagnosed as PitNET or neuroendocrine carcinoma (NEC) {362}. Sparse mitoses and an absence of cell polarity favour paragangliomas over more malignant entities.

## Cytology
FNAB is not advised {7234,6983} but is occasionally performed either deliberately or inadvertently during clinical workup. If performed, smears have moderate to high cellularity with blood, showing cells arranged singly or in small groups, sometimes with acinar formation. Three cell types are interspersed: small to medium-sized polygonal cells with delicate granular cytoplasm, spindled cells with elongated nuclei, and large strap-like cells with eccentric nuclei {1569,3974}.

## Diagnostic molecular pathology
Molecular pathology is not required to diagnose paragangliomas, but germline screening must be considered, guided by the clinical and pathological findings {1509,1903,4995,5541, 7108}.

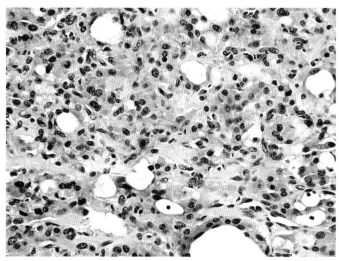

**Fig. 12.52** *SDHB*-related paraganglioma in the neck. This neck paraganglioma from an adolescent boy with an *SDHB* mutation and a history of gastrointestinal stromal tumour has prominent vacuoles and slightly eosinophilic cytoplasm, which is often seen in association with *SDHB* mutation. In this case there is abundant cytoplasm but the Zellballen pattern is poorly formed.

## Essential and desirable diagnostic criteria
*Essential:* nested architecture; round, hyperchromatic nuclei with stippled neuroendocrine chromatin.
*Desirable:* neuroendocrine immunohistochemistry with negative epithelial markers (in selected cases); SDHB immunohistochemistry or relevant genetic evaluation to exclude hereditary risk (as available).

## Staging
There is no TNM system for parasympathetic paragangliomas as published by the Union for International Cancer Control (UICC), but the International Collaboration on Cancer Reporting (ICCR) and other expert-initiated reporting guidelines may be used {4627,6983}.

## Prognosis and prediction
The main putative risk factor is hereditary mutation of *SDHB*, which is associated with metastasis {1925,4513,3289,3602}. Still, risk stratification is suggested, especially with the proliferation index as determined by Ki-67 immunohistochemistry, although no histological finding or biomarker reliably predicts metastatic disease {362,4627,3695,5526,6983}, and none has been validated in paediatric patients.

# Phaeochromocytoma

Mete O
de Krijger RR
Hicks MJ
Kimura N
Tischler AS

## Definition

Phaeochromocytoma is a neuroendocrine neoplasm (NEN) composed of adrenal medulla–derived chromaffin, representing an intra-adrenal paraganglioma.

## ICD-O coding

8700/3 Phaeochromocytoma

## ICD-11 coding

2D11.1 Malignant phaeochromocytoma of adrenal gland

## Related terminology

*Acceptable:* adrenal paraganglioma.

*Not recommended:* chromaffin cell tumour; chromaffinoma; adrenal sympathetic paraganglioma.

## Subtype(s)

None

## Localization

By definition, a paraganglioma within the adrenal gland is called a phaeochromocytoma, even when (rarely) identified in ectopic adrenal tissue {5145}. Direct invasion into adjacent organs may be seen.

## Clinical features

Symptoms are related to catecholamine excess. Unlike most functioning adult tumours, which show episodic or intermittent manifestations, paediatric phaeochromocytomas tend to show sustained symptoms {5411,504}. Hypertension, with associated manifestations including hypertensive crisis, headache, and diaphoresis, is the most common first documented presenting sign of phaeochromocytoma {7310}. Abdominal pain, weight loss, palpitations, seizures, convulsions, tremor, facial pallor, asthenia, fever, hypertensive cardiomyopathy, and other signs of hypertension-induced organ damage have been variably reported in affected patients {1653,7310,5411,4083}.

Approximately 10% of paediatric phaeochromocytomas are discovered incidentally on abdominal imaging studies or during systemic workup of a known familial predisposition syndrome

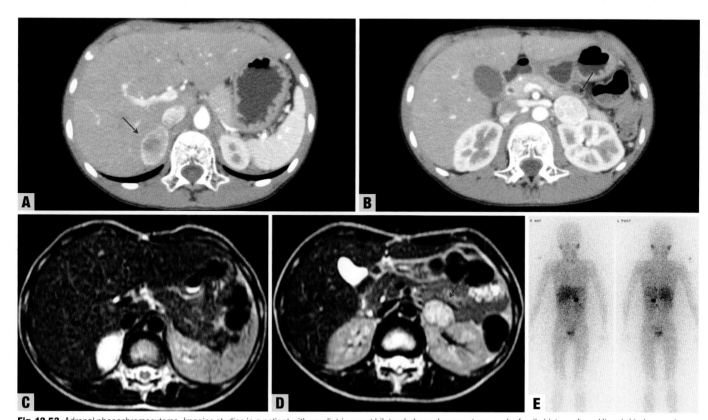

**Fig. 12.53** Adrenal phaeochromocytoma. Imaging studies in a patient with paediatric-onset bilateral phaeochromocytoma and a family history of von Hippel–Lindau syndrome. **A,B** CT shows bilateral adrenal tumours (arrows). **C,D** T2-weighted MRI shows hyperintense tumours (arrows). **E** lobenguane (metaiodobenzylguanidine; 123I-MIBG) scintigraphy shows bilateral uptake in both adrenal tumours.

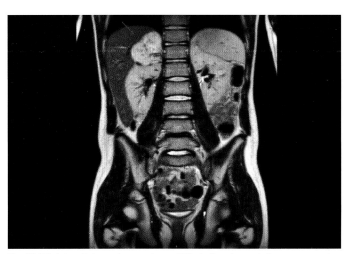

**Fig. 12.54** Adrenal phaeochromocytoma. MRI studies show a heterogeneous adrenal tumour (arrow).

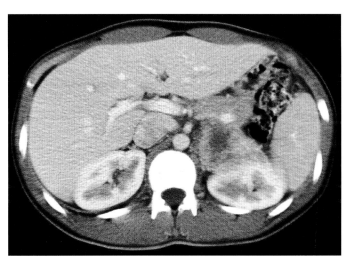

**Fig. 12.55** Phaeochromocytoma. Contrast-enhanced axial CT shows a large mass in the left adrenal gland, which is posterior to the pancreatic tail, with marked contrast enhancement and well-defined internal cystic change.

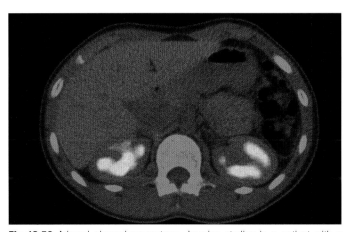

**Fig. 12.56** Adrenal phaeochromocytoma. Imaging studies in a patient with a paediatric-onset phaeochromocytoma with recurrent hypertension. During follow-up, an additional functional tumour was noted on imaging studies using 68Ga-DOTATOC PET-CT. The tumour was not removed from the former surgery site, and histopathological examination confirmed this lesion as a metachronous primary paraganglioma.

{7310,1653,13}. Patients with genetic susceptibility syndromes are predisposed to an increased frequency of bilateral and/ or multifocal phaeochromocytomas, as well as synchronous or metachronous extra-adrenal tumours including paragangliomas, and other characteristic familial manifestations. About 10–60% of paediatric-onset phaeochromocytomas are bilateral {7310,1653,5296,4083,504,3624,1336,432}, with about 60% of tumours in children aged < 10 years being bilateral {504}.

*Biochemical testing*
Biochemical testing includes measuring free catecholamine metabolites (metanephrine, normetanephrine, 3-methoxytyramine) in 24-hour fractionated urine or plasma, which is often preferable to measuring the parent catecholamines, because the metabolites are generated intratumourally by O-methylation of parent amines that leak into the tumour cell cytoplasm from secretory granules. These metabolites are therefore more sensitive biomarkers than catecholamines per se, which are also produced by sympathetic neurons {1903}. The challenges of 24-hour urine collection from paediatric patients makes plasma-based testing preferred {5411,7614}. Serum chromogranin levels are often elevated {6364}. New testing approaches aim to identify succinate or other compounds associated with specific mutations {1903}.

Phaeochromocytomas exhibit a strong correlation between genotype and biochemical phenotype {6364,362,1905,5072, 1080}. Gene mutations involved in hypoxic signalling {3657} cause a cluster 1 phenotype {1529} that manifests with dopaminergic, noradrenergic, mixed dopaminergic and noradrenergic, or non-functioning tumours. Tumours with mutations in the kinase signalling pathway (cluster 2) {1529} and in the recently described WNT-altered pathway (cluster 3) {2133} tend to be either adrenergic or mixed adrenergic and noradrenergic tumours {6364,362}. Paediatric phaeochromocytomas are commonly associated with a noradrenergic secretory phenotype, because they are enriched in molecular alterations that define cluster 1 disease {5296}. Despite the age-dependent, very common (40–80% of cases) germline susceptibility in paediatric phaeochromocytomas {4975,432,5296,1079,550}, a large proportion of children present with apparently sporadic phaeochromocytomas in the setting of germline pathogenic sequence variants {4975,7614,1079,432,6125,6986}. These findings support the need for routine genetic screening. Phaeochromocytomas can secrete ectopic peptides, with ectopic ACTH-secreting phaeochromocytomas causing Cushing syndrome being the most commonly reported {3816,5181}, and with rare reports of elevated testosterone levels and ectopic erythropoietin-producing phaeochromocytomas {7366,1266}.

*Imaging*
Among the available structural/anatomical imaging modalities, CT and MRI equally define tumour size and extent {5411,2688}, but MRI is preferentially used in paediatric-age patients because of CT-related radiation concerns {5411,7614}. Most phaeochromocytomas demonstrate a characteristic delineated hyperintense appearance (lightbulb sign) on T2-weighted imaging {5411,2179, 2688}. However, heterogeneous or lower intensity may also occur {2688}. Whole-body MRI may provide additional value in detecting multifocal extra-adrenal tumours, especially in patients harbouring germline pathogenic sequence variants {2688}. Ultrasound is

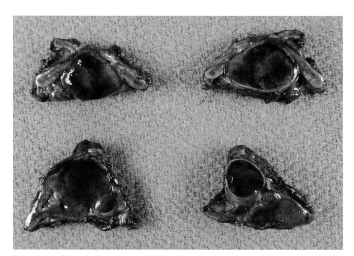

**Fig. 12.57** Gross findings in a paediatric phaeochromocytoma. The cut surface of the adrenal gland shows a phaeochromocytoma.

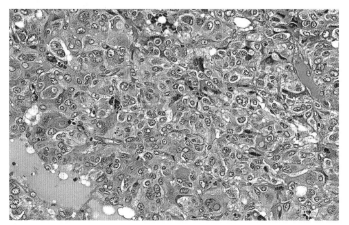

**Fig. 12.58** Conventional cytomorphology in paediatric phaeochromocytoma. Like in adults, conventional phaeochromocytomas in children consist of tumour cells resembling normal chromaffin cells that display basophilic to amphophilic cytoplasmic granularity. The cells in this example show mild nuclear pleomorphism and occasional nuclear pseudoinclusions, which can also be seen in adrenal cortical carcinomas.

considered for children aged < 10 years who cannot tolerate MRI {7104,7614}.

Functional imaging studies – including 18F-fluorodeoxyglucose (FDG), 18F-L-dihydroxyphenylalanine (FDOPA), and 18F-fluorodopamine (FDA) PET-CT; iobenguane (metaiodobenzylguanidine; 123I-MIBG and 131I-MIBG) scintigraphy; and 68Ga-DOTATATE PET-CT – are increasingly employed in the workup and treatment of patients with these tumours, aiding in the assessment of multifocal disease, synchronous or metachronous extra-adrenal paragangliomas, and staging {1616,3720,3261,1497,432,362,6364}. The mutation status and tumour location appear to impact the detection by a given functional imaging modality {1497,3261}.

## Epidemiology

The incidence of paediatric-onset phaeochromocytoma is difficult to determine; estimates range from < 0.3 to 2 cases per 1 million person-years {7360}. Although as many as 20% of all phaeochromocytomas are estimated to occur in the paediatric population {7360}, recent data from the US National Institutes of Health (NIH) showed that 5.7% of phaeochromocytomas and paragangliomas were diagnosed in patients aged < 20 years {3289}. Meta-analyses demonstrate that the frequency of phaeochromocytoma is three times as high as that of paraganglioma in paediatric-age patients {1653,504,1079,5505,4711,5296,432,550,3602}. Multifocal tumours, including phaeochromocytomas with synchronous or metachronous paragangliomas, are more frequent in paediatric patients than in adults {5296}. Phaeochromocytomas account for 16–30% of paediatric index patients harbouring germline pathogenic SDH gene variants {7614,3289}; 50% of patients with multiple endocrine neoplasia type 2 have a lifelong risk of developing phaeochromocytomas {7360}, with approximately 20% of these affected individuals presenting with phaeochromocytomas in childhood {4340}. As many as 20% of patients with von Hippel–Lindau syndrome (VHL) present with a paediatric-onset phaeochromocytoma {3961, 7360}; however, the overall lifetime frequency of phaeochromocytoma in VHL can be as high as 37% {6125}. The reported mean ages at the time of clinical diagnosis of paediatric phaeochromocytomas and paragangliomas range from 11 to 16 years

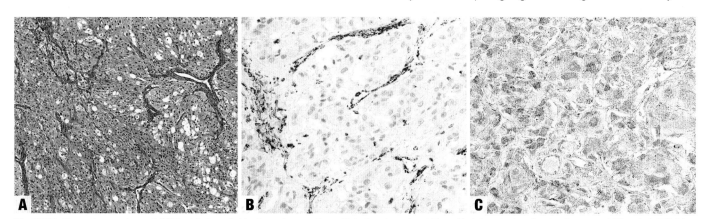

**Fig. 12.59** Phaeochromocytoma. **A** SDH-related paediatric phaeochromocytoma. Cytoplasmic eosinophilia and/or intracytoplasmic vacuoles are variably noted. **B,C** Adrenal phaeochromocytoma. SDHB is a crucial molecular immunohistochemistry biomarker in the detection of SDH-related pathogenesis. Loss of SDHB immunoreactivity (**B**) is regarded as a surrogate biomarker for SDH gene–related tumours, with a loss of cytoplasmic granular staining being a sign of succinate dehydrogenase immunodeficiency. The presence of positive staining in endothelial cells is an obligatory endogenous control. Normal staining (**C**) is characterized by the presence of intracytoplasmic granular reactivity in the neoplastic cells as well as in the non-neoplastic elements including endothelial cells and inflammatory cells. The granularity corresponds to the mitochondrial localization of SDHB.

{1653}. Most clinical series have indicated a male sex predi-lection {7310,1653,4083}, but reporting bias and tumour rarity make definitive conclusions unreliable.

## Etiology

As many as 80% of phaeochromocytomas are associated with germline susceptibility in the paediatric population {432,5296, 4975,1079,550}. The etiology, including environmental factors triggering sporadic disease, is largely unknown. Chronic hypoxia due to cyanotic congenital heart disease has been proposed as a factor in some phaeochromocytomas and paragangliomas in paediatric patients with no apparent underlying germline pathogenic sequence variants {7463,81,3461, 5207,7845}. Early-onset secondary polycythaemia (e.g. Pacak–Zhuang syndrome) is a potential risk factor for the development of these tumours {1567,4164,5310,13}.

## Pathogenesis

Genetic and/or epigenetic alterations are responsible for tumour development. As many as 80% of paediatric phaeochromocy-tomas are associated with germline pathogenic sequence vari-ants {432,550,5296}. Germline pathogenic sequence variants in phaeochromocytomas and paragangliomas encompass many mutually exclusive susceptibility genes, with the most common including *RET*, *NF1*, *TMEM127*, *MAX*, *KIF1B*, *VHL*, *FH*, *MDH2*, *EPAS1* (*HIF2A*), SDH genes (*SDHA*, *SDHB*, *SDHC*,

*SDHD*, and *SDHAF2*), *EGLN2* (*PHD1*), *EGLN1* (*PHD2*), *GOT2*, *SLC25A11*, *BAP1*, *MEN1*, *KMT2D* (*MLL2*), *DLST*, *IDH3B*, and *DNMT3A* {2857,385,3215,3349,1078,929,5834,5835,950,7717, 386,5488,4223,5836}. According to the transcriptional profile, most alterations are linked to either pseudohypoxia (cluster 1 disease) or kinase signalling pathways (cluster 2 disease) {6364,362,2133}.

At the molecular level, mutations related to the Krebs cycle (e.g. SDH genes, *FH*) and the HIF pathway (e.g. *VHL*, *EPAS1* [*HIF2A*], *EGLN2* [*PHD1*], *EGLN1* [*PHD2*]) determine cluster 1 disease, in which different cellular mechanisms cause stabiliza-tion of HIFα as well as upregulation of hypoxia signalling target genes with distinct methylation signatures and hypoxia-related microRNA profiles (e.g. miR-210) {5072,1080,2133}. Alterations related to cluster 2 disease (e.g. *RET*, *NF1*, *TMEM127*, *KIF1B*) result in kinase signalling pathway activation via different mech-anisms involving the MAPK and PI3K/AKT/mTOR pathways {5072,1080,2133}. The Cancer Genome Atlas (TCGA) project revealed rare somatic *MAML3* oncogene fusions and *CSDE1* and *ATRX* mutations that defined the WNT-altered pathway (cluster 3 disease) in sporadic adult phaeochromocytomas {2133}. The TCGA series suggested a cortical admixture sub-type (cluster 4 disease), but samples contained histologically confirmed normal cortical tissue {2133}.

Compared with their adult counterparts, paediatric phaeo-chromocytomas are typically enriched in cluster 1 disease and

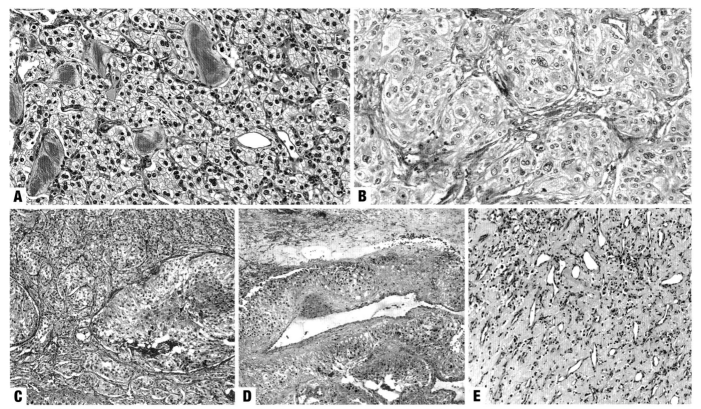

**Fig. 12.60** Adrenal phaeochromocytoma. **A** Clear cell change in a phaeochromocytoma should not be mistaken for an adrenal cortical neoplasm. The spectrum of clear cell change varies in phaeochromocytomas. This composite photomicrograph illustrates an example of diffuse zona fasciculata–like clear cell change in a von Hippel–Lindau syn-drome–related phaeochromocytoma. **B–E** Spectrum of morphological changes in a von Hippel–Lindau syndrome–related paediatric phaeochromocytoma: **B** A nested Zellballen pattern can be identified. **C** A range of cytological and architectural variations is identified in von Hippel–Lindau syndrome–related phaeochromocytomas. Trabecular or diffuse growth with large confluent nests can also occur. This case also shows comedonecrosis. **D** Pseudorosettes can occur. **E** Increased stromal vascularity and degenerative changes can feature in von Hippel–Lindau syndrome–related tumours.

show a 2-fold higher frequency of noradrenergic and/or dopaminergic tumours {5296}. Germline pathogenic sequence variants are most common in *VHL*, followed by SDH genes (most commonly in *SDHB*, followed by *SDHD*, and rarely in *SDHC* and *SDHA*), *RET*, *NF1*, and (rarely) *MAX* {432,5296,1079,1632,550}. Although the genomic landscape of paediatric phaeochromocytomas without germline alterations has not been extensively studied, genomic correlates of cluster 1 disease including somatic *EPAS1* (*HIF2A*) and *VHL* mutations have been variably documented in paediatric tumours {5296}. To date, there are no data pertaining to cluster 3 disease in paediatric patients.

Elevated levels of HIF2α and erythropoietin as a result of somatic mosaicism or rare germline alterations involving *EPAS1* (*HIF2A*) are known to lead to early-onset secondary polycythaemia {4164,13,1567} and also increase the risk of paediatric phaeochromocytomas and paragangliomas, as seen in Pacak–Zhuang syndrome {13,1567}. A report of a phaeochromocytoma harbouring a somatic *ACO1* (*IRP1*) mutation in a patient with *JAK2* p.V617F–associated polycythaemia vera further highlights primary polycythaemia as a risk factor for sporadic tumour development {5310}.

Synchronous or metachronous bilateral disease in paediatric phaeochromocytomas has been associated with germline pathogenic sequence variants in *VHL* (most frequently), *RET*, SDH genes, and *MAX* {432,4340,3624,1079}. Rare examples of bilateral paediatric disease are also reported in Pacak–Zhuang syndrome (somatic *EPAS1* [*HIF2A*] mutation) {13}, in association with Beckwith–Wiedemann syndrome {469,1111,7195}, and in a paediatric patient with hemihyperplasia caused by mosaic chromosome 11p16 paternal uniparental isodisomy {3383}. These observations raise a link to the IGF2 pathway in some paediatric phaeochromocytomas.

## Macroscopic appearance

Phaeochromocytomas originate from the adrenal medulla and may extend into adjacent structures. A tumour pseudocapsule may be present; a thick, vascularized capsule in association with degenerative vascular stroma raises the possibility of VHL {1084}. Sampling of the non-tumorous adrenal gland is required to assess for the presence of

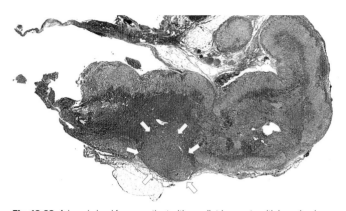

**Fig. 12.62** Adrenal gland from a patient with paediatric-onset multiple endocrine neoplasia type 2A syndrome with a microphaeochromocytoma arising in the background of adrenal medullary hyperplasia. Arrows indicate a microtumour in the background of expanded (hyperplastic) adrenal medulla.

adrenal medullary hyperplasia as well as additional adrenal medullary micronodules.

## Histopathology

Paediatric phaeochromocytomas are indistinguishable from their adult counterparts and have a range of cytological and architectural variations. Most phaeochromocytomas show a nested, Zellballen pattern, although trabecular or diffuse growth with large confluent nests and/or pseudorosettes variably occur. Conventional tumours consist of tumour cells resembling normal chromaffin cells that display basophilic to amphophilic granular cytoplasm. Variable intracytoplasmic eosinophilia and/or intracytoplasmic vacuoles may be seen, especially in patients with SDH-related tumours. Clear cell change, especially in association with other morphological findings (such as a thick, vascular tumour capsule; myxoid and hyalinized stroma; rich vascular network; and absence of cytoplasmic hyaline globules) raises the possibility of an association with VHL {3679,1084}.

Bilateral (multicentric) and/or multifocal tumours and adrenal medullary hyperplasia should prompt exclusion of germline disease {432,4340,3624,1079}. Adrenal medullary hyperplasia is defined when medulla tissue extends into the alae of the gland {4620,4627} and/or involves more than one third of the gland

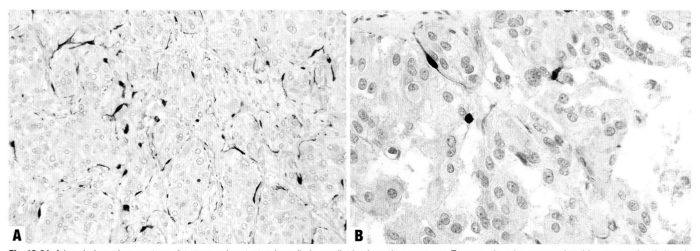

**Fig. 12.61** Adrenal phaeochromocytoma. Intratumoural sustentacular cells in paediatric phaeochromocytoma. Tumours show intertumoural and intratumoural variations in sustentacular cells (S100-positive and SOX10-positive), ranging from a well-developed sustentacular cell network (**A**) to sustentacular cells that are reduced or disorganized (**B**).

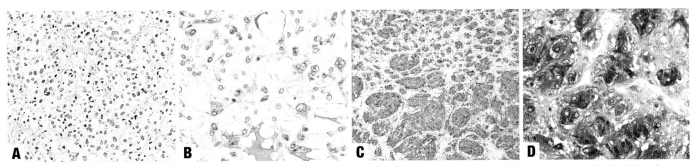

**Fig. 12.63** Adrenal phaeochromocytoma. Biomarkers of phaeochromocytomas. **A** Positivity for GATA3 is variably reported. **B,C** Several immunohistochemical biomarkers can be used to confirm the diagnosis of phaeochromocytoma. The tumour cells are negative for cytokeratins (AE1/AE3) (**B**) and strongly and diffusely positive for chromogranin A (**C**). **D** DBH, which converts dopamine into norepinephrine, has also been found useful in supporting the diagnosis.

thickness. The concept of nodular medullary hyperplasia is no longer acceptable, because distinct micronodules represent microphaeochromocytomas {4620,4627}. Although the frequency of adrenal medullary hyperplasia in paediatric series is unknown, it is seen in patients with pathogenic variants of *RET*, SDH genes, and *MAX* {4620,2563,5960}.

Multifocal primary paragangliomas in various sites must not be mistaken for metastatic spread {362}. Metastasis is defined when tumours are identified at sites where paraganglia do not occur (lymph node, bone), and so familiarity with normal anatomical distribution of autonomic nervous system elements is important {362}. A lung or liver tumour does not automatically equate with metastatic disease, because primary paragangliomas may be seen in these sites {362}. The presence of sustentacular cells may favour primary disease because these cells are often absent or greatly reduced in metastases {7144}.

### Immunohistochemistry

Most tumours are positive for tyrosine hydroxylase, DBH, GATA3, and general neuroendocrine biomarkers (chromogranin A, synaptophysin, INSM1), and negative for keratins {1832, 3598,4328,6983}. S100 and SOX10 mark intratumoural sustentacular cells. Tyrosine hydroxylase expression can be focal or absent in non-functioning tumours. Molecular immunohistochemistry is useful in facilitating genetic triaging. Membranous CAIX staining can identify VHL {5546,2065}; loss of cytoplasmic granular SDHB expression serves as a surrogate biomarker

for tumours caused by SDH gene alterations {2417,5320}. Loss of expression of SDHA correlates with *SDHA* mutations {1869}. Antibodies against 2-succinocysteine or fumarate hydratase and MAX can facilitate screening for *FH*-related and *MAX*-related tumours, respectively {4995,7127}. α-inhibin may be an immunohistochemical biomarker of pseudohypoxia-related paragangliomas and phaeochromocytomas {5286}, but it is expressed in adrenal cortical proliferations and so is not diagnostic of phaeochromocytomas. Alternatively, liquid chromatography / mass spectrometry–based measurements of tumour tissue metabolites may help to detect pathogenic variants of SDH genes {7373}.

### Risk stratification

Like for other NENs, proliferation should be routinely assessed {6983} by performing a formal mitotic count (reported per mm², assessed by counting mitotic figures from areas of 10 mm² with a high mitotic density) and the Ki-67 index as determined using the MIB1 antibody (counting ≥ 1000 tumour cells from hotspots, using either an automated nuclear algorithm or image-captured counting).

### Differential diagnosis

Predominant clear or oncocytic cell change can mimic an adrenocortical neoplasm. Positivity for SF1 and negativity for chromogranin A, GATA3, and/or tyrosine hydroxylase are characteristic of adrenal cortical tumours {4621}.

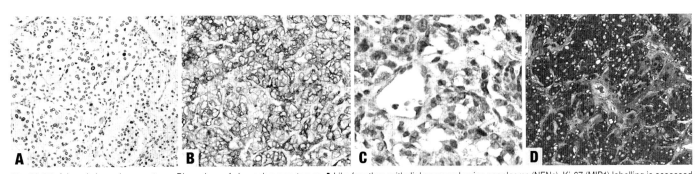

**Fig. 12.64** Adrenal phaeochromocytoma. Biomarkers of phaeochromocytomas. **A** Like for other epithelial neuroendocrine neoplasms (NENs), Ki-67 (MIB1) labelling is assessed by counting ≥ 1000 tumour cells from hotspots. **B** CAIX as a molecular immunohistochemistry biomarker for von Hippel–Lindau syndrome–related pathogenesis. Membranous CAIX reactivity is illustrated in a von Hippel–Lindau syndrome–related phaeochromocytoma. Note that negative staining does not exclude the possibility of von Hippel–Lindau syndrome. **C** The same tumour shows no loss of SDHB immunoreactivity. **D** Several immunohistochemical biomarkers can be used to confirm the diagnosis of phaeochromocytoma. Immunohistochemistry for tyrosine hydroxylase (the rate-limiting enzyme in catecholamine synthesis) is very useful to confirm the diagnosis.

## Cytology

Aspiration sampling is not advised, because of potential bleeding or catecholamine release with a possible life-threatening hypertensive crisis {7234,6983}.

## Diagnostic molecular pathology

Molecular pathology is not required to render the diagnosis of phaeochromocytoma, but germline screening must be considered, guided by the clinical and pathological findings.

## Essential and desirable diagnostic criteria

*Essential:* a nested pattern; basophilic to amphophilic granular cytoplasm; neuroendocrine marker expression by immuno-histochemistry.

*Desirable:* a neuroendocrine medulla-based neoplasm with keratin negativity (in selected cases); routine assessment of cell proliferation (mitotic count, Ki-67 index as determined using MIB1); SDHB immunohistochemistry; assessment of other biomarkers relevant to tumour pathogenesis (in selected cases).

## Staging

Phaeochromocytoma is staged using the TNM system as published by the Union for International Cancer Control (UICC), with clarification by International Collaboration on Cancer Reporting (ICCR) guidelines {6983} and other expert-initiated guidelines {4627}.

## Prognosis and prediction

Several histological findings, such as a high proliferation index, atypical mitoses, tumour comedonecrosis, large cells in a nested to diffuse growth pattern, and high tumour cellularity, suggest a more aggressive biological behaviour {6983}. However, no single histological finding or biomarker reliably predicts metastatic disease {362,4627}. There are currently four multiparameter scoring systems – the phaeochromocytoma of the adrenal gland scaled score (PASS) {6978}, the grading system for adrenal phaeochromocytoma and paraganglioma (GAPP) {3599}, the modified GAPP {3695}, and the composite phaeochromocytoma/paraganglioma prognostic score (COPPS) {5526} – each with variable prognostic-predictive performance {6676,6677} but not formally validated in paediatric patient tumours. Biomarkers of aggressive disease require validation in paediatric patients, although germline *SDHB* mutations have already been confirmed {3289,3602}. Somatic alterations shown to correlate with aggressive disease in adults include somatic *SETD2* or *ATRX* mutations, a high total somatic mutation load, *MAML3* fusions and the WNT-altered pathway {2133}, and *TERT* activation {3288}. All patients with phaeochromocytomas have a lifelong risk of metastases, with a risk of 13% in tumours arising in paediatric patients {1653}. Large tumour size and *SDHB* mutation status are linked to an increased frequency of metastatic spread {3289}.

# Composite phaeochromocytoma/ paraganglioma

Lam AK
Gill AJ

## Definition
Composite phaeochromocytoma/paraganglioma is a tumour composed of a phaeochromocytoma/paraganglioma and one or more developmentally related tumour(s) such as ganglioneuroma, ganglioneuroblastoma, neuroblastoma, or peripheral nerve sheath tumour.

## ICD-O coding
8700/3 Composite paraganglion tumours
8700/3 Composite phaeochromocytoma-ganglioneuroma
8700/3 Composite phaeochromocytoma-ganglioneuroblastoma
8700/3 Composite phaeochromocytoma-neuroblastoma
8700/3 Composite phaeochromocytoma–peripheral nerve sheath tumour
8693/3 Extra-adrenal composite paraganglion tumours
8693/3 Composite paraganglioma-neuroblastoma
8693/3 Composite paraganglioma-ganglioneuroblastoma

## ICD-11 coding
2D11.1 & XH9K97 Malignant phaeochromocytoma of adrenal gland & Composite phaeochromocytoma

## Related terminology
*Not recommended:* composite extra-adrenal phaeochromocytoma; compound adrenal medullary tumour; mixed adrenal medullary tumour; compound paraganglioma; mixed neuroendocrine–neural tumour; ganglioneuromatous paraganglioma.

## Subtype(s)
*Adrenal*
Composite phaeochromocytoma-ganglioneuroma; composite phaeochromocytoma-ganglioneuroblastoma; composite phaeochromocytoma-neuroblastoma; composite phaeochromocytoma–peripheral nerve sheath tumour

*Extra-adrenal*
Composite paraganglioma-neuroblastoma; composite paraganglioma-ganglioneuroblastoma

## Localization
Paediatric composite tumours occur slightly more commonly on the right side, with multiple tumours possible {5613}. The majority of composite tumours in paediatric populations are composite phaeochromocytomas, with only three composite paragangliomas reported {344,5613}. Composite paragangliomas develop in the retroperitoneum and mediastinum in children {344,5613}, different from the retroperitoneal and urinary bladder localization in adults {3897,5318}.

## Clinical features
Most composite tumours are functional, although levels of catecholamines vary. Patients may present with WDHA syndrome (watery diarrhoea, hypokalaemia, and achlorhydria) caused by the production of serum-detected VIP. Paroxysmal high blood pressure may manifest as headache and sweating. An abdominal mass may also be detected {6962}. Diagnosis can be confirmed by endocrinological investigations (increased blood and urine catecholamines) and radiological investigations (CT, MRI, and MIBG), with PET-CT aiding in the detection of metastatic lesions.

## Epidemiology
Composite phaeochromocytoma/paraganglioma is extremely rare {3895,5318,2624,3022}, with about 7% of cases identified in paediatric patients {5613,7044,3557,6962,1411,344,1288, 6908,5027}. Paediatric composite tumours are slightly more common in girls {5318}.

## Etiology
Unknown

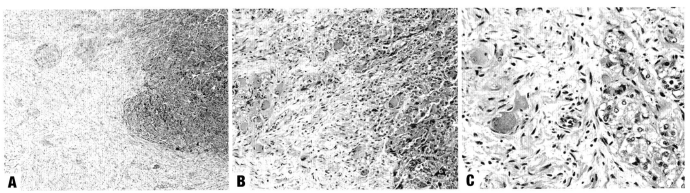

**Fig. 12.65** Adrenal composite tumour. **A** This composite tumour demonstrates a phaeochromocytoma (right) with a well-developed ganglioneuroma, including well-formed ganglion cells. **B** The two elements of this composite tumour show blending, with the phaeochromocytoma Zellballen blending intimately with the ganglioneuroma. The Schwannian cell background is well developed. **C** A high-power view shows a nest of phaeochromocytoma adjacent to well-formed ganglion cells in a background of Schwannian cells (ganglioneuroma) in a composite tumour.

Chapter 12

## Pathogenesis

Both the neuroendocrine and neural elements have a common embryogenic origin in the neural crest. Tumours that have one component initially and later develop another component during the clinical course have been reported {3557,5613, 1288}. Any tumour with a component of phaeochromocytoma/paraganglioma is considered an indication for genetic testing {7108}. With > 25 different genes implicated in the pathogenesis of phaeochromocytoma/paraganglioma, the degree of testing should be determined by local resources and pretest probabilities {5541,7108}. Germline mutations appear to be less common in composite tumours than in pure phaeochromocytoma/paraganglioma. However, NF1 and MAX mutations have been reported {5613,344,5027,1411}, along with SDHB deletion {344, 2415}. Rare composite phaeochromocytoma may be seen in neurofibromatosis type 1 {1411}. MYCN amplification is a poor prognostic factor in neuroblastoma {939} and has been reported in composite phaeochromocytoma-neuroblastoma {7044}.

## Macroscopic appearance

The cut surface is heterogeneous, with distinct components visible that match the different components: brown areas with haemorrhage (chromaffin tumour) mixed with tan areas (neural tumour) {3557}. Cystic change may be seen {6962}. The median tumour diameter is 60 mm (range: 35–150 mm).

## Histopathology

A composite tumour requires the presence of well-developed cytological and architectural features of both a phaeochromocytoma/paraganglioma component and another embryologically related (i.e. not cortical) tumour type. The presence of a few isolated ganglion cells or a small amount of Schwannian stroma in an otherwise typical phaeochromocytoma/paraganglioma does not warrant classification as a composite tumour. A useful rule of thumb is that ≥ 5% of the tumour should be composed of each tumour type. In paediatric populations, the neural component is most often neuroblastoma and less frequently ganglioneuroblastoma or ganglioneuroma. Neuroblastoma is identified by the immature neuroblastic cells with focal rosette-like arrangement and background neuropil. Schwannian stroma and ganglion cells are noted in ganglioneuroblastoma or ganglioneuroma, whereas streaming fascicles of elongated tumour cells with myxoid stroma are noted when the second tumour is malignant peripheral nerve sheath tumour {1288}. Paediatric composite tumours may spread to lymph nodes {5027}, liver, lung, and bones {5027,3557}. Metastatic foci may contain one or both components {5027,7044,5613,3557}, although in composite phaeochromocytoma–malignant peripheral nerve sheath tumour, metastatic foci consisted exclusively of one component or the other, with metastatic phaeochromocytoma in the bones and malignant peripheral nerve sheath tumour in the liver, lungs, and lymph nodes {1288}.

### Immunohistochemistry

Phaeochromocytoma/paraganglioma shows vimentin reactivity, with sustentacular cells positive for GFAP and S100, whereas neuroblastoma is negative or only focally positive for these markers {6908}. VIP protein may be identified in patients with WDHA syndrome.

## Cytology

Not clinically relevant

## Diagnostic molecular pathology

Not relevant

## Essential and desirable diagnostic criteria

Essential: presence of cytologically and architecturally recognizable phaeochromocytoma/paraganglioma differentiation and a neural component; minor component constituting ≥ 5% of tumour volume.

## Staging

Not applicable

## Prognosis and prediction

In contrast to composite tumours in adults, in which metastases are uncommon {3022,1206,2624,3896}, > 55% of paediatric composite tumours have metastases {7044,3557,1288,5027, 5613}.

# Other neuroendocrine tumours

Mete O
Asa SL
de Krijger RR
Hicks MJ

Kimura N
La Rosa S
Tischler AS

## Definition
Neuroendocrine tumours (NETs) are epithelial neuroendocrine neoplasms composed of well-differentiated cells.

## ICD-O coding
8240/3 Neuroendocrine tumour, grade 1
8249/3 Neuroendocrine tumour, grade 2
8151/3 Insulinoma

## ICD-11 coding
Site-specific code &
XH9LV8 Neuroendocrine tumour, grade 1
XH51K1 Neuroendocrine tumour, grade 2

## Related terminology
*Acceptable:* epithelial neuroendocrine neoplasm; well-differentiated neuroendocrine tumour; carcinoid.
*Not recommended:* well-differentiated neuroendocrine carcinoma; benign neuroendocrine tumour; malignant neuroendocrine tumour.

## Subtype(s)
Subtypes according to neuroendocrine cell type and hormone production.

## Localization
Paediatric NETs occur anywhere within the body, including in the pituitary, thyroid, parathyroid, lung, thymus, and gonads; they are most common in the gut and pancreas {3302}. NETs can also arise in paediatric-onset teratomas {93,6948}.

## Clinical features
The clinical features depend on the site of origin and hormonal activity of the tumour. Those involving the gut may cause obstruction or intussusception. They may be detected as a mass. They may cause hormone excess and symptoms such as hypoglycaemia due to insulinoma {6653}, gastrin excess due to gastrinoma {6653}, carcinoid syndrome due to metastatic small bowel NET {173,2187}, and (extremely rarely) Cushing syndrome due to ectopic ACTH {4389}.

## Epidemiology
Gastroenteropancreatic NETs (GEP-NETs) represent < 1% of paediatric tumours and 10.5% of digestive neoplasms, with an annual incidence of about 2.8 cases per 1 million children {7867,4950}. The incidence of hindgut, midgut, and foregut NETs, in cases per 1 million person-years, is 0.2, 0.1, and 0.1, respectively {4950}. The average age of disease onset is about 12–15 years {6653}, and there is a female predominance {173, 4889,2285}. Pancreatic NETs account for about 9% of pancreatic neoplasms diagnosed in the paediatric age group {4889,

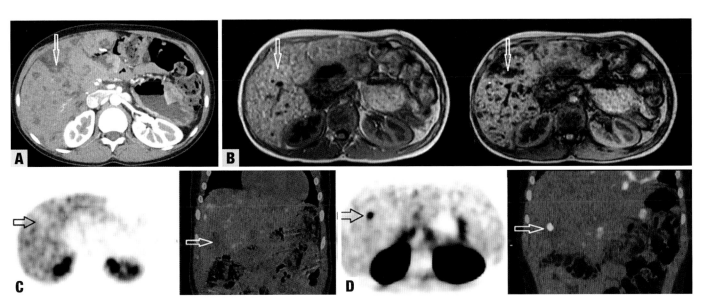

**Fig. 12.66** Structural and functional imaging studies in a paediatric age–onset metastatic insulin-producing well-differentiated pancreatic neuroendocrine tumour (PanNET). An 11-year-old child presented with an insulin-producing well-differentiated PanNET with low-grade proliferative features (G1 NET; insulinoma). Subsequently, the patient developed progressive symptoms related to the insulinoma and was found to have diffuse miliary hypervascular liver metastases in association with massive peritumoural steatosis. The metastatic disease was difficult to see on CT (**A**) and MRI (**B**; in-phase and out-of-phase T1 sequence images are shown), as well as on initial 68Ga-DOTATOC PET-CT imaging (**C**), because of the small size of the tumour deposits. The interim liver biopsy showed only steatosis. During follow-up, the largest metastatic tumour deposit did show uptake using 68Ga-exendin PET-CT (GLP-1–targeted PET) (**D**). Arrows indicate the dominant metastatic tumour deposit in different imaging modalities.

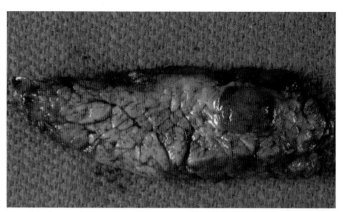

**Fig. 12.67** Pancreatic neuroendocrine tumour (PanNET). Gross findings of a paediatric age–onset PanNET.

1239}. The estimated annual incidence of pulmonary NET is about 0.6 cases per 1 million children {4950}.

## Etiology

The etiology of sporadic paediatric NETs is largely unknown. Genetic susceptibility varies among tumour subtypes {3302}.

## Pathogenesis

Like in adults, anatomical site–specific genetic and epigenetic alterations contribute to tumorigenesis in NETs in children. Germline susceptibility to neuroendocrine neoplasia is summarized in Table 12.06.

## Macroscopic appearance

The consistency and colour of these tumours vary, but most are solid and yellow. Tumours are often confined to the anatomical limits of individual organs, but invasion into adjacent structures also occurs. Sampling of the non-tumorous parenchyma is required to assess microscopic tumour multifocality, associated neuroendocrine cell hyperplasia, or findings related to pathogenesis {4620}.

## Histopathology

Most NETs have an insular/nested architecture and are composed of polygonal cells with smoothly contoured round to oval nuclei with stippled chromatin (salt-and-pepper nuclei). Peripheral palisading is frequently present. Tumour cells express INSM1, synaptophysin, chromogranins, and keratins. NETs are graded as G1, G2, or G3 on the basis of cell proliferation as evaluated using the Ki-67 index or mitoses per 2 mm$^2$ (see Table 12.07, p. 870).

**Table 12.06** Genetic susceptibility in paediatric gastroenteropancreatic, pulmonary, and thymic neuroendocrine tumours (NETs)[a] (continued on next page)

| Syndrome/condition | Gene(s) | Location(s) | Histopathology and immunohistochemistry |
|---|---|---|---|
| Multiple endocrine neoplasia type 1 | MEN1 | Gastric<br>Pancreatic<br>Duodenal<br>Pulmonary<br>Thymic | Global menin loss<br>Multifocal NETs arising in neuroendocrine cell hyperplasia<br>Gastric:<br>• ECL-cell and parietal cell hyperplasia<br>• Multifocal (type 2) ECL-cell NETs<br>Pancreatic:<br>• Glucagon most frequent in pancreatic NETs<br>• Islet dysplasia, ductuloinsular complexes, islet peliosis<br>• Pancreatic neuroendocrine microtumours[b]<br>Duodenal/pancreatic:<br>• Gastrinomas and plurihormonal NETs |
| Multiple endocrine neoplasia type 4 | CDKN1B | Gastric<br>Pancreatic<br>Duodenal<br>Pulmonary<br>Thymic | Global loss of nuclear p27 expression |
| Von Hippel–Lindau syndrome | VHL | Pancreatic<br>Duodenal | Frequent associated cystic disease<br>Multifocal NETs and microtumours[b]<br>Islet dysplasia, ductuloinsular complexes, islet peliosis<br>Clear cell and oncocytic cytomorphology<br>PP-expressing NETs are common<br>Variably positive for CAIX, α-inhibin, HIF1α |
| Neurofibromatosis type 1 | NF1 | Pancreatic<br>Duodenal (ampullary type) | Insulin-producing pancreatic NET<br>Somatostatin-producing duodenal D-cell NET with psammoma bodies |
| Mahvash disease | GCGR | Pancreatic | Glucagon A-cell hyperplasia to neoplasia progression |
| Familial insulinomatosis | MAFA | Pancreatic | Insulin B-cell hyperplasia to neoplasia progression |

Chr, chromosome; del, deletion; EC, enterochromaffin; ECL, enterochromaffin-like; LINE, localized islet nuclear enlargement; NEN, neuroendocrine neoplasm; PGL, paraganglioma; UPD, uniparental disomy.
[a]Data are based on overall experience in adults and children. [b]Neuroendocrine microtumours (also known as neuroendocrine microadenomas). [c]A subset of patients without other characteristic mutations harbour mosaic uniparental isodisomy for chromosome 11p15 in association with Beckwith–Wiedemann syndrome–related congenital hyperinsulinism. [d]Single case report of a pancreatic NET. [e]Often somatic and rarely germline.

**Table 12.06** Genetic susceptibility in paediatric gastroenteropancreatic, pulmonary, and thymic neuroendocrine tumours (NETs)[a] (continued)

| Syndrome/condition | Gene(s) | Location(s) | Histopathology and immunohistochemistry |
|---|---|---|---|
| Congenital hyperinsulinism | ABCC8<br>KCNJ11<br>GCK<br>GLUD1<br>SLC16A1<br>HNF4A<br>HADH<br>UPD (11p15)[c] | Pancreatic | Typical form: partial/diffuse islet hyperplasia, nesidioblastosis, microtumours[b]<br>Atypical forms: LINE, islet proliferations related to Beckwith–Wiedemann syndrome |
| Tuberous sclerosis | TSC1<br>TSC2 | Pancreatic<br>Rectal | Multifocal in pancreas<br>Global loss of tuberin or hamartin |
| Familial small bowel NET | IPMK<br>SMARCB1<br>Chr 18 del | Ileal | Multifocal EC-cell NETs unassociated with other well-known genetic syndromes<br>No underlying neuroendocrine cell hyperplasia |
| SDH-related familial PGL syndromes | SDH genes | Pancreatic[d] | Global loss of SDHB |
| Pacak–Zhuang syndrome | EPAS1<br>(HIF2A)[e] | Duodenal | Duodenal somatostatin-producing D-cell NET |
| Lynch syndrome | MLH1<br>MSH2<br>MSH6<br>PMS2 | Pancreatic | Global loss of MLH1, MSH2, MSH6, or PMS2 |
| DNA repair pathway–related NENs | BRCA2<br>CHEK2<br>MUTYH<br>PALB2<br>NTHL1 | Pancreatic<br>Pulmonary<br>Thymic | Scant morphological data |

Chr, chromosome; del, deletion; EC, enterochromaffin; ECL, enterochromaffin-like; LINE, localized islet nuclear enlargement; NEN, neuroendocrine neoplasm; PGL, paraganglioma; UPD, uniparental disomy.

[a]Data are based on overall experience in adults and children. [b]Neuroendocrine microtumours (also known as neuroendocrine microadenomas). [c]A subset of patients without other characteristic mutations harbour mosaic uniparental isodisomy for chromosome 11p15 in association with Beckwith–Wiedemann syndrome–related congenital hyperinsulinism. [d]Single case report of a pancreatic NET. [e]Often somatic and rarely germline.

Pulmonary and thymic NETs (carcinoids) may be composed of polygonal or spindle-shaped cells, the latter being especially likely in peripheral lung NETs. They tend to be well delineated but locally infiltrative. In addition to general markers of NETs, pulmonary NETs may express thyroid transcription factor 1 (TTF1) (using the SPT24 clone) and can express serotonin, calcitonin, CGRP/bombesin, and focal CEA (using a monoclonal antibody). Ectopic hormone production is more common by thymic NETs than other NETs. The current WHO classification still proposes using mitotic activity and necrosis to distinguish intermediate-grade disease (atypical carcinoid; see Table 12.08, p. 870); however, Ki-67 immunohistochemistry is useful in the distinction of neuroendocrine carcinomas (NECs), especially in small biopsies.

Gastric NETs in children are most often type 2 enterochromaffin-like (ECL)-cell NETs and rarely type 1 tumours {3302}. Like in adults, the distinction among different tumour subtypes in children is based on the patient's clinicopathological background, which includes morphology of the peritumoural mucosa, serum gastrin level, presence or absence of antral PP-cell hyperplasia, and presence or absence of multiple endocrine neoplasia type 1 (MEN1) {7521}. ECL cells are positive for VMAT2 and HDC.

Duodenal NETs in the ampullary region are composed of somatostatin-producing D cells showing a predominant tubuloacinar structure with or without intraluminal psammoma bodies. MEN1-related presentations can show underlying

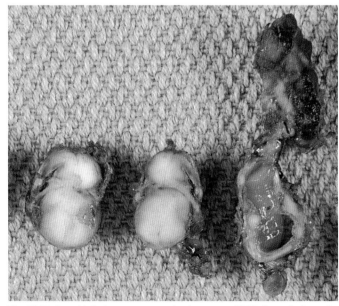

**Fig. 12.68** Bronchial/pulmonary neuroendocrine tumour (NET). Gross findings of a paediatric age–onset bronchial/pulmonary NET.

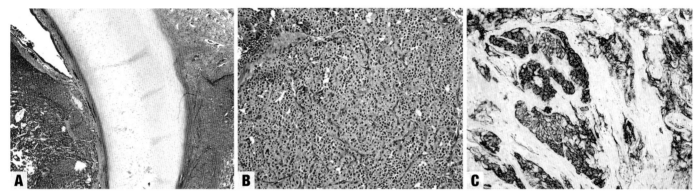

**Fig. 12.69** Histological features in a paediatric age–onset bronchopulmonary neuroendocrine tumour (NET). The tumour consists of a well-differentiated NET involving the bronchus and adjacent lung parenchyma. The tumour shows a mixed growth pattern including nests, sheets, and trabeculae. **A,B** H&E. **C** Chromogranin A.

neuroendocrine cell hyperplasia and multifocality associated with PP-cell and D-cell proliferations. Duodenal gangliocytic paragangliomas that consist of epithelial, spindle, and

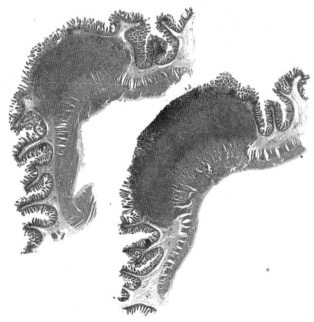

**Fig. 12.70** Ileal enterochromaffin (EC)-cell neuroendocrine tumour (NET). An ileal EC-cell well-differentiated NET in a 17-year-old girl.

ganglion cell–like tumour cells can occur in the paediatric population {5155}. Recent data suggest that these tumours and cauda equina paragangliomas are aligned with epithelial neuroendocrine neoplasms (NENs) and are not true paragangliomas {4359}.

Ileal NETs are composed of enterochromaffin (EC) cells with brightly eosinophilic cytoplasm. Tumour cells are positive for serotonin, substance P, CDX2, and VMAT1.

Rectal NETs are most frequently composed of L cells with a striking trabecular architecture {4023,2338,3585}; they generally infiltrate the mucosa and submucosa. Tumour cells express glicentin, GLP-1 and/or GLP-2 (identified with glucagon antibodies), PP, and PYY {3708}. Chromogranin A may be expressed only focally, and some rectal tumours may preferentially express chromogranin B {3597}. SATB2 and PAP are frequently expressed, whereas CDX2 expression is variable.

Pancreatic NETs (PanNETs) in children are similar to those in adults. Insulinoma is thought to be the most common functional PanNET in children {3302,6653}. Assessment of the non-tumorous pancreatic parenchyma identifies multifocal microscopic lesions including islet cell dysplasia (quantitative and qualitative alteration in the four islet cell types is demonstrated using insulin, glucagon, somatostatin, and PP immunohistochemistry), microtumours/microadenomas (dysplastic islets measuring 0.5–5 mm), ductuloinsular complexes (nesidioblastosis), and peliosis of the non-tumorous islets {4620}. These findings and

**Table 12.07** Grading criteria for neuroendocrine tumours (NETs) of the gastrointestinal tract and pancreas

| Terminology | Differentiation | Grade | Mitotic count (mitoses / 2 mm²) | Ki-67 index |
|---|---|---|---|---|
| **NET G1** | Well differentiated | Low | < 2 | < 3% |
| **NET G2** | Well differentiated | Intermediate | 2–20 | 3–20% |
| **NET G3** | Well differentiated | High | > 20 | > 20% |

Note: The Ki-67 index is calculated by counting ≥ 500 cells in the region of highest labelling (hotspot) identified at scanning magnification. The mitotic count is based on the evaluation of ≥ 50 high-power microscopic fields (10 mm²) and is expressed as mitoses per 2 mm². The final grade is based on whichever proliferative measure (Ki-67 or mitoses) places the neoplasm in the highest-grade category.

**Table 12.08** Classification of neuroendocrine tumours (NETs) of the lung and thymus

| Terminology | Differentiation | Grade | Diagnostic histological criteria | Terminology proposal |
|---|---|---|---|---|
| Typical carcinoid | Well differentiated | Low | • Neuroendocrine morphology<br>• < 2 mitoses / 2 mm²<br>• No necrosis | NET G1 |
| Atypical carcinoid | Well differentiated | Intermediate | • Neuroendocrine morphology<br>• 2–10 mitoses / 2 mm²[a]<br>• Necrosis[a] | NET G2 |

[a]One or both should be present.

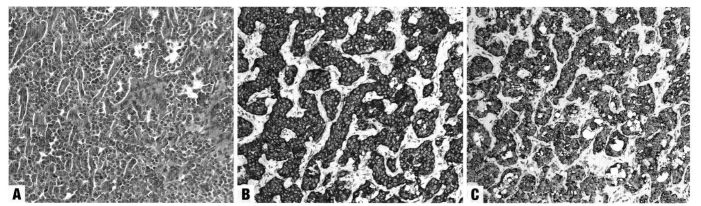

**Fig. 12.71** Metastatic well-differentiated enterochromaffin (EC)-cell neuroendocrine tumour (NET). **A** Liver metastasis in a paediatric patient with a primary ileal EC-cell NET. The tumour is positive for chromogranin A (**B**) and serotonin (**C**), as well as for CAM5.2 and CDX2. The immunohistochemical findings are consistent with a midgut EC-cell origin.

tumour multifocality are a harbinger of germline susceptibility for MEN1, MEN4, and von Hippel–Lindau syndrome {4620, 1084,3656}.

The tumour cells are variably positive for insulin gene enhancer protein ISL1, PDX1, PAX6, polyclonal PAX8, and CDX2, and they show variable expression of pancreatic hormones as well as other hormones (e.g. calcitonin, serotonin, VIP, gastrin). Immunostaining characteristics for hormones can also provide additional value to the distinction of MEN1 (always plurihormonal) and other rare manifestations including Mahvash disease (islet A-cell hyperplasia to neoplasia progression sequence) or inherited forms of insulinomatosis (islet B-cell hyperplasia to neoplasia progression sequence) {3656}.

Non-endocrine cystic disease suggests von Hippel–Lindau syndrome {1084}. The use of immunohistochemical biomarkers can facilitate germline screening {1833} (see Table 12.06, p. 869).

The differential diagnosis at all sites includes paraganglioma. In the pancreas, pancreatoblastoma, acinar cell carcinoma, and solid pseudopapillary neoplasm should be considered.

### Cytology

NETs are composed of loosely cohesive epithelial cells with indistinct cell membranes, displaying cytoplasmic granularity and salt-and-pepper nuclei.

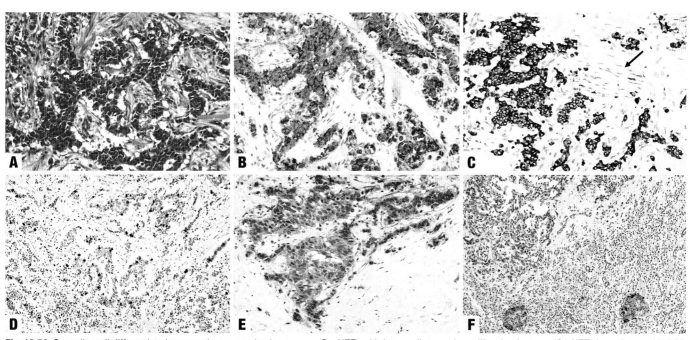

**Fig. 12.72** Sporadic well-differentiated pancreatic neuroendocrine tumour (PanNET) with intermediate-grade proliferative features (G2 NET) in a 12-year-old child. **A** The PanNET shows trabeculae and a cord-like growth pattern with fibrotic stroma. **B** The tumour is diffusely positive for chromogranin A. **C** It is also diffusely positive for CAM5.2 and shows angioinvasion, lymphatic invasion, and perineural invasion (arrow). **D** The Ki-67 index is 14.8% in hotspots. **E** The tumour cells also show positive reactivity for KIT (CD117; shown here) and CK19 (not shown). Both KIT (CD117) and CK19 have been linked to biologically aggressive forms of PanNETs in adults. **F** The non-tumorous pancreas displays a normal distribution of islet A, B, PP, and D cells, as shown by immunohistochemistry for glucagon, insulin, PP, and somatostatin (somatostatin shown here).

### Diagnostic molecular pathology

Molecular pathology is not required to render the diagnosis. Germline testing should be considered in light of clinical and pathological findings.

### Essential and desirable diagnostic criteria

*Essential diagnostic criteria*

*Pathological:* morphological assessment is accompanied by immunohistochemistry to confirm the epithelial nature, neuroendocrine differentiation, and proliferative features (Ki-67 index); assessment of the non-tumorous parenchyma or mucosa for findings relevant to germline susceptibility.

*Clinical:* elevated serum chromogranin levels; other circulating biomarkers for functional tumours as subtyped.

*Desirable diagnostic criteria*

*Pathological:* use of confirmatory immunohistochemistry for cell lineage–specific biomarkers (hormones and transcription factors) and biomarkers relevant to tumour pathogenesis.

*Clinical:* functional imaging studies; routine germline testing.

### Staging

Staging of NETs follows the tumour location and grade–dependent eighth-edition American Joint Committee on Cancer (AJCC) and Union for International Cancer Control (UICC) TNM staging system and the College of American Pathologists (CAP) standardized reporting guidance.

### Prognosis and prediction

The prognosis of paediatric NETs is not unlike that of adult NETs. Complete resection can result in cure {6971}, but metastatic disease requires ongoing therapy. Pancreatic insulinoma and L-cell rectal tumours have better prognosis than other tumours at those sites. Primary tumours arising in the gonads are more aggressive {173}. Patient age < 5 years predicts a worse 5-year survival; Black patients have a lower 5-year survival rate than White patients {173}. Ectopic hormone production is a poor prognostic sign; accordingly, Cushing syndrome due to ectopic ACTH has a poor prognosis {2437}.

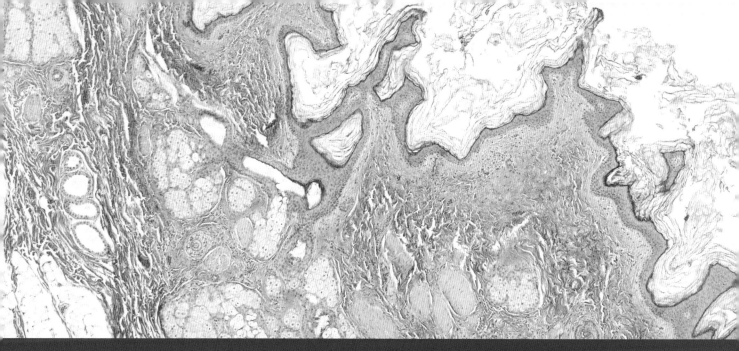

# 13

# Head and neck tumours

Edited by: López-Terrada DH, Pfister SM, Thompson LDR

Benign tumours
    Squamous papilloma and papillomatosis
    White sponge naevus
    Congenital granular cell epulis
    Central giant cell granuloma
    Odontogenic tumours
    Ossifying fibroma
    Sinonasal tract myxoma
    Nasal dermoid cyst
    Nasopharyngeal dermoid
    Nasal chondromesenchymal hamartoma
    Pleomorphic adenoma
Malignant tumours
    Mucoepidermoid carcinoma
    Acinic cell carcinoma
    Sialoblastoma
    Nasopharyngeal carcinoma
    NUT carcinoma
    Melanotic neuroectodermal tumour of infancy

# Head and neck tumours: Introduction

Thompson LDR

Head and neck tumours are uncommon in paediatric patients; however, some tumours occur almost exclusively in the paediatric age group. The exclusively paediatric tumours include congenital granular cell epulis, sialoblastoma, and melanotic neuroectodermal tumour of infancy. Some salivary gland malignancies (mucoepidermoid carcinoma, acinic cell carcinoma) and nasopharyngeal carcinoma represent a relatively large proportion of the overall tumour category; however, of all cancers in children in the USA (incidence: ~168 cases per 1 million person-years), < 1% develop in the head and neck (excluding CNS malignancies, retinoblastoma, thyroid malignancies, and lymphomas) {6473,6474}. Inherited tumour syndromes such as Li–Fraumeni syndrome, von Hippel–Lindau syndrome, and Fanconi anaemia frequently come to light in paediatric patients, but these do not give rise to a significant head and neck tumour burden. A few exceptions are odontogenic lesions, where naevoid basal cell carcinoma syndrome is associated with odontogenic keratocysts, patients with hyperparathyroidism–jaw tumour syndrome have ossifying fibroma {6416}, and patients with *DICER1* syndrome have nasal chondromesenchymal hamartoma {6524}. One of the major differences between cancers in children and adults is that for head and neck epithelial malignancies, there is a significantly better overall outcome for those identified in paediatric patients, with a 5-year survival rate of 95–98% {7723, 7799}. This chapter also contains sections on tumour entities that are not neoplasms, such as nasal dermoid cyst and white sponge naevus, but which have been included because of their clinical manifestations as well as the differential diagnostic considerations they may raise. Also included are several entities that are more common in paediatric patients but also seen in adults, such as NUT carcinoma. For the majority of these head and neck tumours, molecular findings support the diagnosis but are not required for it, potentially allowing for the classification of these entities using more standard techniques. Exceptions are the rule in medicine, and so these topics are presented with humility and with our current understanding of these entities, recognizing that advancements and exceptions are bound to occur.

# Squamous papilloma and papillomatosis

Richardson MS
Flaitz CM

## Definition
Squamous papilloma (SP) and squamous papillomatosis are benign exophytic-papillary squamous epithelial neoplasms usually associated with low-risk HPV.

## ICD-O coding
8052/0 Squamous papilloma of the larynx
8060/0 Squamous papillomatosis of the larynx

## ICD-11 coding
2F00.Y & XH50T2 Other specified benign neoplasm of middle ear or respiratory system & Squamous cell papilloma, NOS
2E90 & XH50T2 Benign neoplasm of lip, oral cavity, or pharynx & Squamous cell papilloma, NOS

## Related terminology
*Acceptable:* recurrent respiratory papillomatosis (RRP); laryngeal papillomatosis; squamous cell papilloma.
*Not recommended:* juvenile papillomatosis; adult papillomatosis.

## Subtype(s)
None

## Localization
The distribution of squamous papillomatosis follows a predictable pattern, with the tumours occurring at sites where ciliated epithelium and squamous epithelium are juxtaposed. Any oral mucosal site may be affected, but solitary lesions have a predilection for the palatal complex and oral tongue {8,2240}. Within the larynx, where multifocal disease is common, the vocal cords and ventricles are most frequently affected, followed by the false cords, epiglottis, subglottic area, hypopharynx, and nasopharynx.

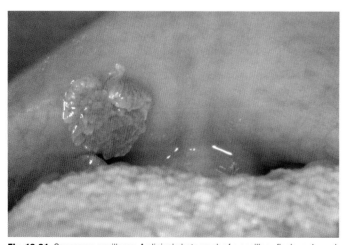

**Fig. 13.01** Squamous papilloma. A clinical photograph of a papillary, fleshy-coloured, pedunculated tumour of the soft palate.

Lower respiratory tract extension is rare (occurring in 1–3% of cases), often associated with high mortality {2347}.

## Clinical features
A painless soft nodule with pink or white finger-like fronds or a pebbly, cauliflower-like surface and pedunculated base are the characteristic findings for SP {2240}. There is clinical overlap with solitary verruca vulgaris and condyloma acuminatum. Laryngeal tumours are associated with symptoms of progressive hoarseness, stridor, chronic cough, and dysphagia.

## Epidemiology
SP is the most common benign epithelial tumour of the larynx and oral cavity in children {8,2240}. Recurrent respiratory papillomatosis (RRP) is a rare disease that occurs in children and adults. The projected annual estimates of RRP incidence are 4.3 cases per 100 000 children and approximately 1.8 cases per 100 000 adults {1042,1710}. There is a bimodal age distribution, with the first peak occurring at < 5 years of age (juvenile cases) and the second peak at 20–40 years (adult cases) {1042,3681}. RRP is more common in children than in adults and is the most aggressive form of SP, with 25% of cases arising during infancy {5812,7525}. There is no sex predilection in children. Although the disease is rare, morbidity is notoriously high, because it compromises functions such as vocalization, swallowing, and breathing {7525,2347}.

## Etiology
HPV6 and HPV11 (identified in 90% of cases) are the genotypes most frequently associated with RRP and solitary oral SP {7525,667}, with a minority of RRP cases (4–5%) showing coinfection. Other HPV genotypes (e.g. 16, 31, 33, 35, and 39) are found in a minority of cases (3–4%) {7525}. The modes of HPV transmission include non-sexual contact, maternal contact (direct or indirect), and sexual contact {3866}. Most neonatal HPV infection occurs by vertical transmission at birth {6816}. A triad of factors (first-born child, vaginal delivery, and maternal age < 20 years) correlates with RRP in children {3463}. An active maternal genital HPV infection at the time of delivery increases exposure to a significant viral load, with a high risk of transmitting infection. Caesarean section provides a lower risk of transmission but is not completely protective against infection {667,6816}.

## Pathogenesis
HPVs are double-stranded DNA viruses, differentiated by the genetic sequence of the outer capsid protein L1. The virions replicate within the nuclei of infected host cells {4199}. More than 40 types affect mucosal epithelium, separated into non-oncogenic types (e.g. HPV6 and HPV11) and oncogenic types (e.g. HPV16 and HPV18). Viral infection occurs at the basal epithelium, frequently in zones of the body lined by squamous

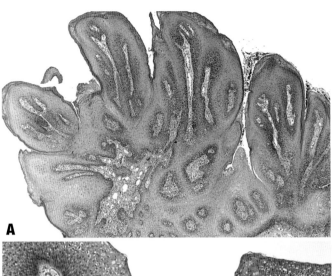

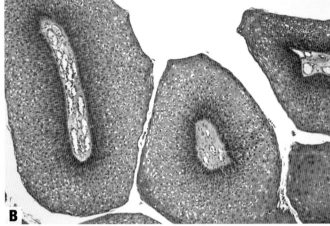

**Fig. 13.02** Squamous papilloma. **A** Histologically, there are multiple papillary projections lined by thickened epithelium with luminal cells showing koilocytic changes. **B** High-power view shows thickened epithelium with orderly maturation to the surface. Crenated nuclei with perinuclear haloes and sharp cell borders are characteristic of koilocytic change in squamous papilloma.

epithelium with a squamocolumnar transition. The transcripts initiated at major viral promoter sites in oncogenic types are not seen in non-oncogenic types.

## Macroscopic appearance
A sessile or pedunculated nodule with a bosselated, papillary surface is characteristic.

## Histopathology
SCPs are exophytic-verrucous, composed of an arborizing fibrovascular network covered by squamous epithelium ranging from non-keratinized to showing varying degrees of keratinization. Koilocytic atypia (crenated nucleus, perinuclear halo, prominent cell borders) may be seen, but epithelial dysplasia is infrequently observed and should be reported if present. Mitoses may be increased in traumatized or inflamed lesions. In RRP, premature keratinization of individual epithelial cells contributes to a disorganized appearance. The distribution of RRP follows a predictable pattern, occurring where ciliated and squamous epithelium is juxtaposed.

## Cytology
Not clinically relevant

## Diagnostic molecular pathology
Specific HPV genotyping is not diagnostically required {5182}, but in situ hybridization can distinguish between episomal or integrated patterns {5182}. Papilloma recurrence in paediatric patients may be more attributable to HPV integration {890}.

## Essential and desirable diagnostic criteria
*Essential:* exophytic multilayered benign squamous cell proliferation; central fibrovascular cores supporting epithelial proliferation.
*Desirable:* isolated koilocytes; low-risk HPV type (in selected cases).

## Staging
Not applicable

## Prognosis and prediction
Most oral and oropharyngeal SPs persist for years without increasing in size or dissemination, with a minimal risk of recurrence (2%) {2240}. The clinical course of RRP, however, is unpredictable and ranges from complete remission, to relatively stable lesions, to an aggressive clinical course of rapid, progressive recurrences associated with potentially life-threatening respiratory obstruction {1710,6816,6561}. Children diagnosed at < 3 years of age are 3.6 times as likely as children diagnosed at an older age to have more than four surgeries per year {5812,5182}. HPV11 is more closely associated with a younger age at diagnosis and sometimes an aggressive clinical course {7525}. A recent systematic review and meta-analysis found that the HPV vaccine significantly reduced the number of surgical procedures and increased the time between surgeries in both children and adults {5986}, with further vaccine effects still to be determined {1042}. Oral SPs do not undergo malignant transformation, but there is a 1–4% rate of malignant transformation of RRP into squamous cell carcinoma, especially in the setting of irradiation, smoking, or another promoter {1710,3396,3479,7365}.

# White sponge naevus

Muller S
Flaitz CM

## Definition
White sponge naevus is an autosomal dominant genodermatosis resulting in leukokeratotic abnormal keratin tonofilament deposition.

## ICD-O coding
None

## ICD-11 coding
DA02.0 Genetic or developmental disorders involving lips or oral mucosa

## Related terminology
Not recommended: Cannon disease; hereditary leukokeratosis; familial white folded mucosal dysplasia.

## Subtype(s)
None

## Localization
The non-keratinized oral mucosa (buccal, ventral tongue, labial, soft palate, alveolar, and floor of the mouth) is the most common site of involvement {5551,969,6584}. Less frequently affected sites include the nasal, laryngeal, oesophageal, and anogenital mucosae.

## Clinical features
The onset of the disorder is typically in infancy or early childhood, but it becomes more prominent during adolescence and persists throughout life. Early lesions appear as non-tender, filmy-white, mildly wrinkled to velvety patches or plaques with a bilateral, symmetrical presentation {4846,6584,969}. During puberty, the adherent plaques are more prominent, with a thickened, spongy, and opaque white surface. The surface architecture varies from mildly irregular and shredded to markedly corrugated. Initially localized, over time they become more diffuse and widespread. When the affected oral mucosa is stretched, the plaques do not disappear. Maceration of the affected intraoral tissue is common along the occlusal plane. Tenderness may occur, especially if the tissue is traumatized.

## Epidemiology
The worldwide prevalence is about 0.5 cases per 100 000 individuals {5551,969}. White sponge naevus exhibits a high degree of penetrance and variable expressivity with a familial distribution. However, sporadic cases have been documented {7510}. There is an equal sex distribution and no racial predilection.

## Etiology
Unknown

## Pathogenesis
Mutations in KRT4 and KRT13 have been found {7510,5551, 969}. These genes are responsible for the production of keratin proteins that normally combine to form intermediate filaments, but mismatched proteins in white sponge naevus result in tissue fragility. This condition is inherited in an autosomal dominant pattern with reduced penetrance, and some people who carry these mutations do not develop white sponge naevus.

## Macroscopic appearance
See Clinical features, above.

## Histopathology
The epithelium displays shaggy hyperparakeratosis and acanthosis with vacuolation of the spinous layer {4846,4415}. Within the parakeratin and spinous cell layer, bright eosinophilic perinuclear condensation, representing keratin tonofilaments, is identified. The basement membrane is intact, and inflammation is sparse.

## Cytology
Exfoliative cytology with Pap staining highlights the eosinophilic perinuclear condensation {4415,4846}.

## Diagnostic molecular pathology
Not relevant

## Essential and desirable diagnostic criteria
Essential: bright eosinophilic perinuclear condensation within the spinous cell layer.
Desirable: parakeratosis and acanthosis with vacuolation of the spinous layer.

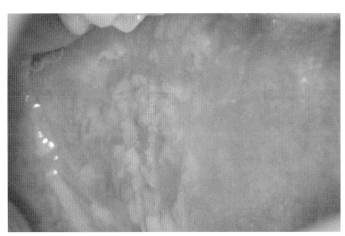

**Fig. 13.03** White sponge naevus. Buccal mucosa with white, adherent, velvety to folded plaques.

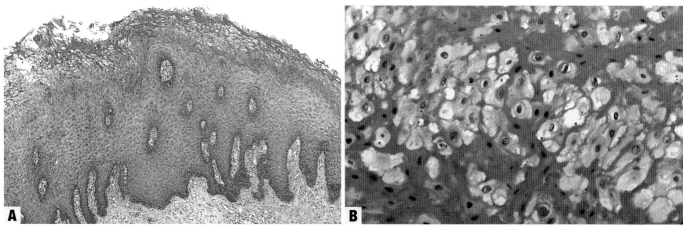

**Fig. 13.04** White sponge naevus. **A** Prominent hyperparakeratosis and acanthosis with spinous cell layer vacuolation. **B** High-power view of bright eosinophilic perinuclear condensation in some of the cells in the spinous layer.

## Staging
Not applicable

## Prognosis and prediction
Episodes of remission and exacerbation are reported, along with intermittent superficial sloughing. Disease progression usually stops after puberty and there are no reports of malignant transformation.

# Congenital granular cell epulis

Muller S
Fuller MY

## Definition
Congenital granular cell epulis is a rare congenital benign tumour, usually occurring on the alveolar ridge of the newborn, composed of granular cells negative for S100.

## ICD-O coding
None

## ICD-11 coding
KC23 Neonatal disorders of the oral mucosa

## Related terminology
*Acceptable:* congenital epulis, congenital epulis of the newborn, congenital gingival granular cell tumour, Neumann tumour.
*Not recommended:* congenital granular cell myoblastoma.

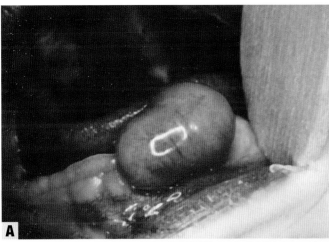

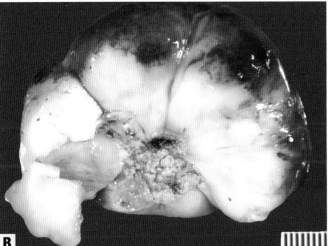

**Fig. 13.05** Congenital granular cell epulis. **A** A polypoid mass in the anterior mandible of a newborn girl. **B** A gross photograph demonstrates a polypoid mass with a tan, smooth, homogeneous surface.

## Subtype(s)
None

## Localization
Most cases of congenital granular cell epulis arise on the anterior maxillary alveolus; they occur at this site three times more often than on the mandibular alveolus {7280}. Rarely, congenital granular cell epulis can be multifocal, involving both the maxilla and mandible, or arise on the tongue {3824,4243,6341,7695, 4104}.

## Clinical features
The lesion manifests as a polypoid, sessile, or pedunculated mass with a smooth, mucosal-coloured surface. Although it is firmly attached to the dental ridge, bone and teeth are uninvolved. Most cases are < 20 mm, but they can be as large as 90 mm {1256}.

### Imaging
Antenatal ultrasonographic findings have been reported {3824}, with T1-weighted MRI showing a homogeneous mass without enhancement and without bone extension {5732}.

## Epidemiology
Congenital granular cell epulis manifests at birth or with the first few weeks. There is an overwhelming female predilection (M:F ratio: 1:7–10) {3824,1419}.

## Etiology
The etiology is unknown, although a mesenchymal origin is favoured {3824}.

## Pathogenesis
Unknown

## Macroscopic appearance
The cut surface is typically tan-yellow, smooth, and homogeneous {1256}.

## Histopathology
The tumour is relatively well delineated and is composed of sheets and nests of polygonal cells with eosinophilic, granular cytoplasm and prominent cell membranes. The bland nuclei are eccentric, small, and uniform. Mitoses are inconspicuous {1256,1419,7280}. A prominent capillary network of dilated vessels traverses the lesion. An attenuated stratified squamous epithelium of uniform thickness lacking pseudoepitheliomatous hyperplasia overlies the tumour.

### Immunohistochemistry
Tumour cells are negative for S100 and/or SOX10, unlike in granular cell tumour {1419,7280,1256}, and reactive for CD68, NSE, and vimentin.

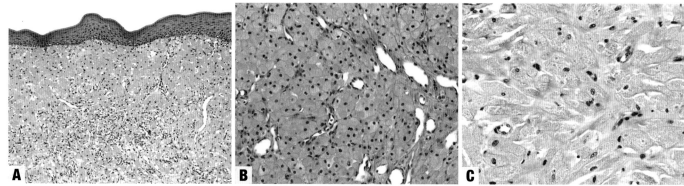

**Fig. 13.06** Congenital granular cell epulis. **A** Uniform atrophic epithelium overlying sheets of tightly packed, medium-sized to large homogeneous polygonal cells with abundant eosinophilic granular cytoplasm, replacing the subepithelial stroma. **B** Cells have abundant eosinophilic granular cytoplasm and basophilic eccentric nuclei. Mitoses are absent but a background vascularity is seen. **C** High-power view shows numerous granules in polygonal cells with small, eccentrically placed nuclei. This is similar to conventional granular cell tumour but lacks S100 immunoreactivity.

### Cytology
Not clinically relevant

### Diagnostic molecular pathology
Not relevant

### Essential and desirable diagnostic criteria
*Essential:* neonatal presentation; soft lump on maxillary or mandibular alveolar ridge; sheets and nests of polygonal cells with eosinophilic, granular cytoplasm.

*Desirable:* attenuated to atrophic stratified squamous epithelium of uniform thickness; negative reaction for S100 protein.

### Staging
Not applicable

### Prognosis and prediction
Respiratory or feeding problems require the tumour to be removed {3824,3707}. The tumour does not recur, even after incomplete excision, and spontaneous regression has been reported {6054}. Malignant transformation has not been reported.

# Central giant cell granuloma

Odell EW
Childers ELB

## Definition
Central giant cell granuloma is a localized destructive jaw lesion characterized by osteoclast-type giant cells in a mononuclear and fibrous vascular stroma without systemic or contiguous diseases causing similar findings.

## ICD-O coding
None

## ICD-11 coding
DA01.20 Giant cell granuloma, central

## Related terminology
Not recommended: reparative giant cell granuloma; central giant cell lesion.

## Subtype(s)
None

## Localization
Central giant cell granuloma arises in the anterior maxilla and mandible, rarely in the condyle {752} or coronoid process {7725}, and usually anterior to the permanent mandibular first molars {1307}.

## Clinical features
Central giant cell granulomas are usually asymptomatic lesions identified as expansile radiolucencies on routine dental radiographs. A few patients may have pain, jaw expansion, or paraesthesia, with root resorption and tooth displacement. Multifocal lesions are usually associated with a syndrome or systemic disease.

## Imaging
Lesions range from small, unilocular, cyst-like radiolucencies to large, multilocular or scalloped/corticated lesions, with thin internal trabeculation or a faint honeycomb pattern {6651}. Osteolysis, root resorption, tooth displacement, and cortical perforation may be seen {6651}.

## Epidemiology
Central giant cell granuloma is a common benign paediatric jaw lesion, identified in about 12% of jaw biopsies {1231,1307}. It has a slight female predilection {1231,1682} and is seen most commonly in the first two decades of life {1307}.

## Etiology
The etiology is unknown, but a few cases arising after granulocyte colony–stimulating factor treatment have been reported {3548}.

## Pathogenesis
Although the pathogenesis is unknown, TRPV4, KRAS, and FGFR1 mutations are reported in sporadic cases, whereas PTPN11 mutations are reported in Noonan-like / multiple giant cell lesion syndrome {6500}. Pathogenesis is distinct from that of giant cell tumour of bone {5636}, solid aneurysmal bone cyst {73}, cherubism (SH3BP2) {3112}, and giant cell epulis.

## Macroscopic appearance
Central giant cell granulomas are unencapsulated and solid, with a reddish-brown, haemorrhagic appearance.

## Histopathology
Central giant cell granuloma is a solid, unencapsulated tumour with vague clustering of numerous multinucleated osteoclast-like giant cells, with a background of haemorrhagic, vascular stroma with bland spindle cells {4005}. Osteoid or woven bone may be extensive. Scattered normal mitoses may be seen. There is no cyst formation. Very rarely, it may contain odontogenic epithelial islands {5120}. The lesion may be the presenting finding of a syndrome. Multifocal lesions especially necessitate clinical and radiographic evaluation to exclude cherubism, hyperparathyroidism, Noonan syndrome, LEOPARD syndrome (multiple lentigines, electrocardiographic conduction abnormalities, ocular hypertelorism, pulmonic stenosis, abnormal genitalia, retardation of growth, and sensorineural deafness), neurofibromatosis type 1, and some RASopathies {1355}. Similar histological findings may be focally present in odontogenic cysts, odontogenic tumours, benign fibro-osseous lesions, brown tumour of hyperparathyroidism, aneurysmal bone cyst, and the reactive gingival lesion peripheral giant cell granuloma.

## Cytology
Not clinically relevant

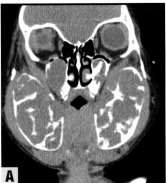
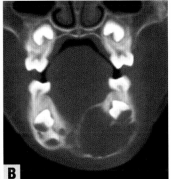

**Fig. 13.07** Differential diagnosis. **A** Cherubism. CT of a 4-year-old boy showing bilateral multilocular, radiolucent areas within the mandibles, a finding considered diagnostic of cherubism. Giant cells are prominent in this lesion and thus are part of the differential for central giant cell granuloma, but the imaging helps greatly in separating between lesions that contain giant cells histologically. **B** Giant cell granuloma. Coronal CT showing a rounded, multilocular, and markedly expansile radiolucent lesion displacing teeth. There is patchy cortical erosion in a background of mixed dentition.

## Diagnostic molecular pathology

Not relevant

## Essential and desirable diagnostic criteria

*Essential:* jaw location; numerous multinucleated osteoclast-like giant cells in a haemorrhagic, vascular stroma with bland spindle cells; no cyst formation; exclusion of hyperparathyroidism.

*Desirable:* lobular structure; osteoid or woven bone; evaluation for syndrome association.

## Staging

Not relevant

## Prognosis and prediction

Recurrent lesions after curettage are labelled aggressive {1307}. Recurrence is associated with a large size, rapid growth, thin or perforated cortex, cortical expansion, tooth displacement, and root resorption {1986,1307}.

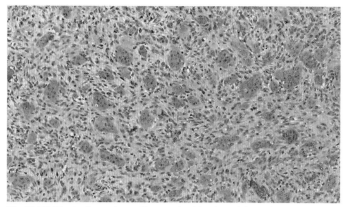

**Fig. 13.08** Giant cell granuloma. Clusters of multinucleated giant cells in a bland spindle cell stroma with haemorrhage.

# Odontogenic tumours

Odell EW
Childers ELB

## Definition
Primarily paediatric odontogenic tumours include hamartomas and neoplasms derived from odontogenic epithelium and mesenchyme, which overlap with the odontogenic cyst category. Entities not listed affect children and adolescents infrequently. Definitions are provided with each entity.

## ICD-O coding
9310/0 Ameloblastoma
9330/0 Ameloblastic fibroma
9300/0 Adenomatoid odontogenic tumour
9280/0 Odontoma
9320/0 Odontogenic myxoma

## ICD-11 coding
2E83.1 & XH1SV4 Benign osteogenic tumours of bone or articular cartilage of lower jaw & Ameloblastoma, NOS

2E83.0 & XH1SV4 Benign osteogenic tumours of bone or articular cartilage of skull or face & Ameloblastoma, NOS

2E83.1 & XH06Y3 Benign osteogenic tumours of bone or articular cartilage of lower jaw & Ameloblastic fibroma

2E83.0 & XH06Y3 Benign osteogenic tumours of bone or articular cartilage of skull or face & Ameloblastic fibroma

2E83.1 & XH2SD0 Benign osteogenic tumours of bone or articular cartilage of lower jaw & Adenomatoid odontogenic tumour

2E83.0 & XH2SD0 Benign osteogenic tumours of bone or articular cartilage of skull or face & Adenomatoid odontogenic tumour

2E83.1 & XH4QJ8 Benign osteogenic tumours of bone or articular cartilage of lower jaw & Odontoma, NOS

2E83.0 & XH4QJ8 Benign osteogenic tumours of bone or articular cartilage of skull or face & Odontoma, NOS

2E83.1 & XH48L4 Benign osteogenic tumours of bone or articular cartilage of lower jaw & Odontogenic myxoma

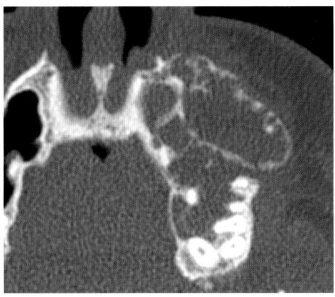

**Fig. 13.10** Odontogenic myxoma. Axial CT showing an expanding mass affecting the maxillary alveolus anteriorly and laterally. The lesion is radiolucent but has irregular thin bony septa at right angles to the cortex, with focal cortical destruction.

2E83.0 & XH48L4 Benign osteogenic tumours of bone or articular cartilage of skull or face & Odontogenic myxoma
DA05.0 Developmental odontogenic cysts

## Related terminology
*Acceptable:* keratocystic odontogenic tumour.

## Subtype(s)
None

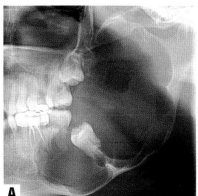
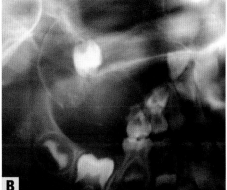
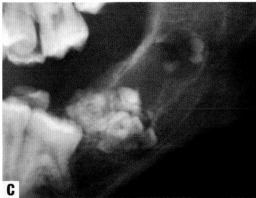

**Fig. 13.09** Odontogenic tumours. **A** Ameloblastoma. A typical multilocular, scalloped, radiolucent expansile lesion with partial cortication extending from the coronoid notch to the posterior body of the mandible, with cortical perforation and a displaced developing tooth and minor tooth root resorption (plain radiograph). **B** Ameloblastic fibroma. A radiolucent posterior maxilla lesion displacing the crown of a developing tooth superiorly and surrounded by a thin expanded cortical bone layer. There is displacement of forming teeth anteriorly (plain radiograph). **C** Odontoma. A corticated mixed radiolucency containing discrete denticles of enamel and dentin, radiopaque mesially and distally, with little cortical expansion but a prominent central unmineralized portion that has not yet matured (plain radiograph).

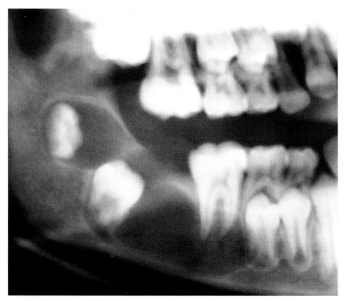

**Fig. 13.11** Odontogenic keratocyst. A multilocular radiolucency extending from the mid-ramus to the premolar region with minimal expansion of the inferior cortex. There is peripheral cortication and little displacement of the associated teeth, which do not show root resorption (plain radiograph).

## Localization

Odontogenic tumours arise in the tooth-bearing segments of the jaws, most frequently posteriorly in the mandible, whereas ameloblastic fibroma and adenomatoid odontogenic tumour are more frequent in the maxilla.

## Clinical features

Most patients present with jaw swelling, expansion of the jaw, asymmetry, displacement, or failure of teeth eruption. Incidental identification by routine dental imaging is common. Adjacent teeth may be missing, displaced, or partially resorbed.

### Imaging

Plain radiographs (including panoramic), CT, or cone beam CT are essential for the diagnosis, to identify internal mineralization. Odontogenic tumours range from cyst-like radiolucencies to dense opacities. Benign lesions are usually corticated. Internal mineralization consistent with dentin or enamel indicates dental induction and a probable hamartoma or benign neoplasm.

## Epidemiology

The incidence rate cannot be determined, because of inconsistent terminology and classification and a lack of population-based studies. Odontogenic cysts (excluding odontogenic keratocyst) are primarily inflammatory and are nearly twice as common as odontogenic tumours {3301}. Dentigerous cysts, rather than radicular cysts, predominate in paediatric populations {5412,3311}. Odontogenic keratocysts appear to be proportionally more frequent in China {4085}.

Within odontogenic tumours, odontoma is the most common {6575,6189,2581}, but as a hamartoma, it is often excluded from epidemiological studies of tumours. The commonest paediatric odontogenic neoplasms are ameloblastomas {2047,2581}, of which approximately half are unicystic {483}. Conventional ameloblastoma has a pooled incidence rate of 0.09 cases per 100 000 person-years. Ameloblastoma is more prevalent in western African populations, where it arises more frequently in anterior jaw sites {55,354}. Calcifying epithelial odontogenic tumour is very rare in the paediatric group {2581} but is reported to be more prevalent in China {2047}. Thus, all odontogenic tumours are rare {3311,6189}, with benign odontogenic neoplasms being much more common than malignant ones {354}; when malignant jaw tumours are identified, they are almost exclusively non-odontogenic.

## Etiology

Unknown

## Pathogenesis

Ameloblastoma is associated with somatic MAPK pathway alterations – usually *BRAF* p.V600E mutations (including in the unicystic subtype), which are thought to be driver mutations, with less frequent mutations in *KRAS*, *NRAS*, *HRAS*, *FGFR2*, and *SMO* {6808,2819}. Syndromic odontogenic keratocysts (in naevoid basal cell carcinoma syndrome, MIM number: 109400) are associated with mutation or inactivation of *PTCH1*, *PTCH2*, or *SUFU*, a finding also seen in sporadic cases {508,3303, 2662}. Odontomas are associated with WNT/β-catenin pathway activation {2249} and are seen in the *APC*-driven Gardner subtype of familial adenomatous polyposis {2478}.

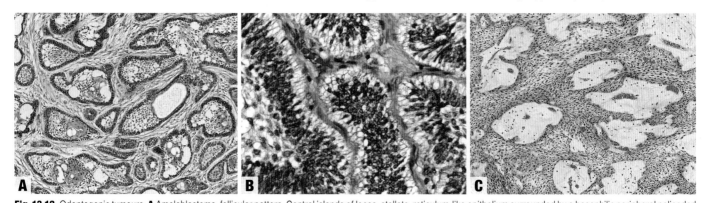

**Fig. 13.12** Odontogenic tumours. **A** Ameloblastoma, follicular pattern. Central islands of loose, stellate, reticulum-like epithelium surrounded by a basophilic peripheral palisaded basal layer of columnar ameloblastic cells. There is focal acanthomatous change, and multiple small cysts are seen forming within the epithelium. **B** Ameloblastoma. Classic ameloblast-like cells at the periphery of follicular ameloblastoma islands, showing elongate palisaded nuclei with reverse polarity and subnuclear vacuolation. **C** Plexiform ameloblastoma. A meshwork of strands of epithelium with peripheral ameloblast-like cells.

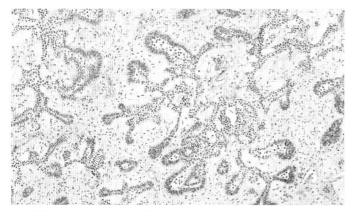

**Fig. 13.13** Ameloblastic fibroma. Strands of epithelium with cuboidal or slightly elongate basophilic basal epithelium without stellate reticulum, lying in a highly cellular uniform fibroblastic stroma. Note the absence of matrix and calcified tissue.

## Macroscopic appearance

Odontogenic tumours range from thin-walled cysts through partly cystic or multicystic masses to solid tissue, depending on type. Some contain gritty or large irregular mineralized masses or malformed teeth. The odontogenic myxoma is gelatinous. Odontogenic keratocysts contain masses of dense white keratin debris.

## Histopathology

Selected odontogenic tumours with a predilection for paediatric patients are presented below; please refer to the WHO classification of head and neck tumours for a comprehensive list. Generally, odontogenic tumours are diagnosed with routine H&E stains, but these must be correlated with radiological findings along with clinical data. Immunohistochemistry and molecular investigations have limited value. Furthermore, mitotic activity is uncommon and tumour necrosis is generally absent.

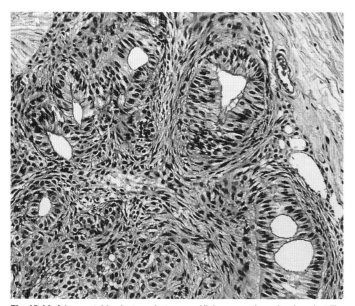

**Fig. 13.14** Adenomatoid odontogenic tumour. High-power view showing duct-like structures surrounded by elongate, ameloblast-like cells and, on the lower right, an array or rosette of ameloblast-like cells with small amounts of eosinophilic enamel matrix secreted between them.

### Ameloblastoma

Ameloblastoma is a benign neoplasm comprising islands (follicular pattern), sheets, or strands (plexiform pattern) of epithelium with peripheral ameloblast-like cells. Ameloblastic cells are elongate and palisaded, and at least focally they show reverse nuclear polarity and peripheral vacuolation. Centrally, the islands contain a loose meshwork of epithelium resembling odontogenic stellate reticulum, sometimes with acanthomatous change and rarely with focal keratinization {697}. Cystic change within the epithelium is common in the follicular pattern and in the stroma in the plexiform pattern. Although benign, islands of ameloblastoma may permeate the adjacent medullary spaces well beyond the apparent bone margin. Follicular-pattern lesions are more likely to recur than lesions of other patterns {5816}. In young patients, mitotic figures may be relatively frequent. Unicystic ameloblastoma is a subtype with a single cyst and no mural component. The tumour shows less obvious ameloblastic differentiation histologically and may be misdiagnosed as a dentigerous cyst without radiological correlation {510}.

### Ameloblastic fibroma

Ameloblastic fibroma is a rare, benign neoplasm of both odontogenic epithelium and mesenchyme. The epithelium forms smaller islands than in ameloblastoma, often as bilaminar strands with peripheral budding but little to absent stellate reticulum. The epithelium lies in a very cellular but cytologically bland stroma, which is myxoid to collagenous {697}. The histological appearance may be identical to early-stage odontoma, which makes clinical and radiological correlation essential for diagnosis. Ameloblastic fibroma is relatively aggressive in the growing facial skeleton and requires excision.

### Adenomatoid odontogenic tumour

Adenomatoid odontogenic tumour is a solid and cystic hamartomatous lesion of odontogenic epithelium that shows an encapsulated lesion usually within the maxilla. Sheets of epithelium are organized in large nodules, within which there are numerous duct-like structures and rosettes or arrays of ameloblast-like cells. The latter may form an enamel matrix–like eosinophilic material that can mineralize; in a minority there may be dentin-like matrix and mineralized tissue. Odontoma may have areas that are histologically identical.

### Odontoma

Odontomas are hamartomatous malformations of odontogenic tissues that show good histodifferentiation to functional ameloblasts and odontoblasts. There is variable morphodifferentiation, from disorganized masses of dental hard tissues (complex pattern) to multiple tooth-like structures (compound pattern). In the early stage, they comprise a cellular or slightly myxoid odontogenic mesenchyme containing budding bilaminar strands of preameloblast-like cells; this appearance is similar to that of ameloblastic fibroma or odontogenic myxoma. Maturation to form both enamel and dentin matrix confirms a diagnosis of odontoma histologically. With time, the lesion becomes heavily mineralized and dental hard tissues dominate. At all stages, a thin capsule of unmineralized tissue is present, with a corticated outline radiologically. Despite their hamartomatous appearance, odontomas may reach > 80 mm. They are frequently

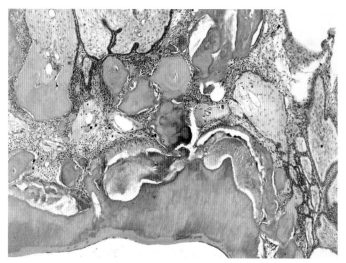

**Fig. 13.15** Odontoma, complex pattern. Typical complex odontoma decalcified section showing a band of tubular dentin inferiorly and eosinophilic enamel matrix on its upper surface, together with a disorganized mass of strands of odontogenic epithelium showing ameloblastic and stellate reticulum differentiation.

misdiagnosed when there are ghost cells, hypercellularity, or amyloid, and when there are patterns almost identical to ameloblastoma, ameloblastic fibroma {922}, and other odontogenic tumours.

## Odontogenic myxoma

Odontogenic myxoma is a benign neoplasm composed of cellular odontogenic mesenchyme dispersed in extensive proteoglycan ground substance arising in a gnathic locale. Collagen content is variable; commonly there is none, but more collagenous lesions may be called odontogenic fibromyxoma. Expansion by secretion of ground substance gives this unencapsulated lesion the ability to permeate adjacent medullary spaces and recur after treatment. Accurate diagnosis with radiological correlation is required to ensure appropriate treatment that is size- and site-dependent. A small proportion of odontogenic myxomas may contain scattered small islands or clusters of mitotically inactive epithelium without ameloblastic differentiation, but these are not required for diagnosis. Occasionally these islands become a predominant feature. Normal odontogenic connective tissue is slightly myxoid, and small areas with similar histological appearances may be seen in developing tooth germs, normal dental follicle, ameloblastic fibroma, primordial odontogenic tumour, and odontoma {3578}. Diagnosis requires radiological correlation and exclusion of other myxoid neoplasms. Odontogenic myxomas are not a feature of Carney complex.

## Odontogenic keratocyst

Odontogenic keratocyst is a benign odontogenic cyst lined by a thin, uniform-thickness epithelium with palisaded hyperchromatic basal cells and (at least focally) reverse nuclear polarity, and a thin layer of corrugated luminal parakeratin {697}. With inflammation, these typical features are obscured. Odontogenic keratocysts are usually multilocular and may have microscopic satellite cysts in the wall that may form keratinized islands. Multiple odontogenic keratocysts with satellite cysts manifesting in the first two decades of life suggest naevoid basal cell carcinoma syndrome. Keratinization may be seen in the linings of other odontogenic cysts, such as orthokeratinized jaw cyst, a separate entity known not to recur.

## Cytology
Not clinically relevant

## Diagnostic molecular pathology
Not relevant

## Essential and desirable diagnostic criteria
See Table 13.01.

## Staging
Not relevant

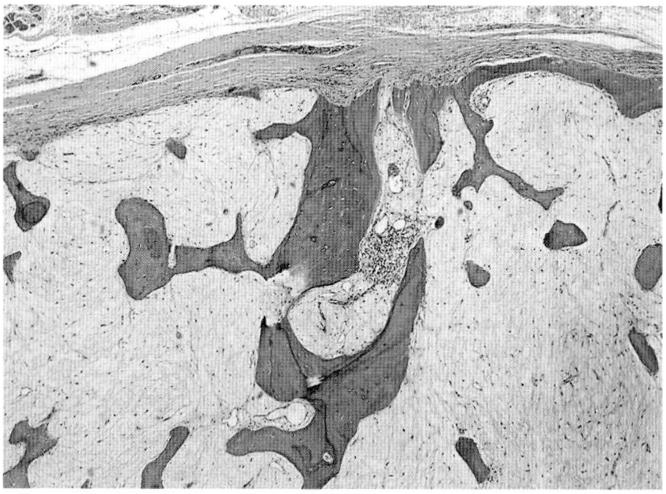

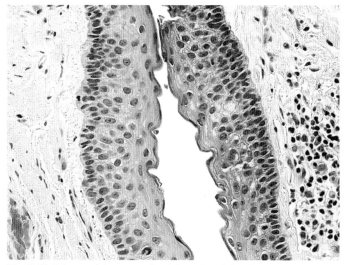

**Fig. 13.16** Odontogenic myxoma. Periphery of an odontogenic myxoma showing microscopic cortical perforation. The sparsely cellular myxoid lesion is contained by the periosteum at the top, with permeative spread around residual bone trabecula and into medullary areas.

**Fig. 13.17** Odontogenic keratocyst. Non-inflamed cyst lining, showing a flat basement membrane with palisaded basal cells, a thin epithelium, and a corrugated, parakeratinized refractile luminal surface.

**Table 13.01** Diagnostic criteria for odontogenic tumours, with radiographic findings indicated in italics

| Category | Essential criteria | Desirable criteria |
|---|---|---|
| Ameloblastoma | Elongate palisaded basal cells with reverse polarity<br>Stellate reticulum<br>Stroma of normal or collagenous fibrous tissue<br>No dental hard tissues<br>No abnormal mitoses<br>*Cyst-like radiolucency, unilocular or multilocular, with cortication* | Basal cell subnuclear vacuolization |
| Ameloblastic fibroma | Budding strands of cuboidal or low columnar epithelium<br>Hypercellular loose myxoid stroma<br>No dental hard tissues<br>*Cyst-like radiolucency, unilocular or multilocular, with cortication* | Minimal stellate reticulum<br>Sparse normal mitoses |
| Adenomatoid odontogenic tumour | Sheets and nodules of bland epithelium<br>Intraepithelial duct-like structures<br>Encapsulated<br>*Cyst-like unilocular radiolucency* | Arrays of ameloblasts<br>Enamel matrix<br>Dentinoid mineralization of connective tissue in the wall of a cyst |
| Odontoma | Odontogenic epithelium and mesenchyme<br>Histologically normal development of hard tissue<br>Enamel matrix and tubular dentin<br>*Sharply demarcated, mixed radiolucency with lucent rim and cortication* | Variable formation of tooth-like denticles |
| Odontogenic myxoma | Myxoid stroma<br>Low cellularity<br>Variable islands of bland epithelium without ameloblastic differentiation<br>No abnormal mitoses<br>*Multilocular radiographic appearance, no mineralization* | |
| Odontogenic keratocyst | Thin-walled cyst without rete ridges<br>Epithelium uniformly 6–8 cells thick<br>Parakeratinized corrugated luminal surface<br>Palisaded basal cells with reverse polarity, at least focally<br>*Cyst-like radiolucency, unilocular or multilocular, with cortication* | No mineralization |

## Prognosis and prediction

There is a risk of recurrence with ameloblastoma, ameloblastic fibroma, odontogenic myxoma, and odontogenic keratocyst, all of which show permeation of adjacent medullary spaces beyond their apparent radiographic margin. Behaviour cannot be predicted on incisional biopsy or with any biomarkers. In general, most odontogenic lesions with a multilocular radiographic appearance are more likely to recur than unilocular lesions or those containing mineralized dental tissues. Malignant odontogenic tumours are extremely rare in paediatric patients {5876}.

# Ossifying fibroma

Odell EW
Childers ELB

## Definition

Ossifying fibromas (OFs) are a distinct group of fibro-osseous benign neoplasms composed of woven bone maturing to dense bone and/or cementum-like masses within a hypercellular stroma of spindle cells.

## ICD-O coding

9262/0 Ossifying fibroma
9262/0 Juvenile trabecular ossifying fibroma
9262/0 Psammomatoid ossifying fibroma

## ICD-11 coding

2E83.1 & XH6M86 Benign osteogenic tumours of bone or articular cartilage of lower jaw & Ossifying fibroma
2E83.0 & XH6M86 Benign osteogenic tumours of bone or articular cartilage of skull or face & Ossifying fibroma

## Related terminology

*Acceptable:* cemento-ossifying fibroma.
*Not recommended:* cementifying fibroma; periodontoma; juvenile active ossifying fibroma; juvenile aggressive ossifying fibroma; juvenile ossifying fibroma.

## Subtype(s)

Juvenile trabecular ossifying fibroma (JTOF); psammomatoid ossifying fibroma (PsOF)

## Localization

OF and JTOF affect the jaws {1308,7623}, with OF usually arising in the mandible and JTOF in the maxilla. PsOF affects facial bones and sinuses more frequently than jaws {7501,1940}.

## Clinical features

All types manifest as asymptomatic bony swellings, limited by the periosteum, that may reach a large size, with disfigurement, displacement, and resorption of tooth roots. Some tumours may show rapid clinical growth {1308,1940,7501}.

### Imaging

OF initially appears as a well-defined corticated radiolucency, maturing to a mixed radiolucency or sometimes to a dense radiopacity with a thin radiolucent rim; the juvenile types are less opaque {4294}.

## Epidemiology

OF is the most common primary non-odontogenic neoplasm of the jaws {6189,7623,1231}. The incidence of PsOF peaks in the second and third decades of life, and JTOF affects children aged 2–12 years {1940,1941,7501,7623}. OF has a strong female predilection. Classic OF is rare in the paediatric population unless syndromic.

## Etiology

Unknown

## Pathogenesis

Multiple OFs are present in hyperparathyroidism–jaw tumour syndrome, caused by a germline mutation of *CDC73*, a mutation also identified in sporadic tumours {7031,5545}. JTOF and PsOF show rearrangements involving *RASAL1* and *MDM2*, and they may show *MDM2* amplification but not MDM2 overexpression by immunohistochemistry {6825}. Despite the histological similarity between OF and fibrous dysplasia, *GNAS* (*GNAS1*) mutations are not seen in OF.

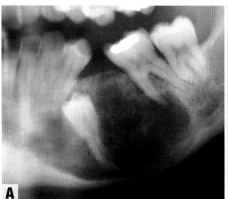 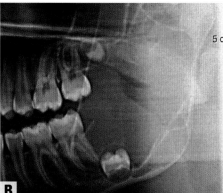 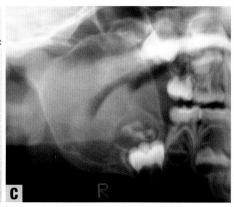

**Fig. 13.18** Ossifying fibroma. **A** Conventional type. A typical well-defined and corticated mixed radiolucency with patchy internal mineralization and displacement of teeth with minor root resorption (dental bitewing). **B** Psammomatoid subtype. A typical large radiolucent lesion with prominent expansion, well-defined margin, and minimal internal mineralization. Developing teeth are displaced (X-ray). **C** Juvenile trabecular subtype. A typical radiolucent lesion with prominent expansion and tooth displacement in a young child (dental imaging).

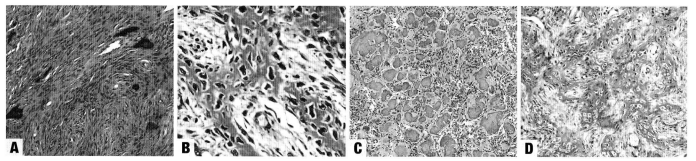

**Fig. 13.19** Ossifying fibroma. **A** A conventional ossifying fibroma with a denser collagenous stroma than the juvenile type, with mineralization ranging from focal (shown) to dense sheets and trabeculae of relatively acellular bone. **B** High-power view of a juvenile trabecular ossifying fibroma showing disorganized woven bone with apparent atypia. **C** A psammomatoid ossifying fibroma showing numerous small, densely mineralized nodules with a thin unmineralized rim set in hypercellular fibrous tissue. **D** Juvenile trabecular ossifying fibroma. Medium-power view showing purposeless osteoid trabeculae with minimal mineralization in a cellular non-collagenous stroma.

## Macroscopic appearance

OF is a soft, gritty, or hard tumour with a well-defined margin.

## Histopathology

OF has woven bone maturing to dense cementum-like masses that coalesce centrally and have a cellular rim, lacking nuclear atypia and with occasional mitoses. JTOF is unencapsulated but well defined, with prominent long and slender osteoid seams (paint-brush strokes), woven bone, and a hypercellular stroma of spindle cells and fibroblasts {1940}. Mineralization is minimal and irregular, sometimes mimicking osteosarcoma. Mitoses are few. PsOF has a similar periphery but has small, rounded, non-coalescing, densely mineralized ossicles with an unmineralized, eosinophilic rim {7501}. Secondary aneurysmal bone cyst or a giant cell reaction may develop {1940}.

## Cytology

Not clinically relevant

## Diagnostic molecular pathology

Not relevant

## Essential and desirable diagnostic criteria

*Essential:* a radiographically well-demarcated lesion; a benign fibro-osseous lesion with variable maturation; a hypercellular stroma of spindle cells.

## Staging

Not relevant

## Prognosis and prediction

PsOF and JTOF often recur after simple curettage but respond to repeated curettage or conservative excision {3295,4366}, with long-term follow-up to exclude recurrence {4294,7359}. Malignant transformation is not seen.

# Sinonasal tract myxoma

Alaggio R

## Definition

Sinonasal tract myxoma is a benign myofibroblastic proliferation within an extensively myxoid ground substance, arising in paranasal sinuses (not gnathic bone).

## ICD-O coding

8840/0 Sinonasal tract myxoma

## ICD-11 coding

2E90.6 & XH6Q84 Benign neoplasm of nasopharynx & Myxoma, NOS

## Related terminology

*Not recommended:* infantile odontogenic myxoma; peripheral odontogenic myxoma.

## Subtype(s)

None

## Localization

Sinonasal myxomas arise in the sinonasal region. They appear to arise in the soft tissue but may expand to involve adjacent bone.

## Clinical features

Sinonasal myxoma manifests as a slow-growing nasolabial swelling. Symptoms may be related to local tumour extension into the palate, orbit, and/or nasal cavity. Radiographically, sinonasal myxomas appear as well-defined, intraosseous, unilocular/multilocular radiolucencies. Tumours can be as large as 50 mm {2812,6102,3363,6008,5623,3513,4631}.

## Epidemiology

Sinonasal myxomas are rare, and they are reported almost exclusively in children aged < 3 years (mean: 15 months). There is a slight male predominance {2813,2812,6102,3363,6008, 3412,5623,4631}.

## Etiology

Unknown

## Pathogenesis

The pathogenetic relationship between odontogenic myxoma and sinonasal myxoma is unclear {6008,3412,6102,4631}.

## Macroscopic appearance

Tumours have a grey-white, glistening surface and a gelatinous to firm consistency.

## Histopathology

Myxomas are similar no matter the site affected, showing a loose hypocellular proliferation of spindled, stellate, or round cells within a myxoid stroma containing arciform thin blood vessels and scattered fine collagen bands. Pleomorphism, mitotic figures, and tumour necrosis are absent {2813,2812}. Odontogenic epithelium is absent {3363,4631}. Immunohistochemistry is noncontributory, with variable SMA and nuclear β-catenin positivity {4631,3412}.

## Cytology

Not relevant

## Diagnostic molecular pathology

Not relevant

## Essential and desirable diagnostic criteria

*Essential:* a hypocellular proliferation of spindled/stellate cells forming a myxoid mass lesion of the sinonasal area not arising in gnathic bones.
*Desirable:* nuclear β-catenin staining.

## Staging

Not clinically relevant

## Prognosis and prediction

These lesions are benign, but recurrence may be seen (in ~10% of cases) when incompletely removed {4631,3412,3363,2812}.

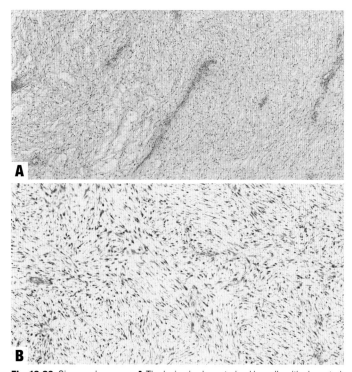

**Fig. 13.20** Sinonasal myxoma. **A** The lesion is characterized by cells with elongated, slender cytoplasm and without atypia, interspersed in an abundant myxoid stroma containing curvilinear blood vessels. **B** There is diffuse nuclear staining for β-catenin.

# Nasal dermoid cyst

Perez-Atayde AR

## Definition
Nasal dermoid cyst is a congenital developmental midline nasal defect histologically containing stratified squamous epithelium (ectoderm) and cutaneous adnexal structures (mesoderm).

## ICD-O coding
None

## ICD-11 coding
DA05.Y & XH9F67 Other specified cysts of oral or facial-neck region & Dermoid cyst, NOS

## Related terminology
*Not recommended:* nasal dermoid sinus; craniofacial dermoid; dermoid; dermal cyst; dermoid cyst.

## Subtype(s)
None

## Localization
Nasal dermoid cysts are commonly found on the nasal dorsum, glabella, or nasal tip {5728,4803,2734,2865,1917}.

## Clinical features
A sinus may be visible centrally over the nasal mass or adjacent to the mass. A nasal pit with protruding hair is pathognomonic. Progressive enlargement of the nasal dermoid cyst may cause lateral orbital displacement and other facial skeletal deformities, with 10% of the patients documented having craniofacial anomalies {7155,5728,4803,2250,7131,7441}. Intermittent drainage and local infection leading to swelling and erythema may occur. A blind tract may be seen, but intracranial extension is present in 10–20% of cases {2250,5728,7131,7441,2865,1917,5671}, necessitating preoperative imaging.

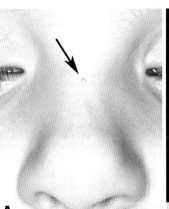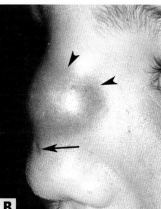

**Fig. 13.21** Nasal dermoid cyst. **A** Protruding hair on the nasal dorsum (arrow). **B** Inflamed dermoid cyst (arrowheads) and nasal pit (arrow).

## Imaging
Preoperative imaging is performed to document deep tissue involvement and cyst extent, and to exclude intracranial extension {5602,5728,7806,6635,4803,2865,5931,5671}. Lesions are classified as with or without intracranial extension, and then as superficial, intraosseous, intracranial extradural, and intracranial intradural, which allows for surgical planning and decreased complications {4803,2734}.

## Epidemiology
The estimated incidence is 2.5–5 cases per 100 000 births, representing about 3% of all dermoids and about 12% of all head and neck dermoids {5602,2865,1917}. There is a slight male predilection (M:F ratio: 1.3:1) {5728,4803,2734,2865, 1917}. Nasal dermoid cysts have a mean age at presentation of about 3 years {5728,4803,2734,2865,1917}.

## Etiology
Unknown

## Pathogenesis
The pathogenesis is embryologically based on the incomplete obliteration of neuroectoderm during the development of the frontonasal process. An autosomal dominant inheritance pattern (~3%) is seen in several kindreds, including those with a solitary median maxillary central incisor (part of holoprosencephaly) {2670,4803}.

## Macroscopic appearance
Not relevant – see *Clinical features* (above)

## Histopathology
The cyst and sinus are lined by keratinizing stratified squamous epithelium with normal-appearing dermal appendages, including hair follicles, hair shafts, and sloughed keratin debris, as well as sweat and sebaceous glands.

### Differential diagnosis
Nasal dermoid cysts are distinguished from epidermoid cysts by the presence of adnexal structures (see above). Also in the differential diagnosis are teratoma, which has endodermal elements; encephalocoele, which has glial/neural tissue; and sinonasal polyps, which are internal oedematous tissues.

## Cytology
Not clinically relevant

## Diagnostic molecular pathology
Not relevant

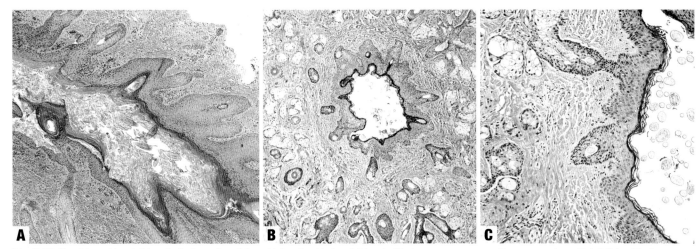

**Fig. 13.22** Nasal dermoid cyst. **A** Longitudinally sectioned dermoid sinus lined by keratinizing stratified squamous mucosa with numerous dermal hair follicles. The lumen contains hair shafts and laminated keratin debris. **B** Cross-section of dermoid sinus lined by keratinizing stratified squamous mucosa associated with numerous dermal appendages including hair follicles, sebaceous glands, and sweat glands. Hair fragments are present within the lumen. **C** Higher-magnification view showing numerous dermal pilosebaceous units and cross-sectioned hair shafts within the lumen.

### Essential and desirable diagnostic criteria

*Essential:* a cyst and/or sinus lined by keratinizing stratified squamous epithelium with normal-appearing dermal appendages.

*Desirable:* a nasal pit with protruding hair; paediatric presentation.

### Staging

Not relevant

### Prognosis and prediction

Recurrences are seen in about 10% of patients, more often in intracranial cases {5728,2865}. Complications (wound infection, meningitis, cavernous sinus thrombosis) are uncommon {2865}.

# Nasopharyngeal dermoid

Nelson BL

## Definition
Nasopharyngeal dermoid is a congenital benign developmental nasopharyngeal anomaly containing ectoderm- and mesoderm-derived tissues.

## ICD-O coding
None

## ICD-11 coding
DA05.Y & XH9F67 Other specified cysts of oral or facial-neck region & Dermoid cyst, NOS

## Related terminology
None

## Subtype(s)
None

## Localization
Nasopharyngeal dermoid usually occurs in the nasopharynx, but it may arise in other areas of the pharynx {2811,1437,1414, 6897}.

## Clinical features
Babies and newborns may present with observable difficulties in breathing, swallowing, or eating due to an often pedunculated mass variably obstructing the nasopharynx {1437,2811,1414}.

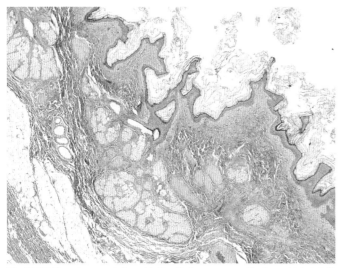

**Fig. 13.23** Nasopharyngeal dermoid. Stratified squamous epithelium with hair follicles and sebaceous glands.

## Imaging
A nasopharyngeal or oropharyngeal mass can be identified by various modalities {7046,5697}.

## Epidemiology
About 7% of dermoids develop in the head and neck, with nasopharyngeal lesions representing about 10% of head and neck dermoids {5697,1437,2811}. Most occur in infants and newborns {5931,5658,6897,2814}, with girls affected more frequently than boys {5329,1437,1414,6897}.

## Etiology
Pharyngeal dermoids are developmental choristomatous anomalies, probably arising from first branchial cleft remnants along embryonic fusion lines {2814,5697}.

## Pathogenesis
Unknown

## Macroscopic appearance
Grossly, nasopharyngeal dermoids are polypoid and covered with hair shafts, and grumous material may be seen. They may reach 120 mm in size {2814,3470,1414,1437}.

## Histopathology
Nasopharyngeal dermoids may be polypoid, solid, or cystic, showing stratified squamous epithelium associated with cutaneous adnexal structures such as hair follicles and sebaceous glands, sometimes creating a hairy polyp, and often with cartilage {2814}. Teratoma, considered a separate entity, is diagnosed when all germ cell layers are represented.

## Cytology
Not clinically relevant

## Diagnostic molecular pathology
Not clinically relevant

## Essential and desirable diagnostic criteria
*Essential:* a polyp in the pharynx of squamous epithelium with associated adnexal structures (including cartilage).

## Staging
Not clinically relevant

## Prognosis and prediction
Recurrences are rare after excision {1437,5697}.

# Nasal chondromesenchymal hamartoma

Thompson LDR

## Definition

Nasal chondromesenchymal hamartoma is a benign mesenchymal sinonasal tract tumour composed of cysts lined by respiratory epithelium associated with nodules of cartilage and a variably myxoid spindle cell stroma.

## ICD-O coding

None

## ICD-11 coding

2E83.0 Benign osteogenic tumours of bone or articular cartilage of skull or face

## Related terminology

*Not recommended:* chondroid hamartoma; nasal hamartoma; congenital mesenchymoma.

## Subtype(s)

None

## Localization

Tumours involve the paranasal sinuses (mostly ethmoid) and nasal cavity, expanding into the orbit and skull base {4074,4452, 4515,5648}. Bilateral tumours are frequent (~25% of cases).

## Clinical features

Symptoms are nonspecific and include nasal obstruction, a mass, and ophthalmological findings, among others {4452, 6690,4515,5648,5268}. Tumours may erode into the cranial cavity. Most cases are part of *DICER1* pleuropulmonary blastoma familial tumour predisposition syndrome {6284,6690,5648,1798}, with the risk of neoplasms being highest in early childhood.

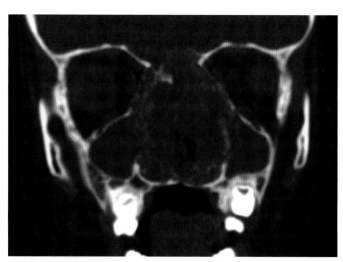

**Fig. 13.24** Nasal chondromesenchymal hamartoma. Coronal CT showing a destructive sinonasal tract mass with intracranial extension.

Pleuropulmonary blastoma in particular is detected before or concurrently with nasal disease. The tumours are analogues of chest wall mesenchymal hamartoma {4515}.

### Imaging

Imaging shows one or more complex, solid and cystic, heterogeneous soft tissue masses, frequent calcifications, and associated bone erosion {4515,7419,3623,2586}.

## Epidemiology

*DICER1* pleuropulmonary blastoma familial tumour predisposition syndrome is rare. By the age of 10 years, 5.3% of non-proband *DICER1* carriers develop a neoplasm, with female patients having an elevated risk over male patients with advancing age {6689}. Only 0.6% of patients with pleuropulmonary blastoma have a nasal chondromesenchymal hamartoma {5648}. When nasal chondromesenchymal hamartoma is diagnosed, germline *DICER1* genetic testing must be considered {6287}. There are twice as many male patients as female patients, and the mean age at presentation is 10 years (range: 1 day to 69 years), with most patients aged < 1 year.

## Etiology

Both inherited susceptibility and acquired mutations in *DICER1* are considered etiological. A t(12;17)(q24.1;q21) translocation has been reported {574}.

## Pathogenesis

*DICER1* tumour predisposition syndrome is characterized by mutations in the gene *DICER1*. Most patients carry an inherited germline mutation that disables one copy of *DICER1*, while within tumours, a second mutation alters the function of the other allele {2586}. The tumour-specific RNase IIIb missense mutations involve one of five hotspot codons: p.E1705, p.D1709, p.G1809, p.D1810, or p.E1813 {6287}. Both germline and somatic pathogenic sequence variants of *DICER1* have been reported in nasal chondromesenchymal hamartomas {5648}.

## Macroscopic appearance

Nasal chondromesenchymal hamartomas are polypoid, fragmented soft tissue masses with a glistening to fibrotic cut surface.

## Histopathology

Nasal chondromesenchymal hamartomas have a collage of histological features that includes well-demarcated nodules of immature to mature cartilage showing variation in the cellular density and maturation of the chondrocytes, set in a loose, myxoid to spindle cell stroma. The cartilage may be primitive to chondromyxoid to well differentiated. Hypocellular fibrous stroma may be seen at the periphery of the cartilaginous nodules. Focal osteoclast-like giant cells may be seen in the stroma

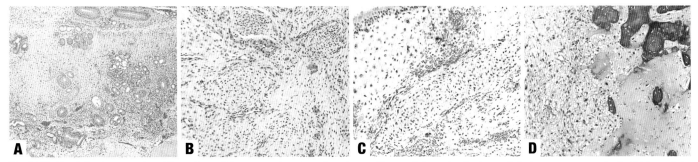

**Fig. 13.25** Nasal chondromesenchymal hamartoma. **A** Low-power view shows immature cartilage and stroma in a background of minor mucoserous glands. **B** Intermediate-power view demonstrates immature islands of cartilage in a cellular background stroma. **C** High-power view shows immature cartilage in a cellular stroma showing mild nuclear pleomorphism. Extravasated erythrocytes are noted with focal cystic changes. **D** Bone, immature cartilage, and a cellular spindled cell stroma are noted in this hamartoma.

near erythrocyte-filled spaces resembling aneurysmal bone cyst {4515,5648,5268,6408}. A fibro-osseous proliferation with ossicles or trabeculae of immature (woven) bone can be seen {3020}. Mature adipose tissue may be focally present. Epithelial elements or proliferations are not present. Concurrent other findings include sinonasal papilloma and chronic rhinosinusitis.

*Immunohistochemistry*
The immature cartilage is highlighted with S100 or SOX9 immunohistochemistry, whereas SMA and MSA highlight stromal myofibroblasts {5268,3020}.

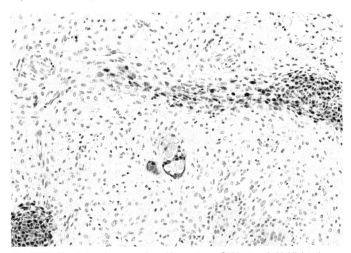

**Fig. 13.26** Nasal chondromesenchymal hamartoma. S100 strongly highlights the nuclei and cytoplasm of the cartilaginous portions of the hamartoma. (The minor mucoserous gland is a good internal control.)

*Differential diagnosis*
The differential diagnosis includes other sinonasal tract hamartomas (respiratory epithelial adenomatoid hamartoma, chondro-osseous and respiratory epithelial hamartoma, seromucinous hamartoma) and biphenotypic sinonasal sarcoma.

## Cytology
Not clinically relevant

## Diagnostic molecular pathology
When nasal chondromesenchymal hamartoma is diagnosed, germline *DICER1* genetic testing is suggested {6287}.

## Essential and desirable diagnostic criteria
*Essential:* cysts lined by respiratory epithelium, associated with a composite of immature to mature cartilage within a bland spindled cell stroma.
*Desirable:* biallelic *DICER1* pathogenic sequence variants (in selected cases).

## Staging
Not relevant

## Prognosis and prediction
Local recurrence (seen in ~25% of cases) or persistence (especially after incomplete excision) requires long-term follow-up {4452,4515,4920}. Rare malignant transformation has been reported {4095}.

# Pleomorphic adenoma

Thompson LDR
Alaggio R
López-Terrada DH
Nelson BL
Reyes-Múgica M

## Definition
Pleomorphic adenoma (PA) is a benign neoplasm showing a wide variety of cytological, nuclear, and architectural features reflecting the admixture of ductal and myoepithelial/chondromesenchymal components.

## ICD-O coding
8940/0 Pleomorphic adenoma

## ICD-11 coding
2E91.1 & XH2KC1 Benign neoplasm of other specified major salivary glands & Pleomorphic adenoma

## Related terminology
*Acceptable:* benign mixed tumour.

## Subtype(s)
None

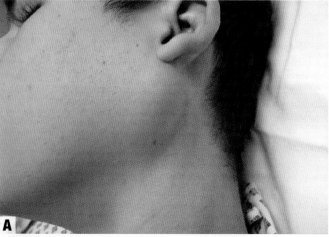

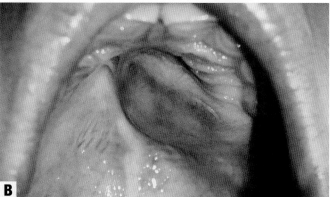

**Fig. 13.27** Pleomorphic adenoma. **A** A clinical photograph showing a smooth, rounded mass in the region of the parotid gland. **B** A 9-year-old girl demonstrates an intact mucosa overlying a left palate mass.

## Localization
The major salivary glands are most commonly affected, especially the parotid gland followed by the submandibular gland. Minor salivary glands in the palate mucosa, buccal mucosa, parapharyngeal space, and upper lip are less commonly involved {1780,4612,5867}.

## Clinical features
PA manifests as a slow-growing, generally asymptomatic, discrete mass that may become quite large {6629,5843,4287, 4082,3310,4567,171,7017,712,2312,7187,7656}. There is usually an intact overlying skin or mucosa covering a single, irregularly nodular, firm, slightly compressible mass. Clinically recurrent tumours, especially in the neck, usually show multiple nodules. Palate mucosal tumours, mostly lateral, show reduced mobility due to a tightly bound mucosa in this site.

### Imaging
Imaging studies help identify a mass but are not reliable for separating benign from malignant neoplasms. However, a very large asymptomatic mass affecting the deep lobe of the parotid gland is nearly always a PA. Studies show a smooth, sharp margination with a lobulated, homogeneously enhancing, ovoid mass. Dystrophic calcification may be seen, an uncommon finding in other salivary gland neoplasms. MRI usually shows a very uniform high T2-weighted signal (higher signal than cerebrospinal fluid), which is quite characteristic of PA {1310}. Greyscale ultrasound shows a well-demarcated, usually homogeneous hypoechoic mass, often with posterior enhancement {1846}.

## Epidemiology
Salivary gland epithelial neoplasms are relatively rare in children and adolescents. National, regional, and referral centre data, as well as retrospective data from large institutional studies including paediatric PA cases {7432,7367,6998,5843, 3501,3497,3310,3143,2312,2180,2009,1641,1191,209,1780,2008, 7656}, indicate that salivary gland tumours diagnosed in patients from birth to 19 years of age represent about 4.7% of all cases of salivary gland neoplasms. Of all reported salivary gland tumours in paediatric patients, 72% are benign and 28% are malignant. PA represents 97.6% of all benign tumours. In children, 10% of PAs occur between 0 and 9 years of age, and 90% occur between 10 and 19 years. Paediatric PA shows a slight male predominance (M:F ratio: 1.3:1), the inverse of adult PA. Solitary tumours are most common, but rarely, second synchronous or metachronous tumours may develop in the same gland or a different gland {2451,6680,4676,4716}. Familial PAs are exceptional {2791,3629,2367,104}.

## Etiology
Unknown

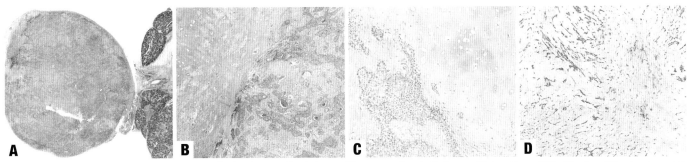

**Fig. 13.28** Pleomorphic adenoma. **A** A well-circumscribed and encapsulated pleomorphic adenoma is noted in the parotid gland tissue. **B** The blending of the chondromesenchymal stroma with the epithelial and myoepithelial components is shown. Fibrous bands are present. **C** Abundant chondroid material blends with the epithelial-myoepithelial proliferation of a pleomorphic adenoma. **D** The stroma-rich pattern is shown here, with only limited epithelial-myoepithelial elements present.

## Pathogenesis

There is very limited molecular work on PA in paediatric patients. Chromosomal abnormalities have been reported in > 70% of PAs studied, often involving chromosomal regions 8q12 (*PLAG1*), 12q13-q15 (*HMGA2*) and 3p21 {7340}. The most common translocation reported in PA, t(3;8)(p21;q12), results in fusion and promoter swapping between *PLAG1* and the β-catenin gene, *CTNNB1* {3459}. *PLAG1* encodes a developmentally regulated transcription factor (zinc finger protein) and proto-oncogene that appears to play an important role in PA pathogenesis, responsible for the induction of target genes and uncontrolled proliferation of PA tumour cells. *PLAG1* may be activated by different mechanisms in PA, including chromosomal translocations involving *PLAG1* and one of its fusion partners (e.g. *CTNNB1*, *CHCHD7*, *LIFR*, and *TCEA1*) {3459,377, 7341,383}.

*HMGA2* gene (12q14.3) rearrangements, with or without amplifications, are the second most common abnormalities reported in PA {5474,3459,383}.

Molecular profiling of carcinoma ex PA demonstrates the presence of genomic instability and activation of other targetable cancer pathways in addition to *PLAG1* and *HMGA2* rearrangements {1299}, but given the length of time required for transformation, the diagnosis of carcinoma ex PA is not meaningful in paediatrics.

## Macroscopic appearance

These tumours form irregular, bosselated to nodular, round to ovoid masses with well-defined borders. Generally, tumours of major glands demonstrate a well-formed capsule, whereas tumours of minor glands have a poorly formed or incomplete capsule. Recurrent tumours have multiple, often discrete, nodules distributed within connective tissue, fat, and/or salivary gland. The cut surface is yellow-tan to grey and glistening {7060}.

## Histopathology

Tumours show a wide cytomorphological and architectural diversity, but with the fundamental epithelial and myoepithelial-chondromesenchymal features. The contour is often bosselated, with filopodial extensions into adjacent tissues. Solid tumours are most common, but cystic changes are seen, most frequently after core sampling or FNAB. A capsule is usually identified, although it is frequently absent in minor salivary gland sites. Variable cellularity is noted, with cellular tumours showing very limited chondromesenchymal stroma and myxoid tumours

showing scant epithelium {6325,6326,3894,1562,1563,108, 2185}. The relative cellularity can be used to separate tumours into classic, myxoid, and cellular {6679}. Architectural and cellular diversity is the norm, with frequent blending between patterns and cellular components. There are anastomosing trabeculae of bilayered or multilayered epithelial cells with well-formed ductal or tubular structures that blend with the chondromyxoid matrix and mesenchymal components. The duct-like structures vary from small structures with compressed, barely discernible lumina to large well-formed duct lumina with contents. These cells are subtended by myoepithelial-type cells showing a cleared, spindled, or even stellate appearance. Plasmacytoid cells tend to be most common in palate tumours, but they may be dominant in any tumour. It is the myoepithelial component that blends into the stroma, lacking distinct demarcation. This is one of the most important findings in PA: a blending, interweaving, and indistinct junction between many of the elements comprising the neoplasm. Spindle and plasmacytoid cells often appear to be in transition from one form to the other. Spindle cells may combine into short interlacing fascicles or nuclear palisades {6846}. It is this fluid-like dynamic between the cells that contributes to the remarkable diversity of epithelial arrangements, cellular components, and stromal elements {3976,1564, 1660,692,3928,758}. The nuclear chromatin is fine to coarse, and the nucleoli are small. A variety of alterations may be seen de novo or after sampling or treatment, including squamous, oncocytic, apocrine, mucinous, sebaceous, and fatty metaplasia. Mitoses are seen, increased (3–5 mitoses/2 mm$^2$) most often in tumours previously manipulated by either core sampling or

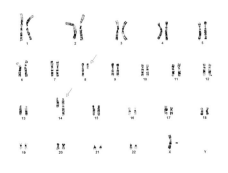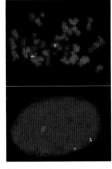

**Fig. 13.29** Pleomorphic adenoma. G-banded karyotype from a patient with a pleomorphic adenoma showing a reciprocal translocation, t(8;14)(q12;q32). *PLAG1* rearrangement is detected in metaphase (upper right) and interphase (lower right) cells using dual-colour break-apart probes (green, 5′ *PLAG1*; red, 3′ *PLAG1*). Arrows indicate der(8) and der(14) chromosomes.

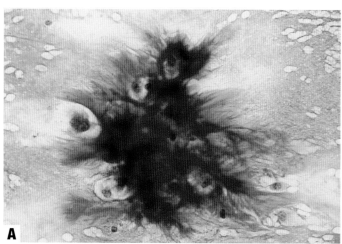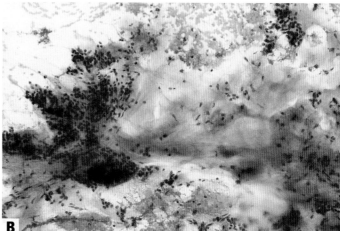

**Fig. 13.30** Pleomorphic adenoma. **A** The fibrillar stroma stains a deep magenta in this Romanowsky (Diff-Quik)-stained smear with embedded plasmacytoid epithelial elements. **B** There is a fibrillar quality to the myxoid matrix material seen in this Pap-stained smear, with embedded myoepithelial cells.

FNAB {3976,1149,5558,7298,751,4087,4840,554,7285}. Infarction or degeneration may be seen {3976}. The mesenchymal-like stroma ranges from chondroid to myxoid, hyaline, fibrous, or even osseous. True hyaline cartilage may be seen. Calcifications are common {2772,4105,3844}. Hyaline stroma, whether amorphous or more fibrillar, appears as delicate fibres between epithelial cells or as large swaths of eosinophilic stroma in epithelium-poor tumours. Extensive hyalinization is a potential predictor of malignant progression {406,4066}, although it is not seen frequently in paediatric patients. Crystalloids are seen in about 20% of cases but are not unique to PA {7176,1173}. When PA is recurrent (in about 8–10% of cases, depending on surgical technique {7432}) there are multiple minute to sizeable separate nodules of entirely benign PA, showing the same morphological diversity seen in the primary tumour. Perineural involvement may be seen in this haphazard architecture, along with a scar from the previous surgery {5512,5844,2844,3735,7585}.

*Immunohistochemistry*
Differential staining is seen in the epithelial and modified myoepithelial cells. There is usually strong and diffuse reactivity for pancytokeratin, AE1/AE3, CAM5.2, and CK7, which is often accentuated in the ductal or luminal cell areas. Various muscle, myoepithelial, and basal markers will be reactive, including calponin (most sensitive), SMA, MSA, SMMHC, S100, SOX10, p40 (better than p63), and CK5/6 {6200,5621,7810,7466,5257,5146,4665,4667}. GFAP is usually more strongly expressed in myxoid and myoepithelial areas, and reduced to absent in cellular areas or plasmacytoid cells {6363,6172,1506,5125}. The combination of pancytokeratin, p40, and GFAP may help to narrow the differential diagnosis in basaloid and myoepithelial cell–rich tumours. PLAG1 is seen in about 80–90% of tumours {1660,3471}, and HMGA2 in as many as 40% {3469,1281,4716}, although neither protein is unique to PA.

*Differential diagnosis*
Basal cell adenoma, canalicular adenoma, and adenoid cystic carcinoma are the most important differential diagnoses in paediatric PA. Nuclear β-catenin reactivity is seen in basal cell adenoma {3287,1102}, whereas strong, luminal KIT (CD117) is more likely in adenoid cystic carcinoma. Canalicular adenoma lacks p63 and shows only peripheral GFAP reactivity.

## Cytology
FNAB smears are usually hypercellular, with the cells dispersed in clusters and singly, and intimately blended with a variable amount of chondromyxoid stroma. The stroma appears fibrillar or frayed at the borders, with easily identified embedded cells, seen as a deep-magenta material in Romanowsky-stained smears {3651, 1951}. The myoepithelial cells vary from polygonal and plasmacytoid to spindled and stellate, and are usually embedded in the stroma. The nuclei of both cell types are round and monotonous.

## Diagnostic molecular pathology
Documentation of *PLAG1* rearrangements by FISH or other methods may rarely be used to confirm a diagnosis in selected cases {4434} but can be seen in carcinomas derived from PA {3469,447,4434}.

## Essential and desirable diagnostic criteria
*Essential:* an architecturally diverse proliferation of epithelial and myoepithelial elements; ductal structures within the neoplasm; chondromyxoid matrix material at least focally; no destructive invasion/infiltration.
*Desirable:* metaplastic changes; epithelial and myoepithelial immunohistochemistry (in selected cases); FISH for *PLAG1* or *HMGA2* (in selected cases).

## Staging
Not relevant

## Prognosis and prediction
Complete excision reduces the possibility of recurrence {3181}. Breach of the capsule or intraoperative spillage is associated with a high risk of recurrence {7187}. When enucleation is performed instead of partial parotidectomy, there is a high recurrence rate {7040,4892,1790,4057,1985,7581,7187}. Tumour management and the preservation of facial nerve function are more difficult with recurrent tumours. The risk of malignant transformation to carcinoma ex PA increases with time, from 0.15% to 13.3% {2553, 1282,7552,1281,7187,7126,4716}. A PA diagnosis in childhood therefore establishes a much greater overall risk of malignant transformation, because of the generally longer lifespan of a child than an older adult initially diagnosed with PA {7582,4211}.

# Mucoepidermoid carcinoma

Chiosea S
Williams MD
Xu B

## Definition

Mucoepidermoid carcinoma (MEC) is a malignant salivary gland neoplasm characterized by mucous, intermediate, and epidermoid (squamoid) tumour cells forming cystic and solid growth patterns, usually associated with *MAML2* rearrangement.

## ICD-O coding

8430/3 Mucoepidermoid carcinoma
8430/3 Oncocytic mucoepidermoid carcinoma
8430/3 Warthin-like mucoepidermoid carcinoma

## ICD-11 coding

2B67.0 & XH1J36 Adenocarcinoma of parotid gland & Mucoepidermoid carcinoma
2B68.0 & XH1J36 Adenocarcinoma of submandibular or sublingual glands & Mucoepidermoid carcinoma

## Related terminology

*Not recommended:* mucoepidermoid tumour.

## Subtype(s)

Oncocytic mucoepidermoid carcinoma; Warthin-like mucoepidermoid carcinoma; central intraosseous mucoepidermoid carcinoma

## Localization

Tumours in paediatric patients most commonly affect the parotid gland {5213,7656}, followed by the submandibular gland and the minor salivary glands in the oral cavity (especially the palate) {5213,7656,4781}, with rare central (intraosseous) cases.

## Clinical features

Patients usually present with a solitary painless mass or mucosal ulceration, which is present for a mean duration of about 1 year {5445,2884}. Some cystic masses may fluctuate, clinically mimicking a mucocoele.

## Epidemiology

Although rare, MEC is the most common salivary gland malignancy in paediatric patients {4185,7656,5213}. It most commonly affects adolescents (reported median ages: 12–15 years) {6935,7656,7259}. There is no sex predilection {7259,6078}.

## Etiology

Treatment with chemotherapy and/or radiation (usually for leukaemia, lymphoma, or sarcoma) may place children at a higher risk of developing a MEC, from several years later (for chemoradiation) to decades later (for radiation alone) {7284}, although tumour characteristics are similar to those of non–treatment-associated tumours. Increased occurrence of childhood MEC has been reported after nuclear disasters and chemotherapy {1779A}.

## Pathogenesis

The majority of MECs are characterized by the t(11;19)(q21;p13) translocation, which results in the *CRTC1::MAML2* fusion, followed in frequency by the t(11;15)(q21;q26) translocation, which results in the *CRTC3::MAML2* fusion {7014,6320,2072,5061, 3238,6321}. There is no association with tumour grade and/or patient outcome and fusion status {4003,4949,701,3404,6091}. *TP53* mutations are commonly identified, more often in intermediate- and high-grade tumours {3404}.

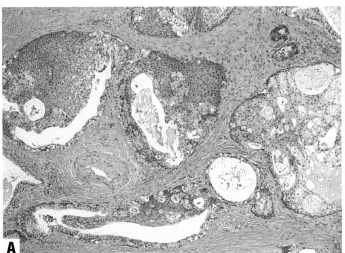
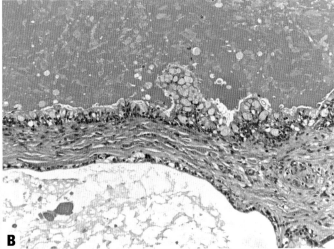

**Fig. 13.31** Mucoepidermoid carcinoma. **A** An intermediate-grade soft palate tumour showing predominantly microcystic and solid growth with an abundance of epidermoid cells. Tumour nests vary in size and shape and infiltrate around an arteriole. **B** The cyst lining is represented by numerous mucous cells.

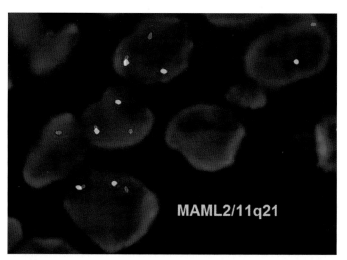

**Fig. 13.32** Mucoepidermoid carcinoma. *MAML2* translocation FISH. Examples of neoplastic cells with one rearranged and one normal *MAML2* signal. The *MAML2* gene without rearrangement is characterized by an overlapping pair of green and red signals (resulting in yellow). The rearranged *MAML2* gene is characterized by separate green and red signals.

## Macroscopic appearance
MEC typically manifests as a well-defined or infiltrative cystic or multicystic white to tan mass, frequently with viscous content.

## Histopathology
The tumour is composed of epidermoid, intermediate, and mucinous cells in varying proportions. The mucinous cells contain intracytoplasmic mucin compressing a peripherally located nucleus. The epidermoid cells are polygonal, have abundant eosinophilic or clear cytoplasm, and (rarely) may show small foci of overt keratinization (extensive keratinization is not seen in MEC). The intermediate (in size) cells are round to oval and are larger than normal basal cells but smaller than epidermoid cells. Clear cell {6836A}, oncocytic {6516A}, Warthin-like {3145A,705A}, and ciliated {705A} patterns/subtypes of MEC have been described.

### Immunohistochemistry
Mucicarmine or PAS stains highlight mucous cells. Immunohistochemically, clusters of epidermoid cells are highlighted by p63, p40, and CK5/6, whereas CEA(m) and EMA (MUC1) highlight mucocytes {5257}. S100 and SOX10 are negative.

### Grading
Grading is defined by the growth pattern and cellular features {6321,839,1341}. Low-grade tumours are well circumscribed and cystic, whereas intermediate-grade tumours are well circumscribed and mixed cystic and solid. High-grade tumours are typically infiltrative and solid. Scant mucous cells, increased mitosis, and profound nuclear anaplasia are characteristic of high-grade tumours.

### Differential diagnosis
Pleomorphic adenoma with mucinous metaplasia, necrotizing sialometaplasia, lymphoepithelial cysts, mucocoele, Warthin tumour, and clear cell carcinoma can mimic MEC {831,3018}.

## Cytology
The cellularity of aspirates varies with tumour grade. Low-grade tumours (common in paediatric patients) are hypocellular, with an abundant mucinous background, macrophages, and debris, admixed with scattered sheets of epidermoid and mucous cells {5968}.

## Diagnostic molecular pathology
The presence of *MAML2* rearrangements (and rarely other gene fusions) is an important diagnostic marker {6320}; their absence raises the possibility of other lesions in the differential diagnosis (mucocoele, chronic sialadenitis, lymphoepithelial cyst, sclerosing polycystic adenoma {6320,1236,2452,707}).

## Essential and desirable diagnostic criteria
*Essential:* a mixture of mucous, intermediate, and epidermoid cells.
*Desirable: MAML2* rearrangement (in selected cases).

## Staging
MECs are staged using the TNM system as published by the Union for International Cancer Control (UICC).

## Prognosis and prediction
The prognosis in paediatric patients is excellent {5727,2884, 7259,7656}, with 5- and 10-year overall survival rates of 98% and 94%, respectively {6078}. Nearly all patients who develop distant metastasis have high-grade tumours {2884,7259,6078, 7656}.

# Acinic cell carcinoma

Fonseca I
Bell D

## Definition

Acinic cell carcinoma is a malignant epithelial neoplasm composed of multiple cell types including acinar (zymogen granule) differentiation.

## ICD-O coding

8550/3 Acinic cell carcinoma

## ICD-11 coding

2B67.0 Adenocarcinoma of parotid gland
2B68.0 Adenocarcinoma of submandibular or sublingual glands

## Related terminology

*Acceptable:* acinic cell adenocarcinoma.

## Subtype(s)

None

## Localization

Nearly all tumours occur in the parotid gland, with a minority arising in the submandibular gland {2639,6770,1274,7656,4801, 7799,7723}.

## Clinical features

Clinically, a slow-growing mass is present, with other symptoms rarely reported.

## Epidemiology

Paediatric salivary gland tumours are rare (annual incidence: ~1 case per 1 million children {7744,174}) with about 6% of acinic cell carcinomas occurring in patients aged < 18 years {6770,7723,7799}. Acinic cell carcinoma accounts for about 30–40% of malignant salivary neoplasms in children {7656, 6770,174,4801,1103,7799}. Paediatric acinic cell carcinoma affects children in their second decade of life, with a female predominance {6770,3223}. One familial case has been reported {1707}.

## Etiology

Unknown

## Pathogenesis

Acinic cell carcinomas usually harbour a recurrent rearrangement, t(4;9)(q13;q31), that translocates active enhancer regions from the secretory calcium-binding phosphoprotein (SCPP) gene cluster at 4q13 to the region upstream of *NR4A3* (*NOR1*) {2671}. NR4A3 is specifically upregulated via enhancer hijacking in acinic cell carcinoma, and active chromatin regions and gene expression signatures are highly correlated with the *NR4A3* transcription binding motif {2671}. The *HTN3::MSANTD3* gene fusion is seen in tumours with prominent serous differentiation {2674}.

## Macroscopic appearance

Tumours range from rounded to lobulated, with a circumscribed variable periphery, which is rarely infiltrative into soft tissue. Most tumours are 10–40 mm, although large tumours have been described {7233}. Tumours affecting minor salivary gland sites are rare, and tumours at these sites may represent secretory carcinoma or other tumour types. The cut surface appears rubbery, solid, or variably cystic, with variegated grey-white, tan, and/or haemorrhagic areas. Necrosis and/or destructively infiltrative growth is usually seen in recurrent or high-grade tumours.

## Histopathology

Classically, these neoplasms (called "blue-dot tumours") appear as a circumscribed/encapsulated haematoxyphilic tumour. Various patterns of growth (solid, microcystic, macrocystic, follicular, papillary, and cystic) may be seen in each tumour, often with one pattern predominating {6300,7233}. Tumour-associated lymphoid proliferation at the advancing tumour edge is common, and cholesterol granulomas are also noted. Various morphological components are present, including serous acinar cells (blue cells with dark cytoplasmic granules), intercalated duct cells (in microcystic and other architectural patterns), clear

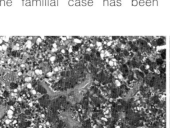
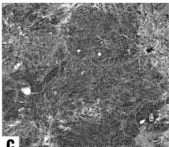
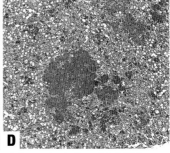

**Fig. 13.33** Acinic cell carcinoma. **A** Low-power view demonstrates an infiltrative tumour with areas of cystic degeneration. A lymph node is noted at the lower left. **B** High-power view showing numerous blue cytoplasmic granules in the acinar cells. Secretory vacuoles are noted. **C** A more solid pattern is noted in this example, but serous acinar differentiation is still easily identified. **D** Acinar differentiation is seen as small blue granules in the cytoplasm. There is an overall fenestrated tumour pattern.

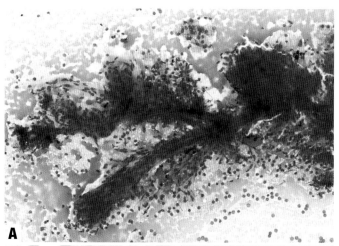

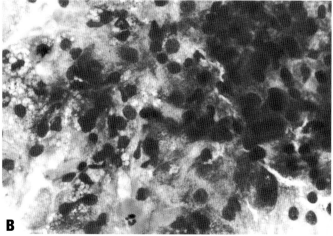

**Fig. 13.34** Acinic cell carcinoma. **A** A Romanowsky (Diff-Quik)-stained cellular smear with cohesive clusters and sheets of serous acinar cells without ducts. Numerous naked tumour nuclei are in the background, created when fragile cytoplasm is stripped away. **B** High-power view of a Romanowsky (Diff-Quik)-stained FNAB smear showing a cohesive cluster of serous acinar cells. These are large, uniform cells with round, centrally placed nuclei and cytoplasmic azurophilic serous granules.

cells, and nonspecific glandular cells (negative for glycogen). High-grade transformation is not seen in paediatric patients {6979,4964}. Tumours are not graded.

*Immunohistochemistry*
PAS stain with digestion highlights dark-blue diastase-resistant cytoplasmic granules. Pancytokeratins AE1/AE3 and CK8/18 stain acinar and ductal components, with CK7 and CK19 seen in the intercalated duct-like cells. Amylase, 1-antitrypsin, lactoferrin, and lysozyme are variably expressed, although they are identified at least focally in most tumours {7445}. DOG1 shows luminal plasmalemmal expression, with nuclear SOX10 {6300,7233}. Nuclear expression of NR4A3 (NOR1) {2674}, NR4A2 (NURR1) {2673}, and MIST1 {3016} are positive immunohistochemistry findings representing corresponding molecular results.

*Differential diagnosis*
When non-serous architecture predominates, the variegated architectural patterns raises a differential that includes neoplasms of intercalated duct origin.

## Cytology
Frequently misinterpreted as normal, smears are usually cellular, with cohesive clusters and sheets of serous acinar cells lacking ducts and adipocytes. The fragile cytoplasm is often stripped away, leaving naked nuclei. Subpopulations show large, uniform cells with round, centrally placed nuclei and cytoplasmic azurophilic serous granules, whereas other cells have granular to vacuolated cytoplasm without granules {7233,1553,4469,1906}. Binucleation may aid in the diagnosis. Cystic tumours may be more hypocellular. Lymphoid cells can be prominent, raising a differential diagnosis with Warthin tumour, as well as with metastatic carcinoma in a lymph node.

## Diagnostic molecular pathology
Typically not needed

## Essential and desirable diagnostic criteria
*Essential:* multiple cellular components with at least one showing serous acinar differentiation.
*Desirable:* prominent tumour-associated lymphoid proliferation; NR4A3/NR4A2 (nuclear) and/or DOG1 immunoreactivity (in selected cases).

## Staging
Acinic cell carcinoma is staged using the TNM system as published by the Union for International Cancer Control (UICC).

## Prognosis and prediction
The vast majority are low-grade tumours with an excellent long-term prognosis (5-year survival rate: 98%), irrespective of stage {2639,6770,1274,7656,4801,7799,7385,7723}. Regional lymph node metastasis is rare {7233,4964,370,7723}.

# Sialoblastoma

Katabi N
Perez-Atayde AR

## Definition
Sialoblastoma is a low-grade malignant primitive salivary gland anlage neoplasm.

## ICD-O coding
8974/1 Sialoblastoma

## ICD-11 coding
2B67.Y & XH0G00 Other specified malignant neoplasms of parotid gland & Sialoblastoma

## Related terminology
*Not recommended:* embryoma; basaloid adenocarcinoma; congenial basal cell adenoma; congenital hybrid basal cell adenoma–adenoid cystic carcinoma.

## Subtype(s)
None

## Localization
Tumours arise most commonly in the parotid gland (in two thirds of cases) followed by the submandibular gland, with only rare reports in minor salivary gland sites {5330,1303,6508,6409, 1736}.

## Clinical features
Patients present with painless facial swelling, with rare cases showing nerve involvement or skin ulceration {58,838,3033, 6912,1303}. Other tumours (naevi and hepatoblastoma) may be coexistent {5265,6307,2541,6576}. Elevated AFP has been reported {5265}.

### Imaging
This lesion is usually diagnosed in the neonatal period but is occasionally seen on antenatal imaging.

## Epidemiology
The vast majority of tumours are identified at birth or within the few months of life, with only rare reports in adults. There is no sex predilection {1303,7418}.

## Etiology
Unknown

## Pathogenesis
The tumour may originate from retained blastema cells rather than basal reserve cells {6508}.

## Macroscopic appearance
Tumours are lobulated, well defined, and encapsulated, or they may show infiltration into the surrounding tissue. The cut surface is usually grey or yellow and solid. Tumours range from 15 to 150 mm in size. Focal haemorrhage or necrosis may be present {6923,6492,6009}.

## Histopathology
Sialoblastoma typically exhibits solid organoid nests composed of primitive basaloid epithelial cells, separated by dense fibrous stroma. Tumour cells have indistinct cell borders, scant cytoplasm, a high N:C ratio, and round to oval vesicular nuclei with occasional nucleoli. In addition, differentiated budding ducts lined by cuboidal to columnar epithelium with intraluminal basophilic secretions or a cribriform pattern may be present. Peripheral nuclear palisading is occasionally present. Tumour cells may exhibit apoptosis, necrosis, and nuclear pleomorphism, with increased mitoses. Tumours are not graded.

### Immunohistochemistry
By immunohistochemistry, tumours are reactive for SOX10, p63, nuclear β-catenin, and KIT (CD117), and variably reactive for cytokeratins including CK5/6, CK7, and CK19, along with SMA and calponin {4069}.

### Differential diagnosis
The primitive histological features and the young ages of patients help to differentiate sialoblastoma from other basaloid salivary gland tumours such as basal cell adenoma/adenocarcinoma, adenoid cystic carcinoma, and adamantinoma-like Ewing sarcoma {7296,3017,7418,5223,5971,4069}.

## Cytology
Aspirations are often not tolerated by infants. When performed, smears are cellular and show arrangements of tight, solid sheets or clusters of basaloid cells with scant cytoplasm, round to oval vesicular nuclei, and occasional nucleoli. The cellular clusters may contain ductal cells and dense, metachromatic, magenta

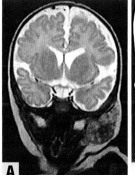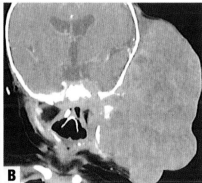

**Fig. 13.35** Sialoblastoma. **A** MRI of the head of a 2-month-old boy with a 30 × 30 mm left parotid, well-defined, lobulated mass. At birth, the mass was 10 mm in size (not shown here). **B** CT of the head of the same boy at 5 months of age. The mass has grown considerably and protrudes from the left side of the face.

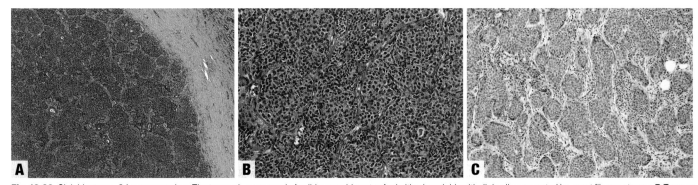

**Fig. 13.36** Sialoblastoma. **A** Low-power view. The tumour is composed of solid organoid nests of primitive basaloid epithelial cells, separated by scant fibrous stroma. **B** Tumour cells exhibit round to oval nuclei with single small nucleoli and scant, poorly outlined cytoplasm. Occasional differentiated ducts are noted within the tumour nests. **C** Sialoblastoma composed of solid organoid nests of tumour cells with a primitive basaloid appearance.

hyaline globular material with smooth, rounded outlines {3472, 3033}.

## Diagnostic molecular pathology
Not relevant

## Essential and desirable diagnostic criteria
*Essential:* primitive, solid, organoid nests; basaloid epithelial cells with vesicular chromatin; cuboidal to columnar ductal cells.
*Desirable:* dividing fibrous stroma; peripheral palisading.

## Staging
Sialoblastoma is staged using the TNM system as published by the Union for International Cancer Control (UICC).

## Prognosis and prediction
Local recurrence is seen in about one third of patients, and regional and distant metastases are seen in about 15% {3136}. Death from disease is rare {2331,6912,1303,3136,7418,1736}. A less aggressive behaviour is suggested for tumours in the submandibular gland versus other anatomical sites. Histological features associated with a worse prognosis include tumour necrosis and increased mitoses or a high Ki-67 proliferation index.

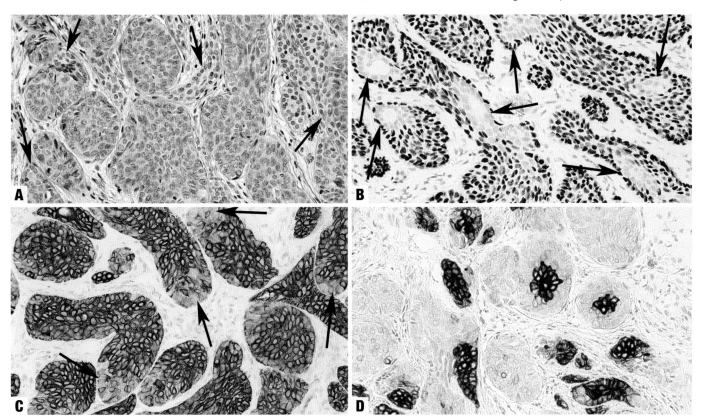

**Fig. 13.37** Sialoblastoma. **A** Tumour cells show round to oval vesicular nuclei with single small nucleoli and scant, poorly outlined cytoplasm. Differentiated ductules (arrows) are present around and within the nests. Occasional mitoses are observed. **B–D** Immunostaining for p63 (**B**), CK19 (**C**), and CK7 (**D**). Tumour cells are strongly immunoreactive for p63 (nuclear) and CK19 (cytoplasmic), consistent with a myoepithelial differentiation. Differentiated ductules (arrows) are negative for p63 and weakly positive for CK19. Expression of CK7 is only present in the differentiated ductules.

# Nasopharyngeal carcinoma

Chan JKC
Lee AWM
Seethala R

## Definition
Nasopharyngeal carcinoma (NPC) is a malignant mucosal epithelial neoplasm usually showing evidence of squamous differentiation.

## ICD-O coding
8070/3 Nasopharyngeal carcinoma
8071/3 Squamous cell carcinoma, keratinizing, NOS
8072/3 Squamous cell carcinoma, non-keratinizing, NOS
8083/3 Basaloid squamous cell carcinoma

## ICD-11 coding
2B6B.0 Squamous cell carcinoma of nasopharynx

## Related terminology
*Not recommended:* lymphoepithelioma-like carcinoma; lymphoepithelial carcinoma.

## Subtype(s)
Non-keratinizing squamous cell carcinoma; keratinizing squamous cell carcinoma; basaloid squamous cell carcinoma

## Localization
The lateral nasopharynx wall, especially the fossa of Rosenmüller, is the most commonly affected site, followed by the superior posterior wall.

## Clinical features
In young patients, the most common presenting symptom is unilateral or bilateral upper cervical lymphadenopathy, which is often bulky and sometimes painful {1807}. Other common symptoms include nasal obstruction, epistaxis, postnasal drip, tinnitus, serous otitis media, hearing impairment, headache, and cranial nerve palsy. A higher proportion of paediatric patients with NPC have locoregionally advanced disease (> 90% stage III/IV or T3/T4) at the time of diagnosis than adults {1807,6768,1253,5873,7693,423,6371}. EBV serology is positive in most patients with non-keratinizing NPC {2651A}.

### Imaging
MRI is widely preferred as the imaging modality of choice in the assessment and staging of NPC because of to its superior soft tissue resolution and ability to visualize perineural extension, bone marrow involvement, and intracranial spread.

## Epidemiology
NPC is common among certain ethnic groups, including ethnic Chinese populations in south-eastern Asia, the Arctic Inuit, and northern Africans. The incidence in southern China is 15–50 cases per 100 000 person-years. NPCs occur most commonly in adults, with only 0.1–2.3% of all NPCs affecting paediatric patients {1807,3042,6398,4167,1214}. In Hong Kong SAR, China, where NPC is endemic, the overall age-standardized incidence rates from 1983 to 2017 for ages 0–4, 5–9, 10–14, and 15–19 years were 0, 0, 0.2, and 0.7 cases per 100 000 person-years, respectively {2969}. In non-endemic regions, cases in children aged < 16 years account for 2.4% of all NPCs in the United Kingdom, 7.2% in Türkiye, and 10% in the USA {423}, with an age-adjusted incidence of < 1 case per 100 000 person-years {1807,423}. The reported median ages of paediatric patients with NPC range from 13 to 16 years. There is a male predilection (M:F ratio: 2–3:1) {4167,7693,6371,1807, 1214,3939}.

## Etiology
Etiological factors include viral, genetic, and environmental factors. Paediatric NPC shows a near-consistent association with EBV, irrespective of ethnic background {1807,5394}. The striking ethnic differences in the prevalence of NPC indicate a major influence of genetic susceptibility {7084,5394}. People with certain HLA class I genes have a higher risk of developing NPC (Asians with HLA-A*02, B*46, and B*16 types; White people with HLA-B*05). Studies have suggested that *GABBR1*, *HCG9*, *TNFRSF19*, *MECOM* (*MDS1-EVI1*), and *CDKN2A* and/or *CDKN2B* may also be implicated {5394}. Studies of familial NPC have identified several germline pathogenic variants involved in NPC predisposition, such as *MST1R*, *NIPAL1*, and *ITGB6* {7084,5394}. Consumption of food containing volatile nitrosamines (e.g. salted dried fish, fermented foods, and rancid butter, especially during weaning and early childhood) and smoking have been reported to be risk factors for NPC {7084, 5394,3266}.

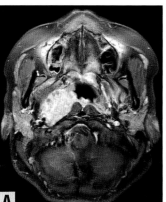 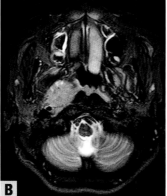

**Fig. 13.38** Nasopharyngeal carcinoma. **A** Contrast-enhanced T1-weighted axial MRI shows heterogeneous enhancement of both the primary nasopharynx carcinoma and the large right retropharyngeal node. **B** T2-weighted fat-suppressed axial MRI shows mildly hyperintense mucosal thickening over the roof of the nasopharynx and a large metastatic right retropharyngeal node.

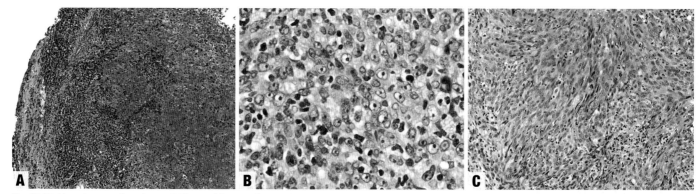

**Fig. 13.39** Nasopharyngeal carcinoma. **A** Biopsy of the nasopharynx shows the tumour beneath an intact epithelium. **B** Undifferentiated carcinoma characterized by large tumour cells that have indistinct cell borders and crowded nuclei with vesicular chromatin and prominent nucleoli. **C** In undifferentiated carcinoma, the tumour cells can be spindly, forming sweeping fascicles.

## Pathogenesis

Data from NPC cases as a whole (not exclusively from paediatric patients) demonstrate that the most common genetic aberrations include negative regulators of chromatin modification genes and the NF-κB, PI3K, and MAPK pathways {4993,4098,4126}.

## Macroscopic appearance

The tumour can produce a smooth bulge in the mucosa, a discrete raised nodule with or without ulceration, or a frankly infiltrative fungating mass. Sometimes there is no grossly visible tumour.

## Histopathology

Although there are several histological subtypes of NPC, including non-keratinizing squamous cell carcinoma (undifferentiated or differentiated subtypes), keratinizing squamous cell carcinoma, and basaloid squamous cell carcinoma, practically all paediatric NPCs fall into the non-keratinizing group.

Nasopharyngeal biopsies vary in appearance, from a frank tumour with surface ulceration to subtle involvement of the mucosa beneath an intact epithelium {6378,7486,1140}. The tumour comprises solid sheets, irregular islands, and trabeculae, often intermingled with variable numbers of lymphocytes and plasma cells. The carcinoma cells are large, often with indistinct cell borders, and crowded, with round to oval vesicular nuclei and large nucleoli. Some foci may show squamous differentiation, where the tumour cells exhibit a greater amount of eosinophilic cytoplasm, distinct cell borders, and vague intercellular

bridges. The carcinoma cells can appear spindly, with formation of streaming fascicles {1140}. In some cases, interspersed amyloid globules are present among the carcinoma cells {5627}. Scattered epithelioid granulomas may be present {1207}. In some cases, interspersed intracellular or extracellular small spherical amyloid globules are present.

Lymph nodes are involved extensively or subtly. Islands and strands of carcinoma cells are intermingled with variable numbers of lymphocytes, plasma cells, and eosinophils {4201}. Tumour cells can be scattered, resembling the Reed–Sternberg or lacunar cells of Hodgkin lymphoma {1035,4039}. Epithelioid granulomas may be present {4039}. NPC may also metastasize as a wholly or partly cystic lesion containing necrotic tumour cells.

### Immunohistochemistry

The tumour cells are positive for pancytokeratin, high-molecular-weight cytokeratins, and p63 or p40. In situ hybridization for EBV-encoded small RNA (EBER) is almost invariably positive {1140}.

## Cytology

FNAB smears, obtained from involved cervical lymph nodes, show irregular clusters of large cells with overlapping vesicular nuclei and large nucleoli, occurring in a background of lymphocytes and plasma cells. The cytoplasm of the tumour cells is fragile and barely visible, resulting in many naked nuclei {3712,1150,4741}. The presence of dispersed large tumour cells

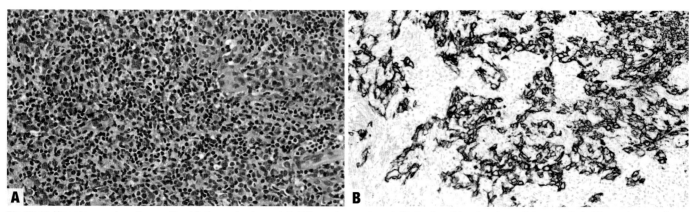

**Fig. 13.40** Nasopharyngeal carcinoma with subtle tumour involvement. **A** A biopsy shows a dense infiltrate of small lymphocytes and plasma cells, but the carcinoma cells can barely be appreciated. **B** Immunostaining for cytokeratin may highlight a surprising number of carcinoma cells.

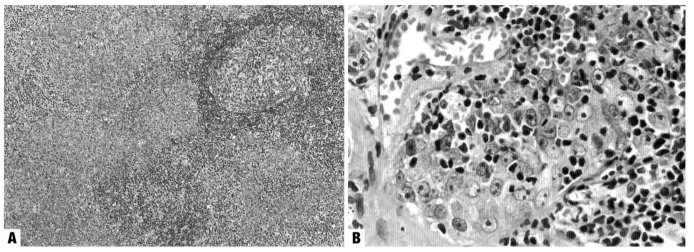

**Fig. 13.41** Metastatic nasopharyngeal carcinoma in lymph node. **A** The node shows extensive replacement by sheets of carcinoma cells. **B** The carcinoma cells have a syncytial appearance, with vesicular nuclei and prominent nucleoli.

among many lymphoid cells may result in a pattern mimicking Hodgkin lymphoma {3712}.

### Diagnostic molecular pathology
Positive in situ hybridization for EBER may aid in confirming the diagnosis of NPC, in particular for specimens obtained from metastatic sites.

### Essential and desirable diagnostic criteria
*Essential:* an infiltrative, poorly differentiated carcinoma with loosely cohesive growth; absence of obvious differentiation or limited squamous differentiation.
*Desirable:* immunoreactivity for cytokeratins or squamous markers and positive labelling for EBER (in selected cases).

### Staging
NPC is staged using the TNM system as published by the Union for International Cancer Control (UICC).

### Prognosis and prediction
NPC is highly radiosensitive, but the prognosis of locoregionally advanced paediatric NPC is poor when treated by radiotherapy alone, with 5-year overall survival rates of 20–40% {1807}. Addition of induction chemotherapy or concomitant chemotherapy has substantially improved the outcome, with 5-year progression-free survival rates of 73–91% {6768,5873,1807,4167}. The mortality rate from NPC is reported to be lower in children/adolescents than in adults {6768,5873}. The presenting TNM stage is the most important prognostic factor {1253,3021}.

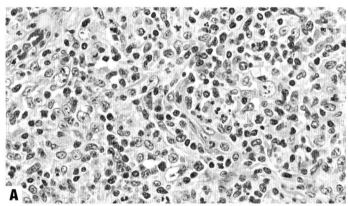
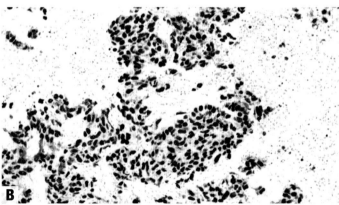

**Fig. 13.42** Metastatic nasopharyngeal carcinoma in lymph node. **A** In this example, the carcinoma cells are intimately intermingled with lymphocytes, plasma cells, and eosinophils, mimicking Hodgkin lymphoma. **B** In a metastatic carcinoma of uncertain origin, positive labelling for EBV-encoded small RNA (EBER) strongly suggests a nasopharyngeal primary.

# NUT carcinoma

Bishop JA
French CA
Stelow EB

## Definition

NUT carcinoma is an epithelial malignancy with a relatively monotonous appearance genetically defined by a rearrangement of the nuclear protein in testis gene (*NUTM1*).

## ICD-O coding

8023/3 NUT carcinoma

## ICD-11 coding

2D42 & XH2855 Malignant neoplasms of ill-defined sites & Nuclear protein in testis (NUT)-associated carcinoma

## Related terminology

*Not recommended:* NUT midline carcinoma; *NUT*-rearranged carcinoma; t(15;19) carcinoma; carcinoma with t(15;19) translocation; aggressive t(15;19)-positive carcinoma; midline lethal carcinoma; midline carcinoma of children and young adults with *NUT* rearrangement.

## Subtype(s)

None

## Localization

NUT carcinoma usually occurs in the lung/mediastinum (in 51% of cases) or the head and neck region (41%) {1188}, although it has been reported in nearly all body sites, including the salivary glands {7397}, thyroid gland {3913}, pancreas {6396}, bone / soft tissue {1188}, kidney {706}, and bladder {2227}.

## Clinical features

Symptoms are nonspecific and mass-related, depending on the tumour location. Tumours are locally aggressive, with a high metastatic rate locally or to distant sites {542,1188}. Bone

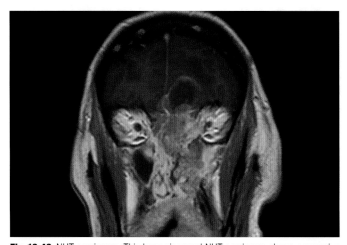

**Fig. 13.43** NUT carcinoma. This large sinonasal NUT carcinoma shows aggressive behaviour, with growth into the brain and orbit.

metastases are often seen early, whereas multiorgan dissemination occurs later in the disease course {7245,6396,6868, 5664,5593}.

## Epidemiology

This rare neoplasm has an equal sex distribution and a broad age range (0–82 years), but it is most frequently seen in children and young adults (median age: 23.6 years) {2227,2226,6396, 6671,2428,1188}.

## Etiology

Unknown

## Pathogenesis

NUT carcinoma is defined by a chromosomal translocation and fusion of *NUTM1*. In most cases (78%), *NUTM1* is fused to *BRD4*, but fusions with *BRD3* (15%), *NSD3* (6%), other genes (*ZNF532*, *ZNF592*; 2%), or unidentified genes (7%) are also seen. NUT fusion oncoproteins act as single drivers that function by blocking differentiation and maintaining proliferation {2228}.

## Macroscopic appearance

Tumours are often unresectable, but when removed they have a tan-white, fleshy gross appearance, with necrosis {6868}.

## Histopathology

NUT carcinoma grows as widely infiltrative nests and sheets of primitive-appearing, medium-sized undifferentiated cells. There is a high mitotic count and frequent necrosis. Tumour nuclei are strikingly monotonous, and round to oval, with vesicular chromatin and prominent nucleoli. Tumour cells have moderate amounts of eosinophilic to amphophilic cytoplasm, which may appear granular. Areas of abrupt keratinization, although diagnostically useful, are only identified in about 30% of cases {1188}. A neutrophilic infiltrate is common. Rare cases with mesenchymal differentiation have been described {1699, 1743}.

### Immunohistochemistry

The monoclonal NUT antibody is highly sensitive (87%), and 100% specific, when staining is seen in > 50% of tumour cells with a dot-like nuclear pattern {2645}. Tumour cells are usually positive for pancytokeratin and p63 or p40 {1988,7861}. CD34 is positive in about half of all cases {2227}. Some cases are positive for synaptophysin, chromogranin, thyroid transcription factor 1 (TTF1), and/or AFP {6868,5797}.

### Differential diagnosis

The differential diagnosis includes other primitive round cell tumours such as rhabdomyosarcoma, Ewing sarcoma, squamous cell carcinoma (when keratinized), and neuroendocrine

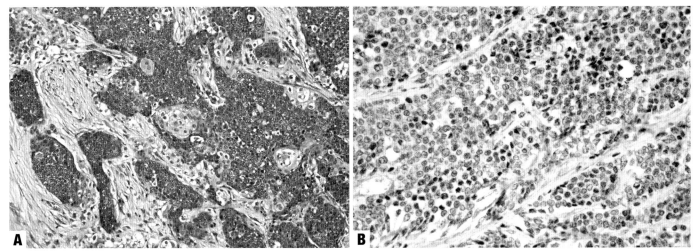

**Fig. 13.44** NUT carcinoma. **A** Infiltrative nests of undifferentiated, monotonous round cells with numerous foci of abrupt keratinization. **B** Diffuse, dot-like immunostaining with NUT monoclonal antibody is diagnostic for NUT carcinoma.

carcinoma (NEC; particularly small cell carcinoma, when aberrant TTF1 and neuroendocrine expression is seen). Particularly challenging is adamantinoma-like Ewing sarcoma, which may show squamous differentiation by histology and immunohistochemistry {5971}, but NUT immunohistochemistry resolves most diagnostic challenges.

## Cytology
Cytology features are nonspecific, with cellular smears of discohesive clusters and single monotonous cells of intermediate size with irregular nuclear contours, granular to vesicular chromatin, and discrete nucleoli {706}. Cytoplasm varies from pale to eosinophilic and may be vacuolated but lacks mucin. Mitotic figures, necrotic debris, and crush artefact are common {591, 7861,706}.

## Diagnostic molecular pathology
Demonstration of *NUTM1* rearrangement is required for the diagnosis, either by NUT immunohistochemistry or by a variety of other molecular techniques.

## Essential and desirable diagnostic criteria
*Essential:* demonstration of *NUTM1* rearrangement (by immunohistochemistry or a molecular technique) in a monotonous, undifferentiated epithelioid malignancy.

*Desirable:* abrupt keratinization; intralesional acute inflammatory infiltrate; in selected cases, identification of the NUT carcinoma–related *NUTM1* fusion partner gene to distinguish NUT carcinoma from other rare *NUTM1*-rearranged neoplasms of either cutaneous or bone / soft tissue origin.

## Staging
NUT carcinoma is staged using the TNM system as published by the Union for International Cancer Control (UICC).

## Prognosis and prediction
NUT carcinoma is an extremely aggressive malignancy, with an overall median survival time of 6.5 months {1188}. Survival is particularly poor in thoracic cases and in cases with non-*BRD4* fusions {1188}. Improved survival is seen with complete resection or initial treatment with radiotherapy, and in cases without metastases {542}.

# Melanotic neuroectodermal tumour of infancy

Prasad ML
Alaggio R

## Definition

Melanotic neuroectodermal tumour of infancy is a biphasic tumour of small neuroblast-like cells and larger melanin-producing epithelial cells.

## ICD-O coding

9363/1 Melanotic neuroectodermal tumour, NOS
9363/3 Melanotic neuroectodermal tumour, malignant

## ICD-11 coding

2D42 & XH6C72 Malignant neoplasms of ill-defined sites & Melanotic neuroectodermal tumour

## Related terminology

*Not recommended:* melanotic progonoma; retinal anlage tumour.

## Subtype(s)

None

## Localization

Most tumours (> 90%) occur in the craniofacial bones affecting the maxilla (> 60%), skull (~15%), or mandible (~8%) {5841, 4786,5711}; soft tissue tumours are rare. Rarely, tumours develop in the testis and epididymis, ovary, uterus, mediastinum, scapula, and the bones and soft tissues of the extremities {2023,5711,191}.

## Clinical features

Typically, the tumour manifests as a sessile, painless, rapidly enlarging mass in the upper alveolus, causing facial deformity and feeding disruption. The mass is usually bluish-black, owing to its melanin content. Some tumours produce vanillylmandelic acid (VMA) (34%) and AFP {4786,1309,5711}.

## Imaging

Imaging shows destruction of cortical bone, with entrapment of developing tooth buds and extension into the sinus, nasal cavity, or orbit {4952}.

## Epidemiology

This rare tumour usually affects infants aged 3–6 months, although it has been diagnosed in utero, at birth, in older children, and in adults. There is a slight male predilection {1309, 4786,5841,5711}.

## Etiology

Unknown

## Pathogenesis

This tumour of neural crest cell origin has no defined pathogenesis {1309}, although germline *CDKN2A* and somatic *BRAF* p.V600E pathogenic sequence variants have been reported {498,2475}.

## Macroscopic appearance

Tumours are pigmented, firm, unencapsulated, and lobulated, without necrosis or ulceration, and can be as large as 200 mm (mean: 30 mm) {5711,1309}.

## Histopathology

Melanotic neuroectodermal tumour of infancy comprises a biphasic population of small neuroblastic cells and larger melanin-producing epithelial cells arranged in alveolar nests, cords, and trabeculae, infiltrating a dense, vascularized, fibrocollagenous stroma. The melanotic epithelial cells typically surround the small cells and may form tubuloglandular structures. The small neuroblast-like cells may rarely produce a neurofibrillary matrix {4786}. Infiltration of bone and entrapped

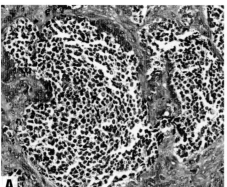 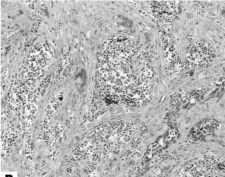 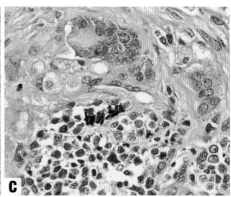

**Fig. 13.45** Melanotic neuroectodermal tumour of infancy. **A** Small primitive cells with associated larger epithelioid cells. **B** Aggregates of tumour cells separated by fibrous stroma. There are small blue cells, with larger epithelial cells at the periphery, some of which contain melanin pigment. **C** High-power view of small neuroblast-like cells with hyperchromatic nuclei and scant cytoplasm, which are associated with larger epithelial cells with vesicular nuclei and cytoplasmic pigment.

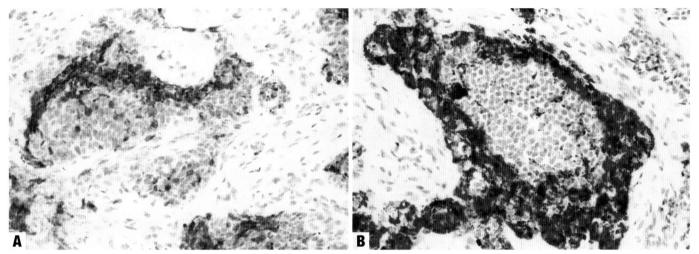

**Fig. 13.46** Melanotic neuroectodermal tumour of infancy. **A** The small neuroblast-like cells are highlighted with synaptophysin, but the melanin-containing epithelial cells are not. **B** Epithelial cells at the periphery of the tumour cell nests are highlighted by HMB45.

odontogenic tissue is frequently present. Mitoses and necrosis are generally absent.

### Immunohistochemistry

Seldom necessary for diagnosis, immunohistochemistry demonstrates that both small and large tumour cells express vimentin and synaptophysin but are typically negative for chromogranin, neurofilaments, S100, and desmin. The large cells coexpress pancytokeratin, HMB45, and melan-A, confirming dual epithelial and melanocytic features, but are negative for other melanoma markers. Rarely, membranous expression of CD99, as well as focal rhabdomyoblastic and glial differentiation, may be seen {4786,5493,1926}.

### Differential diagnosis

The differential diagnosis includes other malignant small round cell tumours, usually with worse prognoses, such as Ewing sarcoma, rhabdomyosarcoma, and lymphoma. However, these other tumours lack the characteristic biphasic melanin-producing, keratin-positive epithelial cells and the synaptophysin-positive neuroblast-like cells.

### Cytology

Smears are cellular with discrete biphasic populations of tumour cells composed of monomorphic small cells with scant cytoplasm and round nuclei with fine chromatin, and large epithelioid cells with vesicular nuclei and intracytoplasmic melanin pigment {3486,2454,191}.

### Diagnostic molecular pathology

Not relevant

### Essential and desirable diagnostic criteria

*Essential:* biphasic small neuroblast-like cells and large melanotic epithelial cells arranged in lobules separated by fibro-collagenous stroma.

*Desirable:* patient aged < 1 year; jaw location; bone destruction; epithelial cells positive for keratin and HMB45.

### Staging

Not relevant

### Prognosis and prediction

Approximately 20–30% of tumours recur, usually within 6 months {1309,4786,5882,5597}, especially in patients aged < 4.5 months at diagnosis {5711,1309}. Rarely, melanotic neuroectodermal tumour of infancy behaves in a malignant fashion (in ~2% of cases), with metastases of the neuroblast-like cells, and death {1309}. Predictive factors are unknown {4786}.

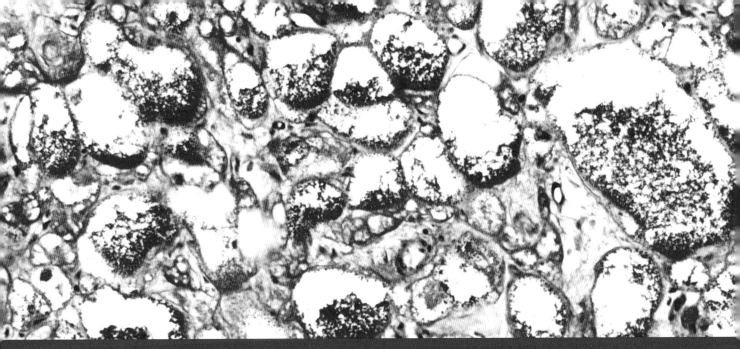

# 14

# Thoracic tumours

Edited by: López-Terrada DH, Reyes-Múgica M, Tsao MS

Lung tumours
    Fetal lung interstitial tumour
    Congenital peribronchial myofibroblastic tumour
    Pleuropulmonary blastoma
Heart tumours
    Cardiac rhabdomyoma

# Fetal lung interstitial tumour

Hill DA
Dishop MK

## Definition
Fetal lung interstitial tumour (FLIT) is a benign tumour of lung interstitial mesenchymal cells, manifesting as a solid or spongy lung mass in neonates.

## ICD-O coding
None

## ICD-11 coding
2F00.Y Other specified benign neoplasm of middle ear or respiratory system

## Related terminology
None

## Subtype(s)
None

## Localization
Lung

## Clinical features
FLIT manifests in the first 3 months of life as a solid or microcystic lung mass {1765}. Most infants present with respiratory difficulties. Imaging studies show well-circumscribed solid or partially cystic masses. Some cases are detectable by prenatal ultrasound. One prenatally diagnosed infant presented with hydrops {3979}.

## Epidemiology
Insufficient data

## Etiology
Unknown

## Pathogenesis
The pathogenesis is unknown. A subset of cases are associated with *ALK* gene fusions {5191,6869}.

## Macroscopic appearance
FLIT appears as well-circumscribed, intraparenchymal, solid or spongy microcystic masses ranging from 20 to 70 mm in size.

## Histopathology
FLIT consists of immature-appearing airspaces with widened septa containing uniform, bland, evenly spaced mesenchymal cells {1765}. These cells have round to ovoid nuclei with dispersed chromatin and a rim of clear or pale-pink cytoplasm and well-defined cell borders. Airway spaces are lined by flattened or cuboidal epithelium with clear cytoplasm. Some cases show areas of fibroblastic or myofibroblastic cells that expand the septa and overgrow the airspaces. These areas may have scattered inflammatory cells including plasma cells and resemble inflammatory myofibroblastic tumour. It is notable that foci resembling inflammatory myofibroblastic tumour appear to arise as the patient (tumour) ages {1765,6869}. The tumour is well demarcated from normal lung with or without a

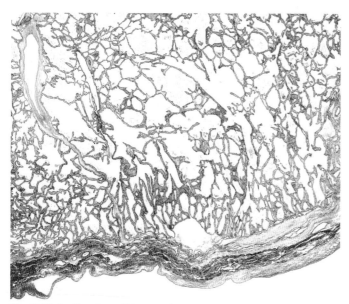

**Fig. 14.01** Fetal lung interstitial tumour. A localized mass showing spongiform alveolus-like structures resembling lung of 20–24 weeks' gestation. Note the thick capsule.

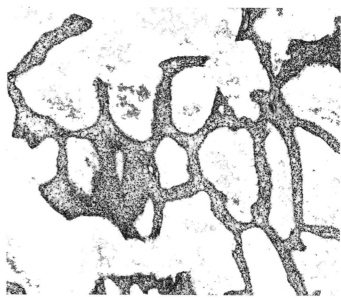

**Fig. 14.02** Fetal lung interstitial tumour. Interstitial cells are monotonous and uniformly distributed, with the walls covered by native epithelium.

thin fibrous capsule. Tumour cells show positivity for vimentin with variable staining for SMA and desmin. Both the interstitial mesenchymal cells and the lining cells contain abundant glycogen. FLIT resembles type I pleuropulmonary blastoma in that it shows proliferation of interstitial mesenchymal cells and arises in early infancy. FLIT tumour cells are more uniformly distributed in the septa and have smaller airspaces than those in type I pleuropulmonary blastoma. Cytologically, FLIT cells lack nuclear hyperchromatism and mitotic activity and have better-defined cytoplasm than type I pleuropulmonary blastoma cells.

## Cytology
Not relevant

## Diagnostic molecular pathology
Some cases of FLIT have shown *ALK* fusions, specifically *A2M::ALK* {5191,6869}.

## Essential and desirable diagnostic criteria
*Essential:* a well-circumscribed, solid or spongy lung mass in an infant; histology shows widened alveolar septa containing bland, uniform mesenchymal cells.

## Staging
Not relevant

## Prognosis and prediction
With the caveat that FLIT is rare and follow-up is limited, there have been no reports of local recurrence or metastatic disease.

# Congenital peribronchial myofibroblastic tumour

Vargas SO
Hill DA

## Definition

Congenital peribronchial myofibroblastic tumour is a solid fibroblastic/myofibroblastic tumour developing in utero or in infancy and composed of mitotically active but histologically bland myofibroblasts arranged in fascicles and resembling congenital mesoblastic nephroma / infantile fibrosarcoma.

## ICD-O coding

8827/1 Congenital peribronchial myofibroblastic tumour

## ICD-11 coding

2F00.Y & XH85R1 Other specified benign neoplasm of middle ear or respiratory system & Myofibroblastic tumour, peribronchial

## Related terminology

*Acceptable:* NTRK-rearranged mesenchymal tumour (for a subset of cases).
*Not recommended:* bronchopulmonary fibrosarcoma; congenital bronchopulmonary leiomyosarcoma.

## Subtype(s)

None

## Localization

Lung, with peribronchovascular distribution

## Clinical features

The tumour may be evident on antenatal imaging, and it may be associated with hydrops fetalis. Other presentations range from fetal demise or respiratory distress in the newborn period to an incidental radiological mass in an asymptomatic infant. Large size (> 50 mm) and unilateral involvement are typical.

## Epidemiology

The tumour is extremely rare, documented only in case reports. There are no known predisposing factors or syndromic associations.

## Etiology

Unknown

## Pathogenesis

The resemblance to NTRK-rearranged mesenchymal tumour suggests the possibility of an NTRK or other kinase gene fusion. To date, three lung tumours called "congenital peribronchial myofibroblastic tumours" have been reported to harbour *ETV6::NTRK3* rearrangement {6655}, but these tumours were not illustrated histologically, and the finding has not been confirmed in other histologically convincing cases {1154}. Of note, there is debate about whether such a finding should automatically instead classify this tumour as a primary pulmonary infantile fibrosarcoma {1154,6655,2999}. Although congenital peribronchial myofibroblastic tumour bears some morphological similarity to congenital *A2M::ALK*-fused tumours reported as "fetal lung interstitial tumour" {5191} and "inflammatory myofibroblastic tumour" {6869}, cartilage proliferation has not been described in these congenital *ALK*-fused mesenchymal tumours, and their relationship to peribronchial myofibroblastic tumour remains unknown at the moment.

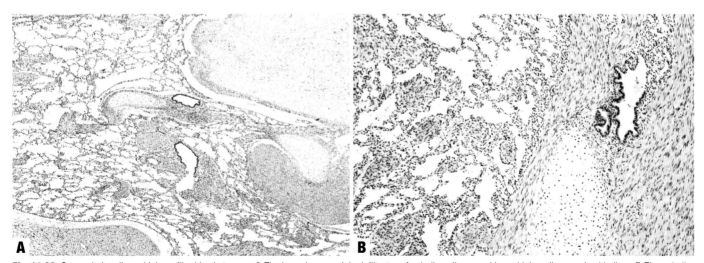

**Fig. 14.03** Congenital peribronchial myofibroblastic tumour. **A** The lung shows nodular infiltrates of spindle cells around bronchial cartilage and epithelium. **B** The spindle-shaped tumour cells are cytologically bland and infiltrate around the bronchial epithelium and cartilage. There is also extension of tumour cells into the interstitium of surrounding alveolar walls.

## Macroscopic appearance
The tumour is pale-tan and firm, and it typically occupies a substantial portion of a lobe or lobes of fetal/infant lung; it surrounds large airways and may connect to the pleura.

## Histopathology
The tumour is composed of interlacing fascicles of uniform spindle cells with eosinophilic cytoplasm and poorly defined cell borders. Nuclei are mitotically active but histologically bland; rare atypical mitoses have been reported {201,3070,4518,1640}. Growth mainly surrounds bronchi and extends along interlobular septa and pleura; there is some extension into alveolar septa. Large islands of benign cartilage located mainly within peribronchial regions are characteristic. The spindle cells are generally positive for SMA; they may also be positive for desmin and S100. Congenital peribronchial myofibroblastic tumour lacks the epithelium-lined cysts and small islands of primitive cartilage that can be observed in the cyst walls of type I pleuropulmonary blastoma; it also lacks the subepithelial condensation of cells (cambium layer), areas of dense cellularity, myogenic differentiation, and anaplasia that can be observed in type II and type III pleuropulmonary blastoma. The cells of congenital peribronchial myofibroblastic tumour lack the pulmonary interstitial glycogenosis–like appearance of the spindle cells of fetal lung interstitial tumour, which have small, delicate nuclei and variably clear cytoplasm {1765}.

## Cytology
Not relevant

## Diagnostic molecular pathology
No firm molecular diagnostic criteria are available, although demonstration of *ETV6::NTRK3* rearrangement may be helpful.

## Essential and desirable diagnostic criteria
*Essential:* interlacing fascicles of uniform, histologically bland spindle cells that are mitotically active; peribronchial accentuation of growth; an associated proliferation of benign-appearing bronchial cartilage.

## Staging
Not relevant

## Prognosis and prediction
The tumour is proposed to be benign because of a lack of documented recurrence; however, there are a limited number of reported patients, and it is difficult to rule out the possibility of borderline malignant / rarely metastasizing behaviour as can be observed in soft tissue infantile fibrosarcoma, cellular mesoblastic nephroma of the kidney, and other NTRK-associated mesenchymal tumours.

# Pleuropulmonary blastoma

Hill DA

## Definition

Pleuropulmonary blastoma (PPB) is an embryonal tumour that manifests as a cystic and/or solid mass in the lung in infants and young children.

## ICD-O coding

8973/3 Pleuropulmonary blastoma
8973/3 Pleuropulmonary blastoma, type I
8973/3 Pleuropulmonary blastoma, type Ir
8973/3 Pleuropulmonary blastoma, type II
8973/3 Pleuropulmonary blastoma, type III

## ICD-11 coding

2C25.Y & XH2FY9 Other specified malignant neoplasms of bronchus or lung & Pleuropulmonary blastoma

## Related terminology

*Not recommended:* rhabdomyosarcoma arising in congenital cystic adenomatoid malformation; pulmonary blastoma of childhood; pulmonary sarcoma arising in mesenchymal cystic hamartoma; embryonal rhabdomyosarcoma arising within congenital bronchogenic cyst; pulmonary blastoma associated with cystic lung disease; pleuropulmonary blastoma in congenital cystic adenomatoid malformation.

## Subtype(s)

Pleuropulmonary blastoma types I, Ir, II, and III

## Localization

PPB occurs in the lung and derives from lung mesenchyme or subpleural mesenchyme {4372}.

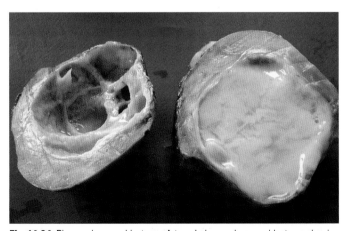

**Fig. 14.04** Pleuropulmonary blastoma. A type I pleuropulmonary blastoma showing a typical loculated cystic architecture (left) after removal of purulent fluid from superimposed infection (right).

## Clinical features

### Signs and symptoms

The clinical presentation of PPB varies by age and tumour type. Children with type I PPB present at a median age of 9 months with shortness of breath with or without pneumothorax secondary to cyst rupture. Some children are asymptomatic, and a cyst is diagnosed as an incidental finding on chest X-ray. Children with type II or type III PPB are typically older (median age: 36 and 42 months, respectively) and present with shortness of breath, weight loss, and fever {4615}.

### Imaging

CT is the preferred imaging modality for detecting tumours/cysts, determining site(s) of disease, and helping to classify tumours as purely cystic (type I), cystic and solid (type II), or purely solid (type III). Plain X-ray images are insensitive to small changes and cannot reliably distinguish between masses and consolidations.

## Epidemiology

The prevalence of germline pathogenic *DICER1* variation is between 1 in 3 000 and 1 in 10 600 individuals {3579}. There are no known ethnic or geographical differences in the incidence of PPB. According to the more conservative estimate, there are probably > 38 000 individuals in the USA and > 765 000 individuals worldwide with a pathogenic *DICER1* variation. Thyroid neoplasia and lung cysts appear to be the most common phenotype for these individuals {3541,6689}. In addition to individuals with pathogenic germline variation, approximately 16% of children with PPB develop these cancers in the absence of an identifiable genetic predisposition, through biallelic tumour-specific *DICER1* mutations {860}. The malignant component derives from immature lung mesenchyme, which has the capacity to differentiate into multiple sarcomatous lineages including rhabdomyosarcoma, fibrosarcoma, and chondrosarcoma.

## Etiology

PPB was first recognized as a distinct clinicopathological entity in 1988 {4372}, and the International Pleuropulmonary Blastoma/*DICER1* Registry (https://www.ppbregistry.org/) was subsequently created to register and study cases. One of the early observations in children with PPB was that disease could be multifocal, could run in families, and co-occurred with other uncommon conditions such as cystic nephroma, embryonal rhabdomyosarcoma, and Sertoli–Leydig cell tumour {5646}. A linkage study of families with multiple affected individuals led to the identification of germline mutations in *DICER1* (MIM number: 606241) as the major genetic factor in this predisposition, now known as *DICER1* syndrome {2892}. *DICER1* encodes a key enzyme that is required to cleave precursor microRNAs into their mature, active form. MicroRNAs modulate gene expression and are critical in organ formation in the embryo and in

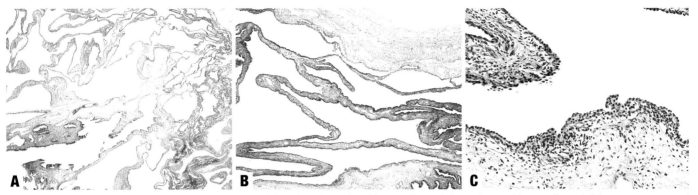

**Fig. 14.05** Type I pleuropulmonary blastoma. **A** Low-power view of the multilocular cystic architecture of a type I pleuropulmonary blastoma. Expanded airspaces are separated by septa of variable thickness. **B** Medium-power view showing intersecting septa lined by bronchiolar epithelium. Small areas of subepithelial mesenchyme in the cyst wall are seen at the bottom of the image. **C** High-power view of a cyst wall shows focal subepithelial collections of primitive cells in a pale-blue matrix. This portion of the cyst is lined by cuboidal alveolar type II pneumocytes.

the prevention of cancer {637}. *DICER1* syndrome thus became the first familial cancer predisposition syndrome linked to a systemic defect in microRNA biogenesis. This gene discovery has led to imaging-based surveillance of children/families that carry the pathogenic *DICER1* variation {541}.

## Pathogenesis

PPB is the most common primary lung neoplasm of childhood and is analogous to other organ-based tumours of childhood, such as Wilms tumour, neuroblastoma, and hepatoblastoma. Germline pathogenic *DICER1* variants that define the syndrome are always loss-of-function (mostly nonsense or frameshift) mutations that truncate the *DICER1* coding sequence {2892,860}. Like other tumour suppressor genes, germline allelic loss-of-function mutations in *DICER1* create tumour susceptibility but appear to be insufficient for initiating tumorigenesis. In addition to the germline allelic loss of function, virtually all PPBs acquire a pathogenic *DICER1* missense variant in the second *DICER1* allele affecting one of five codons – p.E1705, p.D1709, p.G1809, p.D1810, or p.E1813 – in the RNase IIIb domain of DICER1 protein {2849, 6329,5661}. Amino acid substitutions at any one of these five positions can disable the RNase IIIb catalytic domain and prevent an entire class of microRNAs, those from the 5p arm of the precursor hairpin, from being produced {5661}. Among the 5p microRNAs lacking in PPB is the let-7 family that modulates the expression of oncofetal gene networks during early development. In addition to this unique combination of biallelic loss-of-function plus hotspot mutations in *DICER1*, mutations and/or loss of *TP53* are also very common {5661,6329}.

## Macroscopic appearance

There are three main pathological types of PPB, defined by their macroscopic appearance {4372,5645}. Type I PPB is completely cystic in nature. Grossly, the cysts are air-filled and multilocular, with thin, delicate septa. About 40% of type I tumours are multifocal. Type II tumours are composed of a cystic component but in addition have grossly visible thickening of the septa or formation of a solid mass. Type III PPB is purely solid.

## Histopathology
### Pathology of type I PPB
Microscopically, type I PPB has a characteristic architecture of expanded airspaces and wider-than-normal alveolar septa

lined by alveolar- or bronchiolar-type epithelium {2893}. In classic cases, small nodules of primitive mesenchymal cells are found beneath the epithelium in the cyst wall. These cells may be a localized to a single focus or several foci, or they can be arranged more diffusely in layers beneath the epithelium, like they are in botryoid-type embryonal rhabdomyosarcoma. The primitive small cells may display cytoplasmic tails of pink cytoplasm with striations (rhabdomyosarcomatous differentiation), which is more prominent in the layers most distant from the epithelium. Small nodules of immature cartilage or mature spindle cells may also be found in the septa and are not necessarily accompanied by the small primitive cells. Because the small primitive cells or nodules of cartilage are present only focally in some cases, it may be necessary to submit an entire cyst specimen for microscopic examination.

### Pathology of type Ir PPB
In the course of the family linkage study it became apparent that there were relatives of children with PPB who had had lung cysts for years, sometimes decades, without malignant transformation. Some of these cysts from older relatives had been resected and were available for microscopic examination {2893}. These purely cystic lesions show the architecture of type I PPB but lack primitive mesenchymal elements. These cysts were termed "type I regressed", although it is not known if these lesions ever contained a primitive mesenchymal component. Lacking a primitive mesenchymal component, type Ir PPB is thought to have limited biological potential. Differentiating type Ir PPB from blebs or postinfectious cysts can be difficult.

### Pathology of type II and type III PPB
Type II PPBs differ from type I tumours in that the primitive tumour cells are no longer limited to a subepithelial distribution, and they expand the septa and form solid sarcomatous nodules {2893}. Type III tumours represent a complete overgrowth of the cystic portions of the tumour and are purely solid. Microscopically, the solid portions of a type II PPB and a type III PPB appear as a multipatterned sarcoma that typically includes areas with (1) solid, cohesive nests of undifferentiated cells with nuclear hyperchromatism and high N:C ratios (blastemal pattern); (2) spindle-shaped, stellate, and ovoid cells with variable amounts of eosinophilic cytoplasm in a pale-blue myxoid matrix (embryonal rhabdomyosarcoma pattern); (3) compact

arrangements of spindle cells with hyperchromatic nuclei in a fascicular or herringbone pattern (spindle cell or fibrosarcoma pattern); and/or (4) cartilage, often with immature or overtly chondrosarcomatous features. One or more of these elements may predominate in any one tumour. Anaplasia, defined in the same way as in Wilms tumour, occurs in 75% of type II tumours and 90% of type III tumours.

*Differential diagnosis*

Chest wall or mediastinal rhabdomyosarcoma can be challenging to distinguish from PPB. Limited core biopsies of PPB may show a rhabdomyosarcomatous pattern. Attention to the primary location of the mass in the chest wall, diaphragm, or mediastinum – rather than in the lung parenchyma – may help guide the diagnosis, because the lung parenchyma is a rare site for a primary embryonal rhabdomyosarcoma. *DICER1* mutation testing of tumour tissue can also be used to confirm a diagnosis of PPB. Almost all PPBs in infancy are purely cystic. Nevertheless, spongy tumours such as the fetal lung interstitial tumour {1765} and solid tumours such as the congenital peribronchial myofibroblastic tumour, which occur in infants, may present a diagnostic challenge. One of the more common diagnostic dilemmas occurs when encountering a cystic mass with a subepithelial spindle cell component in an adolescent. It is uncommon for PPBs with a primitive cell component to occur in adolescence and adults. The primary differential diagnosis for this situation is with cystic synovial sarcoma. PPBs are typically more heterogeneous than synovial sarcomas, but the spindle cell components of PPB and synovial sarcoma can be remarkably similar. Immunohistochemistry demonstrating epithelial markers or identification of a fusion protein involving the gene *SS18* (*SYT*) is helpful for making a diagnosis of synovial sarcoma.

## Cytology

FNAB has been used to diagnose PPB, typically showing primitive malignant mesenchymal and small ovoid blastemal elements {6441}. Pleural effusion cytology is rarely helpful in making a diagnosis, because tumour cells are rarely shed except in cases of tumour rupture {5006}.

## Diagnostic molecular pathology

Identification of pathogenic loss-of-function and RNase IIIb missense *DICER1* variations in tumour tissue is diagnostic of PPB. In older children with cystic sarcomatous masses, RT-PCR or FISH for synovial sarcoma gene fusions may also be helpful to rule out PPB.

## Essential and desirable diagnostic criteria

*Purely cystic tumours*
*Essential:*
- Young patient age (usually < 1 year)
- Identification of a subepithelial collection of primitive cells or a nodule of cartilage in a multilocular cyst that has been adequately sampled (for type Ir tumours, which lack a primitive cellular component, the diagnosis may remain challenging)

*Desirable:*
- Identification of the *DICER1* pathogenic variant in the germ line, tumour tissue, or both

*Cystic and solid / solid lung mass*
*Essential:*
- Young patient age
- A primitive sarcoma with multiple patterns including rhabdomyosarcoma, spindle cell sarcoma, cartilage, blastemal nodules, and anaplasia

*Desirable:*
- Identification of the *DICER1* pathogenic variant in the germ line, tumour tissue, or both

## Staging

There is no formal staging system for PPB. For patients with type II or type III PPB, head MRI and bone scan are both recommended for the evaluation of metastatic disease; plain radiographs can be used for areas of concern seen on the bone scan. Echocardiography may be necessary to define intracardiac extension of the tumour, tumour thrombi, or pericardial effusion.

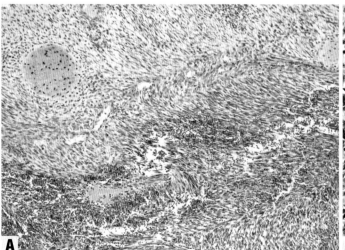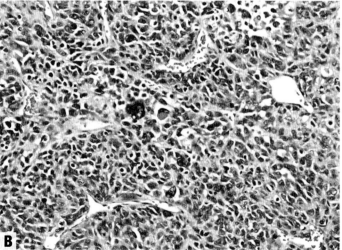

**Fig. 14.06** Solid pleuropulmonary blastoma. **A** Spindle cell sarcoma and malignant cartilage are two other patterns seen in solid portions of type II and type III pleuropulmonary blastomas. **B** High-grade malignant cells with hyperchromatic and enlarged nuclei are common in solid portions of type II and type III pleuropulmonary blastomas. Regions of anaplasia seen here are associated with *TP53* mutations.

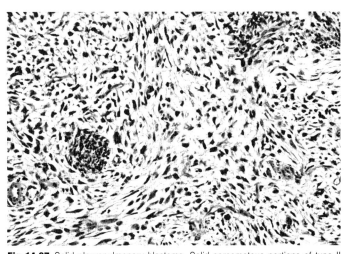

**Fig. 14.07** Solid pleuropulmonary blastoma. Solid sarcomatous portions of type II and type III pleuropulmonary blastomas commonly have spindled, ovoid, and stellate cells in a pale-blue matrix, resembling embryonal rhabdomyosarcoma. These areas are often associated with more tightly packed blastemal nests of cells with hyperchromatic nuclei and high N:C ratios. A small round blastemal nest is seen in the lower-left portion of this photomicrograph.

### Prognosis and prediction

The pathological type is the only independent prognostic factor currently known. Survival rates decrease as PPB type progresses.

Type I PPBs are limited to the lung and are treated with complete surgical resection with or without adjuvant chemotherapy.

Type II and type III tumours are treated with complete surgical excision whenever possible and with high-dose sarcoma-based chemotherapy. Type II and type III tumours can recur locally after incomplete or piecemeal excision. The most common metastatic site is the brain; as many as 40% of children with type III tumours experience brain metastasis. Tumours may also metastasize to bone, but tumour spread to other sites is rare {4615}. Radiation is typically reserved for local recurrence and brain metastatic disease.

For type I tumours, the survival rate is 91%. However, survival rates decrease to 74% for type II tumours and 53% for type III tumours {4615}.

# Cardiac rhabdomyoma

Basso C

## Definition
Rhabdomyoma is a benign tumour of striated cardiac myocytes.

## ICD-O coding
8900/0 Cardiac rhabdomyoma

## ICD-11 coding
2E86.2 & XH8WG9 Rhabdomyoma & Rhabdomyoma, NOS
2E86.2 & XH4729 Rhabdomyoma & Fetal rhabdomyoma
2E86.2 & XH4BG5 Rhabdomyoma & Adult rhabdomyoma

## Related terminology
*Not recommended:* congenital glycogenic tumour.

## Subtype(s)
None

## Localization
The most frequent location for cardiac rhabdomyomas is the ventricular myocardium, but they may occur in atria as well. Although mostly intramural, they may also appear as intracavitary pedunculated or sessile masses {6365,2949,571}.

## Clinical features
The clinical features depend on the localization, number, and dimensions of the tumour(s). The frequency of prenatal detection is increasing dramatically and usually occurs when arrhythmia, hydrops, delayed fetal growth, or a family history of tuberous sclerosis is reported {2949,2902}. Children may be asymptomatic or mildly symptomatic, presenting with a cardiac murmur {560,571,2224}. Haemodynamic impairment can occur, either due to the intracavitary protrusion of a large mass causing outflow obstruction and valve impairment or in the setting of extensive intramural growth with systolic and diastolic dysfunction {5013,5276,5277}. Both atrial and ventricular arrhythmias have been described, as well as conduction abnormalities due to direct compression of the specialized conduction system {3111}. When located in the atrioventricular junction, the tumour may serve as an accessory pathway with pre-excitation {4442}.

### Imaging
Two-dimensional echocardiography remains the main diagnostic tool, and rhabdomyomas manifest with a homogeneous echogenicity, unlike other cardiac masses. By cardiac MRI, the signal characteristics are almost identical to those of the normal myocardium {2224,528}.

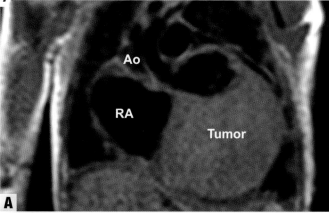

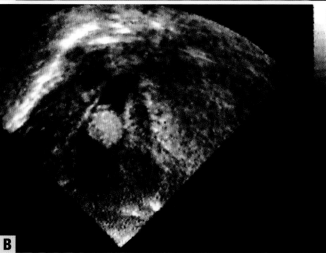

**Fig. 14.08** Cardiac rhabdomyoma. **A** Electrocardiogram-triggered breath-hold proton density (PD)-weighted and T1-weighted fast spin echo MRI in the coronal plane, showing a large homogeneous isointense mass involving the left ventricle wall. **B** 2D echocardiography showing an intracavitary rhabdomyoma of the right ventricular outflow tract.

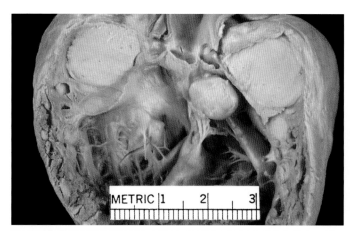

**Fig. 14.09** Cardiac rhabdomyoma. Autopsy specimen demonstrating multiple cardiac rhabdomyomas involving the left ventricle. The masses can be seen obstructing the ventricular outflow tract.

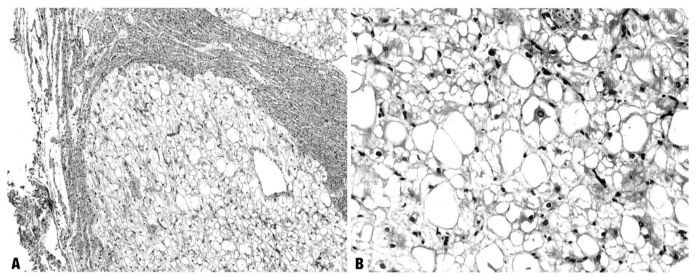

**Fig. 14.10** Cardiac rhabdomyoma. **A** Panoramic view showing the border between tumour and normal cardiac myocytes. **B** At high magnification, enlarged swollen myocytes with clear cytoplasm are visible. Strands of cytoplasm are connected to the peripheral cell membrane.

## Epidemiology

Rhabdomyoma is the most common heart neoplasm in the paediatric age, accounting for > 60% of cardiac tumours {560,571, 2224}. It is also the most common tumour diagnosed prenatally {2949}. Although its prevalence in surgical series is lower than that of other cardiac tumours, because it does not necessarily represent an indication to resection, in a multicentre surgical series of paediatric cardiac tumours, rhabdomyoma was the most frequent (36% of cases) {5277}. As many as 70–90% of cardiac rhabdomyomas have been reported in association with tuberous sclerosis {799,2714,6365,2902}, and > 50% of children with tuberous sclerosis are diagnosed with a cardiac rhabdomyoma by echocardiography {7461}. However, its true prevalence in patients with tuberous sclerosis probably remains underestimated.

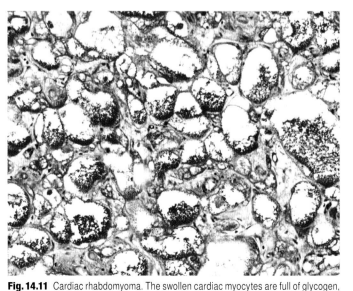

**Fig. 14.11** Cardiac rhabdomyoma. The swollen cardiac myocytes are full of glycogen, shown on PAS stain.

## Etiology

Two genes have been identified in tuberous sclerosis (an autosomal dominant disease with variable penetrance and expression): *TSC1* (9q34), which encodes the protein hamartin; and *TSC2* (16p13.3), which encodes the protein tuberin {2902}. These two proteins normally combine to suppress the growth-promoting mTORC1. Consequently, dysregulation of the TSC1-TSC2 complex is a molecular driver of tumorigenesis.

## Pathogenesis

Rhabdomyoma is a lesion of striated muscle without proliferative activity and as such it is considered to be a hamartoma of developing cardiac myocytes (i.e. embryonic cardiac myoblasts) {6790}.

## Macroscopic appearance

Rhabdomyomas are well-defined, unencapsulated, typically multiple, white-yellow masses of variable size {2902}.

## Histopathology

They consist of well-demarcated but not encapsulated nodules, easily distinguished from the surrounding myocardium, with enlarged vacuolated cells. Abundant glycogen accounts for the clear sarcoplasm of the myocytes, and the characteristic spider-cell feature is the consequence of radial sarcoplasmic extensions emanating from the centrally placed nucleus to the sarcoplasmic membrane {2902,6790}. Transmission electron microscopy shows myocytes with abundant glycogen, rare mitochondria, and peripherally distributed intercalated discs {2078}. Positive expression of markers of striated muscle cells (myoglobin, desmin, actin, and vimentin) is detected by immunohistochemistry {4963}.

## Cytology

Not relevant

## Diagnostic molecular pathology

Not clinically relevant

## Essential and desirable diagnostic criteria

*Essential:* a collection of vacuolated cells with radial sarcoplasmic extensions extending from the nucleus to the sarcoplasmic membrane.

*Desirable:* a diagnosis of tuberous sclerosis.

## Staging

Not relevant

## Prognosis and prediction

The most common symptoms necessitating intervention are ventricular arrhythmia or obstruction. Despite what can be considered rather dramatic presentations, cardiac rhabdomyomas are peculiar in that they have a propensity to resolve spontaneously with age. For this reason, a conservative approach is typically warranted unless the patient is symptomatic and refractory to medical therapy. Partial resection, aimed at preserving adjacent vital cardiac structures, can still be successful owing to this time-based regression {5277}. mTOR pathway inhibitors (such as everolimus) have been used with success to hasten tumour regression {1697}.

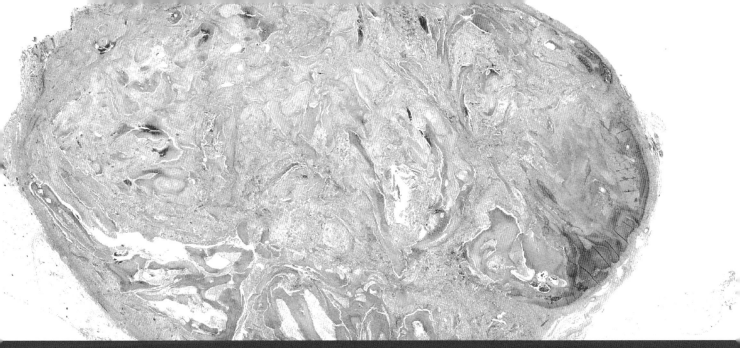

# 15

# Skin tumours

Edited by: Reyes-Múgica M, Singh R

Hamartomas
    Hamartomas
Epithelial neoplasms
  Squamous neoplasms
    Angiokeratoma
    Epidermal naevi
    Pilomatricoma
Melanocytic neoplasms
  Naevi
    Congenital naevi
    Junctional, compound, and dermal naevi
    Blue naevus
    Spitz naevus
    Pigmented spindle cell naevus (Reed naevus)
  Melanoma
    Melanoma

# Skin tumours: Introduction

Singh R
Jarzembowski JA
Lazar AJ

Skin tumours in children are generally infrequent, and the predominant types are benign or metastatic lesions. This results in a pitfall created by a low index of suspicion for malignant paediatric skin tumours, leading to possible delays in diagnosis and treatment {1405}.

Most of the conventional cutaneous tumours are extensively covered in the fourth-edition WHO classification of skin tumours. In this chapter, emphasis is placed on lesions that are particularly frequent in children, in which a developmental perspective has been provided, given their specific genetic basis, such as mosaicism in epidermal naevi or neural crest migration in congenital melanocytic naevi. Benign and malignant melanocytic proliferations have received considerable attention, because these are among the most frequent paediatric skin tumours and their diagnosis may be quite challenging.

Some entities are not mentioned, and readers are referred to the corresponding chapter of the *Skin tumours* volume.

## *BAP1*-inactivated melanocytic naevus/tumour

An entity not included is *BAP1*-inactivated melanocytic naevus/tumour (BIMN/T), which is characterized by mutations in *BAP1* {7539} and which most studies to date suggest has an indolent course, although long-term data are still needed {957}. Acceptable related terms include "BAPoma", "BAP-deficient naevus", and "BAP1-deficient tumour"; the term "melanocytic *BAP1*-associated intradermal tumour" is not recommended. No subtypes have been described. Clinically, BIMN/Ts can be single or multiple cutaneous lesions, sometimes mimicking dermal naevi or Spitz tumours. Some patients report a sudden change in the colour or size of a longstanding naevus {7538, 958}. Epidemiologically, most lesions appear during the first two decades of life, but they can occur at any age {958}. BIMN/T may be sporadic or arise in patients with germline mutations in *BAP1* (*BAP1* tumour predisposition syndrome; MIM number: 614327) {7539}. BIMN/Ts typically have an initiating *BRAF* mutation (although *NRAS*-mutated cases exist {957}), followed by biallelic mutation and/or deletion involving the *BAP1* gene {7374}. In most cases, BIMN/T manifests as well-circumscribed dome-shaped or pedunculated papules that are skin-coloured, reddish, or light-brown, averaging 5 mm in size {4861}. Histologically, BIMN/T is a predominantly dermal lesion composed of epithelioid naevomelanocytes with well-defined, abundant eosinophilic cytoplasm; vesicular nuclei; and prominent nucleoli. A conventional naevus is frequently seen in the background {957}. Some cases show marked atypical features and are classified as intermediate-grade melanocytic tumours. Most tumours lose nuclear BAP1 staining in the epithelioid component and have *BRAF* mutations {957,2326,7539}. In rare cases with retained nuclear BAP1 staining, DNA sequencing may confirm *BAP1* mutation. Essential diagnostic criteria include large epithelioid cells and loss of BAP1 by immunohistochemistry. Desirable diagnostic criteria include molecular demonstration of *BAP1* and *BRAF* mutations. Staging is not relevant. Regarding prognosis and prediction, BIMN/T has a low risk of recurrence, but rare cases have progressed to melanoma {2326}. Comparative genomic hybridization and FISH may help to discriminate between benign and malignant tumours. Patients with multiple lesions require testing for germline *BAP1* mutations {7537}.

# Hamartomas

Torrelo A
Colmenero I
Kozakewich HP

## Definition

A hamartoma is a benign proliferation of tissues native to the area where the growth occurs. Hamartomas are considered to be developmental abnormalities, often caused by postzygotic mutations (mosaicism). Skin hamartomas can be classified according to their predominant tissue or their genetic somatic mutation. Epidermal hamartomas (naevi) and vascular hamartomas (malformations) are discussed in other sections of this volume.

## ICD-O coding

None

## ICD-11 coding

LD2D Phakomatoses or hamartoneoplastic syndromes
LC2Y Other specified hamartomata derived from dermal connective tissue

## Related terminology

*Acceptable:* naevus; malformation; choristoma.

## Subtype(s)

See Table 15.01 (p. 928).

## Localization

Hamartomas occur anywhere in the skin, but some types favour specific locations. Connective tissue naevi (CTNs) are predominantly solitary, although they may be multiple, with symmetrical distribution over the back, buttocks, arms, and thighs. Congenital smooth muscle hamartoma (CSMH) involves the trunk or extremities. Becker naevus (BN) occurs frequently in the shoulder or trunk and less commonly in the legs.

## Clinical features

Most cases are congenital, but onset may be delayed in certain types.

CTN is usually an asymptomatic, flesh-coloured dermal plaque composed of closely grouped papules. Often congenital, it may appear during the first few years of life. Lesions may be subtle or associated with a surface texture described as "peau d'orange", "pigskin", or "cobblestone", with marked thickening {7134}. As with other naevi, a linear arrangement occasionally occurs {243,

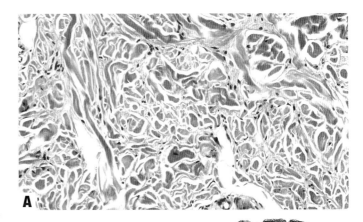

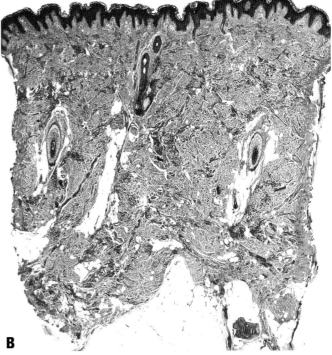

**Fig. 15.02** Collagen naevus. **A** Thick and haphazardly oriented collagen bundles. **B** Thickened reticular dermis.

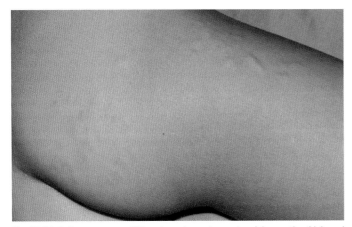

**Fig. 15.01** Collagen naevus. Skin-coloured papules and nodules on the thigh and buttock.

**Table 15.01** The most common types of cutaneous hamartoma (continued on next page)

| Type of naevus | Molecular basis | Distribution | Clinical features | Main histological features |
|---|---|---|---|---|
| **Connective tissue naevi, collagen** | | | | |
| Familial collagenoma {2868} | LEMD3 | Usually plaque; rarely linear | Skin-coloured plaque with confluent papules | Increased dermal collagen bundles |
| Solitary collagenoma | | Usually plaque with confluent papules; rarely linear | Skin-coloured plaque; peau d'orange and thickened plaque | Increased dermal collagen bundles |
| Fibroblastic connective tissue naevus (probably neoplastic) {4785,5441,5900,7264} | | Usually plaque with confluent papules; rarely linear | Red to brownish plaque with confluent papules | Poorly defined proliferation of interlacing bundles of bland spindle cells; entrapped skin adnexa; elastic tissue diminished and fragmented; CD34+ and focal SMA+ |
| Plantar collagenoma of Proteus syndrome {4133} | AKT1 | Localized mass on the foot | Large nodule with cerebriform surface | Increased dermal collagen bundles |
| Shagreen patch, fibrous plaques in tuberous sclerosis {778,3616} | TSC1, TSC2 | Usually small plaques; large plaques usually segmental | Papules or nodules with irregular surface and colour ranging from skin-colour to orange | Increased dermal collagen bundles |
| Facial angiofibromas in tuberous sclerosis {3343} | TSC1, TSC2 | Centrally located on the face | Multiple discrete red papules | Collagenous stroma with concentric orientation around hair follicles and blood vessels, or perpendicular to the epidermis; increased spindled to stellate fibroblasts and increased and dilated blood vessels |
| Folliculocystic and collagen naevus in tuberous sclerosis {7030} | TSC1, TSC2 | Localized mass | Large nodule with comedones, epidermoid cysts, and peau d'orange surface | Thick collagen deposition, concentric perifollicular fibrosis, and keratin-filled infundibular cysts |
| **Connective tissue naevi, elastic tissue** | | | | |
| Juvenile elastoma {5596, 2829} | LEMD3 | Isolated; rarely lines of Blaschko | Small yellowish papules | Increased elastic fibres |
| Pseudoxanthoma elasticum {619} | ABCC6 | Isolated or multiple lesions | Yellow papules, grouped, with pebbly appearance | Fragmentation and mineralization of elastic fibres |
| **Fibrous hamartomas** | | | | |
| Fibrous hamartoma of infancy (probably neoplastic) {166} | EGFR exon 20 insertion/duplication mutations | Localized mass, mostly in the trunk | Subcutaneous nodule | Subcutaneous lesion composed of three elements: (1) myofibroblasts arranged in broad fascicles, (2) nests of small immature mesenchymal cells in a myxoid stroma, and (3) mature adipocytes |
| Precalcaneal congenital fibrolipomatous hamartoma {1944,5222} | | Bilateral plantar nodules | Subcutaneous lesion on the anterior precalcaneal region | Mature adipose tissue enveloped in collagen-fibrous sheaths; there may be an increased number of blood vessels |
| **Subcutaneous naevi** | | | | |
| Naevus psiloliparus (encephalocraniocutaneous lipomatosis) {2703,610,788} | FGFR1, KRAS | Cranial mass with oval/linear shape | Lipomatous lesion on the scalp with partial alopecia; associated features of encephalocraniocutaneous lipomatosis | Abundance of unencapsulated mature adipose tissue producing compression and thinning of the dermis; paucity or absence of mature hair follicles; normal quantities of orphaned arrector pili muscle bundles arranged in a row parallel to the epidermis |
| Naevus lipomatosus superficialis {3319} | | Irregular patch; rarely linear | Clustered skin-coloured, pink, or yellowish papules | Islands of mature adipose tissue in the dermis interposed among the collagen bundles |
| **Smooth muscle hamartomas** | | | | |
| Congenital smooth muscle hamartoma {404,7894} | ACTB | Usually oval patch; rarely linear | Congenital hairy plaque with slight hyperpigmentation; follicular papules | Large and well-defined bundles of smooth muscle randomly oriented in the dermis |
| Becker naevus {967,5390} | ACTB | Localized macule with irregular borders; if large, usually segmental, block-like | Hyperpigmented patch; thick hair develops in adolescence | Increased basal layer pigmentation, mild acanthosis, hyperkeratosis, and regular elongation of rete ridges; variable hypertrichosis; dermal smooth muscle proliferation |
| Michelin tire baby syndrome {2449} | | Generalized | Subcutaneous hypertrophy with regular skin folds | Fragmentation of elastic fibres along with increased smooth muscle mass; increased adipose tissue |

**Table 15.01** The most common types of cutaneous hamartoma (continued)

| Type of naevus | Molecular basis | Distribution | Clinical features | Main histological features |
|---|---|---|---|---|
| **Striated muscle hamartomas** | | | | |
| Naevus of striated muscle {5220} | PIK3CA | Usually segmental, block-like | Segmental overgrowth of the palm with furrowed surface; bone hypertrophy may be associated | Bundles of mature striated muscle replacing the subcutis and extending into the dermis, without any other mesenchymal component |
| Rhabdomyomatous mesenchymal hamartoma {7514, 4689,2836} | | Localized; may be related to branchiae | Irregularly shaped skin tag | Deep dermal and subcutaneous collection of disorganized skeletal muscle fibres, adipose tissue, nerves and adnexal structures |
| **Other skin hamartomas** | | | | |
| Plaque-type CD34+ dermal fibroma (dendrocyte medallion hamartoma) {5948,3850, 6737,4412,1248} | | Localized | Yellow to brown round or oval patch or plaque | CD34+ dermal and hypodermal spindle cell infiltration |

7894}. Unusual clinical forms, including exophytic lesions, have been described.

CSMH appears in the trunk or extremities as a slightly hyperpigmented plaque with thick, dark hairs. Pinpoint follicular papules may also be present. Piloerection often occurs after rubbing (pseudo–Darier sign) {7894,404}.

BN manifests as a unilateral, well-circumscribed, hyperpigmented patch or slightly thickened plaque with irregular borders;

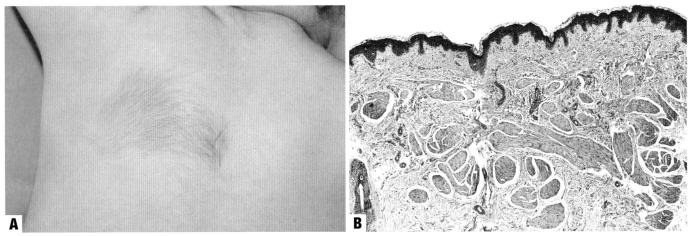

**Fig. 15.03** Congenital smooth muscle hamartoma. **A** A hypertrichotic patch on the back of an infant. **B** Well-defined bundles of randomly oriented bland smooth muscle cells, with a characteristic cleft between the bundles and the surrounding dermis.

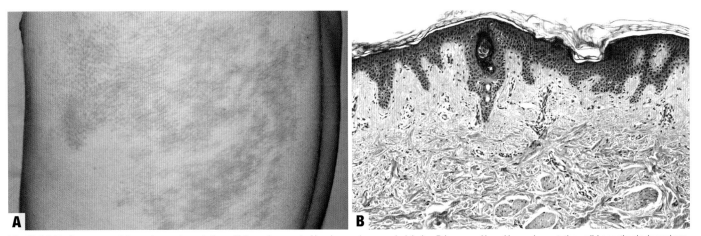

**Fig. 15.04** Becker naevus. **A** Brown hyperpigmentation with irregular serrated borders and coarse dark hairs. **B** Increased basal layer pigmentation, mild acanthosis, hyperkeratosis, and regular elongation of rete ridges together with smooth muscle bundles irregularly dispersed within the dermis.

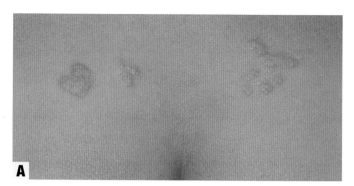

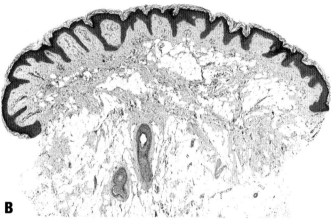

**Fig. 15.05** Naevus lipomatosus superficialis. **A** Soft, skin-coloured papules and nodules on a girl's buttocks. **B** Nests of ectopic mature adipose tissue within the dermis.

hypertrichosis often develops during childhood or adolescence. Lesions are often large, usually > 100 mm in diameter. BN may be present in infancy as light-brown patches or become visible only in later childhood (by adolescence) {5390}. BN syndrome combines BN and muscular or skeletal defects, breast hypoplasia (most frequently ipsilateral), pectoral muscle hypoplasia, and variable thoracic bone anomalies {2702}.

### Epidemiology
CTN is rare worldwide. BN has an estimated prevalence of 0.5% in the male population, and an M:F ratio of 5:1 {7122}. The estimated

prevalence of CSMH is 1 in 2600 live births, with a slight male predominance.

### Etiology
The etiology of most hamartomas remains unclear. CTNs may be isolated (either sporadic or hereditary) or part of a syndrome (see Table 15.02). The shagreen patch of tuberous sclerosis is a CTN. Another form of CTN, dermatofibrosis lenticularis disseminata, is associated with Buschke–Ollendorff syndrome, caused by loss-of-function mutations in *LEMD3* {2829}. Cerebriform CTN of the plantar surface is typically seen in Proteus syndrome {4996,4133}.

### Pathogenesis
See Table 15.01 (p. 929) for mutations identified in different skin hamartomas. The genetic mechanisms are variable, including activating lethal autosomal dominant mutations (e.g. CTNs of Proteus syndrome, or BN), or disseminated mosaicism from second hits in non-lethal autosomal dominant mutations (e.g. CTN in tuberous sclerosis or in Buschke–Ollendorff syndrome).

### Macroscopic appearance
In most cases, biopsies are small and do not allow macroscopic assessment. The clinical features are described above.

### Histopathology
*CTN:* One or more components of extracellular connective tissue (collagen, elastic fibres, or glycosaminoglycans) are present in abnormal amounts. The histopathology of CTN depends on the main component of the naevus {6194,352,5525,7134}. Pure collagenoma is a poorly demarcated area of increased dermal collagen bundles; pure elastoma shows increased elastic fibres only; mixed-type CTN shows both collagen and elastic changes; proteoglycan CTN shows an increased deposition of mucin; and fibroblastic CTN (cellular) is associated with an increased number of fibroblasts {1669,5900,7264,5441}. Many cutaneous lesions in Buschke–Ollendorff syndrome tend to have increased numbers of elastic fibres, but some appear to be primarily collagenous {1762}. Shagreen patches in tuberous sclerosis and Proteus syndrome naevus are collagenomas {2829}.

**Table 15.02** Connective tissue naevi associated with syndromes

| Syndrome | Molecular basis | Type of connective tissue naevus | Other features |
|---|---|---|---|
| Tuberous sclerosis {3183} | Autosomal dominant, biallelic *TSC1*, *TSC2* | Shagreen patch<br>Cephalic fibrous plaque<br>Facial angiofibromas<br>Folliculocystic collagen hamartoma {7030} | CNS tumours, neuropsychological manifestations, kidney tumours, pulmonary cysts, cardiac rhabdomyomas, retinal hamartomas, hypomelanotic macules |
| Buschke–Ollendorff syndrome {1762} | Autosomal dominant, biallelic *LEMD3* | Collagen naevus<br>Dermatofibrosis lenticularis disseminata<br>Elastic tissue naevus | Osteopoikilosis, metaphyseal anomalies |
| Proteus syndrome {2829,4133} | Mosaic *AKT1* | Plantar cerebriform collagenoma | Asymmetrical, disproportionate overgrowth; tumours (ovarian cystadenoma, parotid monomorphic adenoma); lung cysts; dysregulated adipose tissue; epidermal naevus; vascular malformations; facial phenotype |
| Encephalocraniocutaneous lipomatosis {2703,610,788} | Mosaic *FGFR1* or *KRAS* | Naevus psiloliparus | Intracranial lipomas, CNS structural abnormalities, epibulbar choristoma, skin tags |

*CSMH:* Histopathology shows disorganized fascicles of mature smooth muscle in the dermis, often reaching the subcutaneous fat.

*BN:* This is a complex hamartoma showing dermal fascicles of hyperplastic smooth muscle and variable hypertrichosis, elongation of the rete pegs, and increased melanization of basal and suprabasal keratinocytes.

## Cytology
Not relevant

## Diagnostic molecular pathology
Molecular diagnosis can help to classify atypical cases. Because many of these lesions represent mosaicisms, the genetic alteration will only be present in the lesion and not in unaffected skin.

## Essential and desirable diagnostic criteria
*Essential:* variable clinical and histological features (see Table 15.01, p. 929).

*Desirable:* demonstration of a genetic alteration in the affected skin.

## Staging
Not relevant

## Prognosis and prediction
Most hamartomas are stable lesions that do not tend to increase or decrease in size and will persist for life. Treatment is often not necessary.

# Angiokeratoma

Singh V
Calonje JE
Sangüeza OP

## Definition

Angiokeratoma is a cutaneous vascular lesion comprising ectatic, thin-walled vessels in the superficial dermis, associated with epidermal hyperplasia.

## ICD-O coding

9141/0 Angiokeratoma

## ICD-11 coding

EF20.1 Angiokeratoma

## Related terminology

None

## Subtype(s)

*Clinical subtypes*

Angiokeratoma of Mibelli (multiple papules on the digits); angiokeratoma of Fordyce (multiple papules on the external genitalia and upper thighs); angiokeratoma circumscriptum (rare, solitary plaque with confluent smaller papules); angiokeratoma corporis diffusum (multiple papules in a bathing-trunks distribution); solitary and multiple angiokeratomas

## Localization

Location is the defining characteristic in angiokeratoma of Mibelli, angiokeratoma of Fordyce (AF), and angiokeratoma corporis diffusum (AD). Angiokeratoma circumscriptum (AC) has a predilection for the lower extremities.

## Clinical features

Angiokeratoma occurs in localized or diffuse form with solitary or multiple red to black papules, 2–5 mm in size, that may have a scaly or verrucous surface. Rarely, the papules coalesce, forming large (20–70 mm) plaques of AC {3120}. The AD subtype frequently associates with inherited enzyme defects and lysosomal storage disease that affect other organ systems {6234}. Fabry disease was the first enzymatic defect described in association with AD, but many other enzyme defects or lysosomal disorders occur in patients with AD. It is a provisionally unclassified vascular anomaly according to the International Society for the Study of Vascular Anomalies (ISSVA) {7454}.

## Epidemiology

AC frequently manifests at birth or infancy, whereas AF frequently occurs in adults. Other subtypes can arise during childhood and adolescence. Angiokeratoma of Mibelli has a female predominance, and AF has a male predominance. The solitary subtype is the most common, and AC is the least common.

## Etiology

Angiokeratoma is a vascular anomaly, probably representing a congenital or acquired malformation. Solitary paediatric angiokeratoma shows immunohistochemical expression of lymphatic markers in the vascular endothelium {5653,7064},

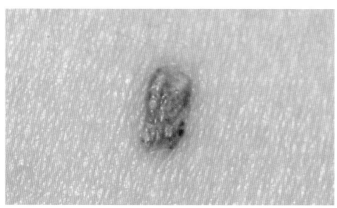

**Fig. 15.06** Angiokeratoma. Clinical appearance.

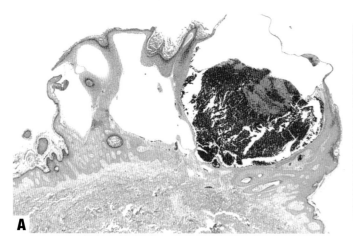

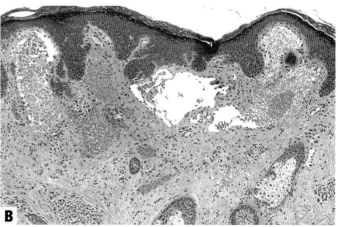

**Fig. 15.07** Angiokeratoma. **A** Exophytic lesion with ectatic vessels showing a thrombus. **B** Vessels abutting epidermis that is variably thick.

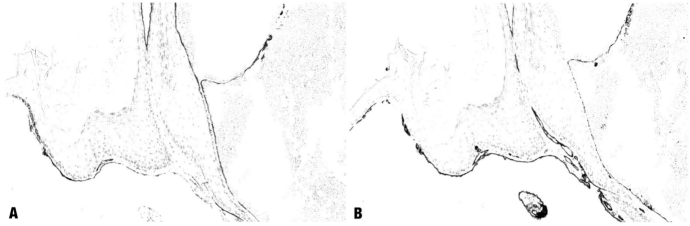

**A**

**B**

**Fig. 15.08** Angiokeratoma. **A** D2-40 is positive by immunohistochemistry. **B** CD31 is positive in vascular endothelium by immunohistochemistry.

suggesting aberrant protein expression by the lesional vessels or a lymphatic-capillary malformation.

## Pathogenesis

The distended capillaries are the primary pathology, whereas the epidermal changes are secondary. Vascular ectasia has been postulated to be due to increased venous pressure in AF and weakening of vessel walls in AD.

## Macroscopic appearance

The papular lesions resemble pigmented lesions owing to the congested or thrombosed capillaries, and they may have a verruciform appearance.

## Histopathology

All subtypes share a common histological appearance that features ectatic thin-walled vessels in the papillary and very superficial reticular dermis, as well as variable epidermal hyperplasia (often absent in AD) comprising acanthosis, elongation of rete ridges, and hyperkeratosis. The lesional endothelium of solitary angiokeratoma is diffusely positive for CD31, ERG, PROX1, and D2-40, and negative for WT1. In AD, the endothelium and the smooth muscle of vessel walls and arrector pili show lipid accumulation, highlighted by Sudan Black B and PAS. The

differential diagnosis includes verrucous venous malformation, lymphangioma circumscriptum, and acral pseudolymphomatous angiokeratoma of children; the first two entities display a deep dermal–subcutaneous component, and the last shows a prominent lymphocytic infiltrate.

## Cytology

Not relevant

## Diagnostic molecular pathology

Not relevant

## Essential and desirable diagnostic criteria

*Essential:* dilated thin-walled vascular channels, mainly in the papillary or very superficial reticular dermis.
*Desirable:* epidermal hyperplasia.

## Staging

Not relevant

## Prognosis and prediction

Angiokeratoma shows no regression and persists without intervention. Malignant transformation has not been reported.

# Epidermal naevi

Colmenero I
Torrelo A

## Definition
Epidermal naevi (ENs) are circumscribed, long-lasting hamartomatous lesions of the skin or neighbouring mucosa, reflecting genetic mosaicism.

## ICD-O coding
None

## ICD-11 coding
LC00.0 Epidermal naevus
LC02 Complex epidermal hamartoma

## Related terminology
*Not recommended:* organoid naevus; naevus sebaceus of Jadassohn; porokeratotic adnexal ostium naevus; porokeratotic eccrine ostial and dermal duct naevus.

## Subtype(s)
See Table 15.03.

## Localization
EN arises anywhere in the skin; some types favour particular locations.

## Clinical features
Most ENs are congenital; certain types show delayed onset. Four types are recognized:

*Common keratinocyte naevus (CKN):* These appear as soft, brown, velvety, slightly elevated streaks or plaques, most often following the lines of Blaschko. CKNs in flexural and bony prominence locations may become more hyperkeratotic. CKNs can occur anywhere, but they rarely affect the scalp; in such cases, a woolly hair naevus is often seen {2476}.

*Naevus sebaceus (NS):* This is a congenital, orange/yellow, round/oval, hairless, slightly elevated plaque, usually on the scalp, with progressive flattening until puberty, when it becomes elevated and hyperkeratotic. Less frequently, the lesions can be large and involve the scalp and face, following the lines of Blaschko. When multiple, they frequently associate

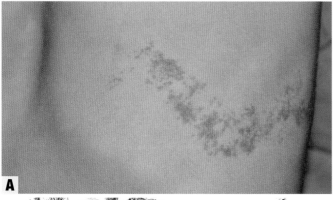

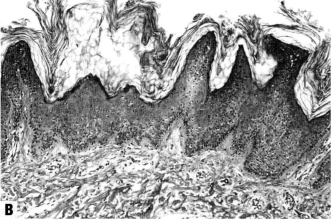

**Fig. 15.09** Common keratinocyte naevus. **A** Hyperkeratotic, brown, velvety papules with a linear arrangement, following the lines of Blaschko. **B** The biopsy shows acanthosis, papillomatosis, elongation of the rete ridges, and hyperkeratosis.

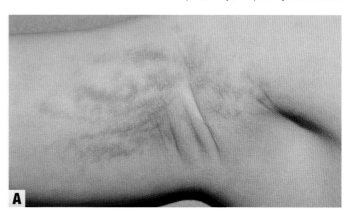

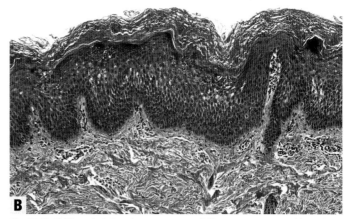

**Fig. 15.10** Epidermolytic keratinocyte naevus. **A** Linear arrangement of hyperkeratotic lesions with scaling. **B** The hallmark is epidermolytic hyperkeratosis characterized by hyperkeratosis and vacuolar degeneration with hypergranulosis of the stratum granulosum and stratum spinosum.

with extracutaneous abnormalities. NS rarely occurs outside the head and neck.

*Naevus comedonicus:* This is a congenital linear arrangement of multiple comedones, often with cutaneous atrophy. Lesions may be short or involve a whole limb. The most common locations are the face, neck, upper arm, and chest. The palms and soles are rarely involved {4893,6217,2102}.

*Porokeratotic eccrine naevus:* These are keratotic or verrucous papules with punctate pits and keratin plugs; they always follow the lines of Blaschko. They occur anywhere in the skin, with a striking involvement of the palms and soles. One or multiple lines of Blaschko can be affected {2456,4174}.

## Epidemiology
CKN is the most common type, followed by NS and naevus comedonicus {2660,2322}. Other EN types are much less frequent.

## Etiology
Most ENs originate from postzygotic mutations in epidermal or appendageal cells (see Table 15.03).

## Pathogenesis
ENs result from postzygotic mosaic mutations, usually with a segmental pattern following the lines of Blaschko. Most are activating

**Table 15.03** Most common types of epidermal naevi (continued on next page)

| Name of naevus | Molecular basis | Distribution | Clinical features | Main histological features |
|---|---|---|---|---|
| **Keratinocyte naevi** | | | | |
| Common keratinocyte naevus {2660,2561,2659,2660} | *FGFR3, KRAS, FGFR2, PIK3CA* | Lines of Blaschko | Velvety, brown, slightly elevated streaks or plaques (see text) | Hyperkeratosis, acanthosis, and papillomatosis (see text) |
| Keratinocyte naevus of the Proteus type {1388,4134,7534} | *AKT1* | Lines of Blaschko | Velvety, brown, slightly elevated streaks or plaques | Hyperkeratosis, acanthosis, and papillomatosis |
| Linear PTEN naevus {2697} | *PTEN* | Lines of Blaschko | Verrucous, elevated streaks or plaques | Hyperkeratosis, acanthosis, and papillomatosis |
| Epidermolytic epidermal naevus {5292,7091,1761} | *KRT1, KRT10* | Lines of Blaschko | Light-brown or hypopigmented verrucous or warty papules | Variable acanthosis and papillomatosis; epidermolytic hyperkeratosis usually seen |
| CHILD naevus {5765,2310, 414,3572} | *NSDHL* | Lines of Blaschko, usually unilateral | Erythematous or yellowish warty plaques; hypertrophic yellowish lesions on main skin folds in chronic lesions | Hyperkeratosis, acanthosis, and papillomatosis; parakeratosis with rounded nuclei; chronic lesions show verruciform xanthoma |
| Acantholytic and dyskeratotic epidermal naevus (linear Darier disease) {4489,6154,6122} | *ATP2A2* | Lines of Blaschko | Crusted keratotic papules | Acantholysis with dyskeratosis |
| Linear Hailey–Hailey disease {4489,2320} | *ATP2C1* | Lines of Blaschko | Erythematous plaques, vesicles, erosions, and crusting | Acantholysis with dyskeratosis |
| Linear porokeratosis {6131, 2698,403} | *MVK, PMVK, MVD, SLC17A9* | Lines of Blaschko | Erythematous-brown papulosquamous plaques with hyperkeratotic rims | Cornoid lamella |
| Papular epidermal naevus with skyline basal cell layer {7029, 4263} | Unknown | Round papules; occasionally lines of Blaschko | Hyperkeratotic papules with flat surface | Regular hyperkeratosis and acanthosis; skyline sign in the basal cell layer |
| **Sebaceous naevi** | | | | |
| Common sebaceous naevus {2699,4060,2560,375} | *HRAS, KRAS, NRAS* | Lines of Blaschko; small lesions are round | Congenital, orange or yellowish, round, hairless patch (see text) | Acanthosis, rudimentary hair follicles, prominent sebaceous glands, and increased apocrine glands (see text) |
| Pedunculated sebaceous naevus {3805} | *FGFR2* | Round tumour | Pink to yellow exophytic fleshy masses | Acanthosis, rudimentary hair follicles, prominent sebaceous glands, and increased apocrine glands |
| **Follicular naevi** | | | | |
| Hair follicle naevus {3938,2363} | Unknown | Isolated | Skin-coloured papule on face and neck | Clusters of mature hair follicles with associated sebaceous glands and arrector pili muscles |
| Follicular mucinous naevus {6832} | Unknown | Lines of Blaschko | Red plaques | Mucin in the follicular units |
| Naevus comedonicus {4893, 6217,2102,4059} | *NEK9* | Lines of Blaschko | Multiple comedones with slight skin atrophy (see text) | Invaginations of epidermis filled with keratin (see text) |
| Munro acne naevus {7020, 4573} | *FGFR2* | Lines of Blaschko | Acne-like lesions | Acne-like histology |
| Naevus trichilemmocysticus {6890,3935} | Unknown | Lines of Blaschko | Trichilemmal cysts, filiform hyperkeratoses, and comedones | Multiple trichilemmal cysts |

CHILD, congenital hemidysplasia with ichthyosiform erythroderma and limb defects.

**Table 15.03** Most common types of epidermal naevi (continued)

| Name of naevus | Molecular basis | Distribution | Clinical features | Main histological features |
|---|---|---|---|---|
| **Eccrine naevi** | | | | |
| Pure eccrine and mucinous eccrine naevus {6942,3496} | Unknown | Isolated; rarely lines of Blaschko | Localized patch of hyperhidrosis; rarely, localized patches or skin tags; sometimes part of an organoid naevus | Increased number or size of eccrine glands; mucin deposits surrounding eccrine glands in the mucinous type |
| Eccrine angiomatous hamartoma {5392,6173} | Unknown | Isolated or multiple lesions | Variable; papules, plaques, or nodules; colour may be red, bluish, brown, or yellowish | Eccrine gland hamartoma associated with blood vessel proliferation |
| Porokeratotic eccrine naevus {4174,2456,1877} | GJB2 | Lines of Blaschko | Verrucous yellowish papules with punctate pits and comedo-like plugs (see text) | Cornoid lamella centred on acrosyringia or acrotrichia (see text) |
| **Apocrine naevi** | | | | |
| Pure apocrine naevus {1439, 3409} | Unknown | Isolated | Nodule on the scalp | Prominent apocrine glands |
| Syringocystadenoma papilliferum {2108,4438,3503} | Unknown | Lines of Blaschko; small lesions are round | Nodule on the scalp; often within sebaceous naevus | Epidermal invagination with papillae covered by tall columnar cells surrounded by myoepithelial cuboid cells; numerous stromal plasma cells |

CHILD, congenital hemidysplasia with ichthyosiform erythroderma and limb defects.

mutations affecting genes of the PI3K and RAS/MAPK pathways that regulate cell growth and survival {4941,2658,375}. Other mutations involve structural epidermal proteins or enzymes of lipid or cholesterol metabolism necessary for keratinization.

The extent of skin involvement depends on the time at which mutations occur during embryonic development: earlier mutations result in more extensive involvement. Very early mutations lead to extracutaneous involvement, termed "epidermal naevus syndrome" {2322,2323,2700,2701}.

## Macroscopic appearance
See *Clinical features* (above).

## Histopathology
*CKN:* Findings are limited to the epidermis. CKNs are usually well demarcated, featuring acanthosis, papillomatosis, elongation of the rete ridges, and hyperkeratosis. They sometimes resemble seborrhoeic keratosis or acanthosis nigricans. Keratin-filled pseudocysts can be seen {6745}.

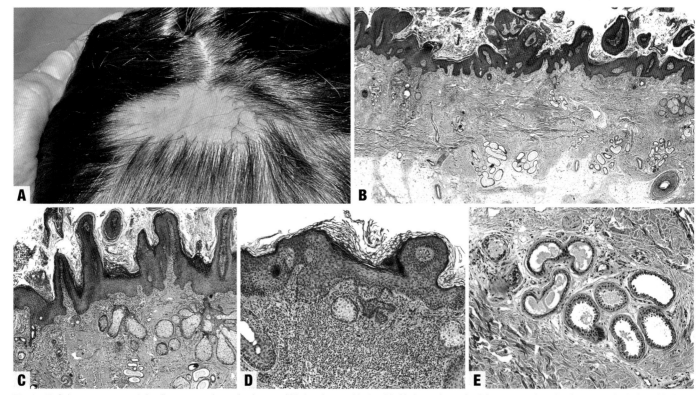

**Fig. 15.11** Sebaceous naevus. **A** A yellow-orange plaque that has a pebbled surface and is devoid of hairs on the scalp. **B** Low-power view showing a complex lesion with abnormal epidermis, sebaceous glands, hair follicles, and sweat glands. **C** The epidermis shows features reminiscent of an epidermal naevus. Note the enlarged and abnormally located sebaceous glands. **D** Follicles are abnormal and represented by germ-like proliferations of basaloid epithelium. **E** Increased numbers of apocrine glands are seen in some cases.

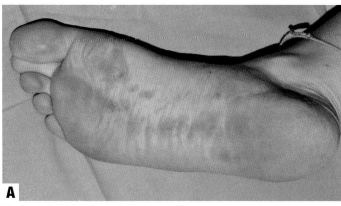
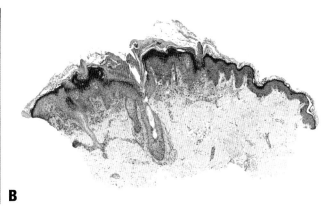

**Fig. 15.12** Porokeratotic eccrine naevus. **A** Linear arrangement of yellowish papules on the sole, with hyperkeratosis on the sweat pores. **B** Cornoid lamellae overlying acrosyringia and acrotrichia together with marked epidermal acanthosis.

*NS:* This is a complex lesion, showing abnormalities in the epidermis, sebaceous glands, hair follicles, and sweat glands. Epidermal findings are similar to those of CKN. Sebaceous glands show hyperplasia and hypertrophy, particularly in early infancy or adolescence, but can also be diminished or even absent. Abnormal sebaceous glands are superficially located, frequently opening to the skin surface independently of hair follicles. Hair follicles are reduced in number, frequently primitive-looking, and abortive. Ectopic apocrine glands within the deep dermis occur in many cases. Associated neoplasms include syringocystadenoma papilliferum, trichoblastoma-like lesions, and viral warts {3227,1490}.

*Naevus comedonicus:* These feature multiple dilated and atrophic hair follicles filled with keratinous debris, as well as dilated infundibula. The epidermis can be either acanthotic or atrophic. Associated epidermolytic hyperkeratosis has been reported {6217}. Cyst rupture induces a foreign body–type reaction.

*Porokeratotic eccrine naevus:* These appear as multiple small dermal invaginations with overlying cornified lamellae. Invaginations correspond to dilated acrosyringia and acrotrichia.

## Cytology
Not relevant

## Diagnostic molecular pathology
The identification of specific mosaic mutations (e.g. in *FGFR3*) is useful for classifying some lesions, particularly in EN syndrome.

## Essential and desirable diagnostic criteria
*Essential:* a mosaic pattern distribution; for CKN: acanthosis, papillomatosis, elongation of the rete ridges, and hyperkeratosis; for NS: abnormalities in the epidermis, sebaceous glands, hair follicles, and sweat glands; for naevus comedonicus: multiple dilated and atrophic hair follicles filled with keratinous debris; for porokeratotic eccrine naevus: cornified lamellae overlying acrosyringia and acrotrichia.

## Staging
Not relevant

## Prognosis and prediction
Most ENs remain stable; some may progressively enlarge. Different tumours, most commonly benign, can develop over NS (trichoblastomas, viral warts, and trichilemmomas) {3227,1490}. Malignant tumours occur rarely; malignancy developing in CKN is extremely unusual {5862,7294}.

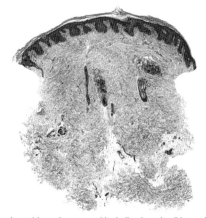
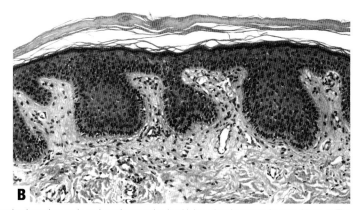

**Fig. 15.13** Papular epidermal naevus with skyline basal cell layer. **A** Punch biopsy showing hyperkeratosis and regular acanthosis with broad and rectangular rete ridges. **B** The basal cell layer shows a striking palisaded arrangement of the nuclei (skyline sign).

# Pilomatricoma

Singh R
Rossi S

## Definition
Pilomatricoma is a benign cutaneous adnexal tumour differentiating towards the matrix and the hair cortex.

## ICD-O coding
8110/0 Pilomatricoma

## ICD-11 coding
2F22 & XH9E37 Benign neoplasms of epidermal appendages & Pilomatricoma, NOS

## Related terminology
*Acceptable:* pilomatrixoma.
*Not recommended:* calcifying epithelioma of Malherbe.

## Subtype(s)
None

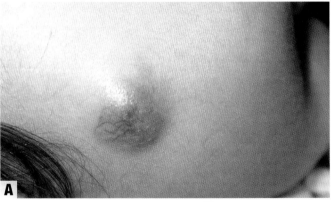

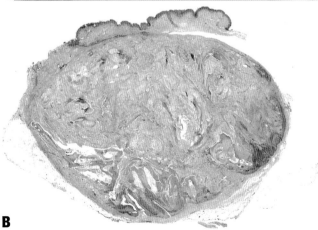

**Fig. 15.14** Pilomatricoma. **A** Clinical picture of a 3-year-old girl with a pilomatricoma of the face. **B** Low-power view of a classic pilomatricoma from the forearm of an 8-year-old child.

## Localization
The predominant localization is the head and neck region (affected in 50% of cases), followed by the extremities (upper: 25% of cases, lower: 10% of cases) and the trunk (15% of cases) {2595}.

## Clinical features
Pilomatricomas manifest as firm or hard, dermal or hypodermal, slow-growing, usually asymptomatic, solitary nodules measuring 10–30 mm {2861}. The overlying skin may look normal, show a red or bluish discolouration, or be anetodermic or bullous/lymphangiectatic {4081,4723}. Giant and perforating forms exist {1027,4723}. As many as 5% of patients have multiple pilomatricomas, usually in association with genetic syndromes (see below).

## Epidemiology
Pilomatricoma is common, accounting for about 1% of all pathologically diagnosed benign skin lesions {2595}. It is the most common non-melanocytic cutaneous tumour excised in children {4214}. It can occur at any age (reported patient age range: 3 months to 93 years), but nearly half of all cases are diagnosed during the first two decades of life {2595}. Most studies have noted a modest female predominance {2759,5117,6301}.

## Etiology
The vast majority of cases are sporadic; however, pilomatricomas can also be familial {2861} or multiple {1768}, often in the setting of complex genetic syndromes such as myotonic dystrophy, familial adenomatous polyposis, Turner syndrome, Rubinstein–Taybi syndrome, Goldenhar syndrome, Kabuki syndrome, Sotos syndrome, trisomy 9, and *DICER1* syndrome.

## Pathogenesis
Most pilomatricomas harbour activating mutations in exon 3 of the gene encoding β-catenin (*CTNNB1*); the 92 kDa protein encoded by this gene is involved in cell–cell adhesion and in the WNT signalling pathway, which regulates cell proliferation, differentiation, and survival {3771}. Basaloid cells often harbour trisomy of chromosome 18, which carries the antiapoptotic gene *BCL2*, suggesting that the BCL2 oncoprotein may play a role in the growth and differentiation of pilomatricoma {88}.

## Macroscopic appearance
Pilomatricoma is a cystic lesion with a thick pale or white wall.

## Histopathology
Pilomatricomas consist of one or several dermal nodules, sometimes extending to the hypodermis. They are made of cells with a variable appearance. The peripheral cells are monomorphic, small, deeply basophilic, and mitotically active, with indistinct borders. Peripheral cells keratinize towards the shadow cells (also called ghost or mummified cells) found towards the centre

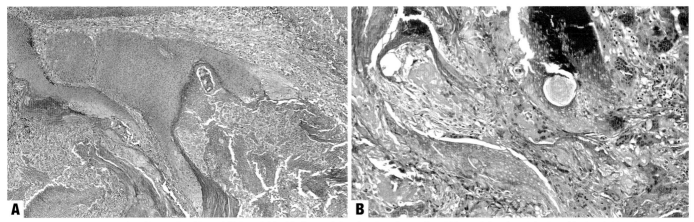

**Fig. 15.15** Pilomatricoma. **A** Note the small and basophilic basaloid epithelium and the abundant ghost cells, which result from keratinization of the basaloid proliferative component. **B** The ghost cells become calcified, eliciting a vigorous foreign body cell reaction.

of the nodules; these are cells with distinct borders, an eosinophilic cytoplasm, and an empty space where the nucleus was once located. The transition occurs via an intermediate zone of cells with a small, pyknotic, basophilic nucleus and pale cytoplasm. The ratio of basophilic cells to shadow cells decreases with increasing age/maturation of the lesion. Pilomatricomas are sometimes cystic (most commonly those associated with familial adenomatous polyposis). Calcification and ossification occur in old lesions, accounting for their stone-hard consistency. The surrounding dermis is fibrotic and often contains a foreign body granulomatous infiltration. Pathological patterns include pigmented and proliferating pilomatricoma (consisting predominantly of mitotically active basaloid cells). Pilomatricoma (basaloid) cells express β-catenin {3150,4081}.

### Differential diagnosis

Pilomatricoma should be differentiated from other pilar tumours that may show (focally) matrical differentiation (i.e. basal cell carcinoma, trichoblastoma, and melanocytic matricoma) and from its malignant counterpart, pilomatrical carcinoma. Pathological features favouring pilomatrical carcinoma include poor circumscription, an asymmetrical silhouette, frequent atypical mitoses, and lymphovascular invasion {2866}.

### Cytology

Not relevant

### Diagnostic molecular pathology

Not relevant

### Essential and desirable diagnostic criteria

*Essential:* a cystic tumour with stratified squamous epithelial elements, ghost cells, and dense keratin.

### Staging

Not relevant

### Prognosis and prediction

Pilomatricomas are benign tumours. Rarely, they may recur, most commonly when incompletely excised {2595,2759}.

# Congenital naevi

Salgado CM
Adameyko I
Etchevers HC
Reyes-Múgica M

### Definition
Congenital melanocytic naevi (CMNs) are benign melanocytic neoplasms that start in utero and appear at birth, or in the first few years of life (late or tardive congenital naevus). Some CMNs fall into the category of blue or cellular naevi and are discussed in a separate section.

### ICD-O coding
8761/0 Congenital naevus
8761/0 Congenital naevus present at birth
8761/0 Late/tardive congenital naevus

### ICD-11 coding
2F20.20 Giant congenital melanocytic naevus
2F20.2Y Other specified congenital melanocytic naevus
2F20.2Z Congenital melanocytic naevus, unspecified

### Related terminology
*Acceptable:* congenital naevocytic naevus; giant naevus.

### Subtype(s)
Congenital naevus present at birth; late/tardive congenital naevus

### Localization
Anywhere on the body

### Clinical features
CMNs are classified according to the projected adult diameter of the largest lesion as small (< 15 mm); medium (M1: 15–100 mm, M2: > 100–200 mm); large (L1: > 200–300 mm, L2: > 300–400 mm); or giant (G1: > 400–600 mm, G2: > 600 mm) {3783}. This classification also includes other clinical characteristics of the naevi: location, number of satellite lesions, colour heterogeneity, surface rugosity, hairiness, and nodule location (dermal or subcutaneous). In addition to benign nodules, other features of large/giant CMN can include neurofibroma-like overgrowths and limb and soft tissue atrophy {3168,6520,1032}. CMN may also be associated with many other clinical problems, including pruritus, skin barrier fragility, decreased sweating, and/or perceived cosmetic impairment {5642,4973}.

### Epidemiology
The frequency of CMNs is inversely related to their size. About 1% of newborns have a small CMN, whereas giant CMN is rare and only affects an estimated 1 in 500 000 newborns {167}.

### Etiology
Unknown

### Pathogenesis
Melanocyte progenitors include neural crest cells delaminating from the prospective CNS during the second gestational month, as well as their persistent derivatives, nerve-associated Schwann cell precursors. Nerve-assisted generation of melanocytes from Schwann cell precursors is an important pathway in delivering melanocytic clones to circumscribed skin areas {49}. Such progenitors may carry a somatic mutation, leading to local clonal expansion and formation of CMN in a permissive physical context like the maturing skin or leptomeninges. Cellular lineage commitment at the moment of mutation onset can account for the variation in size, number, and spatial distribution of CMNs, including segmental and non-segmental types. Multiple or large CMN examples may associate with structural and/or functional CNS abnormalities, and/or with a number of different tumours including lipoma, rhabdomyosarcoma, and others {3206,5568}, supporting the

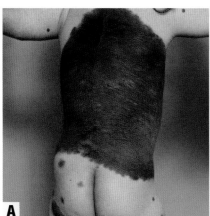 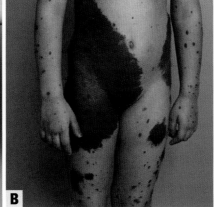 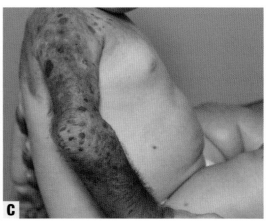

**Fig. 15.16** Congenital melanocytic naevus. **A** A giant congenital melanocytic naevus (projected adult size of the largest naevus: > 400 mm) and multiple satellite naevi. **B** Another example of a giant congenital melanocytic naevus with multiple satellite naevi. **C** A large congenital melanocytic naevus associated with atrophy of the soft tissues of the arm.

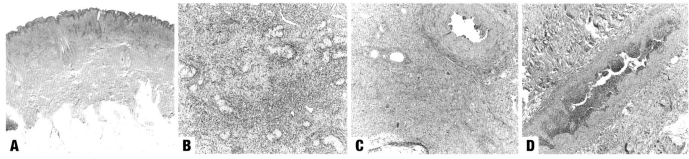

**Fig. 15.17** Congenital melanocytic naevus. **A** Low-power view of a congenital melanocytic naevus. Note the depth of the dermal component and the skin adnexa surrounded by naevus cells. **B** A giant congenital melanocytic naevus with Wagner–Meissner or Masson bodies, characteristic of neurotization. **C** Subendothelial infiltration of naevus cells. **D** Another example (at higher magnification) of subendothelial infiltration of naevus cells in a congenital melanocytic naevus.

early embryonic origin of a corresponding mutation (including possible germline-transmitted cases) {49,48,2267,1984}. The emergence of CMNs from immature neurovascular bundles has been recognized in paediatric specimens {1473,1474}.

## Macroscopic appearance
CMNs are hyperpigmented, flat to rugous, variably hairy, sometimes nodular, thick skin lesions.

## Histopathology
The malformative and hamartomatous appearance of CMNs varies according to their clinical presentation and the patient's age. At birth, they usually are highly cellular. Neuroid features (or neurotization) in the form of Wagner–Meissner or Masson bodies are common. Most naevocytes (naevus cells) invest deeper dermal layers and even subcutaneous tissue. Here, the spindly type C naevocytes have a still-immature, neuroid phenotype, with poorly defined cytoplasm and infrequent pigmentation. Midway through these usually thick lesions, compact groups of round type B naevocytes appear in single file between collagen bundles and intervening lobules of fat, infiltrating adnexal structures, and subendothelial spaces. Superficially, type A naevocytes are larger and more epithelioid, with abundant cytoplasm, and they may have intracytoplasmic melanin. Commonly, these superficial naevocytes are surrounded by clusters of heavily pigmented melanophages {1475}.

CMNs commonly have a compound histological architecture with a prominent band-like pattern, but many feature a grenz zone in the papillary dermis. The epidermis shows variable atrophy of rete ridges, but papillomatosis or verrucoid features are relatively common. Most CMNs show no marked atypia or pleomorphism. However, large CMNs in newborns may have impressive pagetoid patterns, atypia, mitoses and ulceration; therefore, the diagnosis of melanoma in newborns should be made with caution (see *Melanoma*, p. 952).

Large/giant CMNs can show mast cell hyperplasia associated with significant pruritus {6134,4699}. A challenging but frequent observation in large CMNs is the proliferative nodule, a well-delimited compact aggregate of naevocytes surrounded by conventional naevus areas. Features commonly indicative of malignant behaviour in melanocytic lesions of adults (ulceration, pagetoid spreading, and brisk mitoses) are common in proliferative nodules, and when present, the nodule is classified as atypical, raising the need for additional genetic analyses such as comparative genomic hybridization and FISH. Occasionally, large/giant CMNs involving the perineal region manifest as striking tumours composed of naevocytes, termed "bulky perineal naevocytoma" {5859, 2077}, a pattern of congenital naevus that may be confused with malignancy.

## Cytology
Not clinically relevant

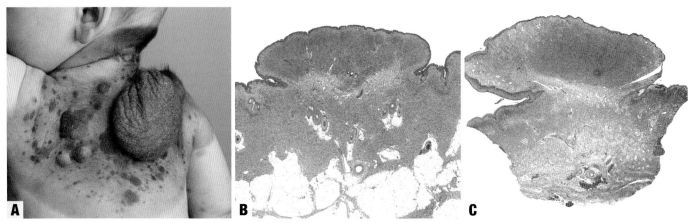

**Fig. 15.18** Congenital melanocytic naevus. **A** Multiple benign nodules (some resembling neurofibromas) within a large congenital melanocytic naevus. **B** A congenital melanocytic naevus with a well-delimited and compact aggregate of naevus cells, characteristic of a proliferative nodule. **C** Another example of a proliferative nodule in a congenital melanocytic naevus.

## Diagnostic molecular pathology

Molecular investigation may be required in difficult cases. CMN may have different genetic signatures that lead to the constitutive activation of MAPK intracellular signalling. The majority of large CMNs harbour *NRAS* p.Q61 somatic mutations {543, 1179}, but *BRAF* p.V600 mutations are present in as many as 8% of cases {6133,1719,5594}. *BRAF* mutations are more common in small CMNs {1179}. Chromosomal rearrangements affecting these and other MAPK pathway genes such as *RAF1* have also been reported {1719,4435,479}.

## Essential and desirable diagnostic criteria

*Essential:* presentation at birth or within the first few years of childhood; single-file pattern of infiltrative naevus cells; frequent band-like arrangement and neurotization; entrapment and/or infiltration of adnexa; bland histological features.

## Staging

Not clinically relevant

## Prognosis and prediction

CMNs are themselves benign, although patients may develop psychosocial problems {5642,4450}. However, large or multiple naevi are associated with a significantly greater risk of melanoma {3609,3782}. Approximately one quarter of patients with large/giant CMNs have neurocutaneous melanocytosis, where abnormal melanocytes are also found in meninges and/or CNS parenchyma. These patients frequently (but not always) develop neurological symptoms such as epilepsy or hydrocephalus {5858,4397,6133,3206}. See the corresponding sections on CNS tumours. No definitive clinical or molecular predictors of any outcome have been identified to date.

# Junctional, compound, and dermal naevi

de la Fouchardière A
Bastian BC
Elder DE

## Definition
Naevi are benign melanocytic proliferations that microscopically can be located in the epidermis (junctional naevi), dermis (dermal naevi), or both (compound naevi).

## ICD-O coding
8740/0 Junctional naevus
8760/0 Compound naevus
8750/0 Dermal naevus

## ICD-11 coding
2F20.0Y & XH1M79 Other specified common acquired melanocytic naevus & Junctional naevus, NOS
2F20.0Y & XH27A6 Other specified common acquired melanocytic naevus & Compound naevus
2F20.0Y & XH2MQ5 Other specified common acquired melanocytic naevus & Dermal naevus

## Related terminology
*Acceptable:* common acquired naevi.
*Not recommended:* banal naevi.

## Subtype(s)
None

## Localization
Naevi can arise in all sites, but they predominate on the trunk.

## Clinical features
Acquired naevi are mostly small (< 5 mm), symmetrical, uniformly pigmented lesions. Junctional naevi are often flat/macular, whereas compound or dermal naevi are more often elevated. They grow slowly during childhood/adolescence and remain stable in size for some time afterwards.

## Epidemiology
Acquired naevi arise during early childhood, with a peak at adolescence, after which they slowly decline in number and size throughout adulthood {369}.

## Etiology
The number and size of acquired naevi in an individual is influenced by ultraviolet (UV) radiation exposure, tanning ability, and heritable genetic factors {1845,4988}.

## Pathogenesis
Naevi are clonal proliferations of melanocytes that are partially transformed by proliferation-inducing somatic mutations in MAPK pathway genes (mainly *BRAF*) {1473}.

## Macroscopic appearance
Naevi are well-circumscribed, homogeneously pigmented papules or macules. Junctional and compound naevi are typically brown, whereas dermal naevi can be pink or skin-coloured.

## Histopathology
Lesions appear as circumscribed and symmetrical proliferations of cytologically bland melanocytes with oval to round nuclei and a mildly pigmented cytoplasm. If a junctional component is present it can assume a lentiginous or nested pattern. The lentiginous architecture is defined by melanocytes distributed as individual units along elongated hyperpigmented rete ridges. In the nested pattern, naevus cells are arranged in small clusters of relatively uniform size along the dermoepidermal junction, with larger nests in the centre of the lesion. No pagetoid spreading is visible, except in examples of irritated naevi where it is present in a limited fashion below zones of parakeratosis.

A dermal component can vary in extent and tends to be situated in the central part of the lesion. When the dermal

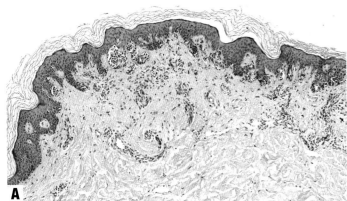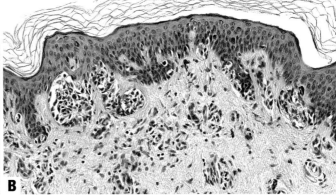

**Fig. 15.19** Junctional naevus. **A** Junctional nests of bland melanocytes in a slightly hyperplastic epidermis. **B** Junctional nests of bland melanocytes (HPS stain).

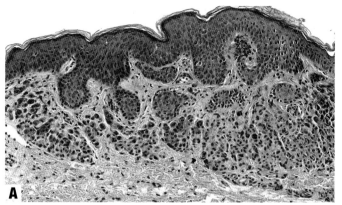

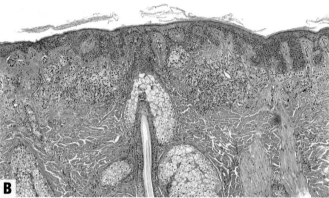

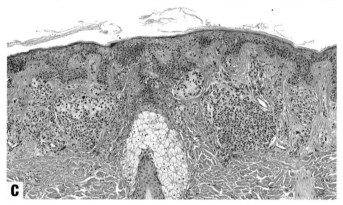

**Fig. 15.20** Compound naevus. **A** Predominantly dermal / compound dermal. **B** Nests of bland melanocytes in a slightly hyperplastic epidermis and in the upper dermis (HPS stain). **C** Nests of bland melanocytes in the junction and upper dermis (HPS stain).

component is more abundant, it may elevate the epidermis and expand the superficial dermis to form a papule. When the melanocytic proliferation extends deeper into the reticular dermis, lesions assume a so-called congenital pattern, which is not indicative of a true congenital origin. The dermal nests and their constituting melanocytes become smaller and less pigmented, with descent into the dermis, dispersing as single cells at the base. The cytology of the superficial cells in the dermis is usually similar to that observed in any overlying junctional component (type A or epithelioid cells), with maturation or senescent change resulting in small type B (lymphocyte-like) cells and often spindled type C cells at the base. Mitoses are usually absent.

## Cytology
Not relevant

## Diagnostic molecular pathology
Acquired naevi frequently have *BRAF* mutations and sometimes have *NRAS* mutations. They do not have chromosomal copy-number changes. They have a low Ki-67 proliferation index and strongly express p16 and other senescence markers {5591}.

## Essential and desirable diagnostic criteria
*Essential:* a bland morphological appearance; absence of pleomorphism or mitotic activity, particularly in deeper areas.
*Desirable:* symmetrical architecture.

## Staging
By definition, naevi are benign and do not require staging.

## Prognosis and prediction
Naevi are stable proliferations with a very low risk of progression to melanoma; the estimated lifetime risk is 0.03% (1 in 3164) for men and 0.009% (1 in 10 800) for women. Progression to melanoma occurs via secondary and tertiary genetic alterations such as *CDKN2A* loss and *TERT* promoter mutations {6367}.

# Blue naevus

de la Fouchardière A
Scolyer RA

## Definition
Blue naevus is a benign dermal melanocytic proliferation characterized by spindled and dendritic melanocytes in a fibrous background.

## ICD-O coding
8780/0 Blue naevus, NOS
8790/0 Cellular blue naevus
8780/0 Dendritic blue naevus

## ICD-11 coding
2F20.Y & XH7QJ7 Other specific types of melanocytic naevus
& Blue naevus, NOS
2F20.Y & XH3X84 Other specific types of melanocytic naevus
& Cellular blue naevus

## Related terminology
*Acceptable:* for dendritic blue naevus: common blue naevus; dermal dendritic melanocytic naevus; naevus of Jadassohn; Tièche naevus; Jadassohn–Tièche blue naevus.

## Subtype(s)
Cellular blue naevus; dendritic blue naevus

## Localization
Blue naevi can occur at any cutaneous site, but dendritic blue naevi (DBNs) are more frequently located on the back of the hands and feet, and cellular blue naevi (CBNs) are predominantly found on the buttocks or the scalp area {4860}. Congenital examples predominate in the scalp.

## Clinical features
DBNs are small, rounded papules with a blue shade. CBNs are larger (often > 10 mm in diameter) and appear as slightly elevated, indurated blue nodules.

## Epidemiology
Blue naevi are most frequent in children and young adults {4860}. They are less frequent than common acquired naevi but are not rare. Familial/syndromic aggregation exists, such as in LAMB syndrome (lentigines, atrial myxoma, mucocutaneous myoma, and blue naevus) or NAME syndrome (naevi, atrial myxoma, myxoid neurofibromas, and ephelides) of Carney complex {7822,4860}.

## Etiology
Blue naevi are considered neural crest lesions derived from primitive Schwann cell and melanocyte precursors. In contrast to common acquired naevi and cutaneous melanomas, ultraviolet (UV) sunlight irradiation is not an important etiological factor for blue naevi {529}.

## Pathogenesis
Blue naevi usually contain activating mutations in *GNAQ*, *GNA11*, or *PLCB4* (or less frequently, in *CYSLTR2*) in a mutually exclusive pattern {4748}. They lack *BRAF*, *NRAS*, and *NF1* mutations and, in contrast to many blue naevus–like melanomas, also lack

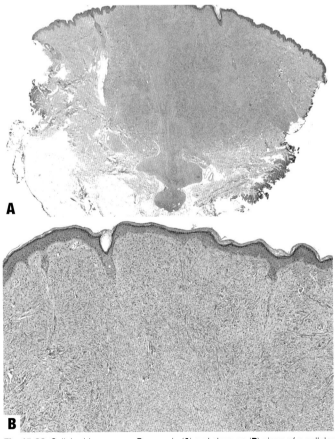

**Fig. 15.22** Cellular blue naevus. Panoramic (**A**) and close-up (**B**) views of a cellular blue naevus in a 5-year-old.

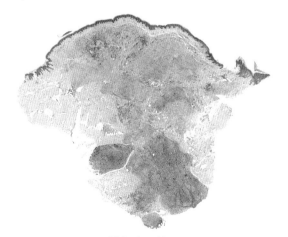

**Fig. 15.21** Cellular blue naevus. Biphasic architecture.

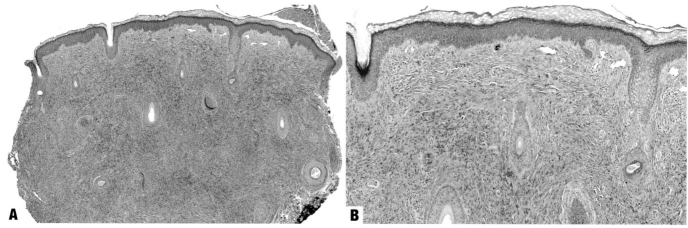

**Fig. 15.23** Cellular blue naevus. Panoramic (**A**) and higher-magnification (**B**) views of a cellular blue naevus in a 12-year-old.

*BAP1* mutations {2551}. Deep-seated dermal melanin pigment appears blue because of the Tyndall effect {7222,7223,4748}.

## Macroscopic appearance

Typically, a blue naevus manifests as a symmetrical homogeneous pigmented papule or nodule. Cut sections of CBN often demonstrate deep involvement of the subcutis.

## Histopathology

DBN and CBN have overlapping features. In DBN, the melanocytic proliferation is mainly situated in the reticular dermis, with occasional extension into the subcutis and upper dermis. Junctional participation (compound blue naevus) is exceptional with isolated dendritic melanocytes or small nests {3226}. The intradermal proliferation is poorly limited, with a fibrosing

background and frequent periadnexal and perivascular tropism. Small, bland dendritic melanocytes of variable density are admixed with melanophages and arranged in short fascicles without deep maturation. Intracytoplasmic pigment is of variable density. No cytonuclear atypia or mitotic activity is usually present. In some cases, the collagenic fibrotic background is predominant, erasing the entrapped follicular/hair shaft structures in a pseudodestructive pattern, often termed "sclerosing blue naevus". In CBN, dense nests and sheets are intricated within a classic DBN pattern. They frequently form vertically oriented expansions that extend deeply into the subcutis. The melanocytes in these CBN areas are medium-sized and often mildly pigmented, with bland oval nuclei that sometimes have central longitudinal nuclear grooves. The cytoplasmic membrane is difficult to visualize. No atypia or notable mitotic activity is present in these areas. A central myxoid/cystic pattern can be found in large lesions in which the nests appear to float in an oedematous background. No areas of necrosis are visible {7820,3060,4860}.

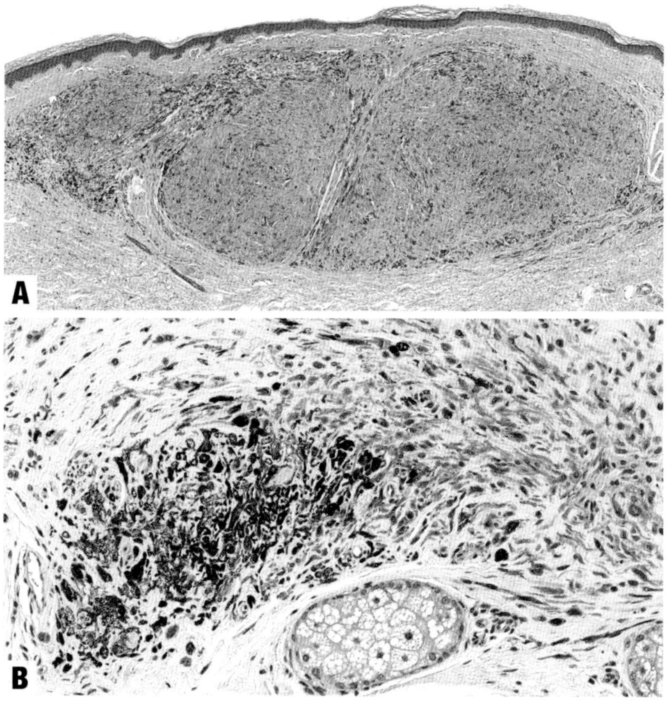

## Cytology

Not clinically relevant

## Diagnostic molecular pathology

Molecular pathology may be helpful for diagnosis in occasional difficult cases (see *Pathogenesis*, above).

## Essential and desirable diagnostic criteria

*Essential:* for DBN: a poorly circumscribed dermal proliferation of dendritic melanocytes with fibroplasia; for CBN: dense nests and sheets of bland melanocytes often within a DBN.

## Staging

Not clinically relevant

## Prognosis and prediction

DBN and CBN are benign lesions. Rarely, malignant transformation (melanoma) may occur, usually in adults. The intermediate-grade lesions (atypical cellular blue naevus / melanocytoma) represent an intermediate state between naevus and melanoma (and as such are classified in the broad group of melanocytomas) {7823}.

**Fig. 15.24** Dendritic blue naevus. **A** At low magnification. **B** Dendritic and spindled melanocytes in a fibrous background.

# Spitz naevus

Colmenero I
Gerami P

## Definition
Spitz naevus (SN) is a benign melanocytic neoplasm that usually appears in childhood and is composed of large epithelioid and/or spindled cells. Spitz melanocytoma (atypical Spitz tumour) is distinguished by the presence of atypical histological features that are insufficient to support a diagnosis of melanoma.

## ICD-O coding
8770/0 Spitz naevus
8770/0 Intradermal Spitz naevus
8770/0 Pagetoid Spitz naevus
8770/0 Dysplastic Spitz naevus
8770/0 Desmoplastic Spitz naevus
8770/0 Angiomatoid Spitz naevus
8770/0 Hyalinizing Spitz naevus
8770/0 Plexiform Spitz naevus
8770/0 Tubular Spitz naevus
8770/0 Myxoid Spitz naevus
8770/0 Balloon cell Spitz naevus
8770/0 Pigmented epithelioid cell Spitz naevus
8770/0 Combined Spitz naevus
8770/0 Recurrent/persistent Spitz naevus

## ICD-11 coding
2F20.Y & XH2HG8 Other specific types of melanocytic naevus & Epithelioid and spindle cell naevus
2F20.Y & XH9WF4 Other specific types of melanocytic naevus & Spitz naevus, atypical

## Related terminology
*Acceptable:* Spitz tumour of uncertain malignant potential.
*Not recommended:* benign juvenile melanoma; epithelioid cell naevus; spindle cell naevus; spindle and epithelioid cell naevus; naevus of large spindle and/or epithelioid cells.

## Subtype(s)
See Box 15.01.

## Localization
Most SNs in children are located in the head and neck or in the lower extremities {5847,7471}. Mucosal involvement is very rare {7160,7291}.

## Clinical features
SNs are usually solitary lesions that grow rapidly and then stabilize; they can remain static in size for years. Some SNs ultimately acquire the aspect of a common melanocytic naevus, and others completely regress {340,6214}. SNs are frequently interpreted as vascular tumours. Multiple SNs are rare and can appear grouped or disseminated {7814}. Spitz melanocytoma (atypical Spitz tumour) can be clinically indistinguishable from melanoma {500,6541,6608}.

## Epidemiology
About 1% of all naevi excised from children are SNs {4544}. They occur in all racial groups and have a similar incidence in both sexes {4226}. Forty per cent of affected patients are aged < 15 years {5847}. Congenital SNs are exceedingly rare {3692}. Spitz melanocytoma (atypical Spitz tumour) is most common in adolescents and young adults {500,6541,6608}.

## Etiology
Cases have been reported after sunburn, perioperative stress, pregnancy, drug abuse, Addison disease, chemotherapy, and

**Box 15.01** Spitz naevus subtypes

**Clinical subtypes**
Polypoid {2024}
Agminated {3050,7814}
Eruptive disseminated {4065,5871}
Halo {2741}
Flat
Pigmented
Fibrosing

**Histological subtypes**
Intradermal {5578}
Pagetoid {954,2087}
Dysplastic
Desmoplastic {507}
Angiomatoid {1738}
Hyalinizing {6791}
Plexiform {3062}
Tubular {937,7870}
Myxoid {2923}
Balloon cell {7171}
Pigmented epithelioid cell {7171}
Combined {488,3671}
Recurrent/persistent {2740}

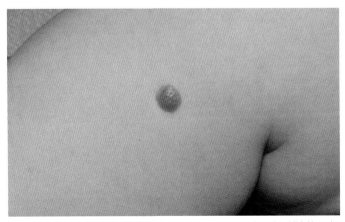

**Fig. 15.25** Spitz naevus. A well-defined rounded papule in the leg of a child. Note the pink colour and smooth surface.

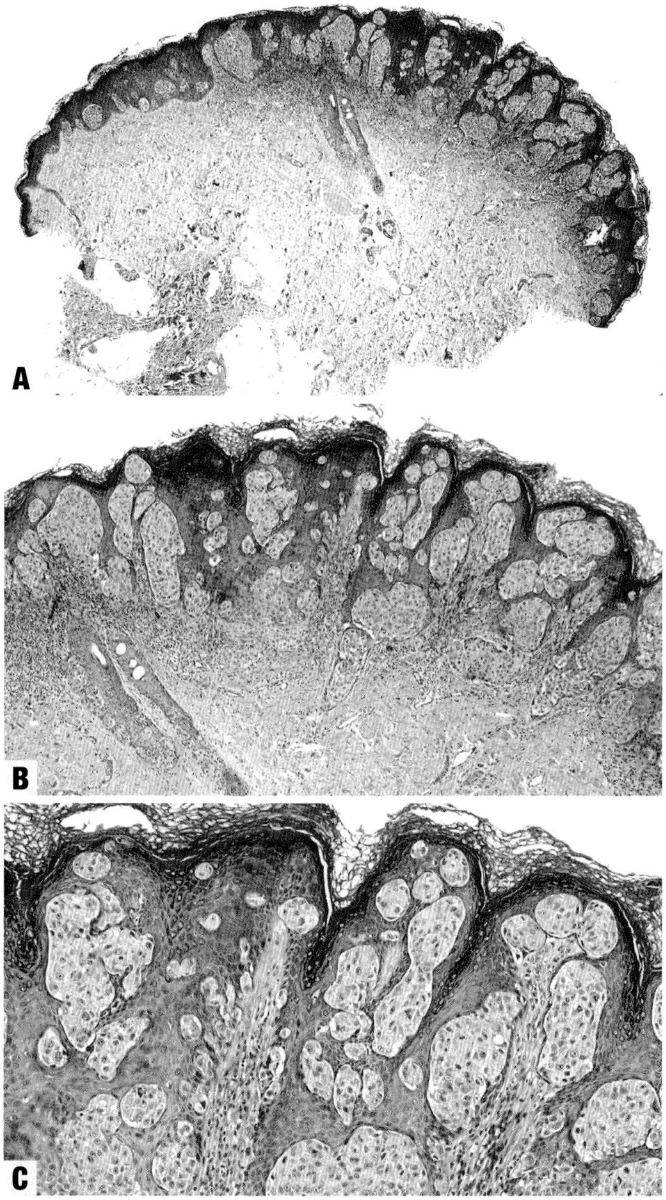

**Fig. 15.26** Spitz naevus. **A** Predominantly epithelioid Spitz naevus with well-circumscribed, mainly intraepidermal nests. **B** Pagetoid migration of naevomelanocytes should not be interpreted as a sign of malignancy in Spitz naevus. **C** Plump epithelioid naevomelanocytes with large nuclei and prominent nucleoli are typically seen.

allogeneic haematopoietic stem cell transplantation {7814}. The presence of a naevus spilus and exposure to ultraviolet (UV) radiation could predispose patients to *HRAS*-mutated SN {530, 6179,786}.

## Pathogenesis

Most SNs are the result of activating structural rearrangements such as chimeric fusions and truncations (see Table 15.04). Kinase genes involved are *ROS1*, *ALK*, *BRAF*, *NTRK1*, *NTRK3*, *MET*, *RET*, and *MAP3K8* {5690,4016,5689,4985,955,7716,7715, 5688}. Mutations in *HRAS* result in a separate subtype of SN {530}. Most eruptive SNs and agminated SNs are the result of mosaic mutations in *HRAS* {6179}. Cases classified as Spitz melanocytoma (atypical Spitz tumour) may have additional mutations

in other genes such as *CDKN2A*, as well as some chromosomal copy-number aberrations {7712}.

## Macroscopic appearance

SNs are well-defined, dome-shaped papules, generally measuring < 5–6 mm and ranging in colour from pink-red to brown. Spitz melanocytomas (atypical Spitz tumours) are often > 6 mm and can show asymmetry, irregular borders, or colour variegation.

## Histopathology

SNs are sharply circumscribed and symmetrical lesions composed of nests of plump epithelioid and/or spindle melanocytes. They are usually compound, but dermal or junctional cases are also seen. Deep maturation is present in compound and intradermal cases, with single cell dispersion at the base. Rare mitoses may be found, usually limited to the superficial portion (< 2 mitoses/mm$^2$). Many SNs are amelanotic or paucimelanotic, but pigmented patterns exist. Other features commonly found are epidermal hyperplasia, clefting around junctional nests, Kamino bodies {3392}, stromal oedema, vascular ectasia, and dermal lymphocytic aggregates. Pagetoid migration of lesional cells into the epidermis may be quite marked, especially in young children {954}. Like other melanocytic naevi, SNs express S100, SOX10, melan-A, tyrosinase, and MITF. SN stains diffusely for S100A6, and p16 is preserved {5866,120}. HMB45 expression is top-heavy {621}, and MIB1 expression is low and shows a gradient, with absent staining at the base of the lesion {622}.

## Cytology
Not relevant

## Diagnostic molecular pathology

Most SNs can be diagnosed by standard histopathology. In cases with less typical morphology, a definitive diagnosis may require confirmatory FISH analysis or next-generation sequencing studies with mRNA sequencing {5690}. In the case of ALK

**Table 15.04** Specific fusion frequency in a study of 80 Spitz naevi {5690}

| Initiating genomic event | | Spitz naevi (*N* = 80) | |
|---|---|---|---|
| **Fusions** | | | |
| Total: | | 54 | (68%) |
| *ALK* | | 14 | (18%) |
| *NTRK1* | | 9 | (11%) |
| *ROS1* | | 7 | (9%) |
| *BRAF* | | 6 | (8%) |
| *MAP3K8* | | 6 | (8%) |
| *NTRK3* | | 4 | (5%) |
| *RET* | | 3 | (4%) |
| *ERBB4* | | 1 | (1%) |
| *FGFR1* | | 1 | (1%) |
| *MAP3K3* | | 1 | (1%) |
| *MET* | | 1 | (1%) |
| *RASGRF1* | | 1 | (1%) |

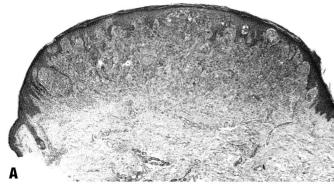

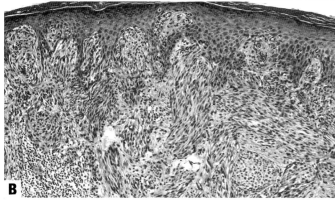

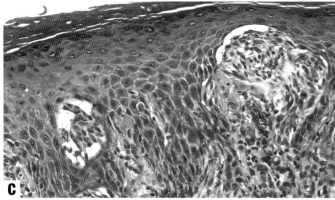

**Fig. 15.27** Spitz naevus. **A** Spitz naevus with predominantly spindle cell morphology, well circumscribed, and with a symmetrical compound pattern. **B** Fascicles of plump spindle naevomelanocytes filling the dermis. **C** Kamino bodies and clefting around intraepidermal nests are relatively frequent.

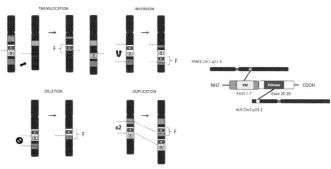

**Fig. 15.28** Chimeric fusions in Spitz naevus. Chimeric fusions of kinase genes involved in Spitz naevi lead to the loss of regulatory and autoinhibitory domains, resulting in constitutive kinase activation.

fusion–positive Spitz, immunohistochemistry is highly reliable in verifying an *ALK* translocation {955}. A pan-NTRK antibody is available, but a positive result should be verified by NTRK break-apart FISH {5690,4016,5689,4985,955,7716}. If Spitz melanoma is a concern, molecular testing with comparative genomic hybridization or FISH to look for multiple chromosomal copy-number aberrations or homozygous deletions of 9p21, as well as mutation analysis for *TERT* promoter mutation, may help identify cases better classified as Spitz melanoma {531}. Such cases may have an increased risk of recurrence or metastasis {4016,2361}. None of the above tests is completely diagnostic, and chromosomal copy-number aberrations can also be seen in cases best classified as Spitz melanocytoma (atypical Spitz tumour).

### Essential and desirable diagnostic criteria

*Essential:* for SN: epithelioid and/or spindle naevomelanocytes; no atypical features; for Spitz melanocytoma (atypical Spitz tumour): one or more atypical histological features.

*Desirable:* Kamino bodies; nest clefting; immunohistochemistry, FISH, and/or next-generation sequencing if malignancy is a concern.

### Staging

Not relevant

### Prognosis and prediction

Although SN and Spitz melanocytoma (atypical Spitz tumour) mimic melanoma clinically and histologically, they have a low risk of recurrence and are rarely precursors to melanoma.

# Pigmented spindle cell naevus (Reed naevus)

Reyes-Múgica M

## Definition
Pigmented spindle cell naevus, also termed Reed naevus (RN), is a benign proliferation of spindle naevomelanocytes that can show clinical and histological features mimicking a melanoma. Genomic studies have demonstrated that RN is a subtype of Spitz naevus.

## ICD-O coding
8770/0 Pigmented spindle cell naevus (Reed naevus)

## ICD-11 coding
2F20.Y & XH2P88 Other specific types of melanocytic naevus & Pigmented spindle cell naevus of Reed

## Related terminology
*Acceptable:* naevus of Reed; pigmented spindle cell Spitz naevus.

## Subtype(s)
Atypical pigmented spindle cell tumour

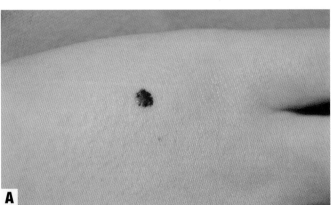

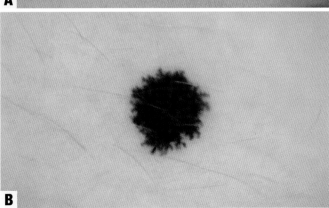

**Fig. 15.29** Reed naevus. **A** A well-delimited rounded black papule in the hand of a child. **B** On dermatoscopy, a starburst pattern is frequently observed in Reed naevus.

## Localization
RN most commonly involves the extremities, particularly the thigh, followed by the trunk and the head and neck {501,6103, 6191}.

## Clinical features
RN usually manifests as an acquired asymptomatic, dome-shaped, dark-brown or black macule or papule {501}. A hypopigmented appearance has also been described {5848}.

## Epidemiology
RN preferentially affects young people (mean age: 25 years, range: 3–66 years) and shows a female preponderance {501, 6103,6191}.

## Etiology
Unknown

## Pathogenesis
RN is caused by chromosomal structural rearrangements resulting in constitutively activated chimeric fusion proteins. Over half of the cases are the result of fusions involving *NTRK3* {7232, 5849}.

## Macroscopic appearance
RN is a well-circumscribed, dark papule measuring < 10 mm.

## Histopathology
RN is a symmetrical and well-circumscribed melanocytic neoplasm characterized by junctional nests of uniform and heavily pigmented spindle cells without atypia, limited to the epidermis or papillary dermis. Nests are vertically oriented, whorled, or concentric. In some cases the nests can extend to the papillary dermis and involve adnexa. Kamino bodies (sometimes pigmented) and pagetoid melanocytosis may be seen. Dermal melanophages are usually present {6191,5810}.

## Cytology
Not relevant

## Diagnostic molecular pathology
See the *Diagnostic molecular pathology* subsection of *Spitz naevus* (p. 947). A break-apart FISH probe for *NTRK3* can confirm rearrangement of *NTRK3*, the most common fusion in RN {7232}.

## Essential and desirable diagnostic criteria
*Essential:* junctional nests of spindle naevomelanocytes; no atypical features.
*Desirable:* abundant melanin in naevomelanocytes and macrophages; break-apart FISH for *NTRK3* or next-generation sequencing to verify an associated fusion {7232}.

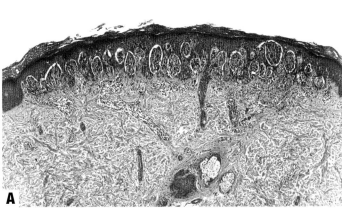 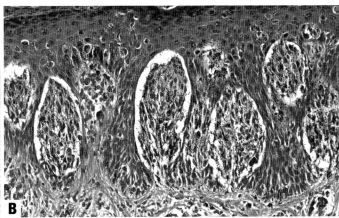

**Fig. 15.30** Reed naevus. **A** A well-circumscribed junctional lesion. **B** Large nests of spindle naevomelanocytes with abundant intracytoplasmic melanin.

## Staging
Not relevant

## Prognosis and prediction
RN is a benign lesion with a low risk of recurrence after adequate excision.

# Melanoma

Fraitag Spinner S
Bastian BC
de la Fouchardière A
Elder DE

## Definition

Melanoma is a malignant neoplasm of melanocytic cells. It is rare in children.

## ICD-O coding

8761/3 Congenital naevus–associated melanoma
8770/3 Spitz melanoma
8743/3 Conventional low-CSD melanoma
8780/3 Melanoma arising in blue naevus
8728/0 Meningeal melanocytosis
8728/3 Meningeal melanomatosis

## ICD-11 coding

2C30.Y & XH5L25 Other specified melanoma of skin & Malignant melanoma arising in giant congenital naevus
2C30.Y & XH8HA2 Other specified melanoma of skin & Mixed epithelioid and spindle cell melanoma
2C30.0 Superficial spreading melanoma, primary
2C30.1 Nodular melanoma, primary
2C30.Z Melanoma of skin, unspecified

## Related terminology

*Acceptable:* childhood melanoma; congenital/infantile melanoma; spitzoid melanoma; conventional/adult melanoma.

## Subtype(s)

Congenital naevus–associated melanoma; Spitz melanoma; conventional melanoma in skin with a low degree of cumulative sun damage (low-CSD melanoma); melanoma arising in blue naevus; meningeal melanocytosis; meningeal melanomatosis

## Localization

Congenital naevus–associated melanoma can occur at any site. Spitz melanomas are located mostly on the limbs and head, and low-CSD melanomas on the torso and legs {1057}. Large naevi localized on the scalp and back, in particular those with satellite naevi, can involve the CNS (a condition called neurocutaneous melanosis) {167,7520}.

## Clinical features

Most congenital naevus–associated melanomas emerge as rapidly growing tumours within the naevus. Spitz melanomas often manifest as rapidly growing unpigmented nodules on normal skin and can mimic a lobular capillary haemangioma (pyogenic granuloma) or xanthogranuloma. Conventional melanomas manifest as irregularly pigmented macules and/or papules meeting the ABCDE criteria for the clinical diagnosis of adult melanoma: asymmetry, border irregularity, colour variegation, diameter enlargement, and evolution (history of change).

Melanoma can be associated with a congenital naevus (commonly large), occasionally even before birth. Very rarely it can occur de novo or manifest as transplacental metastases {5877}. The most common types are Spitz melanomas in prepubescent children, and conventional melanomas, which are similar to the low-CSD melanomas in adults, in older children (mainly after puberty) {445}. A subset of melanomas arise in blue naevi.

## Epidemiology

Melanoma accounts for 3% of all paediatric cancers, with both sexes affected equally. Although 2% of melanomas are reported to occur in patients aged < 20 years, only 0.3% occur in prepubertal children {6656}. The lifetime risk of melanoma for patients with large or giant congenital naevi is 2–10%, with most arising before the age of 10 years {3865}. The incidence of melanoma in adolescents has recently started to decrease, whereas in younger children it has remained stable {1003,431,3374}.

## Etiology

Most paediatric melanomas develop de novo, with no known underlying condition. Large congenital naevus (≥ 200 mm) or

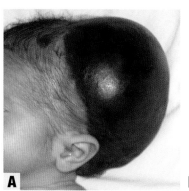
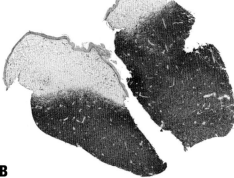
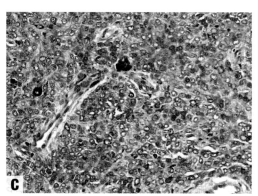

**Fig. 15.31** Congenital melanoma. **A** The child died at the age of 8 months (CHU Béni Messous, Algiers). **B** Cells are positive for HMB45 by immunohistochemistry. **C** Rounded, irregularly pigmented atypical cells with clear nuclei.

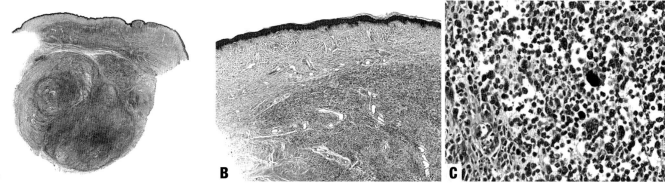

**Fig. 15.32** Congenital naevus–associated melanoma occurring at the age of 8 years. **A** A large tumour is located in the dermis and the subcutis, with no connection to the overlying epidermis. **B** At the top left, in the superficial dermis, there is a congenital junctional melanocytic naevus. **C** Very atypical epithelioid melanocytic cells. The child developed lung metastases at the age of 18 years and was alive without disease at the age of 22 years.

multiple congenital naevi (≥ 2, irrespective of size) and abnormal MRI screening of the CNS in the first few months of life are predisposing factors for congenital naevus–associated melanoma {3609}.

Conventional melanoma is linked to genetic factors such as a light complexion, poor tanning ability, sun exposure, xeroderma pigmentosum, or germline mutation of the *CDKN2A* gene {2474}. *BAP1* tumour predisposition syndrome is also associated with melanoma (see *BAP1 tumour predisposition syndrome*, p. 1012).

### Pathogenesis

Congenital naevus–associated melanomas frequently have *NRAS* mutations. Amplification of mutated *NRAS* has been reported to lead to congenital melanoma arising in the setting of neurocutaneous melanocytosis {6132}. Spitz melanomas are defined as having similar oncogenic alterations to those of Spitz naevi, including kinase fusions involving *ROS1*, *NTRK1*, *NTRK3*, *ALK*, *RET*, *MET*, or *BRAF* and *HRAS*, but no *BRAF* mutations. During progression they acquire inactivation of *CDKN2A* and possibly *TERT* promoter mutations. The low-CSD melanomas in adolescents have similar genetic alterations to those in adults: frequent *BRAF* p.V600 mutations, inactivations of *CDKN2A*, and *TERT* promoter mutations {5709,4245}. Melanomas associated with blue naevi have mutations in the $G_q\alpha$ pathway, mostly at the level of *GNAQ* or *GNA11*.

### Macroscopic appearance

See *Clinical features* (above).

### Histopathology

Melanoma that arises in association with a large congenital naevus often manifests as a nodule in the deep dermis or subcutis, distinct from the background naevus. It can be composed of epithelioid, spindle, or round lymphoblastic-like cells resembling a malignant small blue round cell tumour {3865}. It must be differentiated from proliferative nodules (see *Congenital naevi*, p. 940). Worrisome features are sharp demarcation, expansile growth, pleomorphism, necrosis, and mitotic figures (except in neonates). Immunohistochemistry is of limited utility {5407,956, 7283}.

#### Differential diagnosis

Spitz melanoma usually has irregular epidermal hyperplasia and Kamino bodies. It is characterized by the presence of large epithelioid and fusiform melanocytes arranged in vertically oriented confluent and cellular aggregates. Usually, it is ≥ 6 mm in diameter, asymmetrical, and poorly circumscribed, with a lack of maturation. It shows marked pleomorphism, deep extension, numerous dermal mitoses, and can be ulcerated. HMB45 is often expressed throughout, p16 expression is often lost (see *Spitz naevus*, p. 947).

Low-CSD melanomas are often superficial spreading or nodular, showing pagetoid scatter of enlarged melanocytes, often with dusty melanin pigmentation. However, the presence of pagetoid melanocytic proliferation, which is a helpful criterion in the diagnosis of adult melanoma, should be interpreted with caution when observed in paediatric cases.

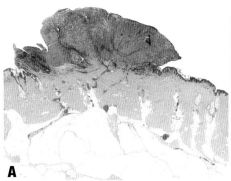
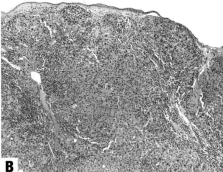
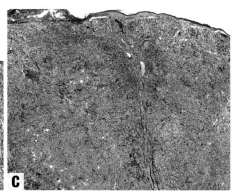

**Fig. 15.33** Small congenital naevus–associated melanoma arising in a 16-year-old adolescent. **A,B** A conventional melanoma arising at the upper part of the dermis. At the periphery there is a junctional naevus. **C** Immunohistochemistry shows inactivation of p16 (CDKN2A).

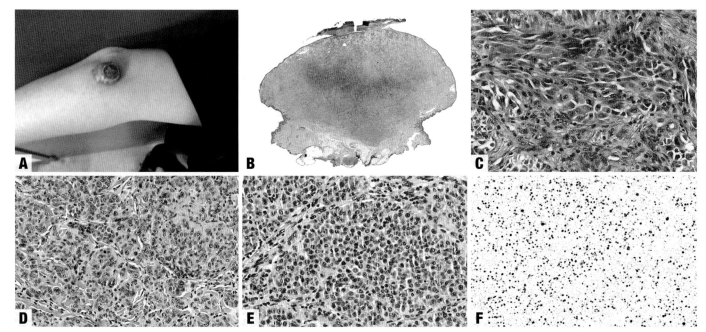

**Fig. 15.34** Spitz melanoma. **A** Spitz melanoma on the right elbow of an 11-year-old girl. There were no distant metastases or local recurrences after a large excision (5 years of follow-up). **B** The tumour infiltrates the whole thickness of the dermis and the superficial subcutis. The lesion seems well circumscribed and symmetrical at first glance. There is an ectopic or invasive nodule deep in the subcutis. **C** High-power view of the deep part of the tumour showing dense cellularity with epithelioid cells and scattered mitotic figures. This tumour showed rearrangement of *ALK*. **D** Some areas are composed of large epithelioid cells simulating a Spitz naevus. **E** Other areas display a denser cellularity with atypical, medium-sized cells with mitotic figures. **F** The Ki-67 proliferation index reaches 40%.

## Cytology
Not clinically relevant

## Diagnostic molecular pathology
Melanomas tend to have multiple DNA copy-number changes, which can be detected by comparative genomic hybridization, FISH, or next-generation sequencing.

Proliferative nodules in congenital naevi tend to have chromosomal aberrations affecting whole chromosomes {532,7283}.

Multiple copy-number changes suggest the diagnosis of Spitz melanoma rather than atypical Spitz naevus, in particular biallelic loss/inactivation of *CDKN2A* at 9p21, especially when associated with *TERT* inactivation {2361}.

Mutation analysis may be helpful in some cases.

## Essential and desirable diagnostic criteria
*Essential:* epithelioid, spindle, or round lymphoblastic-like cells.

*Desirable:* pigmentation (may be absent); immunoreactivity for melanocytic markers.

*Note:* For the diagnosis of Spitz melanoma, fulfilment of a combination of clinical, histological, and molecular criteria is essential, because it overlaps with atypical Spitz tumour and conventional melanoma, some of which may have spitzoid features. Homozygous deletion of *CDKN2A* and/or *TERT* promoter mutation or rearrangement are found in both Spitz subtypes.

## Staging
Melanomas in children are staged in the same way as those in adults. However, high tumour thickness and the presence of nodal metastases in Spitz melanomas do not have the same adverse prognostic role as they do in adult melanomas {3061, 3887}.

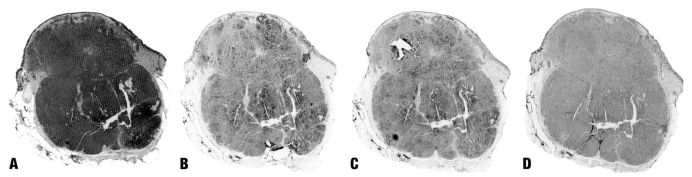

**Fig. 15.35** Spitz melanoma. **A** A well-delimited dermal and subcutaneous tumour with replacement of the skin. **B** Melan-A immunohistochemistry shows heterogeneous staining. **C** HMB45 immunohistochemistry shows heterogeneous and deep staining, emphasizing the absence of vertical maturation. **D** p16 immunohistochemistry shows a total loss of expression.

## Prognosis and prediction

The clinical and histological variables influencing survival in children with melanoma are the same as in adults: ulceration, tumour thickness, and disease stage {850,413,2093}. Paediatric patients with stage I or II disease have a 10-year survival rate of 90% {5328}. Patients aged < 10 years have been reported to have a higher survival rate than adolescents. The prognosis for congenital naevus–associated melanoma is clearly related to melanoma thickness {3865}.

Spitz melanomas are thicker than conventional melanomas and are more frequently ulcerated {4974}, and nodal melanocyte deposits are observed in approximately 50% of cases. Nevertheless, the majority do not develop distant metastases {5327,3887,516,3010}. Therefore, the utility of sentinel lymph node biopsy is questionable for melanomas in childhood other than conventional melanomas {413}.

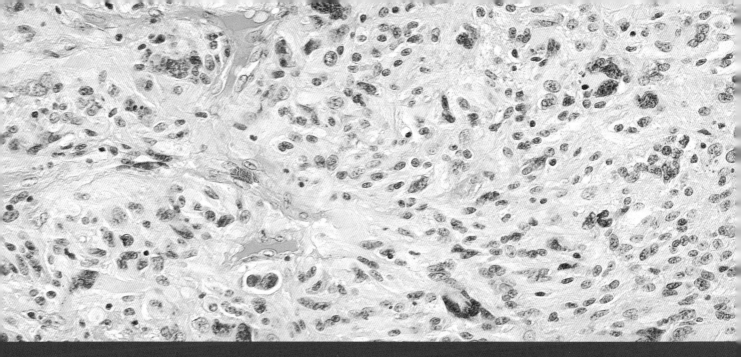

# 16

# Genetic tumour syndromes

Edited by: López-Terrada DH, Lazar AJ

Syndromes predisposing primarily to neural tumours
    Neurofibromatosis type 1
    Neurofibromatosis type 2
    Tuberous sclerosis
    Naevoid basal cell carcinoma syndrome (Gorlin syndrome)
    Retinoblastoma syndrome
Syndromes predisposing primarily to endocrine tumours
    Von Hippel–Lindau syndrome
    Hereditary phaeochromocytoma–paraganglioma syndromes
Syndromes predisposing primarily to Wilms tumours
    WAGR syndrome
    Beckwith–Wiedemann and related overgrowth syndromes
Syndromes predisposing primarily to gastrointestinal tumours
    Familial adenomatous polyposis
    Lynch syndrome
Other syndromes
    Xeroderma pigmentosum
    Rothmund–Thomson syndrome
    Li–Fraumeni syndrome
    DICER1 syndrome
    BAP1 tumour predisposition syndrome
    Constitutional mismatch repair deficiency syndrome
    Rhabdoid tumour predisposition syndrome

# Selected tumour predisposition syndromes: Introduction

López-Terrada DH
Lazar AJ

Advances in our understanding of cancer biology have demonstrated that neoplasms develop as a result of multiple genetic and epigenetic alterations, including mutations, copy-number changes, and gene silencing. The majority of cancers seen in children arise when these abnormalities occur in somatic cells, with only a minority being recognized as clearly caused by germline alterations {881}. Genetic causes of cancer predisposition include germline mutations (either inherited or de novo) and genetic mosaicism, which confer a higher likelihood of developing cancer early in life, compared with the general population. The majority of responsible genes are tumour suppressors, and approximately 10% are oncogenes {6232,6130}. Abnormalities in these genes result in a spectrum of clinical manifestations (including degree of penetrance, age at onset, and associated cancer frequencies) that depend greatly on the tumour type and underlying genetic cause.

Implementation of high-throughput genetic and genomic profiling technologies in the clinical laboratory has accelerated the identification of abnormalities and mechanisms associated with cancer susceptibility syndromes in children. Recent paediatric genomic germline sequencing studies showed that ≥ 10% of paediatric cancer patients, with or without a family history, carry a mutation in a known cancer predisposition gene {881,5365, 2559}, including previously unrecognized associations {4295}. Given the early onset of paediatric tumours and the fact that children are not usually exposed to environmental carcinogens, one would speculate that the number of paediatric cancers attributable to germline mutations in cancer-predisposing genes (including some that may remain unrecognized) may be much higher than previously estimated {3806,5581}.

Clinical tumour sequencing of paediatric cancers is becoming widely used for diagnosis, risk stratification, and selection of appropriate therapies, leading to the routine identification of underlying cancer predisposition germline variants. Pathologists have a very important role in recognizing the paediatric tumour types and syndromes described in this chapter, because for certain histological tumour types, a high proportion are associated with specific syndromes and germline mutations in cancer predisposition genes. Specialized clinical diagnosis, appropriate testing to characterize pathogenic or probably pathogenic mutations, and subsequent surveillance are of utmost importance for early diagnosis in these individuals, and for improving outcomes. Paediatric cancer teams should take into consideration the wide heterogeneity of paediatric genetic susceptibility as well as technical and interpretative challenges {5901}. A multidisciplinary approach should always be attempted, and comprehensive genetic counselling should be available for every patient {6305}.

This chapter will focus on the most common syndromes and conditions that predispose patients to the development of cancer in the first two decades of life, including Li–Fraumeni syndrome, neurofibromatoses (type 1 and type II), overgrowth syndromes (Beckwith–Wiedemann syndrome, WAGR syndrome [Wilms tumour, aniridia, genitourinary anomalies, and a range of developmental delays]), neural tumour syndromes (hereditary retinoblastoma, hereditary neuroblastoma, Gorlin syndrome, malignant rhabdoid tumour syndrome), gastrointestinal cancer syndromes (familial adenomatous polyposis, Lynch syndrome), neuroendocrine syndromes (von Hippel–Lindau syndrome, hereditary phaeochromocytoma–paraganglioma syndrome), DNA instability syndromes (xeroderma pigmentosum, Rothmund–Thomson syndrome), and other miscellaneous syndromes (e.g. *DICER1* syndrome). Table 16.01 includes cancer predisposition syndromes most often diagnosed in children, as well as information regarding their patterns of inheritance, causative gene(s), normal function of the encoded protein(s), and disease/phenotype. Unfortunately, because of space limitations, many other syndromes and conditions that predispose children to cancer are not included in the table or discussed in this chapter. Syndromes associated with specific organ systems (digestive, endocrine, breast, CNS, female genital tract, skin, bone, and soft tissue) can be found in the corresponding volumes of the WHO Classification of Tumours series.

**Table 16.01** Major childhood tumour syndromes (continued on next page)

| Syndrome | Gene | Inheritance | MIM number | Locus | Inheritance | Normal protein function | Neoplasms |
|---|---|---|---|---|---|---|---|
| **Ataxia telangiectasia** | *ATM* | AR | 208900 | 11q22.3 | Point mutation (biallelic), haploinsufficiency | DNA damage response (DNA repair, apoptosis, cell cycle, stress response) | Leukaemia, lymphoma, breast and ovarian cancers |
| **Naevoid basal cell carcinoma syndrome (Gorlin syndrome)** | *PTCH1, PTCH2, SUFU* | AD | 109400 | 1p34.1, 9q22.32, 10q24.32 | Point mutation, deletion | Component of the hedgehog signalling pathway important in embryonic development and tumorigenesis | Basal cell carcinoma, medulloblastoma |
| **Beckwith–Wiedemann syndrome** | *CDKN1C, H19, IGF2, KCNQ1OT1* | AD | 130650 | 11p15.4 | Paternal segmental isodisomy, deletions | Several | Wilms tumour, neuroblastoma, hepatoblastoma, rhabdomyosarcoma |

AD, autosomal dominant; AML, acute myeloid leukaemia; AR, autosomal recessive; CMML, chronic myelomonocytic leukaemia; JMML, juvenile myelomonocytic leukaemia; WAGR syndrome: Wilms tumour, aniridia, genitourinary anomalies, and a range of developmental delays.

| Syndrome | Gene | Inheritance | MIM number | Locus | Inheritanoc | Normal protein function | Neoplasms |
|---|---|---|---|---|---|---|---|
| Birt–Hogg–Dubé syndrome | FLCN | AD | 135150 | 17p11.2 | Small insertions, deletions | GAP that plays a key role in the cellular response to amino acid availability | Renal neoplasms |
| Bloom syndrome | BLM | AR | 210900 | 15q26.1 | Point mutations, deletions | ATP-dependent DNA helicase that unwinds single- and double-stranded DNA; participates in DNA replication and repair | Leukaemia, lymphoma, Wilms tumour, colon cancer, breast cancer, cervical cancer |
| Congenital central hypoventilation syndrome | PHOX2B, others | AD | 209880 | 4p13 | Frameshift or missense | Transcription factor involved in the development of noradrenergic neuron populations and the determination of neurotransmitter phenotype | Neuroblastoma, ganglioneuroma, ganglioneuroblastoma |
| Costello syndrome | HRAS | AD | 218040 | 11p15.5 | Activating missense | Proto-oncogene involved in the activation of RAS protein signal transduction | Papilloma, rhabdomyosarcoma, neuroblastoma, transitional cell carcinoma |
| Cowden syndrome | PTEN, SDHB, SDHD, KLLN | AD | 158350 | 10q23.31 | Point mutations, deletions, promoter mutations | Regulation of cell division; tumour suppression | Breast, thyroid, and renal cancers; glioblastoma |
| Dyskeratosis congenita | DKC1, TERC, TERT | AD | 127550 | 3q26.2 | Point mutations | Telomerase stabilization and maintenance (other) | Leukaemia, oesophageal cancer |
| Dysplastic naevus syndrome | CDKN2A, others | AD | 155600 | 9p21.3, 1p36 | Point mutations, deletions, insertions | Cell-cycle control; stabilizer of the tumour suppressor protein p53 | Melanoma, pancreatic cancer |
| Hereditary breast/ovarian cancer | BRCA1, BRCA2, others | AD, multifactorial | 604370, 612555 | 17q21, 13q13.1 | Point mutations, deletions | Maintenance of genome stability, specifically the homologous recombination pathway for double-strand DNA repair | Breast, ovarian, prostate, and pancreatic cancers |
| Lynch syndrome | MLH1 | AD | 609310 | 3p22.2 | Point mutations | DNA mismatch repair | Colon, uterine, gastric, endometrial, small bowel, and sebaceous gland neoplasms |
| | MSH2 | AD | 120435 | 2p21-p16.3 | | DNA mismatch repair | |
| | MSH6 | AD | 614350 | 2p16.3 | | DNA mismatch repair | |
| | PMS2 | AD | 614337 | 7p22.1 | | DNA mismatch repair | |
| | EPCAM | AD | 613244 | 2p21 | | Calcium-independent cell–cell adhesion; mutation results in epigenetic changes | |
| Fanconi anaemia | Many FANCA, FANCB, FANCC, BRCA2 (FANCD1), FANCD2, FANCE, FANCF, FANCG, FANCI, BRIP1 (FANCJ), FANCL, FANCM, PALB2 (FANCN), RAD51C, SLX4 (BTBD12) | AR | 227650 | 16q24.3 | Truncating, frameshift, missense | DNA repair, postreplication repair or a cell-cycle checkpoint function, interstrand DNA crosslink repair and in maintenance of normal chromosome stability; others | Colon, thyroid, gastric, and intestinal neoplasms; hepatoblastoma; desmoid tumours; medulloblastoma |

AD, autosomal dominant; AML, acute myeloid leukaemia; AR, autosomal recessive; CMML, chronic myelomonocytic leukaemia; JMML, juvenile myelomonocytic leukaemia; WAGR syndrome: Wilms tumour, aniridia, genitourinary anomalies, and a range of developmental delays.

**Table 16.01** Major childhood tumour syndromes (continued from previous page, continued on next page)

| Syndrome | Gene | Inheritance | MIM number | Locus | Inheritance | Normal protein function | Neoplasms |
|---|---|---|---|---|---|---|---|
| **Familial AML** | *RUNX1*, others | AD | 601626 | 21q22.12 | Point mutations | Transcription factor involved in the generation and differentiation of haematopoietic stem cells | Leukaemia |
| **Familial paraganglioma phaeochromocytoma syndrome** | *SDHB, SDHAF2, SDHC, SDHD* | AD | 115310, others | 1p36.13, others | Splice-site, frameshift, nonsense | Complex II of the respiratory chain specifically involved in the oxidation of succinate; others | Paraganglioma, phaeochromocytoma, neuroblastoma |
| **Li–Fraumeni syndrome** | *TP53* | AD | 151623 | 17p13.1 | Point mutations | Regulation of cell division; tumour suppression | Soft tissue sarcoma, osteosarcoma, breast cancer, adrenocortical carcinoma, leukaemia, brain tumours (glioblastoma multiforme, high-grade astrocytoma / primitive neuroectodermal tumour, medulloblastoma, choroid plexus carcinoma) |
| **Multiple endocrine neoplasia type 1** | *MEN1* | AD | 131100 | 11q13 | Point mutations, insertions, deletions | DNA repair and regulation of apoptosis; tumour suppression | Pancreatic islet cell tumours, pituitary adenoma, parathyroid adenoma |
| **Multiple endocrine neoplasia type 2A** | *RET* | AD | 171400 | 10q11.21 | Point mutations | Normal development of nerve cells | Medullary thyroid carcinoma, phaeochromocytoma, parathyroid hyperplasia |
| **Multiple endocrine neoplasia type 2B** | *RET* | AD | 162300 | 10q11.21 | Point mutations | Normal development of nerve cells | Medullary thyroid carcinoma, phaeochromocytoma, mucosal neuromas |
| **Multiple endocrine neoplasia type 4** | *CDKN1B* | AD | 610755 | 12p13.1 | Point mutation | Prevention of aberrant cell division; tumour suppression | Parathyroid, pituitary, adrenal, kidney, and reproductive organ tumours |
| **Neurofibromatosis type 1** | *NF1, SPRED1* | AD | 162200 | 17q11.2, 15q14 | Point mutations, deletions, translocations | Negative regulation of RAS | Neurofibroma, optic pathway glioma, peripheral nerve sheath tumour, astrocytoma, paraganglioma/phaeochromocytoma, CMML/JMML, AML |
| **Neurofibromatosis type 2** | *NF2* | AD | 101000 | 22q12.2 | Point mutations | Regulation of the Hippo signalling pathway; tumour suppression | Astrocytoma, meningioma, melanoma |
| **Noonan syndrome / Noonan-like syndrome** | *PTPN11, HRAS, KRAS, NRAS, RAF1, SOS1, BRAF, SHOC2, MAPK1* | AD, other | 163950, others | 12q24.13 | Activating missense | Several | Leukaemia, neuroblastoma, rhabdomyosarcoma |
| **Nijmegen breakage syndrome** | *NBN* | AR | 251260 | 8q21.3 | Point mutations | Cellular response to DNA damage; maintenance of chromosome integrity | Lymphoma, leukaemia |
| **Peutz–Jeghers syndrome** | *STK11 (LKB1)* | AD | 175200 | 19p13.3 | Point mutations | Suppression of cell division; tumour suppression | Gastric, small intestine, colon, pancreatic, uterine, and breast cancers |
| **Familial adenomatous polyposis** | *APC* | AD | 175100 | 5q22.2 | Point mutations leading to truncations | Tumour suppressor protein that acts as an antagonist of the WNT signalling pathway | Colon, small intestine, thyroid, and pancreatic cancers; hepatoblastoma; medulloblastoma |

AD, autosomal dominant; AML, acute myeloid leukaemia; AR, autosomal recessive; CMML, chronic myelomonocytic leukaemia; JMML, juvenile myelomonocytic leukaemia; WAGR syndrome: Wilms tumour, aniridia, genitourinary anomalies, and a range of developmental delays.

**Table 16.01** Major childhood tumour syndromes (continued)

| Syndrome | Gene | Inheritance | MIM number | Locus | Inheritance | Normal protein function | Neoplasms |
|---|---|---|---|---|---|---|---|
| Retinoblastoma | RB1 (RB) | AD | 180200 | 13q14.2 | Deletions, point mutations | Negative regulation of the cell cycle; tumour suppression | Retinoblastoma, osteosarcoma, melanoma, pineoblastoma, lung cancers |
| Von Hippel–Lindau syndrome | VHL | AD | 193300 | 3p25.3 | Point mutations, deletions | Ubiquitination and degradation of HIF; tumour suppression | Renal cell carcinoma, pancreatic islet cell tumours, phaeochromocytoma |
| Werner syndrome | WRN | AR | 277700 | 8p12 | Point mutations | DNA helicase protein, maintenance of genome stability, DNA repair, replication, transcription and telomere maintenance | Leukaemia, melanoma, osteosarcoma, thyroid cancer |
| Xeroderma pigmentosum | Many | AR, AD, variable | Several | Several | Point mutations | Several | Basal cell neoplasms, melanoma, stomach cancer, leukaemia |
| WAGR syndrome | WT1 | AD | 194072 | 11p13 | Deletions | Transcription factor; normal development of the urogenital system | Neuroblastoma |
| Weaver syndrome | EZH2 | AD | 277590 | 7q36.1 | Missense and truncating | Histone methyltransferase | Neuroblastoma |
| Wiskott–Aldrich syndrome | WAS | X-linked recessive | 301000 | Xp11.23 | Point mutations | Transduction of signals from receptors on the cell surface to the actin cytoskeleton | Leukaemia, lymphoma |

AD, autosomal dominant; AML, acute myeloid leukaemia; AR, autosomal recessive; CMML, chronic myelomonocytic leukaemia; JMML, juvenile myelomonocytic leukaemia; WAGR syndrome: Wilms tumour, aniridia, genitourinary anomalies, and a range of developmental delays.

Chapter 16

# Neurofibromatosis type 1

Fisher MJ
Gutmann DH
Perry A
Reuss DE
Rodriguez FJ

## Definition

Neurofibromatosis type 1 (NF1) is an autosomal dominant disorder caused by mutation of the gene *NF1*, diagnosed clinically when at least two of the following are present: multiple café-au-lait macules, skinfold freckling, iris hamartomas (Lisch nodules), optic pathway glioma / pilocytic astrocytoma (OPG), multiple neurofibromas or one plexiform neurofibroma, specific osseous lesions, and an affected first-degree relative.

## MIM numbering

162200 Neurofibromatosis type 1; NF1

## ICD-11 coding

LD2D.10 Neurofibromatosis type 1

## Related terminology

*Not recommended:* von Recklinghausen disease; peripheral neurofibromatosis.

## Subtype(s)

Mosaic neurofibromatosis type 1, including segmental neurofibromatosis type 1; spinal neurofibromatosis; neurofibromatosis–Noonan syndrome; 17q11.2 microdeletion syndrome

## Localization

NF1 affects many different cell types and tissues in the body, including the central and peripheral nervous systems.

## Clinical features

Multiple café-au-lait macules are usually present at birth, and they increase in number during the first 2 years of life. Skinfold freckling in the axillary, inguinal, and submammary regions occurs in > 80% of adults with NF1. Lisch nodules (iris hamartomas), present in > 90% of adults with NF1, are best detected by slit-lamp examination. Both Lisch nodules and skinfold freckling usually develop before puberty. Cutaneous neurofibromas, present in > 85% of adults with NF1 {2636}, typically develop during puberty. In contrast, plexiform neurofibromas are probably congenital lesions, arising in 30–50% of children with NF1 {2636}. Individual plexiform neurofibromas have variable growth rates, which can be relatively constant for long periods of time but exhibit the highest growth potential during infancy and childhood. A subset of plexiform neurofibromas transform into atypical neurofibroma / atypical neurofibromatous neoplasm of uncertain biological potential (ANNUBP), which can be a premalignant lesion with an increased risk of progression to high-grade malignant peripheral nerve sheath tumour (MPNST) {4672,569}. Possible transformation to ANNUBP or MPNST should be considered in patients with growing nodular plexiform neurofibromas, patients with plexiform neurofibromas in which an isolated portion exhibits disproportionate growth relative to the rest of the tumour, and individuals with continued growth of a plexiform neurofibroma into adulthood.

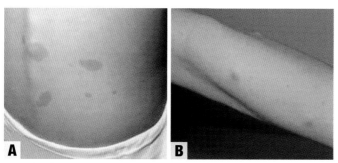

**Fig. 16.01** Neurofibromatosis type 1. **A** Multiple café-au-lait spots on the back of a child with neurofibromatosis type 1. **B** Left arm of an adult with neurofibromatosis type 1, showing cutaneous neurofibromas.

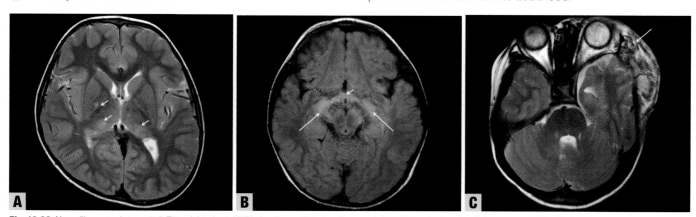

**Fig. 16.02** Neurofibromatosis type 1. **A** T2-weighted axial MRI showing multiple focal areas of signal intensity (previously known as "unidentified bright objects") present in the basal ganglia and thalamic nuclei (arrows). These are common CNS findings in neurofibromatosis type 1. **B** FLAIR MRI showing increased signal intensity at the optic chiasm (short arrow) and bilateral optic radiations (long arrows) consistent with optic pathway glioma / pilocytic astrocytoma. **C** T2-weighted axial MRI showing left sphenoid wing dysplasia (arrow) and mild protrusion of the left eye globe.

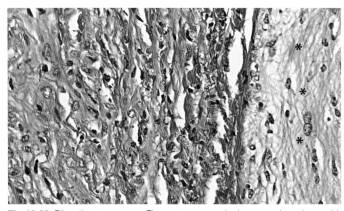

**Fig. 16.03** Pilocytic astrocytoma. The most common brain tumour in patients with neurofibromatosis type 1 is pilocytic astrocytoma, which is frequently located in association with the optic nerve (asterisks).

Specific bone abnormalities can be present in individuals with NF1, including severe scoliosis, sphenoid wing dysplasia, non-ossifying fibromas, and congenital tibial bowing. Progressive tibial bowing can result in pathological fracture, with the development of a pseudarthrosis {6235}.

Many children with NF1 exhibit learning disabilities, attention deficit hyperactivity disorder (ADHD), and problems with reciprocal social interactions {4798}. Brain MRI morphometry shows a larger grey matter volume and a larger corpus callosum, both of which may be associated with learning disabilities {4776}.

Fifteen per cent of children with NF1 will develop an OPG, which can cause progressive vision loss in > 50% of affected individuals {4149}. The second most common location for a glioma is the brainstem {4330}; however, gliomas can develop in other locations {4329}. Young adults with NF1 are also prone to malignant gliomas {5275}. Brain MRI in children shows focal areas of high signal intensity on T2-weighted sequences, which tend to disappear with age and are sometimes difficult to differentiate from low-grade gliomas {2554}.

Epilepsy is more common in individuals with NF1, and drug-resistant epilepsy requiring surgery is often associated with dysembryoplastic neuroepithelial tumours in these patients {5236}. Sleep disturbances are also common in people with NF1 {4109}.

Other neoplasms observed at increased frequency are juvenile myelomonocytic leukaemia, rhabdomyosarcoma, glomus tumours of the digits, gastrointestinal stromal tumours, phaeochromocytoma, breast cancer in female patients, and duodenal neuroendocrine tumours (somatostatinomas) {854}.

## Epidemiology
NF1 is a common autosomal dominant disorder with an incidence of 33.3 cases per 100 000 births {7159}.

## Etiology
NF1 is caused by heterozygous pathogenic variants in the gene *NF1* on chromosome 17q11.2, which encodes neurofibromin (NF1) {7372,1109,7312}. Half of all individuals with NF1 have unaffected parents; such cases represent de novo mutations.

## Pathogenesis
Neurofibromin (NF1) primarily functions as a GAP for the RAS oncogenes {4029}. The EVH1 domain of SPRED1 (the protein implicated in Legius syndrome) binds to neurofibromin (NF1) on both sides of the GAP-related domain and recruits neurofibromin (NF1) to the membrane, where it can accelerate RAS inactivation {6724,2907,1854}.

Most clinical features of NF1, including café-au-lait macules, bony abnormalities, and benign tumours, result from a complete loss of neurofibromin (NF1) function (biallelic *NF1* inactivation), leading to increased RAS and RAS-effector (MEK/ERK or AKT/mTOR) signalling. Atypical neurofibromas / ANNUBPs harbour additional genetic alterations, including loss of the *CDKN2A* and/or *CDKN2B* and *SMARCA2* regions on chromosome 9p {569, 5433,7698}. MPNSTs have a highly rearranged karyotype and frequently show additional aberrations in PRC2 genes and (to a lesser extent) in *TP53* {1647,4024,7839}. Low-grade gliomas in NF1 are typically characterized by biallelic *NF1* loss alone, although other mutations are occasionally seen. Alterations in *CDKN2A*, *CDKN2B*, and/or *ATRX* have been detected in some NF1 low-grade gliomas, where they are often associated with worrisome histological features (anaplasia and increased proliferation) and more aggressive tumour behaviour. In the absence of a low-grade precursor such as pilocytic astrocytoma, high-grade gliomas in NF1 are also characterized by *TP53* mutations, as well as mutations in *CDKN2A* and/or *CDKN2B* and in *ATRX* {1554}.

In both neurofibromas and OPGs, murine studies have revealed that non-neoplastic (stromal) cells with a heterozygous *NF1* mutation, including mast cells, macrophages, neurons, T cells, and microglia, are critical for tumorigenesis and continued growth.

## Macroscopic appearance
The macroscopic appearances of nerve sheath neoplasms affecting people with NF1 include small sessile or pedunculated growths of the skin (cutaneous neurofibromas); plaque-like thickening of the skin (diffuse neurofibroma); fusiform segmental expansions of individual peripheral nerve fascicles (intraneural neurofibromas); and multinodular/multifascicular nerve expansions, described as a "bag of worms" (plexiform neurofibromas). Massive soft tissue neurofibromas occur exclusively in individuals with NF1 and are characterized by large neurofibromatous involvement of anatomical segments (even entire limbs) with infiltration of soft tissue and skeletal muscle. Fleshy masses and areas of necrosis and haemorrhage characterize MPNST.

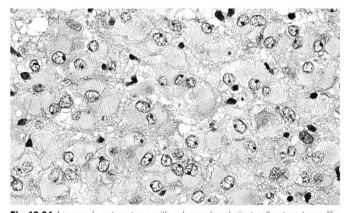

**Fig. 16.04** Low-grade astrocytoma with subependymal giant cell astrocytoma–like morphology. A variety of gliomas may also affect patients with neurofibromatosis type 1, including low-grade astrocytomas that are difficult to classify, occasionally demonstrating subependymal giant cell astrocytoma–like morphology.

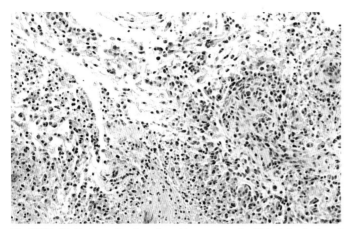

**Fig. 16.05** Glioblastoma. Overtly malignant tumours usually afflict adult patients and may contain infiltration, mitotic activity, and palisading necrosis typical of glioblastoma.

## Histopathology

Nerve sheath tumours in NF1 are predominantly neurofibromas, which resemble their sporadic counterparts. Cells of the haematopoietic lineage (including histiocytes and mast cells) are also encountered and contribute to the tumour microenvironment {3449}.

Recently proposed criteria for ANNUBP are used to describe premalignant or worrisome changes in neurofibromas. They include at least two of the following: cytological atypia, hypercellularity, loss of neurofibroma architecture, and increased mitotic count (< 1.5 mitoses/mm², equating to 3 mitoses/10 HPF of 0.51 mm in diameter and 0.20 mm² in area) {4672}. These changes may be present in clinically designated atypical neurofibromas, which in a subset of cases later transform into MPNST {2888}.

Most MPNSTs in individuals with NF1 are high-grade malignant spindle cell neoplasms with brisk mitotic activity and necrosis, which either develop in a pre-existing plexiform neurofibroma or arise de novo. A wide spectrum of heterologous differentiation (cartilaginous, osseous, rhabdomyoblastic, glandular) may be present.

Immunohistochemical analyses frequently demonstrate p16 and H3 p.K27me3 loss {1354}, as well as decreased or absent expression of Schwann cell markers (S100, SOX10).

Individuals with NF1 are also predisposed to a variety of glial neoplasms, with pilocytic astrocytomas being the predominant histological subtype. Difficult-to-classify gliomas with ambiguous features may also be encountered, as well as low-grade gliomas with morphological similarities to subependymal giant cell astrocytomas {5293}. High-grade astrocytomas in NF1 tend to affect young adults and are similar in aggressiveness to their sporadic counterparts. High-grade astrocytomas in NF1 frequently have loss of ATRX expression, resulting in an alternative-lengthening-of-telomeres phenotype {5934,1554}.

## Cytology

Not clinically relevant

## Diagnostic molecular pathology

Although no mutation hotspots have been identified, a pathogenic *NF1* variant is detected in 95% of people with NF1 {4614}.

Nonsense, frameshift, and splice-site mutations, as well as small insertions, small deletions, or small duplications, all result in *NF1* inactivation. In 5–10% of cases, a 17q11.2 microdeletion is identified, in which multiple genes are codeleted along with *NF1*. One of these deleted genes, *SUZ12*, a component of the polycomb repressive complex 2, has been implicated in MPNST development {1647,4024,7839}.

To date, the most striking genotype–phenotype correlations involve individuals with a specific 3 bp deletion in *NF1* (c.2970_2972del) or with a missense mutation affecting codon p.R1809. These individuals do not develop neurofibromas or OPGs {3682,5958,5552,7150}. In addition, patients with *NF1* missense mutations involving codons 844–848 appear to exhibit a more severe disease symptomatology, including a higher incidence of externally visible plexiform neurofibromas, symptomatic spinal nerve root neurofibromas, OPG, and MPNST {3683}.

### Essential and desirable diagnostic criteria

*Essential:* a clinical diagnosis of NF1 requires the presence of at least two of the following features: six or more café-au-lait macules (> 5 mm diameter in children, > 15 mm in adults); two or more cutaneous or subcutaneous neurofibromas or one plexiform neurofibroma; axillary/inguinal freckling; an OPG; two or more iris hamartomas (Lisch nodules); a distinctive bony abnormality (tibial dysplasia, pseudarthrosis, orbital dysplasia); a first-degree relative with NF1 (by the above criteria).

*Note:* in the future, these criteria may be revised to include genetic testing and other common newly recognized clinical features. In young children, multiple café-au-lait macules are usually the only clinical sign of NF1, such that in the absence of an affected parent, a diagnosis of NF1 cannot be rendered. Multiple café-au-lait spots with or without skinfold freckling can be seen in other conditions, including Legius syndrome (MIM number: 611431). Multiple neurofibromas can also be associated with certain forms of Noonan syndrome, making molecular analysis of the gene *NF1* increasingly more important for diagnostic purposes {4613,5370,1412}. In children with multiple café-au-lait spots and malignant tumours (e.g. leukaemia), constitutive mismatch repair deficiency should also be considered {6752}.

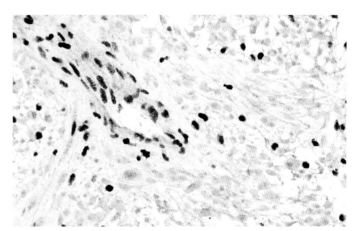

**Fig. 16.06** Neurofibromatosis type 1–associated high-grade glioma. *ATRX* mutations lead to loss of ATRX protein staining by immunohistochemistry, with preservation in blood vessels and other non-neoplastic cells.

## Staging

Not relevant

## Prognosis and prediction

NF1 is an autosomal dominant disorder; affected parents harbour a 50% risk of disease transmission with each pregnancy. Individuals often have a shortened lifespan, which is mainly due to malignant disease and stroke {7159,1999,5784}. The standard mortality ratio for many complications is higher in women aged < 50 years {7159}. Genetic counselling is recommended and includes the possibility of prenatal and/or preimplantation genetic testing.

MEK inhibitors are approved for use in children aged 2–18 years with NF1 who have symptomatic, inoperable plexiform neurofibromas, and they are currently being evaluated for adults with plexiform neurofibromas as well as children with low-grade glioma {2567,5463,3649}.

# Neurofibromatosis type 2

Kratz CP
Louis DN
Perry A
Schuhmann MU
Stemmer-Rachamimov AO

## Definition

Neurofibromatosis type 2 (NF2) is an autosomal dominant disease caused by a pathological variant of the gene *NF2* at 22q12.2 and characterized by multiple benign tumours and dysplastic/hamartomatous lesions in the nervous system, including multiple schwannomas (particularly bilateral vestibular schwannomas), meningiomas, and spinal ependymomas.

## MIM numbering

101000 Neurofibromatosis type 2; NF2

## ICD-11 coding

LD2D.11 Neurofibromatosis type 2

## Related terminology

*Acceptable:* bilateral acoustic neurofibromatosis; central neurofibromatosis.
*Not recommended:* von Recklinghausen disease.

## Subtype(s)

Wishart phenotype (severe); Gardner phenotype (mild)

## Localization

Tumours and hamartomas associated with NF2 affect all locations of the central and peripheral nervous system, with predilections for cranial, paraspinal, and peripheral nerves, as well as the meninges and the spinal cord.

## Clinical features

Patients with NF2 often present in early adulthood (~20 years of age), although the disease can manifest in childhood. The most common presentation in adults is with symptoms referable to a

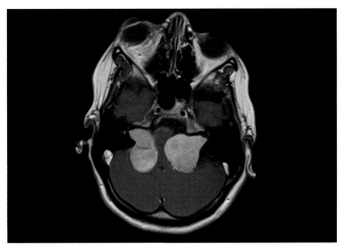

**Fig. 16.07** Neurofibromatosis type 2 schwannomas. MRI of bilateral vestibular schwannomas, the hallmark of neurofibromatosis type 2. When large, vestibular schwannomas may compress the brain stem.

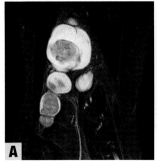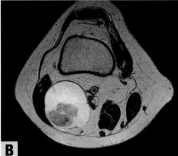

**Fig. 16.08** Plexiform schwannoma. **A,B** MRI showing a large plexiform schwannoma in a patient with neurofibromatosis type 2.

vestibular schwannoma (hearing loss, tinnitus, or imbalance). Presentation with vestibular schwannomas is uncommon in children (seen in only 15% of children with *NF2*), whereas cutaneous schwannomas (NF2 plaques) and ocular abnormalities are more frequent {1991}. NF2 mosaicism, in which a somatic mutation occurs during embryogenesis, appears to be more prevalent than previously thought and has variable phenotypes depending on the cell lineages involved {1993}. It may be challenging to diagnose, and the clinical symptoms may overlap with those of schwannomatosis {5583}.

### Clinical diagnostic criteria

The original clinical diagnostic criteria for NF2 were established at the US National Institutes of Health (NIH) Consensus Development Conference on Neurofibromatosis in 1987 {4945}. Several revisions of these criteria have since been proposed, including the NIH 1991, Manchester (see Box 16.01, p. 970), National Neurofibromatosis Foundation (NNFF), Baser, and Smith criteria. Each of these revisions expanded the original criteria, aiming also to identify patients with multiple NF2 features who do not present with bilateral vestibular schwannomas and have no family history {525,1996,2634}.

When based on clinical features, the diagnosis of NF2 may be challenging because of the wide variability of symptoms and time of onset. Particularly difficult to diagnose is genetic mosaicism (accounting for as many as 60% of sporadic cases {1993}), in which segmental involvement or milder disease may occur {3662}, and paediatric cases in which the full manifestations of the disease have not yet developed. The distinction from other forms is difficult in some cases. There is clinical phenotypic overlap between mosaic NF2, early NF2, and schwannomatosis; some cases that fulfil the clinical diagnostic criteria for schwannomatosis are later proved to be NF2 {5583}. Molecular testing for mutations in *LZTR1* and *SMARCB1* (the two schwannomatosis genes) and in *NF2* is helpful when a patient does not meet the clinical criteria for a definite diagnosis and/or demonstrates overlapping clinical features of NF2 and schwannomatosis.

## Schwannomas

NF2-associated schwannomas differ from sporadic tumours in several ways. They arise in younger patients (in the third versus sixth decades of life), and many patients develop bilateral vestibular schwannomas by their fourth decade of life {1996,4440}. Recent studies with high-resolution MRI showed that in many cases patients have multiple discrete tumour nodules along both the superior and inferior vestibular nerve branches, as well as the cochlear and facial nerves {6701}. This finding refutes the previous hypothesis of schwannoma originating at the junction of central and peripheral myelination in the internal auditory meatus proposed by H. Cushing. In some cases, tumours are a coalescence of multiple nodules/tumours, each with its own somatic *NF2* mutation or deletion {1723}. This explains the characteristic gross and microscopic feature of multinodularity {6564}, as well as the observed lower rates of treatment efficacy and higher rates of surgical complications compared with sporadic vestibular schwannomas {1296,1990}. In addition to the eighth cranial nerve, other sensory nerves may be affected, including the fifth cranial nerve and spinal dorsal roots. However, motor nerves such as the twelfth cranial nerve may also be involved {1996,4230}. In addition to larger schwannomas, peripheral nerves and spinal nerves of patients with NF2 may have numerous small Schwann cell tumourlets, which despite their small size show biallelic *NF2* inactivation suggestive of precursor neoplastic lesions {6674}. Plexiform schwannomas are common and may involve large plexuses (brachial, sacral), skin, or subcutaneous tissues. Cutaneous plexiform schwannomas are common in paediatric patients and are characteristically associated with a pigmented plaque-like lesion {1996,4440, 1091}.

## Meningiomas

Multiple meningiomas represent the second hallmark of NF2, affecting half of all patients {4230}. NF2-associated meningiomas can occur throughout the meninges but are more common in the intracranial compartment (including along the falx cerebri) than the spinal compartment {1004,1466} and may affect sites such as the cerebral ventricles. NF2-associated meningiomas occur earlier in life than sporadic meningiomas {5364} and may be the presenting feature, especially in paediatric patients {1991,1996,4440}.

## Gliomas

Ependymomas account for most of the histologically diagnosed gliomas in NF2, and for almost all spinal gliomas {5943,6061}. In most cases, NF2 spinal ependymomas are multiple, intramedullary, slow-growing, asymptomatic masses {5943,6061}. Most (70–80%) occur in the cervicomedullary junction or cervical spine; a minority occur in the thoracic spine {5391,4484}. Diffuse and pilocytic astrocytomas have been reported in NF2 but probably constitute misdiagnosed tanycytic ependymomas {2661}.

## Meningioangiomatosis

Meningioangiomatosis is a cortical lesion characterized by a plaque-like proliferation of perivascular meningothelial and fibroblast-like cells. It occurs both sporadically and in NF2. Sporadic meningioangiomatosis is a single lesion that usually occurs in young adults or children, who present with seizures or persistent headaches. In contrast, NF2-associated meningioangiomatosis may be multifocal and often asymptomatic, diagnosed only at autopsy {6673}. Meningioangiomatosis may be predominantly vascular (resembling a vascular malformation) or predominantly meningothelial, sometimes with an associated meningioma, although most of the latter probably represent meningiomas with perivascular spread along Virchow–Robin spaces instead {5471}.

## Glial hamartias (also called microhamartomas)

These are circumscribed cellular clusters of the neocortex with medium to large atypical nuclei. They are scattered throughout the cortex and basal ganglia and show strong S100 immunoreactivity but only focal GFAP positivity. Glial hamartias are common in and pathognomonic of NF2 {6034,7540}, and they are not associated with developmental delays or gliomas. The hamartias are usually intracortical, with a predilection for the molecular and deeper cortical layers, but they have also been observed in the basal ganglia, thalamus, cerebellum, and spinal cord {7540}. The fact that merlin (NF2) expression is retained in glial hamartias suggests the possibility that haploinsufficiency during development underlies these malformations {6672}.

## Peripheral neuropathies

Neuropathies not related to tumour masses are increasingly recognized as a common feature of NF2 {1449,4230}. Mononeuropathies may be the presenting symptom in children {1991}, whereas progressive polyneuropathies are more common in adults. Sural nerve biopsies from patients with NF2 suggest that NF2 neuropathies are mostly axonal and may be secondary to focal nerve compression by Schwann cell tumourlets or may be onion bulb–like Schwann cell or perineurial cell proliferations without associated axons {6620,6976}.

## Ophthalmological manifestations

Posterior lens opacities are common in children (juvenile posterior cataract) and highly characteristic of NF2. A variety of retinal abnormalities, including hamartomas, tufts, dysplasias, and epiretinal membranes, may also be found {1133,2582}.

## Neurofibromas

Cutaneous neurofibromas have been reported in NF2. However, on histological review, many such neurofibromas prove to be schwannomas, including plexiform schwannomas and hybrid schwannomas/neurofibromas.

## Skin manifestations

Café-au-lait spots may be present in patients with NF2, but they are fewer in number than in neurofibromatosis type 1 and not associated with freckling.

## Epidemiology

NF2 affects 1 in 25 000–40 000 individuals {1998}. There is no evidence of racial or sex preference.

## Etiology

NF2 is an autosomal dominant disease caused by inactivation of the *NF2* gene. About half of all NF2 cases are sporadic, occurring in individuals with no family history and caused by

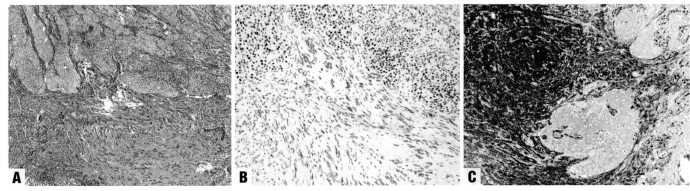

**Fig. 16.09** Schwannoma/meningioma. **A** A collision tumour of schwannoma (lower half) and meningioma (upper half) is characteristic of neurofibromatosis type 2. **B** The meningioma component is highlighted with PR immunostaining. **C** The schwannoma component is highlighted with S100 immunostaining.

newly acquired germline mutations. More than 50% of de novo cases are somatic mosaics, in which the pathogenic variant is present only in some of the individual's cells {1993,3662,7071}.

## Pathogenesis
### The NF2 gene
The *NF2* gene maps to chromosome 22 {6022,7071}, spans 110 kb, and consists of 17 exons. *NF2* mRNA transcripts encode at least two protein forms generated by alternative splicing at the C-terminus. The predominant gene product, merlin (NF2), encoded by exons 1–15 and 17, is a cytoskeletal protein with similar intramolecular interactions to those of the ERM proteins (ezrin, radixin, and moesin) {2629,7658}.

### Gene mutations
Numerous germline and somatic *NF2* mutations have been detected, supporting the hypothesis that *NF2* functions as a tumour suppressor gene {2630,4230}. Germline *NF2* mutations differ somewhat from the somatic mutations identified in sporadic schwannomas and meningiomas. The most frequent germline mutations are point mutations that alter splice junctions or create new stop codons {813,4230,4293,4601,6022,6114,7071}. Germline mutations occur preferentially in exons 1–8 {4601}.

### Gene expression
*NF2* is expressed in most normal human tissues, including brain {6022,7071}. The structural similarity of merlin (NF2) to the ERM proteins suggests that it links membrane-associated proteins and the actin cytoskeleton, thus regulating signal transmission from the extracellular environment to the cell {4498} and influencing multiple downstream pathways including the MAPK, FAK/SRC, PI3K/AKT, RAC/PAK/JNK, mTOR, and WNT/β-catenin pathways. Many merlin (NF2) binding partners have been identified, including integrins and TRKs {3622, 4875}. In addition to its tumour suppression function at the cell membrane, merlin (NF2) translocates to the nucleus where it suppresses the E3 ubiquitin ligase IL-17RB, which is involved in transcription activity {4090}.

## Macroscopic appearance
NF2 schwannomas may have a multilobular (cluster-of-grapes) appearance on both gross and microscopic examination {7516}. Multiple Schwann cell tumourlets may develop along individual nerves, particularly on spinal roots and the cauda equina {4230, 6674}. The gross appearance of meningiomas and ependymomas in NF2 is similar to that of non-syndromic tumours.

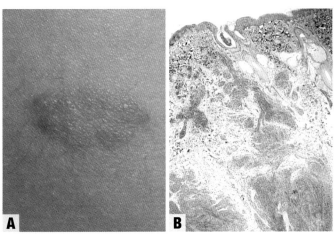

**Fig. 16.10** Cutaneous schwannoma. **A** Cutaneous schwannoma is a common manifestation in children with neurofibromatosis type 2 and is often associated with a raised pigmented lesion of the skin (neurofibromatosis type 2 plaque). **B** S100 immunostaining highlighting a cutaneous plexiform schwannoma.

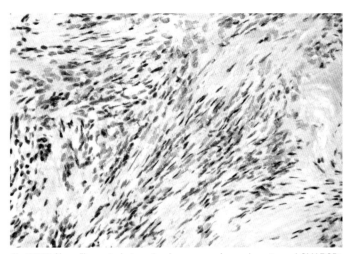

**Fig. 16.11** Neurofibromatosis type 2 schwannoma. A mosaic pattern of SMARCB1 (INI1) staining is common in syndromic (neurofibromatosis type 2 and schwannomatosis) schwannomas.

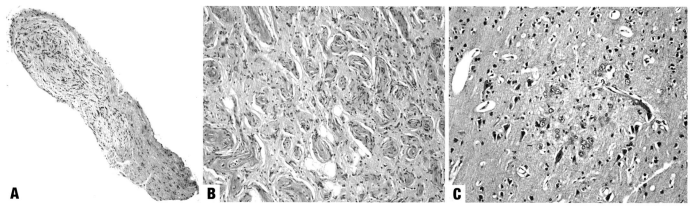

**Fig. 16.12** Other lesions in neurofibromatosis type 2. **A** A Schwann cell tumourlet embedded in a peripheral nerve. **B** Meningioangiomatosis histologically consists of an intracortical proliferation of small capillaries with a cuff of perivascular meningothelial cells, separated by brain parenchyma. In neurofibromatosis type 2, most cases are asymptomatic. **C** Small clusters of atypical large cells, known as glial microhamartomas. They are asymptomatic and pathognomonic of neurofibromatosis type 2.

## Histopathology

NF2 schwannomas may have a multilobular appearance on microscopic examination {7516}, which may reflect a multicentric origin. NF2 schwannomas may entrap seventh cranial nerve fibres {3179} and have a high proliferative activity {276}, although these features do not necessarily connote more aggressive behaviour. A mosaic pattern of immunostaining for SMARCB1 expression (indicating patchy loss) has been reported in most syndrome-associated schwannomas, including in both NF2 and schwannomatosis {5387}. Hybrid schwannoma/neurofibroma tumours are common in NF2 (30% of NF2 schwannomas) {2713, 4771}.

All major subtypes of meningioma can occur in patients with NF2, but the most common subtype is fibroblastic {275,4230}. Although many NF2-associated meningiomas are CNS WHO grade 1 tumours, a wide spectrum of tumours are encountered, including aggressive subtypes {275,5469}. Some reports have characterized their growth as saltatory {1763}. Collision tumours of meningioma and schwannoma are characteristic of NF2.

## Cytology

Not relevant

## Diagnostic molecular pathology

A pathogenic sequence variant of the *NF2* gene is detected in 70–90% of patients with NF2, with lower detection rates in de novo cases (60%), which is most likely due to somatic mosaicism {7371,2001}. The risk of transmission to offspring in familial cases is 50%. Risk of transmission in individuals with mosaicism is unknown. Prenatal diagnosis by mutation analysis and testing of the children of patients with NF2 is possible when the mutation is known.

## Essential and desirable diagnostic criteria

*Essential:* clinical criteria as previously outlined (see Box 16.01, p. 970) OR a demonstrable germline pathological variant of the *NF2* gene in addition to one of the clinical criteria.

## Staging

Not relevant

## Prognosis and prediction

The clinical course in patients with NF2 varies widely between and (to a lesser extent) within families {1996,4440}. Some families feature early onset with diverse tumours and a high tumour

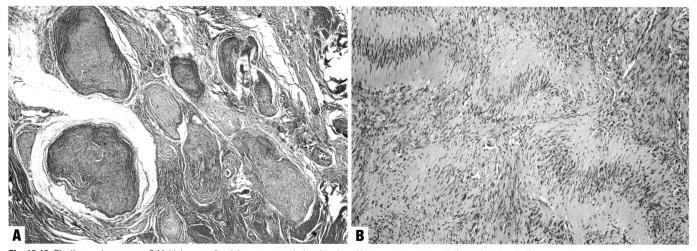

**Fig. 16.13** Plexiform schwannoma. **A** Multiple nerve fascicles are expanded and replaced by tumour, a pattern similar to that of a plexiform neurofibroma. **B** Examination at high magnification shows the typical histological features of schwannoma, including Verocay bodies.

load (Wishart type), whereas others present later, with only vestibular schwannomas (Gardner type). An effect of maternal inheritance on severity has been noted, as have families with genetic anticipation. Genotype–phenotype correlations have been identified wherein truncating mutations are associated with a more severe phenotype, whereas missense mutations, large deletions, and somatic mosaicism have been associated with milder disease {526,2002,3663,4601}. In addition to the mutation type, the position of the mutation within the gene also affects the phenotype: splice-site mutations upstream from exon 7 have more severe phenotypes {3661}, and mutations towards the 5′ end of the gene are associated with a higher risk of intracranial meningiomas {6546}. The life expectancy of patients with NF2 is shortened, compared with the lifespan of a White control population (69 vs 80 years, respectively) {7541}.

**Box 16.01** Clinical diagnostic criteria for neurofibromatosis type 2 (revised Manchester criteria) {1996A}

1. Bilateral vestibular schwannomas
**OR**
2. Family history of neurofibromatosis type 2 **AND**
   a. Unilateral vestibular schwannoma **OR**
   b. Any two of: meningioma, ependymoma, schwannoma, posterior subcapsular opacities
**OR**
3. Unilateral vestibular schwannoma **AND**
   • Any two of: meningioma, ependymoma, schwannoma, posterior subcapsular opacities
**OR**
4. Multiple meningiomas **AND**
   a. Unilateral vestibular schwannoma **OR**
   b. Any two of: ependymoma, schwannoma, posterior subcapsular opacities

# Tuberous sclerosis

Kratz CP
Lopes MBS
Perry A
Rodriguez FJ
Santosh V
Sharma MC
Stemmer-Rachamimov AO

## Definition

Tuberous sclerosis (TS) is a group of autosomal dominant disorders caused by a pathogenic variant of *TSC1* on chromosome 9q34 or *TSC2* on 16p13 and characterized by hamartomas and benign neoplastic lesions that affect the CNS and various non-neural tissues, including the skin, heart, kidneys, and lung.

## MIM numbering

191100 Tuberous sclerosis 1; TSC1
613254 Tuberous sclerosis 2; TSC2

## ICD-11 coding

LD2D.2 Tuberous sclerosis

## Related terminology

None

## Subtype(s)

Tuberous sclerosis 1; tuberous sclerosis 2

## Localization

Major CNS manifestations of TS include cortical dysplasias (tubers and white matter glioneuronal hamartomas), subependymal nodules, and subependymal giant cell astrocytomas (SEGAs). Major extraneural manifestations include cutaneous angiofibromas, shagreen patches, subungual fibromas, cardiac rhabdomyomas, pulmonary lymphangioleiomyomatosis, and renal angiomyolipomas.

## Clinical features

Cardiac rhabdomyomas are often a presenting feature of TS in newborns and infants aged < 2 years, and more than half of all cardiac rhabdomyomas are associated with TS {5908}. Cutaneous

manifestations include hypomelanotic nodules (evident from birth), facial angiofibromas, and shagreen patches. Ungual (or subungual) fibromas often develop in childhood. Renal angiomyolipomas develop in as many as 80% of people with TS by the age of 10 years. Renal cysts are present in as many as 20% of affected individuals, but polycystic kidney disease occurs in only 3–5%. Lymphangioleiomyomatosis severely impairs lung function and may be fatal; it is present in as many as 40% of women with TS. All the phenotypic features of TS can also occur sporadically in individuals without the genetic condition {5908}. About 50% of patients with lymphangioleiomyomatosis do not have TS. Sporadic angiomyolipomas are typically solitary, whereas TS-associated angiomyolipomas are often multiple or bilateral.

Neurological symptoms are among the most frequently observed and serious (sometimes life-threatening) manifestations of TS {1491,6963}. The most common initial signs of TS are intractable epilepsy (including infantile spasms), seen in 80–90% of cases, and cognitive impairment (in 50%); these are followed by the development of a combination of neurobehavioral disorders known as TS-associated neuropsychiatric disorders (TAND) (in > 60% of cases), including autism spectrum disorder (in as many as 40%) {2477,6963,5092}. Both cortical tubers and white matter glioneuronal hamartomas (see *CNS manifestations*, below) are commonly associated with intractable epilepsy and learning difficulties in TS {5093}, although meticulous autopsy studies on small numbers of patients have also suggested that there may be more subtle degrees of cortical and white matter disorganization {4395}.

### CNS manifestations

CNS lesions in TS include cerebral cortical tubers, white matter glioneuronal heterotopia, subependymal hamartomatous nodules, and subependymal giant cell astrocytomas (SEGAs)

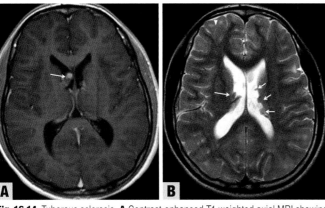

**Fig. 16.14** Tuberous sclerosis. **A** Contrast-enhanced T1-weighted axial MRI showing an enhancing mass (arrow) near the foramen of Monro. It was subsequently confirmed to be a subependymal giant cell astrocytoma. **B** T2-weighted axial MRI showing multiple tiny T2-hypointense, calcified subependymal nodules (arrows) along the lining of bilateral lateral ventricles.

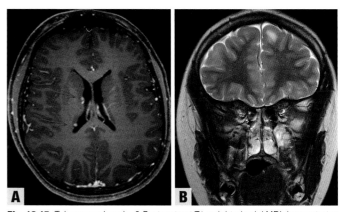

**Fig. 16.15** Tuberous sclerosis. **A** Postcontrast T1-weighted axial MRI demonstrates two small enhancing subependymal nodules along the right caudate nucleus (arrows). **B** T2-weighted coronal MRI demonstrates a minimally expansile hyperintense lesion in the left frontal white matter compatible with a cortical/subcortical tuber (arrow).

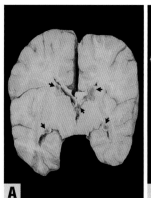
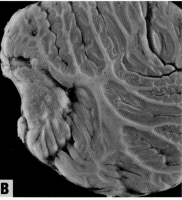

**Fig. 16.16** Tuberous sclerosis. **A** Gross autopsy section from a patient with tuberous sclerosis illustrates axially cut cerebral hemispheric parenchyma with multiple subependymal nodules in the lateral and third ventricles (arrows). **B** Gross image of the brain from a 57-year-old man showing an unusual tuber in the cerebellar hemisphere with extensive calcification.

(for details, see *Subependymal giant cell astrocytoma*, p. 218). Schizencephaly, agenesis of the corpus callosum, and cerebellar dysplasia are rare abnormalities. Cortical tubers can involve the cortex, subcortical white matter, or both. They are both detected by CT or MRI, although MRI is considered the reference method for defining CNS involvement in TS {6063}. Diffusion tensor imaging and metabolic brain studies using AMT PET or FDG PET {6403,6063}, in addition to intraoperative electrocorticography, can identify epileptogenic tubers, facilitating tuberectomy as a reasonable surgical approach to treating intractable seizures in these patients. Tubers resemble sporadic cortical dysplasias of cortex not associated with TS, classified as focal cortical dysplasia type 2b in the classification proposed by the International League Against Epilepsy (ILAE) {746}.

## Epidemiology
The variability of the clinical manifestations of TS previously led to underdiagnosis. Recent data indicate that the disorder affects as many as 25 000–40 000 individuals in the USA and about 1–2 million individuals worldwide, with an estimated incidence of 1 case per 6000–10 000 live births and a population prevalence of about 1 in 20 000 individuals {5093}.

## Etiology
TS is caused by a pathogenic variant of *TSC1* on chromosome 9q or *TSC2* on 16p.

### TSC1
The gene *TSC1* maps to chromosome 9q34 {1418} and contains 23 exons {7225}, 21 of which carry coding information (exons 3–23).

*Gene expression:* The *TSC1*-encoded protein, hamartin, has a molecular weight of 130 kDa. Hamartin is strongly expressed in the brain, kidney, and heart, all of which are tissues frequently affected in TS {5574}. Its pattern of expression overlaps with that of its product, tuberin.

*Gene mutations:* Mutation analyses of large cohorts {1199, 7226} showed that the most common mutations in *TSC1* are small deletions and nonsense mutations (each accounting for ~30% of all mutations in the gene). Virtually all mutations result in a truncated gene product, and more than half of the changes affect exons 15 and 17 {7226}. Large deletions of *TSC1* are rare.

### TSC2
The gene *TSC2* maps to chromosome 16p13.3 {3397} and contains 42 exons, with exons 2–42 encoding the functional protein.

*Gene expression:* *TSC2* encodes a large transcript of 5.5 kb that shows widespread expression in many tissues, including the brain and other organs affected in TS. Alternatively spliced mRNAs have been reported {7649}. A portion of the 180 kDa protein product tuberin bears significant homology with the catalytic domain of RAP1GAP, a member of the RAS family.

*Gene mutations:* The mutation spectrum of *TSC2* is wider than that of *TSC1*; it includes large deletions and missense mutations, and less frequently, splice-site mutations {159,1518,3309}. Exons 16, 33, and 40 have the highest number of mutations. Large deletions in *TSC2* may extend into the adjacent gene *PKD1*, with a resulting phenotype of TS and polycystic kidney disease {760,7226}. Multiple studies of genotype–phenotype correlations have demonstrated that *TSC2* mutations are associated with a more severe phenotype overall, with an earlier seizure onset, a higher number of tubers, and a lower cognition index. However, within that spectrum, *TSC2* missense mutations are associated with milder phenotypes {405,6147}.

Like in other tumour suppressor gene syndromes, somatic inactivation of the wildtype allele (i.e. loss of heterozygosity for the *TSC1* or *TSC2* locus) has been reported in kidney and cardiac lesions associated with TS, as well as in SEGAs {1139}. However, there is conflicting evidence as to whether a second hit is required for cortical tuber formation, raising the possibility that some lesions in TS may be due to haploinsufficiency {5028,7563}. Recent studies have found predominantly activating *MTOR* mutations in focal

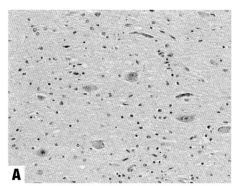
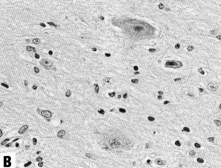
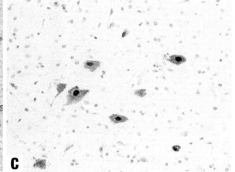

**Fig. 16.17** Tuberous sclerosis. **A,B** Cortical tuber with dysmorphic enlarged neurons embedded in a densely fibrillary background. **C** Cortical tuber with large neuronal cells highlighted by NeuN.

cortical dysplasias, but rarely in combination with *TSC1* and/ or *TSC2* mutations {466,4120}. In recent studies, loss of *TSC1* in periventricular zone neuronal stem cells was sufficient to cause aberrant migration and a giant cell phenotype, supportive of the two-hit hypothesis for tuber formation {2074,7853}.

Most of the cases in which no mutation was identified (15% of patients with TS) {1518,3309} were found to be somatic mosaics when newer sequencing methods were used {7121}. Clinical features of TS are milder in individuals with mosaicism and may have limited distribution (for example involve only one organ).

### Inheritance and genetic heterogeneity
Most TS cases (~60%) are sporadic, with no family history, indicating a high rate of de novo mutations {6144}; familial cases are inherited in an autosomal dominant fashion. In affected kindreds, the disease follows an autosomal dominant pattern of inheritance, with high penetrance but considerable phenotypic variability {6459}.

### Pathogenesis
The impact of *TSC1* and *TSC2* sequence variants is mediated by effects on signalling pathways involving tuberin and hamartin. These proteins, together with TBC1D7, form a heteromeric complex (TSC), which functions as a signalling node that integrates growth factor and stress signals from the upstream PI3K/ AKT pathway and transmits signals downstream to coordinate multiple cellular processes, including cell proliferation and cell size {5683,1418,3397,5575}. The complex negatively regulates the mTOR pathway {382,2313,6937}. Disruption of TSC causes upregulation of the mTOR pathway and increases proliferation and cell growth through two effector molecules: 4E-BP1 and S6K1 {382,6937}. The understanding of the basic mechanism of mTOR pathway activation in TS lesions has led to the use of mTOR inhibitors in the treatment of manifestations of TS. Several TS-associated tumours, renal angiomyolipomas, SEGAs, and lymphangioleiomyomas show a significant size reduction in response to treatment with mTOR inhibitors (everolimus) and regrow when treatment is stopped. mTOR inhibitors were also shown to be effective in reducing seizure frequency in children with refractory epilepsy {1505,1504}.

### Macroscopic appearance
See individual tumour types within the WHO classification.

### Histopathology
Microscopically, CNS tubers consist of a disorganized cortex with disrupted cortical lamination and containing dysmorphic, markedly enlarged neurons, balloon cells (also designated by some authors as giant cells {4733,4395}), dense fibrillary gliosis, calcification of blood vessel walls and/or parenchyma, and myelin loss. The surrounding cortex, which usually appears normal in cytoarchitecture, shows changes on more detailed immunohistochemical and morphometric investigation {3083,4395}. Dysmorphic neurons and balloon cells may be seen in all cortical layers and in the underlying white matter. The dysmorphic neurons show altered radial orientation in the cortex, aberrant dendritic arborization, and an accumulation of perikaryal fibrils. The perikaryal fibrils can be highlighted using silver impregnation techniques, which show many neurons with a neurofibrillary tangle–like morphology. Although the dysmorphic neurons express neuronal-associated proteins, they display cytoarchitectural features of immature or poorly differentiated neurons, such as reduced axonal projections and spine density {2912,3083}. The other frequently observed element in tubers and in adjacent cortex and white matter is the characteristic balloon cell {4317,2912,3083}. Balloon cells may resemble gemistocytic astrocytes with glassy eosinophilic cytoplasm and eccentric, often multinucleated nuclei; however, immunohistochemical markers characteristic of glial and neuronal phenotypes suggest that these cells have a mixed glioneuronal origin. Many balloon cells express nestin mRNA and protein {1492}. Some balloon cells demonstrate immunoreactivity for vimentin and GFAP {2912}, whereas others with an identical morphological phenotype express neuronal markers, including connexins 26 and 32, neurofilaments, class III β-tubulin, MAP2, and α-internexin {1492,2912,7684}. However, the formation of well-defined synapses between balloon cells and adjacent neurons is not a consistent finding. As previously mentioned, cortical dysplasias morphologically indistinguishable from tubers may occur in chronic focal epilepsies without clinical or genetic evidence of an underlying TS condition {742,746}. The pathogenesis of these sporadic lesions is unclear.

White matter glioneuronal heterotopias and radial migration lines are linear or flame-shaped bands radiating from the periventricular zone to the subcortical white matter. They are composed of dysplastic glioneuronal cells and can extend from the cortex down to the periventricular region. Subependymal nodules are elevated, often calcified nodules. They are composed of enlarged glioneuronal cells indistinguishable from those found in SEGA, but are smaller than those in cortical tubers.

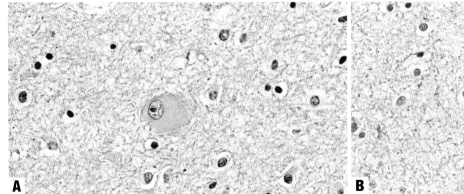
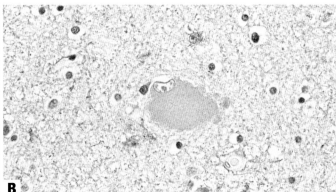

**Fig. 16.18** Tuberous sclerosis. **A** Balloon cells, with eosinophilic cytoplasm, large nuclei, and prominent nucleoli, dispersed in the white matter. **B** Cortical tuber showing a balloon cell with a ganglion-like nucleus and strong immunoreactivity for S100.

The proteins tuberin and hamartin are identifiable by immunohistochemistry and western blotting in many organs and tissues throughout the body {3300}; both proteins are widely expressed throughout the CNS of the normal developing brain {3299,7308}. Immunostaining a given tuber with anti-hamartin or anti-tuberin antibodies does not provide evidence of which mutation is present in a given individual, and therefore is not of diagnostic value.

*Extraneural manifestations*

The extraneural manifestations of TS and the frequencies at which they occur are summarized in Table 16.02.

**Table 16.02** Major manifestations of tuberous sclerosis {5093}

| Manifestation | Frequency |
|---|---|
| **CNS** | |
| Cortical dysplasias (tubers and white matter heterotopias) | ~90% |
| Subependymal nodule | 80% |
| Subependymal giant cell astrocytoma | 5–15% |
| **Skin** | |
| Facial angiofibroma | 75% |
| Hypomelanotic macule | 90% |
| Shagreen patch | 50% |
| Forehead plaque | 25% |
| Confetti skin (hypopigmented macules) | 58% |
| Subungual fibroma | 20% |
| **Eye** | |
| Retinal hamartoma | 30–50% |
| Retinal giant cell astrocytoma | 20–30% |
| Retinal achromic patch | 40% |
| **Kidney** | |
| Angiomyolipoma[a] | 80% |
| Isolated renal cyst | 10–20% |
| Polycystic kidney cysts | 2–3% |
| **Heart** | |
| Cardiac rhabdomyoma | 50% |
| **Digestive system** | |
| Liver angiomyolipomas | 10–15% |
| **Lung** | |
| Lymphangioleiomyomatosis | 30–40% (female patients) |
| Pulmonary cysts | 10–12% (male patients) |
| Micronodular pulmonary pneumocyte hyperplasia | 40–58% |
| **Other** | |
| Intraoral fibroma | 20–50% |
| Dental enamel pits | Variable (up to 100%) |
| Bone cyst | 40% |
| Non-renal hamartomas | Rare |

[a]May occur in other locations besides kidneys.

## Cytology

Not relevant

## Diagnostic molecular pathology

In the revised diagnostic criteria, a pathogenic variant of *TSC1* or *TSC2* is an independent diagnostic criterion and is sufficient for a definitive diagnosis of TS {3798}. Therefore, genetic testing is recommended when TS is suspected but cannot be clinically confirmed. Molecular testing identifies 75–90% of patients with TS as positive for a pathogenic variant, so a negative result does not rule out a diagnosis {3798}. Genetic testing is recommended for family members of an affected patient, especially in babies, and may be offered as a preimplantation or prenatal test.

## Essential and desirable diagnostic criteria

Clinical and genetic diagnostic criteria are summarized in Box 16.02.

## Staging

Not relevant

## Prognosis and prediction

TS tends to shorten the lifespan slightly (as compared with lifespan in a White control population) {6402}. The most common causes of death in the second decade of life are brain tumours and status epilepticus, followed by renal abnormalities {5093, 240}. In patients aged > 40 years, mortality is most commonly associated with renal abnormalities (i.e. cystic disease or neoplasm) or lymphangioleiomyomatosis.

**Box 16.02** Diagnostic criteria for tuberous sclerosis (2012) {5093}

**A. Genetic diagnostic criteria**
Identification of either a *TSC1* or a *TSC2* pathogenic mutation in DNA from normal tissue is sufficient to make a definitive diagnosis of tuberous sclerosis according to strict criteria {4033A,4033B}.

**B. Clinical diagnostic criteria**
Major features:
1. Hypomelanotic macules (≥ 3, at least 5 mm in diameter)
2. Angiofibromas (≥ 3) or fibrous cephalic plaque
3. Ungual fibromas (≥ 2)
4. Shagreen patch
5. Multiple retinal hamartomas
6. Cortical dysplasias (including tubers and cerebral white matter migration lines)
7. Subependymal nodules
8. Subependymal giant cell astrocytoma
9. Cardiac rhabdomyoma
10. Lymphangioleiomyomatosis[a]
11. Angiomyolipomas (≥ 2)[a]
Minor features:
1. Confetti-like skin lesions
2. Dental enamel pits (≥ 3)
3. Intraoral fibromas (≥ 2)
4. Retinal achromic patch
5. Multiple renal cysts
6. Non-renal hamartomas

**Definite diagnosis:** Two major features[a] **OR** one major feature with at least two minor features

**Possible diagnosis:** One major feature **OR** at least two minor features

[a]A combination of the two major clinical features lymphangioleiomyomatosis and angiomyolipomas without other features does not meet the criteria for a definite diagnosis.

# Naevoid basal cell carcinoma syndrome (Gorlin syndrome)

Pajtler KW
Eberhart CG
Kratz CP
Perry A
Pietsch T

## Definition

Naevoid basal cell carcinoma syndrome (NBCCS) is an autosomal dominant disease associated with developmental disorders and predisposition to benign and malignant tumours, including cutaneous basal cell carcinomas, odontogenic keratocysts, palmar/plantar dyskeratotic pits, intratarsal keratinous eyelid cysts, intracranial calcifications, macrocephaly, and medulloblastomas (desmoplastic/nodular subtypes). NBCCS is caused by germline pathogenic variants of genes encoding members of the hedgehog signalling pathway, including *PTCH1*, *SUFU*, and (very rarely) *PTCH2*.

## MIM numbering

109400 Basal cell naevus syndrome; BCNS

## ICD-11 coding

LD2D.4 Gorlin syndrome

## Related terminology

*Acceptable:* Gorlin syndrome; Gorlin–Goltz syndrome.
*Not recommended:* basal cell naevus syndrome; fifth phakomatosis.

## Subtype(s)

None

## Localization

NBCCS sites of disease include the skin (basal cell carcinomas, sebaceous cysts, palmoplantar pits, epidermal inclusion cysts, multiple naevi), jaw (keratocysts, cleft palate/lip), bone (congenital anomalies), CNS (macrocephaly, falx calcification, medulloblastoma, meningioma, craniopharyngioma), and eyelid (cysts). Mesenteric cystic lymphangiomas (lymphomesenteric cysts) and ovarian or cardiac fibromas may also occur.

## Clinical features

The most frequent manifestations of NBCCS are multiple basal cell carcinomas (including in non–sun-exposed skin) and odontogenic keratocysts of the jaw. In one study, basal cell carcinomas and odontogenic keratocysts were found together in > 90% of affected individuals by the age of 40 years {1997}. Other frequent manifestations include calcification of the falx cerebri, palmar and plantar pits, and bifid

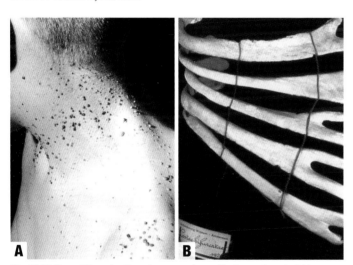

**Fig. 16.19** Naevoid basal cell carcinoma syndrome (Gorlin syndrome). **A** Numerous basal cell carcinomas in the head and neck area and upper trunk. **B** Multiple bifid ribs.

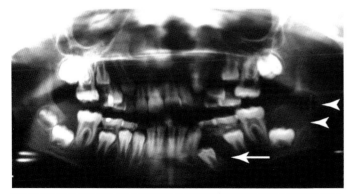

**Fig. 16.20** Naevoid basal cell carcinoma syndrome (Gorlin syndrome). Multiple odontogenic keratocysts are highlighted by the presence of displaced teeth.

**Box 16.03** Diagnostic criteria for naevoid basal cell carcinoma syndrome

**Major criteria:**
Lamellar (sheet-like) calcification of the falx
Jaw keratocyst
Palmar or plantar pits (≥ 2)
Multiple basal cell carcinomas (> 5 in a lifetime) or a basal cell carcinoma in a patient aged < 30 years
First-degree relative with naevoid basal cell carcinoma syndrome

**Minor criteria:**
Childhood medulloblastoma[a]
Mesenteric cystic lymphangiomas (lymphomesenteric cysts) or pleural cysts
Macrocephaly (occipitofrontal circumference > 97th percentile)
Cleft lip or palate
Vertebral or rib anomalies
Preaxial or postaxial polydactyly
Ovarian or cardiac fibromas
Ocular anomalies

**Requirements for diagnosis:**
Two major diagnostic criteria and one minor diagnostic criterion
**OR**
One major and three minor diagnostic criteria
**OR**
Identification of a heterozygous germline *PTCH1* or *SUFU* pathogenic variant on molecular genetic testing and supporting clinical criteria

[a]Medulloblastoma with sonic hedgehog activation, mostly desmoplastic/nodular or extensive nodular types.

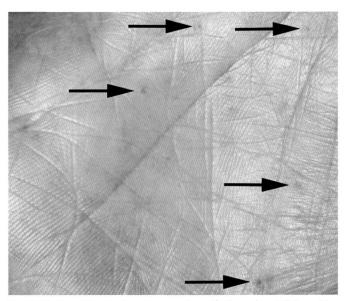

**Fig. 16.21** Naevoid basal cell carcinoma syndrome (Gorlin syndrome). Palmar pitting can be extremely subtle; it is easier to detect in less-clean hands, because dirt tends to become trapped in the pits.

or fused ribs {3595,6376}. These findings are considered major diagnostic criteria (see Box 16.03, p. 975). Minor criteria include medulloblastoma {244}, ovarian fibroma, macrocephaly, congenital facial abnormalities (e.g. cleft lip or palate, frontal bossing, hypertelorism), skeletal abnormalities (e.g. digit syndactyly), and radiological bone abnormalities (e.g. bridging of the sella turcica) {244,3595}. The clinical features manifest at different points in life. Macrocephaly and rib anomalies can be detected at birth, and medulloblastoma typically develops within the first 3 years of life. Jaw cysts do not usually become evident before the age of about 8 years, and basal cell carcinomas are usually found 10 years later {2247}. Radiation treatment of patients with NBCCS (e.g. craniospinal irradiation for the treatment

of cerebellar medulloblastoma) induces multiple basal cell carcinomas of the skin as well as various other tumour types (e.g. meningioma) within the radiation field {1137,5176,6652}.

*NBCCS-associated medulloblastoma:* In a review of 33 reported medulloblastoma cases associated with NBCCS, all but 1 tumour had developed in children aged < 5 years, and 22 cases (66%) had manifested in patients aged < 2 years {244}. Medulloblastomas associated with NBCCS seem to be exclusively the extensively nodular or desmoplastic/nodular types {244,2330,6264,6545}. It has been proposed that desmoplastic/nodular medulloblastomas in young children should serve as a major criterion for the diagnosis of NBCCS {244, 2330}. About 1–2% of patients with NBCCS with germline *PTCH1* pathogenic sequence variants develop medulloblastoma, compared with about 20% of patients with germline *SUFU* pathogenic sequence variants {6545}.

## Epidemiology

In the United Kingdom, a prevalence of 1 in 30 827 individuals and an incidence of 5.3 cases per 100 000 births have been reported {1994}, although lower prevalence rates have been published in Italy (1 in 256 000) {7286}, in Japan (1 in 235 800) {2247}, and Australia (1 in 164 000) {6376}. Of 131 children with medulloblastomas, 6% had germline *SUFU* mutations {913}.

## Etiology

NBCCS results from inactivating germline mutations in the human homologue of the *Drosophila* segment polarity patched gene (*PTCH1*) located on chromosome 9q22 {2662,3303}, *SUFU* on 10q24 {6545}, or exceptionally *GPR161* on 1q24.2.

Numerous different *PTCH1* germline pathogenic variants associated with NBCCS have been reported {2247,4138}. The detection rate of specific pathogenic variants has increased greatly in recent years (with as many as 93% of cases found to be positive in one study), owing to the development of improved methods of detection {2247}. The mostly truncating mutations are distributed over the entire *PTCH1* coding region, with no mutation hotspots {7529}. Missense mutations cluster in a highly

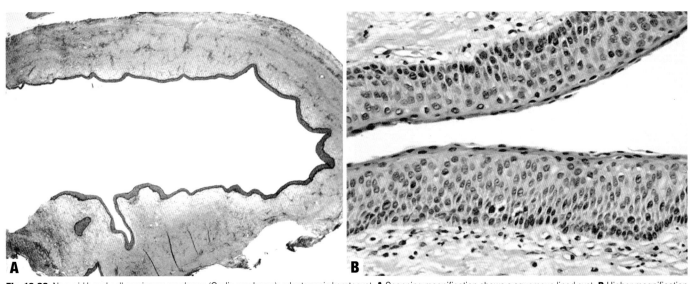

**Fig. 16.22** Naevoid basal cell carcinoma syndrome (Gorlin syndrome): odontogenic keratocyst. **A** Scanning magnification shows a squamous lined cyst. **B** Higher magnification shows expansion of the basal and parabasal layers and parakeratosis.

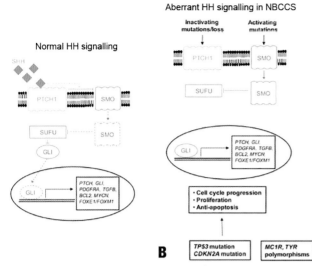

**Fig. 16.23** Naevoid basal cell carcinoma syndrome (Gorlin syndrome). Hedgehog (HH) signalling pathway. Normal HH signalling and aberrant HH signalling in naevoid basal cell carcinoma syndrome (NBCCS). **A** In the normal HH signalling pathway, in the presence of the sonic hedgehog signalling protein (SHH), PTCH1 suppresses smoothened (SMO), which in turn allows SUFU to inhibit GLI transcription factors; in the absence of SHH, SMO is released from inhibition by PTCH1 and translocates to the cytosol, where it inhibits SUFU, thereby relieving inhibition of GLI transcription factors. **B** In NBCCS, *PTCH1* mutations lead to constitutive activation of GLI transcription factors; in rare NBCCS cases, *SMO* mutations (which are common in sporadic basal cell carcinoma) or *SUFU* mutations may lead to the same result.

conserved region (the sterol-sensing domain), and particularly in transmembrane domain 4. *SUFU* pathogenic variants are only detected in approximately 5–6% of tested probands, and most are truncating {6545}.

The rate of new *PTCH1* pathogenic variants has not been precisely determined, but it has been estimated that a high proportion (14–81%) of cases are the result of de novo pathogenic variants {1997,2503,6376,7528}. In 4 of 6 cases of NBCCS reported with a germline *SUFU* pathogenic variant, the mutation was inherited from an unaffected, healthy parent. In the other 2 cases, the mutation was new {6545}. Germline pathogenic variants in *GPR161* have been detected in SHH subgroup medulloblastomas, suggesting possible NBCCS association {570}.

## Pathogenesis

The gene *PTCH1* encodes a 12-transmembrane protein expressed on many progenitor cell types that functions as a receptor for members of the secreted hedgehog protein family of signalling molecules (sonic hedgehog, IHH, and DHH) and represses the transcription of genes encoding members of the TGF-β and WNT signalling pathways {4401,6714}. PTCH1 controls another transmembrane protein, SMO {149,6714}. In the absence of ligand, PTCH1 inhibits the activity of SMO {149, 6714}. Hedgehog signalling takes place in the primary cilium {392}. Binding of hedgehog proteins to PTCH1 can relieve its inhibition of SMO, allowing it to translocate to the tip of the primary cilium, which results in the activation and translocation of GLI transcription factors into the cell nucleus and transcription of a set of specific target genes controlling the survival, differentiation, and proliferation of progenitor cells. In vertebrates,

this pathway is critically involved in the development of various tissues and organ systems, such as limbs, gonads, bone, and the CNS {2491,3126}. *SUFU* is located downstream in the hedgehog pathway. SUFU has been found to directly interact with GLI proteins and is a negative regulator of hedgehog signalling {6715}. *PTCH1* and *SUFU* represent classic tumour suppressor genes; the second allele of the mutant gene is lost in most NBCCS-related tumours. The inactivation of these genes leads to the pathological activation of the sonic hedgehog signalling pathway.

## Macroscopic appearance

Syndromic tumours appear grossly similar to their sporadic counterparts.

## Histopathology

Practically all medulloblastomas associated with NBCCS have the morphological features of desmoplastic tumours, including desmoplastic/nodular medulloblastoma and medulloblastoma with extensive nodularity {6264,244,2330,913,6545}. Basal cell carcinomas do not show any unique histological features, and all subtypes are represented, including pigmented subtypes. NBCCS-associated odontogenic keratocysts are typically multifocal and develop in younger patients than do non-syndromic cases; basal budding and microcysts in the wall are more common in syndromic lesions {840A,4293A,7622B, 7622A}.

## Cytology

Not relevant

## Diagnostic molecular pathology

A comprehensive mutation analysis of *PTCH1* and *SUFU* by DNA sequencing and search for deletions or duplications by appropriate methods (e.g. multiplex ligation-dependent probe amplification, targeted array-based analysis) is able to identify most NBCCS-related germline pathogenic variants {1992}. To detect more complex alterations, additional analysis at the transcript level may be necessary in some cases. Despite the fact that the variant detection rate has increased greatly owing to improved diagnostic methods {2247}, in 15–27% of index cases neither *PTCH1* nor *SUFU* pathogenic variants can be identified {2000}.

Because germline pathogenic variants are frequent in children aged < 5 years who have extensive nodular or desmoplastic/nodular medulloblastomas, human genetic counselling should be offered to the families, and early pathogenic variant analysis of *PTCH1* and *SUFU* should be performed using appropriate methods. The detection of a germline condition is important for appropriate treatment planning, avoiding radiation therapy {2330,913,6545,2579,7456}.

## Essential and desirable diagnostic criteria

The major and minor diagnostic criteria are listed in Box 16.03 (p. 975).

## Staging

Malignancies are staged in accordance with the Union for International Cancer Control (UICC) TNM classification.

## Prognosis and prediction

The prognosis of NBCCS-associated medulloblastomas seems to be better than that of sporadic cases, and it has been suggested that therapy protocols be adjusted in patients aged < 5 years with NBCCS, to prevent radiation-induced secondary tumours {244,6652}. However, a recent analysis of patients with medulloblastoma and a *SUFU* germline pathogenic variant indicated a worse prognosis {2579}. In another retrospective series, no difference in survival was found between patients with medulloblastoma carrying a *PTCH1* pathogenic variant and those carrying a *SUFU* pathogenic variant {7456}.

Surveillance guidelines are well established, including surveillance during childhood {2201,2579A}. For patients carrying a *SUFU* pathogenic variant, these include a recommendation for repeated brain MRI screening for medulloblastoma development within the first 5 years of life {2201}.

# Retinoblastoma syndrome

Chevez-Barrios P
Chintagumpala M
Eagle RC Jr
Jones DTW
Ketteler P
Perry A

## Definition
Retinoblastoma syndrome is a heritable cancer predisposition syndrome associated with a constitutional heterozygous pathogenic *RB1* variant, with the development of retinoblastoma and other extraocular malignancies.

## MIM numbering
180200 Retinoblastoma; RB1

## ICD-11 coding
2D02.2 Retinoblastoma

## Related terminology
*Acceptable:* heritable retinoblastoma; familial retinoblastoma.

## Subtype(s)
Heritable unilateral and bilateral retinoblastoma; trilateral retinoblastoma (associated with primary intracranial tumour [pineal or suprasellar tumour]); second primary non-ocular malignancies

## Localization
Retinoblastoma develops in the retina of one or both eyes; it is most frequently bilateral in retinoblastoma syndrome. In 5% of children with bilateral retinoblastoma, synchronous or metachronous malignant intracranial (pineal or suprasellar) tumours develop. Later in life these patients may develop second primary malignancies (SPMs), most frequently in the soft tissues, bone, endometrium, lung, or skin {7611,3639}.

## Clinical features
MRI of the orbits and brain is performed during the initial diagnosis of intraocular retinoblastoma to exclude extraocular extension and brain involvement. CT should be avoided to prevent radiation exposure. A pineal or sellar tumour with *RB1* alterations in the presence of bilateral retinoblastoma is diagnostic of trilateral retinoblastoma and frequently occurs with leptomeningeal involvement.

The initial therapy for synchronous trilateral retinoblastoma should address both ocular and intracranial disease (see *Retinoblastoma*, p. 385). For pineal tumours, maximal safe surgical resection is encouraged at diagnosis, followed by intensive chemotherapy, often requiring autologous haematopoietic cell rescue. External beam radiation therapy (EBRT) is adapted for age with craniospinal irradiation deferred in early infancy {14}.

Survivors of heritable retinoblastoma may develop SPMs. They should receive counselling and be enrolled in long-term

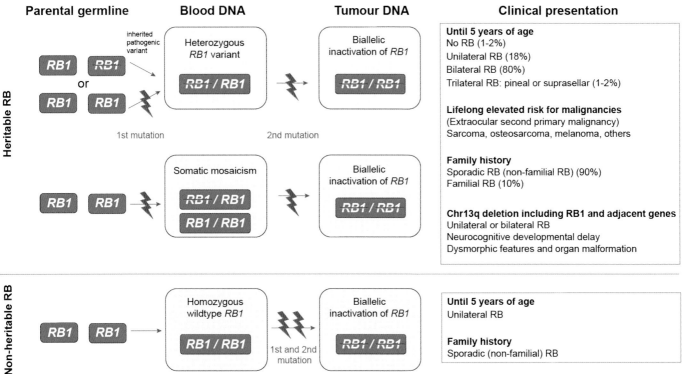

| Parental germline | Blood DNA | Tumour DNA | Clinical presentation |
|---|---|---|---|

**Heritable RB**

Inherited pathogenic variant → Heterozygous *RB1* variant (RB1 / RB1) → Biallelic inactivation of *RB1* (RB1 / RB1)

or

1st mutation / 2nd mutation

Somatic mosaicism (RB1 / RB1, RB1 / RB1) → Biallelic inactivation of *RB1* (RB1 / RB1)

**Clinical presentation (Heritable RB):**

**Until 5 years of age**
No RB (1–2%)
Unilateral RB (18%)
Bilateral RB (80%)
Trilateral RB: pineal or suprasellar (1–2%)

**Lifelong elevated risk for malignancies**
(Extraocular second primary malignancy)
Sarcoma, osteosarcoma, melanoma, others

**Family history**
Sporadic RB (non-familial RB) (90%)
Familial RB (10%)

**Chr13q deletion including RB1 and adjacent genes**
Unilateral or bilateral RB
Neurocognitive developmental delay
Dysmorphic features and organ malformation

**Non-heritable RB**

RB1 / RB1 → Homozygous wildtype *RB1* (RB1 / RB1) → (1st and 2nd mutation) → Biallelic inactivation of *RB1* (RB1 / RB1)

**Until 5 years of age**
Unilateral RB

**Family history**
Sporadic (non-familial) RB

**Fig. 16.24** Retinoblastoma syndrome. Heritable retinoblastoma results from inheritance from a heterozygote or from somatic mosaicism, with both cases leading to the loss of both alleles. In sporadic cases, both alleles are lost by mutation. Chr, chromosome; RB, retinoblastoma.

survivor programmes that have access to specific screening, follow-up, and treatment.

## Epidemiology

Most children with heritable retinoblastoma develop ocular retinoblastoma between 0 and 5 years of age (median: 10 months) and have a 5% risk of developing trilateral retinoblastoma (see *Retinoblastoma*, p. 385) {6941,1622,1623}.

The incidence, localization, and type of SPM depends on the type of retinoblastoma treatment. In particular, EBRT is associated with a 36% cumulative incidence of sarcoma arising in the irradiation field {3640,1195}. Chemotherapy plus EBRT further increases the risk of SPMs {7611}.

## Etiology

See *Retinoblastoma* (p. 385). Most heritable retinoblastomas are sporadic (no family history); only 10% of heritable retinoblastomas are familial.

Constitutional pathogenic *RB1* gene variants are heterogeneous. Low- and regular-penetrance variants show variation of phenotypic expression for retinoblastoma and for SPM in families {3537}. Patients with somatic mosaicism often develop a milder phenotype and unilateral retinoblastoma {6057}. Large deletions on chromosome 13q that include *RB1* and neighbouring genes cause a rare genetic disorder referred to as "13q deletion syndrome". Depending on the location and size of the deletion, these patients may show a neurodevelopmental delay, characteristic facial features, organ malformation, and/or retinoblastoma {4722,1671}.

## Pathogenesis

See *Retinoblastoma* (p. 385).

## Macroscopic appearance

For retinal tumours, see *Retinoblastoma* (p. 385).

Intracranial tumours are poorly demarcated, soft, and friable. The adequacy of surgical resection of intracranial tumours may be defined using postoperative imaging studies when the surgical specimen is representative of the amount of tumour resected (see *Pineoblastoma*, p. 323).

## Histopathology

The histological features of the intracranial tumour in trilateral retinoblastoma are identical to those of retinoblastoma (see *Retinoblastoma*, p. 385). Pineoblastoma is a high-grade embryonal tumour (CNS WHO grade 4) (see *Pineoblastoma*, p. 323).

## Cytology

Not clinically relevant

## Diagnostic molecular pathology

Identification of the specific *RB1* gene variant and genetic counselling should be considered for trilateral retinoblastoma and any patient with retinoblastoma. Intracranial (pineal) retinoblastoma, whether somatic or germline-associated, has a different DNA methylation profile from that of other pineal tumours and shares common characteristics with ocular retinoblastoma (e.g. chromosome 16 loss and 1q gain) {4070, 5498}.

## Essential and desirable diagnostic criteria

*Essential:* confirmation of diagnosis from ocular tumour(s); degree of differentiation for any intracranial tumours; association with meningeal involvement if present.
*Desirable:* demonstration of presence of germline pathogenic variants in *RB1*.

## Staging

The American Joint Committee on Cancer (AJCC) developed a clinical and pathological TNM classification, and in the eighth edition heritability factors were added for retinoblastoma (making it cTNMH). The heredity category comprises HX (unknown or insufficient evidence of a constitutional pathogenic *RB1* gene variant), H0 (normal *RB1* alleles in tested blood), and H1 (bilateral retinoblastoma, trilateral retinoblastoma, patient with a family history of retinoblastoma, or molecular identification of a constitutional pathogenic *RB1* gene variant).

## Prognosis and prediction

Trilateral retinoblastoma has a poor prognosis. Prognosis is related to age at presentation, with children aged < 6 years having the worst outcomes (~6% survival) {14}. The mortality rate of patients with heritable retinoblastoma syndrome and SPMs is about 50% {3275,7777}. Current screening recommendations for patients with retinoblastoma syndrome include annual history and physical examinations with a focus on bony structures and radiotherapy field, and regular skin examination {7015}. Each tumour type manifests at a different age – osteosarcomas in the first and second decades of life, soft tissue sarcomas 10–50 years after retinoblastoma diagnosis, and epithelial tumours and melanoma after the second decade of life. Screening should continue through the life of the patient because they may develop more than one SPM.

# Von Hippel–Lindau syndrome

Aldape KD
Neumann HPH
Perry A
Plate KH
Vortmeyer AO
Zagzag D

## Definition

Von Hippel–Lindau syndrome (VHL) is an autosomal dominant disorder caused by pathogenic germline variants of the tumour suppressor gene *VHL* (located on chromosome 3p25.3) and characterized by the development of haemangioblastoma of the CNS and retina, clear cell renal cell carcinoma (RCC), phaeochromocytoma, pancreatic neuroendocrine tumour (PanNET), and endolymphatic sac tumour (ELST).

## MIM numbering

193300 Von Hippel–Lindau syndrome; VHLS

## ICD-11 coding

None

## Related terminology

None

## Subtype(s)

Von Hippel–Lindau syndrome types 1, 2A, 2B, and 2C

## Localization

Haemangioblastomas most often involve the retina, cerebellum, and spinal cord (especially paraspinal nerve roots) but can occur anywhere along the craniospinal axis, including peripheral nerves and even tissues outside the nervous system {7338, 7337,246,1809,704,4878}. ELST arises from the vestibular aqueduct and may invade through the temporal bone and into the cerebellopontine angle {2440,1828}.

## Clinical features

Retinal haemangioblastomas manifest earlier than RCC (mean age: 25 years) and thus offer the possibility of an early diagnosis {3961}.

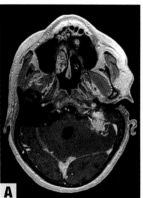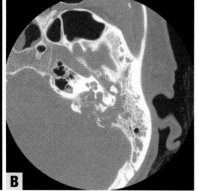

**Fig. 16.25** Endolymphatic sac tumour in a patient with von Hippel–Lindau syndrome. **A** This contrast-enhancing tumour (seen here by postcontrast T1-weighted MRI) arose in the cerebellopontine angle and was therefore resected by a neurosurgeon. **B** CT of the same tumour shows destruction of the temporal bone, which essentially excludes the diagnostic consideration of choroid plexus papilloma.

CNS haemangioblastomas develop mainly in young adults (mean age: 29 years). They are predominantly located in the cerebellum, followed by the brain stem and spinal cord {1797}. Approximately 25% of all cases of CNS haemangioblastoma are associated with hereditary VHL.

Renal cysts and clear cell RCCs are typically multifocal and bilateral. The mean patient age at manifestation is 37 years (vs 61 years for sporadic clear cell RCC) and the patient age at onset is 16–67 years. There is a 70% chance of developing clear cell RCC by the age of 70 years. Metastatic RCC is the leading cause of death from VHL.

Adrenal phaeochromocytomas arise in 20% of patients with VHL. The mean age of onset is 30 years.

Pancreatic manifestations are predominantly multiple cysts but also neuroendocrine tumours (NETs) {3781}.

Other VHL-associated tumours include ELSTs associated with hearing loss, tinnitus, and vertigo, as well as epididymal and broad ligament cystadenomas.

Type 1 VHL is characterized by haemangioblastomas and RCCs but rare or absent phaeochromocytomas, and it is typically caused by deletions, truncations, and missense mutations. Type 2A is characterized by haemangioblastomas and phaeochromocytomas (RCCs are rare) and is caused by missense mutations. Type 2B is characterized by a high frequency of haemangioblastomas, RCCs, and phaeochromocytomas, and it is mainly caused by missense mutations. Type 2C is characterized by phaeochromocytomas and an absence of haemangioblastomas and of RCCs; it is mainly caused by *VHL* missense mutations.

## Epidemiology

VHL is estimated to have an incidence rate of 2.8 cases per 100 000 person-years.

## Etiology

VHL is caused by heterozygous germline pathogenic sequence variants of the *VHL* gene on chromosome 3p25.3. These are spread over the three exons. Missense mutations are most common, but nonsense mutations, microdeletions/insertions, splice-site mutations, and large deletions also occur. In total, > 1000 mutations have been described in the *VHL* gene. The heterogeneous clinical manifestations of VHL are a reflection of the diversity of germline mutations.

## Pathogenesis

Mutational inactivation of the *VHL* tumour suppressor gene in affected family members is responsible for their genetic susceptibility to tumour development at various organ sites, but the mechanisms by which the inactivation or loss of the suppressor gene product (VHL protein) causes neoplastic transformation are only partly understood {2507}. The cell of origin (haemangioblast, stromal cell) is not well defined, but current evidence

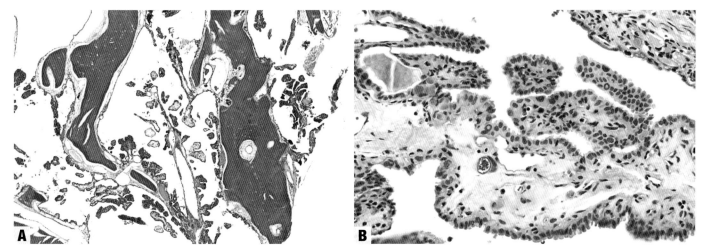

**Fig. 16.26** Endolymphatic sac tumour in a patient with von Hippel–Lindau syndrome. **A,B** The histopathology is reminiscent of choroid plexus papilloma, but the bone invasion essentially excludes that diagnosis.

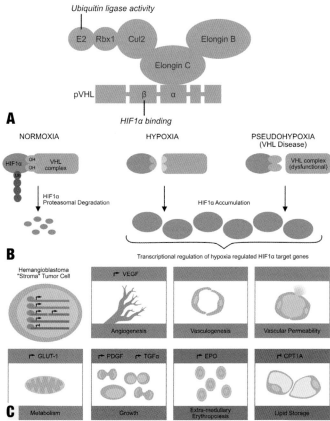

**Fig. 16.27** Von Hippel–Lindau syndrome pathogenesis. **A** The β domain of VHL protein (pVHL) interacts with HIF1α, whereas the α domain interacts with other partners of the VHL complex. In von Hippel–Lindau syndrome, alterations in the α domain prevent the formation of a functional VHL complex. **B** In normoxia, the VHL complex binds to HIF1α and promotes ubiquitination and proteasomal degradation in an oxygen-dependent manner. In hypoxia, binding of VHL protein to HIF1α is impaired, resulting in an accumulation of HIF1α and increased activation of target genes. In von Hippel–Lindau syndrome, HIF1α accumulation results from failed binding of HIF1α to the dysfunctional VHL complex. **C** HIF accumulation in haemangioblastoma stroma tumour cells leads to altered gene expression of HIF-responsive genes and results in increased vascularization due to angiogenesis and vasculogenesis, cyst formation due to increased vascular permeability, metabolic adaptation, growth stimulation, extramedullary haematopoiesis, and lipid deposition (clear cell phenotype).

points to a developmentally arrested haemangioblast precursor {7336}. In accordance with the function of *VHL* as a tumour suppressor gene, mutations are also common in sporadic haemangioblastomas (occurring in as many as 78% of cases) and are ubiquitous in clear cell RCCs.

VHL protein has many different functions and is critically involved in protein degradation. The α domain of VHL protein forms a complex with elongin B (transcription elongation factor B, TCEB2), elongin C (TCEB1), cullin-2, and RBX1 (in conjunction called the VHL complex) that has ubiquitin ligase activity, thereby targeting cellular proteins for ubiquitination and proteasome-mediated degradation. The α domain of the gene involved in the binding to elongin B is frequently mutated in neoplasms associated with VHL.

VHL protein plays a key role in cellular oxygen sensing, via the ubiquitination and proteasomal degradation of hypoxia-inducible factors (HIF1α and HIF2α) {2144,7791}, which mediate cellular responses to hypoxia. This leads to loss of VHL protein function with a pseudohypoxic state characterized by altered expression of genes that drive vascularization, cyst formation, lipid storage, metabolic adaptation, and extramedullary erythropoiesis. The β domain of VHL protein interacts with HIF1α. The hydroxylation of HIF1α on proline residues by oxygen-dependent prolyl hydroxylases generates a binding site for VHL protein. Recruitment of the VHL ubiquitin ligase complex leads to the polyubiquitination and proteasomal degradation of HIF1α. In the absence of functional VHL protein, HIF1α accumulates and activates the transcription of several hypoxia-inducible genes, including *VEGFA*, *PDGFB*, *TGFA*, and *EPO*, by binding to the respective hypoxia-responsive elements in the promoter region (leading to pseudohypoxia). Constitutive overexpression of VEGF-A {7586,6728} explains the extraordinary vascularization of neoplasms associated with VHL due to increased angiogenesis/vasculogenesis, as well as the formation of cysts due to increased vascular permeability (VEGF-A is also known as vascular permeability factor, VPF) {4299}. Increased erythropoietin expression is common in haemangioblastomas {3788} and is responsible for intratumoural (extramedullary) haematopoiesis and for the paraneoplastic erythrocytosis syndrome that can occur in patients with VHL. HIF-dependent downregulation of carnitine palmitoyltransferase 1A leads to enhanced lipid storage, a characteristic of VHL-dependent tumours.

## Macroscopic appearance
The macroscopic appearance of VHL-associated tumours is similar to that of their sporadic tumour counterparts.

## Histopathology
The histopathology of VHL-associated tumours is similar to that of their sporadic tumour counterparts. However, ELSTs arising in the cerebellopontine angle may closely mimic choroid plexus papilloma; neuroimaging is helpful in this differential because only ELSTs invade and destroy temporal bone.

## Cytology
The cytology of VHL-associated tumours is similar to that of their sporadic tumour counterparts.

## Diagnostic molecular pathology
Demonstration of a *VHL* germline sequence variant is desirable to confirm the diagnosis.

## Essential and desirable diagnostic criteria
*Essential:* a capillary haemangioblastoma in the CNS or retina; presence of one of the typical extraneural tumours or a pertinent family history.

*Desirable:* identification of a *VHL* germline pathogenic variant by genetic testing (in virtually all cases).

## Staging
Not relevant

## Prognosis and prediction
The median life expectancy of patients with VHL is 49 years. Clinical surveillance guidance has been published {698,5807}.

# Hereditary phaeochromocytoma–paraganglioma syndromes

de Krijger RR
Asa SL
Brandner S
Perry A
Toledo RA

## Definition
Hereditary phaeochromocytoma–paraganglioma syndromes are a group of inherited cancer syndromes characterized by succinate dehydrogenase (SDH)-deficient neoplasia, usually associated with germline pathogenic sequence variants in one of the genes encoding the subunits of SDH (*SDHA*, *SDHB*, *SDHC*, *SDHD*, *SDHAF2*) or with epimutation (promoter hypermethylation) of the *SDHC* gene.

## MIM numbering
168000 Paragangliomas 1; PGL1
601650 Paragangliomas 2; PGL2
605373 Paragangliomas 3; PGL3
115310 Paragangliomas 4; PGL4
614165 Paragangliomas 5; PGL5

## ICD-11 coding
None

## Related terminology
*Acceptable:* familial paraganglioma–phaeochromocytoma syndromes; hereditary paraganglioma–phaeochromocytoma syndromes; hereditary phaeochromocytoma–paraganglioma.

## Subtype(s)
See Table 16.03.

## Localization
Sympathetic-derived paragangliomas are most commonly located in the adrenal gland (phaeochromocytoma) and retroperitoneum, alongside the infrarenal aorta, near the inferior mesenteric artery, and above the aortic bifurcation.

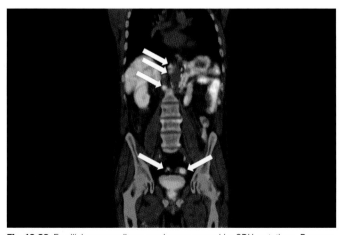

**Fig. 16.28** Familial paraganglioma syndromes caused by SDH mutations. Paragangliomas in familial paraganglioma syndrome. Multiple para-aortic and pelvic paragangliomas (arrows) are identified with 68Ga-DOTATATE PET-CT in a patient with a pathogenic germline *SDHB* mutation.

Parasympathetic-derived paragangliomas commonly occur in the head and neck region, arising from the carotid body and from cervical branches of the glossopharyngeal and vagus nerves {6461}. Familial paragangliomas may be multifocal; they can occur anywhere in the body except in bone, brain, and lymph nodes {362}. Nearly all well-characterized SDH-deficient gastrointestinal stromal tumours have arisen in the stomach {2418, 4671,1951A}. Renal cell carcinomas arise in the kidneys, pituitary neuroendocrine tumours (PitNETs) / pituitary adenomas in the sella turcica (with the exception of ectopic manifestations), and pulmonary chondromas in the lungs.

## Clinical features
Clinical manifestations may be due to catecholamine excess and/or mass effects, with variations according to both genotype and tumour location. Symptoms of epinephrine/norepinephrine excess include sweating, palpitations, and anxiety; signs include hypertension and tachycardia. These are generally associated with sympathetic paragangliomas in the abdomen and with phaeochromocytoma. Some parasympathetic paragangliomas secrete dopamine with minimal clinical manifestations, whereas others, mainly those of the head and neck and cauda equina, are non-secretory. There is a strong genotype–phenotype correlation in the tumour catecholamine profile. Tumours with SDH gene mutations have a pseudohypoxic pathogenesis. They tend to be clinically silent and nonsecretory or dopamine-secreting.

## Epidemiology
Overall, 30–40% of paragangliomas and phaeochromocytomas in adults arise in the context of hereditary disease, and cascade testing of index patients facilitates risk reduction strategies across entire kindreds {759,4436}. A younger age at presentation, multiple tumours, and the presence of extraadrenal tumours are significantly associated with the presence of a germline pathogenic variant {4975}. Other SDH-deficient tumours (gastrointestinal stromal tumours, renal cell carcinoma, PitNETs, and pulmonary chondromas) disproportionately affect children / young adults.

## Etiology
The etiology of these tumours is attributed to the inheritance of mutations in one of the SDH-family genes (see Table 16.03) that predispose individuals to tumour development {2133,7108}.

## Pathogenesis
See Table 16.03.

## Macroscopic appearance
Tumours with SDH pathogenic variants grossly resemble their sporadic counterparts, although multifocality and multicentricity are important clues to syndrome association.

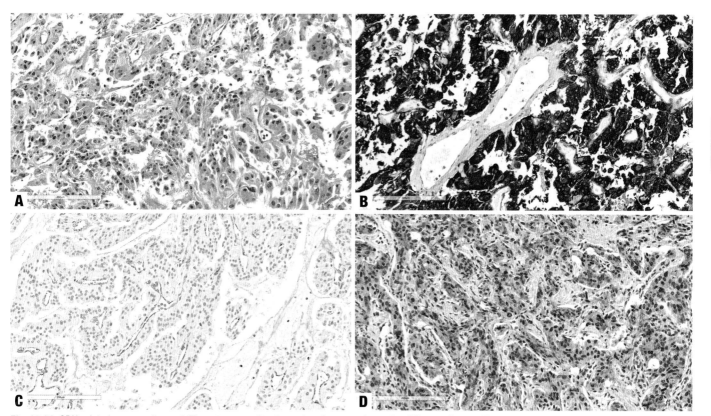

**Fig. 16.29** SDH-related paraganglioma. **A** These tumours often have abundant granular eosinophilic cytoplasm. **B** The tumours express cytoplasmic tyrosine hydroxy-lase. **C** A lack of cytoplasmic SDHB with intact stromal positivity indicates SDH-related disease. **D** Tumours associated with a pseudohypoxia pathway alteration also express inhibin.

## Histopathology

Some SDH gene–associated tumours have a distinct pseudoro-sette pattern {3600}. SDH gene–related paragangliomas from the head and neck usually have small cells with clear cytoplasm. Other unique features include a prominent nested architecture with well-formed, almost circular nests and monotonous cells with vacuolated eosinophilic cytoplasm {7110}. Unlike sporadic paragangliomas, they are rarely associated with a spindled morphology or densely granular cytoplasm {7110}.

Immunohistochemical staining identifies neuroendocrine markers including synaptophysin and chromogranin. S100 or SOX10 staining highlights the sustentacular cells. Paragangli-omas express nuclear GATA3 {6563} and cytoplasmic tyrosine hydroxylase {362}. Most paragangliomas, with the exception of spinal paragangliomas, are immunonegative for cytokeratins {1712}. Loss of SDHB immunoreactivity in tumour cells with granular cytoplasmic staining of stromal cells supports the diag-nosis of SDH disease {2417,7217}; in tumours that lack SDHB immunoreactivity, the addition of SDHA staining can identify loss in patients with *SDHA* mutations {3743}.

## Cytology

Not relevant

## Diagnostic molecular pathology

Mutations in any of the SDH subunit genes (*SDHA*, *SDHB*, *SDHC*, *SDHD*) or related genes (*SDHAF2*) can be detected by any mutation detection system currently used, including Sanger sequencing, targeted next-generation sequencing, and whole-exome sequencing. Immunohistochemistry for SDHA and SDHB may be used for confirming the pathogenicity of variants of unknown significance.

**Table 16.03** SDH-related familial paraganglioma (PGL) syndromes

| Gene | Chromosome location | Syndrome | Commonest PGL locations | Associated lesions |
|------|---------------------|----------|-------------------------|--------------------|
| *SDHA* | 5p15.33 | PGL type 5 (PGL5) | Adrenal and extra-adrenal | RCC, gastrointestinal stromal tumour, PitNET |
| *SDHB* | 1p36.13 | PGL type 4 (PGL4) | Abdominal and thoracic; head and neck | RCC, gastrointestinal stromal tumour, PitNET |
| *SDHC* | 1q23.3 | PGL type 3 (PGL3) | Head and neck | RCC, gastrointestinal stromal tumour |
| *SDHD* | 11q23.1 | PGL type 1 (PGL1) | Adrenal and extra-adrenal | RCC, gastrointestinal stromal tumour, PitNET |
| *SDHAF2* | 11q12.2 | PGL type 2 (PGL2) | Head and neck | Unknown |

PitNET, pituitary neuroendocrine tumour; RCC, renal cell carcinoma.
Note: PGL syndromes with associated gastrointestinal stromal tumour are also known as Carney–Stratakis syndrome.

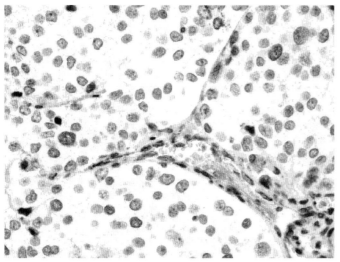

**Fig. 16.30** SDH-related paraganglioma. Familial head and neck paraganglioma immunostained for SDHB, showing succinate dehydrogenase deficiency, with granular cytoplasmic staining of endothelial cells and completely negative tumour cells.

### Essential and desirable diagnostic criteria

*Essential:* manifestation in multiple locations; germline pathogenic variant in one of the SDH genes.

*Desirable:* loss of SDHB immunoreactivity has a high predictive value for SDH gene mutations.

### Staging

The eighth-edition American Joint Committee on Cancer (AJCC) staging system is used. Although many elements are difficult to reconcile with the unique characteristics of these tumours, implementation of this system will increase the data available for a better understanding of prognostic indicators.

### Prognosis and prediction

Most paragangliomas can be surgically resected; however, large tumours and some extra-adrenal tumour locations may preclude complete excision. Familial lesions are often multifocal; the presentations may be asynchronous, mimicking metastasis. Catecholamine profile and *SDHB* mutation increase risk of metastasis, but other genetic causes may be involved. The 5-year overall survival rate in patients with metastatic paraganglioma ranges from 50% to 70% {422,366,2134,2680}.

---

Chromogranin

Dopamine/Methoxytyramine

Noradrenaline/Normetanephrine

| **Cluster 1**<br>**Krebs cycle-related**<br>**Pseudohypoxia pathway** | **Cluster 1**<br>**VHL/EPAS1-related**<br>**Pseudohypoxia pathway** |
|---|---|

Adrenaline/Metanephrine

- *Immature biochemical phenotype*
  - Silent
  - Dopamine
  - Dopamine&Noradrenaline

- Most common cause of germline disease and highest rate of metastatic disease

- *Genotypic prototypes:*
  *SDHx, FH*

- *Immature secretory phenotype*
  - Noradrenaline

- *Genotypic prototypes:*
  *VHL, EPAS1*

| **Wnt-pathway** | **Cluster 2**<br>**Kinase signaling pathway** |
|---|---|

- *Mature secretory phenotype*
  - Adrenaline&Noradrenaline

- *Genotypic prototypes:*
  *MAML3 fusions, CSDE1*
  *All somatic alterations*
  *Identified in pheochromocytomas*

- *Mature secretory phenotype*
  - Adrenaline&Noradrenaline
  - Adrenalie

- *Genotypic prototypes:*
  *RET, NF1, MAX, TMEM127*

**Risk of Metastatic spread**

**Fig. 16.31** Familial paraganglioma syndromes caused by SDH mutations. Biochemical and genetic clusters of paragangliomas {362}.

# WAGR syndrome

Tomlinson GE
Vujanic GM

## Definition

WAGR syndrome (Wilms tumour, aniridia, genitourinary anomalies, and a range of developmental delays) is a contiguous gene syndrome caused by de novo constitutional deletion on chromosome band 11p13 that results in a predisposition to Wilms tumour, the presence at birth of aniridia, genitourinary anomalies, and a range of developmental delays (previously "mental retardation"). Responsible genetic deletions underlying WAGR syndrome include *WT1* deletion, predisposing to the abnormal development of the genitourinary system and to Wilms tumour, and *PAX6* deletion, predisposing to abnormal ocular development.

## MIM numbering

194072 WAGR syndrome; WAGR
612469 WAGRO syndrome; WAGRO

## ICD-11 coding

LD2A.Y Other specified malformative disorders of sex development

## Related terminology

*Not recommended:* Wilms, aniridia, genitourinary abnormalities, mental retardation.

## Subtype(s)

None

## Localization

WAGR syndrome manifests in the eye (including abnormal development of the iris, cornea, and optic nerve), kidney and renal system (including small glomeruli, glomerulosclerosis, and duplicated ureters), gonads (including cryptorchidism, hypospadias, ambiguous genitalia, streak ovaries, and gonadoblastoma), and CNS (including developmental delays, autism, attention deficit hyperactivity disorder [ADHD], hypotonia, and seizures).

## Clinical features

WAGR syndrome can be diagnosed at birth, based on the finding of aniridia, and confirmed by either traditional cytogenetics or microarray demonstrating deletion at 11p13 including both *PAX6* and *WT1*. Aniridia is a pan-ocular disorder and in addition to affecting iris development can cause foveal hypoplasia, cataracts, lens dislocation, and optic nerve coloboma or hypoplasia {2898}. The severity of ocular effects varies among patients. Wilms tumours occur at an earlier age in patients with WAGR syndrome than in those without (22 vs 39 months) and can be detected by serial abdominal ultrasound initiated from infancy and repeated every 3–4 months until 8 years of age. Wilms tumours are often bilateral (17–37%) and low-stage at presentation. Survivors of Wilms tumour have a high incidence of proteinuria in the second decade of life, leading to renal failure {863}.

## Epidemiology

The National Wilms Tumor Study (NWTS) reported that 64 (0.75%) of 8553 patients with Wilms tumour had features of WAGR syndrome. Of the patients with WAGR syndrome, 42% were female {863}.

## Etiology

WAGR syndrome is caused by a de novo interstitial deletion of chromosome 11p13.

WAGRO syndrome (Wilms tumour, aniridia, genitourinary anomalies, a range of developmental delays, and obesity) arises from deletion of chromosome 11p14.1, containing *WT1*, *PAX6*, and *BDNF*.

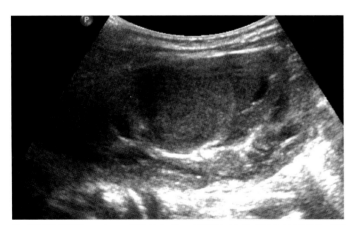

**Fig. 16.32** WAGR syndrome (Wilms tumour, aniridia, genitourinary anomalies, and a range of developmental delays). Greyscale ultrasound of a patient with WAGR syndrome shows a fairly well-circumscribed hypoechoic mass in the middle region of the left kidney, which was subsequently confirmed to be a Wilms tumour.

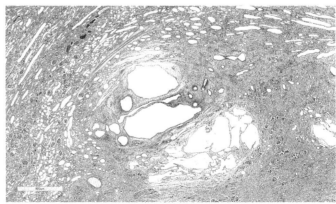

**Fig. 16.33** Intralobar nephrogenic rest. An intralobar nephrogenic rest, rich in stroma and with small cysts, blending with the surrounding renal parenchyma.

WAGRO syndrome includes the physical features of WAGR syndrome in addition to features resulting from *BDNF* haploinsufficiency (altered energy balance, hyperphagia, and obesity) {2596,2683}.

## Pathogenesis

Hemizygous *PAX6* deletion results in abnormal ocular development. Affected infants have aniridia and may also have increased ocular pressure resulting in glaucoma.

Hemizygous *WT1* deletion is responsible for impaired renal development, persistence of intralobar rests, and a predisposition to Wilms tumour. Ambiguous genitalia, also observed with point mutations in *WT1*, can also be seen in WAGR syndrome.

## Macroscopic appearance

See *Nephroblastoma* (p. 697).

## Histopathology

Histologically, WAGR syndrome is associated with stromal features (observed in ~50% of cases) and mixed Wilms tumour, with no anaplastic cases. Intralobar nephrogenic rests are a very frequent finding, observed in as many as 80% of cases {863,2131}. Glomeruli in patients with WAGR syndrome are small (110 ± 37 μm, compared with 125 ± 18.5 μm in controls), a feature that may contribute to renal failure {1528}.

## Cytology

Not relevant

## Diagnostic molecular pathology

Diagnosis is by high-resolution cytogenetics or microarray demonstration of interstitial deletion on chromosome 11p13 involving genomic coordinates 11:31 000 000–36 400 000. In an infant with aniridia, if a contiguous deletion is not detected, then molecular analysis for a point mutation or deletion involving *PAX6* can indicate sporadic aniridia, which substantially reduces the subsequent risk of Wilms tumour.

## Essential and desirable diagnostic criteria

The diagnosis of WAGR syndrome is based on physical features and heterozygous deletion of chromosome 11p13, containing both *PAX6* and *WT1*.

## Staging

WAGR syndrome–related Wilms tumours are staged similarly to non-WAGR Wilms tumours, according to the Children's Oncology Group (COG) criteria if treated initially by surgery, or the International Society of Paediatric Oncology (SIOP) criteria if treated initially with chemotherapy {1783}.

## Prognosis and prediction

Wilms tumours in WAGR syndrome as reported by the NWTS have typically favourable histology and are low-stage, with only 2% being metastatic, and have a high 5-year survival rate, reported as 95%. However, long-term survival (at 27 years after diagnosis of Wilms tumour) is 48% in patients with WAGR syndrome, compared to 86% in patients without. End-stage renal disease, occurring in 52% of patients at 20 years after diagnosis, is the most common cause of death {863}.

# Beckwith–Wiedemann and related overgrowth syndromes

Tomlinson GE
Kratz CP

## Definition
Beckwith–Wiedemann syndrome (BWS) is an overgrowth and cancer predisposition syndrome caused by genetic or epigenetic defects on chromosome 11p15.5, with physical features occurring in infancy and early childhood.

## MIM numbering
130650 Beckwith–Wiedemann syndrome; BWS

## ICD-11 coding
LD2C Overgrowth syndromes

## Related terminology
None

## Subtype(s)
The molecular subtypes of BWS are listed in Box 16.04.

## Localization
Most malignant tumours associated with BWS occur in the abdomen, including in the kidney (Wilms tumour), liver (hepatoblastoma), and adrenal gland (neuroblastoma or adrenocortical carcinoma).

## Clinical features
Beckwith–Wiedemann spectrum comprises BWS and isolated lateralized overgrowth with 11p15.5 genetic or epigenetic defects. BWS predisposes primarily to nephroblastoma and hepatoblastoma. Rarely, other cancer types occur, such as acute lymphoblastic leukaemia, haemangioendothelioma, melanoma, neuroblastoma, pancreatoblastoma, phaeochromocytoma, and rhabdomyosarcoma. Differential diagnoses include Costello, Malan, Perlman, *PTEN* hamartoma tumour, Simpson–Golabi–Behmel, Sotos, and Weaver syndromes, as well as *PIK3CA*-related overgrowth spectrum {4880,3384,875, 1393,876}.

**Box 16.04** The molecular subtypes of Beckwith–Wiedemann syndrome

1. *KCNQ1OT1*:TSS DMR (IC2) loss of methylation (IC2-LOM)
2. *H19/IGF2*:IG DMR (IC1) gain of methylation (IC1-GOM)
3. Chromosome 11p15.5 paternal uniparental disomy (upd(11p)pat)
4. Deletions/duplications of 11p15.5
5. Pathogenic variants on the maternal allele in *CDKN1C*

IC1, imprinting centre 1; IC2, imprinting centre 2; IG DMR, intergenic differentially methylated region; TSS DMR, transcriptional start site differentially methylated region.

Of the molecular subtypes, upd(11p)pat and IC1-GOM are associated with the highest childhood cancer risk (mainly hepatoblastoma and nephroblastoma). Pathogenic variants of *CDKN1C* are associated with neuroblastoma. Children with IC2-LOM have the lowest cancer risk.

See also the clinical diagnostic criteria and scoring system below.

## Epidemiology
BWS occurs in 1 in 10 000–13 700 births {4881}. One third of children with BWS are born prematurely. BWS is observed more frequently in multiple births, although usually only one infant is affected. BWS is slightly more common in children conceived through the use of assisted reproductive technology {4880}.

## Etiology
BWS results from the aberrant expression of imprinted genes located on the chromosomal region 11p15, including *KCNQ1OT1*, *H19*, *CDKN1C*, and *IGF2*. Imprinting of these genes results in only the paternal allele (*KCNQ1OT1* and *IGF2*) or the maternal allele (*H19* and *CDKN1C*) being normally expressed {7505,1898}.

The characteristic overgrowth seen in BWS patients may be partially explained by inappropriate *IGF2* expression of both parental alleles or loss of expression of the *CDKN1C* maternal allele {1082}. *CDKN1C* and *IGF2* are protein-encoding genes. *CDKN1C* encodes a cell cycle, cell division, and growth regulator that acts as a tumour suppressor gene, and *IGF2* encodes

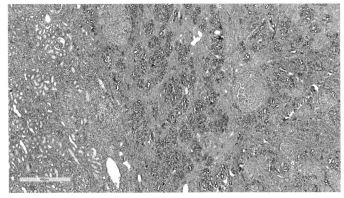

**Fig. 16.34** Perilobar nephrogenic rests. These are in the kidney of a young child with Beckwith–Wiedemann syndrome.

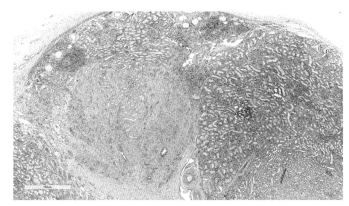

**Fig. 16.35** Medullary ray nodules. These are seen in the kidneys of patients with Wilms tumour and Beckwith–Wiedemann syndrome.

an insulin-like growth-promoting factor. *KCNQ1OT1* and *H19* are transcribed but not translated, and their RNA suppresses the expression of the maternal copy of *IGF2* and the paternal copy of *CDKN1C*, respectively {7403}.

## Pathogenesis

Dysregulated expression of genes on the chromosomal region 11p15 may occur through a number of different epigenetic and genetic mechanisms {7403,1898}.

Chromosomal abnormalities detectable by karyotyping, such as duplications of the paternal 11p15 region, or translocations or inversions of the maternal chromosome 11 region, are identified only in a minority (1–2%) of patients with BWS. Aberrant imprinting of *KCNQ1OT1* or *H19* can be detected in a large proportion of patients with BWS, with 50–60% of them exhibiting *KCNQ1OT1* hypomethylation, *H19* hypermethylation, or (rarely) microdeletions of *KCNQ1OT1* or *H19* {875}.

Other mechanisms responsible for BWS are *CDKN1C* mutations (in 5–10% of sporadic cases of BWS and 40% of families with autosomal dominant BWS) or, more commonly, a lack of expression of the maternal *CDKN1C* allele due to abnormal imprinting. In 10–20% of patients, loss of *CDKN1C* expression and increased *IGF2* expression occurs as a result of paternal isodisomy of the 11p15 chromosomal region. Paternal isodisomy results from somatic recombination after conception; such BWS cases are often mosaic and may require testing of tissues other than blood {7403}.

It is believed that the aberrant *IGF2* and/or *H19* expression contributes to the increased tumour risk in most patients with BWS {4302}.

## Macroscopic appearance

See relevant tumour sections.

## Histopathology

Perilobar nephrogenic rests are seen in the kidneys of infants and young children with BWS and are considered precursor lesions of Wilms tumour. These perilobar rests and also medullary ray nodules are seen in patients with Wilms tumour and BWS.

## Cytology

Not relevant

## Diagnostic molecular pathology

Molecular analyses include methylation at imprinting loci, mutation screening of *CDKN1C*, and copy-number analysis at 11p15.5. Because of mosaicism, analyses of different tissues may be necessary to establish the diagnosis {1393}.

## Essential and desirable diagnostic criteria

The clinical diagnosis is based on a clinical scoring system. For a clinical diagnosis of classic BWS, a patient requires a score of ≥ 4. A score of ≥ 2 merits BWS molecular testing {875,458}.

*Cardinal features (2 points per feature)*
- Macroglossia
- Exomphalos
- Lateralized overgrowth
- Multifocal and/or bilateral Wilms tumour or nephroblastomatosis
- Hyperinsulinism (lasting > 1 week and requiring escalated treatment)
- Pathology findings: adrenal cortex cytomegaly, placental mesenchymal dysplasia, or pancreatic adenomatosis

*Suggestive features (1 point per feature)*
- Birthweight > 2 standard deviations above the mean
- Facial naevus simplex
- Polyhydramnios and/or placentomegaly
- Ear creases and/or pits
- Transient hypoglycaemia (lasting < 1 week)
- Typical Beckwith–Wiedemann spectrum tumours (neuroblastoma, rhabdomyosarcoma, unilateral Wilms tumour, hepatoblastoma, adrenocortical carcinoma, or phaeochromocytoma)
- Nephromegaly and/or hepatomegaly
- Umbilical hernia and/or diastasis recti

## Staging

Staging of embryonal tumours is similar to that of their non-BWS counterparts and includes pretreatment extent of disease (PRE-TEXT) staging for hepatoblastoma and Children's Oncology Group (COG) or International Society of Paediatric Oncology (SIOP) staging for Wilms tumour {7042,7344}.

## Prognosis and prediction

The prognosis largely depends on clinical complications (such as tumours) and the quality of care. Cancer surveillance protocols and clinical guidelines have been developed, and patients should be followed up by a physician with knowledge of this condition {875,3384}.

# Familial adenomatous polyposis

Frayling IM
Abedalthagafi MS
Brosens LAA
Gupta A
Hawkins CE
Perry A

Pfister SM
Pietsch T
Solomon DA
Tabori U
Tomlinson GE
Varlet P

## Definition

Classic familial adenomatous polyposis (FAP) is an autosomal dominant syndrome caused by pathogenic *APC* mutations. It is typically characterized by > 100 adenomatous polyps in the colorectum, extracolonic manifestations (including polyps) elsewhere in the gastrointestinal tract, and desmoid tumours.

## MIM numbering

175100 Familial adenomatous polyposis 1; FAP1

## ICD-11 coding

2B90.Y Other specific malignant neoplasms of colon

## Related terminology

*Acceptable:* adenomatous polyposis coli.

*Not recommended:* Gardner syndrome (obsolete; almost all patients with FAP have such features); Turcot syndrome (acceptable in some cases, but most cases of Turcot syndrome are due to constitutional mismatch repair deficiency syndrome; see *Lynch syndrome*, p. 994).

## Subtype(s)

Attenuated familial adenomatous polyposis

## Localization

Classic FAP is characterized by the development during adolescence of hundreds of colorectal adenomas, a small proportion of which progress to colorectal adenocarcinoma. Most patients also develop gastric and duodenal polyps, leading to an increased risk of duodenal adenocarcinoma. Desmoid tumours occur in about 10% of patients with FAP, mostly in the small bowel mesentery, abdominal wall, or extremities. Less frequent extraintestinal malignancies are hepatoblastoma and cancers of the thyroid, biliary tree, pancreas, and CNS. Frequent benign extraintestinal features are osteomas, dental abnormalities (supernumerary teeth and odontomas), and congenital hypertrophy of the retinal pigment epithelium {893}.

## Clinical features

In the gastrointestinal tract, classic FAP is characterized by numerous (usually > 100 and as many as several thousand) adenomatous polyps of the large bowel. The onset of colorectal adenomatous polyps usually occurs in the second decade of life. If colectomy is not performed, patients have a near-100% risk of developing colorectal adenocarcinoma by the age of 45 years {7253}.

Attenuated FAP is distinguished from classic FAP by fewer (20–100) colorectal adenomas and a slightly reduced risk (of 80%) and later onset (mean age: 56 years) of colorectal cancer {6471,3669}.

Almost all patients with FAP develop duodenal adenomas, mostly in the periampullary region and distal duodenum. Small bowel polyps and cancer typically arise a decade later than colon polyps and cancer. About 4–10% of patients develop duodenal adenocarcinoma {892}. More than 60% of patients with FAP develop gastric polyps, which are mainly benign fundic gland polyps (FGPs), but adenomas may also occur {894}. Severe and predominant fundic gland polyposis without duodenal or colorectal polyposis is defined as gastric adenocarcinoma and proximal polyposis of the stomach (GAPPS), a syndrome currently considered a rare subtype of FAP (see the section on GAPPS and other fundic gland polyposes in the fifth-edition *Digestive system tumours* volume of this series) {4075}. The severity of gastrointestinal features is variable {1469}.

Desmoid tumours occur in about 10% of patients with FAP, mostly in the small intestinal mesentery, abdominal wall, or extremities. The risk of desmoid fibromatosis in FAP is increased by clinical features such as prior surgery and certain types of *APC* mutations {6116}. Although desmoid tumours have no metastatic potential, they cause severe morbidity and mortality in a substantial proportion of patients with FAP {4652,1346}.

The presence of benign extragastrointestinal features is variable, but almost all patients with FAP have some on close inspection {7253}. Some benign extraintestinal manifestations can be used as clinical markers for asymptomatic carriers in families with FAP. In addition, FAP has been associated with a slightly increased risk of papillary carcinoma of the thyroid gland, hepatobiliary tree tumours, childhood hepatoblastoma, adrenocortical adenomas and carcinomas, and brain tumours – i.e. medulloblastoma {5190,2220,2219}.

## Epidemiology

The prevalence of FAP is 1 in 8000–10 000 individuals. It affects both sexes equally and accounts for < 1% of all colorectal cancers {7253}.

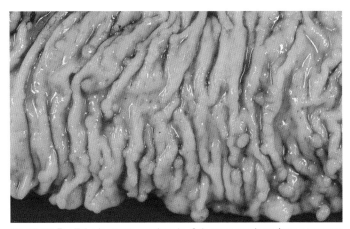

**Fig. 16.36** Familial adenomatous polyposis. Colectomy specimen from a teenager with an *APC* mutation, showing the classic appearance of the resected colon, with several hundred polypoid lesions.

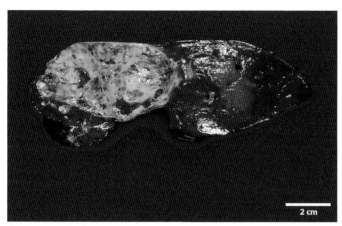

**Fig. 16.37** Hepatoblastoma. Liver explant from an 18-month-old boy with hepatoblastoma status after chemotherapy and with multiple β-catenin–activated adenomas, who was found to have a germline *APC* mutation.

## Etiology

FAP is a Mendelian autosomal dominant syndrome caused by germline (constitutional) mutations in the *APC* gene (chromosome 5q22.2) that result in a truncated or absent APC protein. The severity of disease varies with the position of the mutation in the *APC* gene. Inherited *APC* mutations located in or around the mutation cluster region (around codon / amino acid 1309) are associated with the highest number of adenomas (thousands – severe polyposis) and the greatest risk of cancer at a younger age, whereas mutations outside this region are mostly associated with many hundreds of adenomas and a slightly lower cancer risk {3910,2568}. Attenuated FAP-associated inherited mutations (associated with < 100 adenomas) are located nearer to the N-terminus or within the alternatively spliced section of exon 9 (9a), and these patients develop fewer polyps at a later age {3669}. Desmoid tumours are associated with germline mutations in *APC* involving codons 1310–2011 in the middle to C-terminal portion of the encoded protein {6527}.

*APC* acts as a classic tumour suppressor gene, and a tumour phenotype arises when the non-mutant allele is spontaneously lost or mutated by a somatic event (second hit). When the inherited mutation is in the mutation cluster region, the second somatic mutation may be either a point mutation or a complete deletion or loss of heterozygosity of the second allele. However, loss of heterozygosity is never observed with inherited mutations outside the mutation cluster region, and in attenuated FAP second hits are only observed in the mutation cluster region. Therefore, for a colorectal adenoma/cancer to develop, at least one mutation must be within the mutation cluster region. Interestingly, patients with constitutional deletions of the entire *APC* gene do not always exhibit a low number of colorectal adenomas (i.e. < 100).

In about 20–30% of FAP cases, there is no known family history of the condition; most of these cases probably represent either de novo mutations or cases of the recessive syndrome *MUTYH*-associated polyposis (see the section on other adenomatous polyposes in the fifth-edition *Digestive system tumours* volume of this series). Despite the variations in phenotype, it is very rare for any carrier of a pathogenic *APC* mutation not to develop multiple bowel polyps and cancer if preventive measures are not taken. Mosaic de novo *APC* mutation carriers also exist, and they typically have milder and/or localized polyposis {2874}.

## Pathogenesis

The classic APC protein isoform is 2843 amino acids long (several isoforms exist as a result of alternative splicing), and it is centrally involved in regulating WNT signalling. Normal APC restrains colorectal epithelial cell proliferation through its role as a scaffold protein that binds critical components that tag (by phosphorylation and ubiquitination) the WNT effector protein β-catenin for proteasomal destruction. With APC protein truncation (or absence), the loss of critical APC functions (especially its binding of the AXIN and β-catenin proteins) results in greatly impaired degradation of β-catenin with upregulation of WNT signalling, effectively rendering the WNT pathway constitutively switched on {5420,4960}. Adenomas arise owing to somatically acquired second hits to the non-mutant *APC* gene. The adenomas subsequently progress in a very similar way to sporadic adenomas of the large bowel, through mutations in genes such as *KRAS*, *SMAD4*, and *TP53* (see the section on colorectal adenocarcinoma in the fifth-edition *Digestive system tumours* volume of this series) {3613}.

Children with FAP have an 847-fold increase in relative risk of hepatoblastoma {2407}. *APC* is a tumour suppressor gene involved in regulating the WNT/β-catenin pathway, which regulates liver growth and tumorigenesis. About 50–90% of hepatoblastomas have somatic β-catenin mutations and deletions. Multifocal β-catenin–activated adenomas and hepatoblastomas can occur in the same liver in a child with an *APC* gene mutation {2610}. There is a relatively high incidence of pathogenic *APC* variants and other variants of uncertain significance (VUSs) occurring sporadically in hepatoblastoma {7696}; therefore, the current clinical recommendation is for the routine testing of all patients with hepatoblastoma for *APC* mutations, even in the context of no significant family history of FAP {7696}.

## Macroscopic appearance

There are large numbers of polypoid or villous adenomas. Most patients with FAP also develop duodenal adenomas.

## Histopathology

The large bowel polyps are almost always classic adenomas of varying type (tubular, tubulovillous, or villous), grade (low or high), and size; they are similar to sporadic adenomas in appearance. The same features are observed in duodenal adenomas. However, characteristic of FAP is the frequent presence of monocryptal adenomas and oligocryptal adenomas (microadenomas) in otherwise normal-looking colorectal mucosa, including in the stalk mucosa of resected larger adenomatous polyps.

Most gastric polyps (80%) are FGPs. FGPs in FAP are often multiple and may cause fundic gland polyposis. Low-grade dysplasia has been described in nearly 40% of FAP-associated FGPs, but high-grade dysplasia and malignant transformation are rare {894}. About 20% of gastric polyps are adenomas – mostly foveolar-type adenomas (17%), some pyloric gland adenomas (3%), and rarely intestinal-type adenomas {894}.

Desmoid tumours appear as bland, indolent, invasive fibroblastic tumours of connective tissue that expand relentlessly and are difficult to excise completely (sometimes called "aggressive fibromatosis"). Immunohistochemistry reveals nuclear expression of β-catenin.

## Cytology

Not clinically relevant

## Diagnostic molecular pathology

About 80–90% of sporadic colorectal cancers carry acquired mutations in the *APC* gene, and this is considered to be the tumour-initiating event in most cases {3613}. Although APC has other functions (including regulation of cell polarity, cell–cell adhesion, cytoskeletal organization, and spindle formation), its WNT pathway function of controlling intracellular levels of β-catenin is key to its effects on adenomagenesis {3740}.

## Essential and desirable diagnostic criteria

The presence of > 100 colorectal adenomas is indicative of a probable diagnosis of classic FAP. However, given the phenotypic variability of FAP, several other polyposis conditions can have near-identical features. These other conditions include *MUTYH*-associated polyposis, polymerase proofreading–associated polyposis, *NTHL1*-associated polyposis, hereditary mixed polyposis syndrome, constitutional mismatch repair deficiency syndrome, and multiple polyps associated with mutations in other genes (e.g. *MSH3*, *BUB1*, *AXIN2*, and *FAN1*) {47}, although the number of colorectal polyps is usually lower in these other syndromes and there may be a different pattern of inheritance and other extracolonic features to provide diagnostic clues (see the section on other adenomatous polyposes in the fifth-edition *Digestive system tumours* volume of this series). Another group of patients with a phenotype mimicking FAP have multiple colonic adenomas, usually without extracolonic

features or a strong family history; these individuals may have a polygonic form of polyposis. The essential molecular criterion is the presence of a pathogenic germline (constitutional) *APC* mutation – and this is the gold standard for FAP diagnosis, although a small number of cases have undetectable *APC* mutations and may be regarded as presumed FAP if typical clinical features are present and molecular evidence of the other conditions is absent.

## Staging

FAP tumours are staged in the same way as equivalent sporadic tumours at each site.

## Prognosis and prediction

Approaches to the management of FAP cases are guided by their clinical presentation and severity. Colorectal screening by endoscopy and chemoprevention are in use {41,3569,893}. Colectomy is often required to prevent the development of colorectal adenocarcinoma. Upper gastrointestinal endoscopy is indicated for patients with FAP who are aged 25–30 years and is guided by the Spigelman stage of duodenal polyposis {6624, 892}. Duodenal polyposis is treated endoscopically for as long as possible, but surgery is often required. In addition, screening for extraintestinal manifestations is recommended by some {41, 6815}.

People with FAP have a 3.35-fold elevated risk of dying, compared with the general population {5101}. The main causes of death are upper gastrointestinal malignancy, perioperative complications, desmoid tumours, and suicide {5101,2290}.

# Lynch syndrome

Frayling IM
Gupta A
Tomlinson GE

## Definition

Lynch syndrome (LS) is an autosomal dominant disorder resulting from constitutional pathogenic mutations affecting the DNA mismatch repair genes *MLH1*, *MSH2*, *MSH6*, and *PMS2*.

## MIM numbering

609310 Colorectal cancer, hereditary nonpolyposis, type 2; HNPCC2

120435 Lynch syndrome 1 (colorectal cancer, hereditary nonpolyposis, type 1; HNPCC1)

614350 Colorectal cancer, hereditary nonpolyposis, type 5; HNPCC5

614337 Colorectal cancer, hereditary nonpolyposis, type 4; HNPCC4

613244 Colorectal cancer, hereditary nonpolyposis, type 8; HNPCC8

158320 Muir–Torre syndrome; MRTES

276300 Mismatch repair cancer syndrome 1; MMRCS1

## ICD-11 coding

None

## Related terminology

*Not recommended:* cancer family syndrome {4275}; hereditary non-polyposis colorectal cancer.

## Subtype(s)

Muir–Torre syndrome {4276}; constitutional mismatch repair deficiency syndrome and Turcot syndrome; allelic conditions due to biallelic mismatch repair gene mutations

## Localization

Depending on which gene is involved, cancers occurring in LS can arise in the colon, rectum, endometrium, stomach, small bowel, gallbladder, hepatobiliary tract, pancreas, renal pelvis and/or ureter, bladder, kidney, ovary, brain, or prostate.

## Clinical features

LS is characterized by a predisposition to a wide variety of cancers. Tumours occurring in this setting can develop at any age but often arise in young people. Some individuals with LS develop multiple tumours; others develop no tumours at all, so personal history is important. Family history alone has poor predictive value (both positive and negative). Cases of LS due to de novo germline mutations are well described.

The cancers that occur in LS include tumours of the colorectum, endometrium, stomach, small bowel, ovary, gallbladder, hepatobiliary tract, pancreas, urinary tract (renal pelvis, ureter, and bladder), kidney, brain, and prostate, as well as sebaceous skin tumours. Factors that affect the risk of an individual with LS include sex, age, the affected gene, and history of cancer {4922,4751,4752,4753,6342}. The risk of cancer is highest with

mutations of *MSH2* and *MLH1*, somewhat lower (and with later onset) when *MSH6* is affected, and lower still with *PMS2* mutations. Patients with LS can develop any cancer, which may or may not be due to their LS.

Muir–Torre syndrome is the co-occurrence of a sebaceous skin tumour (i.e. sebaceous adenoma, sebaceoma, sebaceous carcinoma, or keratoacanthoma) with any internal cancer {6298}. Many patients with LS have such skin tumours {53} and therefore may be diagnosed with Muir–Torre syndrome, but not all patients with Muir–Torre syndrome have LS. Sebaceous skin tumours have been reported in some patients with *MUTYH*-associated adenomatous polyposis due to recessive *MUTYH* mutations.

Individuals with LS do not develop large numbers of colorectal adenomas unless they have some other predisposing condition {7518}. However, individuals who inherit a mismatch repair mutation in the same gene from each parent, and therefore have constitutional mismatch repair deficiency syndrome (CMMRD) due to biallelic mismatch repair gene mutations, develop multiple adenomas at a very young age {351} (see also the section on other adenomatous polyposes in the fifth-edition *Digestive system tumours* volume of this series). CMMRD also predisposes individuals to colorectal cancer (CRC), brain tumours, leukaemia, lymphoma, neurofibromatosis type 1–like skin features, and a wide variety of other DNA repair deficiency–related abnormalities {7568}. Turcot described a syndrome of multiple colorectal adenomas and brain cancer {2681,7112}. Most cases are actually due to CMMRD; therefore, Turcot syndrome is an allelic variant of CMMRD. However, similar cases can be due to familial adenomatous polyposis (caused by inherited *APC* mutations).

Although Warthin was the first to describe what is now known as LS, Lynch redescribed it, calling it "the cancer family syndrome" {7453,4275}. Endeavours to study families with the syndrome in order to identify the responsible genes resulted in the Amsterdam criteria, which were intended merely to identify families suitable for participation in research involving genetic linkage analysis (in ignorance of the spectrum and penetrance of the disease). The term "hereditary non-polyposis CRC" was then coined, as an umbrella term to help in the education of clinicians (still before the genes responsible for LS had been identified and the full clinical spectrum had become apparent) {4274}. The subsequent Bethesda guidelines for testing of colorectal tumours for microsatellite instability were developed in an attempt to help select tumours to test for possible LS, again in ignorance of the syndrome's full clinical characteristics. Both the Amsterdam criteria and the Bethesda guidelines suffer from poor sensitivity. The Amsterdam criteria suffer from overly stringent specificity (excluding many individuals from testing), and the Bethesda guidelines suffer from nonspecificity at the cost of poor sensitivity. Later, the term "hereditary non-polyposis CRC" was no longer recommended (because it was inaccurate and confusing), and LS was defined as being caused by a constitutional pathogenic mismatch repair mutation {7251}.

## Epidemiology

Systematic testing of CRC cases suggests that LS is a cause of CRC in approximately 1 in 30 cases. From the weighted mean extrapolated penetrance to age 85 years of LS as CRC (0.25) and the country-specific lifetime risks of CRC, the prevalence of LS in the general population can be estimated to be approximately 1 in 125 (range: 1 in 100–180) {3253,7784,6559,4753}. Founder mutations causing LS have been found in many populations; for example, Finland has a higher prevalence of LS as a result of this effect {5106,2709,2540,7333,1870}. In addition, certain mutations are relatively more common {1714}.

## Etiology

The primary cause of LS is a constitutional pathogenic mutation affecting a mismatch repair gene (*MLH1*, *MSH2*, *MSH6*, or *PMS2*). Some individuals with LS have mutations involving adjacent genes that affect or extend into a mismatch repair gene; for example, a mutation in *EPCAM* (*TACSTD1*) affecting *MSH2*, or a mutation in *LRRFIP2* affecting *MLH1* {7251,4114,3810,4782}. Some individuals may have epigenetic mechanism (DNA methylation) mutations affecting *MLH1* or *MSH2*, some of which may be caused by rearrangements involving adjacent genes {2916, 2464,4114,3810,4782}.

The International Society for Gastrointestinal Hereditary Tumours (InSiGHT) curates a public database of mismatch repair genes {4965}, interprets genetic variants according to published criteria, and is recognized by the Clinical Genome Resource (ClinGen) / Global Alliance for Genomics and Health (GA4GH) as the sole definitive worldwide resource {6977,3131}.

A number of environmental and lifestyle factors have been identified as modifiers of LS. Cigarette smoking, increased body mass index, and alcohol consumption are associated with an increased risk, whereas acetylsalicylic acid, ibuprofen, multivitamin and calcium supplements, hormone replacement therapy (but not oral contraceptive pill use), and increasing parity in women are associated with a reduction of cancer risk in LS {5306,7569,4824,110}.

## Pathogenesis

Cells do not lose their mismatch repair function unless both alleles of a given mismatch repair gene are inactivated. Therefore, it is not until a normal cell in a person with LS acquires a somatic hit in the corresponding normal mismatch repair allele that that cell becomes mismatch repair–deficient (dMMR). This deficiency has several important consequences. Firstly, dMMR cells escape from the normal control of apoptosis and gain a relative growth advantage, although this may be dependent on subsequent mutations in other genes {5607}. Secondly, mismatch repair deficiency leads to an increase in the point mutation rate, especially within repetitive stretches of DNA called microsatellites; this manifests as microsatellite instability (MSI). Thirdly, mismatch repair deficiency may also lead to abnormal mismatch repair protein expression, which is identifiable by immunohistochemistry.

In the normal colonic mucosa of people with LS, mismatch repair deficiency is present in approximately 1 crypt/cm$^2$ (i.e. in ~10 000 crypts per individual) {100}. These crypts can lead to immediately invasive lesions with mutations in *CTNNB1* (encoding β-catenin, which activates the WNT pathway) rather than *APC*, and with flat rather than polypoid morphology; such lesions are thought to account for the interval cancers that occur between seemingly normal colonoscopies. Patients with LS can

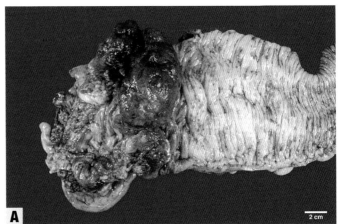

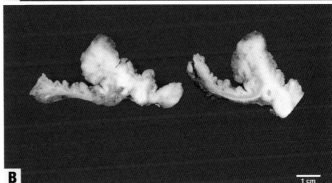

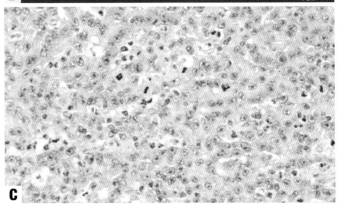

**Fig. 16.38** Lynch syndrome. **A** A segment of proximal ascending colon with a large (110 mm) polypoid mass (tumour) adjacent to several tan-pink mucosal nodules of 2–3 mm (superficial lymphoid aggregates on histology, not shown here) in a 16-year-old with Lynch syndrome who underwent a subtotal colectomy for a colonic adenocarcinoma. **B** Cross-section of the tumour demonstrates a white cut surface abutting the serosal surface. **C** The tumour comprises sheets of poorly differentiated tumour cells with basophilic cytoplasm, increased N:C ratio, irregular nuclear contours, and conspicuous nucleoli. Numerous mitotic figures are present.

undoubtedly develop CRC from adenomas, but some of the flat lesions can also acquire secondary *APC* mutations and become adenomatous and polypoid. Therefore, there are at least three pathways to CRC in LS: (1) dMMR crypts can give rise to flat lesions with mutations in *CTNNB1* rather than *APC*, which develop into flat cancers; (2) these flat lesions may then acquire secondary *APC* mutations and turn into adenomatous polypoid lesions; and (3) patients with LS can develop adenomas with primary *APC* mutations (like people without LS), and these secondarily acquire mismatch repair deficiency during progression {99}.

It is important to note that rectal cancers with MSI are usually due to LS, even though they do not harbour *CTNNB1* mutations, suggesting that pathway only occurs in the colon {5037,1651,5038}.

A substantial proportion (~15%) of non-LS colon cancers have mismatch repair deficiency. Most are due to sporadic somatic biallelic hypermethylation of the *MLH1* gene promoter as part of the right-sided sessile serrated lesion pathway. Usually (in ~85% of cases), these tumours acquire specific *BRAF* oncogene mutations (p.V600E), which can be used to distinguish them from CRCs that are not sporadic. The occasional CRC in patients with LS can arise along this other pathway; therefore, an age-dependent proportion of CRCs show sporadic mismatch repair deficiency (see Table 16.04) {6470,7216}. In some sporadic CRC cases, mismatch repair deficiency is due to two somatic mismatch repair gene mutations. In a proportion of these cases, this may be due to another predisposition to CRC from a hereditary condition affecting DNA repair, such as *MUTYH*-associated polyposis or polymerase proofreading–associated polyposis (PPAP) {7246}. Because these tumours have the characteristics of LS and may occur in individuals with personal and family histories also consistent with LS, some authors use the term "Lynch-like syndrome" to describe such cases (see Table 16.05) {1753,1041,4449}.

Constitutional hypermethylation of the *MLH1* promoter can also cause LS. This is usually sporadic and not heritable, but some cases have heritable chromosomal rearrangements that cause *MLH1* promoter methylation by involving the *LRRFIP2* gene adjacent to *MLH1* on chromosome 3.

Recently, recessive inheritance of mutations in the mismatch repair gene *MSH3* has also been identified as a cause of adenomatous polyposis {47} (see also the section on other adenomatous polyposes in the fifth-edition *Digestive system tumours* volume of this series). With increasing gene panel sequence testing, individuals are also being found with mutations in more than one mismatch repair gene (digenic LS) {4783,7518}, but it is unclear whether this is more severe than LS due to one mismatch repair mutation.

## Macroscopic appearance

The gross appearance is related to the tumour type and is not distinctive.

**Table 16.04** The proportions of colon cancers, by age, caused by microsatellite instability (MSI) overall, MSI due to Lynch syndrome (LS), and sporadic MSI, and the resulting probability that MSI in a colon cancer is due to LS

| Age (years) | Proportion of colon cancers caused by MSI | | | Probability that MSI in a colon cancer is due to LS[a] |
|---|---|---|---|---|
| | Overall | Due to LS | Sporadic | |
| 35 | 23% | 22% | 2% | 92% |
| 40 | 16% | 14% | 2% | 90% |
| 45 | 10% | 9% | 2% | 87% |
| 50 | 7% | 6% | 2% | 79% |
| 55 | 6% | 4% | 2% | 60% |
| 60 | 10% | 3% | 7% | 28% |
| 65 | 11% | 3% | 8% | 32% |
| 70 | 14% | 3% | 11% | 23% |

[a]Assuming that all LS tumours have MSI.
Derived from van Lier et al. {7216}.

## Histopathology

The typical histological features in CRC with MSI include the presence of tumour-infiltrating lymphocytes, Crohn-like peritumoural lymphocytic reaction, poor differentiation, mucinous and signet-ring cell features, and a medullary growth pattern {151, 3593,7080,6412}. These features are identified both in sporadic cancers with MSI and in those that occur in the setting of LS. Although these histological findings are commonly seen, they are not specific enough by themselves to distinguish between microsatellite-stable and MSI cases.

Limited data are available about non-colorectal LS-associated cancers. Most LS-associated gastric carcinomas are of the intestinal type {4,2642,1024}, < 13% are of the diffuse type, and mucinous carcinomas are very rare. The presence of intraepithelial lymphocytes is not described. LS-associated small bowel carcinomas {7648} show frequently mucinous, signet-ring cell or medullary differentiation, often in combination with tumour-infiltrating lymphocytes and Crohn-like reaction, similarly to ampullary carcinomas {6484}. Other types of LS-associated biliary carcinomas do not have any distinguishing features {6484}. Pancreatic cancers strongly associated with LS are acinar cell carcinomas {4166} and medullary carcinomas {7542}.

Although patients with these specific subtypes do present with an increased incidence of MSI and LS, the histological features of LS-associated cancers are not specific. Testing of (selections of) patients with CRC and/or other types of cancer is recommended by a large number of professional organizations, based on either the presence of MSI or the absence of mismatch repair proteins in the tumour. There is no consensus as to whether immunohistochemistry or molecular testing is the preferred first test, and they can be used in combination {4944,6559,6558,6470}. In cases with a low tumour cell percentage or intense inflammatory reaction, immunohistochemistry is the better option. Subsequent determination of hypermethylation and somatic mutations can be applied to estimate the risk of germline mutations in patients. *BRAF* mutation analysis is an alternative to *MLH1* hypermethylation testing. The use of larger targeted mutation panels that combine microsatellite testing and mutation analyses is under investigation.

Immunohistochemistry for the mismatch repair proteins (MLH1, PMS2, MSH2, and MSH6) is a common first step in screening CRCs for mismatch repair deficiency. The presence of all four proteins suggests microsatellite stability. Loss of nuclear staining for any of the proteins indicates MSI and suggests the most likely involved gene and the need for additional testing. Loss of MSH2 alone or loss of both MSH2 and MSH6 suggests a mutation in *MSH2*. Similarly, loss of MLH1 alone or loss of both MLH1 and PMS2 suggests an underlying mutation or methylation in *MLH1*. Concomitant loss of both MSH2 and MSH6 (or of both MLH1 and PMS2) reflects the heterodimeric binding of MSH2 with MSH6 (or of MLH1 with PMS2) in mismatch repair complexes, such that loss of the first partner leads to relative instability and loss of the second {4073}. The typical expression pattern includes diffuse staining in the tumour nuclei and many benign cells, including epithelial and stromal cells and lymphocytes. A pattern such as loss of nuclear expression of MLH1 and PMS2 and intact staining for MSH2 and MSH6 could be seen either in a sporadic tumour (most commonly due to methylation of the *MLH1* promoter) or in the setting of LS.

The interpretation of mismatch repair protein immunohistochemistry is typically straightforward, but it should always be

**Table 16.05** The term "Lynch-like syndrome (LLS)" is used to describe tumours with mismatch repair (MMR) deficiency (and therefore microsatellite instability and/or abnormal immunohistochemistry) due to somatic mutations in both alleles of the same MMR gene, occurring in the setting of other features suggestive of Lynch syndrome (LS), such as young age of onset, other LS-associated tumour types, and a related family history; patients with LLS may have heritable mutations in other (often DNA repair or maintenance) genes that have predisposed them to somatic MMR gene mutations; these are important to recognize and are listed below

| Syndrome | Gene(s) | Mode of inheritance | Characteristic distinguishing clinical features |
|---|---|---|---|
| Polymerase proofreading–associated polyposis | POLE and POLD1 | Autosomal dominant | Multiple colorectal adenomas; personal and/or family history of endometrial, brain, or other LS-associated tumours; hypermutant phenotype on DNA sequencing {3407A} |
| MUTYH-associated polyposis | MUTYH | Autosomal recessive | Multiple colorectal adenomas; frequent G>T mutations on DNA sequencing {1091A} |
| NTHL1-associated polyposis | NTHL1 | Autosomal recessive | {7502A} |
| n/a | FAN1 | Autosomal dominant | {6321A,7246} |
| n/a | BUB1 and BUB3 | Autosomal dominant | {7246} |
| n/a | SETD2 | Autosomal dominant | {7246} |
| None | None | None | Coincidental sporadic MMR mutations; no underlying cause |

n/a, not applicable.

Notes: Synonyms for LLS include "LS mimic", "LS-like", and "mutation-negative LS". Patients with LLS may represent a heterogeneous group. LLS has a mean age of onset similar to that of LS. At least 50–60% of LLS-associated colorectal cancers exhibit biallelic somatic inactivation of the MMR genes within the tumour through somatic mutations (nonsense, missense, or frameshift mutations; splice-site deletions; gene deletions; or loss of heterozygosity). LS tumours may themselves have somatic mutations in the same genes in which heritable mutations cause the syndromes that in turn give rise to LLS. The overarching term "familial colorectal cancer X (FCC-X)" has been used for familial colorectal cancer in which the tumours are microsatellite-stable (i.e. do not have MMR deficiency). Mutations in LLS-associated genes can also be the cause of FCC-X. The potential value of multiple gene test panels and tumour DNA sequencing will be apparent.

Sources: {3407A,1091A,7183A,2692A,1040A}

performed with adequate internal control staining. Some pitfalls and unusual patterns of expression can occur, but awareness will prevent misinterpretation. Patchy intact staining can occur due to uneven antibody diffusion, variable fixation, or tissue hypoxia {1156,4674}. Cytoplasmic staining may occur, but it is considered abnormal and therefore deficient, because there is no staining in the nuclei and cytoplasmic staining has been described with mutations {6331}. Weak, patchy, nucleolar, or even absent MSH6 expression has been reported in a substantial number of rectal tumours after neoadjuvant treatment without MSI or mutation confirmed by molecular testing {484,5716}. In occasional cases, heterogeneous staining or loss of MSH6 expression can be due to a secondary (non-germline) mutation in the MSH6 coding mononucleotide tract {2521,6413}. Approximately 3–10% of LS tumours that have mismatch repair deficiency with MSI show no abnormality on immunohistochemistry (presumably because of mutations that disable protein function but leave the protein detectable by immunohistochemistry) {518}.

## Cytology

Not clinically relevant

## Diagnostic molecular pathology

LS results from autosomal dominant inheritance of a constitutional mutation affecting one of four DNA mismatch repair genes: MSH2 (2p21-p16.3), MLH1 (3p22.2), MSH6 (2p16.3, only 300 kb from MSH2), and PMS2 (7p22.1) {4278}. InSiGHT curates a public database of mismatch repair genes {4965}, interprets genetic variants according to published criteria, and is recognized by ClinGen/GA4GH as the sole definitive worldwide resource {6977,3131}.

Patients with deletions of the 3' (terminal) end of EPCAM that do not extend into MSH2 are at risk of gastrointestinal cancers but seemingly not of the non-gastrointestinal cancers characteristic of LS {3514,4277,4114}. In contrast, patients with EPCAM deletions that extend into MSH2 have a phenotype indistinguishable from that of patients with mutations in MSH2.

Defective mismatch repair in a tumour prevents recognition and repair of insertions or deletions that naturally occur during DNA replication within repetitive DNA sequences. This can be detected as MSI, which is defined as the presence of extra alleles at a microsatellite compared with normal DNA (from normal tissue or blood) from the same individual {2218}. Microsatellites vary in their propensity to show instability, and therefore the frequency with which the same microsatellite is affected in different tumour types varies. Instability is best observed at mononucleotide repeats (e.g. AAAAAAAAA…), with this being more substantial than at dinucleotide repeats (e.g. CACACACA…). Like any laboratory test, MSI tests balance sensitivity against specificity. Current markers used in colon cancer MSI diagnosis are known to have reduced sensitivity for detecting MSI in non-colonic tumours, such as endometrial, small bowel, or gastric cancers, and in tumours from patients with MSH6 mutations. Therefore, a small number of LS-associated tumours may not appear to have MSI using this test (although they might be recognized by abnormal mismatch repair immunohistochemistry).

It is important to note that dMMR tumours do not always have abnormal immunohistochemistry or test positive for MSI. Immunohistochemistry and MSI testing of carcinomas at sites other than the colon, carcinomas due to constitutional mutations in MSH6 or PMS2, or adenomas, has reduced sensitivity. Immunohistochemistry and MSI tests must be interpreted bearing in mind the tumour type, the patient's personal and family history, and other test results (e.g. BRAF mutation status); a multidisciplinary approach is recommended.

The value of mismatch repair immunohistochemistry and MSI testing is considerably enhanced by testing more than one tumour from the same family and/or individual, especially if the tumours are rare (e.g. rectal cancers, colorectal adenomas, small bowel cancers, and sebaceous skin tumours). Consistent immunohistochemical abnormality of one mismatch repair protein is excellent evidence for the pathogenicity of a mutation in that gene, which is important given the number of missense and other difficult-to-interpret mutations that occur in LS. MSI in rectal cancers is rare and strongly associated with LS; this can be exploited clinically, because the finding therefore has excellent positive and negative predictive values for LS. Similarly, MSI is rare in adenomas outside of LS, again providing good positive and negative predictive values {4238}. Some CRCs due to MUTYH-associated polyposis or PPAP may exhibit both MSI and abnormal immunohistochemistry due to somatic mismatch repair gene mutations; they therefore appear to be due to LS but are Lynch-like syndrome cases (see Table 16.05, p. 997).

About 15% of sporadic colon cancers have MSI, usually due to epigenetic silencing of MLH1 by promoter hypermethylation at both alleles. Therefore, unselected colon cancers with MSI have a poor positive predictive value for LS, although an absence of MSI has a good negative predictive value for LS. Further tests (BRAF mutation and MLH1 methylation tests) are required for MSI cancers with loss of MLH1 on immunohistochemistry, to distinguish between LS and sporadic origin. Because sporadic MLH1 promoter hypermethylation in colon cancers is strongly age-dependent, age is a useful discriminator in its interpretation.

Somatic mutations in CRCs in the proto-oncogene BRAF, usually resulting in activating missense p.V600E mutations or similar mutations at this codon, occur in ≥ 85% of sporadic colon cancers with MSI, but not in those due to LS; therefore, such mutations are highly predictive of the tumour being of sporadic origin and not due to LS. However, sporadic tumours harbouring BRAF mutations can occasionally occur in patients with LS, so the absence of BRAF p.V600E mutations does not definitively diagnose LS, although it does indicate that LS is more likely. Alternatively, detection of MLH1 gene promoter hypermethylation in a tumour provides good (although not unequivocal) evidence that the tumour is sporadic in origin, for two reasons: (1) very occasional sporadic tumours do occur in LS and (2) constitutional MLH1 promoter methylation can be found in a few patients with LS (in some cases, this constitutional MLH1 methylation is due to a rearrangement and is therefore transmissible) {2916}. Good practice for testing for MLH1 promoter methylation in tumours is to include testing of the patient's normal DNA (e.g. from normal tissue surrounding a cancer or from blood), then MLH1 promoter methylation will be readily apparent when it occurs.

LS can be definitively diagnosed after tumour testing by constitutional mismatch repair gene sequencing to identify the pathogenic constitutional mutation. It is often useful to have samples from more than one individual in the family, because case segregation studies may be required in order to determine pathogenicity or whether an individual is a phenocopy. If the family is likely to have a mutation but no point mutation is found, then large-scale mutations, such as deletion of a whole exon (or more), should be considered. In cases with an early onset (e.g. at age < 35 years), LS is likely even in the absence of a family history, although mutations in genes (e.g. BUB1 and BUB3) encoding mitotic spindle checkpoint proteins should be considered, especially in teenage patients. Tumours from such individuals do not exhibit MSI, nor (usually) do those from families with specific POLD1 and POLE proofreading mutations (in PPAP), although the family histories may be Lynch-like. In such cases, some tumours may acquire two mismatch repair gene mutations due to a non-LS underlying syndrome (including PPAP

due to mutations in POLD1 and/or POLE), and therefore appear to be due to LS on tumour testing. Rare, characteristic tumours (e.g. small bowel cancer, ureteric transitional cell carcinoma, or skin sebaceous adenoma/carcinoma) have a high positive predictive value for LS and are therefore clinically significant. Synchronous or metachronous bowel cancers are also clinically significant, as is the development of any two LS-related tumours (e.g. CRC and endometrial cancer).

Mismatch repair deficiency causes frequent insertion and deletion mutations. When these occur in the protein-coding regions of genes, they result in frameshifts, which in turn result in the expression of novel, antigenic frameshift peptides that stimulate the immune system {5852}. Local immunosuppression in such tumours enables their survival; therefore, immune checkpoint inhibitors such as PD1/PDL1 blockers, which inhibit such suppression, are effective in dMMR tumours {3983}.

As tumour sequencing becomes more widespread, data on specific mutations in cancer-associated genes, as well as mutation spectra, are becoming available in individual cases. This will both guide treatment and identify more causes of hereditary predisposition, including Lynch-like syndrome and multilocus inherited neoplasia alleles syndrome (multiple constitutional mutations in the same patient). It is also likely that mutation spectra (or signatures), being more sensitive and specific, will replace MSI testing. Although gene panel testing may remove the need for mismatch repair immunohistochemistry as a way of selecting which genes to test, mismatch repair immunohistochemistry will remain critically important in providing phenotypic data to enable the interpretation of genetic variants {7518,154}.

### Essential and desirable diagnostic criteria
A suggested algorithm for CRC tumour testing for LS is shown in Fig. 16.39.

### Staging
Not clinically relevant

### Prognosis and prediction
Not clinically relevant

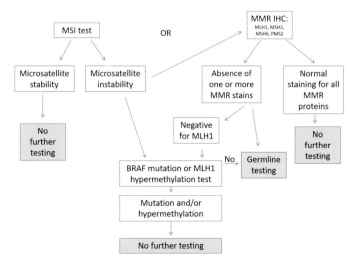

**Fig. 16.39** Lynch syndrome. A suggested algorithm for colorectal cancer tumour testing for Lynch syndrome. MMR, mismatch repair; MSI, microsatellite instability.

# Xeroderma pigmentosum

Tomlinson GE
Kraemer KH

## Definition

Xeroderma pigmentosum (XP) is an autosomal recessive disease characterized by sensitivity to sunlight, photophobia, and early-onset freckling followed by neoplastic changes in sun-exposed sites. There is cellular hypersensitivity to ultraviolet (UV) radiation due to deficient nucleotide excision repair (NER) of DNA damage. There are seven complementation groups of XP (XPA–XPG), each caused by mutations in one of seven NER genes. There is also a variant form of XP (XPV), in which NER is normal but there is a defect in a translesion DNA polymerase.

## MIM numbering

278700 Xeroderma pigmentosum, complementation group A; XPA
610651 Xeroderma pigmentosum, complementation group B; XPB
278720 Xeroderma pigmentosum, complementation group C; XPC
278730 Xeroderma pigmentosum, complementation group D; XPD
278740 Xeroderma pigmentosum, complementation group E; XPE
278760 Xeroderma pigmentosum, complementation group F; XPF
278780 Xeroderma pigmentosum, complementation group G; XPG
278750 Xeroderma pigmentosum, variant type; XPV

## ICD-11 coding

LD27.1 Xeroderma pigmentosum

## Related terminology

*Not recommended:* DeSanctis–Cacchione syndrome.

## Subtype(s)

Xeroderma pigmentosum complementation groups XPA–XPG; variant form XPV

## Localization

In addition to skin lesions, patients may present with tumours of the eye, CNS, lung, uterus {3879}, breast, pancreas, stomach, kidney, or testicle {3770}, or with leukaemia (see Box 16.05).

## Clinical features

Diagnosis is based on clinical features and confirmed by DNA sequencing and by tests of cellular hypersensitivity to (and DNA repair after) UV radiation–induced damage {3769}.

*Skin:* Approximately half of the patients with XP have a history of acute sunburn after minimal sun exposure {835}. The other half have a history of almost-normal tanning. However, in all patients, numerous freckle-like hyperpigmented macules appear on sun-exposed skin, usually before the age of 2 years. Eyelid papillomas may be present. Basal cell carcinoma and squamous cell carcinoma are common, as is melanoma in the UV radiation–exposed portions of the eye {889}.

*Eyes:* Ocular findings are limited to the anterior (UV radiation–exposed) structures {5761}. Photophobia may be associated with prominent conjunctival redness. UV irradiation of the eye may result in severe keratitis, leading to corneal opacification and vascularization. Patients may have loss of eyelashes, ectropion, entropion, or complete loss of the lids. Benign conjunctival inflammatory masses have been reported.

*Nervous system:* Neurological abnormalities have been reported in approximately 25% of cases {835}. Onset may occur early in infancy or may be delayed until the second decade of life. The neurological abnormalities may initially be mild (e.g. isolated hyporeflexia), but they often lead to progressive sensorineural deafness (beginning with high-frequency hearing loss)

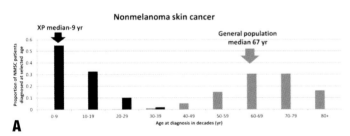

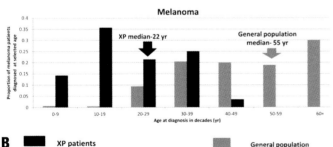

**Fig. 16.40** Skin cancer in the setting of xeroderma pigmentosum (XP). The graphs show the proportions of non-melanoma skin cancer cases (**A**) and melanoma cases (**B**) first diagnosed within each of the age groups indicated, among patients with XP (black bars) and in the general population of the USA (grey bars); individuals with both non-melanoma skin cancer and melanoma are included in both graphs. The median age at first diagnosis of non-melanoma skin cancer was 9 years among the patients with XP versus 67 years in the general population. The median age at first diagnosis of melanoma was 22 years among the patients with XP versus 55 years in the general population.

**Box 16.05** Cancers in patients with xeroderma pigmentosum

**Ultraviolet (UV) radiation (i.e. sunlight)-induced neoplasms**
Skin: basal cell carcinoma, squamous cell carcinoma, melanoma {835}
Eyes (lids, conjunctiva, cornea): squamous cell carcinoma, basal cell carcinoma, melanoma {889,5761}
Tongue (tip): squamous cell carcinoma {3770}

**Internal neoplasms**
CNS (brain, spinal cord): astrocytoma, glioblastoma 3770,3879}
Thyroid: papillary carcinoma {2654}
Lung: carcinoma (in smokers) {3770}
Uterus: adenocarcinoma {3879}
Blood and bone marrow: myelodysplastic syndrome, leukaemia, lymphoma {5122A,6177}

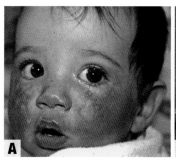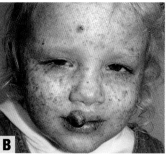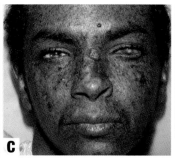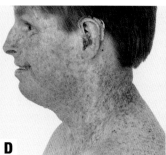

**Fig. 16.41** Xeroderma pigmentosum (XP). **A** A 9-month-old girl with XP complementation group D (XPD) with severe blistering erythema of the cheeks following minimal sun exposure. Note the sparing of her forehead and eyes, which were protected by a hat. **B** A 2-year-old girl with XP complementation group C (XPC) who did not sunburn easily but developed multiple hyperpigmented macules on her face. A rapidly growing keratoacanthoma or other squamous cell carcinoma grew on her upper lip and a precancerous lesion appeared on her forehead. **C** A 23-year-old northern African man with XPC with numerous hyperpigmented macules on his face. A nodular basal cell carcinoma is present on his left nasal root and a pigmented basal cell carcinoma on his left cheek. His eyes show corneal scarring from unprotected sun exposure. **D** A 35-year-old man with XP complementation group A (XPA) with neurological degeneration. He has numerous hyperpigmented macules on the sun-exposed areas of his face and neck. Progressive sensorineural deafness necessitates the use of a hearing aid.

{7037}, developmental delays, microcephaly, spasticity, and/ or seizures. In one study, the predominant neuropathological abnormality found at autopsy was loss of neurons, particularly in the cerebrum and cerebellum {3879}.

*Cancer:* Among XP patients aged < 20 years, the risk of skin cancer (basal cell carcinoma, squamous cell carcinoma, and melanoma) in sun-exposed sites, including the anterior eye and the tip of the tongue, is > 10 000 times as high as the risk in the general population {835,1063}. Multiple primary skin cancers are common. The reported median age of onset of non-melanoma skin cancer in patients with XP in the USA is 9 years – this is 50 years earlier than in the general population. Tumours of the brain (glioma and medulloblastoma) {835,3770}, spinal cord astrocytoma {1751}, and tumours of the lung, uterus {3879}, breast, pancreas, stomach, kidney, and testicle {3770}, as well as leukaemia {3770}, have also been reported in small numbers of patients. These reports suggest an overall risk of internal neoplasms that is about 10–20 times as high as that in the general population {835,3879}.

### Epidemiology

The incidence of XP is about 1 case per 1 million live births in Europe {3633} and the USA, 4.5 cases per 100 000 live births in Japan {2904}, and 20 cases per 100 000 live births in the archipelago of the Comoros {1063}. Patients (of all races) have been reported worldwide.

### Etiology

XP has been associated with mutations in seven NER genes: *XPA*, *ERCC3* (*XPB*), *XPC*, *ERCC2* (*XPD*), *DDB2* (*XPE*), *ERCC4* (*XPF*), and *ERCC5* (*XPG*) {1750,5678}. *XPC* and *DDB2* (*XPE*) code for proteins that recognize bulky DNA lesions produced by UV radiation and some other DNA-damaging agents. *ERCC3* (*XPB*) and *ERCC2* (*XPD*) code for helicases necessary to open the double helix at the site of the lesion. *ERCC4* (*XPF*) and *ERCC5* (*XPG*) code for endonucleases that cut the damaged strand at the 5′ and 3′ sites, respectively. There is marked clinical and molecular heterogeneity in XP. Patients with XPC, XPE, or XPV do not have neurological involvement, whereas patients with XPA, XPB, XPD, or XPG may have neurological abnormalities in addition to skin involvement. Patients with XPD may have one of at least five known clinical phenotypes: XP with skin disease, XP with neurological disease, XP–Cockayne syndrome complex, trichothiodystrophy (a disorder characterized by sulfur-deficient brittle hair), and XP–trichothiodystrophy complex {1750}.

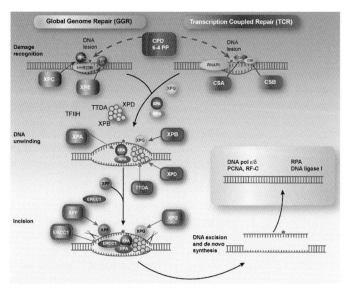

**Fig. 16.42** The nucleotide excision repair pathway. Transcription-coupled repair removes damage from actively transcribed genes, and global genome repair removes damage from the remainder of the genome. In global genome repair, DNA damage such as ultraviolet (UV) radiation–induced cyclobutane pyrimidine dimers (CPDs) and 6–4 photoproducts (6–4 PPs) is recognized by proteins including the *DDB2* (*XPE*) and *XPC* gene products. In transcription-coupled repair, the lesion appears to block the progress of RNA polymerase II (RNAPII) in a process involving the *ERCC8* (*CSA*) and *ERCC6* (*CSB*) gene products. Following initial damage recognition, the two pathways converge. The XPB (ERCC3) and XPD (ERCC2) helicases unwind the DNA region surrounding the lesion, along with the *XPA* and *ERCC5* (*XPG*) gene products and replication protein A (RPA). The XPF and XPG (ERCC5) endonucleases perform incisions to excise the lesion in a fragment of B30 nucleotides. The resulting gap is filled via de novo DNA synthesis. If any individual part of this highly coordinated system is mutated, the entire pathway fails to function normally. Mutations in the genes shown in rounded rectangles have been associated with clinical disease. DNA pol ε/δ, DNA polymerase ε/δ; PCNA, proliferating cell nuclear antigen; RF-C, replication factor C.

### Pathogenesis

Patients with XP have defective repair of UV radiation damage to DNA {1857,6859}. In sun-exposed portions of the body (skin, anterior eyes, tip of tongue) unrepaired DNA repaired damage manifests as severe actinic damage and increased skin pigmentation. Repeated UV radiation exposure leads to the accumulation of mutations and to premalignant and malignant changes. Internal neoplasms are presumably also the result of DNA damage, but the source is not known.

## Macroscopic appearance
The macroscopic appearance of tumours in XP is similar to that of their sporadic counterparts.

## Histopathology
The histopathology of tumours in XP is similar to that of their sporadic counterparts.

## Cytology
The cytology of tumours in XP is similar to that of their sporadic counterparts.

## Diagnostic molecular pathology
Sequencing of *XPA* is helpful for diagnosis {1750,6859}, and in some cases the diagnosis is first suspected by exome sequencing and then confirmed by clinical evaluation.

## Essential and desirable diagnostic criteria
*Essential:* clinical abnormalities of the skin and eyes (see above); a family history of XP.

*Desirable:* confirmation of clinical suspicion by specialized testing including cellular hypersensitivity to UV radiation and chromosomal breakage studies; DNA sequencing to identify the specific gene complementation group (this may require the identification of pathogenic variants of specific genes, i.e. *DDB2*, *ERCC1*, *ERCC2*, *ERCC3*, *ERCC4*, *ERCC5*, *POLH*, *XPA*, or *XPC*); hypersensitivity of cultured skin fibroblasts to killing by UV radiation.

## Staging
Staging of tumours in XP is similar to that of their sporadic counterparts.

## Prognosis and prediction
Management of XP is based on early diagnosis, lifelong protection from UV radiation exposure, and early detection and treatment of neoplasms {6858}. Gene therapy using corrected XP skin cells is being investigated {1857,1858,7451}.

# Rothmund–Thomson syndrome

Tomlinson GE
Hicks MJ
Wang LL (Lisa L.)

## Definition

Rothmund–Thomson syndrome (RTS) is an autosomal recessive genodermatosis and cancer predisposition disorder, with the diagnostic hallmark of poikiloderma. Germline pathogenic variants in *RECQL4* are present in about two thirds of patients and associated with RTS type 2, and mutations in *ANAPC1* are associated with RTS type 1.

## MIM numbering

618625 Rothmund–Thomson syndrome type 1; RTS1
268400 Rothmund–Thomson syndrome type 2; RTS2

## ICD-11 coding

LD2B Syndromes with premature ageing appearance as a major feature

## Related terminology

*Acceptable:* poikiloderma congenitale; poikiloderma atrophicans and cataract.

## Subtype(s)

Rothmund–Thomson syndrome type 1 (*ANAPC1* mutations in a subset, notably intronic splice mutations; absence of *RECQL4* mutations; absence of osteosarcoma); Rothmund–Thomson syndrome type 2 (*RECQL4* mutations, osteosarcoma predisposition)

## Localization

- *Skin and appendages:* rash and pigmentation changes (see below), hyperkeratosis, sparse hair, skin cancers
- *Bone:* skeletal abnormalities, osteosarcoma (associated with RTS type 2)
- *Eye:* juvenile cataracts (associated with RTS type 1)
- *Constitutional:* small stature

## Clinical features

The dermatological hallmark of RTS is an erythematous rash that starts on the cheeks in infancy and then spreads to the extremities, typically with truncal and abdominal sparing. The rash enters a chronic lifelong phase with reticulated hypopigmentation and hyperpigmentation, telangiectasia, and atrophy (collectively, poikiloderma) {3933,7413,7410,3932}. Additional findings include small stature; sparse scalp hair, eyebrows, and eyelashes; dental and nail abnormalities; skeletal defects including fused or missing bones, osteoporosis, radial ray defects, and brachymesophalangy {1021}; gastrointestinal disturbance (feeding problems, emesis, diarrhoea) in early childhood; cataracts; and an increased risk of malignancy, most commonly osteosarcoma in RTS type 2 {7409} and squamous or basal cell carcinoma of the skin {3204}. Melanoma, although rare in RTS, has been reported {3004}. In the absence of death from cancer, patients appear to have a normal lifespan, although further natural history studies are needed {7413}. Patients with RTS type 1 more commonly show juvenile cataracts as well as poikiloderma and sparse hair, eyebrows, or eyelashes, but they do not have an increased risk of osteosarcoma {111}.

## Epidemiology

RTS is a rare disorder, with approximately 300 cases reported worldwide, affecting all ethnic and racial groups {3933,7413, 7410,7409}.

## Etiology

Germline pathogenic variants in the *RECQL4* gene (8q24.3) are present in about two thirds of patients; these patients are designated as having RTS type 2 {7409}, which is associated with an increased risk of osteosarcoma and other bone abnormalities {4555}. Most of these mutations are nonsense or frameshift mutations and occur within the helicase domain, and less frequently within the N-terminus and C-terminus of the gene {3933}.

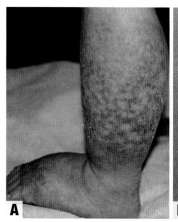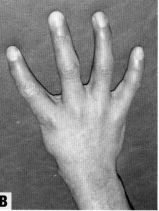

**Fig. 16.43** Rothmund–Thomson syndrome. **A** Poikiloderma. Extensor surface of the lower leg demonstrating the chronic phase, with skin atrophy, marbleized mixed hypopigmentation, and hyperpigmentation with telangiectasia. **B** Radial ray defect manifesting as a missing thumb.

**Fig. 16.44** Rothmund–Thomson syndrome, Baller–Gerold syndrome, and RAPADILINO syndrome. The overlapping clinical features of Rothmund–Thomson syndrome, Baller–Gerold syndrome, and RAPADILINO syndrome (radial ray malformations, patella and palate abnormalities, diarrhoea and dislocated joints, limb abnormalities and little size, slender nose, and normal intelligence; associated with *RECQL4* pathogenic variants).

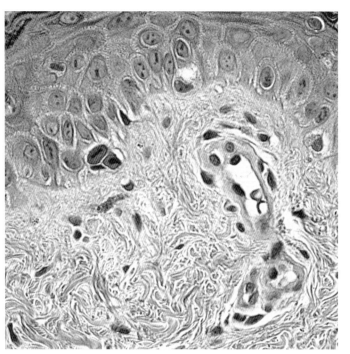

**Fig. 16.45** Rothmund–Thomson syndrome. Histopathological features of poikiloderma characteristically seen in Rothmund–Thomson syndrome, with prominent superficial dermal vessels, minimal basal cell vacuolization, and intraepidermal dyskeratotic cells.

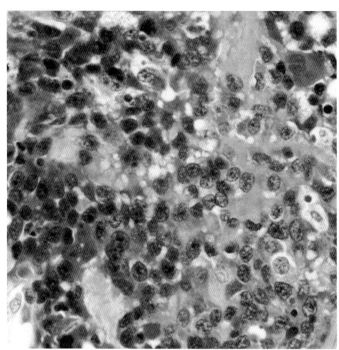

**Fig. 16.46** Rothmund–Thomson syndrome. Osteoblastic osteosarcoma, the most common malignancy seen in Rothmund–Thomson syndrome, displays pleomorphic osteoblasts and eosinophilic malignant osteoid.

Patients with RTS type 1 lack *RECQL4* pathogenic variants; this form is more commonly associated with bilateral juvenile cataracts. A subset of RTS type 1 cases are due to mutations in *ANAPC1*, encoding the protein APC1, a component of the anaphase-promoting complex/cyclosome (APC/C) {111, 7413}.

## Pathogenesis
RECQL4 is a member of the highly conserved RECQ DNA helicase family that shares sequence homology in the helicase domain. RECQ helicases are able to unwind duplex DNA to provide single-stranded templates for basic cellular processes such as replication, repair, recombination, and transcription {1498}. RECQL4 is a multifunctional protein that has been implicated in several processes, including DNA replication, DNA damage repair, and maintenance of telomeres and of mitochondrial DNA integrity {1315,4734}. Pathogenic variants in *RECQL4* have also been identified in patients with RAPADILINO syndrome (radial ray malformations, patella and palate abnormalities, diarrhoea and dislocated joints, limb abnormalities and little size, slender nose, and normal intelligence) {6483} and Baller–Gerold syndrome {7242}, both of which have clinical features overlapping those of RTS.

APC1 is a component of APC/C, which is an E3 ubiquitin ligase important for cell-cycle transition. Molecular studies have shown that the intron splice mutation of *ANAPC1* found in RTS type 1 results in a 95 bp pseudoexon causing premature protein termination of APC1 {111}. Both APC1 and RECQL4 are involved in DNA replication and repair.

## Macroscopic appearance
Patients with RTS type 2 are at increased risk of developing osteosarcoma (mean age: 11 years) {2885} and basal cell and squamous carcinomas (mean age: 34 years) at a younger age than the general population {6698,5564}. Reported sites of RTS osteosarcoma are the distal femur (50%), proximal tibia (25%), proximal humerus (25%), distal fibula (7%), distal ulna (7%), distal radius (7%), and patella (7%) {2885}.

## Histopathology
Routine skin biopsies from individuals with RTS demonstrate characteristic histological features of poikiloderma, which can include hyperkeratosis, epidermal atrophy, intraepidermal dyskeratotic cells, basal cell vacuolization, melanin incontinence, and prominent superficial dermal vessels {7411}.

## Cytology
Not clinically relevant

## Diagnostic molecular pathology
A definitive diagnosis of RTS type 2 can be made by molecular testing for biallelic pathogenic variants in the *RECQL4* gene. In approximately 40% of individuals with a clinical diagnosis of RTS, molecular genetic testing fails to identify a pathogenic variant in *RECQL4*; these individuals are designated as having RTS type 1. A proportion of probands with RTS type 1 will have pathogenic variants in *ANAPC1* (7 of 9 families tested in 1 study {111}). Therefore, an absence of pathogenic variants does not rule out a diagnosis of RTS, because there remain patients with RTS type 1 (~30% of all patients with RTS) who have neither *RECQL4* nor *ANAPC1* mutations. The existence of one or more additional causative genes for RTS type 1 is likely {7409,111,7413}. Additional information on genetic testing was reviewed by Wang and Plon {7413} and is included in the US National Institutes of Health (NIH) Genetic Testing Registry (GTR) {7413}.

## Essential and desirable diagnostic criteria

*Clinical diagnostic criteria:* Poikiloderma is a hallmark of RTS, and all patients with RTS have some form of this skin finding. If the rash follows the classic pattern, consisting of an acute phase that starts in infancy and progresses to a chronic phase {7411}, then a diagnosis of RTS is highly likely. If the rash is atypical, either in pattern of spread or appearance, then two additional features of RTS are needed to make a diagnosis of probable RTS, including sparse scalp hair, eyelashes, or eyebrows; short stature; gastrointestinal disturbance; radial ray defects; radiological bone abnormalities (radial ray and ulnar defects, absent or hypoplastic patella, osteopenia, abnormal trabeculation; dental abnormalities; nail abnormalities; hyperkeratosis; cataracts; and cancer, including basal cell carcinoma, squamous cell carcinoma, or osteosarcoma {7410,7413}. Additional details on diagnostic criteria may be found in the RTS entry on the GeneReviews website {7413}.

A definitive diagnosis of RTS is established in a proband with the classic rash of RTS (with onset, spread, and appearance as previously described {7413}) and/or biallelic pathogenic variants in *ANAPC1* (RTS type 1) or *RECQL4* (RTS type 2) identified by molecular genetic testing.

See also Box 16.06.

## Staging

Not clinically relevant

## Prognosis and prediction

Patients with RTS type 2 (i.e. with *RECQL4* pathogenic variants) are at increased risk of developing osteosarcoma {7409} and of having bone defects {4555}, and therefore must be counselled and followed up closely. Some patients who develop osteosarcoma may have increased chemotherapy toxicity, and this should be anticipated and monitored closely during treatment. To date, osteosarcoma is not thought to be associated with RTS

type 1. Patients should have regular eye and skin examinations to check for cataracts and skin cancer, respectively.

---

**Box 16.06** Diagnosis of Rothmund–Thomson syndrome (RTS)

**Suggestive findings**

RTS should be suspected in individuals with the classic rash of RTS.
Acute phase:
- Starts in infancy, usually between the ages of 3 and 6 months
- Erythema on the cheeks and face
- Spreads to involve the extensor surfaces of the extremities
- Typically sparing of the trunk and abdomen; may involve the buttocks
Chronic phase:
- Gradually develops over a period of months to years
- Reticulated hyperpigmentation and hypopigmentation, telangiectasias, and areas of punctate atrophy (i.e. poikiloderma)
- Persists throughout life

If the rash is atypical (in appearance, distribution, and/or pattern of onset and spread), a diagnosis of *probable* RTS can be made if two of the following additional features of RTS are present:
- Sparse scalp hair, eyelashes, and/or eyebrows
- Small size, usually symmetrical for height and weight
- Gastrointestinal disturbance as young children, usually consisting of chronic vomiting and diarrhoea, sometimes requiring feeding tubes
- Dental abnormalities that include rudimentary or hypoplastic teeth, enamel defects, delayed tooth eruption
- Nail abnormalities such as dysplastic or poorly formed nails
- Hyperkeratosis, particularly of the soles of the feet
- Cataracts, usually juvenile, bilateral
- Skeletal abnormalities including radial ray defects, ulnar defects, absent or hypoplastic patella, osteopenia, abnormal trabeculation
- Cancers including skin cancers (basal cell carcinoma and squamous cell carcinoma) and in particular osteosarcoma

**Establishing the diagnosis**

The diagnosis of RTS is established in a proband with the classic rash of RTS (with onset, spread, and appearance as described above) and/or biallelic pathogenic variants in *ANAPC1* (RTS type 1) or *RECQL4* (RTS type 2) identified on molecular genetic testing.

# Li–Fraumeni syndrome

Lax SF  
Hawkins CE  
Kratz CP  
Malkin D  

Orr BA  
Perry A  
Solomon DA

## Definition
*TP53*-associated Li–Fraumeni syndrome (LFS) is an autosomal dominant cancer predisposition syndrome caused by germline mutations of the *TP53* gene.

## MIM numbering
151623 Li–Fraumeni syndrome; LFS

## ICD-11 coding
None

## Related terminology
*Not recommended:* sarcoma family syndrome of Li and Fraumeni.

## Subtype(s)
None

## Localization
*TP53*-associated LFS is associated with cancers of the breast, soft tissue, bone, brain, and adrenal glands.

## Clinical features
LFS is characterized by the early onset of a broad spectrum of cancers and a high lifetime cancer risk.

Tumour patterns and penetrance demonstrate distinct phases by age {217}. The mean age at which tumours develop is about 25 years, and in about 40% of cases, tumours occur before the age of 18 years, with brain tumours, adrenocortical carcinomas, soft tissue sarcomas, and osteosarcomas being the most common {806}. Adrenocortical carcinoma associated with a

*TP53* germline mutation develops almost exclusively in children {2059}. In addition, leukaemias, lymphomas, germ cell tumours, nephroblastoma, and neuroblastoma preferably occur in childhood and adolescence {806}. Malignant breast tumours, which are generally the most common LFS-associated neoplasm, rarely occur before the age of 18 years and are more frequently sarcomas or phyllodes tumours than carcinomas. Other malignant tumours of adults with LFS involving the gastrointestinal, urogenital, and female genital tracts also rare in children {4443}.

The clinical definition of LFS has been expanded to allow a broader recognition of individuals and families with LFS {6267}. If any of the tumours mentioned above occur in childhood, LFS should be excluded among other hereditary cancer syndromes.

Patients and families without the full spectrum of classic criteria have been designated as having Li–Fraumeni–like syndrome (LFL), which has been further defined clinically by two sets of criteria, proposed by Birch and by Eeles {6267}. The Birch criteria are close to those of classic LFS but do not require a sarcoma, whereas the Eeles definition of LFL includes two first- or second-degree relatives with LFS component tumours at any age, rather than the three required by the classic criteria {6267}. The investigation of other family genes and non-coding regions of the *TP53* gene may explain the occurrence of LFL {5439}.

## Epidemiology
*TP53* germline variants have been estimated to occur at a rate of about 1 in 500 to 1 in 5000 births and account for as many as 17% of all familial cancer cases {2483,5130,803,3889,1605, 1604}. There is a variant-dependent gradient of phenotype severity, with the most functionally severe mutations associated with early tumour onset {1603}. Tumour patterns are generally

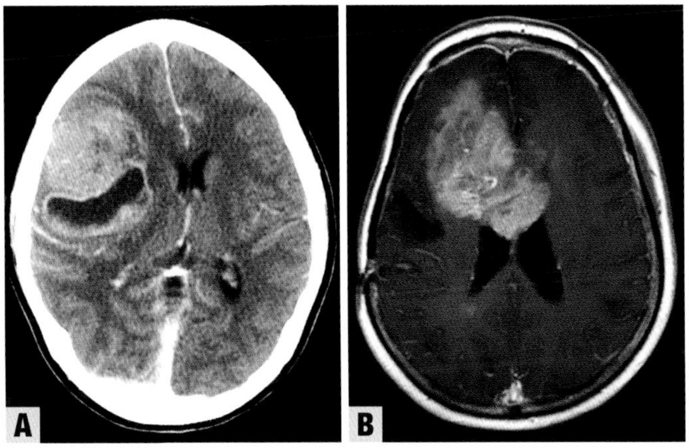

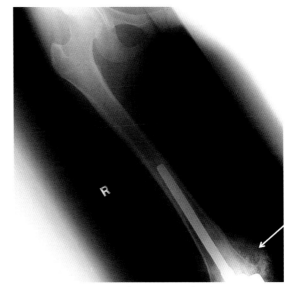

**Fig. 16.47** Li–Fraumeni syndrome. **A** Contrast-enhanced axial CT shows a mixed solid-cystic tumour over the right frontal region. There is marked contrast enhancement of the solid component, associated with mass effect and midline shift. This was confirmed to be a high-grade glioma. **B** Contrast-enhanced T1-weighted axial MRI of the same patient, 2 years after resection of the first high-grade glioma in the right frontal region, showing local recurrence with an avidly enhancing mass.

**Fig. 16.48** Li–Fraumeni syndrome. Osteosarcoma of the femur.

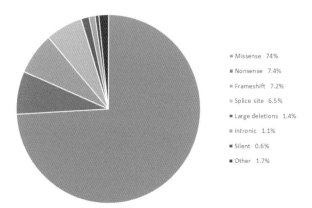

**Fig. 16.49** Li–Fraumeni syndrome. *TP53* mutations. The vast majority of mutations are missense sequence alterations.

stable regardless of geographical or population demographics, with the only notable exceptions being an excess of gastric cancers in south-eastern Asia, soft tissue sarcomas in the western Pacific region {1603}, and an excess of a low-penetrance mutation at codon 334 of *TP53* in patients of Ashkenazi Jewish descent {5610}. In southern Brazil, a specific germline mutation at codon 337 (p.R337H) occurs with an incidence of 154 cases per 100 000 person-years and is found in 0.3% of the general population {40,2395}. There is recent evidence of the occurrence of de novo *TP53* mutations in about 10–20% of individuals with LFS; about 20% of these mutations seem to occur during embryogenesis {5842}.

### Etiology

The genetic basis of LFS is a heterozygous germline alteration (mutation, rearrangement, or partial/complete deletion) of the *TP53* gene on chromosome 17p13 {4349,6638}.

In the International Agency for Research on Cancer (IARC) *TP53* Database, more than 1500 different germline mutations are listed, with only 4 patterns accounting for about 80% of the mutations: G:C>A:T at CpG islands in almost 50%, followed by A:T>G:C, G:C>A:T, and deletions (in ~10% each) that predominantly involve 11 codons within the coding regions of exons 5–8, most commonly codons 175, 245, 248, 273, and 282 {3100,803}.

### Pathogenesis

*TP53* encodes the transcription factor p53, one of the most prominent tumour suppressors. Its activation stimulates downstream pathways leading to protective cellular processes, including cell-cycle arrest, apoptosis, and senescence, to prevent the propagation of genetically altered cells {7321}. Evidence indicates that p53 also regulates other important processes, such as cell oxidative metabolism, the cellular response to nutrient deprivation, fertility, ferroptosis, and stem cell maintenance. The extent and consequences of the biological response elicited by p53 vary according to stress and cell type {3467}. The functions of p53 rely mainly on its transcriptional activity, but it can also act via interactions with various proteins {4390,3761}. Cells from individuals with LFS exhibit genomic instability, telomere dysfunction, and spontaneous immortalization {5313}.

A broad spectrum of *TP53* germline mutations involving the coding regions of the gene has been found in families with LFS,

but 20–40% of individuals with LFS and the majority of families with LFL may lack detectable mutations {5165,7248}. Most germline *TP53* mutations are spread over exons 5–8, with major hotspots at codons 133, 175, 245, 248, 273 (all within the DNA-binding domain) and 337 (within the tetramerization domain). Missense mutations are most common – accounting for > 85% of all germline *TP53* pathogenic variants – but nonsense mutations, deletions/insertions, and splice-site mutations also occur. Structural variants (SVs) with breakpoints located in intron 1 have also been identified in families fulfilling the clinical criteria for LFS but lacking *TP53* point mutations {5870}. Mutations observed at hotspot codons consist of missense mutations that result in mutant proteins with complete loss of function, dominant negative phenotypes, and oncogenic (gain-of-function) activities.

The lack of 100% concordance between *TP53* mutations and the classic LFS phenotype may be explained in several ways, including posttranslational alterations, complete deletion, the effects of modifier genes, and alterations of other genes influencing the phenotype generated by the presence of specific germline alterations {4348}. Mutations may occur at specific hotspot codons that either interfere with DNA binding or disrupt the structure of the binding surface, thus interfering with its ability to modulate the transcription of target genes {5166}. Missense mutations lead to a codon change, posing challenges to the functional interpretation of new variants {4046}. Further mutations may occur outside of the DNA-binding domain and include rearrangements and deletions {7168}. Lesions within introns or the regulatory regions of the gene have been identified, although their functional significance is unclear and there are open questions about the significance of some *TP53* variants occurring in cancer {4045}.

### Macroscopic appearance

Not clinically relevant

### Histopathology

Brain tumours in children with LFS are mainly sonic hedgehog medulloblastomas, IDH-wildtype high-grade gliomas, and choroid plexus carcinomas. The most frequent types of soft tissue sarcomas are leiomyosarcomas, rhabdomyosarcomas, liposarcomas, and undifferentiated sarcomas that can be challenging to classify. Osteosarcoma is the most frequent bone tumour {3100,803}.

### Cytology

Not clinically relevant

### Diagnostic molecular pathology

Candidates for *TP53* germline testing are identified on the basis of the 2015 Chompret criteria (see Box 16.07) {806} and the recommendations of the National Comprehensive Cancer Network (NCCN; see Box 16.08) {7320}. In the era of testing by next-generation sequencing, it may be necessary to further broaden the criteria to find a greater number of *TP53* germline mutations {5232}.

### Essential and desirable diagnostic criteria

*Essential:* a pathogenic germline alteration (mutation, rearrangement, or partial/complete deletion) in *TP53*.

### Staging

Not clinically relevant

**Box 16.07** Patients with cancer who should be tested for germline disease-causing *TP53* variants[a] {2222}

### Recommendation 1
All patients who meet the modified Chompret criteria should be tested for germline *TP53* variants:
- *familial presentation:* proband with a *TP53* core tumour (breast cancer, soft tissue sarcoma, osteosarcoma, CNS tumour, adrenocortical carcinoma) before the age of 46 years AND at least one first-degree or second-degree relative with a core tumour before the age of 56 years; *or*
- *multiple primitive tumours:* proband with multiple tumours, including two *TP53* core tumours, the first of which occurred before the age of 46 years, irrespective of family history; *or*
- *rare tumours:* patient with adrenocortical carcinoma, choroid plexus carcinoma, or rhabdomyosarcoma of embryonal anaplastic subtype, irrespective of family history; *or*
- *very early onset breast cancer:* breast cancer before the age of 31 years, irrespective of family history

### Recommendation 2
Children and adolescents should be tested for germline *TP53* variants if presenting with:
- hypodiploid acute lymphoblastic leukaemia; *or*
- otherwise unexplained sonic hedgehog–driven medulloblastoma; *or*
- jaw osteosarcoma

### Recommendation 3
Patients who develop a second primary tumour within the radiotherapy field of a first core *TP53* tumour that occurred before the age of 46 years should be tested for germline *TP53* variants.

### Recommendation 4
- Patients older than 46 years presenting with breast cancer without personal or familial history fulfilling the Chompret criteria should not be tested for germline *TP53* variants.
- Any patient presenting with isolated breast cancer and not fulfilling the Chompret criteria, in whom a disease-causing *TP53* variant has been identified, should be referred to an expert multidisciplinary team for discussion.

### Recommendation 5
Children with any cancer from southern and south-eastern Brazilian families should be tested for the p.R337H Brazilian founder germline *TP53* variant.

[a]Testing for disease-causing *TP53* variants should be performed before starting treatment in order to avoid in variant carriers, if possible, radiotherapy and genotoxic chemotherapy and to prioritize surgical treatments.

---

**Box 16.08** Testing criteria for Li–Fraumeni syndrome as recommended by the National Comprehensive Cancer Network (NCCN) {7320}

Person diagnosed with sarcoma at < 45 years of age AND a first-degree relative diagnosed with cancer at < 45 years of age AND an additional first- or second-degree relative with cancer diagnosed at < 45 years of age or sarcoma diagnosed at any age[a]

Person with a tumour associated with Li–Fraumeni syndrome diagnosed before the age of 46 years AND at least one first- or second-degree relative with a tumour associated with Li–Fraumeni syndrome[b] (other than breast cancer if the proband has breast cancer) before the age of 56 years or with multiple primaries at any age[c]

Person with multiple primaries (except multiple breast primaries), with at least two primaries associated with Li–Fraumeni syndrome[b], before the age of 46 years[c]

Person with adrenocortical carcinoma, choroid plexus carcinoma, or rhabdomyosarcoma of embryonal anaplastic subtype diagnosed at any age, regardless of family history[c]

Person with breast cancer before the age of 31 years[c]

Person from a family with known *TP53* mutation

[a]Classic Li–Fraumeni syndrome criteria. [b]Cancers associated with Li–Fraumeni syndrome: soft tissue sarcoma, osteosarcoma, CNS tumour, breast cancer, and adrenocortical carcinoma. [c]Chompret criteria.

## Prognosis and prediction
The specific cancer risks at ≤ 15 years are 19% in boys and 12% in girls, respectively {7629}. Clinical surveillance has been associated with early tumour detection and improved survival in patients with LFS {7303,3778}.

Medulloblastomas and choroid plexus carcinomas arising in the setting of LFS are associated with a poor prognosis {7456, 6827,2515,4604}. IDH-wildtype high-grade gliomas that arise during childhood in the setting of LFS are associated with a poor prognosis, whereas the IDH-mutant diffuse astrocytic gliomas arising in teenagers and young adults with LFS are associated with a more favourable course {6526}.

Mutated *TP53* as seen in LFS confers an elevated risk of radiation-induced secondary malignancies and possibly increased sensitivity to low-dose radiation exposure by diagnostic methods such as mammography {6595}.

# *DICER1* syndrome

Hill DA
Alexandrescu S
Brenton JD
Kölsche C

Korshunov A
Perry A
Solomon DA

## Definition

*DICER1* syndrome is an autosomal dominant tumour predisposition syndrome caused by heterozygous germline pathogenic sequence variants in *DICER1*, which encodes a microRNA processing enzyme. It is characterized by an increased incidence of benign and malignant neoplasms involving multiple organ systems, including pleuropulmonary blastoma, thyroid cancers, paediatric cystic nephroma, embryonal rhabdomyosarcoma of the uterine cervix, ovarian Sertoli–Leydig cell tumour, pineoblastoma, embryonal tumour with multilayered rosettes, pituitary blastoma, and *DICER1*-mutant primary intracranial sarcoma.

## MIM numbering

606241 DICER 1, Ribonuclease III; DICER1

## ICD-11 coding

None

## Related terminology

*Not recommended*: pleuropulmonary blastoma-family tumour and dysplasia syndrome.

## Subtype(s)

None

## Localization

The most common organs of involvement are the lungs, kidneys, thyroid, sinonasal tract, ovaries, uterine cervix, liver, gastrointestinal tract, eyes, and brain.

## Clinical features

The clinical features are listed in Table 16.06. Some tumours are either so rare or so characteristic that any affected individual is likely to carry a germline *DICER1* mutation {2202}, including pleuropulmonary blastoma, cystic nephroma {449, 774}, nasal chondromesenchymal hamartoma {6690}, ciliary body medulloepithelioma {449,1631,5647}, pituitary blastoma, embryonal rhabdomyosarcoma of the cervix {1626,2199}, and anaplastic sarcoma of the kidney {1799}. Affected individuals

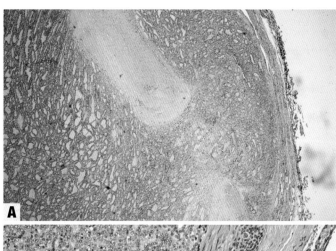

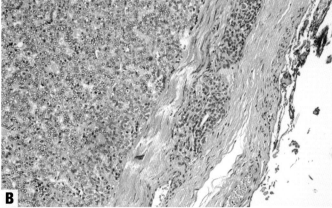

**Fig. 16.51** Differentiated thyroid carcinoma (DTC) arising in *DICER1* syndrome. **A** The diagnosis of thyroid carcinoma in *DICER1* syndrome should be restricted to lesions showing invasive growth. Here, a follicular carcinoma shows mushrooming growth into the adjacent thyroid. **B** DTCs arising in *DICER1* syndrome usually demonstrate a follicular or solid architecture. The nuclei may show subtle nuclear atypia.

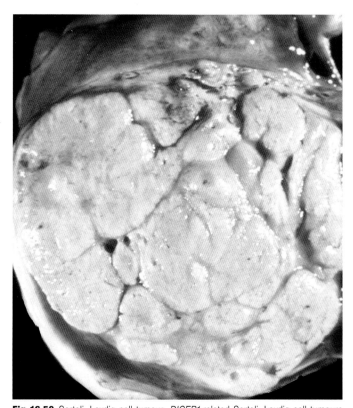

**Fig. 16.50** Sertoli–Leydig cell tumour. *DICER1*-related Sertoli–Leydig cell tumours are usually poorly differentiated, solid and cystic, and pale tan.

**Table 16.06** Key clinical phenotypes associated with germline *DICER1* pathogenic variants

| Phenotype and relative frequency | Approximate ages of susceptibility, range (peak) | Malignant (M) or benign (B) | Deaths in *DICER1*-mutated cases? |
|---|---|---|---|
| **Most frequent phenotypes** | | | |
| Pleuropulmonary blastoma (PPB) | | | |
| Type I (cystic) PPB | 0–24 months (8 months) | M | Yes, if it progresses to type II or III |
| Type II (cystic/solid) PPB | 12–60 months (31 months) | M | Yes, ~40% |
| Type III (solid) PPB | 18–72 months (44 months) | M | Yes, ~60% |
| Type Ir (cystic) PPB | Any age | B or M | None observed |
| Multinodular goitre[a] | 5–40 years (10–20 years) | B | No |
| Cystic nephroma | 0–48 months (undetermined) | B | No (see anaplastic sarcoma of the kidney, below) |
| Sertoli–Leydig cell tumour of ovary | 2–45 years (10–25 years) | M | Yes, < 5% |
| **Moderate-frequency phenotype** | | | |
| Cervical embryonal rhabdomyosarcoma | 4–45 years (10–20 years) | M | None observed |
| **Rare phenotypes** | | | |
| Differentiated thyroid carcinoma[b] | 5–40 years (10–20 years) | M | None observed |
| Wilms tumour[b] | 3–13 years (undetermined) | M | None observed |
| Juvenile hamartomatous intestinal polyps[b] | 0–4 years (undetermined) | B | No |
| Ciliary body medulloepithelioma | 3–10 years (undetermined) | B or M | None observed |
| Nasal chondromesenchymal hamartoma | 6–18 years (undetermined) | B | No |
| Pituitary blastoma | 0–24 months (undetermined) | Undetermined | Yes, ~50% |
| Pineoblastoma | 2–25 years (undetermined) | M | Yes |
| **Very rare phenotypes** | | | |
| Anaplastic sarcoma of the kidney | Estimated: 2–20 years | M | Yes |
| Embryonal tumour with multilayered rosettes[b] | Undetermined | M | Unknown |
| Primary intracranial sarcoma, *DICER1*-mutant | Median: 6 years | M | Unknown |
| Embryonal rhabdomyosarcoma – bladder | Estimated: < 5 years | M | None observed |
| Embryonal rhabdomyosarcoma – ovary | Undetermined | M | None observed |
| Neuroblastoma[b] | Estimated: < 5 years | M | Yes |
| Congenital phthisis bulbi[b] | Birth | B | No |
| Juvenile granulosa cell tumour[b] | Undetermined | M | None observed |
| Gynandroblastoma | Undetermined | M | None observed |

[a]Multinodular goitre occurring before the age of 18 years may warrant *DICER1* testing, even if occurring in the absence of other syndromic features in the patient or family. [b]These conditions may not be sufficiently associated with *DICER1* mutations to warrant testing in the absence of other personal or family history suggestive of *DICER1* syndrome.

are predominantly children and young adults. Approximately 5% of carriers (female: 4%, male: 7%) develop their first neoplasm by the time they are 10 years old. The average prevalence of neoplasms by the age of 50 years is 19%, with a substantially higher risk in women than in men (27% vs 10%). In contrast to endocrine organ neoplasms, gynaecological neoplasms predominate in older patients {6689}.

## Epidemiology

*DICER1* syndrome is transmitted as an autosomal dominant disorder with reduced/incomplete penetrance. A recent genotype-first study showed that germline *DICER1* pathogenic loss-of-function mutations were observed in 1 in 3700 to 1 in 4600 individuals; this cohort was 98% White and may not be reflective of incidence in all races/ethnicities {4709}.

Penetrance has been difficult to measure precisely, for a variety of reasons. Some benign neoplasms may not produce symptoms (small lung and kidney cysts, small thyroid nodules) and may be detectable only with systematic detailed imaging of carriers. The large genotype-first study did not include many children and probably under-ascertained conditions that may remain asymptomatic. Endocrine organ neoplasms predominate in adolescents and young adults {6689}.

The most common phenotype in an individual carrying a germline pathogenic loss-of-function variant in *DICER1* is thyroid nodules. More than 50% of female *DICER1* variant carriers develop multinodular goitre in their lifetime {3541}.

There is a unique expression of the syndrome in individuals who are mosaic for RNase IIIb hotspot mutations (see below). These individuals present earlier, with multiple neoplasms in

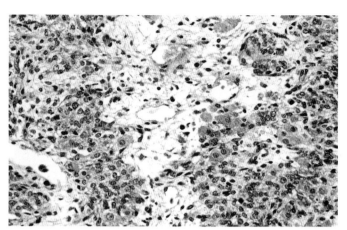

**Fig. 16.52** Sertoli–Leydig cell tumour. An example with intermediate differentiation. These tumours often grow in cellular lobules, as seen in this picture. The lobules are usually predominantly composed of dark-staining Sertoli cells, with fewer Leydig cells. The latter are often conspicuous at the periphery of the lobules, as seen to some degree in this picture at the 3 o'clock position.

multiple organ systems and additional rare manifestations {1631,3638}.

## Etiology

*DICER1* syndrome is caused by heterozygous germline loss-of-function variants in the gene *DICER1* on chromosome 14q32.13 {2892}. Although variants are most often transmitted in a familial manner, approximately 13% of affected individuals with pleuropulmonary blastoma harbour de novo mutations {860}. Additionally, a subset of affected individuals acquire *DICER1* variants during postzygotic development and are mosaic {1631}. Individuals with somatic mosaicism for a *DICER1* RNase IIIb hotspot mutation show a higher tumour incidence and a younger age at presentation than those with germline loss-of-function truncating variants {860}, which may also arise de novo or cause somatic mosaicism.

## Pathogenesis

DICER1 is an RNase IIIb endoribonuclease and is essential for processing microRNAs in the RNA interference pathway. MicroRNAs are small RNAs that regulate gene expression at the post-transcriptional level. They are very important in regulating gene expression programmes for cellular functions including proliferation and differentiation. As a result, microRNAs are necessary for normal development. The unique constellation of tumours, age at presentation, and organ types in *DICER1* syndrome reflects the unique roles of microRNAs during development and in organ functioning. Some tumours, such as pleuropulmonary blastoma, cystic nephroma, and ocular medulloepithelioma, arise during organ development and growth, and manifest at a young age. Other tumours in endocrine-responsive organs, such as thyroid nodules, Sertoli–Leydig cell tumour, and embryonal rhabdomyosarcoma of the uterine cervix, have a broader age range and occur most often when the organ is responding to endocrine signals.

Most *DICER1* syndrome tumours have biallelic pathogenic variation. In addition to the germline *DICER1* loss-of-function pathogenic variant, *DICER1* syndrome–related tumours typically harbour an additional somatically acquired missense mutation in exon 24 or 25, encoding the RNase IIIb

cleavage domain. These missense mutations are limited to one of the following codons, also called hotspots: p.E1705, p.D1709, p.G1809, p.D1810, or p.E1813 (RefSeq transcript ID: NM_177438). The combination of loss-of-function plus RNase IIIb hotspot mutations abrogates the cleavage of the 5p mature microRNA from the precursor hairpin while the 3p mature microRNA is cleaved normally. The expressivity of biallelic mutations is dependent on the gene expression programme active in the cell at the time, i.e. during early development; cells lacking 5p mature microRNAs cannot turn off oncofetal gene expression, resulting in continued cell proliferation.

Biallelic *DICER1* mutations may not be sufficient to drive malignant progression, because similar patterns of mutations are seen in both benign and malignant tumours. Additional oncogenic alterations, such as *TP53*, *NRAS*, or *BRAF* variants {5661,4151,4070}, may be required for malignant transformation in specific tumour types.

## Macroscopic appearance

The macroscopic appearance of *DICER1* syndrome–associated tumours is similar to that of their sporadic counterparts.

## Histopathology

These tumours are not histologically distinct from their non-syndromic counterparts. Sertoli–Leydig cell tumours in patients with *DICER1* germline mutations are often moderately to poorly differentiated {1630,2849}. Difficult-to-classify or mixed sex cord stromal tumours may be a clue to *DICER1* syndrome. Other rare tumours include gynandroblastoma and cervical embryonal rhabdomyosarcoma.

## Cytology

The cytology of *DICER1* syndrome–associated tumours is similar to that of their sporadic counterparts.

## Diagnostic molecular pathology

The presence of heterozygous germline loss-of-function pathogenic variants in *DICER1* is diagnostic. Most pathogenic variants are nonsense mutations, small insertions/deletions (indels), or splice-site substitutions resulting in the truncation

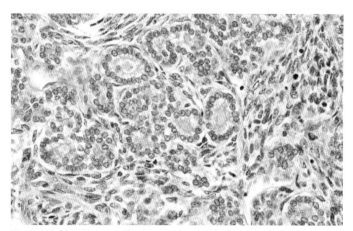

**Fig. 16.53** Thyroblastoma. This is an underrecognized *DICER1*-associated tumour with primitive thyroid follicles surrounded by primitive spindle cell stroma, mimicking thyroid in development.

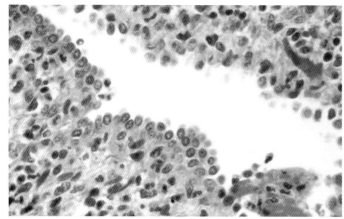

**Fig. 16.54** *DICER1*-related pleuropulmonary blastoma. Type I cysts are lined by epithelial cells beneath which lie primitive mesenchymal tumour cells.

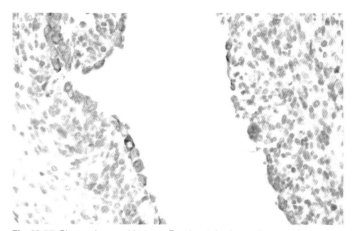

**Fig. 16.55** Pleuropulmonary blastoma. Type I cysts in pleuropulmonary blastoma are lined by keratin-positive epithelial cells.

of the protein. Larger deletions and pathogenic missense variants make up a small percentage of causative sequence variants {860}.

## Essential and desirable diagnostic criteria
*Essential:* demonstration of a pathogenic germline variant in *DICER1*.
*Desirable:* personal or family history of pathologically confirmed syndrome-related lesions, particularly those with high specificity for *DICER1* syndrome.

## Staging
Staging is the same as for other neoplasms at the corresponding sites.

## Prognosis and prediction
There are no data to suggest that the presence of a germline *DICER1* pathogenic variant influences the prognosis associated with *DICER1*-related tumours as compared with that of their sporadic counterparts. No difference in clinical outcome has been observed for *DICER1* syndrome–associated versus sporadic pineoblastoma, embryonal tumour with multilayered rosettes, or *DICER1*-mutant primary intracranial sarcoma. The outcome after a diagnosis of ovarian sex cord stromal tumour, cystic nephroma, embryonal rhabdomyosarcoma of the cervix, multinodular goitre, differentiated thyroid carcinoma, nasal chondromesenchymal hamartoma, or ciliary body medulloepithelioma is favourable, whereas solid-cystic and solid pleuropulmonary blastoma, pituitary blastoma, and anaplastic sarcoma of the kidney may have survival rates as low as 50% {1629,4615, 7346}. The CNS is the most frequent site of distant pleuropulmonary blastoma metastasis, occurring in 11% of patients with advanced pleuropulmonary blastoma. The International Pleuroblastoma/*DICER1* Registry recommends brain MRI surveillance every 3 months until 36 months after a diagnosis of type II or type III pleuropulmonary blastoma {7208,6287}.

# BAP1 tumour predisposition syndrome

Santagata S

## Definition
BAP1 tumour predisposition syndrome is a hereditary cancer syndrome caused by autosomal dominant inheritance of heterozygous germline pathogenic variants in the gene BAP1 (BRCA1 associated protein 1). The syndrome is characterized by a predisposition to various tumours including uveal melanoma, mesothelioma, cutaneous melanoma, and renal cell carcinoma, with less frequently associated tumours including meningioma, basal cell carcinoma, and cholangiocarcinoma.

## MIM numbering
614327 Tumour predisposition syndrome; TPDS

## ICD-11 coding
None

## Related terminology
None

## Subtype(s)
None

## Localization
Multiple sites and organs systems are involved, including the eyes {2712,16,3198}, pleura, peritoneum {6957}, skin {7539, 7353}, kidney {5599}, liver {5537}, and meninges {16,1258, 7353,6374,7374}.

## Clinical features
BAP1 germline pathogenic variant carriers have an increased risk of cancers, including mesothelioma (with an increased frequency in the peritoneum vs the pleura compared with that seen in sporadic mesothelioma {544,5137,5380}), uveal melanoma, cutaneous melanoma, renal cell carcinoma, cholangiocarcinoma, and basal cell carcinoma {6957,5599,16,7353}. Additionally, many BAP1 germline pathogenic variant carriers develop BAP1-inactivated melanocytic tumours (naevi or melanocytomas) {7539}. Although penetrance information remains limited because of the small number of cases identified and ascertainment bias, in one study of 324 carriers of BAP1 loss-of-function germline variants, 84.9% had developed at least 1 cancer, with the most common malignancies being uveal melanoma, mesothelioma, and cutaneous melanoma, and with 38 of 40 tested tumours showing loss of expression of BAP1 by immunohistochemistry {7374}. In another study, 40 (~75%) of 53 patients who underwent total-body skin examinations were found to have BAP1-inactivated melanocytic tumours {2778,7646}, although these tumours are not specific for the syndrome {966}.

Compared with their sporadic counterparts, mesotheliomas have substantially different clinical features when arising in BAP1 tumour predisposition syndrome: they arise 20 years earlier, lack a male predominance, and are frequently peritoneal rather than pleural {544,5137,5380}. An association between meningioma formation and BAP1 germline pathogenic variants was first reported in 3 affected families {16,1258,7353} and subsequently linked to meningiomas with rhabdoid and papillary morphology {6374,6375,7549}.

## Epidemiology
More than 180 families have been described with 140 unique pathogenic germline BAP1 variants, 104 of which are null variants and 9 of which are missense variants in the UCH domain {7374}. The carrier frequency of germline pathogenic variants is ~1 in 50 000 in people without cancer, and ~1 in 1900 among cancer patients, suggesting that the syndrome is underestimated {4455}. p.L573Wfs*2 is the most prevalent founder variant {7374}. The lifetime risk of developing cancer is reported to be as high as 80–100%, with many carriers developing multiple cancers; most families have at least two types of tumours in first- or second-degree relatives of the proband {5730,7374}. Null variants predispose individuals to earlier tumour formation than missense variants {7374}.

Although BAP1 is the most frequently mutated gene in sporadic mesothelioma {926} and in metastatic uveal melanoma {2712,16,3198}, 1–4% of these BAP1-mutant tumours arise in germline carriers {6957,6053,6375,5846}. This contrasts with meningioma, where half of the BAP1-mutant meningiomas in a small series arose in germline carriers {6374,6375}. BAP1-mutant meningiomas account for < 1% of all meningiomas.

Multiple studies have demonstrated that the median age at diagnosis of germline BAP1-associated mesothelioma is significantly younger (reported as 55–58 years) than that of sporadic mesothelioma (reported as 68–72 years) {544,5137,7374}. In children, 12 years is the youngest reported age for meningioma development {5789} and 15 years is the youngest age for uveal melanoma {7761}.

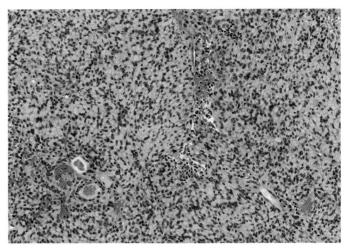

**Fig. 16.56** BAP1 tumour predisposition syndrome. Associated meningioma.

## Etiology

*BAP1* tumour predisposition syndrome is caused by pathogenic germline variants in the *BAP1* tumour suppressor gene on chromosome 3p21.1. To date, most individuals diagnosed with *BAP1* tumour predisposition syndrome have inherited the *BAP1* pathogenic germline variant from a parent. The proportion of *BAP1* tumour predisposition syndrome cases caused by a de novo pathogenic variant arising from a mutation in a germ cell is unknown, although one study found that 2 (9.5%) of 21 probands tested had a probable de novo *BAP1* pathogenic germline variant {7374,1187}. More data are required to evaluate the effect of environmental mutagens (e.g. asbestos, ultraviolet [UV] radiation) on modulating the penetrance of germline mutations.

## Pathogenesis

*BAP1* (on chromosome 3p21.1) comprises 17 exons encoding a protein with UCH activity first identified as interacting with *BRCA1* {3251}, which encodes a nuclear deubiquitinating enzyme {5042,802}. *BAP1* interactors include *ASXL1*, *ASXL2*, *FOXK1*, *FOXK2*, *HCFC1*, and *YY1*, consistent with roles in the DNA damage response, transcriptional regulation, cell-cycle regulation, metabolism, inflammatory responses, and lineage differentiation {6375,1259,7374,3851}. Nuclear localization and deubiquitination activity are both necessary for BAP1-mediated tumour suppression {7273}. *BAP1* tumour predisposition syndrome is caused by heterozygous germline variants in *BAP1* that lead to a loss of protein function {6957}.

## Macroscopic appearance

The macroscopic appearance of tumours in *BAP1* tumour predisposition syndrome is similar to that of their sporadic counterparts.

## Histopathology

*Skin:* Histologically, *BAP1*-inactivated melanocytic tumours of the skin are predominantly composed of intradermal melanocytes with varying degrees of atypia, ranging from clearly benign lesions with naevoid cells and minimal atypia (*BAP1*-inactivated naevi) to highly atypical tumours that have large epithelioid cells with well-defined cytoplasmic borders, abundant amphophilic cytoplasm, pleomorphic vesicular nuclei, and prominent nucleoli (*BAP1*-inactivated melanocytomas). Tumour-infiltrating lymphocytes are often seen. Many of these skin lesions appear as combined melanocytic naevi, with areas of small oval melanocytes (a common naevus component) adjacent to the larger, epithelioid melanocytes. In most lesions, the wildtype *BAP1* allele is inactivated (by various somatic alterations), resulting in a lack of nuclear BAP1 expression on immunohistochemistry. Most lesions also harbour *BRAF* p.V600E mutations {4176,7538}.

*CNS:* The histopathology of *BAP1* tumour predisposition syndrome–associated tumours is similar to that of their sporadic counterparts. Many *BAP1*-mutant meningiomas have overt rhabdoid cytomorphology, but the histology can be diverse, including epithelioid-type cells and papillary growth {6374,6375,7549}.

*Thorax:* The histological features of mesothelioma occurring in the setting of *BAP1* tumour predisposition syndrome are the same as those of tumours occurring sporadically.

## Cytology

The cytology of tumours in *BAP1* tumour predisposition syndrome is similar to that of their sporadic counterparts.

## Diagnostic molecular pathology

*BAP1* genetic sequencing and deletion/duplication analysis performed on peripheral blood can confirm the diagnosis of *BAP1* tumour predisposition syndrome. The vast majority of pathogenic germline variants in *BAP1* reported to date have been sequence variants {5730} as opposed to copy-number changes. In sequencing data, appraising pathogenicity is straightforward for indels and for frameshift, nonsense, and splice-site mutations; guidelines for interpretation of sequence variants can assist in the classification of missense mutations {5875,4084}.

Loss of BAP1 immunoreactivity in tumour nuclei also readily identifies deficient tumours. Concordance between immunohistochemistry and genotyping is high but incomplete {802,3731, 4940,7193}.

## Essential and desirable diagnostic criteria

*Essential:* demonstration of a germline pathogenic variant in *BAP1*.

## Staging

Stage as appropriate for tumour type.

## Prognosis and prediction

Penetrance is incomplete, but the precise risk of an individual patient with *BAP1* tumour predisposition syndrome developing one or more of the associated tumours has not yet been determined. Additional environmental factors may increase the risk; for example, UV radiation and asbestos exposure may increase the risk of melanoma and mesothelioma, respectively. Prognosis depends on the tumour type and stage of the malignancies. *BAP1*-inactivated melanocytic tumours of the skin have a good prognosis and rarely metastasize {4861}.

Some studies suggest that individuals with *BAP1* tumour predisposition syndrome who develop mesothelioma have a longer survival than those with sporadic mesothelioma, and a better 5-year survival rate (47% vs 6.7%) {544,5137,7813}. However, uveal melanomas in *BAP1* germline pathogenic variant carriers may be more aggressive than sporadic cases {2618,5056}. *BAP1*-mutant meningiomas display aggressive behaviour with frequent recurrences {6374,6375}; however, it is unclear whether meningiomas arising in *BAP1* tumour predisposition syndrome have a different prognosis from that of sporadic *BAP1*-mutant meningiomas.

Cancer screening criteria for uveal melanoma, cutaneous melanoma, mesothelioma, cholangiocarcinoma, and renal cell carcinoma have been proposed for carriers of *BAP1* germline pathogenic variants. To identify tumours at early stages, screening includes eye and skin examinations and ultrasound/MRI {5730,6648,7374,1187}. *BAP1*-inactivated melanocytic tumours often precede the onset of other tumours, and their recognition may facilitate early syndrome detection.

# Constitutional mismatch repair deficiency syndrome

Hawkins CE
Frayling IM
Tabori U
Tomlinson GE

## Definition

Constitutional mismatch repair deficiency syndrome (CMMRD) is an autosomal recessive cancer predisposition syndrome caused by biallelic germline mutations in one of four mismatch repair genes (*MLH1*, *PMS2*, *MSH2*, and *MSH6*). Individuals with CMMRD develop ultrahypermutated malignant gliomas, CNS embryonal tumours, and a variety of other cancers during childhood and early adulthood.

## MIM numbering

276300 Mismatch repair cancer syndrome 1; MMRCS1

## ICD-11 coding

None

## Related terminology

*Not recommended:* mismatch repair cancer syndrome; Turcot syndrome; brain tumour polyposis syndrome type 1.
*Acceptable:* biallelic mismatch repair deficiency syndrome.

## Subtype(s)

None

## Localization

The glioblastomas arising in the setting of CMMRD, Lynch syndrome, and polymerase proofreading deficiency can occur both in the cerebral hemispheres and the posterior fossa, including a gliomatosis-like dissemination pattern in a subset. Medulloblastoma centred in the posterior fossa and other embryonal CNS tumours have also been reported {461}.

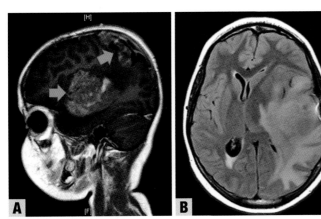

**Fig. 16.57** Representative imaging of replication repair–deficient glioblastomas. **A** T1-weighted postcontrast MRI of a patient with constitutional mismatch repair deficiency syndrome with a homozygous *MSH2* pathogenic germline variant. Note two synchronous tumours (arrows). Both tumours had secondary somatic mutations and ultrahypermutation, one involving *POLE* and one involving *POLD1*. **B** A FLAIR sequence of a patient with Lynch syndrome and *MLH1* heterozygous pathogenic germline variant. This gliomatosis-like pattern is typical for somatic mutation in *IDH1* and hypermutation.

## Clinical features

The combination of café-au-lait skin macules and consanguinity with specific brain, haematological, and gastrointestinal cancers arising during childhood should raise suspicion for CMMRD. A scoring system has been developed for determining those patients in whom genetic testing for CMMRD should be performed {7568}. Importantly, a family history of cancer is often uninformative, especially for those children with biallelic *PMS2* mutations, because of the substantially lower cancer risks associated with heterozygous mutations in this gene compared to the other mismatch repair genes.

### Nervous system neoplasms

Brain tumours, most commonly gliomas, occur in the first two decades of life and account for 25–40% of all CMMRD-associated cancers {461,7568}. Medulloblastoma and CNS embryonal tumours have also been described in patients with CMMRD {2580}. Molecularly, all brain tumours arising in the setting of CMMRD have a unique ultrahypermutation genotype, which distinguishes them from the typically low somatic mutation burdens in their sporadic paediatric counterparts {805,1002}.

### Other CNS manifestations

Agenesis of the corpus callosum and venous anomalies have been reported in children with CMMRD. Developmental venous anomalies are extremely common and may point towards the possibility of CMMRD {6451}.

### Extraneural manifestations

More than 90% of patients with CMMRD have café-au-lait macules and other dermatological abnormalities such as hyperpigmented or hypopigmented areas {461}. These café-au-lait macules can mimic those found in patients with neurofibromatosis type 1. However, patients with CMMRD typically lack other stigmata of neurofibromatosis type 1, such as axillary and groin freckling, cutaneous neurofibromas, and Lisch nodules {7568, 1867}. Haematological malignancies, predominantly T-cell leukaemia/lymphoma, occur mostly in the first two decades of life, in as many as 30% of patients, whereas gastrointestinal polyposis and cancers are present in virtually all patients by the second decade of life. Other cancers (e.g. urinary tract cancers and sarcomas) have also been reported {461,7568}. Multiple pilomatricomas appear to be frequent and might suggest CMMRD in combination with another feature of the condition {1286}. An increased frequency of paediatric systemic lupus erythematosus has been reported in patients with CMMRD; all 5 patients described were girls, and 4 of them had biallelic *MSH6* mutations {7009}.

### Differential diagnosis

CMMRD should not be confused with Lynch syndrome (also known as hereditary non-polyposis colorectal cancer syndrome).

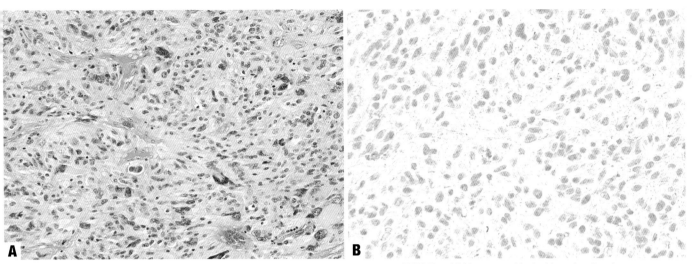

**Fig. 16.58** Glioblastoma arising in the setting of constitutional mismatch repair deficiency syndrome (CMMRD). **A** Glioblastomas arising in this setting often demonstrate severe nuclear pleomorphism with bizarre and multinucleated giant cells. **B** This glioblastoma in the cerebral hemispheres of a child with CMMRD demonstrates a complete absence of PMS2 protein both in tumour cells and in normal cells, resulting from biallelic inactivation of the *PMS2* mismatch repair gene in the germline of this patient.

Whereas CMMRD is an autosomal recessive syndrome resulting from a biallelic germline mutation in one of the mismatch repair genes, Lynch syndrome is an autosomal dominant syndrome resulting from a heterozygous germline mutation. It results in a different cancer spectrum and a different age of onset (mostly colorectal, genitourinary, and sebaceous carcinomas during adulthood). Hypermutant cancers including glioblastomas, accompanied by some of the features of CMMRD including café-au-lait macules, can also occur with germline mutations in *POLE*, encoding DNA polymerase epsilon, which has been termed "polymerase proofreading deficiency" {7184,267}.

## Epidemiology
More than 200 kindreds with CMMRD have been reported {461, 7568}. However, this syndrome is probably underdiagnosed and highly prevalent in populations where consanguinity is high {230,1865}. In countries with a low level of consanguinity, the frequency of this condition has been estimated at 1 case per 1 million children.

## Etiology
CMMRD is caused by the biallelic germline inactivation of one of the four main mismatch repair genes: *MLH1* at chromosome 3p22.2, *MSH2* at 2p16, *MSH6* at 2p16, and *PMS2* at 7p22. This can be the result either of two different mutations present in trans (compound heterozygous) or the same mutation present on both alleles (homozygous), the latter being common in consanguinity.

## Pathogenesis
The genetic defect underlying CMMRD is the inability to recognize and repair DNA mismatches during replication. Recognition and repair of base-pair mismatches in human DNA is mediated by heterodimers of MSH2 and MSH6, which form a sliding clamp on DNA. The C-terminus of PMS2 interacts with MLH1, and this complex binds to MSH2/MSH6 heterodimers to form a functional strand-specific mismatch recognition complex {6499}. Cells that are deficient in any of the above genes are defective in the repair of mismatched bases and insertions/

deletions (indels) of single nucleotides, resulting in high mutation rates and microsatellite instability (MSI). Unlike in heterozygous carriers with Lynch syndrome (in whom MSI is robustly observed in the resultant endometrial and colorectal cancers), glioblastomas arising in patients with CMMRD often lack classic MSI and are characterized instead by extremely high rates of single-nucleotide mutations with a much smaller component of small indels {461,6455}. CMMRD-associated glioblastomas commonly acquire mutations in *POLE* or *POLD1* to create complete replication deficiency and ultrahypermutation {461,6455}. These tumours almost invariably inactivate tumour suppressor genes such as *TP53*.

## Macroscopic appearance
The macroscopic appearance reflects the tumour type.

## Histopathology
Glioblastomas arising in the setting of CMMRD often have severe nuclear pleomorphism and/or bizarre multinucleated giant cells {2580}. Another morphological appearance of brain tumours in CMMRD is sheets of primitive small blue cells, raising the differential diagnosis of a CNS embryonal tumour or medulloblastoma, depending on the location {461,2580}. Whether all the brain tumours that arise in the setting of CMMRD are in fact glioblastomas, or whether true medulloblastomas, pleomorphic xanthoastrocytomas, and other tumour types can occur in this syndrome, remains to be determined.

The finding of a paediatric high-grade glioma or glioblastoma with severe pleomorphism or giant cell features should raise suspicion for possible CMMRD and prompt immunohistochemical testing for the mismatch repair proteins.

## Cytology
Not relevant

## Diagnostic molecular pathology
Detection of biallelic germline mutation (either homozygous or compound heterozygous) in one of the four main mismatch repair genes is required for the diagnosis of CMMRD. The abundance

of variants of unknown significance and the technical problems with sequencing *PMS2*, which has multiple pseudogenes, have led to the development of several functional assays that can aid in the rapid detection of CMMRD. MSI testing on glioblastomas is not reliable because they typically demonstrate only a low level of MSI despite being mismatch repair–deficient and ultrahypermutated. Immunohistochemistry demonstrates a loss of expression of the inactivated mismatch repair protein (and when appropriate, its heterodimer) in both tumour and normal tissue in > 90% of CMMRD-associated cancers {461}. In vitro cell-based assays on normal fibroblasts and lymphoblasts can detect MSI, resistance to several compounds, and failure to repair G–T mismatches {6455,757}. Recently, screening tests based on MSI using next-generation sequencing of normal tissue successfully identified patients with CMMRD {2292,2485}.

### Essential and desirable diagnostic criteria
*Essential:* biallelic pathogenic germline mutation/deletion in one of the four main mismatch repair genes (*MSH2*, *MSH6*, *PMS2*, *MLH1*) or a combination of clinical criteria and two functional assays.
*Desirable:* genomic profiling of the index brain tumour demonstrating an ultrahypermutated genotype with a mutation signature characteristic of mismatch repair deficiency; immunohistochemical absence of expression of mismatch repair proteins in both tumour cells and normal cells.

### Staging
Not relevant

### Prognosis and prediction
Patients with CMMRD and their family members benefit from genetic counselling, because surveillance protocols exist and early detection may result in increased survival for both biallelic and heterozygous carriers {1866,7252}. The inherent resistance of mismatch repair–deficient cells to several common chemotherapies, including temozolomide, makes them ineffective in the management of gliomas in the setting of CMMRD. In contrast, the ultrahypermutation phenotype of CMMRD-associated cancers results in a greatly increased neoantigen burden on cancer cells, which can be therapeutically exploited by immune checkpoint blockade {6455,3983}. Because the prognosis of children with glioblastomas arising in the setting of CMMRD is unfavourable, immunotherapeutic approaches and prevention strategies are now being tested {805,21,2580}.

# Rhabdoid tumour predisposition syndrome

Sredni ST
Biegel JA
Eberhart CG
Huang A
Judkins AR

Kool M
Pawel BR
Perry A
Tabori U
Wesseling P

## Definition
Rhabdoid tumour predisposition syndrome (RTPS) is a disorder characterized by a markedly increased risk of developing malignant rhabdoid tumours (MRTs), including atypical teratoid/rhabdoid tumour (AT/RT), due to constitutional loss or inactivation of *SMARCB1* (rhabdoid tumour predisposition syndrome 1 [RTPS1]) or, rarely, *SMARCA4* (rhabdoid tumour predisposition syndrome 2 [RTPS2]).

## MIM numbering
609322 Rhabdoid tumour predisposition syndrome 1; RTPS1
613325 Rhabdoid tumour predisposition syndrome 2; RTPS2

## ICD-11 coding
None

## Related terminology
*Not recommended:* rhabdoid predisposition syndrome; familial posterior fossa brain tumour syndrome of infancy.

## Subtype(s)
Rhabdoid tumour predisposition syndrome 1; rhabdoid tumour predisposition syndrome 2

## Localization
Both the nervous system and extraneural organs/tissues can be involved.

## Clinical features
The median age of tumour onset in patients with RTPS is younger than that in patients with sporadic tumours. To date, no other clinical features distinguish RTPS-associated tumours from sporadic rhabdoid tumours.

### Nervous system
Individuals with RTPS1 often present with isolated AT/RTs or an AT/RT with a synchronous renal or extrarenal MRT {4004}.

In the past, a variety of other CNS tumours have been reported to be associated with RTPS, including choroid plexus carcinoma {2376}, medulloblastoma, and supratentorial tumours {6350}. However, because these tumours may be hard to distinguish from AT/RTs and because some AT/RTs lack well-developed rhabdoid cells, the occurrence of such tumours in RTPS is controversial {2648,3346,3348,7148}.

### Extraneural manifestations
By far the most common extra-CNS manifestation is MRT of the kidney. Bilateral renal MRTs are almost always associated with a germline *SMARCB1* mutation, but infants with an isolated MRT may carry germline mutations as well. MRTs have been reported to originate in the head and neck region, paraspinal soft tissues, heart, mediastinum, and liver {7513}. Children surviving a primary MRT can develop a second primary in a different location {2188}. *SMARCB1* mutations may occasionally underlie the oncogenesis of other neoplasms, such as proximal-type epithelioid sarcoma {4738}, but to date, these sarcomas have not been described in RTPS. Germline and somatic mutations in *SMARCA4* also give rise to hypercalcaemic-type small cell carcinoma of the ovary – a rare, highly aggressive tumour in adolescents and young adults {2200, 7001}. The incidence of germline mutations is high in hypercalcaemic-type small cell carcinoma of the ovary, and in one family with a *SMARCA4* germline mutation, AT/RT and ovarian cancer were diagnosed in a newborn and his mother, respectively {7576}.

## Epidemiology
AT/RTs generally occur in early childhood but are occasionally found in adults {5731}. RTPS is found in 25–35% of all patients

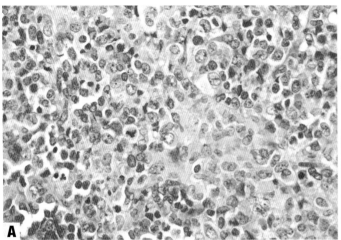
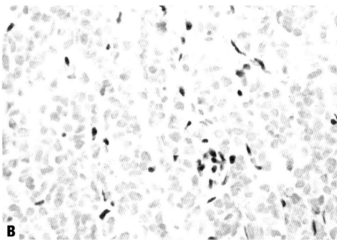

**Fig. 16.59** CNS atypical teratoid/rhabdoid tumour. **A** The tumour nuclei are large and irregular, many with vesicular chromatin and prominent nucleoli. Mitotic figures and apoptotic bodies are numerous. **B** SMARCB1 (INI1) expression is lost in neoplastic cells.

with AT/RT {677,1878}; these patients are more likely to present in their first year of life. Second primary tumours may arise as late as 8 years after the primary diagnosis {673}, suggesting that lifetime surveillance is required.

## Etiology
RTPS1 and RTPS2 are caused by a germline *SMARCB1* or *SMARCA4* mutation, respectively. De novo germline mutations can occur during oogenesis/spermatogenesis, or postzygotically during the early stages of embryogenesis (mosaicism) {1878,2764,3221,6350}. Tumours in rare families with multiple affected children and no parental *SMARCB1* mutation are probably due to gonadal mosaicism. In some families, apparently unaffected carriers develop schwannomas in the fourth or fifth decade of life.

*SMARCB1* has also been identified as a predisposing gene in familial schwannomatosis, germline mutations in *SMARCA4* predispose to hypercalcaemic-type small cell carcinoma of the ovary, and germline mutations in both *SMARCB1* and *SMARCA4* have been identified as contributing to syndromes associated with dysmorphic features and intellectual disability, such as Coffin–Siris syndrome.

## Pathogenesis
### SMARCB1
*SMARCB1* was the first gene encoding a subunit of the SWI/SNF complex found to be mutated in cancer. This gene is located in chromosome region 22q11.23 and contains nine exons spanning 50 kb of genomic DNA {7290}. Alternative splicing of exon 2 results in two transcripts and two proteins with lengths of 385 and 376 amino acid residues, respectively. The SNF5 homology domain in the second half of the protein harbours highly conserved structural motifs through which SMARCB1 interacts with other proteins {6708}. The SMARCB1 protein is a core subunit of mammalian SWI/SNF chromatin-remodelling complexes, which regulate gene expression via ATP-mediated nucleosomal remodelling {7561}. SMARCB1 functions as a tumour suppressor via the repression of *CCND1* gene expression, induction of the *CDKN2A* gene, and hypophosphorylation of RB1, resulting in G0/G1 cell-cycle arrest {665,5917}. Loss of SMARCB1 leads to activation of EZH2, a histone lysine methyltransferase and catalytic component of the PRC2 complex, resulting in increased H3 p. K27me3 marks associated with the repression of polycomb gene targets. The Hippo signalling pathway is involved in the detrimental effects of SMARCB1 deficiency, and its main effector (YAP1) is overexpressed in AT/RT {3242,7562}.

*SMARCB1* is a classic tumour suppressor requiring biallelic loss of function, with the second event typically being loss of heterozygosity / deletion. The types of *SMARCB1* mutations observed in sporadic MRTs are similar to the germline mutations in RTPS. However, single base deletions in exon 9 occur most often in sporadic AT/RTs {677,1878,6810}. The second inactivating event is most frequently a deletion of the wildtype allele, often due to monosomy 22. Schwannomatosis mutations are more likely to occur at either end of the gene and to be non-truncating {6548}.

Germline *SMARCB1* mutations may predispose individuals to the development of rhabdoid tumours or schwannomatosis. In rhabdoid tumours, the two copies of *SMARCB1* are inactivated by a truncating mutation and deletion of the wildtype gene, resulting in total loss of SMARCB1 expression in tumour cells. This is in contrast to the non-truncating *SMARCB1* mutations and mosaic SMARCB1 expression in patients with schwannomas or schwannomatosis {6548}. Because of the high mortality and morbidity rates in patients with rhabdoid tumours, familial inheritance of RTPS is extremely rare {6350,6927}. It has been reported that as many as 35% of patients with rhabdoid tumour carry a germline *SMARCB1* alteration as the first hit {808,1878}. However, a recent study demonstrated a lower incidence, suggesting that prior studies may have been biased by the inclusion of patients with multiple primary tumours, virtually all of whom have a germline *SMARCB1* alteration {5803}. A few families have been reported wherein affected individuals inherited a *SMARCB1* mutation and developed either schwannomatosis or a rhabdoid tumour {1065,1878,6810}. In these families, both the rhabdoid tumours and the schwannomas displayed total SMARCB1 loss {1065,6810}. Recently, a patient with co-occurrence of rhabdoid tumour and schwannomas was reported {3508}.

### SMARCA4
*SMARCA4*, located on chromosome 19p13.2 and encoding a catalytic subunit of the SWI/SNF complex, was the second member of this complex reported in a cancer predisposition syndrome {678,6261}. More recently, other SWI/SNF subunit genes have also been implicated in cancers. Collectively, 20% of all human cancers contain a mutation in SWI/SNF, and because most of these tumours are not classic MRTs, the definition of RTPS may need adjustment in the future {3586}.

## Macroscopic appearance
RTPS-associated tumours are macroscopically similar to their sporadic counterparts.

## Histopathology
RTPS-associated tumours are histopathologically similar to their sporadic counterparts.

## Cytology
RTPS-associated tumours are cytologically similar to their sporadic counterparts.

## Diagnostic molecular pathology
Loss of immunohistochemical staining for SMARCB1 (INI1) or SMARCA4 (BRG1) identifies tumours (MRTs and AT/RTs) associated with RTPS1 and RTPS2, respectively. However, molecular genetic testing of the patient is needed to confirm a suspected germline alteration.

## Essential and desirable diagnostic criteria
*Essential:* demonstration of a germline *SMARCB1* or *SMARCA4* mutation in a patient with MRT or AT/RT.
*Desirable:* multiple MRTs or AT/RTs; siblings or other relatives with MRT or AT/RT.

## Staging
See individual tumour types.

## Prognosis and prediction

Transcriptome and DNA methylation profiling separate AT/RTs into three molecular groups, which by consensus have been designated as AT/RT-TYR, AT/RT-SHH, and AT/RT-MYC {2919}. Although these subgroups show differences in patient age and tumour localization, to date no pattern of germline predisposition and subgroup has been confirmed.

Because only a relatively small number of patients with RTPS have been reported in prospective therapeutic studies, the impact of germline alterations on patient outcomes remains unclear. Although prior data suggested a poorer outcome for patients with germline SMARCB1 alterations, an increasing number of AT/RT survivors with germline SMARCB1 alterations are being seen, suggesting that other variables, such as intensity or type of therapy, as well as specific SMARCB1 genotypes, may influence outcomes.

# Contributors

ABEDALTHAGAFI, Malak S.
Department of Pathology and Laboratory
Medicine
Emory School of Medicine
1364 Clifton Rd
Atlanta GA 30322

ADAMEYKO, Igor
Center for Brain Research
Medical University of Vienna
Spitalgasse 4
1090 Vienna

AGAIMY, Abbas
Erlangen University Hospital
Krankenhausstraße 8-10
91054 Erlangen

AGARAM, Narasimhan P.
Memorial Sloan Kettering Cancer Center
1275 York Ave
New York NY 10065

AL-IBRAHEEMI, Alyaa
Boston Children's Hospital
300 Longwood Ave
Boston MA 02115

ALAGGIO, Rita
Sapienza Università di Roma
IRCCS Ospedale Bambino Gesù
Piazza di Sant'Onofrio, 4
00165 Rome RM

ALDAPE, Kenneth D.
National Cancer Institute
9000 Rockville Pike
Bethesda MD 20892

ALEXANDRESCU, Sanda
Boston Children's Hospital
Harvard Medical School
300 Longwood Ave, Bader 104
Boston MA 02115

AMARY, Fernanda
Royal National Orthopaedic Hospital
Brockley Hill
Greater London HA7 4LP

ANTONESCU, Cristina R.
Memorial Sloan Kettering Cancer Center
1275 York Ave
New York NY 10065

ARGANI, Pedram
Johns Hopkins Hospital
Weinberg 2242, 401 N Broadway
Baltimore MD 21231-2410

ARMON, Subasri
Hospital Kuala Lumpur
Pathology Department
Jalan Pahang 50586
Wilayah Persekutuan Kuala Lumpur

ASA, Sylvia L.*
Case Western Reserve University
11100 Euclid Ave
Cleveland OH 44106

ATTARBASCHI, Andishe
St. Anna Children's Hospital
Kinderspitalgasse 6
1090 Vienna

BACON, Chris M.
Newcastle University
Herschel Building, Brewery Ln
Newcastle upon Tyne NE1 7RU

BAHRAMI, Armita
Emory School of Medicine
1364 Clifton Rd NE, Suite H185A
Atlanta GA 30322

BAKER, Suzanne J.
St. Jude Children's Research Hospital
262 Danny Thomas Pl
Memphis TN 38105

BALE, Allen E.
Yale University
333 Cedar St
New Haven CT 06520

BANDOPADHAYAY, Pratiti*
Dana-Farber/Boston Children's
Cancer and Blood Disorders Center
450 Brookline Ave, Mayer 658
Dana-Farber Cancer Institute
Boston MA 02215

BASSO, Cristina
Pathological Anatomy-Cardiovascular
Pathology
University of Padova Medical School
Via Gabelli, 61
35121 Padua PD

BASTIAN, Boris C.*
University of California, San Francisco
1450 3rd St #281
San Francisco CA 94143-3118

BAUER, Andrew J.
Children's Hospital of Philadelphia;
University of Pennsylvania
3500 Civic Center Blvd
Philadelphia PA 19104

BAUMHOER, Daniel
University Hospital Basel
Schönbeinstrasse 40
4031 Basel

BEISKE, Klaus Hermann
Oslo University Hospital, Radiumhospitalet
Ullernchausseen 64
0379 Oslo

BELL, Diana
City of Hope
1500 E Duarte Rd
Duarte CA 91010

BENNETT, Jennifer A.
University of Chicago Medicine
5841 S Maryland Ave, MC 6101
Chicago IL 60637

BIEGEL, Jaclyn A.
Children's Hospital Los Angeles
Department of Pathology
4650 Sunset Blvd, MS 173
Los Angeles CA 90027

BILLINGS, Steven D.
Cleveland Clinic
9500 Euclid Ave, L25
Cleveland OH 44195

BISHOP, Justin A.
UT Southwestern Medical Center
6201 Harry Hines Blvd
Dallas TX 75390

BISOGNO, Gianni
University of Padova
Via Nicolò Giustiniani, 3
35121 Padua PD

BLACK, Jennifer Olivia
Children's Hospital Colorado
University of Colorado
13123 E 16th Ave
Aurora CO 80045

---

\* Indicates disclosure of interests (see p. 1034).

BLÜMCKE, Ingmar
Institute of Neuropathology
University of Erlangen
Schwabachanlage 6
91054 Erlangen

BODE, Peter Karl
Institute of Pathology
Cantonal Hospital Winterthur
Brauerstrasse 15
8401 Winterthur

BOVÉE, Judith V.M.G.
Department of Pathology
Leiden University Medical Center
Albinusdreef 2
2333 ZA Leiden

BRANDNER, Sebastian
UCL Queen Square Institute of Neurology and
National Hospital for Neurology and
Neurosurgery, University College London
Hospitals NHS Foundation Trust
Queen Square
London WC1N 3BG

BRAT, Daniel J.
Northwestern University
Feinberg School of Medicine
303 E Chicago Ave
Ward Building, Room 3-140
Chicago IL 60611

BRENN, Thomas
Cumming School of Medicine
University of Calgary
9-3535 Research Rd NW
Calgary AB T2L 2K8

BRENTON, James Derek
Cancer Research UK Cambridge Institute
University of Cambridge
Li Ka Shing Centre, Robinson Way
Cambridge CB2 0RE

BRIDGE, Julia A.
ProPath
1355 River Bend Dr
Dallas TX 75247

BROSENS, Lodewijk A.A.
Department of Pathology
University Medical Center Utrecht
Heidelberglaan 100
3584 CX Utrecht

BUI, Marilyn M.
Moffitt Cancer Center
12902 Magnolia Dr
Tampa FL 33612

BUSH, Jonathan Willard
BC Children's and Women's Hospital
University of British Columbia
4480 Oak St
Vancouver BC V6H 3N1

BUZA, Natalia
Yale School of Medicine
310 Cedar St
New Haven CT 06510

CALONJE, Jaime E.
St John's Institute of Dermatology
St Thomas' Hospital
Westminster Bridge Rd
London SE1 7EH

CAMPO, Elias
Hospital Clinic of Barcelona
University of Barcelona
C. de Villarroel, 170
08036 Barcelona

CAPPER, David*
Charité – Universitätsmedizin Berlin
Charitépl. 1
10117 Berlin

CARNEIRO, Fátima
Institute of Molecular Pathology and
Immunology of the University of Porto
(Ipatimup/i3S) and Centro Hospitalar
Universitário de São João (CHUSJ)/Faculty
of Medicine of the University of Porto (FMUP)
Rua Júlio Amaral de Carvalho 45
4200-135 Porto

CATES, Justin M.M.
Vanderbilt University Medical Center
1161 21st Ave S, MCN-3322
Nashville TN 37232

CHAN, John K.C.
Queen Elizabeth Hospital
30 Gascoigne Rd
Kowloon, Hong Kong SAR

CHANG, Kenneth Tou En*
KK Women's and Children's Hospital
100 Bukit Timah Rd
Singapore 229899

CHEN, Lian
Children's Hospital of Fudan University
399 Wanyuan Rd, Minhang District
Shanghai 201102

CHEUNG, Annie Nga-Yin
University of Hong Kong
Queen Mary Hospital
Pok Fu Lam Rd
Hong Kong SAR

CHEVEZ-BARRIOS, Patricia
Houston Methodist Hospital
6565 Fannin St, M227
Houston TX 77030

CHI, Ping
Memorial Sloan Kettering Cancer Center
1275 York Ave
New York NY 10065

CHILDERS, Esther Lynn Blinderman
Howard University College of Dentistry
600 W Street NW
Washington DC 20059

CHINTAGUMPALA, Murali
Baylor College of Medicine
6701 Fannin St, Suite 1510.15
Houston TX 77030

CHIOSEA, Simon
UPMC Presbyterian Hospital
200 Lothrop St, PUH A610.3
Pittsburgh PA 15213

CHO, Soo-Jin
University of California, San Francisco
1825 4th St, Room M2356
San Francisco CA 94143

CHOI, John Kim
University of Alabama at Birmingham
619 19th St S, WP P230N
Birmingham AL 35249

CHU, Winnie Chiu Wing
Chinese University of Hong Kong
Prince of Wales Hospital
G/F, Day Treatment Block and Children
Wards, Room 27026
Shatin
Hong Kong SAR

CIPRIANI, Nicole A.
University of Chicago
5841 S Maryland Ave, MC 6101
Chicago IL 60637

CLIFFORD, Steven C.
Newcastle University Centre for Cancer
Herschel Building
Newcastle upon Tyne NE1 7RU

COLLINI, Paola
Fondazione IRCCS Istituto Nazionale dei
Tumori, Milan
Via Giacomo Venezian, 1
20133 Milan MI

COLMENERO, Isabel
Hospital Infantil Universitario Niño Jesús
Av. de Menéndez Pelayo, 65
28009 Madrid

---

* Indicates disclosure of interests (see p. 1034).

COTTER, Jennifer A.
Children's Hospital Los Angeles and
Keck School of Medicine of USC
4650 Sunset Blvd, Mail Stop #43
Los Angeles CA 90027

COUPLAND, Sarah E.
Institute of Systems, Molecular and
Integrative Biology, University of Liverpool
W Derby St, William Henry Duncan Building,
3rd Floor
Liverpool L7 8TX

CREE, Ian A.
International Agency for Research on Cancer
25 Av. Tony Garnier, CS 90627
69366 Lyon, CEDEX 07

CREYTENS, David
Ghent University Hospital, Ghent University
Department of Pathology
Corneel Heymanslaan 10
9000 Ghent

CULLINANE, Catherine
Department of Histopathology
St James's University Hospital
Beckett St, Level 5, Bexley Wing
Leeds LS9 7TF

CZAUDERNA, Piotr
Medical University of Gdańsk
Mariana Smoluchowskiego 17
80-214 Gdańsk

D'AMORE, Emanuele S.G.
Ospedale San Bortolo di Vicenza
Viale Ferdinando Rodolfi
35123 Vicenza VI

DAVIS, Jessica L.*
Indiana University
350 W 11th St, Mail code CP4010
Indianapolis IN 46202

DAVIS, Kara L.
Department of Pediatrics, Stanford University
Bass Center for Childhood Cancer and Blood
Diseases
2078b Lokey Stem Cell Research Building
269 Campus Dr
Stanford CA 94305

DE ÁLAVA, Enrique
Hospital Universitario Virgen del Rocío-IBiS
University of Seville
Av. Manuel Siurot, S/N
41013 Seville

DE KOCK, Leanne
Children's Hospital of Eastern Ontario
Research Institute
401 Smyth Rd
Ottawa ON K1H 5B2

DE KRIJGER, Ronald R.
Princess Máxima Center for Pediatric
Oncology and Department of Pathology,
University Medical Center Utrecht
Heidelberglaan 25
3584 CS Utrecht

DE LA FOUCHARDIÈRE, Arnaud
Centre Léon Bérard
28 Rue Laennec
69008 Lyon

DE SAINT AUBAIN SOMERHAUSEN, Nicolas
Institut Jules Bordet
Rue Héger-Bordet 1
1000 Brussels

DEI TOS, Angelo Paolo
University of Padua School of Medicine /
Azienda Ospedale-Università Padova
(Department of Pathology)
Via Gabelli, 61
35121 Padua PD

DeNAPOLI, Thomas S.
Children's Hospital of San Antonio /
Baylor College of Medicine
333 N Santa Rosa St
San Antonio TX 78207

DENTON, Erika R.E.
Norfolk and Norwich University Hospitals
NHS Foundation Trust
Colney Ln
Norwich NR4 7UY

DI NAPOLI, Arianna
Sapienza University of Rome
Sant'Andrea Hospital
Via di Grottarossa, 1035
00189 Rome RM

DIEPSTRA, Arjan
University Medical Center Groningen
Hanzeplein 1, Box 30.001
9700 RB Groningen

DIRNHOFER, Stefan
Institute of Medical Genetics and Pathology
University Hospital Basel
Schönbeinstrasse 40
4031 Basel

DISHOP, Megan K.*
Phoenix Children's Hospital
1919 E Thomas Rd
Phoenix AZ 85016

DOYLE, Leona A.
Brigham and Women's Hospital and
Harvard Medical School
75 Francis St
Boston MA 02115

DOZ, François*
Université Paris Cité; and SIREDO (Care,
Innovation & Research in Childhood,
Adolescent & Young-Adult Oncology),
Institut Curie
26 Rue d'Ulm
75005 Paris

DRY, Sarah M.
University of California, Los Angeles (UCLA)
13-222 CHS, 10833 Le Conte Ave
Los Angeles CA 90095

DU, Ming-Qing
University of Cambridge
Cellular and Molecular Pathology, Box 231
Level 3 Lab Block, Addenbrooke's Hospital
Hills Rd
Cambridge CB2 0QQ

EAGLE, Ralph C. Jr
Wills Eye Hospital
840 Walnut St, Suite 1410
Philadelphia PA 19107

EBERHART, Charles G.
Johns Hopkins University
720 Rutland Ave, Ross Building 558
Baltimore MD 21205

ELDER, David E.
Hospital of the University of Pennsylvania
3400 Spruce St
Philadelphia PA 19104

ERICKSON, Lori A.
Mayo Clinic
200 1st St SW
Rochester MN 55905

ETCHEVERS, Heather C.
Marseille Medical Genetics, INSERM
Aix-Marseille Université, Faculté de Médecine
27 Bd Jean Moulin
13005 Marseille

FANBURG-SMITH, Julie C.
Penn State Health
Milton S. Hershey Medical Center
Penn State Health Children's Hospital
Pathology, Pediatrics, Orthopedics
500 University Dr, C7714D
Hershey PA 17044

FAQUIN, William C.
Massachusetts General Hospital
Harvard Medical School
Department of Pathology, Warren 219
55 Fruit St
Boston MA 02114

---

* Indicates disclosure of interests (see p. 1034).

FERRARI, Andrea
Fondazione IRCCS Istituto Nazionale dei
Tumori, Milan
Via Giacomo Venezian, 1
20133 Milan MI

FIELD, Andrew S.
University of NSW Sydney and
University of Notre Dame Medical Schools
Department of Anatomical Pathology
St Vincent's Hospital Sydney
Victoria St
2010 Darlinghurst NSW

FIGARELLA-BRANGER, Dominique
Assistance Publique des Hôpitaux de
Marseille
264 Rue Saint-Pierre
13005 Marseille

FISCHER, Matthias
University Children's Hospital
Kerpener Str. 62
50937 Cologne

FISHER, Kevin E.
Baylor College of Medicine
Texas Children's Hospital
6621 Fannin St
Houston TX 77030

FISHER, Michael J.
Children's Hospital of Philadelphia
3501 Civic Center Blvd
Philadelphia PA 19104

FLAITZ, Catherine Mary
University of Colorado School of Dental
Medicine
13065 E 17th Ave, Room 130J;
Mail Stop F844
Aurora CO 80045

FLUCKE, Uta
Radboudumc
Geert Groteplein 10
6500 HB Nijmegen

FOGELSTRAND, Linda
Institute of Biomedicine, Sahlgrenska
Academy at University of Gothenburg
Sahlgrenska University Hospital
Bruna Stråket 16
413 45 Gothenburg

FOLPE, Andrew L.
Mayo Clinic
200 1st St SW
Rochester MN 55905

FONSECA, Anil Felix Angelo
Gandhi Medical College/TIMS
Hyderabad, Telangana

FONSECA, Daphne
Basavatarakam Indo American Cancer
Hospital and Research Institute
Banjara Hills
Hyderabad 500034

FONSECA, Isabel
Faculdade de Medicina
Universidade de Lisboa
Av. Prof. Egas Moniz
1649-028 Lisbon

FRAITAG SPINNER, Sylvie
Hôpital Necker-Enfants Malades
149 Rue de Sèvres
75015 Paris

FRAYLING, Ian M.
St Mark's Hospital
Northwick Park
Harrow HA1 3UJ

FRENCH, Christopher A.*
Brigham and Women's Hospital and
Harvard Medical School
New Research Building, Room 630G
77 Ave Louis Pasteur
Boston MA 02115

FRITCHIE, Karen J.
Cleveland Clinic
9500 Euclid Ave
Cleveland OH 44195

FULLER, Gregory N.
University of Texas
MD Anderson Cancer Center
1515 Holcombe Blvd, Unit 85
Houston TX 77030

FULLER, Maren Y.
Baylor College of Medicine /
Texas Children's Hospital
6621 Fannin St, AB195
Houston TX 77030

GALLUZZO, Maria Laura
Hospital de Pediatría Garrahan
Combate de los Pozos 1881
1245 Buenos Aires

GALMICHE, Louise
University Hospital of Nantes
9 Quai Moncousu, Plateau technique 1
44093 Nantes, CEDEX 01

GAMBAROTTI, Marco
Department of Pathology
IRCCS, Istituto Ortopedico Rizzoli
Via di Barbiano, 1/10
40136 Bologna BO

GANESAN, Raji
Birmingham Women's and Children's
NHS Foundation Trust
Mindelsohn Way
Birmingham B15 2TG

GANG, David L.
UMMS-Baystate
759 Chestnut St
Springfield MA 01199

GAULARD, Philippe
Henri Mondor Hospital, Inserm U955
51 Av. du Maréchal de Lattre de Tassigny
94010 Créteil

GELLER, James
Cincinnati Children's Hospital Medical Center
3333 Burnet Ave
Cincinnati OH 45229

GEORGE, Tracy I.*
University of Utah
500 Chipeta Way
Salt Lake City UT 84108

GERAMI, Pedram
Feinberg School of Medicine
Northwestern University
NMH Arkes Family Pavilion, Suite 1600
676 N Saint Clair St
Chicago IL 60611

GESSI, Marco
Fondazione Policlinico Universitario
"Agostino Gemelli" IRCCS
Università Cattolica del Sacro Cuore
Largo Agostino Gemelli, 8
00168 Rome RM

GIANGASPERO, Felice
Policlinico Umberto I, Sapienza University
and IRCCS Neuromed (Pozzilli)
Viale Regina Elena, 324
00161 Rome RM

GIANNINI, Caterina
Mayo Clinic
(and Alma Mater Studiorum -
University of Bologna)
200 1st St SW
Rochester MN 55905

GILBERTSON, Richard James*
University of Cambridge
Li Ka Shing Centre, Robinson Way
Cambridge CB2 0RE

GILL, Anthony J.
Royal North Shore Hospital
Pacific Hwy
St Leonards NSW 2065

---

\* Indicates disclosure of interests (see p. 1034).

GIORDANO, Thomas J.
Michigan Medicine
1150 W Medical Center Dr, 4520 MSRB I
Ann Arbor MI 48109

GOLDMAN-LÉVY, Gabrielle
International Agency for Research on Cancer
25 Av. Tony Garnier, CS 90627
69366 Lyon, CEDEX 07

GONZÁLEZ-PERAMATO, Pilar
Hospital Universitario La Paz, UAM
P.° de la Castellana, 261
28046 Madrid

GRAHAM, Rondell P.
Mayo Clinic
200 1st St SW
Rochester MN 55905

GROSSNIKLAUS, Hans E.
Emory Eye Center
1365 Clifton Rd
Atlanta GA 30322

GUDI, Mihir
KK Women's and Children's Hospital
100 Bukit Timah Rd
Singapore 229899

GUETTIER, Catherine
University Paris-Saclay
Hôpital Bicêtre AP-HP
78 Rue du Général Leclerc
94270 Le Kremlin-Bicêtre

GUJRAL, Sumeet
Tata Memorial Hospital, Mumbai
7, Charak, BPT Hospital Campus,
Wadala East
Mumbai 400037

GUPTA, Anita
Ann and Robert H. Lurie Children's Hospital
of Chicago
225 E Chicago Ave, Box 17
Chicago IL 60611-2605

GUPTA, Kirti
Postgraduate Institute of Medical Education
and Research
5th Floor, A Block (Research)
PGIMER, Sector 12
Chandigarh 160012

GUTMANN, David H.*
Washington University School of Medicine
660 S Euclid Ave, Box 8111
St. Louis MO 63110

GWIN, Katja
UT Southwestern Medical Center
Parkland Memorial Hospital
5201 Harry Hines Blvd, Room 02-621
Dallas TX 75235

HABERLER, Christine
Medical University of Vienna
Währinger Gürtel 18–20
1090 Vienna

HAMEED, Meera
Memorial Sloan Kettering Cancer Center
1275 York Ave
New York NY 10065

HARBOUR, J. William
UT Southwestern Medical Center
5323 Harry Hines Blvd, MC 9057
Dallas TX 75390

HARRIS, Marian H.
Boston Children's Hospital
300 Longwood Ave
Boston MA 02115

HASLE, Henrik
Aarhus University Hospital
Palle Juul-Jensens Blvd 99
8200 Aarhus

HASSELBLATT, Martin
University Hospital Münster
Pottkamp 2
48149 Münster

HAWKINS, Cynthia E.
Hospital for Sick Children
555 University Ave
Toronto ON M5G 1X8

HE, Lejian
Beijing Children's Hospital
56 Nanlishi Rd, Xicheng District
Beijing 100045

HEBEDA, Konnie M.
Radboudumc
Box 9101, r. 812
6500 HB Nijmegen

HELLER, Debra S.
Rutgers New Jersey Medical School
Pathology, 185 S Orange Ave
Newark NJ 07103-2757

HERWIG-CARL, Martina C.
Department of Ophthalmology
University Hospital Bonn
Ernst-Abbe-Straße 2
53127 Bonn

HICKS, M. John
Texas Children's Hospital
Baylor College of Medicine
6621 Fannin St, AB1195
Houston TX 77030

HILL, D. Ashley*
Children's National Hospital
111 Michigan Ave NW
Washington DC 20010

HIROSE, Takanori
Kobe University Graduate School of Medicine
7-5-2 Kusunoki-cho, Chuo-ku,
Hyogo Prefecture
Kobe City 650-0017

HITZLER, Johann Karl
Hospital for Sick Children
University of Toronto
555 University Ave
Toronto ON M5G 1X8

HIYAMA, Eiso
Hiroshima University Hospital
1-2-3 Kasumi, Minami-ku
Hiroshima 734-8551

HOGENDOORN, Pancras C.W.
Leiden University Medical Center
Box 9600
2300 RC Leiden

HORNICK, Jason L.*
Brigham and Women's Hospital
Harvard Medical School
75 Francis St
Boston MA 02115

HOWITT, Brooke E.
Stanford University School of Medicine
Department of Pathology, L235
300 Pasteur Dr
Stanford CA 94305

HUANG, Annie
Hospital for Sick Children
555 University Ave
Toronto ON M5G 1X8

HUANG, Shih-Chiang
Chang Gung Memorial Hospital
No. 5, Fuxing St, Guishan District
Taoyuan City 33305

HUNTSMAN, David G.
University of British Columbia
675 W 10th Ave, Room 4.111
Vancouver BC V5Z 1L3

HUSE, Jason T.
University of Texas
MD Anderson Cancer Center
2130 W Holcombe Blvd
LSP9.4009, Unit 2951
Houston TX 77005

IDBAIH, Ahmed*
Sorbonne Université, AP-HP, Institut du
Cerveau - Paris Brain Institute - ICM, Inserm,
CNRS, Hôpital de la Pitié Salpêtrière, DMU
Neurosciences, Service de Neurologie 2
47-83 Bd de l'Hôpital
75013 Paris

IRVING, Julie A.
University of British Columbia
Royal Jubilee Hospital
1952 Bay St
Victoria BC V8R 1J8

IRWIN, Meredith S.
Hospital for Sick Children
555 University Ave
Toronto ON M5G 1A8

ITO, Masafumi
Japanese Red Cross Nagoya Daiichi Hospital
Aichi Medical Center
3-35 Michishita-cho, Nakamura-ku
Nagoya 453-8511

JABADO, Nada
McGill University
1001 Bd Décarie
Montréal QC H4A 3J1

JACQUES, Thomas S.*
UCL GOS Institute of Child Health
30 Guilford St
London WC1N 1EH

JAMBHEKAR, Nirmala A.
Tata Memorial Hospital
4, Aamrai, Arvind
Vishnunagar, Naupada
Thane West 400 602

JARZEMBOWSKI, Jason A.
Medical College of Wisconsin
8701 W Watertown Plank Rd
Milwaukee WI 53226

JO, Vickie Y.*
Brigham and Women's Hospital and
Harvard Medical School
75 Francis St
Boston MA 02115

JOHN, Ivy
University of Pittsburgh School of Medicine
5230 Centre Ave
Pittsburgh PA 15232

JONES, Chris*
Institute of Cancer Research
15 Cotswold Rd
Sutton SM2 5NG

JONES, David T.W.
Hopp Children's Cancer Center
Heidelberg (KiTZ) and German Cancer
Research Center (DKFZ)
Im Neuenheimer Feld 280
69120 Heidelberg

JUDKINS, Alexander R.*
Children's Hospital Los Angeles and
Keck School of Medicine of USC
4650 Sunset Blvd, Mail Stop #43
Los Angeles CA 90027

KAO, Chia-Sui
Stanford University School of Medicine
300 Pasteur Dr, L235
Department of Pathology
Stanford CA 94305

KARANIAN, Marie
Centre Léon Bérard
28 Rue Laennec
69008 Lyon

KARNEZIS, Anthony N.
UC Davis Medical Center
4400 V St #1234
Sacramento CA 95817

KATABI, Nora
Memorial Sloan Kettering Cancer Center
1275 York Ave
New York NY 10065

KAUR, Kavneet
All India Institute of Medical Sciences
Ansari Nagar
New Delhi 110029

KELSEY, Anna
Royal Manchester Children's Hospital
Oxford Rd
Manchester M13 9WL

KETTELER, Petra
Essen University Hospital
Hufelandstraße 55
45147 Essen

KHOURY, Joseph D.
University of Nebraska Medical Center
985900 Nebraska Medical Center
Omaha NE 68198

KILPATRICK, Scott E.
Cleveland Clinic
9500 Euclid Ave, L25
Cleveland OH 44195

KIMURA, Noriko
National Hospital Organization
Hakodate Hospital
18-16 Kawahara
Hakodate, Hokkaido 041-8512

KIVELÄ, Tero
Helsinki University Central Hospital
Haartmaninkatu 4 C PL220
00029 Helsinki

KLAPPER, Wolfram
Department of Pathology
Hematopathology Section
University Hospital Schleswig-Holstein
Arnold-Heller-Straße 3, Haus U33
24105 Kiel

KLCO, Jeffery M.
St. Jude Children's Research Hospital
262 Danny Thomas Pl
Memphis TN 38105

KLEINSCHMIDT-DeMASTERS, Bette K.
University of Colorado
Anschutz Medical Campus
12605 E 16th Ave, Room 3017
Aurora CO 80045

KLETSKAYA, Iryna S.
Russian Children's Clinical Hospital
Leninskiy Prospekt, 117
Moscow 119571

KLIMSTRA, David S.*
Paige AI
New York NY 10036

KOHASHI, Kenichi
Graduate School of Medical Sciences
Kyushu University
3-1-1 Maidashi, Higashi-ku
Fukuoka 812-8582

KÖLSCHE, Christian
Institute of Pathology
University Hospital Heidelberg
Im Neuenheimer Feld 224
69120 Heidelberg

KOMORI, Takashi
Neuropathology
Tokyo Metropolitan Neurological Hospital
2-6-1 Musashidai, Fuchu
Tokyo 183-0042

KONG, Christina S.
Stanford University
300 Pasteur Dr, Room L235
Stanford CA 94305-5324

---

* Indicates disclosure of interests (see p. 1034).

KOOL, Marcel
German Cancer Research Center (DKFZ)
Im Neuenheimer Feld 280
69120 Heidelberg

KORSHUNOV, Andrey
Neuropathology
German Cancer Research Center (DKFZ)
Im Neuenheimer Feld 280
69120 Heidelberg

KOZAKEWICH, Harry P.
Boston Childen's Hospital
300 Longwood Ave
Boston MA 02115

KRAEMER, Kenneth H.
National Cancer Institute
37 Convent Dr, Building 37, Room 4002
Bethesda MD 20892

KRATZ, Christian P.
Hannover Medical School
Carl-Neuberg-Straße 1
30625 Hannover

KRISHNAN, Chandra
Dell Children's Medical Center
University of Texas - Dell Medical School
4900 Mueller Blvd
Austin TX 78723

KRITSANEEPHAIBOON, Supika
Faculty of Medicine
Prince of Songkla University
15 Kanjanavanich Rd, Kho Hong
Hat Yai 90110

KRUIJFF, Schelto
University Medical Center Groningen
Hanzeplein 1a
9713 GZ Groningen

KUREK, Kyle C.
University of Calgary
3330 Hospital Dr NW, HMRB 262
Calgary AB T2N 4N1

KÜSTERS-VANDEVELDE, Heidi V.
Canisius Wilhelmina Hospital
Weg door Jonkerbos 100
6532 SZ Nijmegen

LA ROSA, Stefano
Unit of Pathology, Department of Medicine
and Technological Innovation
University of Insubria
Via Ottorino Rossi, 9
21100 Varese VA

LAKHANI, Sunil R.
University of Queensland and
Pathology Queensland
Royal Brisbane and Women's Hospital
Herston QLD 4029

LAM, Alfred King-yin
Griffith University School of Medicine and
Dentistry
Gold Coast Campus
Gold Coast QLD 4222

LAMANT-ROCHAIX, Laurence
Institut universitaire du cancer de Toulouse
Oncopole
1 Av. Irène Joliot-Curie
31059 Toulouse

LARSSON, Catharina
Karolinska Institutet
Karolinska University Hospital
BioClinicum J6:20
171 64 Solna

LAX, Sigurd F.
General Hospital Graz II
Medical University of Graz
Göstinger Str. 22
8020 Graz

LAZAR, Alexander J.
University of Texas
MD Anderson Cancer Center
1515 Holcombe Blvd, Unit 85
Houston TX 77030

LE LOARER, François*
Université de Bordeaux and
Institut Bergonié
276 Cr de l'Argonne
33000 Bordeaux

LEE, Anne W.M.
HKU-Shenzhen Hospital and
University of Hong Kong
1/F Professorial Block, Queen Mary Hospital
102 Pok Fu Lam Rd
Hong Kong SAR

LESKE, Henning
Department of Pathology
Rikshospitalet (OUS)
Sognsvannsveien 20
0372 Oslo

LEVENTAKI, Vasiliki
University of Texas
MD Anderson Cancer Center
1515 Holcombe Blvd, Unit 0072
Houston TX 77030

LIEBERMAN, Richard W.*
Michigan Medicine
2800 Plymouth Rd, Building 35
Ann Arbor MI 48109

LIEGL-ATZWANGER, Bernadette
Diagnostic and Research Institute of
Pathology
Medical University Graz
Neue Stiftingtalstraße 6
8010 Graz

LIGON, Keith Lloyd*
Dana-Farber Cancer Institute
Harvard Medical School
450 Brookline Ave, JF215
Boston MA 02215

LIM, Megan*
Memorial Sloan Kettering Cancer Center
1275 York Ave
New York NY 10065

LOH, Mignon
Benioff Children's Hospital
1450 3rd St
San Francisco CA 94143

LOKUHETTY, Dilani
University of Colombo
25 Kynsey Rd
Colombo 00800

LOOIJENGA, Leendert H.J.
Princess Máxima Center for Pediatric
Oncology
Heidelberglaan 25
3584 CS Utrecht

LOPES, Maria Beatriz S.
University of Virginia School of Medicine
1215 Lee St
Charlottesville VA 22908-0214

LÓPEZ-TERRADA, Dolores H.
Texas Children's Hospital
Baylor College of Medicine
6621 Fannin St, Suite AB1.195
Houston TX 77030

LOUGHRAN, Thomas P. Jr*
University of Virginia
1300 Jefferson Park Ave
Charlottesville VA 22903

LOUIS, David N.
Massachusetts General Hospital,
Brigham and Women's Hospital, and
Harvard Medical School
55 Fruit St, Warren 225
Boston MA 02114

LUTHERT, Philip J.
UCL Institute of Ophthalmology
11-43 Bath St
London EC1V 9EL

LUZAR, Boštjan
Institute of Pathology, Medical Faculty
University of Ljubljana
Korytkova Ulica 2
1000 Ljubljana

MAGRO, Gaetano
University of Catania
Via Santa Sofia, 87
95123 Catania CT

MAHAR, Annabelle M.
Royal Prince Alfred Hospital
Missenden Rd
Sydney NSW 2050

MAKHLOUF, Hala R.
National Cancer Institute, NIH
9609 Medical Center Dr
Bethesda MD 20892

MALKIN, David
Hospital for Sick Children
University of Toronto
555 University Ave
Toronto ON M5G 1X8

MALPICA, Anais
University of Texas
MD Anderson Cancer Center
1515 Holcombe Blvd, Unit 085
Houston TX 77030

MARCOGLIESE, Andrea Nicole
Baylor College of Medicine
1 Baylor Plaza
Houston TX 77030

MARGO, Curtis
Morsani College of Medicine
University of South Florida
USF Eye Pathology
13330 USF Laurel Dr 4th Floor
Tampa FL 33612

MARTIGNONI, Guido
University of Verona-Pederzoli Hospital
Piazzale L.A. Scuro, 10
37134 Verona VR

MATOSO, Andres
Johns Hopkins University
401 N Broadway, Room 2242
Baltimore MD 21231-2410

McKENNEY, Jesse K.
Cleveland Clinic
9500 Euclid Ave, L25
Cleveland OH 44195

MENTZEL, Thomas D.W.
Dermatopathologie Bodensee
Siemensstraße 6/1
88048 Friedrichshafen

MESHINCHI, Soheil
Fred Hutchinson Cancer Center
1100 Fairview Ave N
Seattle WA 98109

METE, Ozgur
University Health Network and
University of Toronto
200 Elizabeth St, 11th Floor
Toronto General Hospital
Toronto ON M5G 2C4

MILES, Rodney R.
University of Utah
15 Medical Dr N, E JMRB 2100
Salt Lake City UT 84112

MILLOT, Frédéric
Poitiers University Hospital
2 Rue de la Milétrie
86000 Poitiers

MILMAN, Tatyana
Wills Eye Hospital, Sidney Kimmel Medical
College - Thomas Jefferson University
840 Walnut Street, Suite 1410
Philadelphia PA 19107

MIRKOVIC, Jelena
Sunnybrook Health Sciences Centre
2075 Bayview Ave
Toronto ON M4N 3M5

MOCH, Holger
University of Zurich and
University Hospital Zurich
Schmelzbergstrasse 12
8091 Zurich

MONTES-MORENO, Santiago
Hospital Universitario Marqués de
Valdecilla / IDIVAL
Av. de Valdecilla, 25
39008 Santander

MORITANI, Suzuko
Shiga University of Medical Science
Setatsukinowa-cho
Otsu 520-2192

MOULIN, Alexandre
Jules Gonin Eye Hospital
University of Lausanne
Av. de France 15
1004 Lausanne

MUDHAR, Hardeep Singh
E-Floor, Royal Hallamshire Hospital
Glossop Road
Sheffield S10 2JF

MÜLLER, Hermann L.
University Children's Hospital
Klinikum Oldenburg AöR
Rahel-Straus-Straße 10
26133 Oldenburg

MULLER, Susan
Emory University
Emory Decatur Hospital, 2701 N Decatur Rd
Decatur GA 30033

NAJM, Imad
Cleveland Clinic
9500 Euclid Ave
Cleveland OH 44195

NAKAZAWA, Atsuko
Saitama Children's Medical Center
1-2 Shintoshin, Chuo-ku
Saitama 330-8777

NAVARRO, Samuel
University of Valencia Medical School
Av. de Blasco Ibáñez
46010 Valencia

NELSON, Brenda L.
Naval Medical Center San Diego
34800 Bob Wilson Dr
San Diego CA 92134-5000

NEUMANN, Hartmut P.H.
Albert-Ludwigs-Universität Freiburg
Hugstetter Str. 55
79106 Freiburg

NGA, Min En
Yong Loo Lin School of Medicine
National University of Singapore
5 Lower Kent Ridge Rd
Singapore 119074

NIELSEN, G. Petur
Massachusetts General Hospital
55 Fruit St
Boston MA 02114-2696

NIEMEYER, Charlotte M.*
University Medical Center Freiburg
Mathildenstraße 1
79106 Freiburg

NORTH, Paula E.
Medical College of Wisconsin
8700 Watertown Plank Rd
Milwaukee WI 53226

---

* Indicates disclosure of interests (see p. 1034).

NORTHCOTT, Paul A.
St. Jude Children's Research Hospital
262 Danny Thomas Pl, MS325
Memphis TN 38105-3678

NUCCI, Marisa R.
Brigham and Women's Hospital
Harvard Medical School
75 Francis St
Boston MA 02115

OCHIAI, Atsushi
National Cancer Center
6-5-1 Kashiwanoha
Kashiwa 277-8577

ODA, Yoshinao
Department of Anatomic Pathology
Graduate School of Medical Sciences
Kyushu University
3-1-1 Maidashi, Higashi-ku
Fukuoka 812-8582

ODELL, Edward W.
King's College London
Guy's and St Thomas' NHS Foundation Trust
Floor 4 Tower Wing, Guy's Hospital
London SE1 9RT

OHIKE, Nobuyuki
St. Marianna University School of Medicine
2-16-1 Sugao
Miyamae-ku, Kawasaki
Kanagawa 216-8511

OKITA, Hajime
Keio University School of Medicine
35 Shinanomachi, Shinjuku-ku
Tokyo 160-8582

OLIGNY, Luc Laurier
CHU Sainte-Justine, Université de Montréal
3175 Chem. de la Côte-Sainte-Catherine
Montréal QC H3T 1C5

OLIVA, Esther
Massachusetts General Hospital
55 Fruit St
Boston MA 02114

OLIVEIRA, André M.
Mayo Clinic
200 1st St SW
Rochester MN 55905

OLSON, Timothy S.
Children's Hospital of Philadelphia
3615 Civic Center Blvd
Philadelphia PA 19104

ONCIU, Mihaela
St. Jude Children's Research Hospital
262 Danny Thomas Pl
Memphis TN 38105

OOSTERHUIS, J. Wolter
Erasmus University Medical Center
Box 2040
3000 CA Rotterdam

ORR, Brent A.
St. Jude Children's Research Hospital
262 Danny Thomas Pl
Memphis TN 38105

OSAMURA, Robert Y.
Nippon Koukan Hospital and
Keio University School of Medicine
1-2-1 Koukan-dori, Kawasaki-ku, Kawasaki-shi
Kanagawa 210-0852

OSCHLIES, Ilske
Department of Pathology
Hematopathology Section
University Hospital Schleswig-Holstein
Arnold-Heller-Straße 3, Haus U33
24105 Kiel

OTT, German
Department of Clinical Pathology
Robert-Bosch-Krankenhaus
Auerbachstraße 110
70376 Stuttgart

PAJTLER, Kristian W.
Hopp Children's Cancer Center Heidelberg
(KiTZ), German Cancer Research Center
(DKFZ), and Heidelberg University Hospital
Im Neuenheimer Feld 280
69120 Heidelberg

PANTANOWITZ, Liron
University of Michigan
NCRC Building 35, Room 36-1221-35
2800 Plymouth Rd
Ann Arbor MI 48109-2800

PAPADOGIANNAKIS, Nikos
Karolinska Institutet
Karolinska University Hospital, F46
141 86 Stockholm

PARAFIORITI, Antonina
ASST Centro Specialistico Ortopedico
Traumatologico Gaetano Pini - CTO
Piazza Cardinale Andrea Ferrari, 1
20122 Milan MI

PARHAM, David M.
15 Foxfield Cove
Little Rock AR 72211

PAULUS, Werner
University Hospital Münster
Pottkamp 2
48149 Münster

PAWEL, Bruce R.
Children's Hospital Los Angeles
4650 Sunset Blvd
Los Angeles CA 90027

PE'ER, Jacob
Hadassah – Hebrew University Medical
Center
Box 12000
91120 Jerusalem

PEDEUTOUR, Florence
University of Nice-Côte d'Azur /
Nice University Hospital
28 Av. de Valombrose
06107 Nice

PEKMEZCI, Melike
University of California, San Francisco
505 Parnassus Ave, M551
San Francisco CA 94143

PEREZ-ATAYDE, Antonio R.
Boston Children's Hospital
300 Longwood Ave
Boston MA 02115

PERRY, Arie
University of California, San Francisco
505 Parnassus Ave, M551
San Francisco CA 94143-0102

PEUCHMAUR, Michel
Hôpital universitaire Robert-Debré, AP-HP
Université de Paris
48 Bd Sérurier
75019 Paris

PFISTER, Stefan M.*
Hopp Children's Cancer Center Heidelberg
(KiTZ), German Cancer Research Center
(DKFZ), and Heidelberg University Hospital
Im Neuenheimer Feld 280
69120 Heidelberg

PICARSIC, Jennifer
Cincinnati Children's Hospital Medical Center
3333 Burnet Ave, MLC 1035
Cincinnati OH 45229-3026

PIETSCH, Torsten
University of Bonn Medical Center
Venusberg-Campus 1
53127 Bonn

PITTALUGA, Stefania
Center for Cancer Research
National Cancer Institute
Building 10, Room 2S235A
Bethesda MD 20892-1500

---

* Indicates disclosure of interests (see p. 1034).

PLATE, Karl H.
Frankfurt University Hospital
Theodor-Stern-Kai 7
60590 Frankfurt am Main

PRASAD, Manju Lata
Yale School of Medicine
310 Cedar St, Box 208023
New Haven CT 06520-8023

PREUSSER, Matthias*
Medical University of Vienna
Währinger Gürtel 18–20
1097 Vienna

PRITCHARD-JONES, Kathy
University College London
UCL Great Ormond Street Institute of Child
Health
30 Guilford St
London WC1N 1EH

PULS, Florian
Sahlgrenska University Hospital
Gula Stråket 8
413 46 Gothenburg

QUINTANILLA-MARTINEZ, Leticia
University Hospital Tübingen
Eberhard Karls University of Tübingen
Liebermeisterstraße 8
72076 Tübingen

RAMASWAMY, Vijay
Hospital for Sick Children and
University of Toronto
555 University Ave
Toronto ON M5G 1X8

RANGANATHAN, Sarangarajan
Cincinnati Children's Hospital Medical Center
3333 Burnet Ave, MLC 1035
Cincinnati OH 45229

RANGASWAMI, Arun
University of California, San Francisco
550 16th St, 4th Floor
(Pediatric Hematology-Oncology)
San Francisco CA 94158

RAO, B. Vishal
Basavatarakam Indo American Cancer
Hospital and Research Institute
Road No. 10, Banjara Hills
Hyderabad 500034

REIFENBERGER, Guido
Heinrich Heine University Düsseldorf
Moorenstraße 5
40225 Düsseldorf

REKHI, Bharat
Tata Memorial Centre, HBNI University
Dr Ernest Borges Rd, Parel
Mumbai, Maharashtra 400012

REUSS, David Emanuel*
Heidelberg University and
German Cancer Research Center (DKFZ)
Im Neuenheimer Feld 224
69120 Heidelberg

REYES-MÚGICA, Miguel
University of Pittsburgh School of Medicine
UPMC Children's Hospital of Pittsburgh
4401 Penn Ave, Main Hospital B260
One Children's Hospital Drive
Pittsburgh PA 15224

RICHARDSON, Mary S.
Children's Hospital
Medical University of South Carolina
165 Ashley Ave, Room EH303D4
Charleston SC 29425

RIGHI, Alberto
IRCCS, Istituto Ortopedico Rizzoli
Via di Barbiano, 1/10
40136 Bologna BO

ROBERTS, Irene A.G.
University of Oxford
MRC Weatherall Institute of Molecular
Medicine
John Radcliffe Hospital
Oxford OX3 9DS

RODRIGUEZ, Fausto J.
David Geffen School of Medicine at UCLA
10833 Le Conte Ave, CHS 18-170B
Los Angeles CA 90095

ROSENBERG, Andrew E.
Miller School of Medicine
University of Miami
1400 NW 12th Ave
Miami FL 33136

ROSENBLUM, Marc K.
Memorial Sloan Kettering Cancer Center
1275 York Ave
New York NY 10021

ROSSI, Esther D.
Fondazione Policlinico Universitario Agostino
Gemelli IRCCS
Largo Agostino Gemelli
00168 Rome RM

ROSSI, Sabrina
Bambino Gesù Children's Hospital
Piazza Sant'Onofrio, 4
00165 Rome RM

ROTONDO, Fabio
St. Michael's Hospital
30 Bond St
Toronto ON M5B 1W8

ROUS, Brian
NHS Digital
Victoria House, Capital Park
Fulbourn, Cambridge CB21 5XA

ROY, Angshumoy
Baylor College of Medicine
Texas Children's Hospital
1102 Bates Ave, FC830
Houston TX 77030

RUDÀ, Roberta
University of Turin and
City of Health and Science Hospital, Turin
Via Cherasco, 15
10126 Turin TO

RUDZINSKI, Erin R.
Seattle Children's Hospital
4800 Sand Point Way NE
Seattle WA 98105

SAGOO, Mandeep S.
UCL Institute of Ophthalmology /
Moorfields Eye Hospital
162 City Rd
London EC1V 2PD

SAHM, Felix*
Heidelberg University and
German Cancer Research Center (DKFZ)
Im Neuenheimer Feld 224
69120 Heidelberg

SAID, Jonathan William
David Geffen School of Medicine
10833 Le Conte Ave
Los Angeles CA 90095

SALGADO, Claudia M.
University of Pittsburgh School of Medicine
UPMC Children's Hospital of Pittsburgh
4401 Penn Ave, B258
Pittsburgh PA 15224

SANDER, Christian A.
Asklepios Klinik St. Georg
Lohmühlenstraße 5
20099 Hamburg

SANGUEZA, J. Martin
Hospital Obrero No. 1 CNS, Hospital General
Av. 6 de Agosto 2700, Edificio Torre Cadeco
6541 La Paz

SANGÜEZA, Omar P.
Wake Forest University School of Medicine
Medical Center Blvd
Winston-Salem NC 27157-1072

* Indicates disclosure of interests (see p. 1034).

SANTAGATA, Sandro
Brigham and Women's Hospital
60 Fenwood Rd, Hale 8002P
Boston MA 02115

SANTOSH, Vani
National Institute of Mental Health and
Neurosciences
Hosur Rd
Bengaluru 560029

SARKAR, Chitra
All India Institute of Medical Sciences
Ansari Nagar
New Delhi 110029

SARTELET, Herve
CHRU de Nancy
Rue du Morvan
54511 Vandoeuvre-lès-Nancy

SAXENA, Romil*
Emory University
1364 Clifton Rd NE, Room H182-A
Atlanta GA 30322

SCHMITT, Fernando
CINTESIS@RISE (Health Research Network);
Medical Faculty of the University of Porto;
Molecular Pathology Unit, Ipatimup
Rua Júlio Amaral de Carvalho 45
4200-135 Porto

SCHNEIDER, Dominik T.
Clinic of Pediatrics
Beurhausstraße 40
44137 Dortmund

SCHUHMANN, Martin Ulrich
University Hospital Tübingen
Hoppe-Seyler-Straße 3
72076 Tübingen

SCHÜLLER, Ulrich
University of Hamburg
Martinistraße 52
20246 Hamburg

SCHULTZ, Kris Ann P.
International PPB/DICER1 Registry
Cancer and Blood Disorders
Children's Minnesota
2530 Chicago Ave S
Minneapolis MN 55404

SCOLYER, Richard A.*
Royal Prince Alfred Hospital;
Melanoma Institute Australia; and
University of Sydney
Missenden Rd, Camperdown
Sydney NSW 2050

SEETHALA, Raja
UPMC Presbyterian Hospital
200 Lothrop St, Room A614
Pittsburgh PA 15213

SHARMA, Mehar C.
All India Institute of Medical Sciences
Ansari Nagar
New Delhi 110029

SHIMADA, Hiroyuki
Stanford University
300 Pasteur Dr
Stanford CA 94305

SHIMAMURA, Akiko
Dana-Farber/Boston Children's Cancer and
Blood Disorders Center
1 Blackfan Cir, Karp 8210
Boston MA 02115

SHIN, Sandra J.
Albany Medical College
47 New Scotland Ave
Albany NY 12208

SINGH, Rajendra
Northwell Health
1991 Marcus Ave, Suite 300
Lake Success NY 11042

SINGH, Vivekanand
University of Texas Southwestern
5323 Harry Hines Blvd
Dallas TX 75390

SINGHI, Aatur D.
University of Pittsburgh Medical Center
200 Lothrop St, Scaife Hall A616.2
Pittsburgh PA 15213

SNUDERL, Matija
NYU Langone Health
240 E 38th St, 22nd Floor
New York NY 10016

SOARES, Fernando Augusto
Rede D'Or Hospitals
Rua das Perobas, 266
São Paulo SP 04321-120

SOLARY, Eric*
Gustave Roussy
114 Rue Edouard Vaillant
94805 Villejuif

SOLOMON, David A.
University of California, San Francisco
513 Parnassus Ave, HSW 451
San Francisco CA 94143

SOMERS, Gino Rene
University of Toronto
Hospital for Sick Children
555 University Ave
Toronto ON M5G 1X8

SPUNT, Sheri L.*
Stanford University School of Medicine
1000 Welch Rd, Suite 300, MC 5798
Palo Alto CA 94304

SREDNI, Simone T.*
Ann and Robert H. Lurie Children's Hospital
of Chicago
225 E Chicago Ave
Chicago IL 60611

SRIGLEY, John R.
University of Toronto
Trillium Health Partners
2200 Eglinton Ave W
Mississauga ON L5M 2N1

STELIAROVA-FOUCHER, Eva
International Agency for Research on Cancer
25 Av. Tony Garnier, CS 90627
69366 Lyon, CEDEX 07

STELOW, Edward B.
University of Virginia School of Medicine
Box 800214
Charlottesville VA 22908-0214

STEMMER-RACHAMIMOV, Anat Olga
Massachusetts General Hospital
55 Fruit St
Boston MA 02114

STEWART, Colin J.R.
King Edward Memorial Hospital
Bagot Rd
Perth WA 6008

STONEHAM, Sara J.
University College Hospitals London
250 Euston Rd
London NW1 2PG

STURM, Dominik
Hopp Children's Cancer Center Heidelberg
(KiTZ), German Cancer Research Center
(DKFZ), and Heidelberg University Hospital
Im Neuenheimer Feld 280
69120 Heidelberg

SURREY, Lea F.
Children's Hospital of Philadelphia
3401 Civic Center Blvd
Philadelphia PA 19104

SUTTORP, Meinolf
Faculty of Medicine, TU Dresden
Fiedlerstraße 74
01307 Dresden

---

* Indicates disclosure of interests (see p. 1034).

SUURMEIJER, Albert J.H.
University Medical Center Groningen
Hanzeplein 1
9700 RB Groningen

SUVÀ, Mario L.*
Massachusetts General Hospital
149 13th St, Office 6.010
Boston MA 02129

TABORI, Uri*
Hospital for Sick Children
555 University Ave
Toronto ON M5G 1X8

TAN, Geok Chin
Universiti Kebangsaan Malaysia
Jalan Yaacob Latif, Bandar Tun Razak
56000 Kuala Lumpur

TAN, Puay Hoon
Division of Pathology
Singapore General Hospital
20 College Rd, Academia, Level 7
Diagnostics Tower
Singapore 169856

TANAKA, Yukichi
Kanagawa Children's Medical Center
2-138-4 Mutsukawa, Minami Ward
Yokohama 232-8555

TAY, Timothy Kwang Yong
Department of Anatomical Pathology
Singapore General Hospital
20 College Rd
Academia, Level 10, Diagnostics Tower
Singapore 169856

TAYLOR, Michael D.
Texas Children's Hospital
Baylor College of Medicine
1102 Bates Ave
Houston TX 77030

THOMPSON, Lester D.R.
Head and Neck Pathology Consultations
22543 Ventura Blvd, Ste 22, PMB1034
Woodland Hills CA 91364

THWAY, Khin
Royal Marsden Hospital /
Institute of Cancer Research
203 Fulham Rd
London SW3 6JJ

TIHAN, Tarik
University of California, San Francisco
Helen Diller Family Comprehensive Cancer
Center
505 Parnassus Ave, Moffitt
San Francisco CA 94143-0511

TIRABOSCO, Roberto
Royal National Orthopaedic Hospital
Brockley Hill
Stanmore, London HA7 4LP

TISCHLER, Arthur S.
Tufts Medical Center
800 Washington St, Box 802
Boston MA 02111

TOLEDO, Rodrigo Almeida
Vall d'Hebron Institute of Oncology (VHIO)
Centro Cellex, Carrer de Natzaret, 115-117
08035 Barcelona

TOMLINSON, Gail E.
UT Health San Antonio
7703 Floyd Curl Dr
Dallas TX 78229

TONINI, Gian Paolo
Pediatric Research Institute
Corso Stati Uniti, 4
35127 Padua PD

TORNÓCZKY, Tamás
University of Pécs
Medical School and Clinical Centre
Szigeti út 12
Pécs 7625

TORRELO, Antonio
Hospital Infantil Universitario Niño Jesús
Av. de Menéndez Pelayo, 65
28009 Madrid

TSAO, Ming Sound
University Health Network
200 Elizabeth St, 11th Floor
Toronto ON M5G 2C4

TSUI, Wilson M.
Caritas Medical Centre
Wing Hong St, Shamshuipo
Kowloon, Hong Kong SAR

TSUZUKI, Toyonori
Aichi Medical University Hospital
1-1 Yazakokarimata
Nagakute 480-1195

ULBRIGHT, Thomas M.
Indiana University School of Medicine
350 W 11th St, Room 4014
Indianapolis IN 46202

USUBUTUN, Alp
Hacettepe University Medical School
Hacettepe Üniversitesi Tıp Fakültesi
Patoloji AD, Sıhhıye
06100 Ankara

VAN DER VALK, Paul
VUmc University Medical Center
Postbus 7057
1007 MB Amsterdam

VANG, Russell
Johns Hopkins Hospital
401 N Broadway
Weinberg Building, Room 2242
Baltimore MD 21231

VARGAS, Sara O.*
Boston Children's Hospital and
Harvard Medical School
300 Longwood Ave
Boston MA 02115

VARLET, Pascale
GHU Paris, Site Hôpital Sainte-Anne
1 Rue Cabanis
75014 Paris

VASILJEVIC, Alexandre
Groupement Hospitalier Est
59 Bd Pinel
69677 Bron, CEDEX

VENNETI, Sriram
University of Michigan
1150 W Medical Center Dr
3520E MSRB 1
Ann Arbor MI 48109

VERDIJK, Robert M.
Erasmus University Medical Center; and
Department of Pathology,
Leiden University Medical Center
Box 2040
3000 CA Rotterdam

VERMEER, Maarten H.
Leiden University Medical Center
Albinusdreef 2, Room B1-Q93
2333 ZA Leiden

VILLA, Chiara
Institut Cochin
24 Rue du Faubourg Saint-Jacques
75014 Paris

VOKUHL, Christian
Section of Pediatric Pathology
University of Bonn
Venusberg-Campus 1
53127 Bonn

VOLANTE, Marco
University of Turin, San Luigi Hospital
Regione Gonzole, 10
10043 Orbassano TO

---

\* Indicates disclosure of interests (see p. 1034).

**VON DEIMLING, Andreas\***
Heidelberg University and
German Cancer Research Center (DKFZ)
Im Neuenheimer Feld 224
69120 Heidelberg

**VON HOFF, Katja**
Charité – Universitätsmedizin Berlin
Augustenburger Platz 1
13353 Berlin

**VORTMEYER, Alexander Oliver**
Indiana University–Purdue University
Indianapolis
350 W 11th St
Indianapolis IN 46202

**VUJANIC, Gordan M.**
Sidra Medicine /
Weill Cornell Medicine - Qatar
Al Luqta St, Box 26999
Doha

**WANG, Larry Liang**
Children's Hospital Los Angeles
University of Southern California
4650 Sunset Blvd
Los Angeles CA 90027

**WANG, Lisa L.**
Baylor College of Medicine
1102 Bates Ave, Suite 1200
Houston TX 77030

**WANG, Wei-Lien**
University of Texas
MD Anderson Cancer Center
1515 Holcombe Blvd
Unit 085, Room B3.4611
Houston TX 77030

**WARREN, Katherine E.\***
Dana-Farber/Boston Children's Cancer and
Blood Disorders Center
450 Brookline Ave, DANA 3154
Boston MA 02215

**WASHINGTON, Mary K.**
Vanderbilt University Medical Center
C-3321 MCN
Nashville TN 37232

**WATANABE, Reiko**
National Cancer Center Hospital East
6-5-1 Kashiwanoha, Kashiwa-shi
Chiba 277-8577

**WEIGELT, Britta\***
Memorial Sloan Kettering Cancer Center
1275 York Ave
New York NY 10065

**WELLER, Michael\***
Department of Neurology
University Hospital Zurich and
University of Zurich
Frauenklinikstrasse 26
8091 Zurich

**WESSELING, Pieter**
Princess Máxima Center for Pediatric
Oncology, Utrecht, and
Amsterdam University Medical Centers/VUmc
De Boelelaan 1117
1081 HV Amsterdam

**WHITE, Valerie A.**
International Agency for Research on Cancer
25 Av. Tony Garnier, CS 90627
69366 Lyon, CEDEX 07

**WILLIAMS, Michelle D.**
University of Texas
MD Anderson Cancer Center
1515 Holcombe Blvd, Unit 085
Houston TX 77030

**WILLIAMSON, Sean R.**
Cleveland Clinic
9500 Euclid Ave, L25
Cleveland OH 44195

**WONG, Ivan Y.C.**
Radiology Department, Tuen Mun Hospital
Tuen Mun

Hong Kong SAR

**WONG, Richard Wing-Cheuk**
United Christian Hospital
130 Hip Wo St, Kwun Tong
Hong Kong SAR

**WONG, Tai-Tong**
Taipei Medical University Hospital
Taipei Medical University
250 Wu-Hsing St
Taipei City 110

**WOOD, Brent Lee\***
Children's Hospital Los Angeles
4650 Sunset Blvd
Los Angeles CA 90027

**XU, Bin**
Memorial Sloan Kettering Cancer Center
1275 York Ave
New York NY 10065

**YOSHIDA, Akihiko**
National Cancer Center Hospital
5-1-1 Tsukiji, Chuo-ku
Tokyo 104-0045

**ZAGZAG, David**
NYU Langone Health and
NYU Grossman School of Medicine
550 1st Ave
New York NY 10016

**ZAMBRANO, Eduardo**
University of Pittsburgh Medical Center
UPMC Children's Hospital of Pittsburgh
One Children's Hospital Drive
Pittsburgh PA 15224

**ZERBINI, Maria Claudia Nogueira**
University of São Paulo Medical School
Av. Dr. Arnaldo, 455
São Paulo SP 01246-903

* Indicates disclosure of interests (see p. 1034).

# Declaration of interests

**Dr Asa** reports serving on the medical advisory boards of Leica Biosystems and Ibex Medical Analytics, receiving honoraria from Med Learning Group, and having received personal consultancy fees from Iron Mountain and PathAI.

**Dr Bandopadhayay** reports that her unit at Dana-Farber/Boston Children's Cancer and Blood Disorders Center benefits from research funding from Novartis.

**Dr Bastian** reports having provided expert testimony in relation to melanoma-related litigation.

**Dr Capper** reports being a cofounder and stakeholder of Heidelberg Epignostix GmbH, and receiving royalties for the patents on "Means and methods for diagnosing cancer using an antibody which specifically binds to BRAF V600E" and "Methods for the diagnosis and the prognosis of a brain tumor".

**Dr Chang** reports that his unit at KK Women's and Children's Hospital benefited from non-monetary research support from FoundationOne CDx.

**Dr J.L. Davis** reports receiving personal consultancy fees from Bayer Pharmaceuticals in her capacity as a scientific advisory board member.

**Dr Dishop** reports that she receives personal consultancy fees from Boehringer Ingelheim in her capacity as a disease review committee member.

**Dr Doz** reports participating in a project with Laboratoires Synth-Innove about developing photodynamic therapy for retinoblastoma.

**Dr French** reports receiving personal consultancy fees from Boehringer Ingelheim, and that his unit at Brigham and Women's Hospital and Harvard Medical School benefits from research funding from Boehringer Ingelheim.

**Dr George** reports receiving personal consultancy fees and travel support from Blueprint Medicines; receiving personal consultancy fees from Cogent Biosciences, Celgene/BMS, and Incyte Corporation; and having received honoraria from Novartis.

**Dr Gilbertson** reports holding a patent on an antibody against RELA fusion, licensed to the University of Cambridge and AstraZeneca.

**Dr Gutmann** reports holding a patent on "Neurofibromatosis gene", filed by the University of Michigan.

**Dr Hill** reports having a commercial interest in ResourcePath in her capacity as owner and medical director.

**Dr Hornick** reports having received personal consultancy fees from Aadi Bioscience, Tracon Pharmaceuticals, and Adaptimmune.

**Dr Idbaih** reports that his institution ICM benefits from research funding from Carthera, Transgene, Sanofi, Nutritheragene, and Servier; having received personal consultancy fees from LEO Pharma, Novocure, Novartis, and Boehringer Ingelheim; and having received personal consultancy fees for meetings from Enterome and Carthera.

**Dr Jacques** reports holding shares in Repath Ltd and Neuropath Ltd in his capacity as director, and being editor-in-chief of the journal *Neuropathology and Applied Neurobiology*.

**Dr Jo** reports that her spouse is a salaried employee of Merck & Co.

**Dr C. Jones** reports that his unit at the Institute of Cancer Research benefited from research funding from Hoffmann-La Roche.

**Dr Judkins** reports that his unit at Children's Hospital Los Angeles and the Keck School of Medicine of USC benefits from research funding from Epizyme.

**Dr Klimstra** reports being a founder, employee, and equity holder in Paige AI.

**Dr Le Loarer** reports receiving personal consultancy fees from Blueprint Medicines and AstraZeneca.

**Dr Lieberman** reports that his unit at Michigan Medicine benefits from research support from Inovio Pharmaceuticals.

**Dr Ligon** reports that his unit at Dana-Farber Cancer Institute benefits from research funding from Bristol Myers Squibb, Amgen, and Lilly; having received personal consultancy fees from Bristol Myers Squibb, IntegraGen, BroadBranch, and RareCyte; and holding equity shares in Travera in his capacity as a cofounder.

**Dr Lim** reports being a founding partner of Genomenon; holding patent US20150050274A1; and having provided expert testimony in relation to litigations on lymphoma diagnoses; and that her former unit at the University of Pennsylvania benefits from research funding from Thermo Fisher Scientific.

**Dr Loughran** reports holding shares in Kymera Therapeutics, Dren Bio, Recludix Pharma, Flagship Labs 86, and Keystone Nano in his capacity as a scientific advisory board member.

**Dr Niemeyer** reports having received personal consultancy fees from Celgene / Bristol Myers Squibb in her capacity as a steering committee member.

**Dr Pfister** reports that his unit at the German Cancer Research Center (DKFZ) partners with the Innovative Medicine Initiative (IMI), grant number 116064, and that he is interim CEO of the not-for-profit organization ITCC-P4, the sustainability platform of the IMI project. He also reports being a cofounder and stakeholder of Heidelberg Epignostix GmbH, and holding patent EP3067432A1 on DNA methylation–based tumour classification.

**Dr Preusser** reports having received honoraria for lectures, consultation, or advisory board participation from Bayer, Bristol Myers Squibb, Novartis, Gerson Lehrman Group (GLG), CMC Contrast, GlaxoSmithKline, Mundipharma, Roche, BMJ Journals, MedMedia Group, AstraZeneca, AbbVie, Lilly, Medahead, Daiichi Sankyo, Sanofi, Merck Sharp & Dohme, Tocagen, Adastra, Gan & Lee Pharmaceuticals, and Servier.

**Dr Reuss** reports that his unit at Heidelberg University and the German Cancer Research Center (DKFZ) holds a patent on NF1 antibody clone NFC, licensed to Cell Marque Corporation.

**Dr Sahm** reports being a cofounder and stakeholder of Heidelberg Epignostix GmbH.

**Dr Saxena** reports receiving personal consultancy fees from Arrowhead Pharmaceuticals and Perspectum.

Dr **Scolyer** reports receiving fees for professional services from MetaOptima Technology, F. Hoffmann-La Roche, Evaxion Biotech, Provectus Biopharmaceuticals Australia, QBiotics, Novartis, Merck Sharp & Dohme, NeraCare, Amgen, Bristol Myers Squibb, Myriad Genetics, and GlaxoSmithKline.

Dr **Solary** reports that his unit at Gustave Roussy benefited from research funding from Servier.

Dr **Spunt** reports that her unit at Stanford University School of Medicine has benefited from research funding from Hoffmann-La Roche, Novartis, Sanofi US Services, Loxo Oncology, Incyte Corporation, Bristol Myers Squibb, and Pfizer, and her unit benefits from research funding from Bayer Healthcare Pharmaceuticals.

Dr **Sredni** reports that her unit at Ann and Robert H. Lurie Children's Hospital of Chicago benefited from non-monetary support from Thermo Fisher Scientific.

Dr **Suvà** reports being a scientific cofounder, equity holder, and advisory board member of Immunitas Therapeutics.

Dr **Tabori** reports that his unit at the Hospital for Sick Children benefits from research funding from Bristol Myers Squibb.

Dr **Vargas** reports receiving personal consultancy fees from MilliporeSigma and Vertex Pharmaceuticals, and that she has provided expert testimony pertaining to paediatric and pulmonary pathology.

Dr **von Deimling** reports that his units at Heidelberg University and the German Cancer Research Center (DKFZ) hold patents on IDH antibody clone H09, licensed to Dianova (EP09006620, EP09015511); on BRAF antibody VE1, licensed to Roche (EP11767970); and on DNA methylation–based methods for tumour classification (EP16710700, EP15158660).

Dr **Warren** reports having received fees for advisory board work from Day One Therapeutics and GSK, and that she has received clinical trial support from Celgene/BMS.

Dr **Weigelt** reports that her laboratory at Memorial Sloan Kettering Cancer Center receives research funding from Repare Therapeutics.

Dr **Weller** reports having received personal consultancy fees and remuneration for advisory board participation from Bayer, CureVac, Medac, Novartis, Novocure, Orbus Therapeutics, Philogen, Roche, and Sandoz; and that his institute has received research grants from Quercis Pharma and Versameb.

Dr **Wood** reports receiving personal consultancy fees from Amgen and Beckman Coulter, and that his unit at Children's Hospital Los Angeles benefits from research funding from Novartis, Amgen, MacroGenics, BioSight, and Kite Pharma.

# IARC/WHO Committee for the International Classification of Diseases for Oncology (ICD-O)

**BRAY, Freddie**
International Agency for Research on Cancer
25 Av. Tony Garnier, CS 90627
69366 Lyon, CEDEX 07

**CREE, Ian A.**
International Agency for Research on Cancer
25 Av. Tony Garnier, CS 90627
69366 Lyon, CEDEX 07

**FERLAY, Jacques**
International Agency for Research on Cancer
25 Av. Tony Garnier, CS 90627
69366 Lyon, CEDEX 07

**GOLDMAN-LÉVY, Gabrielle**
International Agency for Research on Cancer
25 Av. Tony Garnier, CS 90627
69366 Lyon, CEDEX 07

**JAKOB, Robert**
Classifications and Terminologies
World Health Organization (WHO)
Av. Appia 20
1211 Geneva

**KRPELANOVA, Eva**
Classifications and Terminologies
World Health Organization (WHO)
Av. Appia 20
1211 Geneva

**LOKUHETTY, Dilani**
University of Colombo
25 Kynsey Rd
Colombo 00800

**ROUS, Brian**
NHS Digital
Victoria House, Capital Park
Fulbourn, Cambridge CB21 5XA

**WATANABE, Reiko**
National Cancer Center Hospital East
6-5-1 Kashiwanoha, Kashiwa-shi
Chiba 277-8577

**WHITE, Valerie A.**
International Agency for Research on Cancer
25 Av. Tony Garnier, CS 90627
69366 Lyon, CEDEX 07

**ZNAOR, Ariana**
International Agency for Research on Cancer
25 Av. Tony Garnier, CS 90627
69366 Lyon, CEDEX 07

# Sources

**TNM staging tables**

## Figures

| | |
|---|---|
| 1.01 | Steliarova-Foucher E; and Ferlay J, Ervik M, Lam F, et al. Global Cancer Observatory: Cancer Today [Internet]. Lyon (France): International Agency for Research on Cancer; 2020. Available from: https://gco.iarc.fr/today; and Adapted, with permission, from: Piñeros M, Mery L, Soerjomataram I, et al. Scaling up the surveillance of childhood cancer: a global roadmap. J Natl Cancer Inst. 2021 Jan 4;113(1):9–15. PMID:32433739. |
| 1.02 | Steliarova-Foucher E; and Adapted, with permission, from: Piñeros M, Mery L, Soerjomataram I, et al. Scaling up the surveillance of childhood cancer: a global roadmap. J Natl Cancer Inst. 2021 Jan 4;113(1):9–15. PMID:32433739. |
| 1.03A,B | Adapted, with permission from Elsevier, from: Steliarova-Foucher E, Colombet M, |

| | |
|---|---|
| | Ries LAG, et al. International incidence of childhood cancer, 2001-10: a population-based registry study. Lancet Oncol. 2017 Jun;18(6):719–31. PMID:28410997. |
| 2.01 | Suttorp M |
| 2.02A,C | Millot F |
| 2.02B | Sabrina Bouyer, Laboratoire d'hématologie, CHU de Poitiers Site de la Milétrie, Poitiers |
| 2.03 | Hans-Heinrich Kreipe, Department of Pathology, Hannover Medical School, Hannover |
| 2.04A,B | Niemeyer CM |
| 2.05 | Adapted, with permission, from: Niemeyer CM. JMML genomics and decisions. Hematology Am Soc Hematol Educ Program. 2018 Nov 30;2018(1):307–12. PMID:30504325. |
| 2.06A–C | Niemeyer CM |
| 2.07A–C | Niemeyer CM |
| 2.08A,B | Rudelius M, Weinberg OK, Niemeyer CM, et al. The International Consensus Classification (ICC) of hematologic neoplasms with germline predisposition, |

| | |
|---|---|
| | pediatric myelodysplastic syndrome, and juvenile myelomonocytic leukemia. Virchows Arch. 2023 Jan;482(1):113–30. PMID:36445482. |
| 2.09 | Ayami Yoshimi-Nöllke, EWOG-MDS/SAA Studienzentrale, University Medical Center Freiburg, Zentrum für Kinder- und Jugendmedizin Klinik IV: Pädiatrische Hämatologie und Onkologie, Freiburg |
| 2.10 | Marcogliese AN |
| 2.11 | Klco JM |
| 2.12 | Marcogliese AN |
| 2.13 | Meshinchi S |
| 2.14 | Fogelstrand L |
| 2.15A–C | Leonie Saft, Department of Clinical Pathology and Cancer Diagnostics, Karolinska University Hospital, Solna, Stockholm |
| 2.16 | Fogelstrand L |
| 2.17A,B | Fogelstrand L |
| 2.18A–C | Fogelstrand L |
| 2.19 | Fogelstrand L |
| 2.20 | Fogelstrand L |
| 2.21A–D | Kratz CP |
| 2.22A–C | Kratz CP |
| 2.23 | Adapted, with permission, from: Behrens YL, Göhring |

| | |
|---|---|
| | G, Bawadi R, et al. A novel classification of hematologic conditions in patients with Fanconi anemia. Haematologica. 2021 Nov 1;106(11):3000–3. PMID:34196171. |
| 2.24A–D | Rita De Vito, Pathology Unit, Department of Laboratories, Bambino Gesù Children's Hospital, Rome |
| 2.25A,B | Roberts IAG |
| 2.26 | Colmenero I |
| 2.27A | Colmenero I |
| 2.27B | Torrelo A |
| 2.28 | Torrelo A |
| 2.29A–C | George TI |
| 2.30A–D | George TI |
| 2.31 | Reprinted, with permission, from: Carter MC, Bai Y, Ruiz-Esteves KN, et al. Detection of KIT D816V in peripheral blood of children with manifestations of cutaneous mastocytosis suggests systemic disease. Br J Haematol. 2018 Dec;183(5):775–82. PMID:30488427. |
| 2.32A,B | Colmenero I |
| 2.33A–C | George TI |
| 2.34A–C | George TI |
| 2.35 | Leventaki V |
| 2.36 | Leventaki V |
| 2.37 | Choi JK |
| 2.38A | Leventaki V |
| 2.38B | Choi JK |
| 2.39A,B | Leventaki V |
| 2.40 | Choi JK |
| 2.41 | Leventaki V |
| 2.42A,C | Chu WCW |
| 2.42B | Birgit Burkhardt, Experimentelle und Translationale päd. Hämatologie u Onkologie, Leitung der Bereiche Lymphome und Stammzelltransplantation, Universitätsklinikum Münster (UKM), Klinik für Kinder- und Jugendmedizin, Pädiatrische Hämatologie und Onkologie, Munich |
| 2.43A,B | Klapper W |
| 2.44A,B | Klapper W |
| 2.45 | Klapper W |

| | |
|---|---|
| 2.46A,B | Oschlies I |
| 2.47A–C | Oschlies I |
| 2.48A,B | Oschlies I |
| 2.49A–D | Pittaluga S |
| 2.50A,B | Oschlies I |
| 2.51A,B | Oschlies I |
| 2.52 | Klapper W |
| 2.53A,B | Oschlies I |
| 2.54A,B | Oschlies I |
| 2.55A,B | Oschlies I |
| 2.56 | Oschlies I |
| 2.57A–F | Di Napoli A |
| 2.58A,B | Di Napoli A |
| 2.59A,D | d'Amore ESG |
| 2.59B,C | Lamant-Rochaix L |
| 2.60A–D | Pittaluga S |
| 2.61A,B | Montes-Moreno S |
| 2.62A–D | Montes-Moreno S |
| 2.63A,B | Montes-Moreno S |
| 2.64A,B | d'Amore ESG |
| 2.65A–F | d'Amore ESG |
| 2.66 | Chu WCW |
| 2.67A | Oschlies I |
| 2.67B–D | Klapper W |
| 2.68A–D | Klapper W |
| 2.69 | Klapper W |
| 2.70 | Alaggio R |
| 2.71 | Klapper W |
| 2.72 | Klapper W |
| 2.73A,B | Klapper W |
| 2.74 | Klapper W |
| 2.75 | Chan JKC |
| 2.76 | Chan JKC |
| 2.77A–D | Chan JKC |
| 2.78A,B | Chan JKC |
| 2.79A–E | d'Amore ESG |
| 2.80A–C | d'Amore ESG |
| 2.81A–E | d'Amore ESG |
| 2.82A | Sander CA |
| 2.82B,C | Alaggio R |
| 2.83A,B | Alaggio R |
| 2.84 | Sander CA |
| 2.85A–D | Alaggio R |
| 2.86A,B | d'Amore ESG |
| 2.86C | Alaggio R |
| 2.87A–C | Lamant-Rochaix L |
| 2.88 | Lamant-Rochaix L |
| 2.89 | Lamant-Rochaix L |
| 2.90A,B | Lamant-Rochaix L |
| 2.91A–D | Lamant-Rochaix L |
| 2.92 | Lamant-Rochaix L |
| 2.93A–C | Joaquín Carrillo-Farga, Institute of Hematopathology, Querétaro |
| 2.94A–D | Quintanilla-Martinez L |

| | |
|---|---|
| 2.95A | Reprinted, with permission, from: Jaffe E, Arber D, Campo E, et al., editors. Hematopathology. 2nd ed. Philadelphia (PA): Elsevier; 2016. Copyright Elsevier 2016. |
| 2.95B | Quintanilla-Martinez L |
| 2.96A–C | Kim WY, Montes-Mojarro IA, Fend F, et al. Epstein-Barr virus-associated T and NK-cell lymphoproliferative diseases. Front Pediatr. 2019 Mar 15;7:71. PMID:30931288. https://creativecommons.org/licenses/by/4.0/ |
| 2.96D | Quintanilla-Martinez L |
| 2.97A–D | Quintanilla-Martinez L |
| 2.98 | Sangueza JM |
| 2.99 | Sangueza JM |
| 2.100A,B | Sangueza JM |
| 2.101 | Sangueza JM |
| 2.102A,B | Chu WCW |
| 2.103A,B | Hebeda KM |
| 2.104A–D | Hebeda KM |
| 2.105A,B | Hebeda KM |
| 2.106A,B | Hebeda KM |
| 2.107A,B | Hebeda KM |
| 2.108A–D | Hebeda KM |
| 2.109 | Arnold Merrow, Emergency and Critical Care Imaging, Cincinnati Children's Hospital Medical Center (CCHMC) and University of Cincinnati College of Medicine, Cincinnati OH |
| 2.110 | Arnold Merrow, Emergency and Critical Care Imaging, Cincinnati Children's Hospital Medical Center (CCHMC) and University of Cincinnati College of Medicine, Cincinnati OH |
| 2.111 | Katherine Hanlon, Medical Photographer, Pediatric Dermatology, Cincinnati Children's Hospital Medical Center, Cincinnati OH |
| 2.112 | Caitlin Treuting, Medical Photographer, Pediatric Dermatology, Cincinnati Children's Hospital Medical Center, Cincinnati OH |
| 2.113A,B,D | Picarsic J |
| 2.113C | © Falini B. Published in: Swerdlow SH, Campo E, Harris NL, et al., editors. WHO classification of tumours of |

haematopoietic and lymphoid tissues. Lyon (France): International Agency for Research on Cancer; 2017. (WHO classification of tumours series, 4th rev. ed.; vol. 2). https://publications.iarc.fr/556.

2.114A–D Picarsic J
2.115A,B Picarsic J
2.116A–C Picarsic J
2.117A–D Krishnan C
2.118 Krishnan C
2.119A–C Krishnan C
2.120A,B Said JW
2.121 Said JW
2.122 Said JW

3.01 Pfister SM
3.02 Capper D
3.03A,B Blümcke I
3.03C,D Perry A
3.04A–D Perry A
3.05A–C David W. Ellison, St. Jude Children's Research Hospital, Memphis TN
3.06 Perry A
3.07A,C,D Perry A
3.07B David W. Ellison, St. Jude Children's Research Hospital, Memphis TN
3.08A,B Chu WCW
3.08C Rosenblum MK
3.09A–D Rosenblum MK
3.10A,B Rosenblum MK
3.11A–C Giannini C
3.12A–D Giannini C
3.13A,B David W. Ellison, St. Jude Children's Research Hospital, Memphis TN
3.14A–C Giannini C
3.15A–D Varlet P
3.16A,B Chu WCW
3.17A–E Leske H
3.18A,C–E Varlet P
3.18B Leske H
3.19A–D Varlet P
3.20A–E Solomon DA
3.21A,B Leske H
3.22 Leske H
3.23A,B Leske H
3.24 Varlet P
3.25A–D Varlet P
3.26A,B Capper D
3.27 Capper D
3.28A,B Hawkins CE

3.29A–C Hawkins CE
3.30A,B Tihan T
3.31A–C,E,F Tihan T
3.31D Perry A
3.32A–C Tihan T
3.33A,B Perry A
3.34A,B Tihan T
3.35A Perry A
3.35B Tihan T
3.36A–D Perry A
3.37 Varlet P
3.38A,B WHO Classification of Tumours Editorial Board. Central nervous system tumours. Lyon (France): International Agency for Research on Cancer; 2021. (WHO classification of tumours series, 5th ed.; vol. 6). https://publications.iarc.fr/601.
3.39A–D Capper D
3.40A–C Capper D
3.41 Philipp Jurmeister, Pathologisches Institut der Ludwig-Maximilian-Universität München, Munich
3.42 Capper D
3.43 Giannini C
3.44A–C Giannini C
3.45 Rachael A. Vaubel, Department of Laboratory Medicine and Pathology, Mayo Clinic, Rochester MN
3.46A–D Giannini C
3.47A–C Giannini C
3.48A–F Giannini C
3.49A–F Giannini C
3.50A,B © Ornan DA. Published in: Louis DN, Ohgaki H, Wiestler OD, et al., editors. WHO classification of tumours of the central nervous system. Lyon (France): International Agency for Research on Cancer; 2016. (WHO classification of tumours series, 4th rev. ed.; vol. 1). https://publications.iarc.fr/543.
3.51A,B Chu WCW
3.52A,B Rodriguez FJ
3.53A–C Perry A
3.54A,B,D Rodriguez FJ
3.54C Sharma MC
3.55A,B,D Rosenblum MK
3.55C,E Perry A
3.56A,B Perry A
3.57A,B Perry A

3.58A Rosenblum MK
3.58B,C Perry A
3.59 Blümcke I
3.60A–C Solomon DA
3.61A © Paul Kleihues. Published in: Louis DN, Ohgaki H, Wiestler OD, et al., editors. WHO classification of tumours of the central nervous system. Lyon (France): International Agency for Research on Cancer; 2016. (WHO classification of tumours series, 4th rev. ed.; vol. 1). https://publications.iarc.fr/543.
3.61B Blümcke I
3.62A–H Solomon DA
3.63A–C Solomon DA
3.64A–F Figarella-Branger D
3.65A,B Figarella-Branger D
3.66A–D Figarella-Branger D
3.67A–C Figarella-Branger D
3.68 Varlet P
3.69A,B Chu WCW
3.70A,B Varlet P
3.71A–C Pietsch T
3.72A–C Sahm F
3.72D,E Adapted, with permission, from: Deng MY, Sill M, Sturm D, et al. Diffuse glioneuronal tumour with oligodendroglioma-like features and nuclear clusters (DGONC) - a molecularly defined glioneuronal CNS tumour class displaying recurrent monosomy 14. Neuropathol Appl Neurobiol. 2020 Aug;46(5):422–30. PMID:31867747.
3.73A–C Sahm F
3.74 Adapted, with permission, from: Deng MY, Sill M, Sturm D, et al. Diffuse glioneuronal tumour with oligodendroglioma-like features and nuclear clusters (DGONC) - a molecularly defined glioneuronal CNS tumour class displaying recurrent monosomy 14. Neuropathol Appl Neurobiol. 2020 Aug;46(5):422–30. PMID:31867747.
3.75A,B Perry A
3.76A–D Perry A
3.77A,B Perry A
3.78A,B Perry A
3.79A Rosenblum MK
3.79B,C Komori T

| | |
|---|---|
| 3.80 | Rosenblum MK |
| 3.81A,B | Rosenblum MK |
| 3.82A–D | Rosenblum MK |
| 3.83A | David W. Ellison, St. Jude Children's Research Hospital, Memphis TN |
| 3.83B | Rudà R |
| 3.84A–D | David W. Ellison, St. Jude Children's Research Hospital, Memphis TN |
| 3.85A–D | David W. Ellison, St. Jude Children's Research Hospital, Memphis TN |
| 3.86A,B | Pietsch T |
| 3.87A,B | Rudà R |
| 3.88A | David W. Ellison, St. Jude Children's Research Hospital, Memphis TN |
| 3.88B | Pietsch T |
| 3.89 | Pajtler KW |
| 3.90A,B | Pietsch T |
| 3.91A,B | Pietsch T |
| 3.92 | Perry A |
| 3.93 | Rosenblum MK |
| 3.94A,C–F | Perry A |
| 3.94B | Rosenblum MK |
| 3.95A | David W. Ellison, St. Jude Children's Research Hospital, Memphis TN |
| 3.95B | Rosenblum MK |
| 3.95C,D | Perry A |
| 3.96 | Ramaswamy V |
| 3.97A,B | David W. Ellison, St. Jude Children's Research Hospital, Memphis TN |
| 3.98A | Rosenblum MK |
| 3.98B | Venneti S |
| 3.99A | David W. Ellison, St. Jude Children's Research Hospital, Memphis TN |
| 3.99B | Venneti S |
| 3.100 | Venneti S |
| 3.101 | WHO Classification of Tumours Editorial Board. Central nervous system tumours. Lyon (France): International Agency for Research on Cancer; 2021. (WHO classification of tumours series, 5th ed.; vol. 6). https://publications.iarc.fr/601. |
| 3.102 | Pietsch T |
| 3.103A,B | Pietsch T |
| 3.104A,B | Giannini C |
| 3.105A | Reuss DE |
| 3.105B–D | Giannini C |

| | |
|---|---|
| 3.106 | Robert B. Jenkins, Department of Laboratory Medicine and Pathology, Mayo Clinic, Rochester MN |
| 3.107A,B | Rosenblum MK |
| 3.108 | Rosenblum MK |
| 3.109 | Rosenblum MK |
| 3.110 | Rosenblum MK |
| 3.111A | Neuroradiological Reference Center for the pediatric brain tumor (HIT) studies of the German Society of Pediatric Oncology and Hematology, Faculty of Medicine, University Augsburg, Augsburg; and Annika Stock, Department of Neuroradiology, University Hospital Würzburg, Würzburg; and Brigitte Bison, Department of Diagnostic and Interventional Neuroradiology, Faculty of Medicine, University Augsburg, Augsburg |
| 3.111B | Martina Messing-Jünger, Department of Pediatric Neurosurgery, Asklepios Children's Hospital, Sankt Augustin |
| 3.112A,C,D | Pietsch T |
| 3.112B | Paulus W |
| 3.113 | Paulus W |
| 3.114A,B | Pietsch T |
| 3.115A,B | Pietsch T |
| 3.116A,B | WHO Classification of Tumours Editorial Board. Central nervous system tumours. Lyon (France): International Agency for Research on Cancer; 2021. (WHO classification of tumours series, 5th ed.; vol. 6). https://publications.iarc.fr/601. |
| 3.117 | Louis DN |
| 3.118A,B | Pietsch T |
| 3.119A,B | Pietsch T |
| 3.120 | Pietsch T |
| 3.121 | Pfister SM |
| 3.122 | David W. Ellison, St. Jude Children's Research Hospital, Memphis TN |
| 3.123 | David W. Ellison, St. Jude Children's Research Hospital, Memphis TN |

| | |
|---|---|
| 3.124 | Zoltán Patay, Diagnostic Imaging Department, St. Jude Children's Research Hospital, Memphis TN |
| 3.125A–C | David W. Ellison, St. Jude Children's Research Hospital, Memphis TN |
| 3.126 | Hawkins CE |
| 3.127 | Hawkins CE |
| 3.128A,B | Doz F |
| 3.128C | © Maria Luisa Garrè. Published in: Louis DN, Ohgaki H, Wiestler OD, et al., editors. WHO classification of tumours of the central nervous system. Lyon (France): International Agency for Research on Cancer; 2016. (WHO classification of tumours series, 4th rev. ed.; vol. 1). https://publications.iarc.fr/543. |
| 3.128D | Chu WCW |
| 3.129A | © Monika Warmuth-Metz. Published in: Louis DN, Ohgaki H, Wiestler OD, et al., editors. WHO classification of tumours of the central nervous system. Lyon (France): International Agency for Research on Cancer; 2016. (WHO classification of tumours series, 4th rev. ed.; vol. 1). https://publications.iarc.fr/543. |
| 3.129B | Perry A |
| 3.130A,B | Giangaspero F |
| 3.130C | © Paul Kleihues. Published in: Louis DN, Ohgaki H, Wiestler OD, et al., editors. WHO classification of tumours of the central nervous system. Lyon (France): International Agency for Research on Cancer; 2016. (WHO classification of tumours series, 4th rev. ed.; vol. 1). https://publications.iarc.fr/543. |
| 3.131A,B | © Paul Kleihues. Published in: Louis DN, Ohgaki H, Wiestler OD, et al., editors. WHO classification of tumours of the central nervous system. Lyon (France): International Agency for Research on Cancer; 2016. (WHO classification of tumours series, 4th rev. ed.; vol. 1). https://publications.iarc.fr/543. |

3.131C   © Lucy Balian Rorke-Adams. Published in: Louis DN, Ohgaki H, Wiestler OD, et al., editors. WHO classification of tumours of the central nervous system. Lyon (France): International Agency for Research on Cancer; 2016. (WHO classification of tumours series, 4th rev. ed.; vol. 1). https://publications.iarc.fr/543.

3.132A,B   David W. Ellison, St. Jude Children's Research Hospital, Memphis TN

3.133A–C   Pietsch T

3.133D   Perry A

3.133E   Giangaspero F

3.134   Pietsch T

3.135A,B   Giangaspero F

3.135C,D   David W. Ellison, St. Jude Children's Research Hospital, Memphis TN

3.136A   David W. Ellison, St. Jude Children's Research Hospital, Memphis TN

3.136B,C   Pietsch T

3.137   Pfister SM; and Adapted, with permission, from: Ho B, Johann PD, Grabovska Y, et al. Molecular subgrouping of atypical teratoid/rhabdoid tumors-a reinvestigation and current consensus. Neuro Oncol. 2020 May 15;22(5):613–624. PMID:31889194.

3.138A,B   Gregor Kasprian, Division of General and Paediatric Radiology, Medical University of Vienna, Vienna

3.139   Judkins AR

3.140A–D   Haberler C

3.141A,C,D   Haberler C

3.141B   Hasselblatt M

3.142   Haberler C

3.143A,B   Hasselblatt M

3.144   Hasselblatt M

3.145A–D   Korshunov A

3.146   Korshunov A

3.147   Korshunov A

3.148A–C   Korshunov A

3.149A   Pietsch T

3.149B   Perry A

3.150A,B   Anna Tietze, Department of Radiation Oncology, on behalf of Charité – Universitätsmedizin Berlin, Berlin

3.151A–D   Pietsch T

3.152A   Haberler C

3.152B–F   Solomon DA

3.153A,B   Solomon DA

3.154A   Haberler C

3.154B–D   Solomon DA

3.155   Wesseling P

3.156A,B   Wesseling P

3.157   WHO Classification of Tumours Editorial Board. Central nervous system tumours. Lyon (France): International Agency for Research on Cancer; 2021. (WHO classification of tumours series, 5th ed.; vol. 6). https://publications.iarc.fr/601.

3.158   WHO Classification of Tumours Editorial Board. Central nervous system tumours. Lyon (France): International Agency for Research on Cancer; 2021. (WHO classification of tumours series, 5th ed.; vol. 6). https://publications.iarc.fr/601.

3.159A,B   Vasiljevic A

3.160A–C   Vasiljevic A

3.161A,B   © Michelle Fèvre-Montange. Published in: Louis DN, Ohgaki H, Wiestler OD, et al., editors. WHO classification of tumours of the central nervous system. Lyon (France): International Agency for Research on Cancer; 2016. (WHO classification of tumours series, 4th rev. ed.; vol. 1). https://publications.iarc.fr/543.

3.162A,B   Küsters-Vandevelde HV

3.163A,B   Küsters-Vandevelde HV

3.164A,C   Adapted and reprinted, with permission from the American Association for Cancer Research, from: Pedersen M, Küsters-Vandevelde HVN, Viros A, et al. Primary melanoma of the CNS in children is driven by congenital expression of oncogenic NRAS in melanocytes. Cancer Discov.

2013 Apr;3(4):458–69. PMID:23303902.

3.164B   Reyes-Múgica M

3.165A–C   Wesseling P

3.166   Pfister SM

3.167A   Lopes MBS

3.167B,C   WHO Classification of Tumours Editorial Board. Central nervous system tumours. Lyon (France): International Agency for Research on Cancer; 2021. (WHO classification of tumours series, 5th ed.; vol. 6). https://publications.iarc.fr/601.

3.168   Reprinted, with permission, from: Mete O, Cintosun A, Pressman I, et al. Epidemiology and biomarker profile of pituitary adenohypophysial tumors. Mod Pathol. 2018 Jun;31(6):900–9. PMID:29434339.

3.169A,B   Villa C

3.170A–C   Adapted, with permission, from: Iacovazzo D, Caswell R, Bunce B, et al. Germline or somatic GPR101 duplication leads to X-linked acrogigantism: a clinico-pathological and genetic study. Acta Neuropathol Commun. 2016 Jun 1;4(1):56. PMID:27245663. https://creativecommons.org/licenses/by/4.0/

3.170D   Lopes MBS

3.171A,B   Adapted, with permission, from: Villa C, Lagonigro MS, Magri F, et al. Hyperplasia-adenoma sequence in pituitary tumorigenesis related to aryl hydrocarbon receptor interacting protein gene mutation. Endocr Relat Cancer. 2011 Jun 8;18(3):347–56. PMID:21450940.

3.172   Lopes MBS

3.173A–D   Lopes MBS

3.174A,B   Mete O

3.175   Asa SL

3.176   Asa SL

3.177   Mete O

| | | | | | |
|---|---|---|---|---|---|
| 3.178A–F | Mete O | 5.10 | Chevez-Barrios P | 6.18A,B | Fritchie KJ |
| 3.179A | Kleinschmidt-DeMasters BK | 5.11 | Chevez-Barrios P | 6.18C | Black JO |
| 3.179B | Chu WCW | 5.12A,B | Chevez-Barrios P | 6.19A–D | Black JO |
| 3.180 | Santagata S | 5.13A,B | Eagle RC Jr | 6.20A–D | Al-Ibraheemi A |
| 3.181A–C | Santagata S | 5.14A,B | White VA | 6.21A–C | Al-Ibraheemi A |
| 3.182A,B | Kleinschmidt-DeMasters BK | 5.15A,B | Mudhar HS | 6.22A,B,D | Black JO |
| 3.183A–F | Kleinschmidt-DeMasters BK | 5.16A–C | Mudhar HS | 6.22C | Alaggio R |
| 3.184A–E | Kleinschmidt-DeMasters BK | 5.17 | Mudhar HS | 6.23 | Reyes-Múgica M |
| 3.185A–C | Kleinschmidt-DeMasters BK | 5.18A,B | Eagle RC Jr | 6.24A–C | Reyes-Múgica M |
| 3.186A–C | Kleinschmidt-DeMasters BK | 5.19 | Sagoo MS | 6.25 | Supika Kritsaneepaiboon, |
| 3.187 | Kleinschmidt-DeMasters BK | 5.20A,B | Margo C | | Section of Pediatric Imaging |
| | | 5.21 | Sagoo MS | | Department of Radiology, |
| 4.01 | Chu WCW | 5.22A,B | Sagoo MS | | Faculty of Medicine, |
| 4.02 | Thompson LDR | 5.23A,B | Sagoo MS | | Songklanagarind Hospital, |
| 4.03A,B | Thompson LDR | 5.24A–D | Chu WCW | | Prince of Songkla University, |
| 4.04 | de Krijger RR | 5.25A–C | Chevez-Barrios P | | Hat Yai |
| 4.05 | Chu WCW | 5.26A–D | Chevez-Barrios P | 6.26A,B | Black JO |
| 4.06 | Chu WCW | 5.27A,B | Chevez-Barrios P | 6.27A–D | Al-Ibraheemi A |
| 4.07A,B | Beiske KH | 5.28A,B | Chevez-Barrios P | 6.28A–C | Thompson LDR |
| 4.08A–D | Beiske KH | 5.29 | Chevez-Barrios P | 6.29A,B | Jo VY |
| 4.09A,B | Chu WCW | 5.30A,B | Chevez-Barrios P | 6.30A–D | Thompson LDR |
| 4.10 | Chu WCW | 5.31 | Eagle RC Jr | 6.31A,B | Thompson LDR |
| 4.11 | Tornóczky T | 5.32 | Eagle RC Jr | 6.32A,B | Fritchie KJ |
| 4.12A–C | Shimada H | 5.33 | Eagle RC Jr | 6.33 | Karanian M |
| 4.13A,B | Shimada H | 5.34 | Eagle RC Jr | 6.34A,B | Karanian M |
| 4.13C | Tornóczky T | 5.35A | White VA | 6.35A,B | Mentzel TDW |
| 4.14A–C | Katia Mazzocco, Department | 5.35B | Eberhart CG | 6.36 | Mentzel TDW |
| | of Pathology, IRCCS Istituto | 5.36 | White VA | 6.37A,B | Karanian M |
| | Giannina Gaslini, Genoa | 5.37 | Eberhart CG | 6.38 | Mentzel TDW |
| 4.15A | Adapted, with permission from | | | 6.39 | Mentzel TDW |
| | Elsevier, from: Peuchmaur M. | 6.01 | Martin Sill, Clinical | 6.40 | Karanian M |
| | Les tumeurs neuroblastiques | | Bioinformatics, Hopp | 6.41A–C | Fritchie KJ |
| | périphériques, classification | | Children's Cancer Center | 6.42A,B | Flucke U |
| | anatomo-pathologique | | Heidelberg (KiTZ) and | 6.42C | Antonescu CR |
| | [Peripheral neuroblastic | | German Cancer Research | 6.43 | Antonescu CR |
| | tumors: anatomo pathological | | Center (DKFZ), Heidelberg | 6.44 | Patrizia Dall'Igna, Pediatric |
| | classification]. Ann Pathol. 2004 | 6.02A,B | Chu WCW | | Surgery, Università di Padova, |
| | Dec;24(6):556–67. French. | 6.03A,B | Black JO | | Padua |
| | PMID:15785402. Copyright | 6.04A,B | Black JO | 6.45A–C | Supika Kritsaneepaiboon, |
| | 2004 Elsevier Masson SAS. All | 6.05 | Chu WCW | | Section of Pediatric Imaging |
| | rights reserved. | 6.06A,C | Alaggio R | | Department of Radiology, |
| 4.15B | Peuchmaur M | 6.06B,D | Black JO | | Faculty of Medicine, |
| 4.16A–C | Peuchmaur M | 6.07A,B | Alaggio R | | Songklanagarind Hospital, |
| | | 6.08A,B | Creytens D | | Prince of Songkla University, |
| 5.01A | Herwig-Carl MC | 6.09A–C | Creytens D | | Hat Yai |
| 5.01B | Verdijk RM | 6.10 | Pedeutour F | 6.46A,B | Davis JL |
| 5.02A,B | Herwig-Carl M.C. | 6.11 | Al-Ibraheemi A | 6.46C | Alaggio R |
| 5.02C | Verdijk RM | 6.12A–D | Rosenberg AE | 6.47A,B | Davis JL |
| 5.03A–D | Moulin A | 6.13A | Rosenberg AE | 6.48A,B | Davis JL |
| 5.04A,B | Verdijk RM | 6.13B | Reyes-Múgica M | 6.49A–E | Davis JL |
| 5.05 | Eagle RC Jr | 6.14A | Rosenberg AE | 6.50A,B | Davis JL |
| 5.06A,B | Milman T | 6.14B | Alaggio R | 6.51A,B | Chu WCW |
| 5.07A–D | Milman T | 6.15A,B | Al-Ibraheemi A | 6.52A,B | Alaggio R |
| 5.08A–D | Milman T | 6.16A–D | Reyes-Múgica M | 6.53 | Billings SD |
| 5.09A,B | Chevez-Barrios P | 6.17A,B | Reyes-Múgica M | 6.54A–C,G | Alaggio R |

| | |
|---|---|
| 6.54D–F | Billings SD |
| 6.55 | Chu WCW |
| 6.56 | Surrey LF |
| 6.57A,B | Surrey LF |
| 6.58A–C | Oscar F. Lopez-Nunez, Division of Pathology and Laboratory Medicine, Cincinnati Children's Hospital Medical Center, Cincinnati OH |
| 6.59A–C | Chan JKC |
| 6.60A–C | Thway K |
| 6.61A–C | Luzar B |
| 6.62 | Luzar B |
| 6.63A,B | Luzar B |
| 6.64A,B | Luzar B |
| 6.65A,B | Luzar B |
| 6.66A,B | Luzar B |
| 6.67A,C,D | Brenn T |
| 6.67B | Davis JL |
| 6.68A–D | de Saint Aubain Somerhausen N |
| 6.69A,B | Kozakewich HP |
| 6.70A,B | Kozakewich HP |
| 6.71 | Kozakewich HP |
| 6.72 | Chu WCW |
| 6.73 | Chu WCW |
| 6.74A,B | Kozakewich HP |
| 6.75A,B | Kozakewich HP |
| 6.76 | Kozakewich HP |
| 6.77A,B | Kozakewich HP |
| 6.78A,B | Kozakewich HP |
| 6.79A,B | Kozakewich HP |
| 6.80 | Chu WCW |
| 6.81A–D | Kozakewich HP |
| 6.82A,B | Kozakewich HP |
| 6.83 | Adapted, with permission, from: Kozakewich HPW, Mulliken JB. Chapter 12: Histopathology of vascular malformations. In: Mulliken JB, Burrows PE, Fishman SJ, editors. Mulliken and Young's vascular anomalies: hemangiomas and malformations. 2nd ed. New York (NY): Oxford University Press; 2013. |
| 6.84A | Adapted, with permission, from: Kozakewich HPW, Mulliken JB. Chapter 12: Histopathology of vascular malformations. In: Mulliken JB, Burrows PE, Fishman SJ, editors. Mulliken and Young's vascular anomalies: hemangiomas and malformations. 2nd ed. New York (NY): Oxford University Press; 2013. |
| 6.84B | Kozakewich HP |
| 6.85A,B | Kozakewich HP |
| 6.86A,B | Kozakewich HP |
| 6.87 | Kozakewich HP |
| 6.88A,B | Kozakewich HP |
| 6.89A,C,D | Kozakewich HP |
| 6.89B | Adapted, with permission, from: Kurek KC, Howard E, Tennant LB, et al. PTEN hamartoma of soft tissue: a distinctive lesion in PTEN syndromes. Am J Surg Pathol. 2012 May;36(5):671–87. PMID:22446940. |
| 6.90A,B | Chu WCW |
| 6.91A,B | Kozakewich HP |
| 6.92 | Kozakewich HP |
| 6.93A–C | Kozakewich HP |
| 6.94A,B | Kozakewich HP |
| 6.95A,B | Kozakewich HP |
| 6.96A,B | Kozakewich HP |
| 6.97A–D | Kozakewich HP |
| 6.98 | Kozakewich HP |
| 6.99A,B | Kozakewich HP |
| 6.100A,B | Papadogiannakis N |
| 6.101A–C | Heller DS |
| 6.102 | Torrelo A |
| 6.103A–C | Calonje JE |
| 6.104A–D | Billings SD |
| 6.105A,B | Supika Kritsaneepaiboon, Section of Pediatric Imaging Department of Radiology, Faculty of Medicine, Songklanagarind Hospital, Prince of Songkla University, Hat Yai |
| 6.106 | Supika Kritsaneepaiboon, Section of Pediatric Imaging Department of Radiology, Faculty of Medicine, Songklanagarind Hospital, Prince of Songkla University, Hat Yai |
| 6.107A–C | Colmenero I |
| 6.108A–C | Colmenero I |
| 6.109A–E | Colmenero I |
| 6.110A–C | Fanburg-Smith JC |
| 6.111 | Fanburg-Smith JC |
| 6.112A–D | Hornick JL |
| 6.113A,B | Hornick JL |
| 6.114A,B | Hornick JL |
| 6.115 | Reprinted, with permission, from: Galluzzo Mutti L, Álvarez M, Siminovich M, et al. Disseminated visceral Kaposi's sarcoma in a pediatric bilateral lung transplant recipient. Pediatr Transplant. 2019 Feb;23(1):e13311. PMID:30362299. |
| 6.116A | Reprinted, with permission, from: Galluzzo Mutti L, Álvarez M, Siminovich M, et al. Disseminated visceral Kaposi's sarcoma in a pediatric bilateral lung transplant recipient. Pediatr Transplant. 2019 Feb;23(1):e13311. PMID:30362299. |
| 6.116B–D | Galluzzo ML |
| 6.117 | Gupta A |
| 6.118A,B,E | Billings SD |
| 6.118C | Colmenero I |
| 6.118D | Gupta A |
| 6.119A,B | Billings SD |
| 6.120A–C | Colmenero I |
| 6.121A–F | Karanian M |
| 6.122A,B | Agaram NP |
| 6.123 | Karanian M |
| 6.124 | Karanian M |
| 6.125A,B | Bode PK |
| 6.126A–D | Carlos Galliani, Pediatric Pathology, Children's and Women's Hospital, University of South Alabama, Mobile AL |
| 6.127A–C | Alaggio R |
| 6.128A,B | Wang LL (Larry Liang) |
| 6.128C | Parham DM |
| 6.129A–C | Wang LL (Larry Liang) |
| 6.130 | Rudzinski ER |
| 6.131A,B | Rudzinski ER |
| 6.132A–C | Rudzinski ER |
| 6.132D | Dry SM |
| 6.133A | Dry SM |
| 6.133B | Kohashi K |
| 6.134A,B | Rudzinski ER |
| 6.134C | Dry SM |
| 6.135A,B | Kelsey A |
| 6.136A–C | Huang SC |
| 6.137 | Huang SC |
| 6.138 | Chu WCW |
| 6.139A–D | Hornick JL |
| 6.140A,B | Hornick JL |
| 6.141 | Hornick JL |
| 6.142 | Reyes-Múgica M |
| 6.143A–D | Reyes-Múgica M |
| 6.144A,B | Chu WCW |
| 6.145A–E | Reyes-Múgica M |

| | | | |
|---|---|---|---|
| 6.146A–D | Reyes-Múgica M | 6.178A,B | Martignoni G |
| 6.147A–C | Alaggio R | 6.179A,B | Chu WCW |
| 6.148 | Reuss DE | 6.180A | Suurmeijer AJH |
| 6.149A–D | Alaggio R | 6.180B–D | Pawel BR |
| 6.150A–D | WHO Classification of Tumours Editorial Board. Soft tissue and bone tumours. Lyon (France): International Agency for Research on Cancer; 2020. (WHO classification of tumours series, 5th ed.; vol. 3). https://publications.iarc.fr/588. | 6.181A,B | Suurmeijer AJH |
| | | 6.181C | Pawel BR |
| | | 6.182A–E | Alaggio R |
| | | 6.183A–C | Oda Y |
| | | 6.184A–C | Oda Y |
| | | 6.185A–D | Oda Y |
| | | 6.186A–F | Jo VY |
| | | 6.187A,B | Jo VY |
| 6.151 | Reyes-Múgica M | 6.188A–C | Reyes-Múgica M |
| 6.152A–D | Reyes-Múgica M | 6.189A,B | Chu WCW |
| 6.153A–C | Alaggio R | 6.190 | Bahrami A |
| 6.154A,B | Chu WCW | 6.191A–C | Bahrami A |
| 6.155 | Rossi S | 6.192A–C | Bahrami A |
| 6.156A–C | Rossi S | 6.192D | Agaram NP |
| 6.157A,B | Rossi S | 6.193A,C | Bahrami A |
| 6.158 | Rossi S | 6.193B | Agaram NP |
| 6.159A,B | Nielsen GP | 6.194A–C | Dei Tos AP |
| 6.160A,B | Magro G | 6.195A,B | Chu WCW |
| 6.161 | WHO Classification of Tumours Editorial Board. Female genital tumours. Lyon (France): International Agency for Research on Cancer; 2020. (WHO classification of tumours series, 5th ed.; vol. 4). https://publications.iarc.fr/592. | 6.196A | Lisa Michelle Rooper, Department of Pathology, Johns Hopkins University School of Medicine, Baltimore MD |
| | | 6.196B | Chang KTE |
| | | 6.197A–D | Chang KTE |
| | | 6.198A–C | Lisa Michelle Rooper, Department of Pathology, Johns Hopkins University School of Medicine, Baltimore MD |
| 6.162 | WHO Classification of Tumours Editorial Board. Female genital tumours. Lyon (France): International Agency for Research on Cancer; 2020. (WHO classification of tumours series, 5th ed.; vol. 4). https://publications.iarc.fr/592. | 6.199A–C | Surrey LF |
| | | 6.200A–D | Le Loarer F |
| | | 6.201 | Daniel Pissaloux, Department of Biopathology, Centre Léon Bérard, Lyon |
| | | 6.202A–C | Somers GR |
| 6.163A–C | Magro G | 6.202A inset | Alaggio R |
| 6.164A,B | Magro G | 6.202D | Yoshida A |
| 6.165A | Rekhi B | 6.203A–C | Puls F |
| 6.165B | Pawel BR | 6.203D | Alessandra Stracuzzi, Department of Anatomical Pathology, Ospedale Pediatrico Bambino Gesù, Rome |
| 6.166A,C–F | Rekhi B | | |
| 6.166B | Pawel BR | | |
| 6.167A–C | Fritchie KJ | 6.204A,B | Puls F |
| 6.168A,B | Fritchie KJ | 6.205A,B | Alessandra Stracuzzi, Department of Anatomical Pathology, Ospedale Pediatrico Bambino Gesù, Rome |
| 6.169A,B | Chu WCW | | |
| 6.170A,B | Fanburg-Smith JC | | |
| 6.171A,B | Fanburg-Smith JC | | |
| 6.172 | Chu WCW | | |
| 6.173A–C | Oda Y | 6.205C,D | Alaggio R |
| 6.174A–D | Oda Y | 6.206 | Alessandra Stracuzzi, Department of Anatomical |
| 6.175 | Biegel JA | | |
| 6.176A,B | Chu WCW | | |
| 6.177A–C | Martignoni G | | |

| | |
|---|---|
| | Pathology, Ospedale Pediatrico Bambino Gesù, Rome |
| 6.207 | Yoshida A |
| 6.208A,B | Zambrano E |
| 6.209A,B | Reyes-Múgica M; and Ana Eugenia Ponciano Castellanos, Laboratorio de Patología y Citología, Guatemala City |
| 6.210A | Reyes-Múgica M; and Ana Eugenia Ponciano Castellanos, Laboratorio de Patología y Citología, Guatemala City |
| 6.210B–D | Zambrano E |
| 6.211A,B | Parafioriti A |
| 6.212A,C | Parafioriti A |
| 6.212B | John I |
| 6.212D | Luzar B |
| 6.213A–C | Parafioriti A |
| 6.214A,B | Parafioriti A |
| 6.215A,B | Doris E. Wenger, Department of Radiology, Mayo Clinic, Rochester MN |
| 6.216A–D | Fritchie KJ |
| 6.217 | Adapted, with permission from Elsevier, from: Chen X, Bahrami A, Pappo A, et al. Recurrent somatic structural variations contribute to tumorigenesis in pediatric osteosarcoma. Cell Rep. 2014 Apr 10;7(1):104–12. PMID:24703847. |
| 6.218 | Adapted, with permission from Elsevier, from: Chen X, Bahrami A, Pappo A, et al. Recurrent somatic structural variations contribute to tumorigenesis in pediatric osteosarcoma. Cell Rep. 2014 Apr 10;7(1):104–12. PMID:24703847. |
| 6.219A–C | Bahrami A |
| 6.220A–E | Bahrami A |
| 6.221 | Bahrami A |
| 6.222 | Bahrami A |
| 6.223A,B | Bahrami A |
| 6.224A,B | Bahrami A |
| 6.225A,B | Bahrami A |
| 6.226A,B | Bahrami A |
| 6.227A,B | Bahrami A |
| 6.228A | Chu WCW |

6.228B–D    Bahrami A
6.229A–C    Bahrami A
6.230A–C    Baumhoer D
6.231A,B    Amary F
6.231C    Paul O'Donnell, Department of Radiology, Royal National Orthopaedic Hospital, Brockley Hill, Stanmore, Middlesex
6.232A–D    Amary F
6.233    Amary F
6.234A,B    Paul O'Donnell, Department of Radiology, Royal National Orthopaedic Hospital, Brockley Hill, Stanmore, Middlesex
6.234C    Supika Kritsaneepaiboon, Section of Pediatric Imaging Department of Radiology, Faculty of Medicine, Songklanagarind Hospital, Prince of Songkla University, Hat Yai
6.235A,B    Tirabosco R
6.236A,B    Tirabosco R
6.237A–C    Chu WCW
6.238    © Ostrowski ML. Published in: Fletcher CDM, Bridge JA, Hogendoorn PCW, et al., editors. WHO classification of tumours of soft tissue and bone. Lyon (France): International Agency for Research on Cancer; 2013. (WHO classification of tumours series, 4th ed.; vol. 5). https://publications.iarc.fr/15; and WHO Classification of Tumours Editorial Board. Soft tissue and bone tumours. Lyon (France): International Agency for Research on Cancer; 2020. (WHO classification of tumours series, 5th ed.; vol. 3). https://publications.iarc.fr/588.
6.239A–C    Bovée JVMG
6.239D    © Ostrowski ML. Published in: Fletcher CDM, Bridge JA, Hogendoorn PCW, et al., editors. WHO classification of tumours of soft tissue and bone. Lyon (France): International Agency for Research on Cancer; 2013. (WHO classification of tumours series, 4th ed.; vol. 5). https://publications.iarc.fr/15; and WHO Classification of Tumours Editorial Board. Soft tissue and bone tumours. Lyon (France): International Agency for Research on Cancer; 2020. (WHO classification of tumours series, 5th ed.; vol. 3). https://publications.iarc.fr/588.
6.240A,B    Paul O'Donnell, Department of Radiology, Royal National Orthopaedic Hospital, Brockley Hill, Stanmore, Middlesex
6.240C    Tirabosco R
6.241A–C    Tirabosco R
6.242    Tirabosco R
6.243A–C    Kilpatrick SE
6.244A,B    Kilpatrick SE
6.245A,B    Kilpatrick SE
6.246A,B    Kilpatrick SE
6.247    Kilpatrick SE
6.248    Kilpatrick SE
6.249A,B    Kilpatrick SE
6.250A,B    Kilpatrick SE
6.251A,B    Rosenberg AE
6.252A,C,D    Rosenberg AE
6.252B    John I
6.253A–C    Rosenberg AE
6.254A,B    Baumhoer D
6.255A–C    Agaram NP
6.256A,B    Agaram NP
6.257A    Perez-Atayde AR
6.257B    Tirabosco R
6.258A,B    Tirabosco R
6.259A,B    Perez-Atayde AR
6.259C    Tirabosco R
6.260A–D    Tirabosco R
6.261A,B    Tirabosco R
6.262    Tirabosco R
6.263A    © Kalil RK. Published in: Fletcher CDM, Bridge JA, Hogendoorn PCW, et al., editors. WHO classification of tumours of soft tissue and bone. Lyon (France): International Agency for Research on Cancer; 2013. (WHO classification of tumours series, 4th ed.; vol. 5). https://publications.iarc.fr/15; and WHO Classification of Tumours Editorial Board. Soft tissue and bone tumours. Lyon (France): International Agency for Research on Cancer; 2020. (WHO classification of tumours series, 5th ed.; vol. 3). https://publications.iarc.fr/588.
6.263B    WHO Classification of Tumours Editorial Board. Soft tissue and bone tumours. Lyon (France): International Agency for Research on Cancer; 2020. (WHO classification of tumours series, 5th ed.; vol. 3). https://publications.iarc.fr/588.
6.264A–D    WHO Classification of Tumours Editorial Board. Soft tissue and bone tumours. Lyon (France): International Agency for Research on Cancer; 2020. (WHO classification of tumours series, 5th ed.; vol. 3). https://publications.iarc.fr/588.
6.265A,B    Gambarotti M
6.266    Gambarotti M
6.267A–C    Nielsen GP
6.268A,B    Nielsen GP
6.269    Nielsen GP
6.270A,B    Chu WCW
6.271A    Alessandra Stracuzzi, Department of Anatomical Pathology, Ospedale Pediatrico Bambino Gesù, Rome
6.271B    Gambarotti M

7.01    Oosterhuis JW
7.02    Oosterhuis JW
7.03A–C    Oosterhuis JW
7.04A,B    Reyes-Múgica M
7.05A,B    Ulbright TM
7.06    González-Peramato P
7.07A–D    Reyes-Múgica M
7.08A    Bode PK
7.08B,C    Chu WCW
7.09    Bode PK
7.10A–C    Bode PK
7.11A,B    Bode PK
7.12    Bode PK
7.13    Bode PK
7.14A,B    Chu WCW
7.15    Vang R
7.16A–C    Ulbright TM
7.17A–C    Vang R
7.18A,B    Bode PK

| | | | | | | |
|---|---|---|---|---|---|
| 7.19 | Bode PK | 7.35 | WHO Classification of Tumours Editorial Board. Female genital tumours. Lyon (France): International Agency for Research on Cancer; 2020. (WHO classification of tumours series, 5th ed.; vol. 4). https://publications.iarc.fr/592. | 8.26A–E | Argani P |
| 7.20A–C | Bode PK | | | 8.27A–C | Tsuzuki T |
| 7.21A,B | Vang R | | | 8.28 | Chu WCW |
| 7.22 | Vang R | | | 8.29A–F | Vujanic GM |
| 7.23 | Vang R | | | 8.30 | Chu WCW |
| 7.24 | Vang R | | | 8.31 | Chang KTE |
| 7.25 | Chu WCW | | | 8.32A–C | Chang KTE |
| 7.26A–C | Vang R | | | 8.33A | Vujanic GM |
| 7.27 | Reyes-Múgica M | 7.36 | Chu WCW | 8.33B,C | Chang KTE |
| 7.28A,B | Williamson SR | 7.37A,B | Reyes-Múgica M | 8.34A | Reprinted from: Aw SJ, Chang KTE. Clear cell sarcoma of the kidney. Arch Pathol Lab Med. 2019 Aug;143(8):1022–6. PMID:30628851. |
| 7.29 | Williamson SR | 7.38A,B | Reyes-Múgica M | | |
| 7.30A–D | WHO Classification of Tumours Editorial Board. Urinary and male genital tumours. Lyon (France): International Agency for Research on Cancer; 2022. (WHO classification of tumours series, 5th ed.; vol. 8). https://publications.iarc.fr/610. | 7.39A–C | Reyes-Múgica M | | |
| | | 7.40A,B | Chu WCW | | |
| | | 7.41A–C | Reyes-Múgica M | | |
| | | 7.42A,B | Reyes-Múgica M | 8.34B | Chang KTE |
| | | 7.43A–C | Reyes-Múgica M | 8.35A,B | Chang KTE |
| | | 7.44 | Reyes-Múgica M | 8.36A,B | Chu WCW |
| | | 7.45A,B | Chu WCW | 8.37A–C | de Krijger RR |
| | | 7.46A,B | Reyes-Múgica M | 8.38A–D | Vujanic GM |
| | | 7.47A–C | Reyes-Múgica M | 8.39A–C | Vujanic GM |
| 7.31A–E | WHO Classification of Tumours Editorial Board. Urinary and male genital tumours. Lyon (France): International Agency for Research on Cancer; 2022. (WHO classification of tumours series, 5th ed.; vol. 8). https://publications.iarc.fr/610. | 7.48A,B | Reyes-Múgica M | 8.40A,B | de Krijger RR |
| | | 7.49A,B | Reyes-Múgica M | 8.41A | Okita H |
| | | 7.50 | Reyes-Múgica M | 8.41B | de Krijger RR |
| | | | | 8.42 | Bode PK |
| | | 8.01 | Chu WCW | 8.43A,B | Bode PK |
| | | 8.02 | Chu WCW | | |
| | | 8.03A–C | Vujanic GM | 9.01A,B | Reyes-Múgica M |
| | | 8.04 | Chu WCW | 9.02A–C | Reyes-Múgica M |
| 7.32A,B | WHO Classification of Tumours Editorial Board. Urinary and male genital tumours. Lyon (France): International Agency for Research on Cancer; 2022. (WHO classification of tumours series, 5th ed.; vol. 8). https://publications.iarc.fr/610. | 8.05A,B | Hill DA | 9.03A,B | Bennett JA |
| | | 8.06A–D | Vujanic GM | 9.04A,B | Chu WCW |
| | | 8.07A,B | Vujanic GM | 9.05 | Stewart CJR |
| | | 8.08A–C | Vujanic GM | 9.06A–C | Stewart CJR |
| | | 8.09A,B | Hill DA | 9.07 | Stewart CJR |
| | | 8.10 | Vujanic GM | 9.08A,B | Stewart CJR |
| | | 8.11 | Hill DA | 9.09A,B | Usubutun A |
| | | 8.12A,B | Chu WCW | 9.10 | Buza N |
| | | 8.13A,C,D | Bode PK | 9.11A–C | Buza N |
| | | 8.13B | Argani P | 9.12A,B | Buza N |
| 7.33A–C | WHO Classification of Tumours Editorial Board. Urinary and male genital tumours. Lyon (France): International Agency for Research on Cancer; 2022. (WHO classification of tumours series, 5th ed.; vol. 8). https://publications.iarc.fr/610. | 8.14A | Matoso A | 9.13 | WHO Classification of Tumours Editorial Board. Female genital tumours. Lyon (France): International Agency for Research on Cancer; 2020. (WHO classification of tumours series, 5th ed.; vol. 4). https://publications.iarc.fr/592. |
| | | 8.14B | Bode PK | | |
| | | 8.15A | Bode PK | | |
| | | 8.15B | Hill DA | | |
| | | 8.15C | Matoso A | | |
| | | 8.16A,B | Matoso A | | |
| | | 8.16C | Argani P | | |
| | | 8.17A | Bode PK | | |
| | | 8.17B | Argani P | 9.14A,B | WHO Classification of Tumours Editorial Board. Female genital tumours. Lyon (France): International Agency for Research on Cancer; 2020. (WHO classification of tumours series, 5th ed.; vol. 4). https://publications.iarc.fr/592. |
| 7.34 | WHO Classification of Tumours Editorial Board. Female genital tumours. Lyon (France): International Agency for Research on Cancer; 2020. (WHO classification of tumours series, 5th ed.; vol. 4). https://publications.iarc.fr/592. | 8.18A–D | Argani P | | |
| | | 8.19A,B | Argani P | | |
| | | 8.20A–F | Argani P | | |
| | | 8.21A,B | Argani P | | |
| | | 8.22A–F | Argani P | | |
| | | 8.23A–D | Argani P | | |
| | | 8.24A–C | Argani P | | |
| | | 8.25 | Argani P | 9.15A–E | Karnezis AN |

| | | | | | |
|---|---|---|---|---|---|
| 9.16A,B | Moritani S | 11.19 | Reprinted, with permission, from: Makhlouf HR, Abdul-Al HM, Wang G, et al. Calcifying nested stromal-epithelial tumors of the liver: a clinicopathologic, immunohistochemical, and molecular genetic study of 9 cases with a long-term follow-up. Am J Surg Pathol. 2009 Jul;33(7):976–83. PMID:19363442. | 11.41A,B | Chu WCW |
| 9.17A,B | Pantanowitz L | | | 11.42A,B | Singhi AD |
| 9.18A,B | Lieberman RW | | | 11.43A–D | Singhi AD |
| 9.19A,B | Lieberman RW | | | 11.44A–C | Singhi AD |
| 9.20A,B | Malpica A | | | 11.45A,B | Thompson LDR |
| | | | | 11.46A,C | Pawel BR |
| 10.01A,B | Gudi M | | | 11.46B | Graham RP |
| 10.02A–C | Gudi M | | | 11.47 | Graham RP |
| 10.03 | Gudi M | | | 11.48 | Reyes-Múgica M |
| 10.04 | Gudi M | | | 11.49A–D | Reyes-Múgica M |
| 10.05 | Gudi M | | | 11.50A,B | Reyes-Múgica M |
| 10.06A,B | Tay TKY | 11.20A–D | Hornick JL | | |
| 10.07A,B | Tay TKY | 11.21 | Chu WCW | 12.01A,B | Seethala R |
| 10.08A,B | Tay TKY | 11.22 | Ranganathan S | 12.02A,B | Seethala R |
| 10.09A | Chu WCW | 11.23A,B,D | Vokuhl C | 12.03A,B | Seethala R |
| 10.09B | Gudi M | 11.23C | Ranganathan S | 12.04 | Seethala R |
| 10.10 | Gudi M | 11.24 | Chu WCW | 12.05 | Thompson LDR |
| 10.11A–D | Tay TKY | 11.25A,B | Gupta A | 12.06A–C | Nga ME |
| 10.12 | Yien Sien Lee, Department of Diagnostic and Interventional Imaging, KK Women's and Children's Hospital, Singapore | 11.26A–C | Gupta A | 12.07A–C | Nga ME |
| | | 11.27 | Kozakewich HP | 12.08A,B | Nga ME |
| | | 11.28A–C | Kozakewich HP | 12.09 | Nga ME |
| | | 11.29 | Chu WCW | 12.10A,B | Nga ME |
| | | 11.30A | Gupta A | 12.11 | Nga ME |
| 10.13 | Gudi M | 11.30B | Reprinted, with permission, from: Gupta A, Sheil A. Chapter 9: Imprint and aspiration cytology of abdominal lesions: liver, biliary tree, pancreas, and GI tract. In: Chou P, Gattuso P, Reddy V, et al., editors. Diagnostic pediatric cytopathology and histopathologic correlation. Cambridge (UK): Cambridge University Press; 2000. pp. 241–78. | 12.12A | Nga ME |
| 10.14A–C | Gudi M | | | 12.12B | Faquin WC |
| | | | | 12.13A,B,D | Nga ME |
| 11.01A–C | Chu WCW | | | 12.13C | Rossi ED |
| 11.02A–D | Ranganathan S | | | 12.14 | José Manuel Cameselle-Teijeiro, Department of Anatomic Pathology, Clinical University Hospital, University of Santiago de Compostela, Santiago de Compostela |
| 11.03A,B | Ranganathan S | | | | |
| 11.04A–C | Ranganathan S | | | | |
| 11.05A,B | Ranganathan S | | | | |
| 11.06 | Czauderna P | | | | |
| 11.07A,B | Ranganathan S | | | | |
| 11.07C,D | Cho SJ | | | 12.15A,B | Erickson LA |
| 11.08A–C | Cho SJ | | | 12.16A,B | Erickson LA |
| 11.09A,B | Ranganathan S | 11.31A,B | Gupta A | 12.17A–C | Nga ME |
| 11.09C,D,F,G | Cho SJ | 11.32 | Gupta A | 12.18A,B | Vania Nosé, Department of Pathology, Massachusetts General Hospital, Harvard Medical School, Boston MA |
| 11.09E | Makhlouf HR | 11.33A–C | Gupta A | | |
| 11.10A,B | Chu WCW | 11.34A,B | Chu WCW | | |
| 11.11A,B | Guettier C | 11.34C | Singhi AD | | |
| 11.12A–D | Guettier C | 11.35 | Singhi AD | 12.18C | José Manuel Cameselle-Teijeiro, Department of Anatomic Pathology, Clinical University Hospital, University of Santiago de Compostela, Santiago de Compostela |
| 11.13 | Guettier C | 11.36A–D | Singhi AD | | |
| 11.14A–D | Ranganathan S | 11.37A,B | Ohike N | | |
| 11.15A–D | Ranganathan S | 11.38A–C | Singhi AD | | |
| 11.16 | Rose Chami, Department of Laboratory Medicine and Pathobiology, Hospital for Sick Children, Toronto ON | 11.38D | Ohike N | | |
| | | 11.39A–D | Luigi Maria Terracciano, Postgraduate School of Anatomic Pathology, Humanitas University, Institute of Medical Genetics and Pathology, University Hospital Basel, Basel | 12.18D,E | Erickson LA |
| 11.17A,B | Derek Tsz Wai Yau, Diagnostix Pathology Laboratories Ltd, Canossa Hospital, Hong Kong SAR | | | 12.19A,B | Melvy Sarah Mathew, Ultrasound Abdominal Imaging Section, Department of Radiology, University of Chicago Medical Center, Chicago IL |
| 11.17C,D | Saxena R | | | | |
| 11.17E,F | Tsui WMS | | | 12.20 | Cipriani NA |
| 11.18A–C | Ranganathan S | 11.40A–D | La Rosa S | 12.21 | Cipriani NA |

12.22 Cipriani NA

12.23A Collini P

12.23B,C Cipriani NA

12.24A,B Collini P

12.25A,B Cipriani NA

12.26A–D Chan JKC

12.27A,B Chan JKC

12.28 Folpe AL

12.29A,B Gill AJ

12.30 Gill AJ

12.31 Gill AJ

12.32A,B Chu WCW

12.33A,B Reprinted, with permission, from: Pinto EM, Chen X, Easton J, et al. Genomic landscape of paediatric adrenocortical tumours. Nat Commun. 2015 Mar 6;6:6302. PMID:25743702.

12.34 Reprinted, with permission, from: Pinto EM, Chen X, Easton J, et al. Genomic landscape of paediatric adrenocortical tumours. Nat Commun. 2015 Mar 6;6:6302. PMID:25743702.

12.35 Giordano TJ

12.36A,B Giordano TJ

12.37A–C Giordano TJ

12.38A–C Giordano TJ

12.39 Giordano TJ

12.40A–C Giordano TJ

12.41A–C Tischler AS

12.42A–C Kozakewich HP

12.43 Tischler AS

12.44A,B Tischler AS

12.45A–C Kozakewich HP

12.46A–C Arthur J.A.T. Braat, Imaging Division, Department of Radiology and Nuclear Medicine, University Medical Center Utrecht and Princess Máxima Center for Pediatric Oncology, Utrecht

12.47 de Krijger RR

12.48A–D Tischler AS

12.49A–C Tischler AS

12.50A–D Tischler AS

12.51A–C Tischler AS

12.52 Kozakewich HP

12.53A–E Takao Sasaki, Department of Pediatric Surgery, Faculty of Medicine, University of Tsukuba, Tsukuba, Ibaraki

12.54 Arthur J.A.T. Braat, Imaging Division, Department of Radiology and Nuclear Medicine, University Medical Center Utrecht and Princess Máxima Center for Pediatric Oncology, Utrecht

12.55 Chu WCW

12.56 Arthur J.A.T. Braat, Imaging Division, Department of Radiology and Nuclear Medicine, University Medical Center Utrecht and Princess Máxima Center for Pediatric Oncology, Utrecht

12.57 Hicks MJ

12.58 Mete O

12.59A de Krijger RR

12.59B,C Mete O

12.60A,E Mete O

12.60B–D Kimura N

12.61A Kimura N

12.61B Mete O

12.62 de Krijger RR

12.63A,B Mete O

12.63C,D Kimura N

12.64A Kimura N

12.64B–D Mete O

12.65A–C Thompson LDR

12.66A–D Arthur J.A.T. Braat, Imaging Division, Department of Radiology and Nuclear Medicine, University Medical Center Utrecht and Princess Máxima Center for Pediatric Oncology, Utrecht

12.67 Hicks MJ

12.68 Hicks MJ

12.69A–C Hicks MJ

12.70 Mete O

12.71A–C Mete O; Asa SL

12.72A–F Mete O

13.01 Flaitz CM

13.02A,B Richardson MS

13.03 Flaitz CM

13.04A,B Muller S

13.05A Muller S

13.05B Reyes-Múgica M

13.06A,B Muller S

13.06C Reyes-Múgica M

13.07A Thompson LDR

13.07B Childers ELB

13.08 Odell EW

13.09A Childers ELB

13.09B,C Odell EW

13.10 Odell EW

13.11 Odell EW

13.12A,C Odell EW

13.12B Thompson LDR

13.13 Odell EW

13.14 Odell EW

13.15 Odell EW

13.16 Odell EW

13.17 Thompson LDR

13.18A–C Odell EW

13.19A–D Odell EW

13.20A,B Alaggio R

13.21A,B Perez-Atayde AR

13.22A–C Perez-Atayde AR

13.23 Nelson BL

13.24 Baumhoer D

13.25A–C Thompson LDR

13.25D Baumhoer D

13.26 Thompson LDR

13.27A Filippo Maria Tucci, UOS Chirurgia Cervicale, Dipartimento Chirurgia UOC ORL, Ospedale Pediatrico Bambino Gesù, IRCCS, Rome

13.27B Roman Carlos (deceased)

13.28A,B Thompson LDR

13.28C,D Reyes-Múgica M

13.29 Pulivarthi H. Rao, Department of Pediatrics, Baylor College of Medicine, Houston TX

13.30A,B Thompson LDR

13.31A,B Chiosea S

13.32 Chiosea S

13.33A–D Bell D

13.34A,B Thompson LDR

13.35A,B Perez-Atayde AR

13.36A,B Katabi N

13.36C Perez-Atayde AR

13.37A–D Perez-Atayde AR

13.38A,B Chu WCW

13.39A–C Chan JKC

13.40A,B Chan JKC

13.41A,B Chan JKC

13.42A,B Chan JKC

13.43 Stelow EB

13.44A,B Bishop JA

13.45A Alaggio R

13.45B,C Thompson LDR

13.46A,B Alaggio R

14.01 Travis WD, Brambilla E, Burke AP, et al., editors. WHO classification of tumours of the lung, pleura, thymus and heart. Lyon (France): International Agency for Research on Cancer; 2015. (WHO classification of tumours series, 4th ed.; vol. 7). https://publications.iarc.fr/17.

14.02 Travis WD, Brambilla E, Burke AP, et al., editors. WHO classification of tumours of the lung, pleura, thymus and heart. Lyon (France): International Agency for Research on Cancer; 2015. (WHO classification of tumours series, 4th ed.; vol. 7). https://publications.iarc.fr/17.

14.03A,B WHO Classification of Tumours Editorial Board. Thoracic tumours. Lyon (France): International Agency for Research on Cancer; 2021. (WHO classification of tumours series, 5th ed.; vol. 5). https://publications.iarc.fr/595.

14.04 Travis WD, Brambilla E, Burke AP, et al., editors. WHO classification of tumours of the lung, pleura, thymus and heart. Lyon (France): International Agency for Research on Cancer; 2015. (WHO classification of tumours series, 4th ed.; vol. 7). https://publications.iarc.fr/17.

14.05A–C Hill DA
14.06A,B Hill DA
14.07 Hill DA
14.08A Adapted, with permission, from: Padalino MA, Vida VL, Bhattarai A, et al. Giant intramural left ventricular rhabdomyoma in a newborn. Circulation. 2011 Nov 15;124(20):2275–7. PMID:22083149.
14.08B Basso C
14.09 WHO Classification of Tumours Editorial Board. Thoracic tumours. Lyon (France): International Agency for Research on Cancer; 2021. (WHO classification of tumours series, 5th ed.; vol. 5). https://publications.iarc.fr/595.
14.10A,B Basso C
14.11 Basso C

15.01 Torrelo A
15.02A,B Torrelo A
15.03A,B Torrelo A
15.04A Torrelo A
15.04B Colmenero I
15.05A,B Torrelo A
15.06 Singh V
15.07A,B Singh V
15.08A,B Singh V
15.09A,B Colmenero I
15.10A Torrelo A
15.10B Colmenero I
15.11A Torrelo A
15.11B–E Colmenero I
15.12A Torrelo A
15.12B Colmenero I
15.13A,B Colmenero I
15.14A Andrea Diociaiuti, UOS "Centro delle Dermatosi Croniche Complesse e Genodermatosi", UOC Dermatologia, Bambino Gesù Children's Hospital, Rome
15.14B Reyes-Múgica M
15.15A,B Reyes-Múgica M
15.16A–C Reyes-Múgica M
15.17A Salgado CM
15.17B–D Reyes-Múgica M
15.18A–C Reyes-Múgica M
15.19A,B de la Fouchardière A
15.20A–C de la Fouchardière A
15.21 de la Fouchardière A
15.22A,B Reyes-Múgica M
15.23A,B Reyes-Múgica M
15.24A,B de la Fouchardière A
15.25 Colmenero I
15.26A–C Colmenero I
15.27A–C Colmenero I
15.28 Reprinted, with permission, from: Quan VL, Panah E, Zhang B, et al. The role of gene fusions in melanocytic neoplasms. J Cutan Pathol. 2019 Nov;46(11):878–87. PMID:31152596.
15.29A,B Colmenero I
15.30A,B Colmenero I
15.31A–C Fraitag Spinner S
15.32A–C Fraitag Spinner S
15.33A–C Fraitag Spinner S
15.34A–F Fraitag Spinner S
15.35A–D Fraitag Spinner S

16.01A,B WHO Classification of Tumours Editorial Board. Soft tissue and bone tumours. Lyon (France): International Agency for Research on Cancer; 2020. (WHO classification of tumours series, 5th ed.; vol. 3). https://publications.iarc.fr/588.
16.02A–C Chu WCW
16.03 Rodriguez FJ
16.04 Rodriguez FJ
16.05 Rodriguez FJ
16.06 Rodriguez FJ
16.07 Schuhmann MU
16.08A,B Schuhmann MU
16.09A–C Perry A
16.10A Schuhmann MU
16.10B Stemmer-Rachamimov AO
16.11 Stemmer-Rachamimov AO
16.12A,B Stemmer-Rachamimov AO
16.12C Perry A
16.13A,B Perry A
16.14A,B Chu WCW
16.15A,B WHO Classification of Tumours Editorial Board. Central nervous system tumours. Lyon (France): International Agency for Research on Cancer; 2021. (WHO classification of tumours series, 5th ed.; vol. 6). https://publications.iarc.fr/601.
16.16A Santosh V
16.16B WHO Classification of Tumours Editorial Board. Central nervous system tumours. Lyon (France): International Agency for Research on Cancer; 2021. (WHO classification of tumours series, 5th ed.; vol. 6). https://publications.iarc.fr/601.
16.17A–C Lopes MBS
16.18A,B Lopes MBS
16.19A,B © Sarasin A. Reproduced from: LeBoit PE, Burg G, Weedon D, et al., editors. Pathology and genetics of skin tumours. Lyon (France): International Agency for Research on Cancer; 2005. (WHO classification of tumours series, 3rd ed.; vol. 6). https://publications.iarc.fr/6.
16.20 Bonnie L. Padwa, Department of Plastic and Oral Surgery, Boston Children's Hospital, Boston MA

16.21    Reprinted, with permission, from: Bresler SC, Padwa BL, Granter SR. Nevoid basal cell carcinoma syndrome (Gorlin syndrome). Head Neck Pathol. 2016 Jun;10(2):119–24. PMID:26971503;
and
Elder DE, Massi D, Scolyer RA, et al., editors. WHO classification of skin tumours. Lyon (France): International Agency for Research on Cancer; 2018. (WHO classification of tumours series, 4th ed.; vol. 11). https://publications.iarc.fr/560.

16.22A,B    Reprinted with permission from Bresler SC, Padwa BL, Granter SR. Nevoid basal cell carcinoma syndrome (Gorlin syndrome). Head Neck Pathol. 2016 Jun;10(2):119–24. PMID:26971503;
and
Elder DE, Massi D, Scolyer RA, et al., editors. WHO classification of skin tumours. Lyon (France): International Agency for Research on Cancer; 2018. (WHO classification of tumours series, 4th ed.; vol. 11). https://publications.iarc.fr/560.

16.23A,B    Adapted, with permission from the Archives of Pathology & Laboratory Medicine, from: Kraft S, Granter SR. Molecular pathology of skin neoplasms of the head and neck. Arch Pathol Lab Med. 2014 Jun;138(6):759–87. PMID:24878016. Copyright 2014 College of American Pathologists;
and
Elder DE, Massi D, Scolyer RA, et al., editors. WHO classification of skin tumours. Lyon (France): International Agency for Research on Cancer; 2018. (WHO classification of tumours series, 4th ed.; vol. 11). https://publications.iarc.fr/560.

16.24    Ketteler P
16.25A,B    Perry A
16.26A,B    Perry A
16.27    Plate KH;
and
Susanne Berger, Visual Science Communication
16.28    Asa SL
16.29A–D    Asa SL
16.30    Asa SL
16.31    Asa SL, Ezzat S, Mete O. The diagnosis and clinical significance of paragangliomas in unusual locations. J Clin Med. 2018 Sep 13;7(9):280. PMID:30217041;
and
Reprinted from: WHO Classification of Tumours Editorial Board. Central nervous system tumours. Lyon (France): International Agency for Research on Cancer; 2021. (WHO classification of tumours series, 5th ed.; vol. 6). https://publications.iarc.fr/601.
16.32    Chu WCW
16.33    Vujanic GM
16.34    Tomlinson GE
16.35    Tomlinson GE
16.36    Gupta A
16.37    Gupta A
16.38A–C    Gupta A
16.39    WHO Classification of Tumours Editorial Board. Digestive system tumours. Lyon (France): International Agency for Research on Cancer; 2019. (WHO classification of tumours series, 5th ed.; vol. 1). https://publications.iarc.fr/579.
16.40    Reprinted, with permission from BMJ Publishing Group Ltd, from: Bradford PT, Goldstein AM, Tamura D, et al. Cancer and neurologic degeneration in xeroderma pigmentosum: long term follow-up characterises the role of DNA repair. J Med Genet. 2011 Mar;48(3):168–76. PMID:21097776;
and

Adapted, with permission from Elsevier, from DiGiovanna JJ, Kraemer KH. Shining a light on xeroderma pigmentosum. J Invest Dermatol. 2012 Mar;132(3 Pt 2):785–96. PMID:22217736. Copyright 2012;
and
Elder DE, Massi D, Scolyer RA, et al., editors. WHO classification of skin tumours. Lyon (France): International Agency for Research on Cancer; 2018. (WHO classification of tumours series, 4th ed.; vol. 11). https://publications.iarc.fr/560.

16.41A–D    Reprinted, with permission from BMJ Publishing Group Ltd, from: Bradford PT, Goldstein AM, Tamura D, et al. Cancer and neurologic degeneration in xeroderma pigmentosum: long term follow-up characterises the role of DNA repair. J Med Genet. 2011 Mar;48(3):168–76. PMID:21097776;
and
Adapted, with permission from Elsevier, from DiGiovanna JJ, Kraemer KH. Shining a light on xeroderma pigmentosum. J Invest Dermatol. 2012 Mar;132(3 Pt 2):785–96. PMID:22217736. Copyright 2012;
and
Elder DE, Massi D, Scolyer RA, et al., editors. WHO classification of skin tumours. Lyon (France): International Agency for Research on Cancer; 2018. (WHO classification of tumours series, 4th ed.; vol. 11). https://publications.iarc.fr/560.

16.42    Adapted, with permission from Elsevier, from: van Steeg H, Kraemer KH. Xeroderma pigmentosum and the role of UV-induced DNA damage in skin cancer. Mol Med Today.

1999 Feb;5(2):86–94.
PMID:10200950. Copyright
1999;
and
Kraemer KH, Patronas
NJ, Schiffmann R, et al.
Xeroderma pigmentosum,
trichothiodystrophy and
Cockayne syndrome:
a complex genotype-
phenotype relationship.
Neuroscience. 2007
Apr 14;145(4):1388–96.
PMID:17276014. Copyright
2007;
and
DiGiovanna JJ, Kraemer KH.
Shining a light on xeroderma
pigmentosum. J Invest
Dermatol. 2012 Mar;132(3 Pt
2):785–96. PMID:22217736.
Copyright 2012;
and
Elder DE, Massi D, Scolyer
RA, et al., editors. WHO
classification of skin tumours.
Lyon (France): International
Agency for Research
on Cancer; 2018. (WHO
classification of tumours
series, 4th ed.; vol. 11).
https://publications.iarc.fr/560.

16.43A,B    Wang LL (Lisa L.)

16.44    Reprinted, with permission,
from: Fletcher CDM, Bridge
JA, Hogendoorn PCW, et al.,
editors. WHO classification
of tumours of soft tissue
and bone. Lyon (France):
International Agency for
Research on Cancer; 2013.
(WHO classification of tumours
series, 4th ed.; vol. 5).
https://publications.iarc.fr/15;
and
Adapted, with permission
from Elsevier, from: Larizza
L, Magnani I, Roversi G.
Rothmund-Thomson syndrome
and RECQL4 defect: splitting
and lumping. Cancer Lett.
2006 Jan 28;232(1):107–20.
PMID:16271439.

16.45    Hicks MJ

16.46    Hicks MJ

16.47A,B    Chu WCW

16.48    Chu WCW

16.49    Adapted from: IARC TP53
Database [Internet]. Lyon
(France): International
Agency for Research on
Cancer; 2018. Version R19,
August 2018. Available from:
http://p53.iarc.fr/.

16.50    Vania Nosé, Department of
Pathology, Massachusetts
General Hospital, Harvard
Medical School, Boston MA

16.51A,B    Gill AJ

16.52    Vania Nosé, Department of
Pathology, Massachusetts
General Hospital, Harvard
Medical School, Boston MA

16.53    Vania Nosé, Department of
Pathology, Massachusetts
General Hospital, Harvard
Medical School, Boston MA

16.54    Vania Nosé, Department of
Pathology, Massachusetts
General Hospital, Harvard
Medical School, Boston MA

16.55    Vania Nosé, Department of
Pathology, Massachusetts
General Hospital, Harvard
Medical School, Boston MA

16.56    Santagata S

16.57A,B    Tabori U

16.58A,B    Solomon DA

16.59A,B    Eberhart CG

**Tables**

Table A    Adapted from: WHO
Classification of Tumours
Editorial Board. Breast
tumours. Lyon (France):
International Agency for
Research on Cancer; 2019.
(WHO classification of tumours
series, 5th ed.; vol. 2).
https://publications.iarc.fr/581.

2.01    Niemeyer CM

2.02    Niemeyer CM

2.03    Klco JM

2.04    Fogelstrand L

2.05    Meshinchi S

2.06    Kratz CP

2.07    Alaggio R

2.08    Alaggio R

2.09    Oschlies I

2.10    Adapted, with permission
from Elsevier, from: Olsen
E, Vondorhcid E, Pimpinclli
N, et al. Revisions to the
staging and classification
of mycosis fungoides and
Sezary syndrome: a proposal
of the International Society
for Cutaneous Lymphomas
(ISCL) and the cutaneous
lymphoma task force of the
European Organization of
Research and Treatment
of Cancer (EORTC). Blood.
2007 Sep 15;110(6):1713–22.
PMID:17540844;
and
Elder DE, Massi D, Scolyer
RA, et al., editors. WHO
classification of skin tumours.
Lyon (France): International
Agency for Research
on Cancer; 2018. (WHO
classification of tumours series,
4th ed.; vol. 11).
https://publications.iarc.fr/560.

2.11    Alaggio R

2.12    Lamant-Rochaix L

2.13    Quintanilla-Martinez L

2.14    Bacon CM

2.15    Krishnan C

2.16    Krishnan C

2.17    Hebeda KM

3.01    Wesseling P

3.02    Published in: Louis DN,
Ohgaki H, Wiestler OD, et al.,
editors. WHO classification of
tumours of the central nervous
system. Lyon (France):
International Agency for
Research on Cancer; 2016.
(WHO classification of tumours
series, 4th rev. ed.; vol. 1).
https://publications.iarc.fr/543;
and
Adapted from: Collins VP,
Jones DT, Giannini C. Pilocytic
astrocytoma: pathology,
molecular mechanisms and
markers. Acta Neuropathol.
2015 Jun;129(6):775–88.
PMID:25792358.

3.03    Capper D

3.04    Blümcke I

3.05  David W. Ellison, St. Jude Children's Research Hospital, Memphis TN

3.06  White VA

3.07  Lloyd RV, Osamura RY, Klöppel G, et al., editors. WHO classification of tumours of endocrine organs. Lyon (France): International Agency for Research on Cancer; 2017. (WHO classification of tumours series, 4th ed.; vol. 10). https://publications.iarc.fr/554.

3.08  Lopes MBS

4.01  Shimada H

4.02  Shimada H

4.03  Reprinted, with permission, from: Cohn SL, Pearson AD, London WB, et al. The International Neuroblastoma Risk Group (INRG) classification system: an INRG Task Force report. J Clin Oncol. 2009 Jan 10;27(2):289–97. PMID:19047291. Copyright 2009 American Society of Clinical Oncology. All rights reserved.

5.01  Chevez-Barrios P

6.01  Martin Sill, Clinical Bioinformatics, Hopp Children's Cancer Center Heidelberg (KiTZ) and German Cancer Research Center (DKFZ), Heidelberg

6.02  Martin Sill, Clinical Bioinformatics, Hopp Children's Cancer Center Heidelberg (KiTZ) and German Cancer Research Center (DKFZ), Heidelberg

6.03  Black JO

6.04  Alaggio R

6.05  Surrey LF

6.06  Wang LL (Larry Liang)

6.07  Reprinted, with permission, from: Miettinen MM, Antonescu CR, Fletcher CDM, et al. Histopathologic evaluation of atypical neurofibromatous tumors and their transformation into malignant peripheral nerve sheath tumor in patients with neurofibromatosis 1-a consensus overview. Hum Pathol. 2017 Sep;67:1–10. PMID:28551330.

7.01  Rao BV

7.02  Srigley JR

7.03  Bode PK

7.04  Bode PK

7.05  Vang R

8.01  Moch H

8.02  Pritchard-Jones K

8.03  Moch H

8.04  Moch H

8.05  Vujanic GM

8.06  Vujanic GM

11.01  Ranganathan S

11.02  Ranganathan S

11.03  Ranganathan S

11.04  Cho SJ

11.05  Cho SJ

11.06  Cho SJ

12.01  Seethala R

12.02  Seethala R

12.03  Bauer AJ

12.04  Bauer AJ

12.05  Gill AJ

12.06  Mete O

12.07  La Rosa S

12.08  La Rosa S

13.01  Thompson LDR

15.01  Reyes-Múgica M

15.02  Reyes-Múgica M

15.03  Reyes-Múgica M

15.04  Gerami P

16.01  López-Terrada DH

16.03  Asa SL

16.04  WHO Classification of Tumours Editorial Board. Digestive system tumours. Lyon (France): International Agency for Research on Cancer; 2019. (WHO classification of tumours series, 5th ed.; vol. 1). https://publications.iarc.fr/579; and Reprinted, with permission, from: Frayling I, Berry I, Wallace A, et al. ACGS best practice guidelines for genetic testing and diagnosis of Lynch syndrome. London (UK): Association for Clinical Genomic Science; 2016 Mar. Available from: https://www.acgs.uk.com/media/10774/ls_bpg_approved.pdf, derived from van Lier et al., 2012 {7216}.

16.05  WHO Classification of Tumours Editorial Board. Digestive system tumours. Lyon (France): International Agency for Research on Cancer; 2019. (WHO classification of tumours series, 5th ed.; vol. 1). https://publications.iarc.fr/579.

16.06  WHO Classification of Tumours Editorial Board. Central nervous system tumours. Lyon (France): International Agency for Research on Cancer; 2021. (WHO classification of tumours series, 5th ed.; vol. 6). https://publications.iarc.fr/601; and WHO Classification of Tumours Editorial Board. Female genital tumours. Lyon (France): International Agency for Research on Cancer; 2020. (WHO classification of tumours series, 5th ed.; vol. 4). https://publications.iarc.fr/592; and Adapted, with permission from Springer Nature, from Nature Reviews Cancer: Foulkes WD, Priest JR, Duchaine TF. DICER1: mutations, microRNAs and mechanisms. Nat Rev Cancer. 2014 Oct;14(10):662–72. PMID:25176334. Copyright 2014.

**Boxes**

2.01  Alaggio R

2.02  Niemeyer CM

2.03  Torrelo A

2.04  Torrelo A

2.05  Alaggio R

3.01  Wesseling P

3.02  Reifenberger G

6.01  Rossi S

6.02  Reprinted, with permission, from: El-Mallawany NK, McAtee CL, Campbell LR, et al. Pediatric Kaposi sarcoma in context of the HIV epidemic in sub-Saharan Africa: current perspectives. Pediatric Health Med Ther. 2018 Apr 19;9:35–46. PMID:29722363. Originally published by, and used with permission from, Dove Medical Press Ltd.

11.01 Ranganathan S

11.02 WHO Classification of Tumours Editorial Board. Digestive system tumours. Lyon (France): International Agency for Research on Cancer; 2019. (WHO classification of tumours series, 5th ed.; vol. 1). https://publications.iarc.fr/579.

11.03 Ranganathan S

15.01 Colmenero I

16.01 Stemmer-Rachamimov AO

16.02 Adapted, with permission from Elsevier, from: Northrup H, Krueger DA, International Tuberous Sclerosis Complex Consensus Group. Tuberous sclerosis complex diagnostic criteria update: recommendations of the 2012 International Tuberous Sclerosis Complex Consensus Conference. Pediatr Neurol. 2013 Oct;49(4):243–54. PMID:24053982.

16.03 Pietsch T

16.05 Kraemer KH

16.06 Adapted, with permission, from: Wang LL, Plon SE. Rothmund-Thomson syndrome. In: Adam MP, Everman DB, Mirzaa GM, et al., editors. GeneReviews. Seattle (WA): University of Washington, Seattle; 1999 Oct 6 [updated 2020 Jun 4]. PMID:20301415.

16.07 Adapted from: Frebourg T, Bajalica Lagercrantz S, Oliveira C, et al. Guidelines for the Li-Fraumeni and heritable TP53-related cancer syndromes. Eur J Hum Genet. 2020 Oct;28(10):1379–86. PMID:32457520. https://creativecommons.org/licenses/by/4.0/

16.08 Reprinted, with permission, from: Vogel WH. Li-Fraumeni syndrome. J Adv Pract Oncol. 2017 Nov-Dec;8(7):742–6. PMID:30333936.

**Images on the cover of Part A**

| | |
|---|---|
| Top left | Fig. 6.229A: Bahrami A |
| Middle left | Fig. 6.220B: Bahrami A |
| Bottom left | Fig. 6.217: Adapted, with permission from Elsevier, from: Chen X, Bahrami A, Pappo A, et al. Recurrent somatic structural variations contribute to tumorigenesis in pediatric osteosarcoma. Cell Rep. 2014 Apr 10;7(1):104–12. PMID:24703847. |
| Top centre | Fig. 4.10: Chu WCW |
| Middle centre | Fig. 4.12A: Shimada H |
| Bottom centre | Fig. 4.14A: Katia Mazzocco, Department of Pathology, IRCCS Istituto Giannina Gaslini, Genoa |
| Top right | Fig. 2.102B: Chu WCW |
| Middle right | Fig. 2.104A: Hebeda KM |
| Bottom right | Fig. 2.105B: Hebeda KM |

**Images on the cover of Part B**

| | |
|---|---|
| Top left | Fig. 8.13B: Argani P |
| Middle left | Fig. 8.14B: Bode PK |
| Bottom left | Fig. 8.17B: Argani P |
| Top centre | Fig. 7.09: Bode PK |
| Middle centre | Fig. 7.10B: Bode PK |
| Bottom centre | Fig. 7.12: Bode PK |
| Top right | Fig. 12.56: Arthur J.A.T. Braat, Imaging Division, Department of Radiology and Nuclear Medicine, University Medical Center Utrecht and Princess Máxima Center for Pediatric Oncology, Utrecht |
| Middle right | Fig. 12.58: Mete O |
| Bottom right | Fig. 12.64B: Mete O |

**Images on the chapter title pages**

| | |
|---|---|
| Chapter 1 | Fig. 4.13C: Tornóczky T |
| Chapter 2 | Fig. 2.121: Said JW |
| Chapter 3 | Fig. 3.181A: Santagata S |
| Chapter 4 | Fig. 4.12B: Shimada H |
| Chapter 5 | Fig. 5.04B: Verdijk RM |
| Chapter 6 | Fig. 6.118D: Gupta A |
| Chapter 7 | Fig. 7.23: Vang R |
| Chapter 8 | Fig. 8.15C: Matoso A |
| Chapter 9 | Fig. 9.09B: Usubutun A |
| Chapter 10 | Fig. 10.02B: Gudi M |
| Chapter 11 | Fig. 11.13: Guettier C |
| Chapter 12 | Fig. 12.59A: de Krijger RR |
| Chapter 13 | Fig. 13.23: Nelson BL |
| Chapter 14 | Fig. 14.11: Basso C |
| Chapter 15 | Fig. 15.14B: Reyes-Múgica M |
| Chapter 16 | Fig. 16.58A: Solomon DA |

# References

1. Aalbers AM, van den Heuvel-Eibrink MM, Baumann I, et al. Bone marrow immunophenotyping by flow cytometry in refractory cytopenia of childhood. Haematologica. 2015 Mar;100(3):315–23. PMID:25425683

2. Aalbers AM, van den Heuvel-Eibrink MM, Baumann I, et al. T-cell receptor Vβ skewing frequently occurs in refractory cytopenia of childhood and is associated with an expansion of effector cytotoxic T cells: a prospective study by EWOG-MDS. Blood Cancer J. 2014 May 2;4:e209. PMID:24786393

3. Aarabi S, Drugas G, Avansino JR. Mesothelial cyst presenting as an irreducible inguinal mass. J Pediatr Surg. 2010 Jun;45(6):e19–21. PMID:20620295

4. Aarnio M, Salovaara R, Aaltonen LA, et al. Features of gastric cancer in hereditary non-polyposis colorectal cancer syndrome. Int J Cancer. 1997 Oct 21;74(5):551–5. PMID:9355980

5. Aaronson NL, Toman JC, Lerner MZ, et al. Fetal rhabdomyoma of the tongue in a newborn. Ear Nose Throat J. 2015 Jul;94(7):266–8. PMID:26214666

6. Aarts WM, Willemze R, Bende RJ, et al. VH gene analysis of primary cutaneous B-cell lymphomas: evidence for ongoing somatic hypermutation and isotype switching. Blood. 1998 Nov 15;92(10):3857–64. PMID:9808579

7. Abate F, Ambrosio MR, Mundo L, et al. Distinct viral and mutational spectrum of endemic Burkitt lymphoma. PLoS Pathog. 2015 Oct 15;11(10):e1005158. PMID:26468873

8. Abbey LM, Page DG, Sawyer DR. The clinical and histopathologic features of a series of 464 oral squamous cell papillomas. Oral Surg Oral Med Oral Pathol. 1980 May;49(5):419–28. PMID:6154913

9. Abbosh PH, Zhang S, Maclennan GT, et al. Germ cell origin of testicular carcinoid tumors. Clin Cancer Res. 2008 Mar 1;14(5):1393–6. PMID:18316560

10. Abbott JJ, Oliveira AM, Nascimento AG. The prognostic significance of fibrosarcomatous transformation in dermatofibrosarcoma protuberans. Am J Surg Pathol. 2006 Apr;30(4):436–43. PMID:16625088

11. Abbott TM, Hermann WJ Jr, Scully RE. Ovarian fetiform teratoma (homunculus) in a 9-year-old girl. Int J Gynecol Pathol. 1984;2(4):392–402. PMID:6724790

12. Abdallah A, Emel E, Gündüz HB, et al. Long-term surgical resection outcomes of pediatric myxopapillary ependymoma: experience of two centers and brief literature review. World Neurosurg. 2020 Apr;136:e245–61. PMID:31899399

13. Abdallah A, Pappo A, Reiss U, et al. Clinical manifestations of Pacak-Zhuang syndrome in a male pediatric patient. Pediatr Blood Cancer. 2020 Apr;67(4):e28096. PMID:31876082

14. Abdelbaki MS, Abu-Arja MH, Davidson TB, et al. Pineoblastoma in children less than six years of age: the Head Start I, II, and III experience. Pediatr Blood Cancer. 2020 Jun;67(6):e28252. PMID:32187454

15. AbdelBaki MS, Boué DR, Finlay JL, et al. Desmoplastic nodular medulloblastoma in young children: a management dilemma. Neuro Oncol. 2018 Jul 5;20(8):1026–33. PMID:29156007

16. Abdel-Rahman MH, Pilarski R, Cebulla CM, et al. Germline BAP1 mutation predisposes to uveal melanoma, lung adenocarcinoma, meningioma, and other cancers. J Med Genet. 2011 Dec;48(12):856–9. PMID:21941004

17. AbdollahiFakhim S, Bayazian G, Notash R. Nasal septal lipoma in a child: Pai syndrome or not? Int J Pediatr Otorhinolaryngol. 2014 Apr;78(4):697–700. PMID:24560239

18. Abdolrahimzadeh S, Plateroti AM, Recupero SM, et al. An update on the ophthalmologic features in the phakomatoses. J Ophthalmol. 2016;2016:3043026. PMID:27493794

19. Abdul-Al HM, Wang G, Makhlouf HR, et al. Fibrolamellar hepatocellular carcinoma: an immunohistochemical comparison with conventional hepatocellular carcinoma. Int J Surg Pathol. 2010 Oct;18(5):313–8. PMID:20444731

20. Abdulhamid I, Rabah R. Granular cell tumor of the bronchus. Pediatr Pulmonol. 2000 Nov;30(5):425–8. PMID:11064434

21. Abedalthagafi M. Constitutional mismatch repair-deficiency: current problems and emerging therapeutic strategies. Oncotarget. 2018 Oct 23;9(83):35458–69. PMID:30459937

22. Abla O, Jacobsen E, Picarsic J, et al. Consensus recommendations for the diagnosis and clinical management of Rosai-Dorfman-Destombes disease. Blood. 2018 Jun 28;131(26):2877–90. PMID:29720485

23. Ablin DS, Jain K, Howell L, et al. Ultrasound and MR imaging of fibromatosis colli (sternomastoid tumor of infancy). Pediatr Radiol. 1998 Apr;28(4):230–3. PMID:9545475

24. Abouzeid H, Balmer A, Moulin AP, et al. Phenotypic variability of retinocytomas: preregression and postregression growth patterns. Br J Ophthalmol. 2012 Jun;96(6):884–9. PMID:22328814

25. Abraham JA, Hornicek FJ, Kaufman AM, et al. Treatment and outcome of 82 patients with angiosarcoma. Ann Surg Oncol. 2007 Jun;14(6):1953–67. PMID:17356953

26. Abraham S, Salama M, Hancock J, et al. Congenital and childhood myeloproliferative disorders with eosinophilia responsive to imatinib. Pediatr Blood Cancer. 2012 Nov;59(5):928–9. PMID:22488677

27. Abraham SC, Klimstra DS, Wilentz RE, et al. Solid-pseudopapillary tumors of the pancreas are genetically distinct from pancreatic ductal adenocarcinomas and almost always harbor beta-catenin mutations. Am J Pathol. 2002 Apr;160(4):1361–9. PMID:11943721

28. Abraham SC, Montgomery EA, Giardiello FM, et al. Frequent beta-catenin mutations in juvenile nasopharyngeal angiofibromas. Am J Pathol. 2001 Mar;158(3):1073–8. PMID:11238055

29. Abraham SC, Wu TT, Hruban RH, et al. Genetic and immunohistochemical analysis of pancreatic acinar cell carcinoma: frequent allelic loss on chromosome 11p and alterations in the APC/beta-catenin pathway. Am J Pathol. 2002 Mar;160(3):953–62. PMID:11891193

30. Abraham SC, Wu TT, Klimstra DS, et al. Distinctive molecular genetic alterations in sporadic and familial adenomatous polyposis-associated pancreatoblastomas : frequent alterations in the APC/beta-catenin pathway and chromosome 11p. Am J Pathol. 2001 Nov;159(5):1619–27. PMID:11696422

31. Abrahamsson J, Forestier E, Heldrup J, et al. Response-guided induction therapy in pediatric acute myeloid leukemia with excellent remission rate. J Clin Oncol. 2011 Jan 20;29(3):310–5. PMID:21149663

32. Abramson DH, Dunkel IJ, Brodie SE, et al. A phase I/II study of direct intraarterial (ophthalmic artery) chemotherapy with melphalan for intraocular retinoblastoma initial results. Ophthalmology. 2008 Aug;115(8):1398–404. PMID:18342944

33. Abramson DH, Dunkel IJ, Marr BP, et al. Incidence of pineal gland cyst and pineoblastoma in children with retinoblastoma during the chemoreduction era. Am J Ophthalmol. 2013 Dec;156(6):1319–20. PMID:24238207

34. Abramson DH, Frank CM, Susman M, et al. Presenting signs of retinoblastoma. J Pediatr. 1998 Mar;132(3 Pt 1):505–8. PMID:9544909

35. Abramson DH, Shields CL, Munier FL, et al. Treatment of retinoblastoma in 2015. JAMA Ophthalmol. 2015 Nov;133(11):1341–7. PMID:26378747

36. Abruzzo LV, Jaffe ES, Cotelingam JD, et al. T-cell lymphoblastic lymphoma with eosinophilia associated with subsequent myeloid malignancy. Am J Surg Pathol. 1992 Mar;16(3):236–45. PMID:1599015

37. Abu J, Nunns D, Ireland D, et al. Malignant progression through borderline changes in recurrent Mullerian papilloma of the vagina. Histopathology. 2003 May;42(5):510–1. PMID:12713630

38. Acharya S, DeWees T, Shinohara ET, et al. Long-term outcomes and late effects for childhood and young adulthood intracranial germinomas. Neuro Oncol. 2015 May;17(5):741–6. PMID:25422317

39. Acharya S, Sarafoglou K, LaQuaglia M, et al. Thyroid neoplasms after therapeutic radiation for malignancies during childhood or adolescence. Cancer. 2003 May 15;97(10):2397–403. PMID:12733137

40. Achatz MI, Olivier M, Le Calvez F, et al. The TP53 mutation, R337H, is associated with Li-Fraumeni and Li-Fraumeni-like syndromes in Brazilian families. Cancer Lett. 2007 Jan 8;245(1-2):96–102. PMID:16494995

41. Achatz MI, Porter CC, Brugières L, et al. Cancer screening recommendations and clinical management of inherited gastrointestinal cancer syndromes in childhood. Clin Cancer Res. 2017 Jul 1;23(13):e107–14. PMID:28674119

42. Achilles E, Padberg BC, Holl K, et al. Immunocytochemistry of paragangliomas–value of staining for S-100 protein and glial fibrillary acid protein in diagnosis and prognosis. Histopathology. 1991 May;18(5):453–8. PMID:1679411

43. Achten R, Debiec-Rychter M, De Wever I, et al. An unusual case of clear cell sarcoma arising in the jejunum highlights the diagnostic value of molecular genetic techniques in establishing a correct diagnosis. Histopathology. 2005 Apr;46(4):472–4. PMID:15810965

44. Ackermann O, Fabre M, Franchi S, et al. Widening spectrum of liver angiosarcoma in children. J Pediatr Gastroenterol Nutr. 2011 Dec;53(6):615–9. PMID:21832953

45. Acquaye AA, Vera E, Gilbert MR, et al. Clinical presentation and outcomes for adult ependymoma patients. Cancer. 2017 Feb 1;123(3):494–501. PMID:27679985

46. Acree SC, Tovar JP, Pattengale PK, et al. Subcutaneous panniculitis-like T-cell lymphoma in two pediatric patients: an HIV-positive adolescent and a 4-month-old infant. Fetal Pediatr Pathol. 2013 Jun;32(3):175–83. PMID:23092204

47. Adam R, Spier I, Zhao B, et al. Exome sequencing identifies biallelic MSH3 germline mutations as a recessive subtype of colorectal adenomatous polyposis. Am J Hum Genet. 2016 Aug 4;99(2):337–51. PMID:27476653

48. Adameyko I, Lallemend F. Glial versus melanocyte cell fate choice: Schwann cell precursors as a cellular origin of melanocytes. Cell Mol Life Sci. 2010 Sep;67(18):3037–55. PMID:20454996

49. Adameyko I, Lallemend F, Aquino JB, et al. Schwann cell precursors from nerve innervation are a cellular origin of melanocytes in skin. Cell. 2009 Oct 16;139(2):366–79. PMID:19837037

50. Adams DM, Brandão LR, Peterman CM, et al. Vascular anomaly cases for the pediatric hematologist oncologists-an interdisciplinary review. Pediatr Blood Cancer. 2018 Jan;65(1). PMID:28727248

51. Adams DM, Hammill A. Other vascular tumors. Semin Pediatr Surg. 2014 Aug;23(4):173–7. PMID:25241094

52. Adams DM, Ricci KW. Vascular anomalies: diagnosis of complicated anomalies and new medical treatment options. Hematol Oncol Clin North Am. 2019 Jun;33(3):455–70. PMID:31030813

53. Adan F, Crijns MB, Zandstra WSE, et al. Cumulative risk of skin tumours in patients with Lynch syndrome. Br J Dermatol. 2018 Aug;179(2):522–3. PMID:29542113

54. Addis BJ, Isaacson PG. Large cell lymphoma of the mediastinum: a B-cell tumour of probable thymic origin. Histopathology. 1986 Apr;10(4):379–90. PMID:2423430

55. Adebayo ET, Ajike SO, Adekeye EO. Odontogenic tumours in children and adolescents: a study of 78 Nigerian cases. J Craniomaxillofac Surg. 2002 Oct;30(5):267–72. PMID:12377198

56. Adeleye AO, Okolo CA, Akang EE, et al. Cerebral pleomorphic xanthoastrocytoma associated with NF1: an updated review with a rare atypical case from Africa. Neurosurg Rev. 2012 Jul;35(3):313–9. PMID:22020543

57. Adeniran A, Al-Ahmadie H, Mahoney MC, et al. Granular cell tumor of the breast: a series of 17 cases and review of the literature. Breast J. 2004 Nov-Dec;10(6):528–31. PMID:15569210

58. Adkins GF. Low grade basaloid adenocarcinoma of salivary gland in childhood–the so-called hybrid basal cell adenoma–adenoid cystic carcinoma. Pathology. 1990 Oct;22(4):187–90. PMID:1965332

59. Adler R, Viehmann S, Kuhlisch E, et al. Correlation of BCR/ABL transcript variants with patients' characteristics in childhood chronic myeloid leukaemia. Eur J Haematol. 2009 Feb;82(2):112–8. PMID:19067742

60. Advani SH, Malhotra H, Kadam PR, et al. T-lymphoid blast crisis in chronic myeloid leukemia. Am J Hematol. 1991 Feb;36(2):86–92. PMID:2012070

61. Aerts I, Sastre-Garau X, Savignoni A, et al. Results of a multicenter prospective study on the postoperative treatment of unilateral retinoblastoma after primary enucleation.

J Clin Oncol. 2013 Apr 10;31(11):1458–63. PMID:23460706
**62.** Agaimy A. Microscopic intraneural perineurial cell proliferations in patients with neurofibromatosis type 1. Ann Diagn Pathol. 2014 Apr;18(2):95–8. PMID:24461704
**63.** Agaimy A, Bieg M, Michal M, et al. Recurrent somatic PDGFRB mutations in sporadic infantile/solitary adult myofibromas but not in angioleiomyomas and myopericytomas. Am J Surg Pathol. 2017 Feb;41(2):195–203. PMID:27776010
**64.** Agaimy A, Michal M, Chiosea S, et al. Phosphaturic mesenchymal tumors: clinicopathologic, immunohistochemical and molecular analysis of 22 cases expanding their morphologic and immunophenotypic spectrum. Am J Surg Pathol. 2017 Oct;41(10):1371–80. PMID:28614212
**65.** Agaimy A, Thiel F, Hartmann A, et al. SMARCA4-deficient undifferentiated carcinoma of the ovary (small cell carcinoma, hypercalcemic type): clinicopathologic and immunohistochemical study of 3 cases. Ann Diagn Pathol. 2015 Oct;19(5):283–7. PMID:26123103
**66.** Agaimy A, Wünsch PH, Schroeder J, et al. Low-grade abdominopelvic sarcoma with myofibroblastic features (low-grade myofibroblastic sarcoma): clinicopathological, immunohistochemical, molecular genetic and ultrastructural study of two cases with literature review. J Clin Pathol. 2008 Mar;61(3):301–6. PMID:17513510
**67.** Agamanolis DP, Katsetos CD, Klonk CJ, et al. An unusual form of superficially disseminated glioma in children: report of 3 cases. J Child Neurol. 2012 Jun;27(6):727–33. PMID:22596013
**68.** Agaram NP, Baren A, Antonescu CR. Pediatric and adult hepatic embryonal sarcoma: a comparative ultrastructural study with morphologic correlations. Ultrastruct Pathol. 2006 Nov-Dec;30(6):403–8. PMID:17182431
**69.** Agaram NP, Chen CL, Zhang L, et al. Recurrent MYOD1 mutations in pediatric and adult sclerosing and spindle cell rhabdomyosarcomas: evidence for a common pathogenesis. Genes Chromosomes Cancer. 2014 Sep;53(9):779–87. PMID:24824843
**70.** Agaram NP, Chen HW, Zhang L, et al. EWSR1-PBX3: a novel gene fusion in myoepithelial tumors. Genes Chromosomes Cancer. 2015 Feb;54(2):63–71. PMID:25231231
**71.** Agaram NP, LaQuaglia MP, Alaggio R, et al. MYOD1-mutant spindle cell and sclerosing rhabdomyosarcoma: an aggressive subtype irrespective of age. A reappraisal for molecular classification and risk stratification. Mod Pathol. 2019 Jan;32(1):27–36. PMID:30181563
**72.** Agaram NP, Laquaglia MP, Ustun B, et al. Molecular characterization of pediatric gastrointestinal stromal tumors. Clin Cancer Res. 2008 May 15;14(10):3204–15. PMID:18483389
**73.** Agaram NP, LeLoarer FV, Zhang L, et al. USP6 gene rearrangements occur preferentially in giant cell reparative granulomas of the hands and feet but not in gnathic location. Hum Pathol. 2014 Jun;45(6):1147–52. PMID:24742829
**74.** Agaram NP, Prakash S, Antonescu CR. Deep-seated plexiform schwannoma: a pathologic study of 16 cases and comparative analysis with the superficial variety. Am J Surg Pathol. 2005 Aug;29(8):1042–8. PMID:16006798
**75.** Agaram NP, Sung YS, Zhang L, et al. Dichotomy of genetic abnormalities in PEComas with therapeutic implications. Am J Surg Pathol. 2015 Jun;39(6):813–25. PMID:25651471
**76.** Agaram NP, Zhang L, Cotzia P, et al. Expanding the spectrum of genetic alterations in pseudomyogenic hemangioendothelioma with recurrent novel ACTB-FOSB gene fusions. Am J Surg Pathol. 2018 Dec;42(12):1653–61. PMID:30256258
**77.** Agaram NP, Zhang L, Dickson BC, et al. A molecular study of synovial chondromatosis. Genes Chromosomes Cancer. 2020 Mar;59(3):144–51. PMID:31589790
**78.** Agaram NP, Zhang L, Jungbluth AA, et al. A molecular reappraisal of glomus tumors and related pericytic neoplasms with emphasis on NOTCH-gene fusions. Am J Surg Pathol. 2020 Nov;44(11):1556–62. PMID:32604167
**79.** Agaram NP, Zhang L, Sung YS, et al. Expanding the spectrum of intraosseous rhabdomyosarcoma: correlation between 2 distinct gene fusions and phenotype. Am J Surg Pathol. 2019 May;43(5):695–702. PMID:30720533
**80.** Agaram NP, Zhang L, Sung YS, et al. Recurrent NTRK1 gene fusions define a novel subset of locally aggressive lipofibromatosis-like neural tumors. Am J Surg Pathol. 2016 Oct;40(10):1407–16. PMID:27259011
**81.** Agarwal S, Jindal I, Balazs A, et al. Catecholamine-secreting tumors in pediatric patients with cyanotic congenital Heart Disease. J Endocr Soc. 2019 Sep 5;3(11):2135–50. PMID:31687640
**82.** Agarwal SK, Munjal M, Rai D, et al. Malignant transformation of vagal nerve schwannoma in to angiosarcoma: a rare event. J Surg Tech Case Rep. 2015 Jan-Jun;7(1):17–9. PMID:27512546
**83.** Agely A, Okromelidze L, Vilanilam GK, et al. Ectopic pituitary adenomas: common presentations of a rare entity. Pituitary. 2019 Aug;22(4):339–43. PMID:30895500
**84.** Aghajan Y, Levy ML, Malicki DM, et al. Novel PPP1CB-ALK fusion protein in a high-grade glioma of infancy. BMJ Case Rep. 2016 Aug 16;2016:bcr2016217189. PMID:27530886
**85.** Aghamohammadi A, Parvaneh N, Tirgari F, et al. Lymphoma of mucosa-associated lymphoid tissue in common variable immunodeficiency. Leuk Lymphoma. 2006 Feb;47(2):343–6. PMID:16321869
**86.** Agnihotri S, Jalali S, Wilson MR, et al. The genomic landscape of schwannoma. Nat Genet. 2016 Nov;48(11):1339–48. PMID:27723760
**87.** Agostinelli C, Akarca AU, Ramsay A, et al. Novel markers in pediatric-type follicular lymphoma. Virchows Arch. 2019 Dec;475(6):771–9. PMID:31686194
**88.** Agoston AT, Liang CW, Richkind KE, et al. Trisomy 18 is a consistent cytogenetic feature in pilomatricoma. Mod Pathol. 2010 Aug;23(8):1147–50. PMID:20495544
**89.** Agrawal D, Singhal A, Hendson G, et al. Gyriform differentiation in medulloblastoma - a radiological predictor of histology. Pediatr Neurosurg. 2007;43(2):142–5. PMID:17337929
**90.** Agrawal M, Uppin MS, Patibandla MR, et al. Teratomas in central nervous system: a clinico-morphological study with review of literature. Neurol India. 2010 Nov-Dec;58(6):841–6. PMID:21150046
**91.** Agrawal P, Srinivasan R, Rajwanshi A, et al. Fine needle aspiration cytology of paediatric soft tissue tumours highlighting challenges in diagnosis of benign lesions and unusual malignant tumours. Cytopathology. 2019 May;30(3):301–8. PMID:30848523
**92.** Agrawal R, Wang J. Pediatric follicular lymphoma: a rare clinicopathologic entity. Arch Pathol Lab Med. 2009 Jan;133(1):142–6. PMID:19123728
**93.** Agrawal T, Blau AJ, Chwals WJ, et al. A unique case of mediastinal teratoma with mature pancreatic tissue, nesidioblastosis, and aberrant islet differentiation: a case report and literature review. Endocr Pathol. 2016 Mar;27(1):21–4. PMID:26318442
**94.** Agretti P, Segni M, De Marco G, et al. Prevalence of activating thyrotropin receptor and Gsα gene mutations in paediatric thyroid toxic adenomas: a multicentric Italian study. Clin Endocrinol (Oxf). 2013 Nov;79(5):747–9. PMID:23346880
**95.** Agrons GA, Lonergan GJ, Dickey GE, et al. Adrenocortical neoplasms in children: radiologic-pathologic correlation. Radiographics. 1999 Jul-Aug;19(4):989–1008. PMID:10464805
**96.** Aguilera D, Flamini R, Mazewski C, et al. Response of subependymal giant cell astrocytoma with spinal cord metastasis to everolimus. J Pediatr Hematol Oncol. 2014 Oct;36(7):e448–51. PMID:24276039
**97.** Aguilera D, Janss A, Mazewski C, et al. Successful retreatment of a child with a refractory brainstem ganglioglioma with vemurafenib. Pediatr Blood Cancer. 2016 Mar;63(3):541–3. PMID:26579623
**98.** Agustsson TT, Baldvinsdottir T, Jonasson JG, et al. The epidemiology of pituitary adenomas in Iceland, 1955-2012: a nationwide population-based study. Eur J Endocrinol. 2015 Nov;173(5):655–64. PMID:26423473
**99.** Ahadova A, Gallon R, Gebert J, et al. Three molecular pathways model colorectal carcinogenesis in Lynch syndrome. Int J Cancer. 2018 Jul 1;143(1):139–50. PMID:29424427
**100.** Ahadova A, von Knebel Doeberitz M, Bläker H, et al. CTNNB1-mutant colorectal carcinomas with immediate invasive growth: a model of interval cancers in Lynch syndrome. Fam Cancer. 2016 Oct;15(4):579–86. PMID:26960970
**101.** Ahlsén G, Gillberg IC, Lindblom R, et al. Tuberous sclerosis in Western Sweden. A population study of cases with early childhood onset. Arch Neurol. 1994 Jan;51(1):76–81. PMID:8274113
**102.** Ahmed MAM, Uehelie MA, Rage AMA, et al. Aggressive angiomyxoma of the penis: the first case report in a 9-month-old infant. Urology. 2017 Jun;104:187–90. PMID:28161377
**103.** Ahn D, Lee GJ, Sohn JH, et al. Fine-needle aspiration cytology versus core-needle biopsy for the diagnosis of extracranial head and neck schwannoma. Head Neck. 2018 Dec;40(12):2695–700. PMID:30457183
**104.** Ahn MS, Hayashi GM, Hilsinger RL Jr, et al. Familial mixed tumors of the parotid gland. Head Neck. 1999 Dec;21(8):772–5. PMID:10562692
**105.** Ahuja A, Iyer VK, Mathur S. Fine needle aspiration cytology and immunocytochemistry of myxopapillary ependymoma. Cytopathology. 2013 Apr;24(2):134–6. PMID:22175883
**106.** Ahuja A, Sharma MC, Suri V, et al. Pineal anlage tumour - a rare entity with divergent histology. J Clin Neurosci. 2011 Jun;18(6):811–3. PMID:21435885
**107.** Aicardi J. Aicardi syndrome. Brain Dev. 2005 Apr;27(3):164–71. PMID:15737696
**108.** Aigner T, Neureiter D, Völker U, et al. Epithelial-mesenchymal transdifferentiation and extracellular matrix gene expression in pleomorphic adenomas of the parotid salivary gland. J Pathol. 1998 Oct;186(2):178–85. PMID:9924434
**109.** Ainsworth KE, Chavhan GB, Gupta AA, et al. Congenital infantile fibrosarcoma: review of imaging features. Pediatr Radiol. 2014 Sep;44(9):1124–9. PMID:24706181
**110.** Ait Ouakrim D, Dashti SG, Chau R, et al. Aspirin, ibuprofen, and the risk of colorectal cancer in Lynch syndrome. J Natl Cancer Inst. 2015 Jun 24;107(9):djv170. PMID:26109217
**111.** Ajeawung NF, Nguyen TTM, Lu L, et al. Mutations in ANAPC1, encoding a scaffold subunit of the anaphase-promoting complex, cause Rothmund-Thomson syndrome type 1. Am J Hum Genet. 2019 Sep 5;105(3):625–30. PMID:31303264
**112.** Ajithkumar T, Mazhari AL, Stickan-Verfürth M, et al. Proton therapy for craniopharyngioma - an early report from a single European centre. Clin Oncol (R Coll Radiol). 2018 May;30(5):307–16. PMID:29459099
**113.** Akakpo PK, Derkyi-Kwarteng L, Quayson SE, et al. Ovarian tumors in children and adolescents: a 10-yr histopathologic review in Korle-Bu Teaching Hospital, Ghana. Int J Gynecol Pathol. 2016 Jul;35(4):333–6. PMID:26630227
**114.** Akhavan A, Richards M, Shnorhavorian M, et al. Renal cell carcinoma in children, adolescents and young adults: a National Cancer Database study. J Urol. 2015 Apr;193(4):1336–41. PMID:25451825
**115.** Akhlaghpoor S, Aziz Ahari A, Ahmadi SA, et al. Histological evaluation of drill fragments obtained during osteoid osteoma radiofrequency ablation. Skeletal Radiol. 2010 May;39(5):451–5. PMID:20204353
**116.** Akirov A, Asa SL, Amer L, et al. The clinicopathological spectrum of acromegaly. J Clin Med. 2019 Nov 13;8(11):E1962. PMID:31766255
**117.** Akiyama S, Ito K, Kim WJ, et al. Prepubertal testicular tumors: a single-center experience of 44years. J Pediatr Surg. 2016 Aug;51(8):1351–4. PMID:26987710
**118.** Akramipour R, Zargooshi J, Rahimi Z. Infant with concomitant presence of hernia/hydrocele and primary paratesticular neuroblastoma: a diagnostic and therapeutic challenge. J Pediatr Hematol Oncol. 2009 May;31(5):349. PMID:19415016
**119.** Akyüz C, Emir S, Büyükpamukçu M, et al. Successful treatment with interferon alfa in infiltrating angiolipoma: a case presenting with Kasabach-Merritt syndrome. Arch Dis Child. 2003 Jan;88(1):67–8. PMID:12495967
**120.** Al Dhaybi R, Agoumi M, Gagné I, et al. p16 expression: a marker of differentiation between childhood malignant melanomas and Spitz nevi. J Am Acad Dermatol. 2011 Aug;65(2):357–63. PMID:21550132
**121.** Al Khader A, Nsour E, Al-Zubi RB, et al. Extraskeletal myxoid chondrosarcoma of the leg in a child: a case report. Medicine (Baltimore). 2019 Apr;98(15):e15207. PMID:30985717
**122.** Al Mahmoud R, Weitzman S, Schechter T, et al. Peripheral T-cell lymphoma in children and adolescents: a single-institution experience. J Pediatr Hematol Oncol. 2012 Nov;34(8):611–6. PMID:23042011
**123.** Al-Abbadi MA, Almasri NM, Al-Quran S, et al. Cytokeratin and epithelial membrane antigen expression in angiosarcomas: an immunohistochemical study of 33 cases. Arch Pathol Lab Med. 2007 Feb;131(2):288–92. PMID:17284115
**124.** Al-Adnani M. Soft tissue perineurioma in a child with neurofibromatosis type 1: a case report and review of the literature. Pediatr Dev Pathol. 2017 Sep-Oct;20(5):444–8. PMID:28812461
**125.** Alagaratnam S, Kurzawinski TR. Aetiology, diagnosis and surgical treatment of primary hyperparathyroidism in children: new trends. Horm Res Paediatr. 2015 May 1. PMID:25966652
**126.** Alaggio R, Amador C, Anagnostopoulos I, et al. The 5th edition of the World Health Organization Classification of Haematolymphoid Tumours: lymphoid neoplasms. Leukemia. 2022 Jul ;36(7):1720–48. PMID:35732829
**127.** Alaggio R, Barisani D, Ninfo V, et al. Morphologic overlap between infantile myofibromatosis and infantile fibrosarcoma: a pitfall in diagnosis. Pediatr Dev Pathol. 2008 Sep-Oct;11(5):355–62. PMID:19006426
**128.** Alaggio R, Bisogno G, Rosato A, et al. Undifferentiated sarcoma: Does it exist? A

clinicopathologic study of 7 pediatric cases and review of literature. Hum Pathol. 2009 Nov;40(11):1600–10. PMID:19647855
**129.** Alaggio R, Cecchetto G, Martignoni G, et al. Malignant perivascular epithelioid cell tumor in children: description of a case and review of the literature. J Pediatr Surg. 2012 Jun;47(6):e31–40. PMID:22703822
**130.** Alaggio R, Coffin CM, Dall'igna P, et al. Myxoinflammatory fibroblastic sarcoma: report of a case and review of the literature. Pediatr Dev Pathol. 2012 May-Jun;15(3):254–8. PMID:22372507
**131.** Alaggio R, Coffin CM, Vargas SO. Soft tissue tumors of uncertain origin. Pediatr Dev Pathol. 2012;15(1 Suppl):267–305. PMID:22420732
**132.** Alaggio R, Coffin CM, Weiss SW, et al. Liposarcomas in young patients: a study of 82 cases occurring in patients younger than 22 years of age. Am J Surg Pathol. 2009 May;33(5):645–58. PMID:19194281
**133.** Alaggio R, Collini P, Randall RL, et al. Undifferentiated high-grade pleomorphic sarcomas in children: a clinicopathologic study of 10 cases and review of literature. Pediatr Dev Pathol. 2010 May-Jun;13(3):209–17. PMID:20055602
**134.** Alaggio R, Ninfo V, Rosolen A, et al. Primitive myxoid mesenchymal tumor of infancy: a clinicopathologic report of 6 cases. Am J Surg Pathol. 2006 Mar;30(3):388–94. PMID:16538060
**135.** Alaggio R, Zhang L, Sung YS, et al. A molecular study of pediatric spindle and sclerosing rhabdomyosarcoma: identification of novel and recurrent VGLL2-related fusions in infantile cases. Am J Surg Pathol. 2016 Feb;40(2):224–35. PMID:26501226
**136.** Al-Agha OM, Huwait HF, Chow C, et al. FOXL2 is a sensitive and specific marker for sex cord-stromal tumors of the ovary. Am J Surg Pathol. 2011 Apr;35(4):484–94. PMID:21378549
**137.** Alahmadi H, Lee D, Wilson JR, et al. Clinical features of silent corticotroph adenomas. Acta Neurochir (Wien). 2012 Aug;154(8):1493–8. PMID:22619024
**138.** Alam FM, Samarasinghe DS, Pillai RG. Myofibroblastoma of the breast in an adolescent. Saudi Med J. 2002 Feb;23(2):232–3. PMID:11938404
**139.** Alassiri AH, Ali RH, Shen Y, et al. ETV6-NTRK3 is expressed in a subset of ALK-negative inflammatory myofibroblastic tumors. Am J Surg Pathol. 2016 Aug;40(8):1051–61. PMID:27259007
**140.** Albani A, Pérez-Rivas LG, Dimopoulou C, et al. The USP8 mutational status may predict long-term remission in patients with Cushing's disease. Clin Endocrinol (Oxf). 2018 Jun 29. PMID:29957855
**141.** Al-Bazzaz S, Karamchandani J, Mocarski E, et al. Ectopic prolactin-producing pituitary adenoma in a benign ovarian cystic teratoma. Endocr Pathol. 2014 Sep;25(3):321–3. PMID:24584638
**142.** Alberghini M, Kliskey K, Krenacs T, et al. Morphological and immunophenotypic features of primary and metastatic giant cell tumour of bone. Virchows Arch. 2010 Jan;456(1):97–103. PMID:20012988
**143.** Albergo JI, Gaston CL, Laitinen M, et al. Ewing's sarcoma: only patients with 100% of necrosis after chemotherapy should be classified as having a good response. Bone Joint J. 2016 Aug;98-B(8):1138–44. PMID:27482030
**144.** Albers P, Siener R, Kliesch S, et al. Risk factors for relapse in clinical stage I nonseminomatous testicular germ cell tumors: results of the German Testicular Cancer Study Group Trial. J Clin Oncol. 2003 Apr 15;21(8):1505–12. PMID:12697874
**145.** Albers P, Ulbright TM, Albers J, et al. Tumor proliferative activity is predictive of pathological stage in clinical stage A nonseminomatous testicular germ cell tumors. J Urol. 1996 Feb;155(2):579–86. PMID:8558664
**146.** Albertini AF, Brousse N, Bodemer C, et al. Retiform hemangioendothelioma developed on the site of an earlier cystic lymphangioma in a six-year-old girl. Am J Dermatopathol. 2011 Oct;33(7):e84–7. PMID:21915027
**147.** Albores-Saavedra J, Simpson KW, Bilello SJ. The clear cell variant of solid pseudopapillary tumor of the pancreas: a previously unrecognized pancreatic neoplasm. Am J Surg Pathol. 2006 Oct;30(10):1237–42. PMID:17001153
**148.** Albrecht S, Rouah E, Becker LE, et al. Transthyretin immunoreactivity in choroid plexus neoplasms and brain metastases. Mod Pathol. 1991 Sep;4(5):610–4. PMID:1758873
**149.** Alcedo J, Noll M. Hedgehog and its patched-smoothened receptor complex: a novel signalling mechanism at the cell surface. Biol Chem. 1997 Jul;378(7):583–90. PMID:9278137
**150.** Alessandri AJ, Pritchard SL, Schultz KR, et al. A population-based study of pediatric anaplastic large cell lymphoma. Cancer. 2002 Mar 15;94(6):1830–5. PMID:11920547
**151.** Alexander J, Watanabe T, Wu TT, et al. Histopathological identification of colon cancer with microsatellite instability. Am J Pathol. 2001 Feb;158(2):527–35. PMID:11159189
**152.** Alexander N, Sullivan K, Shaikh F, et al. Characteristics and management of ganglioneuroma and ganglioneuroblastoma-intermixed in children and adolescents. Pediatr Blood Cancer. 2018 May;65(5):e26964. PMID:29369484
**153.** Alexandrescu S, Korshunov A, Lai SH, et al. Epithelioid glioblastomas and anaplastic epithelioid pleomorphic xanthoastrocytomas–same entity or first cousins? Brain Pathol. 2016 Mar;26(2):215–23. PMID:26238627
**154.** Alexandrov LB, Nik-Zainal S, Wedge DC, et al. Signatures of mutational processes in human cancer. Nature. 2013 Aug 22;500(7463):415–21. PMID:23945592
**155.** Alford KA, Reinhardt K, Garnett C, et al. Analysis of GATA1 mutations in Down syndrome transient myeloproliferative disorder and myeloid leukemia. Blood. 2011 Aug 25;118(8):2222–38. PMID:21715302
**156.** Al-Hajri A, Al-Mughairi S, Somani A, et al. Pathology-MRI correlations in diffuse low-grade epilepsy associated tumors. J Neuropathol Exp Neurol. 2017 Dec 1;76(12):1023–33. PMID:29040640
**157.** Al Hamed R, Bazarbachi AH, Mohty M. Epstein-Barr virus-related post-transplant lymphoproliferative disease (EBV-PTLD) in the setting of allogeneic stem cell transplantation: a comprehensive review from pathogenesis to forthcoming treatment modalities. Bone Marrow Transplant. 2020 Jan;55(1):25–39. PMID:31089285
**158.** Al-Hussaini M, Abuirmeileh N, Swaidan M, et al. Embryonal tumor with abundant neuropil and true rosettes: a report of three cases of a rare tumor, with an unusual case showing rhabdomyoblastic and melanocytic differentiation. Neuropathology. 2011 Dec;31(6):620–5. PMID:22103481
**159.** Ali JB, Sepp T, Ward S, et al. Mutations in the TSC1 gene account for a minority of patients with tuberous sclerosis. J Med Genet. 1998 Dec;35(12):969–72. PMID:9863590
**160.** Ali MJ, Honavar SG, Reddy VA. Orbital retinoblastoma: present status and future challenges - a review. Saudi J Ophthalmol. 2011 Apr;25(2):159–67. PMID:23960917
**161.** Ali MJ, Honavar SG, Vemuganti GK. Ciliary body medulloepithelioma in an adult. Surv Ophthalmol. 2013 May-Jun;58(3):266–72. PMID:23218809
**162.** Ali NM, Niada S, Morris MR, et al. Comprehensive molecular characterization of adamantinoma and OFD-like adamantinoma bone tumors. Am J Surg Pathol. 2019 Jul;43(7):965–74. PMID:31021853
**163.** Ali SZ, Cibas ES, editors. The Bethesda system for reporting thyroid cytopathology: definitions, criteria, and explanatory notes. 2nd ed. New York (NY): Springer; 2018.
**164.** Al-Ibraheemi A, Folpe AL, Perez-Atayde AR, et al. Aberrant receptor tyrosine kinase signaling in lipofibromatosis: a clinicopathological and molecular genetic study of 20 cases. Mod Pathol. 2019 Mar;32(3):423–34. PMID:30310176
**165.** Al-Ibraheemi A, Inwards CY, Zreik RT, et al. Histologic spectrum of giant cell tumor (GCT) of bone in patients 18 years of age and below: a study of 63 patients. Am J Surg Pathol. 2016 Dec;40(12):1702–12. PMID:27526293
**166.** Al-Ibraheemi A, Martinez A, Weiss SW, et al. Fibrous hamartoma of infancy: a clinicopathologic study of 145 cases, including 2 with sarcomatous features. Mod Pathol. 2017 Apr;30(4):474–85. PMID:28059097
**167.** Alikhan A, Ibrahimi OA, Eisen DB. Congenital melanocytic nevi: Where are we now? Part I. Clinical presentation, epidemiology, pathogenesis, histology, malignant transformation, and neurocutaneous melanosis. J Am Acad Dermatol. 2012 Oct;67(4):495.e1–17. PMID:22980258
**168.** Alkatan HM, Al-Arfaj KM, Maktabi A. Conjunctival nevi: clinical and histopathologic features in a Saudi population. Ann Saudi Med. 2010 Jul-Aug;30(4):306–12. PMID:20622349
**169.** Alkhaili J, Cambon-Binder A, Belkheyar Z. Intraneural perineurioma: a retrospective study of 19 patients. Pan Afr Med J. 2018 Aug 14;30:275. PMID:30637060
**170.** Alkhairy OK, Perez-Becker R, Driessen GJ, et al. Novel mutations in TNFRSF7/CD27: clinical, immunologic, and genetic characterization of human CD27 deficiency. J Allergy Clin Immunol. 2015 Sep;136(3):703–712.e10. PMID:25843314
**171.** Al-Khtoum N, Qubilat AR, Al-Zaidaneen S, et al. Clinical characteristics of pleomorphic adenoma of salivary glands among Jordanian patients. J Pak Med Assoc. 2013 Mar;63(3):358–60. PMID:23914638
**172.** Alkonyi B, Nowak J, Gnekow AK, et al. Differential imaging characteristics and dissemination potential of pilomyxoid astrocytomas versus pilocytic astrocytomas. Neuroradiology. 2015 Jun;57(6):625–38. PMID:25666233
**173.** Allan B, Davis J, Perez E, et al. Malignant neuroendocrine tumors: incidence and outcomes in pediatric patients. Eur J Pediatr Surg. 2013 Oct;23(5):394–9. PMID:23444065
**174.** Allan BJ, Tashiro J, Diaz S, et al. Malignant tumors of the parotid gland in children: incidence and outcomes. J Craniofac Surg. 2013 Sep;24(5):1660–4. PMID:24036747
**175.** Allan BJ, Wang B, Davis JS, et al. A review of 218 pediatric cases of hepatocellular carcinoma. J Pediatr Surg. 2014 Jan;49(1):166–71. PMID:24439603
**176.** Allemani C, Matsuda T, Di Carlo V, et al. Global surveillance of trends in cancer survival 2000-14 (CONCORD-3): analysis of individual records for 37 513 025 patients diagnosed with one of 18 cancers from 322 population-based registries in 71 countries. Lancet. 2018 Mar 17;391(10125):1023–75. PMID:29395269
**177.** Allen AL, Siegfried EC. The natural history of condyloma in children. J Am Acad Dermatol. 1998 Dec;39(6):951–5. PMID:9843007
**178.** Allen CE, Kelly KM, Bollard CM. Pediatric lymphomas and histiocytic disorders of childhood. Pediatr Clin North Am. 2015 Feb;62(1):139–65. PMID:25435117
**179.** Allen CE, Ladisch S, McClain KL. How I treat Langerhans cell histiocytosis. Blood. 2015 Jul 2;126(1):26–35. PMID:25827831
**180.** Allen CE, Li L, Peters TL, et al. Cell-specific gene expression in Langerhans cell histiocytosis lesions reveals a distinct profile compared with epidermal Langerhans cells. J Immunol. 2010 Apr 15;184(8):4557–67. PMID:20220088
**181.** Allen CE, Merad M, McClain KL. Langerhans-cell histiocytosis. N Engl J Med. 2018 Aug 30;379(9):856–68. PMID:30157397
**182.** Allen JC, Judkins AR, Rosenblum MK, et al. Atypical teratoid/rhabdoid tumor evolving from an optic pathway ganglioglioma: case study. Neuro Oncol. 2006 Jan;8(1):79–82. PMID:16443951
**183.** Allen PW. Recurring digital fibrous tumours of childhood. Pathology. 1972 Jul;4(3):215–23. PMID:4344937
**184.** Allen PW, Enzinger FM. Juvenile aponeurotic fibroma. Cancer. 1970 Oct;26(4):857–67. PMID:5506609
**185.** Allen U, Hébert D, Moore D, et al. Epstein-Barr virus-related post-transplant lymphoproliferative disease in solid organ transplant recipients, 1988-97: a Canadian multi-centre experience. Pediatr Transplant. 2001 Jun;5(3):198–203. PMID:11422823
**186.** Allen UD, Farkas G, Hébert D, et al. Risk factors for post-transplant lymphoproliferative disorder in pediatric patients: a case-control study. Pediatr Transplant. 2005 Aug;9(4):450–5. PMID:16048596
**187.** Allen UD, Preiksaitis JK, AST Infectious Diseases Community of Practice. Post-transplant lymphoproliferative disorders, Epstein-Barr virus infection, and disease in solid organ transplantation: guidelines from the American Society of Transplantation Infectious Diseases Community of Practice. Clin Transplant. 2019 Sep;33(9):e13652. PMID:31230381
**188.** Allen-Rhoades W, Al-Ibraheemi A, Kohorst M, et al. Cellular variant of kaposiform lymphangiomatosis: a report of three cases, expanding the morphologic and molecular genetic spectrum of this rare entity. Hum Pathol. 2022 Apr;122:72–81. PMID:35202617
**189.** Allison DB, VandenBussche CJ, Rooper LM, et al. Nodular fasciitis of the parotid gland: a challenging diagnosis on FNA. Cancer Cytopathol. 2018 Oct;126(10):872–80. PMID:30311731
**190.** Allolio B, Fassnacht M. Clinical review: adrenocortical carcinoma: clinical update. J Clin Endocrinol Metab. 2006 Jun;91(6):2027–37. PMID:16551738
**191.** Al-Marzooq YM, Al-Bagshi MH, Chopra R, et al. Melanotic neuroectodermal tumor of infancy in the soft tissues of the arm: fine needle aspiration biopsy and histologic correlation-a case report. Diagn Cytopathol. 2003 Dec;29(6):352–5. PMID:14648795
**192.** Al-Mazrou KA, Mansoor A, Payne M, et al. Ossifying fibromyxoid tumor of the ethmoid sinus in a newborn: report of a case and literature review. Int J Pediatr Otorhinolaryngol. 2004 Feb;68(2):225–30. PMID:14725991
**193.** Almefty R, Webber BL, Arnautovic KI. Intraneural perineurioma of the third cranial nerve: occurrence and identification. Case report. J Neurosurg. 2006 May;104(5):824–7. PMID:16703891
**194.** Almeida JP, Stephens CC, Eschbacher JM, et al. Clinical, pathologic, and imaging characteristics of pituitary null cell adenomas as defined according to the 2017 World Health Organization criteria: a case series from two

pituitary centers. Pituitary. 2019 Oct;22(5):514–9. PMID:31401793

**195.** al Moutaery K, Aabed MY, Ojeda VJ. Cerebral and spinal cord myxopapillary ependymomas: a case report. Pathology. 1996 Nov;28(4):373–6. PMID:9007962

**196.** Almstrup K, Hoei-Hansen CE, Nielsen JE, et al. Genome-wide gene expression profiling of testicular carcinoma in situ progression into overt tumours. Br J Cancer. 2005 May 23;92(10):1934–41. PMID:15856041

**197.** Almstrup K, Hoei-Hansen CE, Wirkner U, et al. Embryonic stem cell-like features of testicular carcinoma in situ revealed by genome-wide gene expression profiling. Cancer Res. 2004 Jul 15;64(14):4736–43. PMID:15256440

**198.** Almstrup K, Lippert M, Mogensen HO, et al. Screening of subfertile men for testicular carcinoma in situ by an automated image analysis-based cytological test of the ejaculate. Int J Androl. 2011 Aug;34(4 Pt 2):e21–30. PMID:21696398

**199.** Almstrup K, Lobo J, Mørup N, et al. Application of miRNAs in the diagnosis and monitoring of testicular germ cell tumours. Nat Rev Urol. 2020 Apr;17(4):201–13. PMID:32157202

**200.** Almstrup K, Nielsen JE, Mlynarska O, et al. Carcinoma in situ testis displays permissive chromatin modifications similar to immature foetal germ cells. Br J Cancer. 2010 Oct 12;103(8):1269–76. PMID:20823885

**201.** Alobeid B, Beneck D, Sreekantaiah C, et al. Congenital pulmonary myofibroblastic tumor: a case report with cytogenetic analysis and review of the literature. Am J Surg Pathol. 1997 May;21(5):610–4. PMID:9158688

**202.** Al-Olabi L, Polubothu S, Dowsett K, et al. Mosaic RAS/MAPK variants cause sporadic vascular malformations which respond to targeted therapy. J Clin Invest. 2018 Apr 2;128(4):1496–508. PMID:29461977

**203.** Alomari AI, Spencer SA, Arnold RW, et al. Fibro-adipose vascular anomaly: clinical-radiologic-pathologic features of a newly delineated disorder of the extremity. J Pediatr Orthop. 2014 Jan;34(1):109–17. PMID:24322574

**204.** Alomari MH, Kozakewich HPW, Kerr CL, et al. Congenital disseminated pyogenic granuloma: characterization of an aggressive multisystemic disorder. J Pediatr. 2020 Nov;226:157–66. PMID:32622671

**205.** Al-Qattan MM, El-Shayeb A, Rasool MN. An intramuscular myxoma of the hand. Hand Surg. 2004 Jul;9(1):97–9. PMID:15368634

**206.** Alshaikh OM, Asa SL, Mete O, et al. An institutional experience of tumor progression to pituitary carcinoma in a 15-year cohort of 1055 consecutive pituitary neuroendocrine tumors. Endocr Pathol. 2019 Jun;30(2):118–27. PMID:30706322

**207.** Alsufayan R, Alcaide-Leon P, de Tilly LN, et al. Natural history of lesions with the MR imaging appearance of multinodular and vacuolating neuronal tumor. Neuroradiology. 2017 Sep;59(9):873–83. PMID:28752311

**208.** Alter BP. Fanconi anemia and the development of leukemia. Best Pract Res Clin Haematol. 2014 Sep-Dec;27(3-4):214–21. PMID:25455269

**209.** Altinay S, Taskın U, Sar M, et al. Histopathological diversity in parotidectomy materials in Turkish population: clinicopathologic analysis and demographic features of 136 cases in a tertiary care hospital. Asian Pac J Cancer Prev. 2014;15(14):5701–7. PMID:25081689

**210.** Altman RP, Randolph JG, Lilly JR. Sacrococcygeal teratoma: American Academy of Pediatrics Surgical Section Survey-1973. J Pediatr Surg. 1974 Jun;9(3):389–98. PMID:4843993

**211.** Alvarado-Cabrero I, Hernández-Toriz N, Paner GP. Clinicopathologic analysis of choriocarcinoma as a pure or predominant component of germ cell tumor of the testis. Am J Surg Pathol. 2014 Jan;38(1):111–8. PMID:24145647

**212.** Alvarez-Twose I, González P, Morgado JM, et al. Complete response after imatinib mesylate therapy in a patient with well-differentiated systemic mastocytosis. J Clin Oncol. 2012 Apr 20;30(12):e126–9. PMID:22370312

**213.** Álvarez-Twose I, Jara-Acevedo M, Morgado JM, et al. Clinical, immunophenotypic, and molecular characteristics of well-differentiated systemic mastocytosis. J Allergy Clin Immunol. 2016 Jan;137(1):168–178.e1. PMID:26100086

**214.** Alvarez-Twose I, Vañó-Galván S, Sánchez-Muñoz L, et al. Increased serum baseline tryptase levels and extensive skin involvement are predictors for the severity of mast cell activation episodes in children with mastocytosis. Allergy. 2012 Jun;67(6):813–21. PMID:22458675

**215.** Alver BH, Kim KH, Lu P, et al. The SWI/SNF chromatin remodelling complex is required for maintenance of lineage specific enhancers. Nat Commun. 2017 Mar 6;8:14648. PMID:28262751

**216.** Alwaheeb S, Rambaldini G, Boerner S, et al. Worrisome histologic alterations following fine-needle aspiration of the parathyroid. J Clin Pathol. 2006 Oct;59(10):1094–6. PMID:17021134

**217.** Amadou A, Achatz MIW, Hainaut P. Revisiting tumor patterns and penetrance in germline TP53 mutation carriers: temporal phases of Li-Fraumeni syndrome. Curr Opin Oncol. 2018 Jan;30(1):23–9. PMID:29076966

**218.** Amano K, Kubo O, Komori T, et al. Clinicopathological features of sellar region xanthogranuloma: correlation with Rathke's cleft cyst. Brain Tumor Pathol. 2013 Oct;30(4):233–41. PMID:23322180

**219.** Amar YG, Nguyen LH, Manoukian JJ, et al. Granular cell tumor of the trachea in a child. Int J Pediatr Otorhinolaryngol. 2002 Jan 11;62(1):75–80. PMID:11738699

**220.** Amary F, Berisha F, Ye H, et al. H3F3A (Histone 3.3) G34W Immunohistochemistry: a reliable marker defining benign and malignant giant cell tumor of bone. Am J Surg Pathol. 2017 Aug;41(8):1059–68. PMID:28505000

**221.** Amary F, Markert E, Berisha F, et al. FOS expression in osteoid osteoma and osteoblastoma: a valuable ancillary diagnostic tool. Am J Surg Pathol. 2019 Dec;43(12):1661–7. PMID:31490237

**222.** Amary F, Perez-Casanova L, Ye H, et al. Synovial chondromatosis and soft tissue chondroma: extraosseous cartilaginous tumor defined by FN1 gene rearrangement. Mod Pathol. 2019 Dec;32(12):1762–71. PMID:31273315

**223.** Amary MF, Bacsi K, Maggiani F, et al. IDH1 and IDH2 mutations are frequent events in central chondrosarcoma and central and periosteal chondromas but not in other mesenchymal tumours. J Pathol. 2011 Jul;224(3):334–43. PMID:21598255

**224.** Amary MF, Berisha F, Bernardi FdelC, et al. Detection of SS18-SSX fusion transcripts in formalin-fixed paraffin-embedded neoplasms: analysis of conventional RT-PCR, qRT-PCR and dual color FISH as diagnostic tools for synovial sarcoma. Mod Pathol. 2007 Apr;20(4):482–96. PMID:17334349

**225.** Amary MF, Berisha F, Mozela R, et al. The H3F3 K36M mutant antibody is a sensitive and specific marker for the diagnosis of chondroblastoma. Histopathology. 2016 Jul;69(1):121–7. PMID:26844533

**226.** Amary MF, Damato S, Halai D, et al. Ollier disease and Maffucci syndrome are caused by somatic mosaic mutations of IDH1 and IDH2. Nat Genet. 2011 Nov 6;43(12):1262–5. PMID:22057236

**227.** Amary MF, O'Donnell P, Berisha F, et al. Pseudomyogenic (epithelioid sarcoma-like) hemangioendothelioma: characterization of five cases. Skeletal Radiol. 2013 Jul;42(7):947–57. PMID:23381465

**228.** Amary MF, Pauwels P, Meulemans E, et al. Detection of beta-catenin mutations in paraffin-embedded sporadic desmoid-type fibromatosis by mutation-specific restriction enzyme digestion (MSRED): an ancillary diagnostic tool. Am J Surg Pathol. 2007 Sep;31(9):1299–309. PMID:17721184

**229.** Amato E, Mafficini A, Hirabayashi K, et al. Molecular alterations associated with metastases of solid pseudopapillary neoplasms of the pancreas. J Pathol. 2019 Jan;247(1):123–34. PMID:30306561

**230.** Amayiri N, Tabori U, Campbell B, et al. High frequency of mismatch repair deficiency among pediatric high grade gliomas in Jordan. Int J Cancer. 2016 Jan 15;138(2):380–5. PMID:26293621

**231.** Ambros IM, Zellner A, Roald B, et al. Role of ploidy, chromosome 1p, and Schwann cells in the maturation of neuroblastoma. N Engl J Med. 1996 Jun 6;334(23):1505–11. PMID:8618605

**232.** Ambros PF, Ambros IM, Brodeur GM, et al. International consensus for neuroblastoma molecular diagnostics: report from the International Neuroblastoma Risk Group (INRG) Biology Committee. Br J Cancer. 2009 May 5;100(9):1471–82. PMID:19401703

**233.** Amelio JM, Rockberg J, Hernandez RK, et al. Population-based study of giant cell tumor of bone in Sweden (1983-2011). Cancer Epidemiol. 2016 Jun;42:82–9. PMID:27060625

**234.** Amer HZ, Heller DS. Chorangioma and related vascular lesions of the placenta–a review. Fetal Pediatr Pathol. 2010;29(4):199–206. PMID:20594143

**235.** Amesse LS, Gibbs P, Hardy J, et al. Peritoneal inclusion cysts in adolescent females: a clinicopathological characterization of four cases. J Pediatr Adolesc Gynecol. 2009 Feb;22(1):41–8. PMID:19232301

**236.** Amin HM, McDonnell TJ, Ma Y, et al. Selective inhibition of STAT3 induces apoptosis and G(1) cell cycle arrest in ALK-positive anaplastic large cell lymphoma. Oncogene. 2004 Jul 15;23(32):5426–34. PMID:15184887

**237.** Amin HM, Medeiros LJ, Ma Y, et al. Inhibition of JAK3 induces apoptosis and decreases anaplastic lymphoma kinase activity in anaplastic large cell lymphoma. Oncogene. 2003 Aug 21;22(35):5399–407. PMID:12934099

**238.** Amin MB, Edge S, Greene F, et al., editors. AJCC cancer staging manual. 8th ed. New York (NY): Springer; 2017.

**239.** Amin MB, Patel RM, Oliveira P, et al. Alveolar soft-part sarcoma of the urinary bladder with urethral recurrence: a unique case with emphasis on differential diagnoses and diagnostic utility of an immunohistochemical panel including TFE3. Am J Surg Pathol. 2006 Oct;30(10):1322–5. PMID:17001165

**240.** Amin S, Lux A, Calder N, et al. Causes of mortality in individuals with tuberous sclerosis complex. Dev Med Child Neurol. 2017 Jun;59(6):612–7. PMID:27935023

**241.** Aminudin CA, Sharaf I, Hamzaini AH, et al. Ossifying fibromyxoid tumour in a child. Med J Malaysia. 2004 Dec;59 Suppl F:49–51. PMID:15941162

**242.** Amir G, Mogle P, Sucher E. Case report 729. Myositis ossificans and aneurysmal bone cyst. Skeletal Radiol. 1992;21(4):257–9. PMID:1626294

**243.** Amjadi M, Khorrami-Arani N, Mashman G, et al. Zosteriform connective tissue nevus: a case report. Am J Dermatopathol. 2007 Jun;29(3):303–5. PMID:17519633

**244.** Amlashi SF, Riffaud L, Brassier G, et al. Nevoid basal cell carcinoma syndrome: relation with desmoplastic medulloblastoma in infancy. A population-based study and review of the literature. Cancer. 2003 Aug 1;98(3):618–24. PMID:12879481

**245.** Ammerlaan AC, Ararou A, Houben MP, et al. Long-term survival and transmission of INI1-mutation via nonpenetrant males in a family with rhabdoid tumour predisposition syndrome. Br J Cancer. 2008 Jan 29;98(2):474–9. PMID:18087273

**246.** Ammerman JM, Lonser RR, Dambrosia J, et al. Long-term natural history of hemangioblastomas in patients with von Hippel-Lindau disease: implications for treatment. J Neurosurg. 2006 Aug;105(2):248–55. PMID:17219830

**247.** Amorim-Costa C, Costa A, Baptista P, et al. Sclerosing stromal tumour of the ovary associated with Meigs' syndrome and elevated CA125. J Obstet Gynaecol. 2010;30(7):747–8. PMID:20925634

**248.** Amortegui AJ, Kanbour AI. Compound nevus in a cystic teratoma of the ovary. Arch Pathol Lab Med. 1981 Feb;105(2):115–6. PMID:6893919

**249.** Ampie L, Choy W, DiDomenico JD, et al. Clinical attributes and surgical outcomes of angiocentric gliomas. J Clin Neurosci. 2016 Jun;28:117–22. PMID:26778052

**250.** Amram AL, Rico G, Kim JW, et al. Vitreous seeds in retinoblastoma: clinicopathologic classification and correlation. ophthalmology. 2017 Oct;124(10):1540–7. PMID:28528011

**251.** Amstalden EM, Carvalho RB, Pacheco EM, et al. Chondromatous hamartoma of the chest wall: description of 3 new cases and literature review. Int J Surg Pathol. 2006 Apr;14(2):119–26. PMID:16703172

**252.** Amyere M, Aerts V, Brouillard P, et al. Somatic uniparental isodisomy explains multifocality of glomuvenous malformations. Am J Hum Genet. 2013 Feb 7;92(2):188–96. PMID:23375657

**253.** Amyere M, Revencu N, Helaers R, et al. Germline loss-of-function mutations in ephb4 cause a second form of capillary malformation-arteriovenous malformation (CM-AVM2) deregulating RAS-MAPK signaling. Circulation. 2017 Sep 12;136(11):1037–48. PMID:28687708

**254.** Anazoeze M, Najibah G, Garba U, et al. Is renal medullary carcinoma the seventh nephropathy in sickle cell disease? A multi-center Nigerian survey. Afr Health Sci. 2016 Jun;16(2):490–6. PMID:27605964

**255.** Anderson JR, Armitage JO, Weisenburger DD. Epidemiology of the non-Hodgkin's lymphomas: distributions of the major subtypes differ by geographic locations. Non-Hodgkin's Lymphoma Classification Project. Ann Oncol. 1998 Jul;9(7):717–20. PMID:9739436

**256.** Anderson ND, de Borja R, Young MD, et al. Rearrangement bursts generate canonical gene fusions in bone and soft tissue tumors. Science. 2018 Aug 31;361(6405):eaam8419. PMID:30166462

**257.** Anderson WJ, Jo VY. Pleomorphic liposarcoma: updates and current differential diagnosis. Semin Diagn Pathol. 2019 Mar;36(2):122–8. PMID:30852046

**258.** Andersson AK, Ma J, Wang J, et al. The landscape of somatic mutations in infant MLL-rearranged acute lymphoblastic leukemias. Nat Genet. 2015 Apr;47(4):330–7. PMID:25730765

**259.** Andoniadou CL, Gaston-Massuet C, Reddy R, et al. Identification of novel pathways involved in the pathogenesis of human

adamantinomatous craniopharyngioma. Acta Neuropathol. 2012 Aug;124(2):259–71. PMID:22349813
**260.** Andoniadou CL, Matsushima D, Mousavy Gharavy SN, et al. Sox2(+) stem/progenitor cells in the adult mouse pituitary support organ homeostasis and have tumor-inducing potential. Cell Stem Cell. 2013 Oct 3;13(4):433–45. PMID:24094324
**261.** Andrade NN, Gandhewar T, Aggarwal N, et al. Adult rhabdomyoma of the tongue in a child: report of a case and a literature appraisal. Contemp Clin Dent. 2018 Jan-Mar;9(1):2–4. PMID:29599574
**262.** Andreiuolo F, Lisner T, Zlocha J, et al. H3F3A-G34R mutant high grade neuroepithelial neoplasms with glial and dysplastic ganglion cell components. Acta Neuropathol Commun. 2019 May 20;7(1):78. PMID:31109382
**263.** Andreiuolo F, Varlet P, Tauziède-Espariat A, et al. Childhood supratentorial ependymomas with YAP1-MAMLD1 fusion: an entity with characteristic clinical, radiological, cytogenetic and histopathological features. Brain Pathol. 2019 Mar;29(2):205–16. PMID:30246434
**264.** Andreou D, Bielack SS, Carrle D, et al. The influence of tumor- and treatment-related factors on the development of local recurrence in osteosarcoma after adequate surgery. An analysis of 1355 patients treated on neoadjuvant Cooperative Osteosarcoma Study Group protocols. Ann Oncol. 2011 May;22(5):1228–35. PMID:21030381
**265.** Andresen KJ, Sundaram M, Unni KK, et al. Imaging features of low-grade central osteosarcoma of the long bones and pelvis. Skeletal Radiol. 2004 Jul;33(7):373–9. PMID:15175837
**266.** Andrews JC, Fisch U, Valavanis A, et al. The surgical management of extensive nasopharyngeal angiofibromas with the infratemporal fossa approach. Laryngoscope. 1989 Apr;99(4):429–37. PMID:2538688
**267.** Andrianova MA, Chetan GK, Sibin MK, et al. Germline PMS2 and somatic POLE exonuclease mutations cause hypermutability of the leading DNA strand in biallelic mismatch repair deficiency syndrome brain tumours. J Pathol. 2017 Nov;243(3):331–41. PMID:28805995
**268.** Ang SM, Dalvin LA, Emrich J, et al. Plaque radiotherapy for medulloepithelioma in 6 cases from a single center. Asia Pac J Ophthalmol (Phila). 2019 Jan-Feb;8(1):30–5. PMID:30375203
**269.** Angelini A, Mavrogenis AF, Trovarelli G, et al. Telangiectatic osteosarcoma: a review of 87 cases. J Cancer Res Clin Oncol. 2016 Oct;142(10):2197–207. PMID:27469493
**270.** Angelini P, Baruchel S, Marrano P, et al. The neuroblastoma and ganglion components of nodular ganglioneuroblastoma are genetically similar: evidence against separate clonal origins. Mod Pathol. 2015 Feb;28(2):166–76. PMID:25081755
**271.** Angelini P, London WB, Cohn SL, et al. Characteristics and outcome of patients with ganglioneuroblastoma, nodular subtype: a report from the INRG project. Eur J Cancer. 2012 May;48(8):1185–91. PMID:22137163
**272.** Anglesio MS, Wang Y, Yang W, et al. Cancer-associated somatic DICER1 hotspot mutations cause defective miRNA processing and reverse-strand expression bias to predominantly mature 3p strands through loss of 5p strand cleavage. J Pathol. 2013 Feb;229(3):400–9. PMID:23132766
**273.** Anninga JK, Gelderblom H, Fiocco M, et al. Chemotherapeutic adjuvant treatment for osteosarcoma: Where do we stand? Eur J Cancer. 2011 Nov;47(16):2431–45. PMID:21703851
**274.** Antaya RJ, Cajaiba MM, Madri J, et al. Juvenile hyaline fibromatosis and infantile systemic hyalinosis overlap associated with a novel mutation in capillary morphogenesis protein-2 gene. Am J Dermatopathol. 2007 Feb;29(1):99–103. PMID:17284973
**275.** Antinheimo J, Haapasalo H, Haltia M, et al. Proliferation potential and histological features in neurofibromatosis 2-associated and sporadic meningiomas. J Neurosurg. 1997 Oct;87(4):610–4. PMID:9322850
**276.** Antinheimo J, Haapasalo H, Seppälä M, et al. Proliferative potential of sporadic and neurofibromatosis 2-associated schwannomas as studied by MIB-1 (Ki-67) and PCNA labeling. J Neuropathol Exp Neurol. 1995 Nov;54(6):776–82. PMID:7595650
**277.** Antonelli M, Korshunov A, Mastronuzzi A, et al. Long-term survival in a case of ETANTR with histological features of neuronal maturation after therapy. Virchows Arch. 2015 May;466(5):603–7. PMID:25697539
**278.** Antonelli M, Raso A, Mascelli S, et al. SMARCB1/INI1 Involvement in pediatric chordoma: a mutational and immunohistochemical analysis. Am J Surg Pathol. 2017 Jan;41(1):56–61. PMID:27635948
**279.** Antonescu C. Round cell sarcomas beyond Ewing: emerging entities. Histopathology. 2014 Jan;64(1):26–37. PMID:24215322
**280.** Antonescu CR. Emerging soft tissue tumors with kinase fusions: an overview of the recent literature with an emphasis on diagnostic criteria. Genes Chromosomes Cancer. 2020 Aug;59(8):437–44. PMID:32243019
**281.** Antonescu CR, Chen HW, Zhang L, et al. ZFP36-FOSB fusion defines a subset of epithelioid hemangioma with atypical features. Genes Chromosomes Cancer. 2014 Nov;53(11):951–9. PMID:25043949
**282.** Antonescu CR, Dal Cin P, Nafa K, et al. EWSR1-CREB1 is the predominant gene fusion in angiomatoid fibrous histiocytoma. Genes Chromosomes Cancer. 2007 Dec;46(12):1051–60. PMID:17724745
**283.** Antonescu CR, Dickson BC, Swanson D, et al. Spindle cell tumors with RET gene fusions exhibit a morphologic spectrum akin to tumors with NTRK gene fusions. Am J Surg Pathol. 2019 Oct;43(10):1384–91. PMID:31219820
**284.** Antonescu CR, Kao YC, Xu B, et al. Undifferentiated round cell sarcoma with BCOR internal tandem duplications (ITD) or YWHAE fusions: a clinicopathologic and molecular study. Mod Pathol. 2020 Sep;33(9):1669–77. PMID:32372022
**285.** Antonescu CR, Kawai A, Leung DH, et al. Strong association of SYT-SSX fusion type and morphologic epithelial differentiation in synovial sarcoma. Diagn Mol Pathol. 2000 Mar;9(1):1–8. PMID:10718206
**286.** Antonescu CR, Le Loarer F, Mosquera JM, et al. Novel YAP1-TFE3 fusion defines a distinct subset of epithelioid hemangioendothelioma. Genes Chromosomes Cancer. 2013 Aug;52(8):775–84. PMID:23737213
**287.** Antonescu CR, Owosho AA, Zhang L, et al. Sarcomas with CIC-rearrangements are a distinct pathologic entity with aggressive outcome: a clinicopathologic and molecular study of 115 cases. Am J Surg Pathol. 2017 Jul;41(7):941–9. PMID:28346326
**288.** Antonescu CR, Rosenblum MK, Pereira P, et al. Sclerosing epithelioid fibrosarcoma: a study of 16 cases and confirmation of a clinicopathologically distinct tumor. Am J Surg Pathol. 2001 Jun;25(6):699–709. PMID:11395547
**289.** Antonescu CR, Sung YS, Zhang L, et al. Recurrent SRF-RELA fusions define a novel subset of cellular myofibroma/myopericytoma: a potential diagnostic pitfall with sarcomas with myogenic differentiation. Am J Surg Pathol. 2017 May;41(5):677–84. PMID:28248815
**290.** Antonescu CR, Suurmeijer AJ, Zhang L, et al. Molecular characterization of inflammatory myofibroblastic tumors with frequent ALK and ROS1 gene fusions and rare novel RET rearrangement. Am J Surg Pathol. 2015 Jul;39(7):957–67. PMID:25723109
**291.** Antonescu CR, Yoshida A, Guo T, et al. KDR activating mutations in human angiosarcomas are sensitive to specific kinase inhibitors. Cancer Res. 2009 Sep 15;69(18):7175–9. PMID:19723655
**292.** Antonescu CR, Zhang L, Chang NE, et al. EWSR1-POU5F1 fusion in soft tissue myoepithelial tumors. A molecular analysis of sixty-six cases, including soft tissue, bone, and visceral lesions, showing common involvement of the EWSR1 gene. Genes Chromosomes Cancer. 2010 Dec;49(12):1114–24. PMID:20815032
**293.** Antonescu CR, Zhang L, Shao SY, et al. Frequent PLAG1 gene rearrangements in skin and soft tissue myoepithelioma with ductal differentiation. Genes Chromosomes Cancer. 2013 Jul;52(7):675–82. PMID:23630011
**294.** Antonini SR, Latronico AC, Elias LL, et al. Glucocorticoid receptor gene polymorphisms in ACTH-secreting pituitary tumours. Clin Endocrinol (Oxf). 2002 Nov;57(5):657–62. PMID:12390341
**296.** Aoki A, Shiozaki A, Sameshima A, et al. Beckwith-Wiedemann syndrome with placental chorangioma due to H19-differentially methylated region hypermethylation: a case report. J Obstet Gynaecol Res. 2011 Dec;37(12):1872–6. PMID:21955307
**297.** Aoyama C, Hachitanda Y, Sato JK, et al. Undifferentiated (embryonal) sarcoma of the liver. A tumor of uncertain histogenesis showing divergent differentiation. Am J Surg Pathol. 1991 Jul;15(7):615–24. PMID:1711792
**298.** Apellaniz-Ruiz M, Segni M, Kettwig M, et al. Mesenchymal hamartoma of the liver and DICER1 syndrome. N Engl J Med. 2019 May 9;380(19):1834–42. PMID:31067372
**299.** Appay R, Macagno N, Padovani L, et al. HGNET-BCOR tumors of the cerebellum: clinicopathologic and molecular characterization of 3 cases. Am J Surg Pathol. 2017 Sep;41(9):1254–60. PMID:28704208
**300.** Appay R, Pages M, Colin C, et al. Diffuse leptomeningeal glioneuronal tumor: a double misnomer? A report of two cases. Acta Neuropathol Commun. 2020 Jun 30;8(1):95. PMID:32605662
**301.** Appel BE, Chen L, Buxton AB, et al. Minimal treatment of low-risk, pediatric lymphocyte-predominant Hodgkin lymphoma: a report from the Children's Oncology Group. J Clin Oncol. 2016 Jul 10;34(20):2372–9. PMID:27185849
**302.** Apps JR, Carreno G, Gonzalez-Meljem JM, et al. Tumour compartment transcriptomics demonstrates the activation of inflammatory and odontogenic programmes in human adamantinomatous craniopharyngioma and identifies the MAPK/ERK pathway as a novel therapeutic target. Acta Neuropathol. 2018 May;135(5):757–77. PMID:29541918
**303.** Apps JR, Martinez-Barbera JP. Genetically engineered mouse models of craniopharyngioma: an opportunity for therapy development and understanding of tumor biology. Brain Pathol. 2017 May;27(3):364–9. PMID:28414891
**304.** Apps JR, Stache C, Gonzalez-Meljem JM, et al. CTNNB1 mutations are clonal in adamantinomatous craniopharyngioma. Neuropathol Appl Neurobiol. 2020 Aug;46(5):510–4. PMID:32125720
**305.** Apra C, Enachescu C, Lapras V, et al. Is gross total resection reasonable in adults with craniopharyngiomas with hypothalamic involvement? World Neurosurg. 2019 Sep;129:e803–11. PMID:31203080
**306.** Aqil B, Merritt BY, Elghetany MT, et al. Childhood nodal marginal zone lymphoma with unusual clinicopathologic and cytogenetic features for the pediatric variant: a case report. Pediatr Dev Pathol. 2015 Mar-Apr;18(2):167–71. PMID:25625642
**307.** Aquino VM, Tomlinson G, Weinberg AG, et al. Extraskeletal myxoid chondrosarcoma as a second malignancy after bone marrow transplantation. Med Pediatr Oncol. 2003 May;40(5):336–7. PMID:12652628
**308.** Arachchillage DR, Carr TF, Kerr B, et al. Juvenile myelomonocytic leukemia presenting with features of neonatal hemophagocytic lymphohistiocytosis and cutaneous juvenile xanthogranulomata and successfully treated with allogeneic hemopoietic stem cell transplant. J Pediatr Hematol Oncol. 2010 Mar;32(2):152–5. PMID:20168243
**309.** Arata MA, Peterson HA, Dahlin DC. Pathological fractures through non-ossifying fibromas. Review of the Mayo Clinic experience. J Bone Joint Surg Am. 1981 Jul;63(6):980–8. PMID:7240338
**310.** Arbajian E, Puls F, Antonescu CR, et al. In-depth genetic analysis of sclerosing epithelioid fibrosarcoma reveals recurrent genomic alterations and potential treatment targets. Clin Cancer Res. 2017 Dec 1;23(23):7426–34. PMID:28939748
**311.** Arbajian E, Puls F, Magnusson L, et al. Recurrent EWSR1-CREB3L1 gene fusions in sclerosing epithelioid fibrosarcoma. Am J Surg Pathol. 2014 Jun;38(6):801–8. PMID:24441665
**312.** Arber DA, Orazi A, Hasserjian R, et al. The 2016 revision to the World Health Organization classification of myeloid neoplasms and acute leukemia. Blood. 2016 May 19;127(20):2391–405. PMID:27069254
**313.** Argani P. Metanephric neoplasms: the hyperdifferentiated, benign end of the Wilms tumor spectrum? Clin Lab Med. 2005 Jun;25(2):379–92. PMID:15848742
**314.** Argani P, Antonescu CR, Couturier J, et al. PRCC-TFE3 renal carcinomas: morphologic, immunohistochemical, ultrastructural, and molecular analysis of an entity associated with the t(X;1)(p11.2;q21). Am J Surg Pathol. 2002 Dec;26(12):1553–66. PMID:12459622
**315.** Argani P, Antonescu CR, Illei PB, et al. Primary renal neoplasms with the ASPL-TFE3 gene fusion of alveolar soft part sarcoma: a distinctive tumor entity previously included among renal cell carcinomas of children and adolescents. Am J Pathol. 2001 Jul;159(1):179–92. PMID:11438465
**316.** Argani P, Aulmann S, Illei PB, et al. A distinctive subset of PEComas harbors TFE3 gene fusions. Am J Surg Pathol. 2010 Oct;34(10):1395–406. PMID:20871214
**317.** Argani P, Aulmann S, Karanjawala Z, et al. Melanotic Xp11 translocation renal cancers: a distinctive neoplasm with overlapping features of PEComa, carcinoma, and melanoma. Am J Surg Pathol. 2009 Apr;33(4):609–19. PMID:19065101
**318.** Argani P, Fritsch M, Kadkol SS, et al. Detection of the ETV6-NTRK3 chimeric RNA of infantile fibrosarcoma/cellular congenital mesoblastic nephroma in paraffin-embedded tissue: application to challenging pediatric renal stromal tumors. Mod Pathol. 2000 Jan;13(1):29–36. PMID:10658907
**319.** Argani P, Fritsch MK, Shuster AE, et al. Reduced sensitivity of paraffin-based RT-PCR assays for ETV6-NTRK3 fusion transcripts in morphologically defined infantile fibrosarcoma. Am J Surg Pathol. 2001 Nov;25(11):1461–4. PMID:11684968
**320.** Argani P, Harvey I, Nielsen GP, et al. EWSR1/FUS-CREB fusions define a distinctive malignant epithelioid neoplasm with predilection

for mesothelial-lined cavities. Mod Pathol. 2020 Nov;33(11):2233–43. PMID:32770123
**321.** Argani P, Hawkins A, Griffin CA, et al. A distinctive pediatric renal neoplasm characterized by epithelioid morphology, basement membrane production, focal HMB45 immunoreactivity, and t(6;11)(p21.1;q12) chromosome translocation. Am J Pathol. 2001 Jun;158(6):2089–96. PMID:11395386
**322.** Argani P, Hicks J, De Marzo AM, et al. Xp11 translocation renal cell carcinoma (RCC): extended immunohistochemical profile emphasizing novel RCC markers. Am J Surg Pathol. 2010 Sep;34(9):1295–303. PMID:20679884
**323.** Argani P, Kao YC, Zhang L, et al. Primary renal sarcomas with BCOR-CCNB3 gene fusion: a report of 2 cases showing histologic overlap with clear cell sarcoma of kidney, suggesting further link between BCOR-related sarcomas of the kidney and soft tissues. Am J Surg Pathol. 2017 Dec;41(12):1702–12. PMID:28817404
**324.** Argani P, Laé M, Ballard ET, et al. Translocation carcinomas of the kidney after chemotherapy in childhood. J Clin Oncol. 2006 Apr 1;24(10):1529–34. PMID:16575003
**325.** Argani P, Laé M, Hutchinson B, et al. Renal carcinomas with the t(6;11)(p21;q12): clinicopathologic features and demonstration of the specific alpha-TFEB gene fusion by immunohistochemistry, RT-PCR, and DNA PCR. Am J Surg Pathol. 2005 Feb;29(2):230–40. PMID:15644781
**326.** Argani P, Lal P, Hutchinson B, et al. Aberrant nuclear immunoreactivity for TFE3 in neoplasms with TFE3 gene fusions: a sensitive and specific immunohistochemical assay. Am J Surg Pathol. 2003 Jun;27(6):750–61. PMID:12766578
**327.** Argani P, Lee J, Netto GJ, et al. Frequent BRAF V600E mutations in metanephric stromal tumor. Am J Surg Pathol. 2016 May;40(5):719–22. PMID:26796506
**328.** Argani P, Lewin JR, Edmonds P, et al. Primary renal sclerosing epithelioid fibrosarcoma: report of 2 cases with EWSR1-CREB3L1 gene fusion. Am J Surg Pathol. 2015 Mar;39(3):365–73. PMID:25353281
**329.** Argani P, Lui MY, Couturier J, et al. A novel CLTC-TFE3 gene fusion in pediatric renal adenocarcinoma with t(X;17)(p11.2;q23). Oncogene. 2003 Aug 14;22(34):5374–8. PMID:12917640
**330.** Argani P, Olgac S, Tickoo SK, et al. Xp11 translocation renal cell carcinoma in adults: expanded clinical, pathologic, and genetic spectrum. Am J Surg Pathol. 2007 Aug;31(8):1149–60. PMID:17667536
**331.** Argani P, Pawel B, Szabo S, et al. Diffuse strong BCOR immunoreactivity is a sensitive and specific marker for clear cell sarcoma of the kidney (CCSK) in pediatric renal neoplasia. Am J Surg Pathol. 2018 Aug;42(8):1128–31. PMID:29851702
**332.** Argani P, Perlman EJ, Breslow NE, et al. Clear cell sarcoma of the kidney: a review of 351 cases from the National Wilms Tumor Study Group Pathology Center. Am J Surg Pathol. 2000 Jan;24(1):4–18. PMID:10632483
**333.** Argani P, Reuter VE, Zhang L, et al. TFEB-amplified renal cell carcinomas: an aggressive molecular subset demonstrating variable melanocytic marker expression and morphologic heterogeneity. Am J Surg Pathol. 2016 Nov;40(11):1484–95. PMID:27565001
**334.** Argani P, Yonescu R, Morsberger L, et al. Molecular confirmation of t(6;11)(p21;q12) renal cell carcinoma in archival paraffin-embedded material using a break-apart TFEB FISH assay expands its clinicopathologic spectrum. Am J Surg Pathol. 2012 Oct;36(10):1516–26. PMID:22892601
**335.** Argani P, Zhang L, Reuter VE, et al. RBM10-TFE3 renal cell carcinoma: a potential diagnostic pitfall due to cryptic intrachromosomal Xp11.2 inversion resulting in false-negative TFE3 FISH. Am J Surg Pathol. 2017 May;41(5):655–62. PMID:28296677
**336.** Argani P, Zhang L, Sung YS, et al. A novel RBMX-TFE3 gene fusion in a highly aggressive pediatric renal perivascular epithelioid cell tumor. Genes Chromosomes Cancer. 2019 Aug 13. PMID:31408245
**337.** Argani P, Zhong M, Reuter VE, et al. TFE3-fusion variant analysis defines specific clinicopathologic associations among Xp11 translocation cancers. Am J Surg Pathol. 2016 Jun;40(6):723–37. PMID:26975036
**338.** Argenyi ZB. Immunohistochemical characterization of palisaded, encapsulated neuroma. J Cutan Pathol. 1990 Dec;17(6):329–35. PMID:1705947
**339.** Argenyi ZB, Van Rybroek JJ, Kemp JD, et al. Congenital angiomatoid malignant fibrous histiocytoma. A light-microscopic, immunopathologic, and electron-microscopic study. Am J Dermatopathol. 1988 Feb;10(1):59–67. PMID:2845834
**340.** Argenziano G, Agozzino M, Bonifazi E, et al. Natural evolution of Spitz nevi. Dermatology. 2011;222(3):256–60. PMID:21494025
**341.** Arias-Stella JA 3rd, Benayed R, Oliva E, et al. Novel PLAG1 gene rearrangement distinguishes a subset of uterine myxoid leiomyosarcoma from other uterine myxoid mesenchymal tumors. Am J Surg Pathol. 2019 Mar;43(3):382–8. PMID:30489320
**342.** Aricò M, Mussolin L, Carraro E, et al. Non-Hodgkin lymphoma in children with an associated inherited condition: a retrospective analysis of the Associazione Italiana Ematologia Oncologia Pediatrica (AIEOP). Pediatr Blood Cancer. 2015 Oct;62(10):1782–9. PMID:26011068
**343.** Arivazhagan A, Anandh B, Santosh V, et al. Pineal parenchymal tumors–utility of immunohistochemical markers in prognostication. Clin Neuropathol. 2008 Sep-Oct;27(5):325–33. PMID:18808064
**344.** Armstrong R, Greenhalgh KL, Rattenberry E, et al. Succinate dehydrogenase subunit B (SDHB) gene deletion associated with a composite paraganglioma/neuroblastoma. J Med Genet. 2009 Mar;46(3):215–6. PMID:19251979
**345.** Arndt CA, Hammond S, Rodeberg D, et al. Significance of persistent mature rhabdomyoblasts in bladder/prostate rhabdomyosarcoma: results from IRS IV. J Pediatr Hematol Oncol. 2006 Sep;28(9):563–7. PMID:17006261
**346.** Arndt CA, Stoner JA, Hawkins DS, et al. Vincristine, actinomycin, and cyclophosphamide compared with vincristine, actinomycin, and cyclophosphamide alternating with vincristine, topotecan, and cyclophosphamide for intermediate-risk rhabdomyosarcoma: children's oncology group study D9803. J Clin Oncol. 2009 Nov 1;27(31):5182–8. PMID:19770373
**347.** Arnold MA, Anderson JR, Gastier-Foster JM, et al. Histology, fusion status, and outcome in alveolar rhabdomyosarcoma with low-risk clinical features: a report from the Children's Oncology Group. Pediatr Blood Cancer. 2016 Apr;63(4):634–9. PMID:26756883
**348.** Arnold MA, Arnold CA, Li G, et al. A unique pattern of INI1 immunohistochemistry distinguishes synovial sarcoma from its histologic mimics. Hum Pathol. 2013 May;44(5):881–7. PMID:23245672
**349.** Arnold MA, Stallings-Archer K, Marlin E, et al. Cribriform neuroepithelial tumor arising in the lateral ventricle. Pediatr Dev Pathol. 2013 Jul-Aug;16(4):301–7. PMID:23495723
**350.** Aronica E, Leenstra S, van Veelen CW, et al. Glioneuronal tumors and medically intractable epilepsy: a clinical study with long-term follow-up of seizure outcome after surgery. Epilepsy Res. 2001 Mar;43(3):179–91. PMID:11248530
**351.** Aronson M, Gallinger S, Cohen Z, et al. Gastrointestinal findings in the largest series of patients with hereditary biallelic mismatch repair deficiency syndrome: report from the International Consortium. Am J Gastroenterol. 2016 Feb;111(2):275–84. PMID:26729549
**352.** Arora H, Falto-Aizpurua L, Cortés-Fernandez A, et al. Connective tissue nevi: a review of the literature. Am J Dermatopathol. 2017 May;39(5):325–41. PMID:28426484
**353.** Arora RS, Alston RD, Eden TO, et al. Comparative incidence patterns and trends of gonadal and extragonadal germ cell tumors in England, 1979 to 2003. Cancer. 2012 Sep 1;118(17):4290–7. PMID:22252431
**354.** Arotiba GT. A study of orofacial tumors in Nigerian children. J Oral Maxillofac Surg. 1996 Jan;54(1):34–8. PMID:8530997
**355.** Arriola AG, Taylor LA, Asemota E, et al. Atypical retiform hemangioendothelioma arising in a patient with Milroy disease: a case report and review of the literature. J Cutan Pathol. 2017 Jan;44(1):98–103. PMID:27730656
**356.** Arroyo MR, Green DM, Perlman EJ, et al. The spectrum of metanephric adenofibroma and related lesions: clinicopathologic study of 25 cases from the National Wilms Tumor Study Group Pathology Center. Am J Surg Pathol. 2001 Apr;25(4):433–44. PMID:11257617
**357.** Arslan A, Alíç B, Uzunlar AK, et al. Diffuse lipomatosis of thyroid gland. Auris Nasus Larynx. 1999 Apr;26(2):213–5. PMID:10214903
**358.** Arts FA, Sciot R, Brichard B, et al. PDGFRB gain-of-function mutations in sporadic infantile myofibromatosis. Hum Mol Genet. 2017 May 15;26(10):1801–10. PMID:28334876
**359.** Arva NC, Bonadio J, Perlman EJ, et al. Diagnostic utility of Pax8, Pax2, and NGFR immunohistochemical expression in pediatric renal tumors. Appl Immunohistochem Mol Morphol. 2018 Nov-Dec;26(10):721–6. PMID:28426529
**360.** Asa SL, Bamberger AM, Cao B, et al. The transcription activator steroidogenic factor-1 is preferentially expressed in the human pituitary gonadotroph. J Clin Endocrinol Metab. 1996 Jun;81(6):2165–70. PMID:8964846
**361.** Asa SL, Ezzat S, Kelly DF, et al. Hypothalamic vasopressin-producing tumors: often inappropriate diuresis but occasionally cushing disease. Am J Surg Pathol. 2019 Feb;43(2):251–60. PMID:30379651
**362.** Asa SL, Ezzat S, Mete O. The diagnosis and clinical significance of paragangliomas in unusual locations. J Clin Med. 2018 Sep 13;7(9):E280. PMID:30217041
**363.** Asa SL, Kucharczyk W, Ezzat S. Pituitary acromegaly: not one disease. Endocr Relat Cancer. 2017 Mar;24(3):C1–4. PMID:28122798
**364.** Asa SL, Mete O. Hypothalamic endocrine tumors: an update. J Clin Med. 2019 Oct 20;8(10):E1741. PMID:31635149
**365.** Asa SL, Puy LA, Lew AM, et al. Cell type-specific expression of the pituitary transcription activator pit-1 in the human pituitary and pituitary adenomas. J Clin Endocrinol Metab. 1993 Nov;77(5):1275–80. PMID:8077321
**366.** Asai S, Katabami T, Tsuiki M, et al. Controlling tumor progression with cyclophosphamide, vincristine, and dacarbazine treatment improves survival in patients with metastatic and unresectable malignant pheochromocytomas/paragangliomas. Horm Cancer. 2017 Apr;8(2):108–18. PMID:28108930
**367.** Asano N, Yoshida A, Ogura K, et al. Prognostic value of relevant clinicopathologic variables in epithelioid sarcoma: a multi-institutional retrospective study of 44 patients. Ann Surg Oncol. 2015 Aug;22(8):2624–32. PMID:25663591
**368.** Asanuma M, Aoyama T, Sakai K, et al. Hematogenous extraneural metastasis of the germinomatous component of a pineal mixed germ cell tumor. Brain Tumor Pathol. 2012 Oct;29(4):245–50. PMID:22286191
**369.** Asdigian NL, Barón AE, Morelli JG, et al. Trajectories of nevus development from age 3 to 16 years in the Colorado Kids Sun Care Program cohort. JAMA Dermatol. 2018 Nov 1;154(11):1272–80. PMID:30208471
**370.** Ash S, Yaniv I, Feinmesser R, et al. Acinic cell carcinoma of the parotid gland in children and adolescents. J Pediatr Hematol Oncol. 2018 Mar;40(2):99–103. PMID:29240035
**371.** Ashikari R, Farrow JH, O'Hara J. Fibroadenomas in the breast of juveniles. Surg Gynecol Obstet. 1971 Feb;132(2):259–62. PMID:5547408
**372.** Ashworth M. The pathology of preclinical medullary thyroid carcinoma. Endocr Pathol. 2004 Fall;15(3):227–31. PMID:15640548
**373.** Asioli S, Righi A, Iommi M, et al. Validation of a clinicopathological score for the prediction of post-surgical evolution of pituitary adenoma: retrospective analysis on 566 patients from a tertiary care centre. Eur J Endocrinol. 2019 Feb 1;180(2):127–34. PMID:30481158
**374.** Askan G, Deshpande V, Klimstra DS, et al. Expression of markers of hepatocellular differentiation in pancreatic acinar cell neoplasms: a potential diagnostic pitfall. Am J Clin Pathol. 2016 Aug;146(2):163–9. PMID:27425386
**375.** Aslam A, Salam A, Griffiths CE, et al. Naevus sebaceus: a mosaic RASopathy. Clin Exp Dermatol. 2014 Jan;39(1):1–6. PMID:24341474
**376.** Asmandar S, Ranganathan S, Ramirez R, et al. Myxoid lipoblastoma and mimickers on fine-needle biopsy in a child. Pediatr Dev Pathol. 2019 Mar-Apr;22(2):157–60. PMID:30322346
**377.** Asp J, Persson F, Kost-Alimova M, et al. CHCHD7-PLAG1 and TCEA1-PLAG1 gene fusions resulting from cryptic, intrachromosomal 8q rearrangements in pleomorphic salivary gland adenomas. Genes Chromosomes Cancer. 2006 Sep;45(9):820–8. PMID:16736500
**378.** Asselin BL. Epidemiology of childhood and adolescent cancer. In: Kliegman RM, Stanton BMD, St. Geme J, editors. Nelson Textbook of Pediatrics. Volume 2. 20th ed. Philadelphia (PA): Elsevier; 2016. pp. 2416–8.
**379.** Assmann G, Kappler R, Zeindl-Eberhart E, et al. β-Catenin mutations in 2 nested stromal epithelial tumors of the liver–a neoplasia with defective mesenchymal-epithelial transition. Hum Pathol. 2012 Nov;43(11):1815–27. PMID:22749188
**380.** Assoun J, Richardi G, Railhac JJ, et al. Osteoid osteoma: MR imaging versus CT. Radiology. 1994 Apr;191(1):217–23. PMID:8134575
**380A.** Asthagiri AR, Parry DM, Butman JA, et al. Neurofibromatosis type 2. Lancet. 2009 Jun 6;373(9679):1974–86. PMID:19476995
**381.** Astl J, Dvoráková M, Vlcek P, et al. Thyroid surgery in children and adolescents. Int J Pediatr Otorhinolaryngol. 2004 Oct;68(10):1273–8. PMID:15364498
**382.** Astrinidis A, Henske EP. Tuberous sclerosis complex: linking growth and energy signaling pathways with human disease. Oncogene. 2005 Nov 14;24(50):7475–81. PMID:16288294
**383.** Aström AK, Voz ML, Kas K, et al. Conserved mechanism of PLAG1 activation in salivary gland tumors with and without chromosome 8q12 abnormalities: identification of

SII as a new fusion partner gene. Cancer Res. 1999 Feb 15;59(4):918–23. PMID:10029085

**384.** Astrom K, Cohen JE, Willett-Brozick JE, et al. Altitude is a phenotypic modifier in hereditary paraganglioma type 1: evidence for an oxygen-sensing defect. Hum Genet. 2003 Aug;113(3):228–37. PMID:12811540

**385.** Astuti D, Hart-Holden N, Latif F, et al. Genetic analysis of mitochondrial complex II subunits SDHD, SDHB and SDHC in paraganglioma and phaeochromocytoma susceptibility. Clin Endocrinol (Oxf). 2003 Dec;59(6):728–33. PMID:14974914

**386.** Astuti D, Ricketts CJ, Chowdhury R, et al. Mutation analysis of HIF prolyl hydroxylases (PHD/EGLN) in individuals with features of phaeochromocytoma and renal cell carcinoma susceptibility. Endocr Relat Cancer. 2010 Dec 21;18(1):73–83. PMID:20959442

**387.** Atallah-Yunes SA, Murphy DJ, Noy A. HIV-associated Burkitt lymphoma. Lancet Haematol. 2020 Aug;7(8):e594–600. PMID:32735838

**388.** Ater JL, Xia C, Mazewski CM, et al. Nonrandomized comparison of neurofibromatosis type 1 and non-neurofibromatosis type 1 children who received carboplatin and vincristine for progressive low-grade glioma: a report from the Children's Oncology Group. Cancer. 2016 Jun 15;122(12):1928–36. PMID:27061921

**389.** Ates D, Kosemehmetoglu K, Onder S, et al. Pseudopapillary pattern in intra-operative squash smear preparations of central nervous system germinomas. Cytopathology. 2014 Feb;25(1):45–50. PMID:23551548

**390.** Atesok KI, Alman BA, Schemitsch EH, et al. Osteoid osteoma and osteoblastoma. J Am Acad Orthop Surg. 2011 Nov;19(11):678–89. PMID:22052644

**391.** Athale UH, Razzouk BI, Raimondi SC, et al. Biology and outcome of childhood acute megakaryoblastic leukemia: a single institution's experience. Blood. 2001 Jun 15;97(12):3727–32. PMID:11389009

**392.** Athar M, Li C, Kim AL, et al. Sonic hedgehog signaling in Basal cell nevus syndrome. Cancer Res. 2014 Sep 15;74(18):4967–75. PMID:25172843

**393.** Atiq MA, Davis JL, Hornick JL, et al. Mesenchymal tumors of the gastrointestinal tract with NTRK rearrangements: a clinicopathological, immunophenotypic, and molecular study of eight cases, emphasizing their distinction from gastrointestinal stromal tumor (GIST). Mod Pathol. 2021 Jan;34(1):95–103. PMID:32669612

**394.** Atkin NB, Baker MC. Specific chromosome change, i(12p), in testicular tumours? Lancet. 1982 Dec 11;2(8311):1349. PMID:6128640

**395.** Atra A, Meller ST, Stevens RS, et al. Conservative management of follicular non-Hodgkin's lymphoma in childhood. Br J Haematol. 1998 Oct;103(1):220–3. PMID:9792312

**396.** Attarbaschi A, Abla O, Arias Padilla L, et al. Rare non-Hodgkin lymphoma of childhood and adolescence: a consensus diagnostic and therapeutic approach to pediatric-type follicular lymphoma, marginal zone lymphoma, and nonanaplastic peripheral T-cell lymphoma. Pediatr Blood Cancer. 2020 Aug;67(8):e28416. PMID:32452165

**397.** Attarbaschi A, Beishuizen A, Mann G, et al. Children and adolescents with follicular lymphoma have an excellent prognosis with either limited chemotherapy or with a "watch and wait" strategy after complete resection. Ann Hematol. 2013 Nov;92(11):1537–41. PMID:23665980

**398.** Attarbaschi A, Carraro E, Abla O, et al. Non-Hodgkin lymphoma and pre-existing conditions: spectrum, clinical characteristics and outcome in 213 children and adolescents.

Haematologica. 2016 Dec;101(12):1581–91. PMID:27515251

**399.** Attiyeh EF, London WB, Mossé YP, et al. Chromosome 1p and 11q deletions and outcome in neuroblastoma. N Engl J Med. 2005 Nov 24;353(21):2243–53. PMID:16306521

**400.** Attygalle AD, Cabeçadas J, Gaulard P, et al. Peripheral T-cell and NK-cell lymphomas and their mimics; taking a step forward - report on the lymphoma workshop of the XVIth meeting of the European Association for Haematopathology and the Society for Hematopathology. Histopathology. 2014 Jan;64(2):171–99. PMID:24128129

**401.** Attygalle AD, Liu H, Shirali S, et al. Atypical marginal zone hyperplasia of mucosa-associated lymphoid tissue: a reactive condition of childhood showing immunoglobulin lambda light-chain restriction. Blood. 2004 Nov 15;104(10):3343–8. PMID:15256428

**402.** Atun R, Bhakta N, Denburg A, et al. Sustainable care for children with cancer: a Lancet Oncology Commission. Lancet Oncol. 2020 Apr;21(4):e185–224. PMID:32240612

**403.** Atzmony L, Khan HM, Lim YH, et al. Second-hit, postzygotic PMVK and MVD mutations in linear porokeratosis. JAMA Dermatol. 2019 May 1;155(5):548–55. PMID:30942823

**404.** Atzmony L, Ugwu N, Zaki TD, et al. Post-zygotic ACTB mutations underlie congenital smooth muscle hamartomas. J Cutan Pathol. 2020 Aug;47(8):681–5. PMID:32170967

**405.** Au KS, Williams AT, Roach ES, et al. Genotype/phenotype correlation in 325 individuals referred for a diagnosis of tuberous sclerosis complex in the United States. Genet Med. 2007 Feb;9(2):88–100. PMID:17304050

**406.** Auclair PL, Ellis GL. Atypical features in salivary gland mixed tumors: their relationship to malignant transformation. Mod Pathol. 1996 Jun;9(6):652–7. PMID:8782203

**407.** Auer F, Rüschendorf F, Gombert M, et al. Inherited susceptibility to pre B-ALL caused by germline transmission of PAX5 c.547G>A. Leukemia. 2014 May;28(5):1136–8. PMID:24287434

**408.** Au-Yeung RKH, Arias Padilla L, Zimmermann M, et al. Experience with provisional WHO-entities large B-cell lymphoma with IRF4-rearrangement and Burkitt-like lymphoma with 11q aberration in paediatric patients of the NHL-BFM group. Br J Haematol. 2020 Sep;190(5):753–63. PMID:32239695

**409.** Au-Yeung RKH, Richter J, Iaccarino I, et al. Molecular features of non-anaplastic peripheral T-cell lymphoma in children and adolescents. Pediatr Blood Cancer. 2021 Nov;68(11):e29285. PMID:34390161

**410.** Avedschmidt SE, Stagner AM, Eagle RC Jr, et al. The targetable epigenetic tumor protein EZH2 is enriched in intraocular medulloepithelioma. Invest Ophthalmol Vis Sci. 2016 Nov 1;57(14):6242–6. PMID:27842164

**411.** Aveic S, Pantile M, Seydel A, et al. Combating autophagy is a strategy to increase cytotoxic effects of novel ALK inhibitor entrectinib in neuroblastoma cells. Oncotarget. 2016 Feb 2;7(5):5646–63. PMID:26735175

**412.** Aveic S, Tonini GP. Resistance to receptor tyrosine kinase inhibitors in solid tumors: Can we improve the cancer fighting strategy by blocking autophagy? Cancer Cell Int. 2016 Aug 2;16:62. PMID:27486382

**413.** Averbook BJ, Lee SJ, Delman KA, et al. Pediatric melanoma: analysis of an international registry. Cancer. 2013 Nov 15;119(22):4012–9. PMID:24022819

**414.** Avgerinou GP, Asvesti AP, Katsambas AD, et al. CHILD syndrome: the NSDHL gene and its role in CHILD syndrome, a rare hereditary disorder. J Eur Acad Dermatol Venereol. 2010 Jun;24(6):733–6. PMID:19906044

**415.** Aw SJ, Chang KTE. Clear cell sarcoma of the kidney. Arch Pathol Lab Med. 2019 Aug;143(8):1022–6. PMID:30628851

**416.** Awan S, Davenport M, Portmann B, et al. Angiosarcoma of the liver in children. J Pediatr Surg. 1996 Dec;31(12):1729–32. PMID:8987004

**417.** Axiotis CA, Lippes HA, Merino MJ, et al. Corticotroph cell pituitary adenoma within an ovarian teratoma. A new cause of Cushing's syndrome. Am J Surg Pathol. 1987 Mar;11(3):218–24. PMID:3548446

**418.** Ayadi L, Charfi S, Ben Hamed Y, et al. Pigmented lipofibromatosis in unusual location: case report and review of the literature. Virchows Arch. 2008 Apr;452(4):465–7. PMID:18236073

**419.** Ayadi-Kaddour A, Mlika M, Chaabouni S, et al. Mesenchymal hamartoma of the chest wall in an infant. Pathologica. 2007 Dec;99(6):440–2. PMID:18416338

**420.** Ayala AG, Ro JY, Bolio-Solis A, et al. Mesenchymal hamartoma of the chest wall in infants and children: a clinicopathological study of five patients. Skeletal Radiol. 1993 Nov;22(8):569–76. PMID:8291008

**421.** Ayala AG, Ro JY, Raymond AK, et al. Small cell osteosarcoma. A clinicopathologic study of 27 cases. Cancer. 1989 Nov 15;64(10):2162–73. PMID:2804905

**422.** Ayala-Ramirez M, Feng L, Johnson MM, et al. Clinical risk factors for malignancy and overall survival in patients with pheochromocytomas and sympathetic paragangliomas: primary tumor size and primary tumor location as prognostic indicators. J Clin Endocrinol Metab. 2011 Mar;96(3):717–25. PMID:21190975

**423.** Ayan I, Kaytan E, Ayan N. Childhood nasopharyngeal carcinoma: from biology to treatment. Lancet Oncol. 2003 Jan;4(1):13–21. PMID:12517535

**424.** Aydin F, Ghatak NR, Salvant J, et al. Desmoplastic cerebral astrocytoma of infancy. A case report with immunohistochemical, ultrastructural and proliferation studies. Acta Neuropathol. 1993;86(6):666–70. PMID:7906073

**425.** Aydin H, Young RH, Ronnett BM, et al. Clear cell papillary cystadenoma of the epididymis and mesosalpinx: immunohistochemical differentiation from metastatic clear cell renal cell carcinoma. Am J Surg Pathol. 2005 Apr;29(4):520–3. PMID:15767808

**426.** Ayed A, Tonks AM, Lander A, et al. A review of pregnancies complicated by congenital sacrococcygeal teratoma in the West Midlands region over an 18-year period: population-based, cohort study. Prenat Diagn. 2015 Nov;35(11):1037–47. PMID:26114890

**427.** Aygun B, Kimpo M, Lee T, et al. An adolescent with ovarian osteosarcoma arising in a cystic teratoma. J Pediatr Hematol Oncol. 2003 May;25(5):410–3. PMID:12759630

**428.** Ayturk UM, Couto JA, Hann S, et al. Somatic Activating Mutations in GNAQ and GNA11 Are Associated with Congenital Hemangioma. Am J Hum Genet. 2016 Apr 7;98(4):789–95. PMID:27058448

**429.** Ayturk UM, Couto JA, Hann S, et al. Somatic activating mutations in GNAQ and GNA11 are associated with congenital hemangioma. Am J Hum Genet. 2016 Jun 2;98(6):1271. PMID:27259057

**430.** Azaña JM, Torrelo A, Matito A. Update on mastocytosis (part 2): categories, prognosis, and treatment. Actas Dermosifiliogr. 2016 Jan-Feb;107(1):15–22. PMID:26525106

**431.** Baade PD, Youlden DR, Valery PC, et al. Trends in incidence of childhood cancer in Australia, 1983-2006. Br J Cancer. 2010 Feb 2;102(3):620–6. PMID:20051948

**432.** Babic B, Patel D, Aufforth R, et al. Pediatric patients with pheochromocytoma and

paraganglioma should have routine preoperative genetic testing for common susceptibility genes in addition to imaging to detect extra-adrenal and metastatic tumors. Surgery. 2017 Jan;161(1):220–7. PMID:27865588

**433.** Baccarani M, Castagnetti F, Gugliotta G, et al. The proportion of different BCR-ABL1 transcript types in chronic myeloid leukemia. An international overview. Leukemia. 2019 May;33(5):1173–83. PMID:30675008

**434.** Baccarani M, Saglio G, Goldman J, et al. Evolving concepts in the management of chronic myeloid leukemia: recommendations from an expert panel on behalf of the European LeukemiaNet. Blood. 2006 Sep 15;108(6):1809–20. PMID:16709930

**435.** Bacchini P, Inwards C, Biscaglia R, et al. Chondroblastoma-like osteosarcoma. Orthopedics. 1999 Mar;22(3):337–9. PMID:10192265

**436.** Bacci G, Fabbri N, Balladelli A, et al. Treatment and prognosis for synchronous multifocal osteosarcoma in 42 patients. J Bone Joint Surg Br. 2006 Aug;88(8):1071–5. PMID:16877608

**437.** Bacci G, Ferrari S, Bertoni F, et al. Long-term outcome for patients with nonmetastatic osteosarcoma of the extremity treated at the istituto ortopedico rizzoli according to the istituto ortopedico rizzoli/osteosarcoma-2 protocol: an updated report. J Clin Oncol. 2000 Dec 15;18(24):4016–27. PMID:11118462

**438.** Bacci G, Ferrari S, Ruggieri P, et al. Telangiectatic osteosarcoma of the extremity: neoadjuvant chemotherapy in 24 cases. Acta Orthop Scand. 2001 Apr;72(2):167–72. PMID:11372948

**439.** Bacci G, Longhi A, Versari M, et al. Prognostic factors for osteosarcoma of the extremity treated with neoadjuvant chemotherapy: 15-year experience in 789 patients treated at a single institution. Cancer. 2006 Mar 1;106(5):1154–61. PMID:16421923

**440.** Back MR, Hu B, Rutgers J, et al. Metastasis of an intracranial germinoma through a ventriculoperitoneal shunt: recurrence as a yolk-sac tumor. Pediatr Surg Int. 1997;12(1):24–7. PMID:9035204

**441.** Bader A, Heran M, Dunham C, et al. Radiological features of infantile glioblastoma and desmoplastic infantile tumors: British Columbia's Children's Hospital experience. J Neurosurg Pediatr. 2015 Aug;16(2):119–25. PMID:25955808

**442.** Bader-Meunier B, Tchernia G, Miélot F, et al. Occurrence of myeloproliferative disorder in patients with Noonan syndrome. J Pediatr. 1997 Jun;130(6):885–9. PMID:9202609

**443.** Bague S, Folpe AL. Dermatofibrosarcoma protuberans presenting as a subcutaneous mass: a clinicopathological study of 15 cases with exclusive or near-exclusive subcutaneous involvement. Am J Dermatopathol. 2008 Aug;30(4):327–32. PMID:18645303

**444.** Bahk WJ, Mirra JM. Pseudoanaplastic tumors of bone. Skeletal Radiol. 2004 Nov;33(11):641–8. PMID:15365783

**445.** Bahrami A, Barnhill RL. Pathology and genomics of pediatric melanoma: a critical reexamination and new insights. Pediatr Blood Cancer. 2018 Feb;65(2):10.1002/pbc.26792. PMID:28895292

**446.** Bahrami A, Dalton JD, Krane JF, et al. A subset of cutaneous and soft tissue mixed tumors are genetically linked to their salivary gland counterpart. Genes Chromosomes Cancer. 2012 Feb;51(2):140–8. PMID:22038920

**447.** Bahrami A, Perez-Ordonez B, Dalton JD, et al. An analysis of PLAG1 and HMGA2 rearrangements in salivary duct carcinoma and examination of the role of precursor lesions. Histopathology. 2013 Aug;63(2):250–62. PMID:23738717

**448.** Bahrami A, Weiss SW, Montgomery E, et al. RT-PCR analysis for FGF23 using paraffin

sections in the diagnosis of phosphaturic mesenchymal tumors with and without known tumor induced osteomalacia. Am J Surg Pathol. 2009 Sep;33(9):1348–54. PMID:19609206
**449.** Bahubeshi A, Bal N, Rio Frio T, et al. Germline DICER1 mutations and familial cystic nephroma. J Med Genet. 2010 Dec;47(12):863–6. PMID:21036787
**450.** Bai DY, Xie JL, Zheng YY, et al. [Paediatric nodal marginal zone lymphoma: a clinicopathological study of seven cases]. Zhonghua Bing Li Xue Za Zhi. 2019 May 8;48(5):369–72. Chinese. PMID:31104676
**451.** Bai RY, Dieter P, Peschel C, et al. Nucleophosmin-anaplastic lymphoma kinase of large-cell anaplastic lymphoma is a constitutively active tyrosine kinase that utilizes phospholipase C-gamma to mediate its mitogenicity. Mol Cell Biol. 1998 Dec;18(12):6951–61. PMID:9819383
**452.** Bai RY, Ouyang T, Miething C, et al. Nucleophosmin-anaplastic lymphoma kinase associated with anaplastic large-cell lymphoma activates the phosphatidylinositol 3-kinase/Akt antiapoptotic signaling pathway. Blood. 2000 Dec 15;96(13):4319–27. PMID:11110708
**453.** Baildam AD, Higgins RM, Hurley E, et al. Cyclosporin A and multiple fibroadenomas of the breast. Br J Surg. 1996 Dec;83(12):1755–7. PMID:9038560
**454.** Baisden BL, Brat DJ, Melhem ER, et al. Dysembryoplastic neuroepithelial tumor-like neoplasm of the septum pellucidum: a lesion often misdiagnosed as glioma: report of 10 cases. Am J Surg Pathol. 2001 Apr;25(4):494–9. PMID:11257624
**455.** Baker AC, Rezeanu L, O'Laughlin S, et al. Juxtacortical chondromyxoid fibroma of bone: a unique variant: a case study of 20 patients. Am J Surg Pathol. 2007 Nov;31(11):1662–8. PMID:18059222
**456.** Baker PM, Oliva E, Young RH, et al. Ovarian mucinous carcinoids including some with a carcinomatous component: a report of 17 cases. Am J Surg Pathol. 2001 May;25(5):557–68. PMID:11342766
**457.** Baker PM, Rosai J, Young RH. Ovarian teratomas with florid benign vascular proliferation: a distinctive finding associated with the neural component of teratomas that may be confused with a vascular neoplasm. Int J Gynecol Pathol. 2002 Jan;21(1):16–21. PMID:11781518
**458.** Baker SW, Duffy KA, Richards-Yutz J, et al. Improved molecular detection of mosaicism in Beckwith-Wiedemann Syndrome. J Med Genet. 2021 Mar;58(3):178–84. PMID:32430359
**459.** Bakker NA, van Imhoff GW, Verschuuren EA, et al. Early onset post-transplant lymphoproliferative disease is associated with allograft localization. Clin Transplant. 2005 Jun;19(3):327–34. PMID:15877793
**460.** Bakri A, Shinagare AB, Krajewski KM, et al. Synovial sarcoma: imaging features of common and uncommon primary sites, metastatic patterns, and treatment response. AJR Am J Roentgenol. 2012 Aug;199(2):W208-15. PMID:22826423
**461.** Bakry D, Aronson M, Durno C, et al. Genetic and clinical determinants of constitutional mismatch repair deficiency syndrome: report from the constitutional mismatch repair deficiency consortium. Eur J Cancer. 2014 Mar;50(5):987–96. PMID:24440087
**462.** Bakshi P, Srinivasan R, Rao KL, et al. Fine needle aspiration biopsy in pediatric space-occupying lesions of liver: a retrospective study evaluating its role and diagnostic efficacy. J Pediatr Surg. 2006 Nov;41(11):1903–8. PMID:17101368
**463.** Balachandar S, La Quaglia M, Tuttle RM, et al. Pediatric differentiated thyroid carcinoma of follicular cell origin: prognostic significance of histologic subtypes. Thyroid. 2016 Feb;26(2):219–26. PMID:26854950
**464.** Balachandran K, Allen PW, MacCormac LB. Nuchal fibroma. A clinicopathological study of nine cases. Am J Surg Pathol. 1995 Mar;19(3):313–7. PMID:7872429
**465.** Balakumar R, Farr MRB, Fernando M, et al. Adult-type rhabdomyoma of the larynx in Birt-Hogg-Dubé syndrome: evidence for a real association. Head Neck Pathol. 2019 Sep;13(3):507–11. PMID:29744825
**466.** Baldassari S, Ribierre T, Marsan E, et al. Dissecting the genetic basis of focal cortical dysplasia: a large cohort study. Acta Neuropathol. 2019 Dec;138(6):885–900. PMID:31444548
**467.** Baldauf MC, Orth MF, Dallmayer M, et al. Robust diagnosis of Ewing sarcoma by immunohistochemical detection of super-enhancer-driven EWSR1-ETS targets. Oncotarget. 2017 Aug 4;9(2):1587–601. PMID:29416716
**468.** Baldi GG, Brahmi M, Lo Vullo S, et al. The activity of chemotherapy in inflammatory myofibroblastic tumors: a multicenter, European retrospective case series analysis. Oncologist. 2020 Nov;25(11):e1777–84. PMID:32584482
**469.** Baldisserotto M, Peletti AB, Angelo de Araújo M, et al. Beckwith-Wiedemann syndrome and bilateral adrenal pheochromocytoma: sonography and MRI findings. Pediatr Radiol. 2005 Nov;35(11):1132–4. PMID:15983774
**470.** Baldovini C, Sorrentino S, Alves CA, et al. Congenital myoepithelial carcinoma of soft tissue associated with cystic myoepithelioma. Int J Surg Pathol. 2018 Feb;26(1):78–83. PMID:28675958
**471.** Bale TA. FGFR- gene family alterations in low-grade neuroepithelial tumors. Acta Neuropathol Commun. 2020 Feb 21;8(1):21. PMID:32085805
**472.** Bale TA, Oviedo A, Kozakewich H, et al. Intracranial myxoid mesenchymal tumors with EWSR1-CREB family gene fusions: myxoid variant of angiomatoid fibrous histiocytoma or novel entity? Brain Pathol. 2018 Mar;28(2):183–91. PMID:28281318
**473.** Bale TA, Sait SF, Benhamida J, et al. Malignant transformation of a polymorphous low grade neuroepithelial tumor of the young (PLNTY). Acta Neuropathol. 2021 Jan;141(1):123–5. PMID:33226472
**474.** Balgobind BV, Raimondi SC, Harbott J, et al. Novel prognostic subgroups in childhood 11q23/MLL-rearranged acute myeloid leukemia: results of an international retrospective study. Blood. 2009 Sep 17;114(12):2489–96. PMID:19528532
**475.** Ball A, Wenning J, Van Eyk N. Ovarian fibromas in pediatric patients with basal cell nevus (Gorlin) syndrome. J Pediatr Adolesc Gynecol. 2011 Feb;24(1):e5–7. PMID:20817576
**476.** Ballinger ML, Goode DL, Ray-Coquard I, et al. Monogenic and polygenic determinants of sarcoma risk: an international genetic study. Lancet Oncol. 2016 Sep;17(9):1261–71. PMID:27498913
**477.** Baloch Z, Mete O, Asa SL. Immunohistochemical biomarkers in thyroid pathology. Endocr Pathol. 2018 Jun;29(2):91–112. PMID:29744727
**478.** Balogun JA, Monsalves E, Juraschka K, et al. Null cell adenomas of the pituitary gland: an institutional review of their clinical imaging and behavioral characteristics. Endocr Pathol. 2015 Mar;26(1):63–70. PMID:25403448
**479.** Baltres A, Salhi A, Houlier A, et al. Malignant melanoma with areas of rhabdomyosarcomatous differentiation arising in a giant congenital nevus with RAF1 gene fusion. Pigment Cell Melanoma Res. 2019 Sep;32(5):708–13. PMID:30945443
**480.** Bandopadhayay P, Ramkissoon LA, Jain P, et al. MYB-QKI rearrangements in angiocentric glioma drive tumorigenicity through a tripartite mechanism. Nat Genet. 2016 Mar;48(3):273–82. PMID:26829751
**481.** Bandopadhayay P, Silvera VM, Ciarlini PDSC, et al. Myxopapillary ependymomas in children: imaging, treatment and outcomes. J Neurooncol. 2016 Jan;126(1):165–74. PMID:26468139
**482.** Banet N, Gown AM, Shih IeM, et al. GATA-3 expression in trophoblastic tissues: an immunohistochemical study of 445 cases, including diagnostic utility. Am J Surg Pathol. 2015 Jan;39(1):101–8. PMID:25188865
**483.** Bansal S, Desai RS, Shirsat P, et al. The occurrence and pattern of ameloblastoma in children and adolescents: an Indian institutional study of 41 years and review of the literature. Int J Oral Maxillofac Surg. 2015 Jun;44(6):725–31. PMID:25655766
**484.** Bao F, Panarelli NC, Rennert H, et al. Neoadjuvant therapy induces loss of MSH6 expression in colorectal carcinoma. Am J Surg Pathol. 2010 Dec;34(12):1798–804. PMID:21107085
**485.** Bao PP, Li K, Wu CX, et al. [Recent incidences and trends of childhood malignant solid tumors in Shanghai, 2002-2010]. Zhonghua Er Ke Za Zhi. 2013 Apr;51(4):288–94. Chinese. PMID:23927803
**486.** Bar EE, Lin A, Tihan T, et al. Frequent gains at chromosome 7q34 involving BRAF in pilocytic astrocytoma. J Neuropathol Exp Neurol. 2008 Sep;67(9):878–87. PMID:18716556
**487.** Barakat RMB, Garzon S, Laganà AS, et al. Fetus-in-fetu: a rare condition that requires common rules for its definition. Arch Gynecol Obstet. 2020 Dec;302(6):1541–3. PMID:31175400
**488.** Baran JL, Duncan LM. Combined melanocytic nevi: histologic variants and melanoma mimics. Am J Surg Pathol. 2011 Oct;35(10):1540–8. PMID:21881487
**489.** Baranov E, Hornick JL. Soft tissue special issue: fibroblastic and myofibroblastic neoplasms of the head and neck. Head Neck Pathol. 2020 Mar;14(1):43–58. PMID:31950474
**490.** Baranov E, McBride MJ, Bellizzi AM, et al. A novel SS18-SSX fusion-specific antibody for the diagnosis of synovial sarcoma. Am J Surg Pathol. 2020 Jul;44(7):922–33. PMID:32141887
**491.** Barba C, Jacques T, Kahane P, et al. Epilepsy surgery in Neurofibromatosis type 1. Epilepsy Res. 2013 Aug;105(3):384–95. PMID:23597854
**492.** Barclay SF, Inman KW, Luks VL, et al. A somatic activating NRAS variant associated with kaposiform lymphangiomatosis. Genet Med. 2019 Jul;21(7):1517–24. PMID:30542204
**493.** Bardales RH, Centeno B, Mallery JS, et al. Endoscopic ultrasound-guided fine-needle aspiration cytology diagnosis of solid-pseudopapillary tumor of the pancreas: a rare neoplasm of elusive origin but characteristic cytomorphologic features. Am J Clin Pathol. 2004 May;121(5):654–62. PMID:15151205
**494.** Barker D, Wright E, Nguyen K, et al. Gene for von Recklinghausen neurofibromatosis is in the pericentromeric region of chromosome 17. Science. 1987 May 29;236(4805):1100–2. PMID:3107130
**495.** Barkovich AJ, Guerrini R, Kuzniecky RI, et al. A developmental and genetic classification for malformations of cortical development: update 2012. Brain. 2012 May;135(Pt 5):1348–69. PMID:22427329
**496.** Barksdale EM Jr, Obokhare I. Teratomas in infants and children. Curr Opin Pediatr. 2009 Jun;21(3):344–9. PMID:19417664
**497.** Barletta JA, Bellizzi AM, Hornick JL. Immunohistochemical staining of thyroidectomy specimens for PTEN can aid in the identification of patients with Cowden syndrome. Am J Surg Pathol. 2011 Oct;35(10):1505–11. PMID:21921783
**498.** Barnes DJ, Hookway E, Athanasou N, et al. A germline mutation of CDKN2A and a novel RPLP1-C19MC fusion detected in a rare melanotic neuroectodermal tumor of infancy: a case report. BMC Cancer. 2016 Aug 12;16:629. PMID:27519597
**499.** Barnes DJ, Melo JV. Cytogenetic and molecular genetic aspects of chronic myeloid leukaemia. Acta Haematol. 2002;108(4):180–202. PMID:12432215
**500.** Barnhill RL. The Spitzoid lesion: rethinking Spitz tumors, atypical variants, 'Spitzoid melanoma' and risk assessment. Mod Pathol. 2006 Feb;19 Suppl 2:S21–33. PMID:16446713
**501.** Barnhill RL, Barnhill MA, Berwick M, et al. The histologic spectrum of pigmented spindle cell nevus: a review of 120 cases with emphasis on atypical variants. Hum Pathol. 1991 Jan;22(1):52–8. PMID:1985078
**502.** Barnoud R, Sabourin JC, Pasquier D, et al. Immunohistochemical expression of WT1 by desmoplastic small round cell tumor: a comparative study with other small round cell tumors. Am J Surg Pathol. 2000 Jun;24(6):830–6. PMID:10843285
**503.** Baroni E, Russo BD, Masquijo JJ, et al. Pigmented villonodular synovitis of the knee in skeletally immature patients. J Child Orthop. 2010 Apr;4(2):123–7. PMID:21455469
**504.** Barontini M, Levin G, Sanso G. Characteristics of pheochromocytoma in a 4- to 20-year-old population. Ann N Y Acad Sci. 2006 Aug;1073:30–7. PMID:17102069
**505.** Barr FG, Galili N, Holick J, et al. Rearrangement of the PAX3 paired box gene in the paediatric solid tumour alveolar rhabdomyosarcoma. Nat Genet. 1993 Feb;3(2):113–7. PMID:8098985
**506.** Barr FG, Qualman SJ, Macris MH, et al. Genetic heterogeneity in the alveolar rhabdomyosarcoma subset without typical gene fusions. Cancer Res. 2002 Aug 15;62(16):4704–10. PMID:12183429
**507.** Barr RJ, Morales RV, Graham JH. Desmoplastic nevus: a distinct histologic variant of mixed spindle cell and epithelioid cell nevus. Cancer. 1980 Aug 1;46(3):557–64. PMID:7397626
**508.** Barreto DC, Gomez RS, Bale AE, et al. PTCH gene mutations in odontogenic keratocysts. J Dent Res. 2000 Jun;79(6):1418–22. PMID:10890722
**509.** Barreto MW, Silva LV, Barini R, et al. Alpha-fetoprotein following neonatal resection of sacrococcygeal teratoma. Pediatr Hematol Oncol. 2006 Jun;23(4):287–91. PMID:16621769
**510.** Barrett AW, Sneddon KJ, Tighe JV, et al. Dentigerous cyst and ameloblastoma of the jaws. Int J Surg Pathol. 2017 Apr;25(2):141–7. PMID:27621276
**511.** Barrett MM, Strikwerda AM, Somers K, et al. Lymphomatoid papulosis type D: report of a case in a child and review of the literature. Pediatr Dermatol. 2016 Mar-Apr;33(2):e52–6. PMID:26763888
**512.** Barrionuevo C, Anderson VM, Zevallos-Giampietri E, et al. Hydroa-like cutaneous T-cell lymphoma: a clinicopathologic and molecular genetic study of 16 pediatric cases from Peru. Appl Immunohistochem Mol Morphol. 2002 Mar;10(1):7–14. PMID:11893040
**513.** Barrott JJ, Illum BE, Jin H, et al. Paracrine osteoprotegerin and β-catenin stabilization support synovial sarcomagenesis in periosteal cells. J Clin Invest. 2018 Jan 2;128(1):207–18. PMID:29202462

**514.** Bartek J Jr, Dhawan S, Thurin E, et al. Short-term outcome following surgery for rare brain tumor entities in adults: a Swedish nation-wide registry-based study and comparison with SEER database. J Neurooncol. 2020 Jun;148(2):281–90. PMID:32424575
**515.** Bartenstein DW, Coe TM, Gordon SC, et al. Lipofibromatosis-like neural tumor: case report of a unique infantile presentation. JAAD Case Rep. 2018 Feb 4;4(2):185–8. PMID:29892662
**516.** Bartenstein DW, Fisher JM, Stamoulis C, et al. Clinical features and outcomes of spitzoid proliferations in children and adolescents. Br J Dermatol. 2019 Aug;181(2):366–72. PMID:30467833
**517.** Barth TF, Müller S, Pawlita M, et al. Homogeneous immunophenotype and paucity of secondary genomic aberrations are distinctive features of endemic but not of sporadic Burkitt's lymphoma and diffuse large B-cell lymphoma with MYC rearrangement. J Pathol. 2004 Aug;203(4):940–5. PMID:15258997
**518.** Bartley AN, Luthra R, Saraiya DS, et al. Identification of cancer patients with Lynch syndrome: clinically significant discordances and problems in tissue-based mismatch repair testing. Cancer Prev Res (Phila). 2012 Feb;5(2):320–7. PMID:22086678
**519.** Bartolazzi A, Orlandi F, Saggiorato E, et al. Galectin-3-expression analysis in the surgical selection of follicular thyroid nodules with indeterminate fine-needle aspiration cytology: a prospective multicentre study. Lancet Oncol. 2008 Jun;9(6):543–9. PMID:18495537
**520.** Bartuma H, Domanski HA, Von Steyern FV, et al. Cytogenetic and molecular cytogenetic findings in lipoblastoma. Cancer Genet Cytogenet. 2008 May;183(1):60–3. PMID:18474299
**521.** Baruchel A, Cayuela JM, Ballerini P, et al. The majority of myeloid-antigen-positive (My+) childhood B-cell precursor acute lymphoblastic leukaemias express TEL-AML1 fusion transcripts. Br J Haematol. 1997 Oct;99(1):101–6. PMID:9359509
**522.** Baruffi MR, Volpon JB, Neto JB, et al. Osteoid osteomas with chromosome alterations involving 22q. Cancer Genet Cytogenet. 2001 Jan 15;124(2):127–31. PMID:11172903
**523.** Barut F, Onak Kandemir N, Bektas S, et al. Universal markers of thyroid malignancies: galectin-3, HBME-1, and cytokeratin-19. Endocr Pathol. 2010 Jun;21(2):80–9. PMID:20198455
**524.** Baselga E, Wassef M, Lopez S, et al. Agminated, eruptive pyogenic granuloma-like lesions developing over congenital vascular stains. Pediatr Dermatol. 2012 Mar-Apr;29(2):186–90. PMID:22066576
**525.** Baser ME, Friedman JM, Joe H, et al. Empirical development of improved diagnostic criteria for neurofibromatosis 2. Genet Med. 2011 Jun;13(6):576–81. PMID:21451418
**526.** Baser ME, Kuramoto L, Joe H, et al. Genotype-phenotype correlations for nervous system tumors in neurofibromatosis 2: a population-based study. Am J Hum Genet. 2004 Aug;75(2):231–9. PMID:15190457
**527.** Basquiera AL, Pizzi S, Correas AG, et al. Allogeneic hematopoietic stem cell transplantation in pediatric myelodysplastic syndromes: a multicenter experience from Argentina. Pediatr Blood Cancer. 2015 Jan;62(1):153–7. PMID:25264233
**528.** Basso C, Rizzo S, Valente M, et al. Cardiac masses and tumours. Heart. 2016 Aug 1;102(15):1230–45. PMID:27277840
**528A.** Baste Subia MN, Digoy P, Hum M, et al. Cytologic findings of spindle epithelial tumor with thymus-like elements. Laryngoscope. 2018 Feb;128(2):E78–82. PMID:29193099
**529.** Bastian BC. The molecular pathology of melanoma: an integrated taxonomy of melanocytic neoplasia. Annu Rev Pathol. 2014;9:239–71. PMID:24460190
**530.** Bastian BC, LeBoit PE, Pinkel D. Mutations and copy number increase of HRAS in Spitz nevi with distinctive histopathological features. Am J Pathol. 2000 Sep;157(3):967–72. PMID:10980135
**531.** Bastian BC, Wesselmann U, Pinkel D, et al. Molecular cytogenetic analysis of Spitz nevi shows clear differences to melanoma. J Invest Dermatol. 1999 Dec;113(6):1065–9. PMID:10594753
**532.** Bastian BC, Xiong J, Frieden IJ, et al. Genetic changes in neoplasms arising in congenital melanocytic nevi: differences between nodular proliferations and melanomas. Am J Pathol. 2002 Oct;161(4):1163–9. PMID:12368190
**533.** Bastidas Torres AN, Najidh S, Tensen CP, et al. Molecular advances in cutaneous T-cell lymphoma. Semin Cutan Med Surg. 2018 Mar;37(1):81–6. PMID:29719024
**534.** Bata BM, Pulido JS, Patel SV, et al. Combined intraocular and systemic rituximab for ocular lymphoproliferative disorder with extranodal marginal zone lymphoma-type morphology after heart transplant. J AAPOS. 2018 Apr;22(2):159–61. PMID:29408337
**535.** Batata MA, Chu FC, Hilaris BS, et al. Therapy and prognosis of testicular carcinomas in relation to TNM classification. Int J Radiat Oncol Biol Phys. 1982 Aug;8(8):1287–93. PMID:7141907
**536.** Bates JE, Choi G, Milano MT. Myxopapillary ependymoma: a SEER analysis of epidemiology and outcomes. J Neurooncol. 2016 Sep;129(2):251–8. PMID:27306443
**537.** Batukan C, Holzgreve W, Danzer E, et al. Large placental chorioangioma as a cause of sudden intrauterine fetal death. A case report. Fetal Diagn Ther. 2001 Nov-Dec;16(6):394–7. PMID:11694744
**538.** Bauer AJ. Molecular genetics of thyroid cancer in children and adolescents. Endocrinol Metab Clin North Am. 2017 Jun;46(2):389–403. PMID:28476228
**539.** Bauer AJ. Papillary and follicular thyroid cancer in children and adolescents: current approach and future directions. Semin Pediatr Surg. 2020 Jun;29(3):150920. PMID:32571505
**540.** Bauer AJ. Thyroid nodules in children and adolescents. Curr Opin Endocrinol Diabetes Obes. 2019 Oct;26(5):266–74. PMID:31361657
**541.** Bauer AJ, Stewart DR, Kamihara J, et al. DICER1 and associated conditions: identification of at-risk individuals and recommended surveillance strategies-response. Clin Cancer Res. 2019 Mar 1;25(5):1689–90. PMID:30824630
**542.** Bauer DE, Mitchell CM, Strait KM, et al. Clinicopathologic features and long-term outcomes of NUT midline carcinoma. Clin Cancer Res. 2012 Oct 15;18(20):5773–9. PMID:22896655
**543.** Bauer J, Curtin JA, Pinkel D, et al. Congenital melanocytic nevi frequently harbor NRAS mutations but no BRAF mutations. J Invest Dermatol. 2007 Jan;127(1):179–82. PMID:16888631
**544.** Baumann F, Flores E, Napolitano A, et al. Mesothelioma patients with germline BAP1 mutations have 7-fold improved long-term survival. Carcinogenesis. 2015 Jan;36(1):76–81. PMID:25380601
**545.** Baumann U, Adam R, Duvoux C, et al. Survival of children after liver transplantation for hepatocellular carcinoma. Liver Transpl. 2018 Feb;24(2):246–55. PMID:29222922
**546.** Baumhoer D, Amary F, Flanagan AM. An update of molecular pathology of bone tumors. Lessons learned from investigating samples by next generation sequencing. Genes Chromosomes Cancer. 2019 Feb;58(2):88–99. PMID:30582658
**547.** Baumhoer D, Brunner P, Eppenberger-Castori S, et al. Osteosarcomas of the jaws differ from their peripheral counterparts and require a distinct treatment approach. Oral Oncol. 2014 Feb;50(2):147–53. PMID:24246156
**548.** Baumhoer D, Kovac M, Sperveslage J, et al. Activating mutations in the MAP-kinase pathway define non-ossifying fibroma of bone. J Pathol. 2019 May;248(1):116–22. PMID:30549028
**549.** Baumhoer D, Smida J, Nathrath M, et al. The nature of the characteristic cementum-like matrix deposits in the walls of simple bone cysts. Histopathology. 2011 Sep;59(3):390–6. PMID:22034879
**550.** Bausch B, Wellner U, Bausch D, et al. Long-term prognosis of patients with pediatric pheochromocytoma. Endocr Relat Cancer. 2013 Dec 16;21(1):17–25. PMID:24169644
**551.** Bavle A, Shah R, Gross N, et al. Encephalocraniocutaneous lipomatosis. J Pediatr Hematol Oncol. 2018 Oct;40(7):553–4. PMID:29683947
**552.** Bayle C, Charpentier A, Duchayne E, et al. Leukaemic presentation of small cell variant anaplastic large cell lymphoma: report of four cases. Br J Haematol. 1999 Mar;104(4):680–8. PMID:10192426
**553.** Bayliss J, Mukherjee P, Lu C, et al. Lowered H3K27me3 and DNA hypomethylation define poorly prognostic pediatric posterior fossa ependymomas. Sci Transl Med. 2016 Nov 23;8(366):366ra161. PMID:27881822
**554.** Bayramoğlu H, Düzcan E, Akbulut M, et al. Infarction after fine needle aspiration biopsy of pleomorphic adenoma of the parotid gland. Acta Cytol. 2001 Nov-Dec;45(6):1008–10. PMID:11726095
**555.** Beaty NB, Ahn E. Images in clinical medicine. Adamantinomatous craniopharyngioma containing teeth. N Engl J Med. 2014 Feb 27;370(9):860. PMID:24571758
**556.** Beaumont TL, Godzik J, Dahiya S, et al. Subependymal giant cell astrocytoma in the absence of tuberous sclerosis complex: case report. J Neurosurg Pediatr. 2015 Aug;16(2):134–7. PMID:25978531
**557.** Beaunoyer M, Vanatta JM, Ogihara M, et al. Outcomes of transplantation in children with primary hepatic malignancy. Pediatr Transplant. 2007 Sep;11(6):655–60. PMID:17663690
**558.** Beavon JE, Brown MB, Landau RL, et al. Collaborative education: the Dayton approach. J Nurs Staff Dev. 1990 Jul-Aug;6(4):199–201. PMID:2380776
**559.** Beck SD, Foster RS, Bihrle R, et al. Significance of primary tumor size and preorchiectomy serum tumor marker level in predicting pathologic stage at retroperitoneal lymph node dissection in clinical Stage A nonseminomatous germ cell tumors. Urology. 2007 Mar;69(3):557–9. PMID:17382165
**560.** Becker AE. Primary heart tumors in the pediatric age group: a review of salient pathologic features relevant for clinicians. Pediatr Cardiol. 2000 Jul-Aug;21(4):317–23. PMID:10865004
**561.** Becker RL, Becker AD, Sobel DF. Adult medulloblastoma: review of 13 cases with emphasis on MRI. Neuroradiology. 1995 Feb;37(2):104–8. PMID:7760992
**562.** Becker WF. Pancreatoduodenectomy for carcinoma of the pancreas in an infant; report of a case. Ann Surg. 1957 Jun;145(6):864–72. PMID:13425296
**563.** Beckett JH, Jacobs AH. Recurring digital fibrous tumors of childhood: a review. Pediatrics. 1977 Mar;59(3):401–6. PMID:840560
**564.** Beckwith JB. Nephrogenic rests and the pathogenesis of Wilms tumor: developmental and clinical considerations. Am J Med Genet. 1998 Oct 2;79(4):268–73. PMID:9781906
**565.** Bedi DG, John SD, Swischuk LE. Fibromatosis colli of infancy: variability of sonographic appearance. J Clin Ultrasound. 1998 Sep;26(7):345–8. PMID:9719983
**566.** Bedlow AJ, Sampson SA, Holden CA. Congenital superficial angiomyxoma. Clin Exp Dermatol. 1997 Sep;22(5):237–9. PMID:9536546
**567.** Bedwell C, Rowe D, Moulton D, et al. Cytogenetically complex SEC31A-ALK fusions are recurrent in ALK-positive large B-cell lymphomas. Haematologica. 2011 Feb;96(2):343–6. PMID:21109691
**568.** Beer M, Eckert F, Schmoeckel C. The atrophic dermatofibroma. J Am Acad Dermatol. 1991 Dec;25(6 Pt 1):1081–2. PMID:1810988
**569.** Beert E, Brems H, Daniëls B, et al. Atypical neurofibromas in neurofibromatosis type 1 are premalignant tumors. Genes Chromosomes Cancer. 2011 Dec;50(12):1021–32. PMID:21987445
**570.** Begemann M, Waszak SM, Robinson GW, et al. Germline GPR161 mutations predispose to pediatric medulloblastoma. J Clin Oncol. 2020 Jan 1;38(1):43–50. PMID:31609649
**571.** Beghetti M, Gow RM, Haney I, et al. Pediatric primary benign cardiac tumors: a 15-year review. Am Heart J. 1997 Dec;134(6):1107–14. PMID:9424072
**572.** Bégueret H, Galateau-Salle F, Guillou L, et al. Primary intrathoracic synovial sarcoma: a clinicopathologic study of 40 t(X;18)-positive cases from the French Sarcoma Group and the Mesopath Group. Am J Surg Pathol. 2005 Mar;29(3):339–46. PMID:15725802
**573.** Behdad A, Perry A. Central nervous system primitive neuroectodermal tumors: a clinicopathologic and genetic study of 33 cases. Brain Pathol. 2010 Mar;20(2):441–50. PMID:19725831
**574.** Behery RE, Bedrnicek J, Lazenby A, et al. Translocation t(12;17)(q24.1;q21) as the sole anomaly in a nasal chondromesenchymal hamartoma arising in a patient with pleuropulmonary blastoma. Pediatr Dev Pathol. 2012 May-Jun;15(3):249–53. PMID:22356457
**575.** Behjati S, Tarpey PS, Haase K, et al. Recurrent mutation of IGF signalling genes and distinct patterns of genomic rearrangement in osteosarcoma. Nat Commun. 2017 Jun 23;8:15936. PMID:28643781
**576.** Behjati S, Tarpey PS, Presneau N, et al. Distinct H3F3A and H3F3B driver mutations define chondroblastoma and giant cell tumor of bone. Nat Genet. 2013 Dec;45(12):1479–82. PMID:24162739
**577.** Behjati S, Tarpey PS, Sheldon H, et al. Recurrent PTPRB and PLCG1 mutations in angiosarcoma. Nat Genet. 2014 Apr;46(4):376–9. PMID:24633157
**578.** Behnert A, Lee AG, Young EP, et al. NUP98-NSD1 Driven MDS/MPN in Childhood Masquerading as JMML. J Pediatr Hematol Oncol. 2021 Aug 1;43(6):e808–11. PMID:32815876
**578A.** Behnert A, Meyer J, Parsa JY, et al. Exploring the genetic and epigenetic origins of juvenile myelomonocytic leukemia using newborn screening samples. Leukemia. 2022 Jan;36(1):279–82. PMID:34183765
**579.** Behr GG, Fishman SJ, Caty MG, et al. Hepatic mesenchymal hamartoma and infantile hemangioma: a rare association. J Pediatr Surg. 2012 Mar;47(3):448–52. PMID:22424336
**580.** Behrens YL, Göhring G, Bawadi R, et al. A novel classification of hematologic conditions in patients with Fanconi anemia. Haematologica. 2021 Nov 1;106(11):3000–3. PMID:34196171

581. Beil KM. What Linnaeus saw: a scientist's quest to name every living thing. New York (NY): W. W. Norton & Company; 2019.
582. Bejarano PA, Nikiforov YE, Swenson ES, et al. Thyroid transcription factor-1, thyroglobulin, cytokeratin 7, and cytokeratin 20 in thyroid neoplasms. Appl Immunohistochem Mol Morphol. 2000 Sep;8(3):189–94. PMID:10981870
583. Bejarano PA, Serrano MF, Casillas J, et al. Concurrent infantile hemangioendothelioma and mesenchymal hamartoma in a developmentally arrested liver of an infant requiring hepatic transplantation. Pediatr Dev Pathol. 2003 Nov-Dec;6(6):552–7. PMID:15018455
584. Bekers EM, Groenen PJTA, Verdijk MAJ, et al. Soft tissue angiofibroma: clinicopathologic, immunohistochemical and molecular analysis of 14 cases. Genes Chromosomes Cancer. 2017 Oct;56(10):750–7. PMID:28639284
585. Bekkenk MW, Geelen FA, van Voorst Vader PC, et al. Primary and secondary cutaneous CD30(+) lymphoproliferative disorders: a report from the Dutch Cutaneous Lymphoma Group on the long-term follow-up data of 219 patients and guidelines for diagnosis and treatment. Blood. 2000 Jun 15;95(12):3653–61. PMID:10845893
586. Belfiore A, Sava L, Runello F, et al. Solitary autonomously functioning thyroid nodules and iodine deficiency. J Clin Endocrinol Metab. 1983 Feb;56(2):283–7. PMID:6822638
587. Belhadj K, Reyes F, Farcet JP, et al. Hepatosplenic gammadelta T-cell lymphoma is a rare clinicopathologic entity with poor outcome: report on a series of 21 patients. Blood. 2003 Dec 15;102(13):4261–9. PMID:12907441
588. Bell A, Rickinson AB. Epstein-Barr virus, the TCL-1 oncogene and Burkitt's lymphoma. Trends Microbiol. 2003 Nov;11(11):495–7. PMID:14607063
589. Bell D, Ranganathan S, Tao J, et al. Novel advances in understanding of molecular pathogenesis of hepatoblastoma: a Wnt/β-catenin perspective. Gene Expr. 2017 Feb 10;17(2):141–54. PMID:27938502
589A. Bella GP, Manivel JC, Thompson RC Jr, et al. Intramuscular hemangioma: recurrence risk related to surgical margins. Clin Orthop Relat Res. 2007 Jun;459:186–91. PMID:17438470
590. Bellan C, Lazzi S, Hummel M, et al. Immunoglobulin gene analysis reveals 2 distinct cells of origin for EBV-positive and EBV-negative Burkitt lymphomas. Blood. 2005 Aug 1;106(3):1031–6. PMID:15840698
591. Bellizzi AM, Bruzzi C, French CA, et al. The cytologic features of NUT midline carcinoma. Cancer. 2009 Dec 25;117(6):508–15. PMID:19795508
592. Bellon N, Fraitag S, Miquel C, et al. Cutaneous location of atypical teratoid/rhabdoid tumour. Acta Derm Venereol. 2014 Jul;94(4):454–6. PMID:24284868
593. Beltran B, Castillo J, Salas R, et al. ALK-positive diffuse large B-cell lymphoma: report of four cases and review of the literature. J Hematol Oncol. 2009 Feb 27;2:11. PMID:19250532
594. Beltrán BE, Maza I, Moisés-Alfaro CB, et al. Thalidomide for the treatment of hydroa vacciniforme-like lymphoma: report of four pediatric cases from Peru. Am J Hematol. 2014 Dec;89(12):1160–1. PMID:25196949
595. Beltran H. The N-myc oncogene: maximizing its targets, regulation, and therapeutic potential. Mol Cancer Res. 2014 Jun;12(6):815–22. PMID:24589438
596. Benachi A, Durin L, Vasseur Maurer S, et al. Prenatally diagnosed sacrococcygeal teratoma: a prognostic classification. J Pediatr Surg. 2006 Sep;41(9):1517–21. PMID:16952584
597. Ben-Ami E, Barysauskas CM, von Mehren M, et al. Long-term follow-up results of the multicenter phase II trial of regorafenib in patients with metastatic and/or unresectable GI stromal tumor after failure of standard tyrosine kinase inhibitor therapy. Ann Oncol. 2016 Sep;27(9):1794–9. PMID:27371698
598. Bender AM, Thompson ED, Hackam DJ, et al. Solid pseudopapillary neoplasm of the pancreas in a young pediatric patient: a case report and systematic review of the literature. Pancreas. 2018 Nov/Dec;47(10):1364–8. PMID:30325866
599. Bender S, Tang Y, Lindroth AM, et al. Reduced H3K27me3 and DNA hypomethylation are major drivers of gene expression in K27M mutant pediatric high-grade gliomas. Cancer Cell. 2013 Nov 11;24(5):660–72. PMID:24183680
599A. Benesch M, Frappaz D, Massimino M. Spinal cord ependymomas in children and adolescents. Childs Nerv Syst. 2012 Dec;28(12):2017–28. PMID:22961356
600. Benesch M, Wardelmann E, Ferrari A, et al. Gastrointestinal stromal tumors (GIST) in children and adolescents: a comprehensive review of the current literature. Pediatr Blood Cancer. 2009 Dec 15;53(7):1171–9. PMID:19499582
601. Bengtsson D, Schrøder HD, Andersen M, et al. Long-term outcome and MGMT as a predictive marker in 24 patients with atypical pituitary adenomas and pituitary carcinomas given treatment with temozolomide. J Clin Endocrinol Metab. 2015 Apr;100(4):1689–98. PMID:25646794
602. Benharroch D, Meguerian-Bedoyan Z, Lamant L, et al. ALK-positive lymphoma: a single disease with a broad spectrum of morphology. Blood. 1998 Mar 15;91(6):2076–84. PMID:9490693
603. Benito V, Segura J, Martínez MS, et al. Fibrolamellar hepatocellular carcinoma metastatic to the ovary. J Obstet Gynaecol. 2012 Feb;32(2):200–2. PMID:22296446
604. Bennett JA, Bayerl MG. Epstein-barr virus-associated extranodal marginal zone lymphoma of mucosa-associated lymphoid tissue (MALT Lymphoma) arising in the parotid gland of a child with ataxia telangiectasia. J Pediatr Hematol Oncol. 2015 Mar;37(2):e114–7. PMID:25692616
605. Bennett JA, Braga AC, Pinto A, et al. Uterine PEComas: a morphologic, immunohistochemical, and molecular analysis of 32 tumors. Am J Surg Pathol. 2018 Oct;42(10):1370–83. PMID:30001237
606. Bennett JA, Oliva E, Young RH. Sclerosing stromal tumors with prominent luteinization during pregnancy: a report of 8 cases emphasizing diagnostic problems. Int J Gynecol Pathol. 2015 Jul;34(4):357–62. PMID:25851706
607. Bennett JL, Galetta SL, Frohman LP, et al. Neuro-ophthalmologic manifestations of a paraneoplastic syndrome and testicular carcinoma. Neurology. 1999 Mar 10;52(4):864–7. PMID:10078744
608. Bennett JM, Catovsky D, Daniel MT, et al. Proposals for the classification of the acute leukaemias. French-American-British (FAB) co-operative group. Br J Haematol. 1976 Aug;33(4):451–8. PMID:188440
609. Bennett JM, Catovsky D, Daniel MT, et al. The morphological classification of acute lymphoblastic leukaemia: concordance among observers and clinical correlations. Br J Haematol. 1981 Apr;47(4):553–61. PMID:6938236
610. Bennett JT, Tan TY, Alcantara D, et al. Mosaic activating mutations in FGFR1 cause encephalocraniocutaneous lipomatosis. Am J Hum Genet. 2016 Mar 3;98(3):579–87. PMID:26942290
611. Bennett MH, MacLennan KA, Easterling MJ, et al. The prognostic significance of cellular subtypes in nodular sclerosing Hodgkin's disease: an analysis of 271 non-laparotomised cases (BNLI report no. 22). Clin Radiol. 1983 Sep;34(5):497–501. PMID:6617080
612. Benson VS, Kirichek O, Beral V, et al. Menopausal hormone therapy and central nervous system tumor risk: large UK prospective study and meta-analysis. Int J Cancer. 2015 May 15;136(10):2369–77. PMID:25335165
613. Bentz M, Barth TF, Brüderlein S, et al. Gain of chromosome arm 9p is characteristic of primary mediastinal B-cell lymphoma (MBL): comprehensive molecular cytogenetic analysis and presentation of a novel MBL cell line. Genes Chromosomes Cancer. 2001 Apr;30(4):393–401. PMID:11241792
614. Berbegall AP, Villamón E, Piqueras M, et al. Comparative genetic study of intratumoral heterogenous MYCN amplified neuroblastoma versus aggressive genetic profile neuroblastic tumors. Oncogene. 2016 Mar 17;35(11):1423–32. PMID:26119945
615. Berdjis CC, Mostofi FK. Carcinoid tumors of the testis. J Urol. 1977 Nov;118(5):777–82. PMID:916100
616. Berends AMA, Buitenwerf E, de Krijger RR, et al. Incidence of pheochromocytoma and sympathetic paraganglioma in the Netherlands: a nationwide study and systematic review. Eur J Intern Med. 2018 May;51:68–73. PMID:29361475
617. Berenguer B, Mulliken JB, Enjolras O, et al. Rapidly involuting congenital hemangioma: clinical and histopathologic features. Pediatr Dev Pathol. 2003 Nov-Dec;6(6):495–510. PMID:15018449
618. Berg JC, Scheithauer BW, Spinner RJ, et al. Plexiform schwannoma: a clinicopathologic overview with emphasis on the head and neck region. Hum Pathol. 2008 May;39(5):633–40. PMID:18439936
619. Bergen AA, Plomp AS, Schuurman EJ, et al. Mutations in ABCC6 cause pseudoxanthoma elasticum. Nat Genet. 2000 Jun;25(2):228–31. PMID:10835643
620. Bergh P, Meis-Kindblom JM, Gherlinzoni F, et al. Synovial sarcoma: identification of low and high risk groups. Cancer. 1999 Jun 15;85(12):2596–607. PMID:10375108
621. Bergman R, Dromi R, Trau H, et al. The pattern of HMB-45 antibody staining in compound Spitz nevi. Am J Dermatopathol. 1995 Dec;17(6):542–6. PMID:8599465
622. Bergman R, Malkin L, Sabo E, et al. MIB-1 monoclonal antibody to determine proliferative activity of Ki-67 antigen as an adjunct to the histopathologic differential diagnosis of Spitz nevi. J Am Acad Dermatol. 2001 Mar;44(3):500–4. PMID:11209122
623. Bergmann F, Aulmann S, Sipos B, et al. Acinar cell carcinomas of the pancreas: a molecular analysis in a series of 57 cases. Virchows Arch. 2014 Dec;465(6):661–72. PMID:25298229
624. Berk DR, Lind AC, Tapia B, et al. Atypical fibroxanthoma in a child without xeroderma pigmentosum. Pediatr Dermatol. 2007 Jul-Aug;24(4):450–2. PMID:17845192
625. Berklite L, John I, Ranganathan S, et al. SOX9 Immunohistochemistry in the distinction of angiomatoid fibrous histiocytoma from histologic mimics: diagnostic utility and pitfalls. Appl Immunohistochem Mol Morphol. 2020 Sep;28(8):635–40. PMID:31567275
626. Berklite L, Ozolek J, Wang L, et al. Pediatric benign tumors with a skeletal muscle component: myogenin expression, diagnostic pitfalls, and new molecular insights. Pediatr Dev Pathol. 2021 May-Jun;24(3):213–26. PMID:33683985
627. Berklite L, Ranganathan S, John I, et al. Fibrous histiocytoma/dermatofibroma in children: the same as adults? Hum Pathol. 2020 May;99:107–15. PMID:32246988
628. Berklite L, Witchel SF, Yatsenko SA, et al. Early bilateral gonadoblastoma associated with 45,X/46,XY mosaicism: the spectrum of undifferentiated gonadal tissue and gonadoblastoma in the first months of life. Pediatr Dev Pathol. 2019 Jul-Aug;22(4):380–5. PMID:30646821
629. Berman JN, Greer WL, Archambeault S, et al. JAK2 V617F positive polycythemia Vera in a child with neurofibromatosis type I. Pediatr Blood Cancer. 2008 Nov;51(5):689–91. PMID:18623221
630. Bernard MA, Hall CE, Hogue DA, et al. Diminished levels of the putative tumor suppressor proteins EXT1 and EXT2 in exostosis chondrocytes. Cell Motil Cytoskeleton. 2001 Feb;48(2):149–62. PMID:11169766
631. Bernard O, Franchi-Abella S, Branchereau S, et al. Congenital portosystemic shunts in children: recognition, evaluation, and management. Semin Liver Dis. 2012 Nov;32(4):273–87. PMID:23397528
632. Bernard SA, Murphey MD, Flemming DJ, et al. Improved differentiation of benign osteochondromas from secondary chondrosarcomas with standardized measurement of cartilage cap at CT and MR imaging. Radiology. 2010 Jun;255(3):857–65. PMID:20392983
633. Berney DM, Lee A, Shamash J, et al. The frequency and distribution of intratubular trophoblast in association with germ cell tumors of the testis. Am J Surg Pathol. 2005 Oct;29(10):1300–3. PMID:16160471
634. Berney DM, Shamash J, Pieroni K, et al. Loss of CD30 expression in metastatic embryonal carcinoma: the effects of chemotherapy? Histopathology. 2001 Oct;39(4):382–5. PMID:11683938
635. Berney DM, Warren AY, Verma M, et al. Malignant germ cell tumours in the elderly: a histopathological review of 50 cases in men aged 60 years or over. Mod Pathol. 2008 Jan;21(1):54–9. PMID:17975539
636. Berns S, Pearl G. Review of pineal anlage tumor with divergent histology. Arch Pathol Lab Med. 2006 Aug;130(8):1233–5. PMID:16879032
637. Bernstein E, Caudy AA, Hammond SM, et al. Role for a bidentate ribonuclease in the initiation step of RNA interference. Nature. 2001 Jan 18;409(6818):363–6. PMID:11201747
638. Bernstein J. Renal cystic disease in the tuberous sclerosis complex. Pediatr Nephrol. 1993 Aug;7(4):490–5. PMID:8398665
639. Bernstein KE, Lattes R. Nodular (pseudosarcomatous) fasciitis, a nonrecurrent lesion: clinicopathologic study of 134 cases. Cancer. 1982 Apr 15;49(8):1668–78. PMID:6279273
640. Bernstein ML, Buchino JJ. The histologic similarity between craniopharyngioma and odontogenic lesions: a reappraisal. Oral Surg Oral Med Oral Pathol. 1983 Nov;56(5):502–11. PMID:6196702
641. Bernthal NM, Putnam A, Jones KB, et al. The effect of surgical margins on outcomes for low grade MPNSTs and atypical neurofibroma. J Surg Oncol. 2014 Dec;110(7):813–6. PMID:25111615
642. Berres ML, Lim KP, Peters T, et al. BRAF-V600E expression in precursor versus differentiated dendritic cells defines clinically distinct LCH risk groups. J Exp Med. 2014 Apr 7;211(4):669–83. PMID:24638167
643. Berry M, Mankin H, Gebhardt M, et al. Osteoblastoma: a 30-year study of 99 cases. J Surg Oncol. 2008 Sep 1;98(3):179–83. PMID:18561158
644. Berry T, Luther W, Bhatnagar N, et al. The ALK(F1174L) mutation potentiates the

oncogenic activity of MYCN in neuroblastoma. Cancer Cell. 2012 Jul 10;22(1):117–30. PMID:22789543
**645.** Bertario L, Russo A, Sala P, et al. Genotype and phenotype factors as determinants of desmoid tumors in patients with familial adenomatous polyposis. Int J Cancer. 2001 Mar 20;95(2):102–7. PMID:11241320
**646.** Berte N, Filfilan A, Mainard L, et al. Co-existing infantile hepatic hemangioma and mesenchymal hamartoma in a neonate. J Surg Case Rep. 2018 Jan 23;2018(1):rjx260. PMID:29383241
**647.** Berthelsen JG, Skakkebaek NE, von der Maase H, et al. Screening for carcinoma in situ of the contralateral testis in patients with germinal testicular cancer. Br Med J (Clin Res Ed). 1982 Dec 11;285(6356):1683–6. PMID:6129027
**648.** Bertherat J, Horvath A, Groussin L, et al. Mutations in regulatory subunit type 1A of cyclic adenosine 5'-monophosphate-dependent protein kinase (PRKAR1A): phenotype analysis in 353 patients and 80 different genotypes. J Clin Endocrinol Metab. 2009 Jun;94(6):2085–91. PMID:19293268
**649.** Bertoni F, Bacchini P, Capanna R, et al. Solid variant of aneurysmal bone cyst. Cancer. 1993 Feb 1;71(3):729–34. PMID:8431852
**650.** Bertoni F, Bacchini P, Donati D, et al. Osteoblastoma-like osteosarcoma. The Rizzoli Institute experience. Mod Pathol. 1993 Nov;6(6):707–16. PMID:8302813
**651.** Bertoni F, Bacchini P, Fabbri N, et al. Osteosarcoma. Low-grade intraosseous-type osteosarcoma, histologically resembling parosteal osteosarcoma, fibrous dysplasia, and desmoplastic fibroma. Cancer. 1993 Jan 15;71(2):338–45. PMID:8422626
**652.** Bertoni F, Bacchini P, Staals EL. Giant cell-rich osteosarcoma. Orthopedics. 2003 Feb;26(2):179–81. PMID:12597223
**653.** Bertoni F, Bacchini P, Staals EL. Malignancy in giant cell tumor of bone. Cancer. 2003 May 15;97(10):2520–9. PMID:12733152
**654.** Bertoni F, Bacchini P, Staals EL, et al. Dedifferentiated parosteal osteosarcoma: the experience of the Rizzoli Institute. Cancer. 2005 Jun 1;103(11):2373–82. PMID:15852358
**655.** Bertoni F, Boriani S, Laus M, et al. Periosteal chondrosarcoma and periosteal osteosarcoma. Two distinct entities. J Bone Joint Surg Br. 1982;64(3):370–6. PMID:7096408
**656.** Bertoni F, Present D, Bacchini P, et al. The Istituto Rizzoli experience with small cell osteosarcoma. Cancer. 1989 Dec 15;64(12):2591–9. PMID:2684389
**657.** Bertoni F, Present D, Sudanese A, et al. Giant-cell tumor of bone with pulmonary metastases. Six case reports and a review of the literature. Clin Orthop Relat Res. 1988 Dec;(237):275–85. PMID:3056645
**658.** Bertoni F, Unni KK, Beabout JW, et al. Chondroblastoma of the skull and facial bones. Am J Clin Pathol. 1987 Jul;88(1):1–9. PMID:3604981
**659.** Bertrand A, Rondenet C, Masliah-Planchon J, et al. Rhabdoid component emerging as a subclonal evolution of paediatric glioneuronal tumours. Neuropathol Appl Neurobiol. 2018 Feb;44(2):224–8. PMID:28054381
**660.** Beschorner R, Pantazis G, Jeibmann A, et al. Expression of EAAT-1 distinguishes choroid plexus tumors from normal and reactive choroid plexus epithelium. Acta Neuropathol. 2009 Jun;117(6):667–75. PMID:19283393
**661.** Bessière L, Todeschini AL, Auguste A, et al. A Hot-spot of in-frame duplications activates the oncoprotein AKT1 in juvenile granulosa cell tumors. EBioMedicine. 2015 Mar 6;2(5):421–31. PMID:26137586
**662.** Bessler W, Grauer W, Allemann J. Case report 726. Enchondromatosis of the left femur and hemipelvis (Ollier's disease). Skeletal Radiol. 1992;21(3):201–4. PMID:1604350
**663.** Bettegowda C, Adogwa O, Mehta V, et al. Treatment of choroid plexus tumors: a 20-year single institutional experience. J Neurosurg Pediatr. 2012 Nov;10(5):398–405. PMID:22938081
**664.** Bettegowda C, Agrawal N, Jiao Y, et al. Exomic sequencing of four rare central nervous system tumor types. Oncotarget. 2013 Apr;4(4):572–83. PMID:23592488
**665.** Betz BL, Strobeck MW, Reisman DN, et al. Re-expression of hSNF5/INI1/BAF47 in pediatric tumor cells leads to G1 arrest associated with induction of p16ink4a and activation of RB. Oncogene. 2002 Aug 8;21(34):5193–203. PMID:12149641
**666.** Betz SA, Foucar K, Head DR, et al. False-positive flow cytometric platelet glycoprotein IIb/IIIa expression in myeloid leukemias secondary to platelet adherence to blasts. Blood. 1992 May 1;79(9):2399–403. PMID:1349244
**667.** Betz SJ. HPV-related papillary lesions of the oral mucosa: a review. Head Neck Pathol. 2019 Mar;13(1):80–90. PMID:30693456
**668.** Beyer J. Prognostic factors in metastatic germ-cell cancer. Andrology. 2019 Jul;7(4):475–8. PMID:30969027
**669.** Bhadri VA, Stormon MO, Arbuckle S, et al. Hepatocellular carcinoma in children with Alagille syndrome. J Pediatr Gastroenterol Nutr. 2005 Nov;41(5):676–8. PMID:16254531
**670.** Bhamra JS, Al-Khateeb H, Dhinsa BS, et al. Chondromyxoid fibroma management: a single institution experience of 22 cases. World J Surg Oncol. 2014 Sep 12;12:283. PMID:25217119
**671.** Bhat RA, Lim YK, Chia YN, et al. Sertoli-Leydig cell tumor of the ovary: analysis of a single institution database. J Obstet Gynaecol Res. 2013 Jan;39(1):305–10. PMID:22691037
**672.** Bhatnagar R, Vine AK. Diffuse infiltrating retinoblastoma. Ophthalmology. 1991 Nov;98(11):1657–61. PMID:1800925
**673.** Bhatt MD, Al-Karmi S, Druker H, et al. Second rhabdoid tumor 8 years after treatment of atypical teratoid/rhabdoid tumor in a child with germline SMARCB1 mutation. Pediatr Blood Cancer. 2019 Mar;66(3):e27546. PMID:30393974
**674.** Bi WL, Greenwald NF, Ramkissoon SH, et al. Clinical identification of oncogenic drivers and copy-number alterations in pituitary tumors. Endocrinology. 2017 Jul 1;158(7):2284–91. PMID:28486603
**675.** Bi WL, Larsen AG, Dunn IF. Genomic alterations in sporadic pituitary tumors. Curr Neurol Neurosci Rep. 2018 Feb 2;18(1):4. PMID:29396598
**676.** Bianchi F, Tamburrini G, Massimi L, et al. Supratentorial tumors typical of the infantile age: desmoplastic infantile ganglioglioma (DIG) and astrocytoma (DIA). A review. Childs Nerv Syst. 2016 Oct;32(10):1833–8. PMID:27659826
**677.** Biegel JA. Molecular genetics of atypical teratoid/rhabdoid tumor. Neurosurg Focus. 2006 Jan 15;20(1):E11. PMID:16459991
**678.** Biegel JA, Busse TM, Weissman BE. SWI/SNF chromatin remodeling complexes and cancer. Am J Med Genet C Semin Med Genet. 2014 Sep;166C(3):350–66. PMID:25169151
**679.** Biegel JA, Conard K, Brooks JJ. Translocation (11;22)(p13;q12): primary change in intra-abdominal desmoplastic small round cell tumor. Genes Chromosomes Cancer. 1993 Jun;7(2):119–21. PMID:7687454
**680.** Biegel JA, Zhou JY, Rorke LB, et al. Germline and acquired mutations of INI1 in atypical teratoid and rhabdoid tumors. Cancer Res. 1999 Jan 1;59(1):74–9. PMID:9892189
**681.** Bielack SS, Kempf-Bielack B, Delling G, et al. Prognostic factors in high-grade osteosarcoma of the extremities or trunk: an analysis of 1,702 patients treated on neoadjuvant cooperative osteosarcoma study group protocols. J Clin Oncol. 2002 Feb 1;20(3):776–90. PMID:11821461
**682.** Bielack SS, Kempf-Bielack B, Heise U, et al. Combined modality treatment for osteosarcoma occurring as a second malignant disease. J Clin Oncol. 1999 Apr;17(4):1164. PMID:10561175
**683.** Bielle F, Di Stefano AL, Meyronet D, et al. Diffuse gliomas with FGFR3-TACC3 fusion have characteristic histopathological and molecular features. Brain Pathol. 2018 Sep;28(5):674–83. PMID:28976058
**684.** Bielle F, Fréneaux P, Jeanne-Pasquier C, et al. PHOX2B immunolabeling: a novel tool for the diagnosis of undifferentiated neuroblastomas among childhood small round blue-cell tumors. Am J Surg Pathol. 2012 Aug;36(8):1141–9. PMID:22790854
**685.** Bielle F, Villa C, Giry M, et al. Chordoid gliomas of the third ventricle share TTF-1 expression with organum vasculosum of the lamina terminalis. Am J Surg Pathol. 2015 Jul;39(7):948–56. PMID:25786084
**686.** Bien E, Godzinski J, Dall'igna P, et al. Pancreatoblastoma: a report from the European cooperative study group for paediatric rare tumours (EXPeRT). Eur J Cancer. 2011 Oct;47(15):2347–52. PMID:21696948
**687.** Bien E, Kazanowska B, Dantonello T, et al. Factors predicting survival in childhood malignant and intermediate vascular tumors : retrospective analysis of the Polish and German cooperative paediatric soft tissue sarcoma study groups and review of the literature. Ann Surg Oncol. 2010 Jul;17(7):1878–89. PMID:20333551
**688.** Bienemann K, Borkhardt A, Klapper W, et al. High incidence of Epstein-Barr virus (EBV)-positive Hodgkin lymphoma and Hodgkin lymphoma-like B-cell lymphoproliferations with EBV latency profile 2 in children with interleukin-2-inducible T-cell kinase deficiency. Histopathology. 2015 Nov;67(5):607–16. PMID:25728094
**689.** Bienemann K, Burkhardt B, Modlich S, et al. Promising therapy results for lymphoid malignancies in children with chromosomal breakage syndromes (Ataxia teleangiectasia or Nijmegen-breakage syndrome): a retrospective survey. Br J Haematol. 2011 Nov;155(4):468–76. PMID:21923652
**690.** Biermann K, Stoop H, Looijenga L. c-KIT protein expression does not discriminate neoplastic from non-neoplastic intratubular germ cells. Histopathology. 2012 May;60(6):1017–9. PMID:22340755
**691.** Biggar RJ, Frisch M, Goedert JJ; . Risk of cancer in children with AIDS. JAMA. 2000 Jul 12;284(2):205–9. PMID:10889594
**692.** Bilal H, Handra-Luca A, Bertrand JC, et al. P63 is expressed in basal and myoepithelial cells of human normal and tumor salivary gland tissues. J Histochem Cytochem. 2003 Feb;51(2):133–9. PMID:12533521
**693.** Bildirici K, Yalçin OT, Ozalp SS, et al. Sclerosing stromal tumor of the ovary associated with Meigs' syndrome: a case report. Eur J Gynaecol Oncol. 2004;25(4):528–9. PMID:15285324
**694.** Billeret Lebranchu V. [Granular cell tumor. Epidemiology of 263 cases]. Arch Anat Cytol Pathol. 1999;47(1):26–30. French. PMID:10089680
**695.** Billings SD, Folpe AL, Weiss SW. Epithelioid sarcoma-like hemangioendothelioma. Am J Surg Pathol. 2003 Jan;27(1):48–57. PMID:12502927
**696.** Billings SD, Giblen G, Fanburg-Smith JC. Superficial low-grade fibromyxoid sarcoma (Evans tumor): a clinicopathologic analysis of 19 cases with a unique observation in the pediatric population. Am J Surg Pathol. 2005 Feb;29(2):204–10. PMID:15644777
**697.** Bilodeau EA, Collins BM. Odontogenic cysts and neoplasms. Surg Pathol Clin. 2017 Mar;10(1):177–222. PMID:28153133
**698.** Binderup ML, Bisgaard ML, Harbud V, et al. Von Hippel-Lindau disease (vHL). National clinical guideline for diagnosis and surveillance in Denmark. 3rd edition. Dan Med J. 2013 Dec;60(12):B4763. PMID:24355456
**699.** Binh MB, Sastre-Garau X, Guillou L, et al. MDM2 and CDK4 immunostainings are useful adjuncts in diagnosing well-differentiated and dedifferentiated liposarcoma subtypes: a comparative analysis of 559 soft tissue neoplasms with genetic data. Am J Surg Pathol. 2005 Oct;29(10):1340–7. PMID:16160477
**700.** Binokay F, Balal M, Demir E, et al. Risk of developing fibroadenoma with the use of cyclosporine A in renal transplant recipients. Ren Fail. 2005;27(6):721–5. PMID:16350824
**701.** Birkeland AC, Foltin SK, Michmerhuizen NL, et al. Correlation of Crtc1/3-Maml2 fusion status, grade and survival in mucoepidermoid carcinoma. Oral Oncol. 2017 May;68:5–8. PMID:28438292
**702.** Bisbinas I, De Silva U, Grimer RJ. Pigmented villonodular synovitis of the foot and ankle: a 12-year experience from a tertiary orthopedic Oncology Unit. J Foot Ankle Surg. 2004 Nov-Dec;43(6):407–11. PMID:15605054
**703.** Bisceglia M, D'Angelo VA, Guglielmi G, et al. Dedifferentiated chordoma of the thoracic spine with rhabdomyosarcomatous differentiation. Report of a case and review of the literature. Ann Diagn Pathol. 2007 Aug;11(4):262–73. PMID:17630110
**704.** Bisceglia M, Muscarella LA, Galliani CA, et al. Extraneuraxial hemangioblastoma: clinicopathologic features and review of the literature. Adv Anat Pathol. 2018 May;25(3):197–215. PMID:29189208
**705.** Bishop JA, Alaggio R, Zhang L, et al. Adamantinoma-like Ewing family tumors of the head and neck: a pitfall in the differential diagnosis of basaloid and myoepithelial carcinomas. Am J Surg Pathol. 2015 Sep;39(9):1267–74. PMID:26034869
**705A.** Bishop JA, Cowan ML, Shum CH, et al. MAML2 rearrangements in variant forms of mucoepidermoid carcinoma: ancillary diagnostic testing for the ciliated and Warthin-like variants. Am J Surg Pathol. 2018 Jan;42(1):130–6. PMID:28877061
**706.** Bishop JA, French CA, Ali SZ. Cytopathologic features of NUT midline carcinoma: a series of 26 specimens from 13 patients. Cancer Cytopathol. 2016 Dec;124(12):901–8. PMID:27400194
**707.** Bishop JA, Gagan J, Baumhoer D, et al. Sclerosing polycystic "adenosis" of salivary glands: a neoplasm characterized by PI3K pathway alterations more correctly named sclerosing polycystic adenoma. Head Neck Pathol. 2020 Sep;14(3):630–6. PMID:31605313
**708.** Biskup W, Calaminus G, Schneider DT, et al. Teratoma with malignant transformation: experiences of the cooperative GPOH protocols MAKEI 83/86/89/96. Klin Padiatr. 2006 Nov-Dec;218(6):303–8. PMID:17080331
**709.** Bisogno G, Tagarelli A, Schiavetti A, et al. Myoepithelial carcinoma treatment in children: a report from the TREP project. Pediatr Blood Cancer. 2014 Apr;61(4):643–6. PMID:24136896
**710.** Biswas J, Bhushan B, Jayakumar N, et al. Teratoid malignant medulloepithelioma of the optic nerve: report of a case and review

of the literature. Orbit. 1999 Sep;18(3):191–6. PMID:12045984
**711.** Bitar M, Danish SF, Rosenblum MK. A newly diagnosed case of polymorphous low-grade neuroepithelial tumor of the young. Clin Neuropathol. 2018 Jul-Aug;37(4):178–81. PMID:29701169
**712.** Bittar RF, Ferraro HP, Moraes Gonçalves FT, et al. Neoplasms of the salivary glands: analysis of 727 histopathological reports in a single institution. Otolaryngol Pol. 2015;69(4):28–33. PMID:26388357
**713.** Bixby SD, Hettmer S, Taylor GA, et al. Synovial sarcoma in children: imaging features and common benign mimics. AJR Am J Roentgenol. 2010 Oct;195(4):1026–32. PMID:20858835
**714.** Bizzarro T, Martini M, Marrocco C, et al. The role of CD56 in thyroid fine needle aspiration cytology: a pilot study performed on liquid based cytology. PLoS One. 2015 Jul 17;10(7):e0132939. PMID:26186733
**715.** Bizzozero OJ Jr, Johnson KG, Ciocco A. Radiation-related leukemia in Hiroshima and Nagasaki, 1946-1964. I. Distribution, incidence and appearance time. N Engl J Med. 1966 May 19;274(20):1095–101. PMID:5932020
**716.** Bjerke L, Mackay A, Nandhabalan M, et al. Histone H3.3. mutations drive pediatric glioblastoma through upregulation of MYCN. Cancer Discov. 2013 May;3(5):512–9. PMID:23539269
**717.** Bjornard KL, Leventaki V, Nichols KE, et al. Two-year-old female with EBV-positive diffuse large B-cell lymphoma and subsequent CNS involvement with neurolymphomatosis. Pediatr Blood Cancer. 2018 Dec;65(12):e27415. PMID:30151967
**718.** Björnsson J, McLeod RA, Unni KK, et al. Primary chondrosarcoma of long bones and limb girdles. Cancer. 1998 Nov 15;83(10):2105–19. PMID:9827715
**719.** Bjornsson J, Scheithauer BW, Okazaki H, et al. Intracranial germ cell tumors: pathobiological and immunohistochemical aspects of 70 cases. J Neuropathol Exp Neurol. 1985 Jan;44(1):32–46. PMID:4038412
**720.** Blachar A, Federle MP, Ferris JV, et al. Radiologists' performance in the diagnosis of liver tumors with central scars by using specific CT criteria. Radiology. 2002 May;223(2):532–9. PMID:11997564
**721.** Black J, Coffin CM, Dehner LP. Fibrohistiocytic tumors and related neoplasms in children and adolescents. Pediatr Dev Pathol. 2012;15(1 Suppl):181–210. PMID:22420728
**722.** Blackburn PR, Davila JI, Jackson RA, et al. RNA sequencing identifies a novel USP9X-USP6 promoter swap gene fusion in a primary aneurysmal bone cyst. Genes Chromosomes Cancer. 2019 Aug;58(8):589–94. PMID:30767316
**723.** Blackburn PR, Milosevic D, Marek T, et al. PIK3CA mutations in lipomatosis of nerve with or without nerve territory overgrowth. Mod Pathol. 2020 Mar;33(3):420–30. PMID:31481664
**724.** Blakeley JO, Bakker A, Barker A, et al. The path forward: 2015 International Children's Tumor Foundation conference on neurofibromatosis type 1, type 2, and schwannomatosis. Am J Med Genet A. 2017 Jun;173(6):1714–21. PMID:28436162
**725.** Blakeley JO, Plotkin SR. Therapeutic advances for the tumors associated with neurofibromatosis type 1, type 2, and schwannomatosis. Neuro Oncol. 2016 May;18(5):624–38. PMID:26851632
**726.** Blaser SI, Harwood-Nash DC. Neuroradiology of pediatric posterior fossa medulloblastoma. J Neurooncol. 1996 Jul;29(1):23–34. PMID:8817413
**727.** Blatt K, Cerny-Reiterer S, Schwaab J, et al. Identification of the Ki-1 antigen (CD30) as a novel therapeutic target in systemic mastocytosis. Blood. 2015 Dec 24;126(26):2832–41. PMID:26486787
**728.** Blauvelt A. The role of human herpesvirus 8 in the pathogenesis of Kaposi's sarcoma. Adv Dermatol. 1999;14:167–206. PMID:10643499
**729.** Bleakley M, Lau L, Shaw PJ, et al. Bone marrow transplantation for paediatric AML in first remission: a systematic review and meta-analysis. Bone Marrow Transplant. 2002 May;29(10):843–52. PMID:12058234
**729A.** Bleeker JS, Quevedo JF, Folpe AL. "Malignant" perivascular epithelioid cell neoplasm: risk stratification and treatment strategies. Sarcoma. 2012;2012:541626. PMID:22619565
**730.** Bleiweiss IJ, Klein MJ. Chondromyxoid fibroma: report of six cases with immunohistochemical studies. Mod Pathol. 1990 Nov;3(6):664–6. PMID:2263591
**731.** Blemker AL, Parker CM, Tejada E. Petechial rash in toxic-appearing young man. Rocky Mountain spotted fever (RMSF). Arch Dermatol. 1991 Jul;127(7):1049, 1052–3. PMID:2064408
**732.** Blessing MM, Blackburn PR, Balcom JR, et al. Novel BRAF alteration in desmoplastic infantile ganglioglioma with response to targeted therapy. Acta Neuropathol Commun. 2018 Nov 5;6(1):118. PMID:30396366
**733.** Blessing MM, Blackburn PR, Krishnan C, et al. Desmoplastic infantile ganglioglioma: a MAPK pathway-driven and microglia/macrophage-rich neuroepithelial tumor. J Neuropathol Exp Neurol. 2019 Nov 1;78(11):1011–21. PMID:31562743
**734.** Bloem JL, Mulder JD. Chondroblastoma: a clinical and radiological study of 104 cases. Skeletal Radiol. 1985;14(1):1–9. PMID:4023729
**735.** Blohm ME, Vesterling-Hörner D, Calaminus G, et al. Alpha 1-fetoprotein (AFP) reference values in infants up to 2 years of age. Pediatr Hematol Oncol. 1998 Mar-Apr;15(2):135–42. PMID:9592840
**736.** Blount A, Riley KO, Woodworth BA. Juvenile nasopharyngeal angiofibroma. Otolaryngol Clin North Am. 2011 Aug;44(4):989–1004, ix. PMID:21819885
**737.** Bluebond-Langner R, Pinto PA, Argani P, et al. Adult presentation of metanephric stromal tumor. J Urol. 2002 Oct;168(4 Pt 1):1482–3. PMID:12352423
**738.** Blümcke I, Aronica E, Becker A, et al. Low-grade epilepsy-associated neuroepithelial tumours - the 2016 WHO classification. Nat Rev Neurol. 2016 Dec;12(12):732–40. PMID:27857123
**739.** Blumcke I, Aronica E, Urbach H, et al. A neuropathology-based approach to epilepsy surgery in brain tumors and proposal for a new terminology use for long-term epilepsy-associated brain tumors. Acta Neuropathol. 2014 Jul;128(1):39–54. PMID:24858213
**740.** Blümcke I, Coras R, Wefers AK, et al. Review: Challenges in the histopathological classification of ganglioglioma and DNT: microscopic agreement studies and a preliminary genotype-phenotype analysis. Neuropathol Appl Neurobiol. 2019 Feb;45(2):95–107. PMID:30326153
**741.** Blümcke I, Giencke K, Wardelmann E, et al. The CD34 epitope is expressed in neoplastic and malformative lesions associated with chronic, focal epilepsies. Acta Neuropathol. 1999 May;97(5):481–90. PMID:10334485
**742.** Blümcke I, Löbach M, Wolf HK, et al. Evidence for developmental precursor lesions in epilepsy-associated glioneuronal tumors. Microsc Res Tech. 1999 Jul 1;46(1):53–8. PMID:10402272
**743.** Blümcke I, Luyken C, Urbach H, et al. An isomorphic subtype of long-term epilepsy-associated astrocytomas associated with benign prognosis. Acta Neuropathol. 2004 May;107(5):381–8. PMID:15034726
**744.** Blümcke I, Müller S, Buslei R, et al. Microtubule-associated protein-2 immunoreactivity: a useful tool in the differential diagnosis of low-grade neuroepithelial tumors. Acta Neuropathol. 2004 Aug;108(2):89–96. PMID:15146346
**745.** Blumcke I, Spreafico R, Haaker G, et al. Histopathological findings in brain tissue obtained during epilepsy surgery. N Engl J Med. 2017 Oct 26;377(17):1648–56. PMID:29069555
**746.** Blümcke I, Thom M, Aronica E, et al. The clinicopathologic spectrum of focal cortical dysplasias: a consensus classification proposed by an ad hoc Task Force of the ILAE Diagnostic Methods Commission. Epilepsia. 2011 Jan;52(1):158–74. PMID:21219302
**747.** Blümcke I, Wiestler OD. Gangliogliomas: an intriguing tumor entity associated with focal epilepsies. J Neuropathol Exp Neurol. 2002 Jul;61(7):575–84. PMID:12125736
**748.** Blunt W. The compleat naturalist: a life of Linnaeus. London (UK): Frances Lincoln; 2001.
**749.** Bluteau O, Sebert M, Leblanc T, et al. A landscape of germ line mutations in a cohort of inherited bone marrow failure patients. Blood. 2018 Feb 15;131(7):717–32. PMID:29146883
**750.** Boccara O, Blanche S, de Prost Y, et al. Cutaneous hematologic disorders in children. Pediatr Blood Cancer. 2012 Feb;58(2):226–32. PMID:21445946
**751.** Boccato P, Altavilla G, Blandamura S. Fine needle aspiration biopsy of salivary gland lesions. A reappraisal of pitfalls and problems. Acta Cytol. 1998 Jul-Aug;42(4):888–98. PMID:9684573
**752.** Bocchialini G, Salvagni L, Guerini A, et al. Central giant cell granuloma of the mandibular condyle: a rare case and a literature review. Heliyon. 2019 Dec 28;6(1):e03085. PMID:31909260
**753.** Bode PK, Barghorn A, Fritzsche FR, et al. MAGEC2 is a sensitive and novel marker for seminoma: a tissue microarray analysis of 325 testicular germ cell tumors. Mod Pathol. 2011 Jun;24(6):829–35. PMID:21780320
**754.** Bode-Lesniewska B, Fritz C, Exner GU, et al. EWSR1-NFATC2 and FUS-NFATC2 gene fusion-associated mesenchymal tumors: clinicopathologic correlation and literature review. Sarcoma. 2019 Mar 26;2019:9386390. PMID:31049020
**755.** Bodemer C, Hermine O, Palmérini F, et al. Pediatric mastocytosis is a clonal disease associated with D816V and other activating c-KIT mutations. J Invest Dermatol. 2010 Mar;130(3):804–15. PMID:19865100
**756.** Bodi I, Curran O, Selway R, et al. Two cases of multinodular and vacuolating neuronal tumour. Acta Neuropathol Commun. 2014 Jan 20;2:7. PMID:24444358
**757.** Bodo S, Colas C, Buhard O, et al. Diagnosis of constitutional mismatch repair-deficiency syndrome based on microsatellite instability and lymphocyte tolerance to methylating agents. Gastroenterology. 2015 Oct;149(4):1017–29. e3. PMID:26116798
**758.** Boecker W, Stenman G, Loening T, et al. Squamous/epidermoid differentiation in normal breast and salivary gland tissues and their corresponding tumors originate from p63/K5/14-positive progenitor cells. Virchows Arch. 2015 Jan;466(1):21–36. PMID:25344874
**759.** Boedeker CC, Hensen EF, Neumann HP, et al. Genetics of hereditary head and neck paragangliomas. Head Neck. 2014 Jun;36(6):907–16. PMID:23913591
**760.** Boehm D, Bacher J, Neumann HP. Gross genomic rearrangement involving the TSC2-PKD1 contiguous deletion syndrome: characterization of the deletion event by quantitative polymerase chain reaction deletion assay. Am J Kidney Dis. 2007 Jan;49(1):e11–21. PMID:17185137
**761.** Boekhoff S, Bison B, Eveslage M, et al. Craniopharyngiomas presenting as incidentalomas: results of Kraniopharyngeom 2007. Pituitary. 2019 Oct;22(5):532–41. PMID:31440945
**762.** Boer JM, Valsecchi MG, Hormann FM, et al. Favorable outcome of NUTM1-rearranged infant and pediatric B cell precursor acute lymphoblastic leukemia in a collaborative international study. Leukemia. 2021 Oct;35(10):2978–82. PMID:34211097
**763.** Boghani Z, Husain Q, Kanumuri VV, et al. Juvenile nasopharyngeal angiofibroma: a systematic review and comparison of endoscopic, endoscopic-assisted, and open resection in 1047 cases. Laryngoscope. 2013 Apr;123(4):859–69. PMID:23483486
**764.** Bogusz A, Boekhoff S, Warmuth-Metz M, et al. Posterior hypothalamus-sparing surgery improves outcome after childhood craniopharyngioma. Endocr Connect. 2019 May 1;8(5):481–92. PMID:30925462
**765.** Boikos SA, Pappo AS, Killian JK, et al. Molecular subtypes of KIT/PDGFRA wild-type gastrointestinal stromal tumors: a report from the National Institutes of Health Gastrointestinal Stromal Tumor Clinic. JAMA Oncol. 2016 Jul 1;2(7):922–8. PMID:27011036
**766.** Boisseau W, Euskirchen P, Mokhtari K, et al. Molecular profiling reclassifies adult astroblastoma into known and clinically distinct tumor entities with frequent mitogen-activated protein kinase pathway alterations. Oncologist. 2019 Dec;24(12):1584–92. PMID:31346129
**767.** Bokemeyer C, Kuczyk MA, Dunn T, et al. Expression of stem-cell factor and its receptor c-kit protein in normal testicular tissue and malignant germ-cell tumours. J Cancer Res Clin Oncol. 1996;122(5):301–6. PMID:8609154
**768.** Bokemeyer C, Nichols CR, Droz JP, et al. Extragonadal germ cell tumors of the mediastinum and retroperitoneum: results from an international analysis. J Clin Oncol. 2002 Apr 1;20(7):1864–73. PMID:11919246
**769.** Boland JM, Folpe AL, Hornick JL, et al. Clusterin is expressed in normal synoviocytes and in tenosynovial giant cell tumors of localized and diffuse types: diagnostic and histogenetic implications. Am J Surg Pathol. 2009 Aug;33(8):1225–9. PMID:19542874
**770.** Bolen JW, Thorning D. Benign lipoblastoma and myxoid liposarcoma: a comparative light- and electron-microscopic study. Am J Surg Pathol. 1980 Apr;4(2):163–74. PMID:7377463
**771.** Boley S, Sloan JL, Pemov A, et al. A quantitative assessment of the burden and distribution of Lisch nodules in adults with neurofibromatosis type 1. Invest Ophthalmol Vis Sci. 2009 Nov;50(11):5035–43. PMID:19516012
**772.** Bolouri H, Farrar JE, Triche T Jr, et al. The molecular landscape of pediatric acute myeloid leukemia reveals recurrent structural alterations and age-specific mutational interactions. Nat Med. 2018 Jan;24(1):103–12. PMID:29227476
**773.** Boman F, Bossard C, Fabre M, et al. Mesenchymal hamartomas of the liver may be associated with increased serum alpha foetoprotein concentrations and mimic hepatoblastomas. Eur J Pediatr Surg. 2004 Feb;14(1):63–6. PMID:15024683
**774.** Boman F, Hill DA, Williams GM, et al. Familial association of pleuropulmonary blastoma with cystic nephroma and other renal tumors: a report from the International Pleuropulmonary Blastoma Registry. J Pediatr. 2006 Dec;149(6):850–4. PMID:17137906

775. Bonazzi C, Peccatori F, Colombo N, et al. Pure ovarian immature teratoma, a unique and curable disease: 10 years' experience of 32 prospectively treated patients. Obstet Gynecol. 1994 Oct;84(4):598–604. PMID:7522313
776. Bond SJ, Harrison MR, Schmidt KC, et al. Death due to high-output cardiac failure in fetal sacrococcygeal teratoma. J Pediatr Surg. 1990 Dec;25(12):1287–91. PMID:2286911
777. Bongaarts A, Giannikou K, Reinten RJ, et al. Subependymal giant cell astrocytomas in tuberous sclerosis complex have consistent TSC1/TSC2 biallelic inactivation, and no BRAF mutations. Oncotarget. 2017 Sep 8;8(56):95516–29. PMID:29221145
778. Bongiorno MA, Nathan N, Oyerinde O, et al. Clinical characteristics of connective tissue nevi in tuberous sclerosis complex with special emphasis on shagreen patches. JAMA Dermatol. 2017 Jul 1;153(7):660–5. PMID:28445558
779. Boniuk M, Zimmerman LE. Epibulbar osteoma (episcleral osseous choristoma). Am J Ophthalmol. 1962 Feb;53:290–6. PMID:13871021
780. Bonn BR, Rohde M, Zimmermann M, et al. Incidence and prognostic relevance of genetic variations in T-cell lymphoblastic lymphoma in childhood and adolescence. Blood. 2013 Apr 18;121(16):3153–60. PMID:23396305
781. Bonnin JM, Rubinstein LJ. Astroblastomas: a pathological study of 23 tumors, with a postoperative follow-up in 13 patients. Neurosurgery. 1989 Jul;25(1):6–13. PMID:2755581
782. Bonzheim I, Geissinger E, Roth S, et al. Anaplastic large cell lymphomas lack the expression of T-cell receptor molecules or molecules of proximal T-cell receptor signaling. Blood. 2004 Nov 15;104(10):3358–60. PMID:15297316
783. Boocock GR, Morrison JA, Popovic M, et al. Mutations in SBDS are associated with Shwachman-Diamond syndrome. Nat Genet. 2003 Jan;33(1):97–101. PMID:12496757
784. Boon LM, Burrows PE, Paltiel HJ, et al. Hepatic vascular anomalies in infancy: a twenty-seven-year experience. J Pediatr. 1996 Sep;129(3):346–54. PMID:8804322
785. Boon LM, Mulliken JB, Enjolras O, et al. Glomuvenous malformation (glomangioma) and venous malformation: distinct clinicopathologic and genetic entities. Arch Dermatol. 2004 Aug;140(8):971–6. PMID:15313813
786. Boone SL, Busam KJ, Marghoob AA, et al. Two cases of multiple spitz nevi: correlating clinical, histologic, and fluorescence in situ hybridization findings. Arch Dermatol. 2011 Feb;147(2):227–31. PMID:21339450
787. Booth C, Gilmour KC, Veys P, et al. X-linked lymphoproliferative disease due to SAP/SH2D1A deficiency: a multicenter study on the manifestations, management and outcome of the disease. Blood. 2011 Jan 6;117(1):53–62. PMID:20926771
788. Boppudi S, Bögershausen N, Hove HB, et al. Specific mosaic KRAS mutations affecting codon 146 cause oculoectodermal syndrome and encephalocraniocutaneous lipomatosis. Clin Genet. 2016 Oct;90(4):334–42. PMID:26970110
789. Borchmann S, Engert A. The genetics of Hodgkin lymphoma: an overview and clinical implications. Curr Opin Oncol. 2017 Sep;29(5):307–14. PMID:28697001
790. Borda A, Zahan AE, Piciu D, et al. A 15 year institutional experience of well-differentiated follicular cell-derived thyroid carcinomas; impact of the new 2017 TNM and WHO Classifications of Tumors of Endocrine Organs on the epidemiological trends and pathological characteristics. Endocrine. 2020 Mar;67(3):630–42. PMID:31838728
791. Borer JG, Tan PE, Diamond DA. The spectrum of Sertoli cell tumors in children. Urol Clin North Am. 2000 Aug;27(3):529–41. PMID:10985152
792. Bories N, Thomas L, Phan A, et al. [Lymphomatoid papulosis in childhood: six case reports and a literature review]. Ann Dermatol Venereol. 2008 Oct;135(10):657–62. French. PMID:18929914
793. Borit A, Blackwood W, Mair WG. The separation of pineocytoma from pineoblastoma. Cancer. 1980 Mar 15;45(6):1408–18. PMID:6986979
794. Borit A, Richardson EP Jr. The biological and clinical behaviour of pilocytic astrocytomas of the optic pathways. Brain. 1982 Mar;105(Pt 1):161–87. PMID:7066671
795. Borkhardt A, Bojesen S, Haas OA, et al. The human GRAF gene is fused to MLL in a unique t(5;11)(q31;q23) and both alleles are disrupted in three cases of myelodysplastic syndrome/acute myeloid leukemia with a deletion 5q. Proc Natl Acad Sci U S A. 2000 Aug 1;97(16):9168–73. PMID:10908648
796. Borkowska J, Schwartz RA, Kotulska K, et al. Tuberous sclerosis complex: tumors and tumorigenesis. Int J Dermatol. 2011 Jan;50(1):13–20. PMID:21182496
797. Borowitz MJ, Devidas M, Hunger SP, et al. Clinical significance of minimal residual disease in childhood acute lymphoblastic leukemia and its relationship to other prognostic factors: a Children's Oncology Group study. Blood. 2008 Jun 15;111(12):5477–85. PMID:18388178
798. Borowitz MJ, Rubnitz J, Nash M, et al. Surface antigen phenotype can predict TEL-AML1 rearrangement in childhood B-precursor ALL: a Pediatric Oncology Group study. Leukemia. 1998 Nov;12(11):1764–70. PMID:9823952
799. Bosi G, Lintermans JP, Pellegrino PA, et al. The natural history of cardiac rhabdomyoma with and without tuberous sclerosis. Acta Paediatr. 1996 Aug;85(8):928–31. PMID:8863873
800. Bosisio F, Boi S, Caputo V, et al. Lobular panniculitic infiltrates with overlapping histopathologic features of lupus panniculitis (lupus profundus) and subcutaneous T-cell lymphoma: a conceptual and practical dilemma. Am J Surg Pathol. 2015 Feb;39(2):206–11. PMID:25118815
801. Bosl GJ, Lange PH, Nochomovitz LE, et al. Tumor markers in advanced nonseminomatous testicular cancer. Cancer. 1981 Feb 1;47(3):572–6. PMID:6164464
801A. Boström A, von Lehe M, Hartmann W, et al. Surgery for spinal cord ependymomas: outcome and prognostic factors. Neurosurgery. 2011 Feb;68(2):302–8. PMID:21135741
802. Bott M, Brevet M, Taylor BS, et al. The nuclear deubiquitinase BAP1 is commonly inactivated by somatic mutations and 3p21.1 losses in malignant pleural mesothelioma. Nat Genet. 2011 Jun 5;43(7):668–72. PMID:21642991
803. Bouaoun L, Sonkin D, Ardin M, et al. TP53 Variations in human cancers: new lessons from the IARC TP53 Database and genomics data. Hum Mutat. 2016 Sep;37(9):865–76. PMID:27328919
803A. Bouchoucha Y, Tauziède-Espariat A, Gauthier A, et al. Intra- and extra-cranial BCOR-ITD tumours are separate entities within the BCOR-rearranged family. J Pathol Clin Res. 2022 May;8(3):217–232. PMID:35174661
804. Boué DR, Parham DM, Webber B, et al. Clinicopathologic study of ectomesenchymomas from Intergroup Rhabdomyosarcoma Study Groups III and IV. Pediatr Dev Pathol. 2000 May-Jun;3(3):290–300. PMID:10742419
805. Bouffet E, Larouche V, Campbell BB, et al. Immune checkpoint inhibition for hypermutant glioblastoma multiforme resulting from germline biallelic mismatch repair deficiency. J Clin Oncol. 2016 Jul 1;34(19):2206–11. PMID:27001570
806. Bougeard G, Renaux-Petel M, Flaman JM, et al. Revisiting Li-Fraumeni syndrome from TP53 mutation carriers. J Clin Oncol. 2015 Jul 20;33(21):2345–52. PMID:26014290
807. Bourdeaut F, Fréneaux P, Thuille B, et al. Extra-renal non-cerebral rhabdoid tumours. Pediatr Blood Cancer. 2008 Sep;51(3):363–8. PMID:18506766
808. Bourdeaut F, Lequin D, Brugières L, et al. Frequent hSNF5/INI1 germline mutations in patients with rhabdoid tumor. Clin Cancer Res. 2011 Jan 1;17(1):31–8. PMID:21208904
809. Bourdeaut F, Miquel C, Richer W, et al. Rubinstein-Taybi syndrome predisposing to non-WNT, non-SHH, group 3 medulloblastoma. Pediatr Blood Cancer. 2014 Feb;61(2):383–6. PMID:24115570
810. Bourgeois JM, Knezevich SR, Mathers JA, et al. Molecular detection of the ETV6-NTRK3 gene fusion differentiates congenital fibrosarcoma from other childhood spindle cell tumors. Am J Surg Pathol. 2000 Jul;24(7):937–46. PMID:10895816
811. Bourgois B, Boman F, Nelken B, et al. [Intractable diarrhoea revealing a neuroblastoma hypersecreting the vasoactive intestinal peptide]. Arch Pediatr. 2004 Apr;11(4):340–3. French. PMID:15051093
812. Bourkiza R, Cumberland P, Fabian ID, et al. Role of ethnicity and socioeconomic status (SES) in the presentation of retinoblastoma: findings from the UK. BMJ Open Ophthalmol. 2020 May 15;5(1):e000415. PMID:32432168
813. Bourn D, Carter SA, Mason S, et al. Germline mutations in the neurofibromatosis type 2 tumour suppressor gene. Hum Mol Genet. 1994 May;3(5):813–6. PMID:8081368
814. Bourne TD, Mandell JW, Matsumoto JA, et al. Primary disseminated leptomeningeal oligodendroglioma with 1p deletion. Case report. J Neurosurg. 2006 Dec;105(6 Suppl):465–9. PMID:17184079
815. Bousdras K, O'Donnell P, Vujovic S, et al. Chondroblastomas but not chondromyxoid fibromas express cytokeratins: an unusual presentation of a chondroblastoma in the metaphyseal cortex of the tibia. Histopathology. 2007 Sep;51(3):414–6. PMID:17727486
816. Bouska A, Bi C, Lone W, et al. Adult high-grade B-cell lymphoma with Burkitt lymphoma signature: genomic features and potential therapeutic targets. Blood. 2017 Oct 19;130(16):1819–31. PMID:28801451
817. Boutross-Tadross O, Saleh R, Asa SL. Follicular variant papillary thyroid carcinoma arising in struma ovarii. Endocr Pathol. 2007 Fall;18(3):182–6. PMID:18058267
818. Bouzas EA, Mastorakos G, Chrousos GP, et al. Lisch nodules in Cushing's disease. Arch Ophthalmol. 1993 Apr;111(4):439–40. PMID:8470969
819. Bovée JV, Cleton-Jansen AM, Wuyts W, et al. EXT-mutation analysis and loss of heterozygosity in sporadic and hereditary osteochondromas and secondary chondrosarcomas. Am J Hum Genet. 1999 Sep;65(3):689–98. PMID:10441575
820. Bovée JV, Hogendoorn PC. Non-ossifying fibroma: a RAS-MAPK driven benign bone neoplasm. J Pathol. 2019 Jun;248(2):127–30. PMID:30809793
821. Bovée JV, van der Heul RO, Taminiau AH, et al. Chondrosarcoma of the phalanx: a locally aggressive lesion with minimal metastatic potential: a report of 35 cases and a review of the literature. Cancer. 1999 Nov 1;86(9):1724–32. PMID:10547545
822. Bowe AE, Finnegan R, Jan de Beur SM, et al. FGF-23 inhibits renal tubular phosphate transport and is a PHEX substrate. Biochem Biophys Res Commun. 2001 Jun 22;284(4):977–81. PMID:11409890
823. Bowman RL, Busque L, Levine RL. Clonal hematopoiesis and evolution to hematopoietic malignancies. Cell Stem Cell. 2018 Feb 1;22(2):157–70. PMID:29395053
824. Bown N, Cotterill S, Lastowska M, et al. Gain of chromosome arm 17q and adverse outcome in patients with neuroblastoma. N Engl J Med. 1999 Jun 24;340(25):1954–61. PMID:10379019
825. Bown N, Yule SM, Evans J, et al. Chronic myelomonocytic leukemia with t(13;14) in a child. Cancer Genet Cytogenet. 1992 Jun;60(2):190–2. PMID:1606563
826. Boyd AS. Chromosomal translocation-negative cellular extraskeletal myxoid chondrosarcoma in an adolescent female. J Cutan Pathol. 2012 Sep;39(9):872–6. PMID:22804337
827. Boyd C, Patel K, O'Sullivan B, et al. Pulmonary-type adenocarcinoma and signet ring mucinous adenocarcinoma arising in an ovarian dermoid cyst: report of a unique case. Hum Pathol. 2012 Nov;43(11):2088–92. PMID:23026196
828. Boye E, Yu Y, Paranya G, et al. Clonality and altered behavior of endothelial cells from hemangiomas. J Clin Invest. 2001 Mar;107(6):745–52. PMID:11254674
829. Boyer T, Dorfmann H. Arthroscopy in primary synovial chondromatosis of the hip: description and outcome of treatment. J Bone Joint Surg Br. 2008 Mar;90(3):314–8. PMID:18310752
830. Boyle GJ, Michaels MG, Webber SA, et al. Posttransplantation lymphoproliferative disorders in pediatric thoracic organ recipients. J Pediatr. 1997 Aug;131(2):309–13. PMID:9290623
830A. Boyraz B, Sadow PM, Asa SL, et al. Cribriform-morular thyroid carcinoma is a distinct thyroid malignancy of uncertain cytogenesis. Endocr Pathol. 2021 Sep;32(3):327–35. PMID:34019236
831. Bozdogan O, Kadan E, Bozdogan N. Are there EWSR1 rearranged cutaneous hidradenomas and mucoepidermoid carcinomas of salivary glands? A FISH study and review of the literature. Pol J Pathol. 2020;71(2):99–106. PMID:32729300
832. Bozzai B, Hasselblatt M, Turányi E, et al. Atypical teratoid/rhabdoid tumor arising in a malignant glioma. Pediatr Blood Cancer. 2017 Jan;64(1):96–9. PMID:27472468
833. Braatz B, Evans R, Kelman A, et al. Perinatal evolution of mesenchymal hamartoma of the chest wall. J Pediatr Surg. 2010 Dec;45(12):e37–40. PMID:21129530
834. Brace V, Grant SR, Brackley KJ, et al. Prenatal diagnosis and outcome in sacrococcygeal teratomas: a review of cases between 1992 and 1998. Prenat Diagn. 2000 Jan;20(1):51–5. PMID:10701852
835. Bradford PT, Goldstein AM, Tamura D, et al. Cancer and neurologic degeneration in xeroderma pigmentosum: long term follow-up characterises the role of DNA repair. J Med Genet. 2011 Mar;48(3):168–76. PMID:21097776
836. Brady A, Nayar A, Cross P, et al. A detailed immunohistochemical analysis of 2 cases of papillary cystadenoma of the broad ligament: an extremely rare neoplasm characteristic of patients with von hippel-lindau disease. Int J Gynecol Pathol. 2012 Mar;31(2):133–40. PMID:22317868
837. Brandi ML, Gagel RF, Angeli A, et al. Guidelines for diagnosis and therapy of MEN type 1 and type 2. J Clin Endocrinol Metab. 2001 Dec;86(12):5658–71. PMID:11739416
838. Brandwein M, Said-Al-Naief N, Manwani D, et al. Sialoblastoma: clinicopathological/immunohistochemical study. Am J Surg Pathol. 1999 Mar;23(3):342–8. PMID:10078927

**839.** Brandwein MS, Ivanov K, Wallace DI, et al. Mucoepidermoid carcinoma: a clinicopathologic study of 80 patients with special reference to histological grading. Am J Surg Pathol. 2001 Jul;25(7):835–45. PMID:11420454

**840.** Branford S, Kim DDH, Apperley JF, et al. Laying the foundation for genomically-based risk assessment in chronic myeloid leukemia. Leukemia. 2019 Aug;33(8):1835–50. PMID:31209280

**840A.** Brannon RB. The odontogenic keratocyst. A clinicopathologic study of 312 cases. Part I. Clinical features. Oral Surg Oral Med Oral Pathol. 1976 Jul;42(1):54–72. PMID:1065842

**841.** Branstetter DG, Nelson SD, Manivel JC, et al. Denosumab induces tumor reduction and bone formation in patients with giant-cell tumor of bone. Clin Cancer Res. 2012 Aug 15;18(16):4415–24. PMID:22711702

**842.** Brastianos PK, Shankar GM, Gill CM, et al. Dramatic response of BRAF V600E mutant papillary craniopharyngioma to targeted therapy. J Natl Cancer Inst. 2015 Oct 23;108(2):djv310. PMID:26498373

**843.** Brastianos PK, Taylor-Weiner A, Manley PE, et al. Exome sequencing identifies BRAF mutations in papillary craniopharyngiomas. Nat Genet. 2014 Feb;46(2):161–5. PMID:24413733

**844.** Brat DJ, Aldape K, Colman H, et al. cIM-PACT-NOW update 3: recommended diagnostic criteria for "Diffuse astrocytic glioma, IDH-wildtype, with molecular features of glioblastoma, WHO grade IV". Acta Neuropathol. 2018 Nov;136(5):805–10. PMID:30259105

**845.** Brat DJ, Aldape K, Colman H, et al. cIMPACT-NOW update 5: recommended grading criteria and terminologies for IDH-mutant astrocytomas. Acta Neuropathol. 2020 Mar;139(3):603–8. PMID:31996992

**846.** Brat DJ, Hirose Y, Cohen KJ, et al. Astroblastoma: clinicopathologic features and chromosomal abnormalities defined by comparative genomic hybridization. Brain Pathol. 2000 Jul;10(3):342–52. PMID:10885653

**847.** Bray F, Colombet M, Mery L, et al., editors. Cancer incidence in five continents. Volume XI. Lyon (France): International Agency for Research on Cancer; 2017. (IARC Scientific Publication No. 166). https://ci5.iarc.fr/CI5-XI.

**848.** Brayer KJ, Frerich CA, Kang H, et al. Recurrent fusions in MYB and MYBL1 define a common, transcription factor-driven oncogenic pathway in salivary gland adenoid cystic carcinoma. Cancer Discov. 2016 Feb;6(2):176–87. PMID:26631070

**849.** Brčić I, Brodowicz T, Cerroni L, et al. Undifferentiated round cell sarcomas with CIC-DUX4 gene fusion: expanding the clinical spectrum. Pathology. 2020 Feb;52(2):236–42. PMID:31870501

**850.** Brecht IB, Garbe C, Gefeller O, et al. 443 paediatric cases of malignant melanoma registered with the German Central Malignant Melanoma Registry between 1983 and 2011. Eur J Cancer. 2015 May;51(7):861–8. PMID:25794606

**851.** Bredael JJ, Vugrin D, Whitmore WF Jr. Autopsy findings in 154 patients with germ cell tumors of the testis. Cancer. 1982 Aug 1;50(3):548–51. PMID:6284333

**852.** Breit S, Stanulla M, Flohr T, et al. Activating NOTCH1 mutations predict favorable early treatment response and long-term outcome in childhood precursor T-cell lymphoblastic leukemia. Blood. 2006 Aug 15;108(4):1151–7. PMID:16614245

**853.** Bremer J, Kottke R, Johann PD, et al. A single supratentorial high-grade neuroepithelial tumor with two distinct BCOR mutations, exceptionally long complete remission and survival. Pediatr Blood Cancer. 2020 Jul;67(7):e28384. PMID:32383815

**854.** Brems H, Beert E, de Ravel T, et al. Mechanisms in the pathogenesis of malignant tumours in neurofibromatosis type 1. Lancet Oncol. 2009 May;10(5):508–15. PMID:19410195

**855.** Brems H, Park C, Maertens O, et al. Glomus tumors in neurofibromatosis type 1: genetic, functional, and clinical evidence of a novel association. Cancer Res. 2009 Sep 15;69(18):7393–401. PMID:19738042

**856.** Brennan B, De Salvo GL, Orbach D, et al. Outcome of extracranial malignant rhabdoid tumours in children registered in the European Paediatric Soft Tissue Sarcoma Study Group Non-Rhabdomyosarcoma Soft Tissue Sarcoma 2005 Study-EpSSG NRSTS 2005. Eur J Cancer. 2016 Jun;60:69–82. PMID:27082136

**857.** Brennan B, Stiller C, Bourdeaut F. Extracranial rhabdoid tumours: what we have learned so far and future directions. Lancet Oncol. 2013 Jul;14(8):e329–36. PMID:23816299

**858.** Brennan B, Zanetti I, De Salvo GL, et al. Dermatofibrosarcoma protuberans in children and adolescents: the European Paediatric Soft Tissue Sarcoma Study Group prospective trial (EpSSG NRSTS 2005). Pediatr Blood Cancer. 2020 Oct;67(10):e28351. PMID:32558231

**859.** Brennan B, Zanetti I, Orbach D, et al. Alveolar soft part sarcoma in children and adolescents: the European Paediatric Soft Tissue Sarcoma Study Group prospective trial (EpSSG NRSTS 2005). Pediatr Blood Cancer. 2018 Apr;65(4). PMID:29286582

**860.** Brenneman M, Field A, Yang J, et al. Temporal order of RNase IIIb and loss-of-function mutations during development determines phenotype in pleuropulmonary blastoma / DICER1 syndrome: a unique variant of the two-hit tumor suppression model. F1000Res. 2015 Jul 10;4:214. PMID:26925222

**861.** Bresler SC, Weiser DA, Huwe PJ, et al. ALK mutations confer differential oncogenic activation and sensitivity to ALK inhibition therapy in neuroblastoma. Cancer Cell. 2014 Nov 10;26(5):682–94. PMID:25517749

**862.** Breslow N, Olshan A, Beckwith JB, et al. Epidemiology of Wilms tumor. Med Pediatr Oncol. 1993;21(3):172–81. PMID:7680412

**863.** Breslow NE, Norris R, Norkool PA, et al. Characteristics and outcomes of children with the Wilms tumor-aniridia syndrome: a report from the National Wilms Tumor Study Group. J Clin Oncol. 2003 Dec 15;21(24):4579–85. PMID:14673045

**864.** Bridge JA, Dembinski A, DeBoer J, et al. Clonal chromosomal abnormalities in osteofibrous dysplasia. Implications for histopathogenesis and its relationship with adamantinoma. Cancer. 1994 Mar 15;73(6):1746–52. PMID:8156503

**865.** Bridge JA, Kanamori M, Ma Z, et al. Fusion of the ALK gene to the clathrin heavy chain gene, CLTC, in inflammatory myofibroblastic tumor. Am J Pathol. 2001 Aug;159(2):411–5. PMID:11485898

**866.** Bridge JA, Nelson M, McComb E, et al. Cytogenetic findings in 73 osteosarcoma specimens and a review of the literature. Cancer Genet Cytogenet. 1997 May;95(1):74–87. PMID:9140456

**867.** Bridge JA, Sreekantaiah C, Neff JR, et al. Cytogenetic findings in clear cell sarcoma of tendons and aponeuroses. Malignant melanoma of soft parts. Cancer Genet Cytogenet. 1991 Mar;52(1):101–6. PMID:2009504

**868.** Bridge JA, Sumegi J, Druta M, et al. Clinical, pathological, and genomic features of EWSR1-PATZ1 fusion sarcoma. Mod Pathol. 2019 Nov;32(11):1593–604. PMID:31189996

**869.** Bridge JA, Sumegi J, Royce T, et al. A novel CLTC-FOSB gene fusion in pseudomyogenic hemangioendothelioma of bone. Genes

Chromosomes Cancer. 2021 Jan;60(1):38–42. PMID:32749039

**870.** Brierley JD, Gospodarowicz MK, Wittekind C, editors. TNM classification of malignant tumours. 8th ed. Oxford (UK): Wiley-Blackwell; 2017.

**871.** Brignardello E, Corrias A, Isolato G, et al. Ultrasound screening for thyroid carcinoma in childhood cancer survivors: a case series. J Clin Endocrinol Metab. 2008 Dec;93(12):4840–3. PMID:18812481

**872.** Brinkert F, Arrenberg P, Krech T, et al. Two cases of hepatosplenic T-Cell lymphoma in adolescents treated for autoimmune hepatitis. Pediatrics. 2016 Sep;138(3):e20154245. PMID:27516526

**873.** Brinkman AS, Maxfield B, Gill K, et al. A novel t(3;8)(p13;q21.1) translocation in a case of lipoblastoma. Pediatr Surg Int. 2012 Jul;28(7):737–40. PMID:22488564

**874.** Brinkmeier ML, Bando H, Camarano AC, et al. Rathke's cleft-like cysts arise from Isl1 deletion in murine pituitary progenitors. J Clin Invest. 2020 Aug 3;130(8):4501–15. PMID:32453714

**875.** Brioude F, Kalish JM, Mussa A, et al. Expert consensus document: clinical and molecular diagnosis, screening and management of Beckwith-Wiedemann syndrome: an international consensus statement. Nat Rev Endocrinol. 2018 Apr;14(4):229–49. PMID:29377879

**876.** Brioude F, Toutain A, Giabicani E, et al. Overgrowth syndromes - clinical and molecular aspects and tumour risk. Nat Rev Endocrinol. 2019 May;15(5):299–311. PMID:30842651

**877.** Brivio E, Zwaan CM. ALK inhibition in two emblematic cases of pediatric inflammatory myofibroblastic tumor: efficacy and side effects. Pediatr Blood Cancer. 2019 May;66(5):e27645. PMID:30697903

**878.** Broaddus RR, Herzog CE, Hicks MJ. Neuroendocrine tumors (carcinoid and neuroendocrine carcinoma) presenting at extra-appendiceal sites in childhood and adolescence. Arch Pathol Lab Med. 2003 Sep;127(9):1200–3. PMID:12946222

**879.** Brock JE, Perez-Atayde AR, Kozakewich HP, et al. Cytogenetic aberrations in perineurioma: variation with subtype. Am J Surg Pathol. 2005 Sep;29(9):1164–9. PMID:16096405

**880.** Broder MS, Quock TP, Chang E, et al. The cost of hematopoietic stem-cell transplantation in the United States. Am Health Drug Benefits. 2017 Oct;10(7):366–74. PMID:29263771

**881.** Brodeur GM, Nichols KE, Plon SE, et al. Pediatric cancer predisposition and surveillance: an overview, and a tribute to Alfred G. Knudson Jr. Clin Cancer Res. 2017 Jun 1;23(11):e1–5. PMID:28572261

**882.** Brodeur GM, Pritchard J, Berthold F, et al. Revisions of the international criteria for neuroblastoma diagnosis, staging, and response to treatment. J Clin Oncol. 1993 Aug;11(8):1466–77. PMID:8336186

**883.** Brodeur GM, Seeger RC, Schwab M, et al. Amplification of N-myc in untreated human neuroblastomas correlates with advanced disease stage. Science. 1984 Jun 8;224(4653):1121–4. PMID:6719137

**884.** Brodsky SV, Sandoval C, Sharma N, et al. Recurrent nested stromal epithelial tumor of the liver with extrahepatic metastasis: case report and review of literature. Pediatr Dev Pathol. 2008 Nov-Dec;11(6):469–73. PMID:18338937

**885.** Broehm C, Al-Ibraheemi A, Fritchie KJ. Pediatric non-vestibular schwannoma. Pediatr Dev Pathol. 2017 Jun;20(3):232–9. PMID:28420320

**886.** Broehm CJ, M'Lady G, Bocklage T, et al. Bizarre parosteal osteochondromatous proliferation: a new cytogenetic subgroup

characterized by inversion of chromosome 7. Cancer Genet. 2013 Nov;206(11):402–5. PMID:24412018

**887.** Brohl AS, Solomon DA, Chang W, et al. The genomic landscape of the Ewing sarcoma family of tumors reveals recurrent STAG2 mutation. PLoS Genet. 2014 Jul 10;10(7):e1004475. PMID:25010205

**888.** Broniscer A, Hwang SN, Chamdine O, et al. Bithalamic gliomas may be molecularly distinct from their unilateral high-grade counterparts. Brain Pathol. 2018 Jan;28(1):112–20. PMID:28032389

**889.** Brooks BP, Thompson AH, Bishop RJ, et al. Ocular manifestations of xeroderma pigmentosum: long-term follow-up highlights the role of DNA repair in protection from sun damage. Ophthalmology. 2013 Jul;120(7):1324–36. PMID:23601806

**890.** Brooks EG, Evans MF, Adamson CS, et al. In situ hybridization signal patterns in recurrent laryngeal squamous papillomas indicate that HPV integration occurs at an early stage. Head Neck Pathol. 2012 Mar;6(1):32–7. PMID:22052184

**891.** Brooks GA, Stopfer JE, Erlichman J, et al. Childhood cancer in families with and without BRCA1 or BRCA2 mutations ascertained at a high-risk breast cancer clinic. Cancer Biol Ther. 2006 Sep;5(9):1098–102. PMID:16931905

**892.** Brosens LA, Keller JJ, Offerhaus GJ, et al. Prevention and management of duodenal polyps in familial adenomatous polyposis. Gut. 2005 Jul;54(7):1034–43. PMID:15951555

**893.** Brosens LA, Offerhaus GJ, Giardiello FM. Hereditary colorectal cancer: genetics and screening. Surg Clin North Am. 2015 Oct;95(5):1067–80. PMID:26315524

**894.** Brosens LA, Wood LD, Offerhaus GJ, et al. Pathology and genetics of syndromic gastric polyps. Int J Surg Pathol. 2016 May;24(3):185–99. PMID:26721304

**895.** Brosman SA. Testicular tumors in prepubertal children. Urology. 1979 Jun;13(6):581–8. PMID:377749

**896.** Broughton WL, Zimmerman LE. A clinicopathologic study of 56 cases of intraocular medulloepitheliomas. Am J Ophthalmol. 1978 Mar;85(3):407–18. PMID:655220

**897.** Brouillard P, Boon LM, Mulliken JB, et al. Mutations in a novel factor, glomulin, are responsible for glomuvenous malformations ("glomangiomas"). Am J Hum Genet. 2002 Apr;70(4):866–74. PMID:11845407

**898.** Brouillard P, Boon LM, Revencu N, et al. Genotypes and phenotypes of 162 families with a glomulin mutation. Mol Syndromol. 2013 Apr;4(4):157–64. PMID:23801931

**899.** Brousset P, Rochaix P, Chittal S, et al. High incidence of Epstein-Barr virus detection in Hodgkin's disease and absence of detection in anaplastic large-cell lymphoma in children. Histopathology. 1993 Aug;23(2):189–91. PMID:8406393

**900.** Brown AD, Lopez-Terrada D, Denny C, et al. Promoters containing ATF-binding sites are de-regulated in cells that express the EWS/ATF1 oncogene. Oncogene. 1995 May 4;10(9):1749–56. PMID:7753552

**901.** Brown AE, Leibundgut K, Niggli FK, et al. Cytogenetics of pineoblastoma: four new cases and a literature review. Cancer Genet Cytogenet. 2006 Oct 15;170(2):175–9. PMID:17011992

**902.** Brown DA, Deep NL, Driscoll CL, et al. Synchronous Epstein-Barr virus-associated skull base and adrenal smooth-muscle tumors in an 8-year-old girl with recent Epstein-Barr virus infection. J Neurosurg Pediatr. 2018 Sep;22(3):283–7. PMID:29905497

**903.** Brown NA, Ross CW, Gudjonsson JE, et al. Subcutaneous panniculitis-like T-cell

lymphoma with bone marrow involvement. Am J Clin Pathol. 2015 Feb;143(2):265–73. PMID:25596253
**904.** Brown RJ, Szymula NJ, Loré JM Jr. Neuroblastoma of the head and neck. Arch Otolaryngol. 1978 Jul;104(7):395–8. PMID:666647
**905.** Browne TJ, Fletcher CD. Haemosiderotic fibrolipomatous tumour (so-called haemosiderotic fibrohistiocytic lipomatous tumour): analysis of 13 new cases in support of a distinct entity. Histopathology. 2006 Mar;48(4):453–61. PMID:16487368
**906.** Browning J, Frieden I, Baselga E, et al. Congenital, self-regressing tufted angioma. Arch Dermatol. 2006 Jun;142(6):749–51. PMID:16785378
**907.** Brownstein CA, Adler F, Nelson-Williams C, et al. A translocation causing increased alpha-klotho level results in hypophosphatemic rickets and hyperparathyroidism. Proc Natl Acad Sci U S A. 2008 Mar 4;105(9):3455–60. PMID:18308935
**908.** Brownstone ND, Celie KB, Spigland NA, et al. Pediatric breast fibroadenomas: a systematic review and algorithm for treatment. Ann Plast Surg. 2019 Nov;83(5):601–5. PMID:30628932
**909.** Bruder E, Alaggio R, Kozakewich HP, et al. Vascular and perivascular lesions of skin and soft tissues in children and adolescents. Pediatr Dev Pathol. 2012;15(1 Suppl):26–61. PMID:22420724
**910.** Bruder E, Passera O, Harms D, et al. Morphologic and molecular characterization of renal cell carcinoma in children and young adults. Am J Surg Pathol. 2004 Sep;28(9):1117–32. PMID:15316311
**911.** Bruford EA, Antonescu CR, Carroll AJ, et al. HUGO Gene Nomenclature Committee (HGNC) recommendations for the designation of gene fusions. Leukemia. 2021 Nov;35(11):3040–3. PMID:34615987
**912.** Brugières L, Le Deley MC, Rosolen A, et al. Impact of the methotrexate administration dose on the need for intrathecal treatment in children and adolescents with anaplastic large-cell lymphoma: results of a randomized trial of the EICNHL Group. J Clin Oncol. 2009 Feb 20;27(6):897–903. PMID:19139435
**913.** Brugières L, Remenieras A, Pierron G, et al. High frequency of germline SUFU mutations in children with desmoplastic/nodular medulloblastoma younger than 3 years of age. J Clin Oncol. 2012 Jun 10;30(17):2087–93. PMID:22508808
**914.** Brundler MA, Kurek KC, Patel K, et al. Submucosal colonic lipoblastoma presenting with colo-colonic intussusception in an infant. Pediatr Dev Pathol. 2018 Jul-Aug;21(4):401–5. PMID:28420321
**915.** Brunelli M, Eble JN, Zhang S, et al. Metanephric adenoma lacks the gains of chromosomes 7 and 17 and loss of Y that are typical of papillary renal cell carcinoma and papillary adenoma. Mod Pathol. 2003 Oct;16(10):1060–3. PMID:14559991
**916.** Brunner C, Urbschat S, Jung V, et al. [Chromosomal alterations in juvenile angiofibromas]. HNO. 2003 Dec;51(12):981–5. German. PMID:14647927
**917.** Bubała H, Małdyk J, Włodarska I, et al. ALK-positive diffuse large B-cell lymphoma. Pediatr Blood Cancer. 2006 May 1;46(5):649–53. PMID:15852431
**918.** Buccoliero AM, Bacci S, Mennonna P, et al. Pathologic quiz case: infratentorial tumor in a middle-aged woman. Oncocytic variant of choroid plexus papilloma. Arch Pathol Lab Med. 2004 Dec;128(12):1448–50. PMID:15578895
**919.** Buccoliero AM, Castiglione F, Degl'innocenti DR, et al. Angiocentric glioma: clinical, morphological, immunohistochemical and molecular features in three pediatric cases. Clin Neuropathol. 2013 Mar-Apr;32(2):107–13. PMID:23073165
**920.** Buccoliero AM, Castiglione F, Rossi Degl'Innocenti D, et al. Embryonal tumor with abundant neuropil and true rosettes: morphological, immunohistochemical, ultrastructural and molecular study of a case showing features of medulloepithelioma and areas of mesenchymal and epithelial differentiation. Neuropathology. 2010 Feb 1;30(1):84–91. PMID:19563506
**921.** Buccoliero AM, Franchi A, Castiglione F, et al. Subependymal giant cell astrocytoma (SEGA): Is it an astrocytoma? Morphological, immunohistochemical and ultrastructural study. Neuropathology. 2009 Feb;29(1):25–30. PMID:18564101
**922.** Buchner A, Vered M. Ameloblastic fibroma: a stage in the development of a hamartomatous odontoma or a true neoplasm? Critical analysis of 162 previously reported cases plus 10 new cases. Oral Surg Oral Med Oral Pathol Oral Radiol. 2013 Nov;116(5):598–606. PMID:24055148
**923.** Buczkowicz P, Bartels U, Bouffet E, et al. Histopathological spectrum of paediatric diffuse intrinsic pontine glioma: diagnostic and therapeutic implications. Acta Neuropathol. 2014 Oct;128(4):573–81. PMID:25047029
**924.** Buczkowicz P, Hoeman C, Rakopoulos P, et al. Genomic analysis of diffuse intrinsic pontine gliomas identifies three molecular subgroups and recurrent activating ACVR1 mutations. Nat Genet. 2014 May;46(5):451–6. PMID:24705254
**925.** Buell-Gutbrod R, Ivanovic M, Montag A, et al. FOXL2 and SOX9 distinguish the lineage of the sex cord-stromal cells in gonadoblastomas. Pediatr Dev Pathol. 2011 Sep-Oct;14(5):391–5. PMID:21682576
**926.** Bueno R, Stawiski EW, Goldstein LD, et al. Comprehensive genomic analysis of malignant pleural mesothelioma identifies recurrent mutations, gene fusions and splicing alterations. Nat Genet. 2016 Apr;48(4):407–16. PMID:26928227
**927.** Buetow PC, Buck JL, Pantongrag-Brown L, et al. Solid and papillary epithelial neoplasm of the pancreas: imaging-pathologic correlation on 56 cases. Radiology. 1996 Jun;199(3):707–11. PMID:8637992
**928.** Buettner M, Greiner A, Avramidou A, et al. Evidence of abortive plasma cell differentiation in Hodgkin and Reed-Sternberg cells of classical Hodgkin lymphoma. Hematol Oncol. 2005 Sep-Dec;23(3-4):127–32. PMID:16342298
**929.** Buffet A, Morin A, Castro-Vega LJ, et al. Germline mutations in the mitochondrial 2-oxoglutarate/malate carrier SLC25A11 gene confer a predisposition to metastatic paragangliomas. Cancer Res. 2018 Apr 15;78(8):1914–22. PMID:29431636
**930.** Bühren J, Christoph AH, Buslei R, et al. Expression of the neurotrophin receptor p75NTR in medulloblastomas is correlated with distinct histological and clinical features: evidence for a medulloblastoma subtype derived from the external granule cell layer. J Neuropathol Exp Neurol. 2000 Mar;59(3):229–40. PMID:10744061
**931.** Buijs A, Bruin M. Fusion of FIP1L1 and RARA as a result of a novel t(4;17)(q12;q21) in a case of juvenile myelomonocytic leukemia. Leukemia. 2007 May;21(5):1104–8. PMID:17301809
**932.** Buitenkamp TD, Pieters R, Gallimore NE, et al. Outcome in children with Down's syndrome and acute lymphoblastic leukemia: role of IKZF1 deletions and CRLF2 aberrations. Leukemia. 2012 Oct;26(10):2204–11. PMID:22441210
**933.** Bunin GR, Surawicz TS, Witman PA, et al. The descriptive epidemiology of craniopharyngioma. J Neurosurg. 1998 Oct;89(4):547–51. PMID:9761047
**934.** Bunt AH, Tso MO. Feulgen-positive deposits in retinoblastoma. Incidence, composition, and ultrastructure. Arch Ophthalmol. 1981 Jan;99(1):144–50. PMID:7006579
**935.** Buratti S, Savides TJ, Newbury RO, et al. Granular cell tumor of the esophagus: report of a pediatric case and literature review. J Pediatr Gastroenterol Nutr. 2004 Jan;38(1):97–101. PMID:14676603
**936.** Burford A, Mackay A, Popov S, et al. The ten-year evolutionary trajectory of a highly recurrent paediatric high grade neuroepithelial tumour with MN1:BEND2 fusion. Sci Rep. 2018 Jan 18;8(1):1032. PMID:29348602
**937.** Burg G, Kempf W, Höchli M, et al. 'Tubular' epithelioid cell nevus: a new variant of Spitz's nevus. J Cutan Pathol. 1998 Oct;25(9):475–8. PMID:9821077
**937A.** Bürgi J, Kunz B, Abrami L, et al. CMG2/ANTXR2 regulates extracellular collagen VI which accumulates in hyaline fibromatosis syndrome. Nat Commun. 2017 Jun 12;8:15861. PMID:28604699
**938.** Burger PC, Yu IT, Tihan T, et al. Atypical teratoid/rhabdoid tumor of the central nervous system: a highly malignant tumor of infancy and childhood frequently mistaken for medulloblastoma: a Pediatric Oncology Group study. Am J Surg Pathol. 1998 Sep;22(9):1083–92. PMID:9737241
**939.** Burgues O, Navarro S, Noguera R, et al. Prognostic value of the International Neuroblastoma Pathology Classification in Neuroblastoma (Schwannian stroma-poor) and comparison with other prognostic factors: a study of 182 cases from the Spanish Neuroblastoma Registry. Virchows Arch. 2006 Oct;449(4):410–20. PMID:16941154
**940.** Burke AP, Mostofi FK. Intratubular malignant germ cells in testicular biopsies: clinical course and identification by staining for placental alkaline phosphatase. Mod Pathol. 1988 Nov;1(6):475–9. PMID:2851788
**941.** Burke AP, Mostofi FK. Placental alkaline phosphatase immunohistochemistry of intratubular malignant germ cells and associated testicular germ cell tumors. Hum Pathol. 1988 Jun;19(6):663–70. PMID:2837430
**942.** Burke JP, Leitch RJ, Talbot JF, et al. Choroidal neurofibromatosis with congenital iris ectropion and buphthalmos: relationship and significance. J Pediatr Ophthalmol Strabismus. 1991 Sep-Oct;28(5):265–7. PMID:1955961
**943.** Burkhard C, Di Patre PL, Schüler D, et al. A population-based study of the incidence and survival rates in patients with pilocytic astrocytoma. J Neurosurg. 2003 Jun;98(6):1170–4. PMID:12816259
**944.** Burkhardt B, Hermiston ML. Lymphoblastic lymphoma in children and adolescents: review of current challenges and future opportunities. Br J Haematol. 2019 Jun;185(6):1158–70. PMID:30809797
**945.** Burkhardt B, Oschlies I, Klapper W, et al. Non-Hodgkin's lymphoma in adolescents: experiences in 378 adolescent NHL patients treated according to pediatric NHL-BFM protocols. Leukemia. 2011 Jan;25(1):153–60. PMID:21030984
**946.** Burkhardt B, Zimmermann M, Oschlies I, et al. The impact of age and gender on biology, clinical features and treatment outcome of non-Hodgkin lymphoma in childhood and adolescence. Br J Haematol. 2005 Oct;131(1):39–49. PMID:16173961
**947.** Burkitt D. A sarcoma involving the jaws in African children. Br J Surg. 1958 Nov;46(197):218–23. PMID:13628987
**948.** Burmeister T, Reinhardt R. A multiplex PCR for improved detection of typical and atypical BCR-ABL fusion transcripts. Leuk Res. 2008 Apr;32(4):579–85. PMID:17928051
**949.** Burnelli R, Fiumana G, Rondelli R, et al. Comparison of Hodgkin's lymphoma in children and adolescents. A twenty year experience with MH'96 and LH2004 AIEOP (Italian Association of Pediatric Hematology and Oncology) protocols. Cancers (Basel). 2020 Jun 18;12(6):E1620. PMID:32570974
**950.** Burnichon N, Cascón A, Schiavi F, et al. MAX mutations cause hereditary and sporadic pheochromocytoma and paraganglioma. Clin Cancer Res. 2012 May 15;18(10):2828–37. PMID:22452945
**951.** Burnier MN, McLean IW, Zimmerman LE, et al. Retinoblastoma. The relationship of proliferating cells to blood vessels. Invest Ophthalmol Vis Sci. 1990 Oct;31(10):2037–40. PMID:2211000
**952.** Burt AD, Cooper G, MacKay C, et al. Dermoid cyst of the testis. Scott Med J. 1987 Oct;32(5):146–8. PMID:3441784
**953.** Burton GV, Bullard DE, Walther PJ, et al. Paraneoplastic limbic encephalopathy with testicular carcinoma. A reversible neurologic syndrome. Cancer. 1988 Nov 15;62(10):2248–51. PMID:2460212
**954.** Busam KJ, Barnhill RL. Pagetoid Spitz nevus. Intraepidermal Spitz tumor with prominent pagetoid spread. Am J Surg Pathol. 1995 Sep;19(9):1061–7. PMID:7661280
**955.** Busam KJ, Kutzner H, Cerroni L, et al. Clinical and pathologic findings of Spitz nevi and atypical Spitz tumors with ALK fusions. Am J Surg Pathol. 2014 Jul;38(7):925–33. PMID:24698967
**956.** Busam KJ, Shah KN, Gerami P, et al. Reduced H3K27me3 expression is common in nodular melanomas of childhood associated with congenital melanocytic nevi but not in proliferative nodules. Am J Surg Pathol. 2017 Mar;41(3):396–404. PMID:27849631
**957.** Busam KJ, Sung J, Wiesner T, et al. Combined BRAF(V600E)-positive melanocytic lesions with large epithelioid cells lacking BAP1 expression and conventional nevomelanocytes. Am J Surg Pathol. 2013 Feb;37(2):193–9. PMID:23026932
**958.** Busam KJ, Wanna M, Wiesner T. Multiple epithelioid Spitz nevi or tumors with loss of BAP1 expression: a clue to a hereditary tumor syndrome. JAMA Dermatol. 2013 Mar;149(3):335–9. PMID:23552620
**959.** Bush ZM, Longtine JA, Cunningham T, et al. Temozolomide treatment for aggressive pituitary tumors: correlation of clinical outcome with O(6)-methylguanine methyltransferase (MGMT) promoter methylation and expression. J Clin Endocrinol Metab. 2010 Nov;95(11):E280–90. PMID:20668043
**960.** Buskirk SJ, Schray MF, Podratz KC, et al. Ovarian dysgerminoma: a retrospective analysis of results of treatment, sites of treatment failure, and radiosensitivity. Mayo Clin Proc. 1987 Dec;62(12):1149–57. PMID:3682960
**961.** Buslei R, Hölsken A, Hofmann B, et al. Nuclear beta-catenin accumulation associates with epithelial morphogenesis in craniopharyngiomas. Acta Neuropathol. 2007 May;113(5):585–90. PMID:17221204
**962.** Buslei R, Nolde M, Hofmann B, et al. Common mutations of beta-catenin in adamantinomatous craniopharyngiomas but not in other tumours originating from the sellar region. Acta Neuropathol. 2005 Jun;109(6):589–97. PMID:15891929
**963.** Bussey KJ, Lawce HJ, Olson SB, et al. Chromosome abnormalities of eighty-one pediatric germ cell tumors: sex-, age-, site-, and histopathology-related differences–a

Children's Cancer Group study. Genes Chromosomes Cancer. 1999 Jun;25(2):134–46. PMID:10337997
**964.** Büttner C, Grabbe J, Haas N, et al. Comparison of genetic and immunohistochemical findings in childhood and adult onset urticaria pigmentosa. Int Arch Allergy Immunol. 1999 Feb-Apr;118(2-4):206–7. PMID:10224380
**965.** Byrgazov K, Kastner R, Gorna M, et al. NDEL1-PDGFRB fusion gene in a myeloid malignancy with eosinophilia associated with resistance to tyrosine kinase inhibitors. Leukemia. 2017 Jan;31(1):237–40. PMID:27573554
**966.** Cabaret O, Perron E, Bressac-de Paillerets B, et al. Occurrence of BAP1 germline mutations in cutaneous melanocytic tumors with loss of BAP1-expression: a pilot study. Genes Chromosomes Cancer. 2017 Sep;56(9):691–4. PMID:28560743
**966A.** Cada M, Segbefia CI, Klaassen R, et al. The impact of category, cytopathology and cytogenetics on development and progression of clonal and malignant myeloid transformation in inherited bone marrow failure syndromes. Haematologica. 2015 May;100(5):633–42. PMID:25682607
**967.** Cai ED, Sun BK, Chiang A, et al. Postzygotic mutations in beta-actin are associated with Becker's nevus and Becker's nevus syndrome. J Invest Dermatol. 2017 Aug;137(8):1795–8. PMID:28347698
**968.** Cai M, He H, Zhang B, et al. An ectopic recurrent craniopharyngioma of the temporal lobe: case report and review of the literature. World Neurosurg. 2019 Jun;126:216–22. PMID:30877004
**969.** Cai W, Jiang B, Yu F, et al. Current approaches to the diagnosis and treatment of white sponge nevus. Expert Rev Mol Med. 2015 May 29;17:e9. PMID:26021387
**970.** Cai Z, Thomas J, Alava I 3rd, et al. Fetal type rhabdomyoma of the soft palate in an adult patient: report of one case and review of the literature. Head Neck Pathol. 2019 Jun;13(2):182–7. PMID:29761260
**971.** Cairo MS, Beishuizen A. Childhood, adolescent and young adult non-Hodgkin lymphoma: current perspectives. Br J Haematol. 2019 Jun;185(6):1021–42. PMID:30729513
**972.** Cairo MS, Pinkerton R. Childhood, adolescent and young adult non-Hodgkin lymphoma: state of the science. Br J Haematol. 2016 May;173(4):507–30. PMID:27133800
**973.** Cairo MS, Sposto R, Gerrard M, et al. Advanced stage, increased lactate dehydrogenase, and primary site, but not adolescent age (≥ 15 years), are associated with an increased risk of treatment failure in children and adolescents with mature B-cell non-Hodgkin's lymphoma: results of the FAB LMB 96 study. J Clin Oncol. 2012 Feb 1;30(4):387–93. PMID:22215753
**974.** Cairo S, Armengol C, De Reyniès A, et al. Hepatic stem-like phenotype and interplay of Wnt/beta-catenin and Myc signaling in aggressive childhood liver cancer. Cancer Cell. 2008 Dec 9;14(6):471–84. PMID:19061838
**974A.** Cairo S, Armengol C, Maibach R, et al. A combined clinical and biological risk classification improves prediction of outcome in hepatoblastoma patients. Eur J Cancer. 2020 Dec;141:30–9. PMID:33125945
**975.** Cajaiba MM, Benjamin D, Halaban R, et al. Metastatic peritoneal neurocutaneous melanocytosis. Am J Surg Pathol. 2008 Jan;32(1):156–61. PMID:18162783
**976.** Cajaiba MM, Dyer LM, Geller JI, et al. The classification of pediatric and young adult renal cell carcinomas registered on the children's oncology group (COG) protocol AREN03B2 after focused genetic testing. Cancer. 2018 Aug;124(16):3381–9. PMID:29905933
**977.** Cajaiba MM, Jennings LJ, George D, et al. Expanding the spectrum of ALK-rearranged renal cell carcinomas in children: identification of a novel HOOK1-ALK fusion transcript. Genes Chromosomes Cancer. 2016 Oct;55(10):814–7. PMID:27225638
**978.** Cajaiba MM, Khanna G, Smith EA, et al. Pediatric cystic nephromas: distinctive features and frequent DICER1 mutations. Hum Pathol. 2016 Feb;48:81–7. PMID:26772403
**979.** Cajaiba MM, Sarita-Reyes C, Zambrano E, et al. Mesenchymal hamartoma of the liver associated with features of Beckwith-Wiedemann syndrome and high serum alpha-fetoprotein levels. Pediatr Dev Pathol. 2007 May-Jun;10(3):233–8. PMID:17535089
**980.** Calaminici M, Piper K, Lee AM, et al. CD23 expression in mediastinal large B-cell lymphomas. Histopathology. 2004 Dec;45(6):619–24. PMID:15569053
**981.** Calaminus G, Frappaz D, Kortmann RD, et al. Outcome of patients with intracranial non-germinomatous germ cell tumors-lessons from the SIOP-CNS-GCT-96 trial. Neuro Oncol. 2017 Nov 29;19(12):1661–72. PMID:29048505
**982.** Calaminus G, Kortmann R, Worch J, et al. SIOP CNS GCT 96: final report of outcome of a prospective, multinational nonrandomized trial for children and adults with intracranial germinoma, comparing craniospinal irradiation alone with chemotherapy followed by focal primary site irradiation for patients with localized disease. Neuro Oncol. 2013 Jun;15(6):788–96. PMID:23460321
**983.** Calderon-Garcidueñas AL, Mathon B, Lévy P, et al. New clinicopathological associations and histoprognostic markers in ILAE types of hippocampal sclerosis. Brain Pathol. 2018 Sep;28(5):644–55. PMID:29476662
**984.** Calduch L, Monteagudo C, Martínez-Ruiz E, et al. Familial generalized multiple glomangiomyoma: report of a new family, with immunohistochemical and ultrastructural studies and review of the literature. Pediatr Dermatol. 2002 Sep-Oct;19(5):402–8. PMID:12383095
**985.** Calebiro D, Grassi ES, Eszlinger M, et al. Recurrent EZH1 mutations are a second hit in autonomous thyroid adenomas. J Clin Invest. 2016 Sep 1;126(9):3383–8. PMID:27500488
**986.** Caliò A, Eble JN, Hes O, et al. Distinct clinicopathological features in metanephric adenoma harboring BRAF mutation. Oncotarget. 2016 Aug 8;8(33):54096–105. PMID:28903326
**987.** Calkovsky V, Hajtman A. Thyroid diseases in children and adolescents. Bratisl Lek Listy. 2009;110(1):31–4. PMID:19408827
**988.** Calonje E, Fletcher CD. Aneurysmal benign fibrous histiocytoma: clinicopathological analysis of 40 cases of a tumour frequently misdiagnosed as a vascular neoplasm. Histopathology. 1995 Apr;26(4):323–31. PMID:7607620
**989.** Calonje E, Fletcher CD. Myoid differentiation in dermatofibrosarcoma protuberans and its fibrosarcomatous variant: clinicopathologic analysis of 5 cases. J Cutan Pathol. 1996 Feb;23(1):30–6. PMID:8720984
**990.** Calonje E, Fletcher CD, Wilson-Jones E, et al. Retiform hemangioendothelioma. A distinctive form of low-grade angiosarcoma delineated in a series of 15 cases. Am J Surg Pathol. 1994 Feb;18(2):115–25. PMID:8291650
**991.** Calonje E, Mentzel T, Fletcher CD. Cellular benign fibrous histiocytoma. Clinicopathologic analysis of 74 cases of a distinctive variant of cutaneous fibrous histiocytoma with frequent recurrence. Am J Surg Pathol. 1994 Jul;18(7):668–76. PMID:8017561
**992.** Calonje E, Mentzel T, Fletcher CD. Pseudomalignant perineurial invasion in cellular ('infantile') capillary haemangiomas. Histopathology. 1995 Feb;26(2):159–64. PMID:7737662
**993.** Caltabiano R, Magro G, Polizzi A, et al. A mosaic pattern of INI1/SMARCB1 protein expression distinguishes Schwannomatosis and NF2-associated peripheral schwannomas from solitary peripheral schwannomas and NF2-associated vestibular schwannomas. Childs Nerv Syst. 2017 Jun;33(6):933–40. PMID:28365909
**994.** Caltharp SA, Qayed M, Park SI. Atypical marginal zone hyperplasia is a mimic for lymphoma in pediatric transplant recipients: report of two patients. Pediatr Dev Pathol. 2015 Sep-Oct;18(5):416–21. PMID:25955878
**995.** Bridge JA, Sumegi J, Royce T, et al. A novel CLTC-FOSB gene fusion in pseudomyogenic hemangioendothelioma of bone. Genes Chromosomes Cancer. 2021 Jan;60(1):38–42. PMID:30130629
**996.** Calvo KR, Price S, Braylan RC, et al. JMML and RALD (Ras-associated autoimmune leukoproliferative disorder): common genetic etiology yet clinically distinct entities. Blood. 2015 Apr 30;125(18):2753–8. PMID:25691160
**997.** Cameron BR, Berean KW. Cytokeratin subtypes in thyroid tumours: immunohistochemical study with emphasis on the follicular variant of papillary carcinoma. J Otolaryngol. 2003 Oct;32(5):319–22. PMID:14974863
**998.** Cameron D, Ong TH, Borzi P. Conservative management of mesenchymal hamartomas of the chest wall. J Pediatr Surg. 2001 Sep;36(9):1346–9. PMID:11528603
**998A.** Cameselle-Teijeiro J, Alberte-Lista L, Chiarelli S, et al. CD10 is a characteristic marker of tumours forming morules with biotin-rich, optically clear nuclei that occur in different organs. Histopathology. 2008 Feb;52(3):389–92. PMID:18081818
**998B.** Cameselle-Teijeiro J, Alberte-Lista L, Peteiro-González D, et al. CDX2 expression in some variants of papillary thyroid carcinoma. Am J Clin Pathol. 2012 Dec;138(6):907–9. PMID:23161723
**999.** Cameselle-Teijeiro J, Chan JK. Cribriform-morular variant of papillary carcinoma: a distinctive variant representing the sporadic counterpart of familial adenomatous polyposis-associated thyroid carcinoma? Mod Pathol. 1999 Apr;12(4):400–11. PMID:10229505
**999A.** Cameselle-Teijeiro J, Menasce LP, Yap BK, et al. Cribriform-morular variant of papillary thyroid carcinoma: molecular characterization of a case with neuroendocrine differentiation and aggressive behavior. Am J Clin Pathol. 2009 Jan;131(1):134–42. PMID:19095577
**999B.** Cameselle-Teijeiro JM, Peteiro-González D, Caneiro-Gómez J, et al. Cribriform-morular variant of thyroid carcinoma: a neoplasm with distinctive phenotype associated with the activation of the WNT/β-catenin pathway. Mod Pathol. 2018 Aug;31(8):1168–79. PMID:29785019
**999C.** Cameselle-Teijeiro JM, Sobrinho-Simões M. Cribriform-morular variant of thyroid carcinoma. Pathologica. 2019 Mar;111(1):1–3. PMID:31217615
**1000.** Campanacci M, Baldini N, Boriani S, et al. Giant-cell tumor of bone. J Bone Joint Surg Am. 1987 Jan;69(1):106–14. PMID:3805057
**1001.** Campanacci M, Laus M, Boriani S. Multiple non-ossifying fibromata with extraskeletal anomalies: a new syndrome? J Bone Joint Surg Br. 1983 Nov;65(5):627–32. PMID:6643569
**1002.** Campbell BB, Light N, Fabrizio D, et al. Comprehensive analysis of hypermutation in human cancer. Cell. 2017 Nov 16;171(5):1042–1056.e10. PMID:29056344
**1003.** Campbell LB, Kreicher KL, Gittleman HR, et al. Melanoma incidence in children and adolescents: decreasing trends in the United States. J Pediatr. 2015 Jun;166(6):1505–13. PMID:25866386
**1004.** Campian J, Gutmann DH. CNS tumors in neurofibromatosis. J Clin Oncol. 2017 Jul 20;35(21):2378–85. PMID:28640700
**1005.** Campos AR, Clusmann H, von Lehe M, et al. Simple and complex dysembryoplastic neuroepithelial tumors (DNT) variants: clinical profile, MRI, and histopathology. Neuroradiology. 2009 Jul;51(7):433–43. PMID:19242688
**1006.** Cancer Atlas [Internet]. Atlanta (GA): American Cancer Society; 2019. Cancer in children. Available from: https://canceratlas.cancer.org/the-burden/cancer-in-children/.
**1007.** Cancer Genome Atlas Research Network. Integrated genomic characterization of papillary thyroid carcinoma. Cell. 2014 Oct 23;159(3):676–90. PMID:25417114
**1008.** Cancer Genome Atlas Research Network, Ley TJ, Miller C, et al. Genomic and epigenomic landscapes of adult de novo acute myeloid leukemia. N Engl J Med. 2013 May 30;368(22):2059–74. PMID:23634996
**1009.** Cancer Genome Atlas Research Network, Linehan WM, Spellman PT, et al. Comprehensive molecular characterization of papillary renal-cell carcinoma. N Engl J Med. 2016 Jan 14;374(2):135–45. PMID:26536169
**1010.** Cancer Genome Atlas Research Network. Comprehensive and integrated genomic characterization of adult soft tissue sarcomas. Cell. 2017 Nov 2;171(4):950–965.e28. PMID:29100075
**1011.** Cancer Research UK [Internet]. Oxford (UK): Cancer Research UK; 2020. Cancer incidence by age: All cancers combined incidence by age; last reviewed 2020 Mar 10. Available from: https://www.cancerresearchuk.org/health-professional/cancer-statistics/incidence/age.
**1012.** Cannavo S, Ragonese M, Puglisi S, et al. Acromegaly is more severe in patients with AHR or AIP gene variants living in highly polluted areas. J Clin Endocrinol Metab. 2016 Apr;101(4):1872–9. PMID:26963951
**1013.** Cannavo S, Trimarchi F, Ferraù F. Acromegaly, genetic variants of the aryl hydrocarbon receptor pathway and environmental burden. Mol Cell Endocrinol. 2017 Dec 5;457:81–8. PMID:27998805
**1014.** Cannon DM, Mohindra P, Gondi V, et al. Choroid plexus tumor epidemiology and outcomes: implications for surgical and radiotherapeutic management. J Neurooncol. 2015 Jan;121(1):151–7. PMID:25270349
**1015.** Canté-Barrett K, Spijkers-Hagelstein JA, Buijs-Gladdines JG, et al. MEK and PI3K-AKT inhibitors synergistically block activated IL7 receptor signaling in T-cell acute lymphoblastic leukemia. Leukemia. 2016 Sep;30(9):1832–43. PMID:27174491
**1016.** Cantisani V, Mortele KJ, Levy A, et al. MR imaging features of solid pseudopapillary tumor of the pancreas in adult and pediatric patients. AJR Am J Roentgenol. 2003 Aug;181(2):395–401. PMID:12876017
**1017.** Cantwell CP, Obyrne J, Eustace S. Current trends in treatment of osteoid osteoma with an emphasis on radiofrequency ablation. Eur Radiol. 2004 Apr;14(4):607–17. PMID:14663625
**1018.** Cao D, Guo S, Allan RW, et al. SALL4 is a novel sensitive and specific marker of ovarian primitive germ cell tumors and is particularly useful in distinguishing yolk sac tumor from clear cell carcinoma. Am J Surg Pathol. 2009 Jun;33(6):894–904. PMID:19295406
**1019.** Cao D, Li J, Guo CC, et al. SALL4 is a novel diagnostic marker for testicular germ cell tumors. Am J Surg Pathol. 2009 Jul;33(7):1065–77. PMID:19390421

**1020.** Cao D, Liu A, Wang F, et al. RNA-binding protein LIN28 is a marker for primary extragonadal germ cell tumors: an immunohistochemical study of 131 cases. Mod Pathol. 2011 Feb;24(2):288–96. PMID:21057460
**1021.** Cao F, Lu L, Abrams SA, et al. Generalized metabolic bone disease and fracture risk in Rothmund-Thomson syndrome. Hum Mol Genet. 2017 Aug 15;26(16):3046–55. PMID:28486640
**1022.** Cao Q, Ye Z, Chen S, et al. Undifferentiated embryonal sarcoma of liver: a multi-institutional experience with 9 cases. Int J Clin Exp Pathol. 2014 Dec 1;7(12):8647–56. PMID:25674229
**1023.** Capel E, Vatier C, Cervera P, et al. MFN2-associated lipomatosis: clinical spectrum and impact on adipose tissue. J Clin Lipidol. 2018 Nov-Dec;12(6):1420–35. PMID:30158064
**1024.** Capelle LG, Van Grieken NC, Lingsma HF, et al. Risk and epidemiological time trends of gastric cancer in Lynch syndrome carriers in the Netherlands. Gastroenterology. 2010 Feb;138(2):487–92. PMID:19900449
**1025.** Capp JP. Cancer stem cells: from historical roots to a new perspective. J Oncol. 2019 Jun 11;2019:5189232. PMID:31308849
**1026.** Cappelle S, Pans S, Sciot R. Imaging features of chondromyxoid fibroma: report of 15 cases and literature review. Br J Radiol. 2016 Aug;89(1064):20160088. PMID:27226218
**1027.** Cappellesso R, Bellan A, Saraggi D, et al. YAP immunoreactivity is directly related to pilomatrixoma size and proliferation rate. Arch Dermatol Res. 2015 May;307(4):379–83. PMID:25516090
**1028.** Cappellesso R, d'Amore ES, Dall'Igna P, et al. Immunohistochemical expression of p16 in lipoblastomas. Hum Pathol. 2016 Jan;47(1):64–9. PMID:26514741
**1029.** Capper D, Jones DTW, Sill M, et al. DNA methylation-based classification of central nervous system tumours. Nature. 2018 Mar 22;555(7697):469–74. PMID:29539639
**1030.** Capper D, Reuss D, Schittenhelm J, et al. Mutation-specific IDH1 antibody differentiates oligodendrogliomas and oligoastrocytomas from other brain tumors with oligodendroglioma-like morphology. Acta Neuropathol. 2011 Feb;121(2):241–52. PMID:21069360
**1031.** Capper D, Stichel D, Sahm F, et al. Practical implementation of DNA methylation and copy-number-based CNS tumor diagnostics: the Heidelberg experience. Acta Neuropathol. 2018 Aug;136(2):181–210. PMID:29967940
**1032.** Caradona SA, Skidmore R, Gupta A, et al. Giant congenital melanocytic nevus with underlying hypoplasia of the subcutaneous fat. Pediatr Dermatol. 2000 Sep-Oct;17(5):387–90. PMID:11085669
**1033.** Caraway NP, Fanning CV, Wojcik EM, et al. Cytology of malignant melanoma of soft parts: fine-needle aspirates and exfoliative specimens. Diagn Cytopathol. 1993 Dec;9(6):632–8. PMID:8143535
**1034.** Carbone A, Gloghini A, Gaidano G, et al. AIDS-related Burkitt's lymphoma. Morphologic and immunophenotypic study of biopsy specimens. Am J Clin Pathol. 1995 May;103(5):561–7. PMID:7741100
**1035.** Carbone A, Micheau C. Pitfalls in microscopic diagnosis of undifferentiated carcinoma of nasopharyngeal type (lymphoepithelioma). Cancer. 1982 Oct 1;50(7):1344–51. PMID:7104977
**1036.** Carbone PP, Berard CW, Bennett JM, et al. NIH clinical staff conference. Burkitt's tumor. Ann Intern Med. 1969 Apr;70(4):817–32. PMID:4306129
**1037.** Carcangiu ML, Zampi G, Pupi A, et al. Papillary carcinoma of the thyroid. A clinicopathologic study of 241 cases treated at the University of Florence, Italy. Cancer. 1985 Feb 15;55(4):805–28. PMID:3967175
**1038.** Cardoso CC, Auat M, Santos-Pirath IM, et al. The importance of CD39, CD43, CD81, and CD95 expression for differentiating B cell lymphoma by flow cytometry. Cytometry B Clin Cytom. 2018 May;94(3):451–8. PMID:28509416
**1039.** Cardoso de Almeida PC, Scully RE. Diffuse embryoma of the testis. A distinctive form of mixed germ cell tumor. Am J Surg Pathol. 1983 Oct;7(7):633–42. PMID:6195930
**1040.** Carén H, Kryh H, Nethander M, et al. High-risk neuroblastoma tumors with 11q-deletion display a poor prognostic, chromosome instability phenotype with later onset. Proc Natl Acad Sci U S A. 2010 Mar 2;107(9):4323–8. PMID:20145112
**1040A.** Carethers JM. Differentiating Lynch-like from Lynch syndrome. Gastroenterology. 2014 Mar;146(3):602–4. PMID:24468183
**1041.** Carethers JM, Stoffel EM. Lynch syndrome and Lynch syndrome mimics: the growing complex landscape of hereditary colon cancer. World J Gastroenterol. 2015 Aug 21;21(31):9253–61. PMID:26309352
**1042.** Carifi M, Napolitano D, Morandi M, et al. Recurrent respiratory papillomatosis: current and future perspectives. Ther Clin Risk Manag. 2015 May 5;11:731–8. PMID:25999724
**1043.** Cario G, Rhein P, Mitlöhner R, et al. High CD45 surface expression determines relapse risk in children with precursor B-cell and T-cell acute lymphoblastic leukemia treated according to the ALL-BFM 2000 protocol. Haematologica. 2014 Jan;99(1):103–10. PMID:23911702
**1044.** Carli M, Ferrari A, Mattke A, et al. Pediatric malignant peripheral nerve sheath tumor: the Italian and German soft tissue sarcoma cooperative group. J Clin Oncol. 2005 Nov 20;23(33):8422–30. PMID:16293873
**1045.** Carlinfante G, De Marco L, Mori M, et al. Aggressive angiomyxoma of the spermatic cord. Two unusual cases occurring in childhood. Pathol Res Pract. 2001;197(2):139–44. PMID:11261819
**1046.** Carlo MI, Chaim J, Patil S, et al. Genomic characterization of renal medullary carcinoma and treatment outcomes. Clin Genitourin Cancer. 2017 Dec;15(6):e987–94. PMID:28558987
**1047.** Carlos R, Thompson LD, Netto AC, et al. Epstein-Barr virus and human herpes virus-8 are not associated with juvenile nasopharyngeal angiofibroma. Head Neck Pathol. 2008 Sep;2(3):145–9. PMID:20614308
**1048.** Carlson JW, Fletcher CD. Immunohistochemistry for beta-catenin in the differential diagnosis of spindle cell lesions: analysis of a series and review of the literature. Histopathology. 2007 Oct;51(4):509–14. PMID:17711447
**1049.** Carneiro A, Francis P, Bendahl PO, et al. Indistinguishable genomic profiles and shared prognostic markers in undifferentiated pleomorphic sarcoma and leiomyosarcoma: different sides of a single coin? Lab Invest. 2009 Jun;89(6):668–75. PMID:19290004
**1050.** Carney JA. Gastric stromal sarcoma, pulmonary chondroma, and extra-adrenal paraganglioma (Carney Triad): natural history, adrenocortical component, and possible familial occurrence. Mayo Clin Proc. 1999 Jun;74(6):543–52. PMID:10377927
**1051.** Carney JA, Boccon-Gibod L, Jarka DE, et al. Osteochondromyxoma of bone: a congenital tumor associated with lentigines and other unusual disorders. Am J Surg Pathol. 2001 Feb;25(2):164–76. PMID:11176065
**1052.** Carney JA, Lyssikatos C, Seethala RR, et al. The spectrum of thyroid gland pathology in carney complex: the importance of follicular carcinoma. Am J Surg Pathol. 2018 May;42(5):587–94. PMID:29635258
**1053.** Carney JA, Toorkey BC. Myxoid fibroadenoma and allied conditions (myxomatosis) of the breast. A heritable disorder with special associations including cardiac and cutaneous myxomas. Am J Surg Pathol. 1991 Aug;15(8):713–21. PMID:2069209
**1054.** Caron NR, Sturgeon C, Clark OH. Persistent and recurrent hyperparathyroidism. Curr Treat Options Oncol. 2004 Aug;5(4):335–45. PMID:15233910
**1055.** Carpenter EL, Mossé YP. Targeting ALK in neuroblastoma–preclinical and clinical advancements. Nat Rev Clin Oncol. 2012 May 15;9(7):391–9. PMID:22585002
**1056.** Carpenter TO. Oncogenic osteomalacia–a complex dance of factors. N Engl J Med. 2003 Apr 24;348(17):1705–8. PMID:12711747
**1057.** Carrera C, Scope A, Dusza SW, et al. Clinical and dermoscopic characterization of pediatric and adolescent melanomas: multicenter study of 52 cases. J Am Acad Dermatol. 2018 Feb;78(2):278–88. PMID:29024734
**1058.** Carrillo-Reixach J, Torrens L, Simon-Coma M, et al. Epigenetic footprint enables molecular risk stratification of hepatoblastoma with clinical implications. J Hepatol. 2020 Aug;73(2):328–41. PMID:32240714
**1059.** Carrió M, Gel B, Terribas E, et al. Analysis of intratumor heterogeneity in Neurofibromatosis type 1 plexiform neurofibromas and neurofibromas with atypical features: correlating histological and genomic findings. Hum Mutat. 2018 Aug;39(8):1112–25. PMID:29774626
**1060.** Carroll P, Henshaw RM, Garwood C, et al. Plantar fibromatosis: pathophysiology, surgical and nonsurgical therapies: an evidence-based review. Foot Ankle Spec. 2018 Apr;11(2):168–76. PMID:29310463
**1061.** Carta F, Sionis S, Gerosa C, et al. Endoscopic management of adult-type rhabdomyoma of the glottis: case report and review of the literature. Braz J Otorhinolaryngol. 2016 Mar-Apr;82(2):244–7. PMID:26464107
**1062.** Carta M, Maresi E, Giuffrè M, et al. Congenital hepatic mesenchymal hamartoma associated with mesenchymal stem villous hyperplasia of the placenta: case report. J Pediatr Surg. 2005 May;40(5):e37–9. PMID:15937805
**1063.** Cartault F, Nava C, Malbrunot AC, et al. A new XPC gene splicing mutation has lead to the highest worldwide prevalence of xeroderma pigmentosum in black Mahori patients. DNA Repair (Amst). 2011 Jun 10;10(6):577–85. PMID:21482201
**1064.** Carter JM, Howe BM, Hawse JR, et al. CTNNB1 mutations and estrogen receptor expression in neuromuscular choristoma and its associated fibromatosis. Am J Surg Pathol. 2016 Oct;40(10):1368–74. PMID:27259010
**1065.** Carter JM, O'Hara C, Dundas G, et al. Epithelioid malignant peripheral nerve sheath tumor arising in a schwannoma, in a patient with "neuroblastoma-like" schwannomatosis and a novel germline SMARCB1 mutation. Am J Surg Pathol. 2012 Jan;36(1):154–60. PMID:22082606
**1066.** Carter JM, Wang X, Dong J, et al. USP6 genetic rearrangements in cellular fibroma of tendon sheath. Mod Pathol. 2016 Aug;29(8):865–9. PMID:27125357
**1067.** Carter JM, Wu Y, Blessing MM, et al. Recurrent genomic alterations in soft tissue perineuriomas. Am J Surg Pathol. 2018 Dec;42(12):1708–14. PMID:30303818
**1068.** Carter M, Nicholson J, Ross F, et al. Genetic abnormalities detected in ependymomas by comparative genomic hybridisation. Br J Cancer. 2002 Mar 18;86(6):929–39. PMID:11953826
**1069.** Carter MC, Bai Y, Ruiz-Esteves KN, et al. Detection of KIT D816V in peripheral blood of children with manifestations of cutaneous mastocytosis suggests systemic disease. Br J Haematol. 2018 Dec;183(5):775–82. PMID:30488427
**1070.** Carter MC, Clayton ST, Komarow HD, et al. Assessment of clinical findings, tryptase levels, and bone marrow histopathology in the management of pediatric mastocytosis. J Allergy Clin Immunol. 2015 Dec;136(6):1673–1679.e3. PMID:26044856
**1071.** Carugo A, Minelli R, Sapio L, et al. p53 is a master regulator of proteostasis in SMARCB1-deficient malignant rhabdoid tumors. Cancer Cell. 2019 Feb 11;35(2):204–220.e9. PMID:30753823
**1072.** Carver BS, Bianco FJ Jr, Shayegan B, et al. Predicting teratoma in the retroperitoneum in men undergoing post-chemotherapy retroperitoneal lymph node dissection. J Urol. 2006 Jul;176(1):100–3. PMID:16753380
**1073.** Casadei GP, Komori T, Scheithauer BW, et al. Intracranial parenchymal schwannoma. A clinicopathological and neuroimaging study of nine cases. J Neurosurg. 1993 Aug;79(2):217–22. PMID:8331403
**1074.** Casanova M, Brennan B, Alaggio R, et al. Inflammatory myofibroblastic tumor: the experience of the European pediatric Soft Tissue Sarcoma Study Group (EpSSG). Eur J Cancer. 2020 Mar;127:123–9. PMID:32007712
**1075.** Casanova M, Ferrari A, Collini P, et al. Epithelioid sarcoma in children and adolescents: a report from the Italian Soft Tissue Sarcoma Committee. Cancer. 2006 Feb 1;106(3):708–17. PMID:16353216
**1076.** Casar-Borota O, Bollerslev J, Pontén F. Immunohistochemistry for transcription factor T-Pit as a tool in diagnostics of corticotroph pituitary tumours. Pituitary. 2018 Aug;21(4):443. PMID:29468382
**1077.** Casas-Alba D, Martínez-Monseny A, Pino-Ramírez RM, et al. Hyaline fibromatosis syndrome: clinical update and phenotype-genotype correlations. Hum Mutat. 2018 Dec;39(12):1752–63. PMID:30176098
**1078.** Cascón A, Comino-Méndez I, Currás-Freixes M, et al. Whole-exome sequencing identifies MDH2 as a new familial paraganglioma gene. J Natl Cancer Inst. 2015 Mar 11;107(5):djv053. PMID:25766404
**1079.** Cascón A, Inglada-Pérez L, Comino-Méndez I, et al. Genetics of pheochromocytoma and paraganglioma in Spanish pediatric patients. Endocr Relat Cancer. 2013 May 30;20(3):L1–6. PMID:23404858
**1080.** Cascón A, Tennant DA. From transcriptional profiling to tumor biology in pheochromocytoma and paraganglioma. Endocr Pathol. 2012 Mar;23(1):15–20. PMID:22323008
**1081.** Casey MB, Lohse CM, Lloyd RV. Distinction between papillary thyroid hyperplasia and papillary thyroid carcinoma by immunohistochemical staining for cytokeratin 19, galectin-3, and HBME-1. Endocr Pathol. 2003 Spring;14(1):55–60. PMID:12746563
**1082.** Cassidy FC, Charalambous M. Genomic imprinting, growth and maternal-fetal interactions. J Exp Biol. 2018 Mar 7;221(Pt Suppl 1):jeb164517. PMID:29514882
**1083.** Cassiman C, Casteels I, Jacob J, et al. Choroidal abnormalities in café-au-lait syndromes: a new differential diagnostic tool? Clin Genet. 2017 Apr;91(4):529–35. PMID:27716896
**1084.** Cassol C, Mete O. Endocrine manifestations of von Hippel-Lindau disease. Arch Pathol Lab Med. 2015 Feb;139(2):263–8. PMID:25611110
**1085.** Castagna MG, Fugazzola L, Maino F, et al. Reference range of serum calcitonin in pediatric population. J Clin Endocrinol Metab. 2015 May;100(5):1780–4. PMID:25955324

1086. Castagnetti F, Gugliotta G, Baccarani M, et al. Differences among young adults, adults and elderly chronic myeloid leukemia patients. Ann Oncol. 2015 Jan;26(1):185–92. PMID:25361995
1087. Castedo SM, de Jong B, Oosterhuis JW, et al. Cytogenetic analysis of ten human seminomas. Cancer Res. 1989 Jan 15;49(2):439–43. PMID:2910461
1088. Castel D, Kergrohen T, Tauziède-Espariat A, et al. Histone H3 wild-type DIPG/DMG overexpressing EZHIP extend the spectrum diffuse midline gliomas with PRC2 inhibition beyond H3-K27M mutation. Acta Neuropathol. 2020 Jun;139(6):1109–13. PMID:32193787
1089. Castel D, Philippe C, Calmon R, et al. Histone H3F3A and HIST1H3B K27M mutations define two subgroups of diffuse intrinsic pontine gliomas with different prognosis and phenotypes. Acta Neuropathol. 2015 Dec;130(6):815–27. PMID:26399631
1090. Castel D, Philippe C, Kergrohen T, et al. Transcriptomic and epigenetic profiling of 'diffuse midline gliomas, H3 K27M-mutant' discriminate two subgroups based on the type of histone H3 mutated and not supratentorial or infratentorial location. Acta Neuropathol Commun. 2018 Nov 5;6(1):117. PMID:30396367
1091. Castellanos E, Plana A, Carrato C, et al. Early genetic diagnosis of neurofibromatosis type 2 from skin plaque plexiform schwannomas in childhood. JAMA Dermatol. 2018 Mar 1;154(3):341–6. PMID:29322178
1091A. Castillejo A, Vargas G, Castillejo MI, et al. Prevalence of germline MUTYH mutations among Lynch-like syndrome patients. Eur J Cancer. 2014 Sep;50(13):2241–50. PMID:24953332
1091B. Castillo JJ, Beltran BE, Malpica L, et al. Anaplastic lymphoma kinase-positive large B-cell lymphoma (ALK + LBCL): a systematic review of clinicopathological features and management. Leuk Lymphoma. 2021 Dec;62(12):2845–53. PMID:34151703
1092. Castillo JJ, Bibas M, Miranda RN. The biology and treatment of plasmablastic lymphoma. Blood. 2015 Apr 9;125(15):2323–30. PMID:25636338
1093. Castinetti F, Moley J, Mulligan L, et al. A comprehensive review on MEN2B. Endocr Relat Cancer. 2018 Feb;25(2):T29–39. PMID:28698189
1094. Castrén E, Salminen P, Vikkula M, et al. Inheritance patterns of infantile hemangioma. Pediatrics. 2016 Nov;138(5):e20161623. PMID:27940781
1095. Castro-Malaspina H, Schaison G, Passe S, et al. Subacute and chronic myelomonocytic leukemia in children (juvenile CML). Clinical and hematologic observations, and identification of prognostic factors. Cancer. 1984 Aug 15;54(4):675–86. PMID:6589029
1096. Cates JM, Coffin CM. Extraskeletal cartilaginous, osseous, and chordoid tumors in children and adolescents. Pediatr Dev Pathol. 2012;15(1 Suppl):255–66. PMID:22420731
1097. Cates JM, Coffin CM. Neurogenic tumors of soft tissue. Pediatr Dev Pathol. 2012;15(1 Suppl):62–107. PMID:22420725
1098. Cates JM, Stricker TP, Sturgeon D, et al. Desmoid-type fibromatosis-associated Gardner fibromas: prevalence and impact on local recurrence. Cancer Lett. 2014 Oct 28;353(2):176–81. PMID:25064609
1099. Cates JMM. Modeling continuous prognostic factors in survival analysis: implications for tumor staging and assessing chemotherapy effect in osteosarcoma. Am J Surg Pathol. 2018 Apr;42(4):485–91. PMID:29200101
1100. Cathro HP, Stoler MH. The utility of calretinin, inhibin, and WT1 immunohistochemical staining in the differential diagnosis of ovarian tumors. Hum Pathol. 2005 Feb;36(2):195–201. PMID:15754297
1101. Catic A, Kurtovic-Kozaric A, Johnson SH, et al. A novel cytogenetic and molecular characterization of renal metanephric adenoma: identification of partner genes involved in translocation t(9;15)(p24;q24). Cancer Genet. 2017 Aug;214-215:9–15. PMID:28595733
1102. Cavalcante RB, Nonaka CFW, Santos HBP, et al. Assessment of CTNNB1 gene mutations and β-catenin immunoexpression in salivary gland pleomorphic adenomas and adenoid cystic carcinomas. Virchows Arch. 2018 Jun;472(6):999–1005. PMID:29577164
1103. Cavaliere M, De Luca P, Scarpa A, et al. Acinic cell carcinoma of the parotid gland: from pathogenesis to management: a literature review. Eur Arch Otorhinolaryngol. 2020 Oct;277(10):2673–9. PMID:32367151
1104. Cavalli FMG, Hübner JM, Sharma T, et al. Heterogeneity within the PF-EPN-B ependymoma subgroup. Acta Neuropathol. 2018 Aug;136(2):227–37. PMID:30019219
1105. Cavalli FMG, Remke M, Rampasek L, et al. Intertumoral heterogeneity within medulloblastoma subgroups. Cancer Cell. 2017 Jun 12;31(6):737–754.e6. PMID:28609654
1106. Cavard C, Audebourg A, Letourneur F, et al. Gene expression profiling provides insights into the pathways involved in solid pseudopapillary neoplasm of the pancreas. J Pathol. 2009 Jun;218(2):201–9. PMID:19235837
1107. Cavazzana AO, Schmidt D, Ninfo V, et al. Spindle cell rhabdomyosarcoma. A prognostically favorable variant of rhabdomyosarcoma. Am J Surg Pathol. 1992 Mar;16(3):229–35. PMID:1599014
1108. Cavé H, Caye A, Ghedira N, et al. Mutations in RIT1 cause Noonan syndrome with possible juvenile myelomonocytic leukemia but are not involved in acute lymphoblastic leukemia. Eur J Hum Genet. 2016 Aug;24(8):1124–31. PMID:26757980
1109. Cawthon RM, Weiss R, Xu GF, et al. A major segment of the neurofibromatosis type 1 gene: cDNA sequence, genomic structure, and point mutations. Cell. 1990 Jul 13;62(1):193–201. PMID:2114220
1110. Caye A, Strullu M, Guidez F, et al. Juvenile myelomonocytic leukemia displays mutations in components of the RAS pathway and the PRC2 network. Nat Genet. 2015 Nov;47(11):1334–40. PMID:26457648
1111. Caza T, Manwaring J, Riddell J. Recurrent, bilateral, and metastatic pheochromocytoma in a young patient with Beckwith-Wiedemann syndrome: a genetic link? Can Urol Assoc J. 2017 May;11(5):E240–3. PMID:28503241
1112. Cazes A, Lopez-Delisle L, Tsarovina K, et al. Activated Alk triggers prolonged neurogenesis and Ret upregulation providing a therapeutic target in ALK-mutated neuroblastoma. Oncotarget. 2014 May 15;5(9):2688–702. PMID:24811913
1113. Cazzaniga G, Lanciotti M, Rossi V, et al. Prospective molecular monitoring of BCR/ABL transcript in children with Ph+ acute lymphoblastic leukaemia unravels differences in treatment response. Br J Haematol. 2002 Nov;119(2):445–53. PMID:12406084
1114. Cecchetto G, Alaggio R, Bisogno G, et al. Sex cord-stromal tumors of the testis in children. A clinicopathologic report from the Italian TREP project. J Pediatr Surg. 2010 Sep;45(9):1868–73. PMID:20850634
1114A. Celano E, Salehani A, Malcolm JG, et al. Spinal cord ependymoma: a review of the literature and case series of ten patients. J Neurooncol. 2016 Jul;128(3):377–86. PMID:27154165
1115. Celik SU, Besli Celik D, Yetiskin E, et al. Giant juvenile fibroadenoma of the breast: a clinical case. Arch Argent Pediatr. 2017 Dec 1;115(6):e428–31. PMID:29087128
1116. Centonze G, Mangogna A, Salviato T, et al. Gastroblastoma in adulthood-a rarity among rare cancers-a case report and review of the literature. Case Rep Pathol. 2019 Nov 28;2019:4084196. PMID:31871808
1117. Cerecer-Gil NY, Figuera LE, Llamas FJ, et al. Mutation of SDHB is a cause of hypoxia-related high-altitude paraganglioma. Clin Cancer Res. 2010 Aug 15;16(16):4148–54. PMID:20592014
1118. Cernaianu G, Tannapfel A, Nounla J, et al. Appendiceal carcinoid tumor with lymph node metastasis in a child: case report and review of the literature. J Pediatr Surg. 2010 Nov;45(11):e1–5. PMID:21034920
1119. Cervoni L, Celli P, Caruso R, et al. [Neurinomas and ependymomas of the cauda equina. A review of the clinical characteristics]. Minerva Chir. 1997 May;52(5):629–33. Italian. PMID:9297152
1120. Cesari M, Alberghini M, Vanel D, et al. Periosteal osteosarcoma: a single-institution experience. Cancer. 2011 Apr 15;117(8):1731–5. PMID:21472720
1121. Cesarman E, Damania B, Krown SE, et al. Kaposi sarcoma. Nat Rev Dis Primers. 2019 Jan 31;5(1):9. PMID:30705286
1122. Cessna MH, Zhou H, Sanger WG, et al. Expression of ALK1 and p80 in inflammatory myofibroblastic tumor and its mesenchymal mimics: a study of 135 cases. Mod Pathol. 2002 Sep;15(9):931–8. PMID:12218210
1122A. Cetta F, Curia MC, Montalto G, et al. Thyroid carcinoma usually occurs in patients with familial adenomatous polyposis in the absence of biallelic inactivation of the adenomatous polyposis coli gene. J Clin Endocrinol Metab. 2001 Jan;86(1):427–32. PMID:11232035
1122B. Cetta F, Montalto G, Gori M, et al. Germline mutations of the APC gene in patients with familial adenomatous polyposis-associated thyroid carcinoma: results from a European cooperative study. J Clin Endocrinol Metab. 2000 Jan;85(1):286–92. PMID:10634400
1122C. Cetta F, Ugolini G, Barellini L, et al. FAP associated cribriform morular variant of PTC: striking female prevalence and indolent course. Endocr J. 2011;58(9):817–8. PMID:21878742
1123. Cha YJ, Hong CK, Kim DS, et al. Poorly differentiated chordoma with loss of SMARCB1/INI1 expression in pediatric patients: a report of two cases and review of the literature. Neuropathology. 2018 Feb;38(1):47–53. PMID:28812319
1124. Chadburn A, Chen JM, Hsu DT, et al. The morphologic and molecular genetic categories of posttransplantation lymphoproliferative disorders are clinically relevant. Cancer. 1998 May 15;82(10):1978–87. PMID:9587133
1125. Chai RC, Zhang YW, Liu YQ, et al. The molecular characteristics of spinal cord gliomas with or without H3 K27M mutation. Acta Neuropathol Commun. 2020 Mar 30;8(1):40. PMID:32228694
1126. Chakraborti S, Govindan A, Alapatt JP, et al. Primary myxopapillary ependymoma of the fourth ventricle with cartilaginous metaplasia: a case report and review of the literature. Brain Tumor Pathol. 2012 Jan;29(1):25–30. PMID:21837503
1127. Chakrapani A, Warrick A, Nelson D, et al. BRAF and KRAS mutations in sporadic glomus tumors. Am J Dermatopathol. 2012 Jul;34(5):533–5. PMID:22317887
1128. Chalvardjian A, Scully RE. Sclerosing stromal tumors of the ovary. Cancer. 1973 Mar;31(3):664–70. PMID:4348335
1129. Chamberlain BK, McClain CM, Gonzalez RS, et al. Alveolar soft part sarcoma and granular cell tumor: an immunohistochemical comparison study. Hum Pathol. 2014 May;45(5):1039–44. PMID:24746209
1130. Chami R, Ertresvaag K, Azzie G, et al. Myofibroblastoma: report of a rare entity in the pediatric population. Pediatr Dev Pathol. 2012 Nov-Dec;15(6):499–506. PMID:22901100
1131. Chami R, Yin M, Marrano P, et al. BRAF mutations in pediatric metanephric tumors. Hum Pathol. 2015 Aug;46(8):1153–61. PMID:26014474
1132. Chan AK, Han SJ, Choy W, et al. Familial melanoma-astrocytoma syndrome: synchronous diffuse astrocytoma and pleomorphic xanthoastrocytoma in a patient with germline CDKN2A/B deletion and a significant family history. Clin Neuropathol. 2017 Sep/Oct;36(5):213–21. PMID:28699883
1133. Chan CC, Koch CA, Kaiser-Kupfer MI, et al. Loss of heterozygosity for the NF2 gene in retinal and optic nerve lesions of patients with neurofibromatosis 2. J Pathol. 2002 Sep;198(1):14–20. PMID:12210058
1134. Chan CM, Lindsay AD, Spiguel ARV, et al. Periosteal osteosarcoma: a single-institutional study of factors related to oncologic outcomes. Sarcoma. 2018 Sep 27;2018:8631237. PMID:30363676
1135. Chan CM, Young J, Prager J, et al. Pediatric thyroid cancer. Adv Pediatr. 2017 Aug;64(1):171–90. PMID:28688588
1136. Chan E, Bollen AW, Sirohi D, et al. Angiocentric glioma with MYB-QKI fusion located in the brainstem, rather than cerebral cortex. Acta Neuropathol. 2017 Oct;134(4):671–3. PMID:28776091
1137. Chan GL, Little JB. Cultured diploid fibroblasts from patients with the nevoid basal cell carcinoma syndrome are hypersensitive to killing by ionizing radiation. Am J Pathol. 1983 Apr;111(1):50–5. PMID:6837723
1138. Chan JA, McMenamin ME, Fletcher CD. Synovial sarcoma in older patients: clinicopathological analysis of 32 cases with emphasis on unusual histological features. Histopathology. 2003 Jul;43(1):72–83. PMID:12823715
1139. Chan JA, Zhang H, Roberts PS, et al. Pathogenesis of tuberous sclerosis subependymal giant cell astrocytomas: biallelic inactivation of TSC1 or TSC2 leads to mTOR activation. J Neuropathol Exp Neurol. 2004 Dec;63(12):1236–42. PMID:15624760
1140. Chan JK. Virus-associated neoplasms of the nasopharynx and sinonasal tract: diagnostic problems. Mod Pathol. 2017 Jan;30 s1:S68–83. PMID:28060369
1141. Chan JK, Cheuk W, Shimizu M. Anaplastic lymphoma kinase expression in inflammatory pseudotumors. Am J Surg Pathol. 2001 Jun;25(6):761–8. PMID:11395553
1142. Chan JK, Gardner AB, Chan JE, et al. The influence of age and other prognostic factors associated with survival of ovarian immature teratoma - A study of 1307 patients. Gynecol Oncol. 2016 Sep;142(3):446–51. PMID:27423379
1143. Chan JK, Lamant L, Algar E, et al. ALK+ histiocytosis: a novel type of systemic histiocytic proliferative disorder of early infancy. Blood. 2008 Oct 1;112(7):2965–8. PMID:18660380
1144. Chan JK, Rosai J. Tumors of the neck showing thymic or related branchial pouch differentiation: a unifying concept. Hum Pathol. 1991 Apr;22(4):349–67. PMID:2050369
1145. Chan JK, Sin VC, Wong KF, et al. Nonnasal lymphoma expressing the natural killer cell marker CD56: a clinicopathologic study of 49 cases of an uncommon aggressive neoplasm. Blood. 1997 Jun 15;89(12):4501–13. PMID:9192774
1146. Chan JY, Gooi Z, Wong EW, et al. Low-grade myofibroblastic sarcoma: a

population-based study. Laryngoscope. 2017 Jan;127(1):116–21. PMID:27377169
1147. Chan KM, Fang D, Gan H, et al. The histone H3.3K27M mutation in pediatric glioma reprograms H3K27 methylation and gene expression. Genes Dev. 2013 May 1;27(9):985–90. PMID:23603901
1148. Chan MH, Shing MM, Poon TC, et al. Alpha-fetoprotein variants in a case of pancreatoblastoma. Ann Clin Biochem. 2000 Sep;37(Pt 5):681–5. PMID:11026522
1149. Chan MK, McGuire LJ, King W, et al. Cytodiagnosis of 112 salivary gland lesions. Correlation with histologic and frozen section diagnosis. Acta Cytol. 1992 May-Jun;36(3):353–63. PMID:1580118
1150. Chan MK, McGuire LJ, Lee JC. Fine needle aspiration cytodiagnosis of nasopharyngeal carcinoma in cervical lymph nodes. A study of 40 cases. Acta Cytol. 1989 May-Jun;33(3):344–50. PMID:2543172
1151. Chan V, Marro A, Findlay JM, et al. A systematic review of atypical teratoid rhabdoid tumor in adults. Front Oncol. 2018 Nov 28;8:567. PMID:30547013
1152. Chan WH, Anderson CR, Gonsalvez DG. From proliferation to target innervation: signaling molecules that direct sympathetic nervous system development. Cell Tissue Res. 2018 May;372(2):171–93. PMID:28971249
1153. Chandler JR, Goulding R, Moskowitz L, et al. Nasopharyngeal angiofibromas: staging and management. Ann Otol Rhinol Laryngol. 1984 Jul-Aug;93(4 Pt 1):322–9. PMID:6087710
1154. Chang C, Hung LY, Thanh TT, et al. Congenital peribronchial myofibroblastic tumour with features of maturation in the older infant: report of two cases with a literature review. Histopathology. 2014 Apr;64(5):755–7. PMID:24117734
1155. Chang CH, Housepian EM, Herbert C Jr. An operative staging system and a megavoltage radiotherapeutic technic for cerebellar medulloblastomas. Radiology. 1969 Dec;93(6):1351–9. PMID:4983156
1156. Chang CL, Marra G, Chauhan DP, et al. Oxidative stress inactivates the human DNA mismatch repair system. Am J Physiol Cell Physiol. 2002 Jul;283(1):C148–54. PMID:12055083
1157. Chang HJ, Jin SY, Park C, et al. Mesenchymal hamartomas of the liver: comparison of clinicopathologic features between cystic and solid forms. J Korean Med Sci. 2006 Feb;21(1):63–8. PMID:16479067
1158. Chang JC, Zhang L, Drilon AE, et al. Expanding the molecular characterization of thoracic inflammatory myofibroblastic tumors beyond ALK gene rearrangements. J Thorac Oncol. 2019 May;14(5):825–34. PMID:30550870
1159. Chang MC, Vargas SO, Hornick JL, et al. Embryonic stem cell transcription factors and D2-40 (podoplanin) as diagnostic immunohistochemical markers in ovarian germ cell tumors. Int J Gynecol Pathol. 2009 Jul;28(4):347–55. PMID:19483629
1160. Chang MH. Decreasing incidence of hepatocellular carcinoma among children following universal hepatitis B immunization. Liver Int. 2003 Oct;23(5):309–14. PMID:14708890
1161. Chang MH, You SL, Chen CJ, et al. Decreased incidence of hepatocellular carcinoma in hepatitis B vaccinees: a 20-year follow-up study. J Natl Cancer Inst. 2009 Oct 7;101(19):1348–55. PMID:19759364
1162. Chang MY, Shin HJ, Kim HG, et al. Prepubertal testicular teratomas and epidermoid cysts: comparison of clinical and sonographic features. J Ultrasound Med. 2015 Oct;34(10):1745–51. PMID:26324756
1163. Chang SE, Choi JH, Sung KJ, et al. A case of cutaneous low-grade myofibroblastic sarcoma. J Dermatol. 2001 Jul;28(7):383–7. PMID:11510507
1164. Chang SM, Lillis-Hearne PK, Larson DA, et al. Pineoblastoma in adults. Neurosurgery. 1995 Sep;37(3):383–90. PMID:7501100
1165. Chang W, Oiseth SJ, Orentlicher R, et al. Bilateral sclerosing stromal tumor of the ovaries in a premenarchal girl. Gynecol Oncol. 2006 May;101(2):342–5. PMID:16403568
1166. Chang Y, Cesarman E, Pessin MS, et al. Identification of herpesvirus-like DNA sequences in AIDS-associated Kaposi's sarcoma. Science. 1994 Dec 16;266(5192):1865–9. PMID:7997879
1167. Chant H, Ashleigh R, McCollum C. Thrombectomy for acute internal carotid thrombosis: five thrombectomy devices compared. Eur J Vasc Endovasc Surg. 2004 Apr;27(4):403–8. PMID:15015191
1168. Chao AK, Meyer JA, Lee AG, et al. Fusion driven JMML: a novel CCDC88C-FLT3 fusion responsive to sorafenib identified by RNA sequencing. Leukemia. 2020 Feb;34(2):662–6. PMID:31511612
1169. Chao C, Silverberg MJ, Chen LH, et al. Novel tumor markers provide improved prediction of survival after diagnosis of human immunodeficiency virus (HIV)-related diffuse large B-cell lymphoma. Leuk Lymphoma. 2018 Feb;59(2):321–9. PMID:28610450
1170. Chao L, Tao XB, Jun YK, et al. Recurrence and histological evolution of dysembryoplastic neuroepithelial tumor: a case report and review of the literature. Oncol Lett. 2013 Oct;6(4):907–14. PMID:24137435
1171. Chapel DB, Husain AN, Krausz T, et al. PAX8 expression in a subset of malignant peritoneal mesotheliomas and benign mesothelium has diagnostic implications in the differential diagnosis of ovarian serous carcinoma. Am J Surg Pathol. 2017 Dec;41(12):1675–82. PMID:28877056
1172. Chapel H, Lucas M, Lee M, et al. Common variable immunodeficiency disorders: division into distinct clinical phenotypes. Blood. 2008 Jul 15;112(2):277–86. PMID:18319398
1173. Chaplin AJ, Darke P, Patel S. Tyrosine-rich crystals in pleomorphic adenomas of parotid glands. J Oral Pathol. 1983 Oct;12(5):342–6. PMID:6195320
1174. Chappé C, Padovani L, Scavarda D, et al. Dysembryoplastic neuroepithelial tumors share with pleomorphic xanthoastrocytomas and gangliogliomas BRAF(V600E) mutation and expression. Brain Pathol. 2013 Sep;23(5):574–83. PMID:23442159
1175. Chappell AG, Chase EP, Chang B, et al. Atypical fibroxanthoma in a 13-year-old guatemalan girl with xeroderma pigmentosum. Pediatr Dermatol. 2016 May;33(3):e228–9. PMID:27046537
1176. Chappell T, Creech CB, Parra D, et al. Presentation of pulmonary artery intimal sarcoma in an infant with a history of neonatal valvular pulmonic stenosis. Ann Thorac Surg. 2008 Mar;85(3):1092–4. PMID:18291210
1177. Chapuy B, Stewart C, Dunford AJ, et al. Genomic analyses of PMBL reveal new drivers and mechanisms of sensitivity to PD-1 blockade. Blood. 2019 Dec 26;134(26):2369–82. PMID:31697821
1178. Chapuy B, Stewart C, Dunford AJ, et al. Molecular subtypes of diffuse large B cell lymphoma are associated with distinct pathogenic mechanisms and outcomes. Nat Med. 2018 May;24(5):679–90. PMID:29713087
1179. Charbel C, Fontaine RH, Malouf GG, et al. NRAS mutation is the sole recurrent somatic mutation in large congenital melanocytic nevi. J Invest Dermatol. 2014 Apr;134(4):1067–74. PMID:24129063
1180. Charles SJ, Moore AT, Yates JR, et al. Lisch nodules in neurofibromatosis type 2. Case report. Arch Ophthalmol. 1989 Nov;107(11):1571–2. PMID:2510706
1181. Charlton J, Irtan S, Bergeron C, et al. Bilateral Wilms tumour: a review of clinical and molecular features. Expert Rev Mol Med. 2017 Jul 18;19:e8. PMID:28716159
1182. Charville GW, Wang WL, Ingram DR, et al. EWSR1 fusion proteins mediate PAX7 expression in Ewing sarcoma. Mod Pathol. 2017 Sep;30(9):1312–20. PMID:28643791
1183. Chase DR, Enzinger FM. Epithelioid sarcoma. Diagnosis, prognostic indicators, and treatment. Am J Surg Pathol. 1985 Apr;9(4):241–63. PMID:4014539
1184. Chatterjee A, Ghosh J, Kapur R. Mastocytosis: a mutated KIT receptor induced myeloproliferative disorder. Oncotarget. 2015 Jul 30;6(21):18250–64. PMID:26158763
1185. Chatterjee D, Garg C, Singla N, et al. Desmoplastic non-infantile astrocytoma/ganglioglioma: rare low-grade tumor with frequent BRAF V600E mutation. Hum Pathol. 2018 Oct;80:186–91. PMID:29902580
1186. Chatzellis E, Alexandraki KI, Androulakis II, et al. Aggressive pituitary tumors. Neuroendocrinology. 2015;101(2):87–104. PMID:25571935
1187. Chau C, van Doorn R, van Poppelen NM, et al. Families with BAP1-tumor predisposition syndrome in the Netherlands: path to identification and a proposal for genetic screening guidelines. Cancers (Basel). 2019 Aug 4;11(8):E1114. PMID:31382694
1188. Chau NG, Ma C, Danga K, et al. An anatomical site and genetic-based prognostic model for patients with nuclear protein in testis (NUT) midline carcinoma: analysis of 124 patients. JNCI Cancer Spectr. 2019 Nov 6;4(2):pkz094. PMID:32328562
1189. Chaudhary P, Bhadana U, Singh RA, et al. Primary hepatic angiosarcoma. Eur J Surg Oncol. 2015 Sep;41(9):1137–43. PMID:26008857
1190. Chaudhri AA, Lee L, Das K. Cellular metanephric stromal tumor in a postmenopausal woman: a case report with review of the literature. Int J Surg Pathol. 2013 Apr;21(2):153–60. PMID:22832110
1191. Chaudhry AP, Labay GR, Yamane GM, et al. Clinico-pathologic and histogenetic study of 189 intraoral minor salivary gland tumors. J Oral Med. 1984 Apr-Jun;39(2):58–78. PMID:6330327
1192. Chaudhry IH, Kazakov DV, Michal M, et al. Fibro-osseous pseudotumor of the digit: a clinicopathological study of 17 cases. J Cutan Pathol. 2010 Mar;37(3):323–9. PMID:19678826
1193. Chaudry G. Complex lymphatic anomalies and therapeutic options. Tech Vasc Interv Radiol. 2019 Dec;22(4):100632. PMID:31864531
1194. Chaurasia JK, Afroz N, Maheshwari V, et al. Sclerosing stromal tumour of the ovary presenting as precocious puberty: a rare neoplasm. BMJ Case Rep. 2014 Mar 31;2014:bcr2013201124. PMID:24686794
1195. Chaussade A, Millot G, Wells C, et al. Correlation between RB1germline mutations and second primary malignancies in hereditary retinoblastoma patients treated with external beam radiotherapy. Eur J Med Genet. 2019 Mar;62(3):217–23. PMID:30031154
1196. Chavez JC, Sandoval-Sus J, Horna P, et al. Lymphomatoid granulomatosis: a single institution experience and review of the literature. Clin Lymphoma Myeloma Leuk. 2016 Aug;16 Suppl:S170–4. PMID:27521314
1197. Chavez M, Mafee MF, Castillo B, et al. Medulloepithelioma of the optic nerve. J Pediatr Ophthalmol Strabismus. 2004 Jan-Feb;41(1):48–52. PMID:14974835
1198. Chaweephisal P, Sosothikul D, Polprasert C, et al. Subcutaneous panniculitis-like T-cell lymphoma with hemophagocytic lymphohistiocytosis syndrome in children and its essential role of HAVCR2 gene mutation analysis. J Pediatr Hematol Oncol. 2021 Jan;43(1):e80–4. PMID:33003142
1199. Cheadle JP, Reeve MP, Sampson JR, et al. Molecular genetic advances in tuberous sclerosis. Hum Genet. 2000 Aug;107(2):97–114. PMID:11030407
1200. Cheah AL, Zou Y, Lanigan C, et al. ALK expression in angiomatoid fibrous histiocytoma: a potential diagnostic pitfall. Am J Surg Pathol. 2019 Jan;43(1):93–101. PMID:29877921
1201. Chebib I, Hornicek FJ, Nielsen GP, et al. Cytomorphologic features that distinguish schwannoma from other low-grade spindle cell lesions. Cancer Cytopathol. 2015 Mar;123(3):171–9. PMID:25641870
1202. Chelliah D, Mensah Sarfo-Poku C, Stea BD, et al. Medulloblastoma with extensive nodularity undergoing post-therapeutic maturation to a gangliocytoma: a case report and literature review. Pediatr Neurosurg. 2010;46(5):381–4. PMID:21389751
1203. Cheminant M, Mahlaoui N, Desconclois C, et al. Lymphoproliferative disease in patients with Wiskott-Aldrich syndrome: analysis of the French Registry of Primary Immunodeficiencies. J Allergy Clin Immunol. 2019 Jun;143(6):2311–5.e7. PMID:30796981
1204. Chen AR, Alonzo TA, Woods WG, et al. Current controversies: Which patients with acute myeloid leukaemia should receive a bone marrow transplantation?–An American view. Br J Haematol. 2002 Aug;118(2):378–84. PMID:12139721
1205. Chen CC, Liau CT, Chang CH, et al. Giant cell tumors of the bone with pulmonary metastasis. Orthopedics. 2016 Jan-Feb;39(1):e68–73. PMID:26730686
1206. Chen CH, Boag AH, Beiko DT, et al. Composite paraganglioma-ganglioneuroma of the urinary bladder: a rare neoplasm causing hemodynamic crisis at tumour resection. Can Urol Assoc J. 2009 Oct;3(5):E45–8. PMID:19829717
1207. Chen CL, Su IJ, Hsu MM, et al. Granulomatous nasopharyngeal carcinoma: with emphasis on difficulty in diagnosis and favorable outcome. J Formos Med Assoc. 1991 Apr;90(4):353–6. PMID:1717637
1208. Chen CW, Chang WC, Lee HS, et al. MRI features of lipoblastoma: differentiating from other palpable lipomatous tumor in pediatric patients. Clin Imaging. 2010 Nov-Dec;34(6):453–7. PMID:21092875
1209. Chen D, Hu XJ, Lin XX, et al. Nodules arising within port-wine stains: a clinicopathologic study of 31 cases. Am J Dermatopathol. 2011 Apr;33(2):144–51. PMID:20940617
1210. Chen DH, Below JE, Shimamura A, et al. Ataxia-pancytopenia syndrome is caused by missense mutations in SAMD9L. Am J Hum Genet. 2016 Jun 2;98(6):1146–58. PMID:27259050
1211. Chen G, Folpe AL, Colby TV, et al. Angiomatoid fibrous histiocytoma: unusual sites and unusual morphology. Mod Pathol. 2011 Dec;24(12):1560–70. PMID:21822206
1212. Chen H, Sippel RS, O'Dorisio MS, et al. The North American Neuroendocrine Tumor Society consensus guideline for the diagnosis and management of neuroendocrine tumors: pheochromocytoma, paraganglioma, and medullary thyroid cancer. Pancreas. 2010 Aug;39(6):775–83. PMID:20664475
1213. Chen H, Zhang S, Wen JC, et al. Several types of soft tissue sarcomas originate

from the malignant transformation of adipose tissue-derived stem cells. Mol Med Rep. 2010 May-Jun;3(3):441–8. PMID:21472259

**1214.** Chen J, Hu F. Clinical and prognostic analysis in 32 pediatric nasopharyngeal carcinoma. J Cancer Res Ther. 2015 Oct;11 Suppl 2:C226–9. PMID:26506882

**1215.** Chen J, Jian X, Deng S, et al. Identification of recurrent USP48 and BRAF mutations in Cushing's disease. Nat Commun. 2018 Aug 9;9(1):3171. PMID:30093687

**1216.** Chen JS, Tzeng CC, Tsao CJ, et al. Clonal karyotype abnormalities in EBV-associated hemophagocytic syndrome. Haematologica. 1997 Sep-Oct;82(5):572–6. PMID:9407723

**1217.** Chen L, Al-Kzayer LF, Liu T, et al. IFR4/MUM1-positive lymphoma in Waldeyer ring with co-expression of CD5 and CD10. Pediatr Blood Cancer. 2017 Feb;64(2):311–4. PMID:27616053

**1218.** Chen L, Li Y, Lin JH. Intraneural perineurioma in a child with Beckwith-Wiedemann syndrome. J Pediatr Surg. 2005 Feb;40(2):E12–4. PMID:15750909

**1219.** Chen LJ, Lai IC, Wong TT, et al. Can mixed pure hepatocellular carcinoma and germinoma arise together in the brain? J Chin Med Assoc. 2015 Sep;78(9):562–6. PMID:26299462

**1220.** Chen Q, Zhang B, Dong Y, et al. Comparison between intravenous chemotherapy and intra-arterial chemotherapy for retinoblastoma: a meta-analysis. BMC Cancer. 2018 Apr 27;18(1):486. PMID:29703164

**1221.** Chen RJ, Chen KY, Chang TC, et al. Prognosis and treatment of squamous cell carcinoma from a mature cystic teratoma of the ovary. J Formos Med Assoc. 2008 Nov;107(11):857–68. PMID:18971155

**1222.** Chen S, Deniz K, Sung YS, et al. Ewing sarcoma with ERG gene rearrangements: a molecular study focusing on the prevalence of FUS-ERG and common pitfalls in detecting EWSR1-ERG fusions by FISH. Genes Chromosomes Cancer. 2016 Apr;55(4):340–9. PMID:26690869

**1223.** Chen SJT, Tse JY, Harms PW, et al. Utility of CD123 immunohistochemistry in differentiating lupus erythematosus from cutaneous T cell lymphoma. Histopathology. 2019 May;74(6):908–16. PMID:30597607

**1224.** Chen ST, Lee JC. An inflammatory myofibroblastic tumor in liver with ALK and RANBP2 gene rearrangement: combination of distinct morphologic, immunohistochemical, and genetic features. Hum Pathol. 2008 Dec;39(12):1854–8. PMID:18701132

**1225.** Chen TJ, Chen SS. Effects of non-pathological factors on brain stem auditory evoked potentials in rats. Gaoxiong Yi Xue Ke Xue Za Zhi. 1988 Oct;4(10):553–64. PMID:3230601

**1226.** Chen W, Soon YY, Pratiseyo PD, et al. Central nervous system neuroepithelial tumors with MN1-alteration: an individual patient data meta-analysis of 73 cases. Brain Tumor Pathol. 2020 Oct;37(4):145–53. PMID:32601775

**1227.** Chen X, Bahrami A, Pappo A, et al. Recurrent somatic structural variations contribute to tumorigenesis in pediatric osteosarcoma. Cell Rep. 2014 Apr 10;7(1):104–12. PMID:24703847

**1228.** Chen X, Pan C, Zhang P, et al. BRAF V600E mutation is a significant prognosticator of the tumour regrowth rate in brainstem gangliogliomas. J Clin Neurosci. 2017 Dec;46:50–7. PMID:28986151

**1229.** Chen X, Rutledge JC, Wu D, et al. Chronic myelogenous leukemia presenting in blast phase with nodal, bilineal myeloid sarcoma and T-lymphoblastic lymphoma in a child. Pediatr Dev Pathol. 2013 Mar-Apr;16(2):91–6. PMID:23171293

**1230.** Chen Y, Tian T, Guo X, et al. Polymorphous low-grade neuroepithelial tumor of the young: case report and review focus on the radiological features and genetic alterations. BMC Neurol. 2020 Apr 6;20(1):123. PMID:32252664

**1231.** Chen Y, Zhang J, Han Y, et al. Benign pediatric jaw lesions at Massachusetts General Hospital over 13 years. J Oral Maxillofac Surg. 2020 Jul;78(7):1124–35. PMID:32114009

**1232.** Chen YB, Mirsadraei L, Jayakumaran G, et al. Somatic mutations of TSC2 or MTOR characterize a morphologically distinct subset of sporadic renal cell carcinoma with eosinophilic and vacuolated cytoplasm. Am J Surg Pathol. 2019 Jan;43(1):121–31. PMID:30303819

**1233.** Chen Z, Liu C, Patel AJ, et al. Cells of origin in the embryonic nerve roots for NF1-associated plexiform neurofibroma. Cancer Cell. 2014 Nov 10;26(5):695–706. PMID:25446898

**1234.** Chen Z, Mo J, Brosseau JP, et al. Spatiotemporal loss of NF1 in Schwann cell lineage leads to different types of cutaneous neurofibroma susceptible to modification by the Hippo pathway. Cancer Discov. 2019 Jan;9(1):114–29. PMID:30348677

**1235.** Chen Z, Wang M, Guan P, et al. Comparison of systemic EBV-positive T-cell and NK-cell lymphoproliferative diseases of childhood based on classification evolution: new classification, old problems. Am J Surg Pathol. 2020 Aug;44(8):1061–72. PMID:32317607

**1236.** Chenevert J, Barnes LE, Chiosea SI. Mucoepidermoid carcinoma — a five-decade journey. Virchows Arch. 2011 Feb;458(2):133–40. PMID:21243374

**1237.** Cheng E, D'Alfonso T, Patel A, et al. Mammary juvenile papillomatosis ("Swiss cheese" disease): study of 121 cases reiterates need for long-term follow-up. Breast J. 2018 Nov;24(6):1136–7. PMID:30051564

**1238.** Cheng H, Yang S, Cai S, et al. Clinical and prognostic characteristics of 53 cases of extracranial malignant rhabdoid tumor in children. a single-institute experience from 2007 to 2017. Oncologist. 2019 Jul;24(7):e551–8. PMID:30914466

**1239.** Cheng H, Yang S, Ren Q, et al. Pancreatectomies for pediatric pancreatic tumors: a single institute experience from 2007 to 2018. J Pediatr Surg. 2020 Sep;55(9):1722–6. PMID:31575410

**1240.** Cheng JC, Au AW. Infantile torticollis: a review of 624 cases. J Pediatr Orthop. 1994 Nov-Dec;14(6):802–8. PMID:7814599

**1241.** Cheng JC, Tang SP, Chen TM. Sternocleidomastoid pseudotumor and congenital muscular torticollis in infants: a prospective study of 510 cases. J Pediatr. 1999 Jun;134(6):712–6. PMID:10356139

**1242.** Cheng JC, Wong MW, Tang SP, et al. Clinical determinants of the outcome of manual stretching in the treatment of congenital muscular torticollis in infants. A prospective study of eight hundred and twenty-one cases. J Bone Joint Surg Am. 2001 May;83(5):679–87. PMID:11379737

**1243.** Cheng JX, Tretiakova M, Gong C, et al. Renal medullary carcinoma: rhabdoid features and the absence of INI1 expression as markers of aggressive behavior. Mod Pathol. 2008 Jun;21(6):647–52. PMID:18327209

**1244.** Cheng L, Leibovich BC, Cheville JC, et al. Paraganglioma of the urinary bladder: Can biologic potential be predicted? Cancer. 2000 Feb 15;88(4):844–52. PMID:10679654

**1245.** Cheng L, Thomas A, Roth LM, et al. OCT4: a novel biomarker for dysgerminoma of the ovary. Am J Surg Pathol. 2004 Oct;28(10):1341–6. PMID:15371950

**1246.** Cheng Z, Cheung P, Kuo AJ, et al. A molecular threading mechanism underlies

Jumonji lysine demethylase KDM2A regulation of methylated H3K36. Genes Dev. 2014 Aug 15;28(16):1758–71. PMID:25128496

**1247.** Chentli F, Belhimer F, Kessaci F, et al. Congenital craniopharyngioma: a case report and literature review. J Pediatr Endocrinol Metab. 2012;25(11-12):1181–3. PMID:23329768

**1248.** Cheon M, Jung KE, Kim HS, et al. Medallion-like dermal dendrocyte hamartoma: differential diagnosis with congenital atrophic dermatofibrosarcoma protuberans. Ann Dermatol. 2013 Aug;25(3):382–4. PMID:24003290

**1249.** Chera BS, Olivier K, Morris CG, et al. Clinical presentation and outcomes of lymphocyte-predominant Hodgkin disease at the University of Florida. Am J Clin Oncol. 2007 Dec;30(6):601–6. PMID:18091054

**1250.** Chetty R, Biddolph S, Gatter K. An immunohistochemical analysis of Reed-Sternberg-like cells in posttransplantation lymphoproliferative disorders: the possible pathogenetic relationship to Reed-Sternberg cells in Hodgkin's disease and Reed-Sternberg-like cells in non-Hodgkin's lymphomas and reactive conditions. Hum Pathol. 1997 Apr;28(4):493–8. PMID:9104951

**1251.** Chetty R, Goetsch S, Nayler S, et al. Spindle epithelial tumour with thymus-like element (SETTLE): the predominantly monophasic variant. Histopathology. 1998 Jul;33(1):71–4. PMID:9726052

**1252.** Chetty R, Serra S. Membrane loss and aberrant nuclear localization of E-cadherin are consistent features of solid pseudopapillary tumour of the pancreas. An immunohistochemical study using two antibodies recognizing different domains of the E-cadherin molecule. Histopathology. 2008 Feb;52(3):325–30. PMID:18269583

**1253.** Cheuk DK, Billups CA, Martin MG, et al. Prognostic factors and long-term outcomes of childhood nasopharyngeal carcinoma. Cancer. 2011 Jan 1;117(1):197–206. PMID:20737561

**1254.** Cheuk W, Jacobson AA, Chan JK. Spindle epithelial tumor with thymus-like differentiation (SETTLE): a distinctive malignant thyroid neoplasm with significant metastatic potential. Mod Pathol. 2000 Oct;13(10):1150–5. PMID:11048811

**1255.** Cheung CC, Ezzat S, Freeman JL, et al. Immunohistochemical diagnosis of papillary thyroid carcinoma. Mod Pathol. 2001 Apr;14(4):338–42. PMID:11301350

**1256.** Cheung JM, Putra J. Congenital granular cell epulis: classic presentation and its differential diagnosis. Head Neck Pathol. 2020 Mar;14(1):208–11. PMID:30888637

**1257.** Cheung K, Taghinia AH, Sood RF, et al. Fibroadipose vascular anomaly in the upper extremity: a distinct entity with characteristic clinical, radiological, and histopathological findings. J Hand Surg Am. 2020 Jan;45(1):68.e1–13. PMID:31279623

**1258.** Cheung M, Kadariya Y, Talarchek J, et al. Germline BAP1 mutation in a family with high incidence of multiple primary cancers and a potential gene-environment interaction. Cancer Lett. 2015 Dec 28;369(2):261–5. PMID:26409435

**1259.** Cheung M, Testa JR. BAP1, a tumor suppressor gene driving malignant mesothelioma. Transl Lung Cancer Res. 2017 Jun;6(3):270–8. PMID:28713672

**1260.** Cheung NK, Zhang J, Lu C, et al. Association of age at diagnosis and genetic mutations in patients with neuroblastoma. JAMA. 2012 Mar 14;307(10):1062–71. PMID:22416102

**1261.** Cheung YH, Gayden T, Campeau PM, et al. A recurrent PDGFRB mutation causes familial infantile myofibromatosis. Am J Hum Genet. 2013 Jun 6;92(6):996–1000. PMID:23731537

**1262.** Chévez-Barrios P, Eagle RC Jr, Krailo M, et al. Study of unilateral retinoblastoma with and without histopathologic high-risk features and the role of adjuvant chemotherapy: a Children's Oncology Group study. J Clin Oncol. 2019 Nov 1;37(31):2883–91. PMID:31539297

**1263.** Cheville JC, Rao S, Iczkowski KA, et al. Cytokeratin expression in seminoma of the human testis. Am J Clin Pathol. 2000 Apr;113(4):583–8. PMID:10761461

**1264.** Chhuon Y, Weon YC, Park G, et al. Pituitary blastoma in a 19-year-old woman: a case report and review of literature. World Neurosurg. 2020 Jul;139:310–3. PMID:32339726

**1265.** Chi SN, Zimmerman MA, Yao X, et al. Intensive multimodality treatment for children with newly diagnosed CNS atypical teratoid rhabdoid tumor. J Clin Oncol. 2009 Jan 20;27(3):385–9. PMID:19064966

**1266.** Chiale F, Abrigo E, Lonati L, et al. Severe arterial hypertension and hyperandrogenism in a boy: a rare case of catecholamine- and β-HCG-secreting pheochromocytoma. J Pediatr Endocrinol Metab. 2019 Oct 25;32(10):1193–7. PMID:31490776

**1267.** Chiang AJ, La V, Peng J, et al. Squamous cell carcinoma arising from mature cystic teratoma of the ovary. Int J Gynecol Cancer. 2011 Apr;21(3):466–74. PMID:21430455

**1268.** Chiang J, Dalton J, Upadhyaya SA, et al. Chromosome arm 1q gain is an adverse prognostic factor in localized and diffuse leptomeningeal glioneuronal tumors with BRAF gene fusion and 1p deletion. Acta Neuropathol. 2019 Jan;137(1):179–81. PMID:30465258

**1269.** Chiang J, Harreld JH, Tinkle CL, et al. A single-center study of the clinicopathologic correlates of gliomas with a MYB or MYBL1 alteration. Acta Neuropathol. 2019 Dec;138(6):1091–2. PMID:31595312

**1270.** Chiang J, Li X, Liu APY, et al. Tectal glioma harbors high rates of KRAS G12R and concomitant KRAS and BRAF alterations. Acta Neuropathol. 2020 Mar;139(3):601–2. PMID:31822998

**1271.** Chiang JCH, Harreld JH, Orr BA, et al. Low-grade spinal glioneuronal tumors with BRAF gene fusion and 1p deletion but without leptomeningeal dissemination. Acta Neuropathol. 2017 Jul;134(1):159–62. PMID:28547128

**1272.** Chiang JCH, Harreld JH, Tanaka R, et al. Septal dysembryoplastic neuroepithelial tumor: a comprehensive clinical, imaging, histopathologic, and molecular analysis. Neuro Oncol. 2019 Jun 10;21(6):800–8. PMID:30726976

**1273.** Chiang S, Snuderl M, Kojiro-Sanada S, et al. Primitive neuroectodermal tumors of the female genital tract: a morphologic, immunohistochemical, and molecular study of 19 cases. Am J Surg Pathol. 2017 Jun;41(6):761–72. PMID:28296680

**1274.** Chiaravalli S, Guzzo M, Bisogno G, et al. Salivary gland carcinomas in children and adolescents: the Italian TREP project experience. Pediatr Blood Cancer. 2014 Nov;61(11):1961–8. PMID:25132368

**1275.** Chiarle R, Simmons WJ, Cai H, et al. Stat3 is required for ALK-mediated lymphomagenesis and provides a possible therapeutic target. Nat Med. 2005 Jun;11(6):623–9. PMID:15895073

**1276.** Chibon F, Mairal A, Fréneaux P, et al. The RB1 gene is the target of chromosome 13 deletions in malignant fibrous histiocytoma. Cancer Res. 2000 Nov 15;60(22):6339–45. PMID:11103795

**1277.** Chiechi MV, Smirniotopoulos JG, Mena H. Pineal parenchymal tumors: CT and MR features. J Comput Assist Tomogr. 1995 Jul-Aug;19(4):509–17. PMID:7622675

1278. Chiller KG, Passaro D, Frieden IJ. Hemangiomas of infancy: clinical characteristics, morphologic subtypes, and their relationship to race, ethnicity, and sex. Arch Dermatol. 2002 Dec;138(12):1567–76. PMID:12472344
1279. Chin M, Mugishima H, Takamura M, et al. Hemophagocytic syndrome and hepatosplenic gammadelta T-cell lymphoma with isochromosome 7q and 8 trisomy. J Pediatr Hematol Oncol. 2004 Jun;26(6):375–8. PMID:15167351
1280. Chinnock R, Webber SA, Dipchand AI, et al. A 16-year multi-institutional study of the role of age and EBV status on PTLD incidence among pediatric heart transplant recipients. Am J Transplant. 2012 Nov;12(11):3061–8. PMID:23072522
1281. Chiosea SI, Thompson LD, Weinreb I, et al. Subsets of salivary duct carcinoma defined by morphologic evidence of pleomorphic adenoma, PLAG1 or HMGA2 rearrangements, and common genetic alterations. Cancer. 2016 Oct 15;122(20):3136–44. PMID:27379604
1282. Chiosea SI, Williams L, Griffith CC, et al. Molecular characterization of apocrine salivary duct carcinoma. Am J Surg Pathol. 2015 Jun;39(6):744–52. PMID:25723113
1283. Chisholm KM, Denton C, Keel S, et al. Bone marrow morphology associated with germline RUNX1 mutations in patients with familial platelet disorder with associated myeloid malignancy. Pediatr Dev Pathol. 2019 Jul-Aug;22(4):315–28. PMID:30600763
1284. Chisholm KM, Mohlman J, Liew M, et al. IRF4 translocation status in pediatric follicular and diffuse large B-cell lymphoma patients enrolled in Children's Oncology Group trials. Pediatr Blood Cancer. 2019 Aug;66(8):e27770. PMID:31012208
1285. Chivukula M, Hunt J, Carter G, et al. Recurrent gynandroblastoma of ovary-A case report: a molecular and immunohistochemical analysis. Int J Gynecol Pathol. 2007 Jan;26(1):30–3. PMID:17197894
1286. Chmara M, Wernstedt A, Wasag B, et al. Multiple pilomatricomas with somatic CTNNB1 mutations in children with constitutive mismatch repair deficiency. Genes Chromosomes Cancer. 2013 Jul;52(7):656–64. PMID:23629955
1287. Chmielecki J, Hutchinson KE, Frampton GM, et al. Comprehensive genomic profiling of pancreatic acinar cell carcinomas identifies recurrent RAF fusions and frequent inactivation of DNA repair genes. Cancer Discov. 2014 Dec;4(12):1398–405. PMID:25266736
1288. Ch'ng ES, Hoshida Y, Iizuka N, et al. Composite malignant pheochromocytoma with malignant peripheral nerve sheath tumour: a case with 28 years of tumour-bearing history. Histopathology. 2007 Sep;51(3):420–2. PMID:17727489
1289. Cho BK, Wang KC, Nam DH, et al. Pineal tumors: experience with 48 cases over 10 years. Childs Nerv Syst. 1998 Jan-Feb;14(1-2):53–8. PMID:9548342
1290. Cho H, Kim JY, Lee Y, et al. Renal involvement and favorable outcome in a child with mastocytosis. Clin Nephrol. 2020 Nov;94(5):260–5. PMID:32831156
1291. Cho YJ, Kim JY. Alveolar soft part sarcoma: clinical presentation, treatment and outcome in a series of 19 patients. Clin Orthop Surg. 2014 Mar;6(1):80–6. PMID:24605193
1292. Choi E, Kim SI, Won JK, et al. Clinicopathological and molecular analysis of multinodular and vacuolating neuronal tumors of the cerebrum. Hum Pathol. 2019 Apr;86:203–12. PMID:30550736
1293. Choi EJ, Sloma EA, Miller AD. Kir7.1 immunoreactivity in canine choroid plexus tumors. J Vet Diagn Invest. 2016 Jul;28(4):464–8. PMID:27216721
1294. Choi EK, Chévez-Barrios P. Inflamed conjunctival nevi: histopathological criteria. Arch Pathol Lab Med. 2014 Sep;138(9):1242–6. PMID:25171709
1295. Choi J, Goh G, Walradt T, et al. Genomic landscape of cutaneous T cell lymphoma. Nat Genet. 2015 Sep;47(9):1011–9. PMID:26192916
1296. Choi JW, Lee JY, Phi JH, et al. Clinical course of vestibular schwannoma in pediatric neurofibromatosis Type 2. J Neurosurg Pediatr. 2014 Jun;13(6):650–7. PMID:24724714
1297. Chong EM, Coffee RE, Chintagumpala M, et al. Extensively necrotic retinoblastoma is associated with high-risk prognostic factors. Arch Pathol Lab Med. 2006 Nov;130(11):1669–72. PMID:17076529
1298. Chong PS, Vucic S, Hedley-Whyte ET, et al. Multiple symmetric lipomatosis (Madelung's disease) Caused by the MERRF (A8344G) Mutation: a Report of Two Cases and Review of the Literature. J Clin Neuromuscul Dis. 2003 Sep;5(1):1–7. PMID:19078716
1299. Chooback N, Shen Y, Jones M, et al. Carcinoma ex pleomorphic adenoma: case report and options for systemic therapy. Curr Oncol. 2017 Jun;24(3):e251–4. PMID:28680294
1300. Choong PF, Pritchard DJ, Rock MG, et al. Low grade central osteogenic sarcoma. A long-term followup of 20 patients. Clin Orthop Relat Res. 1996 Jan; (322):198–206. PMID:8542697
1301. Chou A, Brown IS, Kumarasinghe MP, et al. RET gene rearrangements occur in a subset of pancreatic acinar cell carcinomas. Mod Pathol. 2020 Apr;33(4):657–64. PMID:31558784
1302. Chou AJ, Geller DS, Gorlick R. Therapy for osteosarcoma: Where do we go from here? Paediatr Drugs. 2008;10(5):315–27. PMID:18754698
1303. Choudhary K, Panda S, Beena VT, et al. Sialoblastoma: a literature review from 1966-2011. Natl J Maxillofac Surg. 2013 Jan;4(1):13–8. PMID:24163547
1304. Choueiri TK, Cheville J, Palescandolo E, et al. BRAF mutations in metanephric adenoma of the kidney. Eur Urol. 2012 Nov;62(5):917–22. PMID:22727996
1305. Chougule A, Taylor MS, Nardi V, et al. Spindle and round cell sarcoma with EWSR1-PATZ1 gene fusion: a sarcoma with polyphenotypic differentiation. Am J Surg Pathol. 2019 Feb;43(2):220–8. PMID:30379650
1306. Chow E, Jenkins JJ, Burger PC, et al. Malignant evolution of choroid plexus papilloma. Pediatr Neurosurg. 1999 Sep;31(3):127–30. PMID:10708353
1307. Chrcanovic BR, Gomes CC, Gomez RS. Central giant cell lesion of the jaws: an updated analysis of 2270 cases reported in the literature. J Oral Pathol Med. 2018 Sep;47(8):731–9. PMID:29751369
1308. Chrcanovic BR, Gomez RS. Juvenile ossifying fibroma of the jaws and paranasal sinuses: a systematic review of the cases reported in the literature. Int J Oral Maxillofac Surg. 2020 Jan;49(1):28–37. PMID:31285096
1309. Chrcanovic BR, Gomez RS. Melanotic neuroectodermal tumour of infancy of the jaws: an analysis of diagnostic features and treatment. Int J Oral Maxillofac Surg. 2019 Jan;48(1):1–8. PMID:30170777
1310. Christe A, Waldherr C, Hallett R, et al. MR imaging of parotid tumors: typical lesion characteristics in MR imaging improve discrimination between benign and malignant disease. AJNR Am J Neuroradiol. 2011 Aug;32(7):1202–7. PMID:21724574
1311. Christison-Lagay ER, Burrows PE, Alomari A, et al. Hepatic hemangiomas: subtype classification and development of a clinical practice algorithm and registry. J Pediatr Surg. 2007 Jan;42(1):62–7. PMID:17208542
1312. Christoforidis M, Buhl R, Paulus W, et al. Intraneural perineurioma of the VIIIth cranial nerve: case report. Neurosurgery. 2007 Sep;61(3):E652. PMID:17881938
1313. Christopherson WM, Foote FW Jr, Stewart FW. Alveolar soft-part sarcomas; structurally characteristic tumors of uncertain histogenesis. Cancer. 1952 Jan;5(1):100–11. PMID:14886902
1314. Chu PG, Benhattar J, Weiss LM, et al. Intraneural synovial sarcoma: two cases. Mod Pathol. 2004 Feb;17(2):258–63. PMID:14685256
1315. Chu WK, Hickson ID. RecQ helicases: multifunctional genome caretakers. Nat Rev Cancer. 2009 Sep;9(9):644–54. PMID:19657341
1316. Chumas JC, Scully RE. Sebaceous tumors arising in ovarian dermoid cysts. Int J Gynecol Pathol. 1991;10(4):356–63. PMID:1774106
1317. Chun HE, Johann PD, Milne K, et al. Identification and analyses of extra-cranial and cranial rhabdoid tumor molecular subgroups reveal tumors with cytotoxic T cell infiltration. Cell Rep. 2019 Nov 19;29(8):2338–2354.e7. PMID:31708418
1318. Chun HE, Lim EL, Heravi-Moussavi A, et al. Genome-wide profiles of extra-cranial malignant rhabdoid tumors reveal heterogeneity and dysregulated developmental pathways. Cancer Cell. 2016 Mar 14;29(3):394–406. PMID:26977886
1319. Chun KA, Cho IH, Won KJ, et al. Osteoblastoma as a cause of osteomalacia assessed by bone scan. Ann Nucl Med. 2003 Jul;17(5):411–4. PMID:12971642
1320. Chun Y, Kim W, Park K, et al. Pancreatoblastoma. J Pediatr Surg. 1997 Nov;32(11):1612–5. PMID:9396538
1321. Chun YS, Wang L, Nascimento AG, et al. Pediatric inflammatory myofibroblastic tumor: anaplastic lymphoma kinase (ALK) expression and prognosis. Pediatr Blood Cancer. 2005 Nov;45(6):796–801. PMID:15602716
1322. Chung EB. Pitfalls in diagnosing benign soft tissue tumors in infancy and childhood. Pathol Annu. 1985;20(Pt 2):323–86. PMID:3892466
1323. Chung EB, Enzinger FM. Benign lipoblastomatosis. An analysis of 35 cases. Cancer. 1973 Aug;32(2):482–92. PMID:4353020
1324. Chung EB, Enzinger FM. Fibroma of tendon sheath. Cancer. 1979 Nov;44(5):1945–54. PMID:91424
1325. Chung EB, Enzinger FM. Infantile fibrosarcoma. Cancer. 1976 Aug;38(2):729–39. PMID:974993
1326. Chung EB, Enzinger FM. Infantile myofibromatosis. Cancer. 1981 Oct 15;48(8):1807–18. PMID:7284977
1327. Chung EB, Enzinger FM. Malignant melanoma of soft parts. A reassessment of clear cell sarcoma. Am J Surg Pathol. 1983 Jul;7(5):405–13. PMID:6614306
1328. Chung EM, Cube R, Hall GJ, et al. From the archives of the AFIP: breast masses in children and adolescents: radiologic-pathologic correlation. Radiographics. 2009 May-Jun;29(3):907–31. PMID:19448124
1329. Chung EM, Travis MD, Conran RM. Pancreatic tumors in children: radiologic-pathologic correlation. Radiographics. 2006 Jul-Aug;26(4):1211–38. PMID:16844942
1330. Chung J, Turaka K, Shields CL. Retinocytoma shows lack of response to chemoreduction. J Pediatr Ophthalmol Strabismus. 2010 Dec 22;47 Online:e1–3. PMID:21175116
1331. Church AJ, Calicchio ML, Nardi V, et al. Recurrent EML4-NTRK3 fusions in infantile fibrosarcoma and congenital mesoblastic nephroma suggest a revised testing strategy. Mod Pathol. 2018 Mar;31(3):463–73. PMID:29099503
1332. Churg A, Sheffield BS, Galateau-Salle F. New markers for separating benign from malignant mesothelial proliferations: Are we there yet? Arch Pathol Lab Med. 2016 Apr;140(4):318–21. PMID:26288396
1333. Churpek JE, Pyrtel K, Kanchi KL, et al. Genomic analysis of germ line and somatic variants in familial myelodysplasia/acute myeloid leukemia. Blood. 2015 Nov 26;126(22):2484–90. PMID:26492932
1334. Cibull TL, Gleason BC, O'Malley DP, et al. Malignant cutaneous glomus tumor presenting as a rapidly growing leg mass in a pregnant woman. J Cutan Pathol. 2008 Aug;35(8):765–9. PMID:18422692
1335. Ciftci AO, Bingöl-Koloğlu M, Senocak ME, et al. Testicular tumors in children. J Pediatr Surg. 2001 Dec;36(12):1796–801. PMID:11733909
1336. Ciftci AO, Tanyel FC, Senocak ME, et al. Pheochromocytoma in children. J Pediatr Surg. 2001 Mar;36(3):447–52. PMID:11226993
1337. Cilião HL, Camargo-Godoy RBO, Souza MF, et al. Polymorphisms in IMPDH2, UGT2B7, and CES2 genes influence the risk of graft rejection in kidney transplant recipients taking mycophenolate mofetil. Mutat Res Genet Toxicol Environ Mutagen. 2018 Dec;836 Pt B:97–102. PMID:30442353
1338. Cina SJ, Radentz SS, Smialek JE. A case of familial angiolipomatosis with Lisch nodules. Arch Pathol Lab Med. 1999 Oct;123(10):946–8. PMID:10506451
1339. Cingel V, Durdik S, Babala J, et al. Fetus in fetu from newborn's mediastinum: case report and a review of literature. Surg Radiol Anat. 2012 Apr;34(3):197–202. PMID:21901374
1340. Cingolani N, Shaco-Levy R, Farruggio A, et al. Alpha-fetoprotein production by pancreatic tumors exhibiting acinar cell differentiation: study of five cases, one arising in a mediastinal teratoma. Hum Pathol. 2000 Aug;31(8):938–44. PMID:10987254
1341. Cipriani NA, Lusardi JJ, McElherne J, et al. Mucoepidermoid carcinoma: a comparison of histologic grading systems and relationship to MAML2 rearrangement and prognosis. Am J Surg Pathol. 2019 Jul;43(7):885–97. PMID:31021855
1342. Clappier E, Collette S, Grardel N, et al. NOTCH1 and FBXW7 mutations have a favorable impact on early response to treatment, but not on outcome, in children with T-cell acute lymphoblastic leukemia (T-ALL) treated on EORTC trials 58881 and 58951. Leukemia. 2010 Dec;24(12):2023–31. PMID:20861920
1343. Clark AJ, Sughrue ME, Ivan ME, et al. Factors influencing overall survival rates for patients with pineocytoma. J Neurooncol. 2010 Nov;100(2):255–60. PMID:20461445
1344. Clark J, Lu YJ, Sidhar SK, et al. Fusion of splicing factor genes PSF and NonO (p54nrb) to the TFE3 gene in papillary renal cell carcinoma. Oncogene. 1997 Oct;15(18):2233–9. PMID:9393982
1345. Clark RM, Lynch MP, Kolp R, et al. The N-methyl-D-aspartate receptor, a precursor to N-methyl-D-aspartate receptor encephalitis, is found in the squamous tissue of ovarian teratomas. Int J Gynecol Pathol. 2014 Nov;33(6):598–606. PMID:25272299
1346. Clark SK, Phillips RK. Desmoids in familial adenomatous polyposis. Br J Surg. 1996 Nov;83(11):1494–504. PMID:9014661
1347. Clarke BA, Witkowski L, Ton Nu TN, et al. Loss of SMARCA4 (BRG1) protein expression as determined by immunohistochemistry in small-cell carcinoma of the ovary, hypercalcaemic type distinguishes these tumours from their

mimics. Histopathology. 2016 Nov;69(5):727–38. PMID:27100627
**1348.** Clarke M, Mackay A, Ismer B, et al. Infant high grade gliomas comprise multiple subgroups characterized by novel targetable gene fusions and favorable outcomes. Cancer Discov. 2020 Jul;10(7):942–63. PMID:32238360
**1349.** Clarke MJ, Foy AB, Wetjen N, et al. Imaging characteristics and growth of subependymal giant cell astrocytomas. Neurosurg Focus. 2006 Jan 15;20(1):E5. PMID:16459995
**1350.** Classe M, Malouf GG, Su X, et al. Incidence, clinicopathological features and fusion transcript landscape of translocation renal cell carcinomas. Histopathology. 2017 Jun;70(7):1089–97. PMID:28106924
**1351.** Claviez A, Meyer U, Dominick C, et al. MALT lymphoma in children: a report from the NHL-BFM Study Group. Pediatr Blood Cancer. 2006 Aug;47(2):210–4. PMID:16123999
**1352.** Clément A, Wiweger M, von der Hardt S, et al. Regulation of zebrafish skeletogenesis by ext2/dackel and papst1/pinscher. PLoS Genet. 2008 Jul 25;4(7):e1000136. PMID:18654627
**1353.** Cleven AH, Höcker S, Briaire-de Bruijn I, et al. Mutation analysis of H3F3A and H3F3B as a diagnostic tool for giant cell tumor of bone and chondroblastoma. Am J Surg Pathol. 2015 Nov;39(11):1576–83. PMID:26457357
**1354.** Cleven AH, Sannaa GA, Briaire-de Bruijn I, et al. Loss of H3K27 tri-methylation is a diagnostic marker for malignant peripheral nerve sheath tumors and an indicator for an inferior survival. Mod Pathol. 2016 Jun;29(6):582–90. PMID:26990975
**1355.** Cleven AHG, Schreuder WH, Groen E, et al. Molecular findings in maxillofacial bone tumours and its diagnostic value. Virchows Arch. 2020 Jan;476(1):159–74. PMID:31838586
**1356.** Clevenger JA, Foster RS, Ulbright TM. Differentiated rhabdomyomatous tumors after chemotherapy for metastatic testicular germ-cell tumors: a clinicopathological study of seven cases mandating separation from rhabdomyosarcoma. Mod Pathol. 2009 Oct;22(10):1361–6. PMID:19633644
**1357.** Clifford SC, Lusher ME, Lindsey JC, et al. Wnt/Wingless pathway activation and chromosome 6 loss characterize a distinct molecular sub-group of medulloblastomas associated with a favorable prognosis. Cell Cycle. 2006 Nov;5(22):2666–70. PMID:17172831
**1358.** Clifton-Bligh RJ, Hofman MS, Duncan E, et al. Improving diagnosis of tumor-induced osteomalacia with Gallium-68 DOTATATE PET/CT. J Clin Endocrinol Metab. 2013 Feb;98(2):687–94. PMID:23295468
**1359.** ClinicalTrials.gov [Internet]. Bethesda (MD): U.S. National Library of Medicine; 2020. Identifier NCT03017326, Paediatric Hepatic International Tumour Trial (PHITT); first posted 2017 Jan 11 [updated 2020 Nov 6]. Available from: https://clinicaltrials.gov/ct2/show/NCT03017326.
**1360.** Coakley KJ, Huston J 3rd, Scheithauer BW, et al. Pilocytic astrocytomas: well-demarcated magnetic resonance appearance despite frequent infiltration histologically. Mayo Clin Proc. 1995 Aug;70(8):747–51. PMID:7630212
**1361.** Cobellis L, Schürfeld K, Ignacchiti E, et al. An ovarian mucinous adenocarcinoma arising from mature cystic teratoma associated with respiratory type tissue: a case report. Tumori. 2004 Sep-Oct;90(5):521–4. PMID:15656343
**1362.** Coccé MC, Mardin BR, Bens S, et al. Identification of ZCCHC8 as fusion partner of ROS1 in a case of congenital glioblastoma multiforme with a t(6;12)(q21;q24.3). Genes Chromosomes Cancer. 2016 Sep;55(9):677–87. PMID:27121553
**1363.** Coenen EA, Zwaan CM, Reinhardt D, et al. Pediatric acute myeloid leukemia with t(8;16)(p11;p13), a distinct clinical and biological entity: a collaborative study by the International-Berlin-Frankfurt-Munster AML-study group. Blood. 2013 Oct 10;122(15):2704–13. PMID:23974201
**1364.** Coffey AM, Lewis A, Marcogliese AN, et al. A clinicopathologic study of the spectrum of systemic forms of EBV-associated T-cell lymphoproliferative disorders of childhood: a single tertiary care pediatric institution experience in North America. Pediatr Blood Cancer. 2019 Aug;66(8):e27798. PMID:31099136
**1365.** Coffin CM, Alaggio R. Adipose and myxoid tumors of childhood and adolescence. Pediatr Dev Pathol. 2012;15(1 Suppl):239–54. PMID:22420730
**1366.** Coffin CM, Alaggio R. Fibroblastic and myofibroblastic tumors in children and adolescents. Pediatr Dev Pathol. 2012;15(1 Suppl):127–80. PMID:22420727
**1367.** Coffin CM, Alaggio R, Dehner LP. Some general considerations about the clinicopathologic aspects of soft tissue tumors in children and adolescents. Pediatr Dev Pathol. 2012;15(1 Suppl):11–25. PMID:22375909
**1368.** Coffin CM, Dehner LP. Fibroblastic-myofibroblastic tumors in children and adolescents: a clinicopathologic study of 108 examples in 103 patients. Pediatr Pathol. 1991 Jul-Aug;11(4):569–88. PMID:1946077
**1369.** Coffin CM, Dehner LP. Vascular tumors in children and adolescents: a clinicopathologic study of 228 tumors in 222 patients. Pathol Annu. 1993;28(Pt 1):97–120. PMID:8416140
**1370.** Coffin CM, Ewing S, Dehner LP. Frequency of intratubular germ cell neoplasia with invasive testicular germ cell tumors. Histologic and immunocytochemical features. Arch Pathol Lab Med. 1985 Jun;109(6):555–9. PMID:2581525
**1371.** Coffin CM, Hornick JL, Fletcher CD. Inflammatory myofibroblastic tumor: comparison of clinicopathologic, histologic, and immunohistochemical features including ALK expression in atypical and aggressive cases. Am J Surg Pathol. 2007 Apr;31(4):509–20. PMID:17414097
**1372.** Coffin CM, Hornick JL, Zhou H, et al. Gardner fibroma: a clinicopathologic and immunohistochemical analysis of 45 patients with 57 fibromas. Am J Surg Pathol. 2007 Mar;31(3):410–6. PMID:17325483
**1373.** Coffin CM, Jaszcz W, O'Shea PA, et al. So-called congenital-infantile fibrosarcoma: Does it exist and what is it? Pediatr Pathol. 1994 Jan-Feb;14(1):133–50. PMID:8159611
**1374.** Coffin CM, Lowichik A, Putnam A. Lipoblastoma (LPB): a clinicopathologic and immunohistochemical analysis of 59 cases. Am J Surg Pathol. 2009 Nov;33(11):1705–12. PMID:19738456
**1375.** Coffin CM, Neilson KA, Ingels S, et al. Congenital generalized myofibromatosis: a disseminated angiocentric myofibromatosis. Pediatr Pathol Lab Med. 1995 Jul-Aug;15(4):571–87. PMID:8597844
**1376.** Coffin CM, Patel A, Perkins S, et al. ALK1 and p80 expression and chromosomal rearrangements involving 2p23 in inflammatory myofibroblastic tumor. Mod Pathol. 2001 Jun;14(6):569–76. PMID:11406658
**1377.** Coffin CM, Watterson J, Priest JR, et al. Extrapulmonary inflammatory myofibroblastic tumor (inflammatory pseudotumor). A clinicopathologic and immunohistochemical study of 84 cases. Am J Surg Pathol. 1995 Aug;19(8):859–72. PMID:7611533
**1378.** Cogliano VJ, Baan R, Straif K, et al. Preventable exposures associated with human cancers. J Natl Cancer Inst. 2011 Dec 21;103(24):1827–39. PMID:22158127
**1379.** Cohen JI, Iwatsuki K, Ko YH, et al. Epstein-Barr virus NK and T cell lymphoproliferative disease: report of a 2018 international meeting. Leuk Lymphoma. 2020 Apr;61(4):808–19. PMID:31833428
**1380.** Cohen JI, Kimura H, Nakamura S, et al. Epstein-Barr virus-associated lymphoproliferative disease in non-immunocompromised hosts: a status report and summary of an international meeting, 8-9 September 2008. Ann Oncol. 2009 Sep;20(9):1472–82. PMID:19515747
**1381.** Cohen JI, Manoli I, Dowdell K, et al. Hydroa vacciniforme-like lymphoproliferative disorder: an EBV disease with a low risk of systemic illness in whites. Blood. 2019 Jun 27;133(26):2753–64. PMID:31064750
**1382.** Cohen JN, Sabnis AJ, Krings G, et al. EWSR1-NFATC2 gene fusion in a soft tissue tumor with epithelioid round cell morphology and abundant stroma: a case report and review of the literature. Hum Pathol. 2018 Nov;81:281–90. PMID:29626598
**1383.** Cohen M, De Matteo E, Narbaitz M, et al. Epstein-Barr virus presence in pediatric diffuse large B-cell lymphoma reveals a particular association and latency patterns: analysis of viral role in tumor microenvironment. Int J Cancer. 2013 Apr 1;132(7):1572–80. PMID:22987474
**1384.** Cohen M, Guger S, Hamilton J. Long term sequelae of pediatric craniopharyngioma - literature review and 20 years of experience. Front Endocrinol (Lausanne). 2011 Nov 28;2:81. PMID:22645511
**1385.** Cohen M, Narbaitz M, Metrebian F, et al. Epstein-Barr virus-positive diffuse large B-cell lymphoma association is not only restricted to elderly patients. Int J Cancer. 2014 Dec 15;135(12):2816–24. PMID:24789501
**1386.** Cohen M, Pedemonte L, Drut R. Pigmented müllerian papilloma of the vagina. Histopathology. 2001 Nov;39(5):541–3. PMID:11737317
**1387.** Cohen MC, Drut R, Garcia C, et al. Mesenchymal hamartoma of the chest wall: a cooperative study with review of the literature. Pediatr Pathol. 1992 Jul-Aug;12(4):525–34. PMID:1409151
**1388.** Cohen MM Jr. Proteus syndrome review: molecular, clinical, and pathologic features. Clin Genet. 2014 Feb;85(2):111–9. PMID:23992099
**1389.** Cohen O, Avinadav E, Sharon E, et al. Pediatric and adolescent surgical breast clinic: preliminary experience. J Pediatr Adolesc Gynecol. 2020 Feb;33(1):23–6. PMID:31445140
**1390.** Cohen-Gogo S, Cellier C, Coindre JM, et al. Ewing-like sarcomas with BCOR-CCNB3 fusion transcript: a clinical, radiological and pathological retrospective study from the Société Française des Cancers de L'Enfant. Pediatr Blood Cancer. 2014 Dec;61(12):2191–8. PMID:25176412
**1391.** Cohn KH, Silen W. Lessons of parathyroid reoperations. Am J Surg. 1982 Nov;144(5):511–7. PMID:7137458
**1392.** Cohn SL, Pearson AD, London WB, et al. The International Neuroblastoma Risk Group (INRG) classification system: an INRG Task Force report. J Clin Oncol. 2009 Jan 10;27(2):289–97. PMID:19047291
**1393.** Cöktü S, Spix C, Kaiser M, et al. Cancer incidence and spectrum among children with genetically confirmed Beckwith-Wiedemann spectrum in Germany: a retrospective cohort study. Br J Cancer. 2020 Aug;123(4):619–23. PMID:32451468
**1394.** Colafati GS, Voicu IP, Carducci C, et al. MRI features as a helpful tool to predict the molecular subgroups of medulloblastoma: state of the art. Ther Adv Neurol Disord. 2018 Jun 18;11:1756286418775375. PMID:29977341
**1395.** Coleman KM, Doherty MC, Bigler SA. Solid-pseudopapillary tumor of the pancreas. Radiographics. 2003 Nov-Dec;23(6):1644–8. PMID:14615569
**1396.** Coleman R, Sanchez O, Ghattaura H, et al. Tubulocystic anomalies of the mesonephric duct associated with ipsilateral renal dysgenesis. J Pediatr Urol. 2019 Feb;15(1):46.e1–6. PMID:30446299
**1397.** Coli A, Novello M, Tamburrini G, et al. Intracranial neuromuscular choristoma: report of a case with literature review. Neuropathology. 2017 Aug;37(4):341–5. PMID:28168739
**1398.** Colleoni GW, Bridge JA, Garicochea B, et al. ATIC-ALK: a novel variant ALK gene fusion in anaplastic large cell lymphoma resulting from the recurrent cryptic chromosomal inversion, inv(2)(p23q35). Am J Pathol. 2000 Mar;156(3):781–9. PMID:10702393
**1399.** Collini P, Mattavelli F, Pellegrinelli A, et al. Papillary carcinoma of the thyroid gland of childhood and adolescence: morphologic subtypes, biologic behavior and prognosis: a clinicopathologic study of 42 sporadic cases treated at a single institution during a 30-year period. Am J Surg Pathol. 2006 Nov;30(11):1420–6. PMID:17063083
**1400.** Collins MH, Chatten J. Lipoblastoma/lipoblastomatosis: a clinicopathologic study of 25 tumors. Am J Surg Pathol. 1997 Oct;21(10):1131–7. PMID:9331284
**1401.** Collins MH, Montone KT, Leahey AM, et al. Post-transplant lymphoproliferative disease in children. Pediatr Transplant. 2001 Aug;5(4):250–7. PMID:11472603
**1402.** Collins MT, Sarlis NJ, Merino MJ, et al. Thyroid carcinoma in the McCune-Albright syndrome: contributory role of activating Gs alpha mutations. J Clin Endocrinol Metab. 2003 Sep;88(9):4413–7. PMID:12970318
**1403.** Collins VP, Jones DT, Giannini C. Pilocytic astrocytoma: pathology, molecular mechanisms and markers. Acta Neuropathol. 2015 Jun;129(6):775–88. PMID:25792358
**1404.** Colmenero I, Hoeger PH. Vascular tumours in infants. Part II: vascular tumours of intermediate malignancy [corrected] and malignant tumours. Br J Dermatol. 2014 Sep;171(3):474–84. PMID:24965196
**1405.** Colmenero I, McCarville MB, Reyes-Múgica M. Malignant skin tumors in children. In: Parham DM, Khoury JD, McCarville MB, editors. Pediatric malignancies: pathology and imaging. New York (NY): Springer; 2015. pp. 359–82.
**1406.** Colombo C, Bolshakov S, Hajibashi S, et al. 'Difficult to diagnose' desmoid tumours: a potential role for CTNNB1 mutational analysis. Histopathology. 2011 Aug;59(2):336–40. PMID:21884214
**1407.** Colombo C, Foo WC, Whiting D, et al. FAP-related desmoid tumors: a series of 44 patients evaluated in a cancer referral center. Histol Histopathol. 2012 May;27(5):641–9. PMID:22419028
**1408.** Colombo C, Miceli R, Lazar AJ, et al. CTNNB1 45F mutation is a molecular prognosticator of increased postoperative primary desmoid tumor recurrence: an independent, multicenter validation study. Cancer. 2013 Oct 15;119(20):3696–702. PMID:23913621
**1409.** Colomo L, Loong F, Rives S, et al. Diffuse large B-cell lymphomas with plasmablastic differentiation represent a heterogeneous group of disease entities. Am J Surg Pathol. 2004 Jun;28(6):736–47. PMID:15166665
**1410.** Compton JJ, Laack NN, Eckel LJ, et al. Long-term outcomes for low-grade intracranial ganglioglioma: 30-year experience from the Mayo Clinic. J Neurosurg. 2012 Nov;117(5):825–30. PMID:22957524

1411. Comstock JM, Willmore-Payne C, Holden JA, et al. Composite pheochromocytoma: a clinicopathologic and molecular comparison with ordinary pheochromocytoma and neuroblastoma. Am J Clin Pathol. 2009 Jul;132(1):69–73. PMID:19864235
1412. Conboy E, Dhamija R, Wang M, et al. Paraspinal neurofibromas and hypertrophic neuropathy in Noonan syndrome with multiple lentigines. J Med Genet. 2016 Feb;53(2):123–6. PMID:26337637
1413. Conconi A, Bertoni F, Pedrinis E, et al. Nodal marginal zone B-cell lymphomas may arise from different subsets of marginal zone B lymphocytes. Blood. 2001 Aug 1;98(3):781–6. PMID:11468179
1414. Cone BM, Taweevisit M, Shenoda S, et al. Pharyngeal hairy polyps: five new cases and review of the literature. Fetal Pediatr Pathol. 2012 Jun;31(3):184–9. PMID:22413746
1415. Conlon N, Schultheis AM, Piscuoglio S, et al. A survey of DICER1 hotspot mutations in ovarian and testicular sex cord-stromal tumors. Mod Pathol. 2015 Dec;28(12):1603–12. PMID:26428316
1416. Conlon N, Silva A, Guerra E, et al. Loss of SMARCA4 expression is both sensitive and specific for the diagnosis of small cell carcinoma of ovary, hypercalcemic type. Am J Surg Pathol. 2016 Mar;40(3):395–403. PMID:26645725
1417. Conner JR, Hornick JL. SATB2 is a novel marker of osteoblastic differentiation in bone and soft tissue tumours. Histopathology. 2013 Jul;63(1):36–49. PMID:23701429
1418. Connor JM, Pirrit LA, Yates JR, et al. Linkage of the tuberous sclerosis locus to a DNA polymorphism detected by v-abl. J Med Genet. 1987 Sep;24(9):544–6. PMID:2889832
1419. Conrad R, Perez MC. Congenital granular cell epulis. Arch Pathol Lab Med. 2014 Jan;138(1):128–31. PMID:24377822
1420. Contreras AL, Malpica A. Angiosarcoma arising in mature cystic teratoma of the ovary: a case report and review of the literature. Int J Gynecol Pathol. 2009 Sep;28(5):453–7. PMID:19696615
1421. Cook JR, Dehner LP, Collins MH, et al. Anaplastic lymphoma kinase (ALK) expression in the inflammatory myofibroblastic tumor: a comparative immunohistochemical study. Am J Surg Pathol. 2001 Nov;25(11):1364–71. PMID:11684952
1422. Cook JR, Pfeifer JD, Dehner LP. Mesenchymal hamartoma of the liver in the adult: association with distinct clinical features and histological changes. Hum Pathol. 2002 Sep;33(9):893–8. PMID:12378513
1423. Cooke CB, Krenacs L, Stetler-Stevenson M, et al. Hepatosplenic T-cell lymphoma: a distinct clinicopathologic entity of cytotoxic gamma delta T-cell origin. Blood. 1996 Dec 1;88(11):4265–74. PMID:8943863
1424. Cool CD, Bitter MA. The malignant lymphomas of Kenya: morphology, immunophenotype, and frequency of Epstein-Barr virus in 73 cases. Hum Pathol. 1997 Sep;28(9):1026–33. PMID:9308726
1425. Cools J, Wlodarska I, Somers R, et al. Identification of novel fusion partners of ALK, the anaplastic lymphoma kinase, in anaplastic large-cell lymphoma and inflammatory myofibroblastic tumor. Genes Chromosomes Cancer. 2002 Aug;34(4):354–62. PMID:12112524
1426. Cools M, Drop SL, Wolffenbuttel KP, et al. Germ cell tumors in the intersex gonad: old paths, new directions, moving frontiers. Endocr Rev. 2006 Aug;27(5):468–84. PMID:16735607
1427. Cools M, Honecker F, Stoop H, et al. Maturation delay of germ cells in fetuses with trisomy 21 results in increased risk for the development of testicular germ cell tumors. Hum Pathol. 2006 Jan;37(1):101–11. PMID:16360422
1428. Cools M, Looijenga LH. Tumor risk and clinical follow-up in patients with disorders of sex development. Pediatr Endocrinol Rev. 2011 Sep;9 Suppl 1:519–24. PMID:22423509
1429. Cools M, Pleskacova J, Stoop H, et al. Gonadal pathology and tumor risk in relation to clinical characteristics in patients with 45,X/46,XY mosaicism. J Clin Endocrinol Metab. 2011 Jul;96(7):E1171–80. PMID:21508138
1430. Cools M, Stoop H, Kersemaekers AM, et al. Gonadoblastoma arising in undifferentiated gonadal tissue within dysgenetic gonads. J Clin Endocrinol Metab. 2006 Jun;91(6):2404–13. PMID:16608895
1431. Cools M, van Aerde K, Kersemaekers AM, et al. Morphological and immunohistochemical differences between gonadal maturation delay and early germ cell neoplasia in patients with undervirilization syndromes. J Clin Endocrinol Metab. 2005 Sep;90(9):5295–303. PMID:15998778
1432. Cools M, Wolffenbuttel KP, Hersmus R, et al. Malignant testicular germ cell tumors in postpubertal individuals with androgen insensitivity: prevalence, pathology and relevance of single nucleotide polymorphism-based susceptibility profiling. Hum Reprod. 2017 Dec 1;32(12):2561–73. PMID:29121256
1433. Cooper O, Ben-Shlomo A, Bonert V, et al. Silent corticogonadotroph adenomas: clinical and cellular characteristics and long-term outcomes. Horm Cancer. 2010 Apr;1(2):80–92. PMID:20717480
1434. Cooper PH, McAllister HA, Helwig EB. Intravenous pyogenic granuloma. A study of 18 cases. Am J Surg Pathol. 1979 Jun;3(3):221–8. PMID:575269
1435. Copie-Bergman C, Gaulard P, Maouche-Chrétien L, et al. The MAL gene is expressed in primary mediastinal large B-cell lymphoma. Blood. 1999 Nov 15;94(10):3567–75. PMID:10552968
1436. Coppes MJ, Arnold M, Beckwith JB, et al. Factors affecting the risk of contralateral Wilms tumor development: a report from the National Wilms Tumor Study Group. Cancer. 1999 Apr 1;85(7):1616–25. PMID:10193955
1437. Coppit GL 3rd, Perkins JA, Manning SC. Nasopharyngeal teratomas and dermoids: a review of the literature and case series. Int J Pediatr Otorhinolaryngol. 2000 May 30;52(3):219–27. PMID:10841951
1438. Cordero FJ, Huang Z, Grenier C, et al. Histone H3.3K27M represses p16 to accelerate gliomagenesis in a murine model of DIPG. Mol Cancer Res. 2017 Sep;15(9):1243–54. PMID:28522693
1439. Cordero SC, Royer MC, Rush WL, et al. Pure apocrine nevus: a report of 4 cases. Am J Dermatopathol. 2012 May;34(3):305–9. PMID:22317889
1439A. Corean J, Furtado LV, Kadri S, et al. Cribriform-morular variant of papillary thyroid carcinoma with poorly differentiated features: a case report with immunohistochemical and molecular genetic analysis. Int J Surg Pathol. 2019 May;27(3):294–304. PMID:30176755
1440. Cornejo KM, Cheng L, Church A, et al. Chromosome 12p abnormalities and IMP3 expression in prepubertal pure testicular teratomas. Hum Pathol. 2016 Mar;49:54–60. PMID:26826410
1441. Cornejo KM, Frazier L, Lee RS, et al. Yolk sac tumor of the testis in infants and children: a clinicopathologic analysis of 33 cases. Am J Surg Pathol. 2015 Aug;39(8):1121–31. PMID:25828390
1442. Cornejo KM, Hutchinson L, Cosar EF, et al. Is it a primary or metastatic melanocytic neoplasm of the central nervous system?: A molecular based approach. Pathol Int. 2013 Nov;63(11):559–64. PMID:24274719
1443. Corr P, Vaithilingum M, Thejpal R, et al. Parotid MALT lymphoma in HIV infected children. J Ultrasound Med. 1997 Sep;16(9):615–7. PMID:9321782
1444. Corrias A, Cassio A, Weber G, et al. Thyroid nodules and cancer in children and adolescents affected by autoimmune thyroiditis. Arch Pediatr Adolesc Med. 2008 Jun;162(6):526–31. PMID:18524742
1445. Corrias A, Mussa A, Baronio F, et al. Diagnostic features of thyroid nodules in pediatrics. Arch Pediatr Adolesc Med. 2010 Aug;164(8):714–9. PMID:20679162
1446. Corso A, Lazzarino M, Morra E, et al. Chronic myelogenous leukemia and exposure to ionizing radiation–a retrospective study of 443 patients. Ann Hematol. 1995 Feb;70(2):79–82. PMID:7880928
1447. Corson TW, Gallie BL. One hit, two hits, three hits, more? Genomic changes in the development of retinoblastoma. Genes Chromosomes Cancer. 2007 Jul;46(7):617–34. PMID:17437278
1448. Cortes JE, Talpaz M, O'Brien S, et al. Staging of chronic myeloid leukemia in the imatinib era: an evaluation of the World Health Organization proposal. Cancer. 2006 Mar 15;106(6):1306–15. PMID:16463391
1449. Cosar M, Iplikcioglu AC, Bek S, et al. Intracranial falcine and convexity chondromas: two case reports. Br J Neurosurg. 2005 Jun;19(3):241–3. PMID:16455525
1450. Cossu-Rocca P, Zhang S, Roth LM, et al. Chromosome 12p abnormalities in dysgerminoma of the ovary: a FISH analysis. Mod Pathol. 2006 Apr;19(4):611–5. PMID:16554737
1451. Costa MJ, Weiss SW. Angiomatoid malignant fibrous histiocytoma. A follow-up study of 108 cases with evaluation of possible histologic predictors of outcome. Am J Surg Pathol. 1990 Dec;14(12):1126–32. PMID:2174650
1452. Cotelingam JD, Witebsky FG, Hsu SM, et al. Malignant lymphoma in patients with the Wiskott-Aldrich syndrome. Cancer Invest. 1985;3(6):515–22. PMID:3910193
1453. Coulam CB, Annegers JF, Abboud CF, et al. Pituitary adenoma and oral contraceptives: a case-control study. Fertil Steril. 1979 Jan;31(1):25–8. PMID:369889
1454. Coulter TI, Chandra A, Bacon CM, et al. Clinical spectrum and features of activated phosphoinositide 3-kinase δ syndrome: a large patient cohort study. J Allergy Clin Immunol. 2017 Feb;139(2):597–606.e4. PMID:27555459
1455. Cournoyer E, Al-Ibraheemi A, Engel E, et al. Clinical characterization and long-term outcomes in pediatric epithelioid hemangioendothelioma. Pediatr Blood Cancer. 2020 Feb;67(2):e28045. PMID:31724797
1456. Coustan-Smith E, Mullighan CG, Onciu M, et al. Early T-cell precursor leukaemia: a subtype of very high-risk acute lymphoblastic leukaemia. Lancet Oncol. 2009 Feb;10(2):147–56. PMID:19147408
1457. Couto JA, Huang AY, Konczyk DJ, et al. Somatic MAP2K1 mutations are associated with extracranial arteriovenous malformation. Am J Hum Genet. 2017 Mar 2;100(3):546–54. PMID:28190454
1458. Couto JA, Konczyk DJ, Vivero MP, et al. Somatic PIK3CA mutations are present in multiple tissues of facial infiltrating lipomatosis. Pediatr Res. 2017 Nov;82(5):850–4. PMID:28665924
1459. Couto JA, Vivero MP, Kozakewich HP, et al. A somatic MAP3K3 mutation is associated with verrucous venous malformation. Am J Hum Genet. 2015 Mar 5;96(3):480–6. PMID:25728774
1460. Covington DB, Rosenblum MK, Brathwaite CD, et al. Angiocentric glioma-like tumor of the midbrain. Pediatr Neurosurg. 2009;45(6):429–33. PMID:20110754
1461. Cox CM, El-Mallawany NK, Kabue M, et al. Clinical characteristics and outcomes of HIV-infected children diagnosed with Kaposi sarcoma in Malawi and Botswana. Pediatr Blood Cancer. 2013 Aug;60(8):1274–80. PMID:23487320
1462. Cox R, Vang R, Epstein JI. Papillary cystadenoma of the epididymis and broad ligament: morphologic and immunohistochemical overlap with clear cell papillary renal cell carcinoma. Am J Surg Pathol. 2014 May;38(5):713–8. PMID:24441657
1463. Coy S, Du Z, Sheu SH, et al. Distinct patterns of primary and motile cilia in Rathke's cleft cysts and craniopharyngioma subtypes. Mod Pathol. 2016 Dec;29(12):1446–59. PMID:27562488
1464. Coy S, Dubuc AM, Dahiya S, et al. Nuclear CRX and FOXJ1 expression differentiates non-germ cell pineal region tumors and supports the ependymal differentiation of papillary tumor of the pineal region. Am J Surg Pathol. 2017 Oct;41(10):1410–21. PMID:28719464
1465. Coy S, Rashid R, Lin JR, et al. Multiplexed immunofluorescence reveals potential PD-1/PD-L1 pathway vulnerabilities in craniopharyngioma. Neuro Oncol. 2018 Jul 5;20(8):1101–12. PMID:29509940
1466. Coy S, Rashid R, Stemmer-Rachamimov A, et al. An update on the CNS manifestations of neurofibromatosis type 2. Acta Neuropathol. 2020 Apr;139(4):643–65. PMID:31161239
1467. Coyle D, Kutasy B, Han Suyin K, et al. Gonadoblastoma in patients with 45,X/46,XY mosaicism: a 16-year experience. J Pediatr Urol. 2016 Oct;12(5):283.e1–7. PMID:27052295
1468. Coyne C, Nikiforov YE. RAS mutation-positive follicular variant of papillary thyroid carcinoma arising in a struma ovarii. Endocr Pathol. 2010 Jun;21(2):144–7. PMID:19898969
1469. Crabtree MD, Tomlinson IP, Talbot IC, et al. Variability in the severity of colonic disease in familial adenomatous polyposis results from differences in tumour initiation rather than progression and depends relatively little on patient age. Gut. 2001 Oct;49(4):540–3. PMID:11559652
1470. Crago AM, Chmielecki J, Rosenberg M, et al. Near universal detection of alterations in CTNNB1 and Wnt pathway regulators in desmoid-type fibromatosis by whole-exome sequencing and genomic analysis. Genes Chromosomes Cancer. 2015 Oct;54(10):606–15. PMID:26171757
1471. Craig JR, Peters RL, Edmondson HA, et al. Fibrolamellar carcinoma of the liver: a tumor of adolescents and young adults with distinctive clinico-pathologic features. Cancer. 1980 Jul 15;46(2):372–9. PMID:6248194
1472. Craig KM, Poppas DP, Akhavan A. Pediatric renal cell carcinoma. Curr Opin Urol. 2019 Sep;29(5):500–4. PMID:31261184
1473. Cramer SF. The histogenesis of acquired melanocytic nevi. Based on a new concept of melanocytic differentiation. Am J Dermatopathol. 1984 Summer;6 Suppl:289–98. PMID:6528932
1474. Cramer SF. The melanocytic differentiation pathway in congenital melanocytic nevi: theoretical considerations. Pediatr Pathol. 1988;8(3):253–65. PMID:3174507
1475. Cramer SF, Salgado CM, Reyes-Múgica M. A study of dermal melanophages in childhood nevi. Reassessing so-called "pigment incontinence". J Cutan Pathol. 2020 Sep;47(9):809–14. PMID:32314421

**1476.** Crankson SJ, Al Namshan M, Al Mane K, et al. Intramuscular myxoma: a rare neck mass in a child. Pediatr Radiol. 2002 Feb;32(2):120–2. PMID:11819080
**1477.** Crapanzano JP, Cardillo M, Lin O, et al. Cytology of desmoplastic small round cell tumor. Cancer. 2002 Feb 25;96(1):21–31. PMID:11836699
**1478.** Crapanzano JP, Lin O. Cytologic findings of marginal zone lymphoma. Cancer. 2003 Oct 25;99(5):301–9. PMID:14579297
**1479.** Craver R, Dewenter T, Ebran N, et al. COL1A1-PDGFB fusion in a pediatric Bednar tumor with 2 copies of a der(22)t(17;22). Cancer Genet Cytogenet. 2006 Jul 15;168(2):155–7. PMID:16843106
**1480.** Craver RD, Correa H, Kao YS, et al. Aggressive giant cell fibroblastoma with a balanced 17;22 translocation. Cancer Genet Cytogenet. 1995 Mar;80(1):20–2. PMID:7697628
**1481.** Craver RD, Henrich S, Kao YS. Fibrous lipoblastoma with 8q11.2 abnormality. Cancer Genet Cytogenet. 2006 Dec;171(2):112–4. PMID:17116489
**1482.** Crawford JB, Howes EL Jr, Char DH. Combined nevi of the conjunctiva. Trans Am Ophthalmol Soc. 1999;97:170–83. PMID:10703123
**1483.** Cree IA. The WHO classification of haematolymphoid tumours. Leukemia. 2022 Jul;36(7):1701–2. PMID:35732830
**1484.** Cree IA, Tan PH, Travis WD, et al. Counting mitoses: SI(ze) matters! Mod Pathol. 2021 Sep;34(9):1651–7. PMID:34079071
**1485.** Cresswell GD, Apps JR, Chagtai T, et al. Intra-tumor genetic heterogeneity in Wilms Tumor: clonal evolution and clinical implications. EBioMedicine. 2016 Jul;9:120–9. PMID:27333041
**1486.** Creytens D. A contemporary review of myxoid adipocytic tumors. Semin Diagn Pathol. 2019 Mar;36(2):129–41. PMID:30853315
**1487.** Creytens D. SATB2 and TLE1 Expression in BCOR-CCNB3 (Ewing-like) sarcoma, mimicking small cell osteosarcoma and poorly differentiated synovial sarcoma. Appl Immunohistochem Mol Morphol. 2020 Jan;28(1):e10–2. PMID:29084055
**1488.** Creytens D. What's new in adipocytic neoplasia? Virchows Arch. 2020 Jan;476(1):29–39. PMID:31501988
**1489.** Creytens D, van Gorp J, Ferdinande L, et al. Array-based comparative genomic hybridization analysis of a pleomorphic myxoid liposarcoma. J Clin Pathol. 2014 Sep;67(9):834–5. PMID:24970901
**1490.** Cribier B, Scrivener Y, Grosshans E. Tumors arising in nevus sebaceus: a study of 596 cases. J Am Acad Dermatol. 2000 Feb;42(2 Pt 1):263–8. PMID:10642683
**1491.** Crino PB, Mehta R, Vinters HV. Pathogenesis of TSC in the brain. In: Kwiatkowski DJ, Whittemore VH, Thiele EA, editors. Tuberous sclerosis complex: genes, clinical features, and therapeutics. Weinheim (Germany): Wiley-Blackwell; 2010. pp. 161–85.
**1492.** Crino PB, Trojanowski JQ, Dichter MA, et al. Embryonic neuronal markers in tuberous sclerosis: single-cell molecular pathology. Proc Natl Acad Sci U S A. 1996 Nov 26;93(24):14152–7. PMID:8943076
**1493.** Crist WM, Anderson JR, Meza JL, et al. Intergroup rhabdomyosarcoma study-IV: results for patients with nonmetastatic disease. J Clin Oncol. 2001 Jun 15;19(12):3091–102. PMID:11408506
**1494.** Crocoli A, Grimaldi C, Virgone C, et al. Outcome after surgery for solid pseudopapillary pancreatic tumors in children: report from the TREP project-Italian Rare Tumors Study Group. Pediatr Blood Cancer. 2019 Mar;66(3):e27519. PMID:30362240
**1495.** Crompton BD, Stewart C, Taylor-Weiner A, et al. The genomic landscape of pediatric Ewing sarcoma. Cancer Discov. 2014 Nov;4(11):1326–41. PMID:25186949
**1496.** Crona J, Lamarca A, Ghosal S, et al. Genotype-phenotype correlations in pheochromocytoma and paraganglioma: a systematic review and individual patient meta-analysis. Endocr Relat Cancer. 2019 May;26(5):539–50. PMID:30893643
**1497.** Crona J, Taïeb D, Pacak K. New perspectives on pheochromocytoma and paraganglioma: toward a molecular classification. Endocr Rev. 2017 Dec 1;38(6):489–515. PMID:28938417
**1498.** Croteau DL, Popuri V, Opresko PL, et al. Human RecQ helicases in DNA repair, recombination, and replication. Annu Rev Biochem. 2014;83:519–52. PMID:24606147
**1499.** Croteau SE, Gupta D. The clinical spectrum of kaposiform hemangioendothelioma and tufted angioma. Semin Cutan Med Surg. 2016 Sep;35(3):147–52. PMID:27607323
**1500.** Croteau SE, Liang MG, Kozakewich HP, et al. Kaposiform hemangioendothelioma: atypical features and risks of Kasabach-Merritt phenomenon in 107 referrals. J Pediatr. 2013 Jan;162(1):142–7. PMID:22871490
**1501.** Cuglievan B, Subbiah V, Wang H, et al. Response to mammalian target of rapamycin-based therapy and incidental finding of Lynch syndrome in a patient with solid pseudopapillary neoplasm of the pancreas with AKT1_E17K mutation. JCO Precis Oncol. 2018;2:PO.18.00182. PMID:31650099
**1502.** Cummings OW, Ulbright TM, Young RH, et al. Desmoplastic small round cell tumors of the paratesticular region. A report of six cases. Am J Surg Pathol. 1997 Feb;21(2):219–25. PMID:9042290
**1503.** Cunniff C, Djavid AR, Carrubba S, et al. Health supervision for people with Bloom syndrome. Am J Med Genet A. 2018 Sep;176(9):1872–81. PMID:30055079
**1504.** Curatolo P, Franz DN, Lawson JA, et al. Adjunctive everolimus for children and adolescents with treatment-refractory seizures associated with tuberous sclerosis complex: post-hoc analysis of the phase 3 EXIST-3 trial. Lancet Child Adolesc Health. 2018 Jul;2(7):495–504. PMID:30169322
**1505.** Curatolo P, Moavero R. mTOR inhibitors in tuberous sclerosis complex. Curr Neuropharmacol. 2012 Dec;10(4):404–15. PMID:23730262
**1506.** Curran AE, Allen CM, Beck FM, et al. Distinctive pattern of glial fibrillary acidic protein immunoreactivity useful in distinguishing fragmented pleomorphic adenoma, canalicular adenoma and polymorphous low grade adenocarcinoma of minor salivary glands. Head Neck Pathol. 2007 Sep;1(1):27–32. PMID:20614277
**1507.** Curran-Melendez SM, Dasher DA, Groben P, et al. Case report: meningothelial hamartoma of the scalp in a 9-year-old child. Pediatr Dermatol. 2011 Nov-Dec;28(6):677–80. PMID:21906138
**1508.** Currarino G, Coln D, Votteler T. Triad of anorectal, sacral, and presacral anomalies. AJR Am J Roentgenol. 1981 Aug;137(2):395–8. PMID:6789651
**1509.** Currás-Freixes M, Inglada-Pérez L, Mancikova V, et al. Recommendations for somatic and germline genetic testing of single pheochromocytoma and paraganglioma based on findings from a series of 329 patients. J Med Genet. 2015 Oct;52(10):647–56. PMID:26269449
**1510.** Curtis RE, Travis LB, Rowlings PA, et al. Risk of lymphoproliferative disorders after bone marrow transplantation: a multi-institutional study. Blood. 1999 Oct 1;94(7):2208–16. PMID:10498590
**1511.** Cutcutache I, Suzuki Y, Tan IB, et al. Exome-wide sequencing shows low mutation rates and identifies novel mutated genes in seminomas. Eur Urol. 2015 Jul;68(1):77–83. PMID:25597018
**1512.** Czauderna P. Adult type vs. childhood hepatocellular carcinoma–Are they the same or different lesions? Biology, natural history, prognosis, and treatment. Med Pediatr Oncol. 2002 Nov;39(5):519–23. PMID:12228910
**1513.** Czauderna P, Haeberle B, Hiyama E, et al. The Children's Hepatic tumors International Collaboration (CHIC): novel global rare tumor database yields new prognostic factors in hepatoblastoma and becomes a research model. Eur J Cancer. 2016 Jan;52:92–101. PMID:26655560
**1514.** Czauderna P, Mackinlay G, Perilongo G, et al. Hepatocellular carcinoma in children: results of the first prospective study of the International Society of Pediatric Oncology group. J Clin Oncol. 2002 Jun 15;20(12):2798–804. PMID:12065556
**1515.** da Silva Almeida AC, Abate F, Khiabanian H, et al. The mutational landscape of cutaneous T cell lymphoma and Sézary syndrome. Nat Genet. 2015 Dec;47(12):1465–70. PMID:26551667
**1516.** da Silva MA, Edmondson JW, Eby C, et al. Humoral hypercalcemia in seminomas. Med Pediatr Oncol. 1992;20(1):38–41. PMID:1370070
**1517.** Dabner M, McCluggage WG, Bundell C, et al. Ovarian teratoma associated with anti-N-methyl D-aspartate receptor encephalitis: a report of 5 cases documenting prominent intratumoral lymphoid infiltrates. Int J Gynecol Pathol. 2012 Sep;31(5):429–37. PMID:22833082
**1518.** Dabora SL, Jozwiak S, Franz DN, et al. Mutational analysis in a cohort of 224 tuberous sclerosis patients indicates increased severity of TSC2, compared with TSC1, disease in multiple organs. Am J Hum Genet. 2001 Jan;68(1):64–80. PMID:11112665
**1519.** Dabska M. Parachordoma: a new clinicopathologic entity. Cancer. 1977 Oct;40(4):1586–92. PMID:907973
**1520.** Dabska M, Koszarowski T. Clinical and pathologic study of aponeurotic (epithelioid) sarcoma. Pathol Annu. 1982;17(Pt 1):129–53. PMID:6750534
**1521.** DaCambra MP, Gupta SK, Ferri-de-Barros F. Subungual exostosis of the toes: a systematic review. Clin Orthop Relat Res. 2014 Apr;472(4):1251–9. PMID:24146360
**1522.** Dachy G, de Krijger RR, Fraitag S, et al. Association of PDGFRB mutations with pediatric myofibroma and myofibromatosis. JAMA Dermatol. 2019 Aug 1;155(8):946–50. PMID:31017643
**1523.** Dadlani R, Ghosal N, Hegde AS, et al. Giant calvarial desmoplastic fibroblastoma. J Clin Neurosci. 2014 Apr;21(4):696–9. PMID:24262774
**1524.** Dadone B, Refae S, Lemarié-Delaunay C, et al. Molecular cytogenetics of pediatric adipocytic tumors. Cancer Genet. 2015 Oct;208(10):469–81. PMID:26319758
**1525.** Dadone-Montaudié B, Alberti L, Duc A, et al. Alternative PDGFD rearrangements in dermatofibrosarcomas protuberans without PDGFB fusions. Mod Pathol. 2018 Nov;31(11):1683–93. PMID:29955147
**1526.** Dadone-Montaudié B, Burel-Vandenbos F, Soler C, et al. Double minute chromosomes harboring MDM2 amplification in a pediatric atypical lipomatous tumor. Genes Chromosomes Cancer. 2019 Sep;58(9):673–9. PMID:30887579
**1527.** Daghistani R, Miller E, Kulkarni AV, et al. Atypical characteristics and behavior of dysembryoplastic neuroepithelial tumors. Neuroradiology. 2013 Feb;55(2):217–24. PMID:23314798
**1528.** Dahan K, Kamal M, Noël LH, et al. Small glomeruli in WAGR (Wilms tumor, aniridia, genitourinary anomalies and mental retardation) syndrome. Am J Kidney Dis. 2007 Jun;49(6):793–800. PMID:17533022
**1529.** Dahia PL, Ross KN, Wright ME, et al. A HIF1alpha regulatory loop links hypoxia and mitochondrial signals in pheochromocytomas. PLoS Genet. 2005 Jul;1(1):72–80. PMID:16103922
**1530.** Dahiya S, Haydon DH, Alvarado D, et al. BRAF(V600E) mutation is a negative prognosticator in pediatric ganglioglioma. Acta Neuropathol. 2013 Jun;125(6):901–10. PMID:23609006
**1531.** Dahl NA, Sheil A, Knapke S, et al. Gardner fibroma: clinical and histopathologic implications of germline APC mutation association. J Pediatr Hematol Oncol. 2016 Jul;38(5):e154–7. PMID:26840078
**1532.** Dahlin DC, Ivins JC. Benign chondroblastoma. A study of 125 cases. Cancer. 1972 Aug;30(2):401–13. PMID:5051664
**1533.** Daimaru Y, Hashimoto H, Enjoji M. Malignant "triton" tumors: a clinicopathologic and immunohistochemical study of nine cases. Hum Pathol. 1984 Aug;15(8):768–78. PMID:6235165
**1534.** Dal Cin P, Kozakewich HP, Goumnerova L, et al. Variant translocations involving 16q22 and 17p13 in solid variant and extraosseous forms of aneurysmal bone cyst. Genes Chromosomes Cancer. 2000 Jun;28(2):233–4. PMID:10825009
**1535.** Dal Cin P, Pauwels P, Poldermans LJ, et al. Clonal chromosome abnormalities in a so-called Dupuytren's subungual exostosis. Genes Chromosomes Cancer. 1999 Feb;24(2):162–4. PMID:9885985
**1536.** Dal Cin P, Polito P, Van Eyken P, et al. Anomalies of chromosomes 17 and 22 in giant cell fibroblastoma. Cancer Genet Cytogenet. 1997 Sep;97(2):165–6. PMID:9283602
**1537.** Dal Cin P, Sciot R, De Smet L, et al. Translocation 2;11 in a fibroma of tendon sheath. Histopathology. 1998 May;32(5):433–5. PMID:9639118
**1538.** Dal Cin P, Sciot R, de Wever I, et al. Cytogenetic and immunohistochemical evidence that giant cell fibroblastoma is related to dermatofibrosarcoma protuberans. Genes Chromosomes Cancer. 1996 Jan;15(1):73–5. PMID:8824728
**1539.** Dal Cin P, Sciot R, Samson I, et al. Osteoid osteoma and osteoblastoma with clonal chromosome changes. Br J Cancer. 1998 Aug;78(3):344–8. PMID:9703280
**1540.** Dale DC, Person RE, Bolyard AA, et al. Mutations in the gene encoding neutrophil elastase in congenital and cyclic neutropenia. Blood. 2000 Oct 1;96(7):2317–22. PMID:11001877
**1541.** Dale S, Breidahl WH, Baker D, et al. Severe toxic osteoblastoma of the humerus associated with diffuse periostitis of multiple bones. Skeletal Radiol. 2001 Aug;30(8):464–8. PMID:11479753
**1542.** Dall'igna P, Cecchetto G, Bisogno G, et al. Pancreatic tumors in children and adolescents: the Italian TREP project experience. Pediatr Blood Cancer. 2010 May;54(5):675–80. PMID:19998473
**1543.** D'Almeida Costa F, Dias TM, Lombardo KA, et al. Intracranial cellular schwannomas: a clinicopathological study of 20 cases. Histopathology. 2020 Jan;76(2):275–82. PMID:31379028

**1544.** Daluiski A, Seeger LL, Doberneck SA, et al. A case of juxta-articular myxoma of the knee. Skeletal Radiol. 1995 Jul;24(5):389–91. PMID:7570164
**1545.** Daly AF, Rixhon M, Adam C, et al. High prevalence of pituitary adenomas: a cross-sectional study in the province of Liege, Belgium. J Clin Endocrinol Metab. 2006 Dec;91(12):4769–75. PMID:16968795
**1546.** Damania B, Münz C. Immunodeficiencies that predispose to pathologies by human oncogenic γ-herpesviruses. FEMS Microbiol Rev. 2019 Mar 1;43(2):181–92. PMID:30649299
**1547.** Damato S, Alorjani M, Bonar F, et al. IDH1 mutations are not found in cartilaginous tumours other than central and periosteal chondrosarcomas and enchondromas. Histopathology. 2012 Jan;60(2):363–5. PMID:22074484
**1548.** Damm-Welk C, Mussolin L, Zimmermann M, et al. Early assessment of minimal residual disease identifies patients at very high relapse risk in NPM-ALK-positive anaplastic large-cell lymphoma. Blood. 2014 Jan 16;123(3):334–7. PMID:24297868
**1549.** d'Amore ES, Menin A, Bonoldi E, et al. Anaplastic large cell lymphomas: a study of 75 pediatric patients. Pediatr Dev Pathol. 2007 May-Jun;10(3):181–91. PMID:17535098
**1550.** d'Amore ES, Visco C, Menin A, et al. STAT3 pathway is activated in ALK-positive large B-cell lymphoma carrying SQSTM1-ALK rearrangement and provides a possible therapeutic target. Am J Surg Pathol. 2013 May;37(5):780–6. PMID:23588372
**1551.** Dancer JY, Henry SP, Bondaruk J, et al. Expression of master regulatory genes controlling skeletal development in benign cartilage and bone forming tumors. Hum Pathol. 2010 Dec;41(12):1788–93. PMID:21078438
**1552.** Dandurand C, Sepehry AA, Asadi Lari MH, et al. Adult craniopharyngioma: case series, systematic review, and meta-analysis. Neurosurgery. 2018 Oct 1;83(4):631–41. PMID:29267973
**1553.** Daneshbod Y, Daneshbod K, Khademi B. Diagnostic difficulties in the interpretation of fine needle aspirate samples in salivary lesions: diagnostic pitfalls revisited. Acta Cytol. 2009 Jan-Feb;53(1):53–70. PMID:19248555
**1554.** D'Angelo F, Ceccarelli M, Tala, et al. The molecular landscape of glioma in patients with Neurofibromatosis 1. Nat Med. 2019 Jan;25(1):176–87. PMID:30531922
**1555.** Danko G, Chapman RW. Simple, noninvasive method to measure the antibronchoconstrictor activity of drugs in conscious guinea pigs. J Pharmacol Methods. 1988 Apr;19(2):165–73. PMID:3129618
**1556.** Dannenberg H, van Nederveen FH, Abbou M, et al. Clinical characteristics of pheochromocytoma patients with germline mutations in SDHD. J Clin Oncol. 2005 Mar 20;23(9):1894–901. PMID:15774781
**1557.** Dantonello TM, Int-Veen C, Harms D, et al. Cooperative trial CWS-91 for localized soft tissue sarcoma in children, adolescents, and young adults. J Clin Oncol. 2009 Mar 20;27(9):1446–55. PMID:19224858
**1558.** Dantonello TM, Leuschner I, Vokuhl C, et al. Malignant ectomesenchymoma in children and adolescents: report from the Cooperative Weichteilsarkom Studiengruppe (CWS). Pediatr Blood Cancer. 2013 Feb;60(2):224–9. PMID:22535600
**1559.** Darbari A, Sabin KM, Shapiro CN, et al. Epidemiology of primary hepatic malignancies in U.S. children. Hepatology. 2003 Sep;38(3):560–6. PMID:12939582
**1560.** D'Arcy CE, Nobre LF, Arnaldo A, et al. Immunohistochemical and nanoString-based subgrouping of clinical medulloblastoma samples. J Neuropathol Exp Neurol. 2020 Apr 1;79(4):437–47. PMID:32053195
**1561.** Darcy DG, Chiaroni-Clarke R, Murphy JM, et al. The genomic landscape of fibrolamellar hepatocellular carcinoma: whole genome sequencing of ten patients. Oncotarget. 2015 Jan 20;6(2):755–70. PMID:25605237
**1562.** Dardick I, van Nostrand AW, Jeans MT, et al. Pleomorphic adenoma, I: Ultrastructural organization of "epithelial" regions. Hum Pathol. 1983 Sep;14(9):780–97. PMID:6309645
**1563.** Dardick I, Van Nostrand AW, Jeans MT, et al. Pleomorphic adenoma, II: Ultrastructural organization of "stromal" regions. Hum Pathol. 1983 Sep;14(9):798–809. PMID:6309646
**1564.** Dardick I, van Nostrand AW. Myoepithelial cells in salivary gland tumors–revisited. Head Neck Surg. 1985 May-Jun;7(5):395–408. PMID:2833468
**1565.** Darlix A, Zouaoui S, Rigau V, et al. Epidemiology for primary brain tumors: a nationwide population-based study. J Neurooncol. 2017 Feb;131(3):525–46. PMID:27853959
**1566.** D'Aronco L, Rouleau C, Gayden T, et al. Brainstem angiocentric gliomas with MYB-QKI rearrangements. Acta Neuropathol. 2017 Oct;134(4):667–9. PMID:28803398
**1567.** Därr R, Nambuba J, Del Rivero J, et al. Novel insights into the polycythemia-paraganglioma-somatostatinoma syndrome. Endocr Relat Cancer. 2016 Dec;23(12):899–908. PMID:27679736
**1568.** Das A, Bansal D, Chatterjee D, et al. Kaposiform hemangioendothelioma: multifocal involvement, chylothorax, and Kasabach-Merritt phenomenon. J Pediatr Hematol Oncol. 2017 Mar;39(2):153–4. PMID:27820128
**1569.** Das DK, Gupta AK, Chowdhury V, et al. Fine-needle aspiration diagnosis of carotid body tumor: report of a case and review of experience with cytologic features in four cases. Diagn Cytopathol. 1997 Aug;17(2):143–7. PMID:9258623
**1570.** Das P, Iyer VK, Mathur SR, et al. Anaplastic large cell lymphoma: a critical evaluation of cytomorphological features in seven cases. Cytopathology. 2010 Aug;21(4):251–8. PMID:19744187
**1571.** Das S, Sengupta M, Islam N, et al. Weineke criteria, Ki-67 index and p53 status to study pediatric adrenocortical tumors: Is there a correlation? J Pediatr Surg. 2016 Nov;51(11):1795–800. PMID:27567308
**1572.** Dasgupta A, Gupta T, Pungavkar S, et al. Nomograms based on preoperative multiparametric magnetic resonance imaging for prediction of molecular subgrouping in medulloblastoma: results from a radiogenomics study of 111 patients. Neuro Oncol. 2019 Jan 1;21(1):115–24. PMID:29846693
**1573.** Dasgupta B, Li W, Perry A, et al. Glioma formation in neurofibromatosis 1 reflects preferential activation of K-RAS in astrocytes. Cancer Res. 2005 Jan 1;65(1):236–45. PMID:15665300
**1574.** Dashti NK, Wehrs RN, Thomas BC, et al. Spindle cell rhabdomyosarcoma of bone with FUS-TFCP2 fusion: confirmation of a very recently described rhabdomyosarcoma subtype. Histopathology. 2018 Sep;73(3):514–20. PMID:29758589
**1575.** Daugaard G, Gundgaard MG, Mortensen MS, et al. Surveillance for stage I nonseminoma testicular cancer: outcomes and long-term follow-up in a population-based cohort. J Clin Oncol. 2014 Dec 1;32(34):3817–23. PMID:25267754
**1576.** Daumas-Duport C. Dysembryoplastic neuroepithelial tumours. Brain Pathol. 1993 Jul;3(3):283–95. PMID:8293188
**1577.** Daumas-Duport C, Scheithauer BW, Chodkiewicz JP, et al. Dysembryoplastic neuroepithelial tumor: a surgically curable tumor of young patients with intractable partial seizures. Report of thirty-nine cases. Neurosurgery. 1988 Nov;23(5):545–56. PMID:3143922
**1578.** Daumas-Duport C, Varlet P. [Dysembryoplastic neuroepithelial tumors]. Rev Neurol (Paris). 2003 Jul;159(6-7 Pt 1):622–36. French. PMID:12910070
**1579.** Daumas-Duport C, Varlet P, Bacha S, et al. Dysembryoplastic neuroepithelial tumors: nonspecific histological forms – a study of 40 cases. J Neurooncol. 1999 Feb;41(3):267–80. PMID:10359147
**1580.** Dave SS, Fu K, Wright GW, et al. Molecular diagnosis of Burkitt's lymphoma. N Engl J Med. 2006 Jun 8;354(23):2431–42. PMID:16760443
**1581.** d'Avella E, Solari D, Somma T, et al. The endoscopic endonasal approach for pediatric craniopharyngiomas: the key lessons learned. Childs Nerv Syst. 2019 Nov;35(11):2147–55. PMID:31055620
**1582.** Davenport RD. Cytologic diagnosis of fibrolamellar carcinoma of the liver by fine-needle aspiration. Diagn Cytopathol. 1990;6(4):275–9. PMID:1698598
**1583.** David S, András F, Endre K, et al. More cases of benign testicular teratomas are detected in adults than in children. a clinicopathological study of 543 testicular germ cell tumor cases. Pathol Oncol Res. 2017 Jul;23(3):513–7. PMID:27796764
**1584.** Davids A. Childhood psychosis. The problem of differential diagnosis. J Autism Child Schizophr. 1975 Jun;5(2):129–38. PMID:1174116
**1585.** Davids JR, Wenger DR, Mubarak SJ. Congenital muscular torticollis: sequela of intrauterine or perinatal compartment syndrome. J Pediatr Orthop. 1993 Mar-Apr;13(2):141–7. PMID:8459000
**1586.** Davidson A, Wainwright RD, Stones DK, et al. Malignancies in South African children with HIV. J Pediatr Hematol Oncol. 2014 Mar;36(2):111–7. PMID:24552745
**1587.** Davidson TI, Kissin MW, Bradish CF, et al. Angiosarcoma arising in a patient with Maffucci syndrome. Eur J Surg Oncol. 1985 Dec;11(4):381–4. PMID:4065351
**1588.** Davidsson J, Puschmann A, Tedgård U, et al. SAMD9 and SAMD9L in inherited predisposition to ataxia, pancytopenia, and myeloid malignancies. Leukemia. 2018 May;32(5):1106–15. PMID:29535429
**1589.** Davies KA, Cope AP, Schofield JB, et al. A rare mediastinal tumour presenting with systemic effects due to IL-6 and tumour necrosis factor (TNF) production. Clin Exp Immunol. 1995 Jan;99(1):117–23. PMID:7813103
**1590.** Davis CJ Jr, Barton JH, Sesterhenn IA, et al. Metanephric adenoma. Clinicopathological study of fifty patients. Am J Surg Pathol. 1995 Oct;19(10):1101–14. PMID:7573669
**1591.** Davis CJ Jr, Mostofi FK, Sesterhenn IA. Renal medullary carcinoma. The seventh sickle cell nephropathy. Am J Surg Pathol. 1995 Jan;19(1):1–11. PMID:7528470
**1592.** Davis GL. Malignant melanoma arising in mature ovarian cystic teratoma (dermoid cyst). Report of two cases and literature analysis. Int J Gynecol Pathol. 1996 Oct;15(4):356–62. PMID:8886884
**1593.** Davis IJ, Hsi BL, Arroyo JD, et al. Cloning of an Alpha-TFEB fusion in renal tumors harboring the t(6;11)(p21;q13) chromosome translocation. Proc Natl Acad Sci U S A. 2003 May 13;100(10):6051–6. PMID:12719541
**1594.** Davis IJ, Kim JJ, Ozsolak F, et al. Oncogenic MITF dysregulation in clear cell sarcoma: defining the MiT family of human cancers. Cancer Cell. 2006 Jun;9(6):473–84. PMID:16766266
**1596.** Davis JL, Lockwood CM, Stohr B, et al. Expanding the spectrum of pediatric NTRK-rearranged mesenchymal tumors. Am J Surg Pathol. 2019 Apr;43(4):435–45. PMID:30585824
**1597.** Davis JL, Vargas SO, Rudzinski ER, et al. Recurrent RET gene fusions in paediatric spindle mesenchymal neoplasms. Histopathology. 2020 Jun;76(7):1032–41. PMID:31994201
**1598.** Davis KP, Hartmann LK, Keeney GL, et al. Primary ovarian carcinoid tumors. Gynecol Oncol. 1996 May;61(2):259–65. PMID:8626144
**1599.** Davis RI, Hamilton A, Biggart JD. Primary synovial chondromatosis: a clinicopathologic review and assessment of malignant potential. Hum Pathol. 1998 Jul;29(7):683–8. PMID:9670824
**1600.** Davis RJ, D'Cruz CM, Lovell MA, et al. Fusion of PAX7 to FKHR by the variant t(1;13)(p36;q14) translocation in alveolar rhabdomyosarcoma. Cancer Res. 1994 Jun 1;54(11):2869–72. PMID:8187070
**1601.** de Alava E, Ladanyi M, Rosai J, et al. Detection of chimeric transcripts in desmoplastic small round cell tumor and related developmental tumors by reverse transcriptase polymerase chain reaction. A specific diagnostic assay. Am J Pathol. 1995 Dec;147(6):1584–91. PMID:7495283
**1602.** de Almeida Verdolin A, Lamback EB, Ventura N, et al. Collision sellar lesions: coexistence of pituitary adenoma and Rathke cleft cyst-a single-center experience. Endocrine. 2020 Apr;68(1):174–81. PMID:31802354
**1603.** de Andrade KC, Frone MN, Wegman-Ostrosky T, et al. Response to: concern regarding classification of germlineTP53 variants as likely pathogenic. Hum Mutat. 2019 Jun;40(6):832–3. PMID:30997946
**1604.** de Andrade KC, Frone MN, Wegman-Ostrosky T, et al. Variable population prevalence estimates of germline TP53 variants: a gnomAD-based analysis. Hum Mutat. 2019 Jan;40(1):97–105. PMID:30352134
**1605.** de Andrade KC, Mirabello L, Stewart DR, et al. Higher-than-expected population prevalence of potentially pathogenic germline TP53 variants in individuals unselected for cancer history. Hum Mutat. 2017 Dec;38(12):1723–30. PMID:28861920
**1606.** de Andrea CE, Kroon HM, Wolterbeek R, et al. Interobserver reliability in the histopathological diagnosis of cartilaginous tumors in patients with multiple osteochondromas. Mod Pathol. 2012 Sep;25(9):1275–83. PMID:22555180
**1607.** de Andrea CE, Prins FA, Wiweger MI, et al. Growth plate regulation and osteochondroma formation: insights from tracing proteoglycans in zebrafish models and human cartilage. J Pathol. 2011 Jun;224(2):160–8. PMID:21506131
**1608.** de Andrea CE, Wiweger M, Prins F, et al. Primary cilia organization reflects polarity in the growth plate and implies loss of polarity and mosaicism in osteochondroma. Lab Invest. 2010 Jul;90(7):1091–101. PMID:20421870
**1609.** De B, Khakoo Y, Souweidane MM, et al. Patterns of relapse for children with localized intracranial ependymoma. J Neurooncol. 2018 Jun;138(2):435–45. PMID:29511977
**1610.** De Bernardi B, Gambini C, Haupt R, et al. Retrospective study of childhood ganglioneuroma. J Clin Oncol. 2008 Apr 1;26(10):1710–6. PMID:18375900
**1611.** De Beur SM, Finnegan RB, Vassiliadis J, et al. Tumors associated with oncogenic osteomalacia express genes important in bone and mineral metabolism. J Bone Miner Res. 2002 Jun;17(6):1102–10. PMID:12054166
**1612.** de Chadarévian JP, Montes JL, O'Gorman AM, et al. Maturation of cerebellar

neuroblastoma into ganglioneuroma with melanosis. A histologic, immunocytochemical, and ultrastructural study. Cancer. 1987 Jan 1;59(1):69–76. PMID:3539310
**1613.** de Chadarévian JP, Pawel BR, Faerber EN, et al. Undifferentiated (embryonal) sarcoma arising in conjunction with mesenchymal hamartoma of the liver. Mod Pathol. 1994 May;7(4):490–3. PMID:8066077
**1614.** De Diego JI, Prim MP, Hardisson D, et al. Post-transplant lymphoproliferative disease in tonsils of children with liver transplantation. Int J Pediatr Otorhinolaryngol. 2001 Apr 27;58(2):113–8. PMID:11278019
**1615.** De Filippi P, Zecca M, Lisini D, et al. Germ-line mutation of the NRAS gene may be responsible for the development of juvenile myelomonocytic leukaemia. Br J Haematol. 2009 Dec;147(5):706–9. PMID:19775298
**1616.** De Filpo G, Maggi M, Mannelli M, et al. Management and outcome of metastatic pheochromocytomas/paragangliomas: an overview. J Endocrinol Invest. 2021 Jan;44(1):15–25. PMID:32602077
**1617.** de Gouveia Brazao CA, Pierik FH, Oosterhuis JW, et al. Bilateral testicular microlithiasis predicts the presence of the precursor of testicular germ cell tumors in subfertile men. J Urol. 2004 Jan;171(1):158–60. PMID:14665866
**1618.** de Jong D, Roemer MG, Chan JK, et al. B-cell and classical Hodgkin lymphomas associated with immunodeficiency: 2015 SH/EAHP workshop report-part 2. Am J Clin Pathol. 2017 Feb 1;147(2):153–70. PMID:28395108
**1619.** de Jong J, Stoop H, Dohle GR, et al. Diagnostic value of OCT3/4 for pre-invasive and invasive testicular germ cell tumours. J Pathol. 2005 Jun;206(2):242–9. PMID:15818593
**1620.** de Jong J, Stoop H, Gillis AJ, et al. Differential expression of SOX17 and SOX2 in germ cells and stem cells has biological and clinical implications. J Pathol. 2008 May;215(1):21–30. PMID:18348160
**1621.** de Jong J, Stoop H, Gillis AJ, et al. Further characterization of the first seminoma cell line TCam-2. Genes Chromosomes Cancer. 2008 Mar;47(3):185–96. PMID:18050305
**1622.** de Jong MC, Kors WA, de Graaf P, et al. Trilateral retinoblastoma: a systematic review and meta-analysis. Lancet Oncol. 2014 Sep;15(10):1157–67. PMID:25126964
**1623.** de Jong MC, Kors WA, Moll AC, et al. Screening for pineal trilateral retinoblastoma revisited: a meta-analysis. Ophthalmology. 2020 May;127(5):601–7. PMID:32061409
**1624.** De Jong MC, van der Meer FJ, Göricke SL, et al. Diagnostic accuracy of intraocular tumor size measured with MR imaging in the prediction of postlaminar optic nerve invasion and massive choroidal invasion of retinoblastoma. Radiology. 2016 Jun;279(3):817–26. PMID:26690907
**1625.** de Jong S, Itinteang T, Withers AH, et al. Does hypoxia play a role in infantile hemangioma? Arch Dermatol Res. 2016 May;308(4):219–27. PMID:26940670
**1626.** de Kock L, Boshari T, Martinelli F, et al. Adult-onset cervical embryonal rhabdomyosarcoma and DICER1 mutations. J Low Genit Tract Dis. 2016 Jan;20(1):e8–10. PMID:26461232
**1627.** de Kock L, Priest JR, Foulkes WD, et al. An update on the central nervous system manifestations of DICER1 syndrome. Acta Neuropathol. 2020 Apr;139(4):689–701. PMID:30953130
**1628.** de Kock L, Sabbaghian N, Druker H, et al. Germ-line and somatic DICER1 mutations in pineoblastoma. Acta Neuropathol. 2014 Oct;128(4):583–95. PMID:25022261
**1629.** de Kock L, Sabbaghian N, Plourde F, et al. Pituitary blastoma: a pathognomonic feature of germ-line DICER1 mutations. Acta Neuropathol. 2014 Jul;128(1):111–22. PMID:24839956
**1630.** de Kock L, Terzic T, McCluggage WG, et al. DICER1 mutations are consistently present in moderately and poorly differentiated Sertoli-Leydig cell tumors. Am J Surg Pathol. 2017 Sep;41(9):1178–87. PMID:28654427
**1631.** de Kock L, Wang YC, Revil T, et al. High-sensitivity sequencing reveals multi-organ somatic mosaicism causing DICER1 syndrome. J Med Genet. 2016 Jan;53(1):43–52. PMID:26475046
**1632.** De Krijger RR, Petri BJ, Van Nederveen FH, et al. Frequent genetic changes in childhood pheochromocytomas. Ann N Y Acad Sci. 2006 Aug;1073:166–76. PMID:17102083
**1633.** de la Fuente J, Baruchel A, Biondi A, et al. Managing children with chronic myeloid leukaemia (CML): recommendations for the management of CML in children and young people up to the age of 18 years. Br J Haematol. 2014 Oct;167(1):33–47. PMID:24976289
**1634.** de Leval L, Bonnet C, Copie-Bergman C, et al. Diffuse large B-cell lymphoma of Waldeyer's ring has distinct clinicopathologic features: a GELA study. Ann Oncol. 2012 Dec;23(12):3143–51. PMID:22700993
**1635.** de Leval L, Ferry JA, Falini B, et al. Expression of BCL-6 and CD10 in primary mediastinal large B-cell lymphoma: evidence for derivation from germinal center B cells? Am J Surg Pathol. 2001 Oct;25(10):1277–82. PMID:11688462
**1636.** de Leval L, Parrens M, Le Bras F, et al. Angioimmunoblastic T-cell lymphoma is the most common T-cell lymphoma in two distinct French information data sets. Haematologica. 2015 Sep;100(9):e361–4. PMID:26045291
**1637.** De Lima L, Sürme MB, Gessi M, et al. Central nervous system high-grade neuroepithelial tumor with BCOR alteration (CNS HGNET-BCOR)-case-based reviews. Childs Nerv Syst. 2020 Aug;36(8):1589–99. PMID:32542405
**1638.** De Munnynck K, Van Gool S, Van Calenbergh F, et al. Desmoplastic infantile ganglioglioma: a potentially malignant tumor? Am J Surg Pathol. 2002 Nov;26(11):1515–22. PMID:12409729
**1639.** De Noon S, Flanagan AM, Tirabosco R, et al. EWSR1-SMAD3 fibroblastic tumour of bone: expanding the clinical spectrum. Skeletal Radiol. 2021 Feb;50(2):445–50. PMID:32710151
**1640.** de Noronha L, Cecílio WA, da Silva TF, et al. Congenital peribronchial myofibroblastic tumor: a case report. Pediatr Dev Pathol. 2010 May-Jun;13(3):243–6. PMID:20064015
**1641.** de Oliveira FA, Duarte EC, Taveira CT, et al. Salivary gland tumor: a review of 599 cases in a Brazilian population. Head Neck Pathol. 2009 Dec;3(4):271–5. PMID:20596844
**1642.** De Paepe P, Baens M, van Krieken H, et al. ALK activation by the CLTC-ALK fusion is a recurrent event in large B-cell lymphoma. Blood. 2003 Oct 1;102(7):2638–41. PMID:12750159
**1643.** De Palo G, Lattuada A, Kenda R, et al. Germ cell tumors of the ovary: the experience of the National Cancer Institute of Milan. I. Dysgerminoma. Int J Radiat Oncol Biol Phys. 1987 Jun;13(6):853–60. PMID:3583856
**1644.** De Pasquale MD, Diomedi-Camassei F, Serra A, et al. Recurrent metanephric stromal tumor in an infant. Urology. 2011 Dec;78(6):1411–3. PMID:21683990
**1645.** de Peralta-Venturina MN, Ro JY, Ordónez NG, et al. Diffuse embryoma of the testis. An immunohistochemical study of two cases. Am J Clin Pathol. 1994 Oct;102(4):402–5. PMID:7524298
**1646.** de Pontual L, Kettaneh D, Gordon CT, et al. Germline gain-of-function mutations of ALK disrupt central nervous system development. Hum Mutat. 2011 Mar;32(3):272–6. PMID:21972109
**1647.** De Raedt T, Beert E, Pasmant E, et al. PRC2 loss amplifies Ras-driven transcription and confers sensitivity to BRD4-based therapies. Nature. 2014 Oct 9;514(7521):247–51. PMID:25119042
**1648.** de Ribaupierre S, Dorfmüller G, Bulteau C, et al. Subependymal giant-cell astrocytomas in pediatric tuberous sclerosis disease: When should we operate? Neurosurgery. 2007 Jan;60(1):83–9. PMID:17228255
**1649.** de Ridder L, Turner D, Wilson DC, et al. Malignancy and mortality in pediatric patients with inflammatory bowel disease: a multinational study from the Porto Pediatric IBD group. Inflamm Bowel Dis. 2014 Feb;20(2):291–300. PMID:24374875
**1650.** de Rooij JD, Branstetter C, Ma J, et al. Pediatric non-Down syndrome acute megakaryoblastic leukemia is characterized by distinct genomic subsets with varying outcomes. Nat Genet. 2017 Mar;49(3):451–6. PMID:28112737
**1651.** de Rosa N, Rodriguez-Bigas MA, Chang GJ, et al. DNA Mismatch repair deficiency in rectal cancer: benchmarking its impact on prognosis, neoadjuvant response prediction, and clinical cancer genetics. J Clin Oncol. 2016 Sep 1;34(25):3039–46. PMID:27432916
**1652.** de Saint Aubain Somerhausen N, Coindre JM, Debiec-Rychter M, et al. Lipoblastoma in adolescents and young adults: report of six cases with FISH analysis. Histopathology. 2008 Feb;52(3):294–8. PMID:18269579
**1653.** de Tersant M, Généré L, Freyçon C, et al. Pheochromocytoma and paraganglioma in children and adolescents: experience of the French Society of Pediatric Oncology (SFCE). J Endocr Soc. 2020 Apr 3;4(5):bvaa039. PMID:32432211
**1654.** de Visser E, Veth RP, Pruszczynski M, et al. Diffuse and localized pigmented villonodular synovitis: evaluation of treatment of 38 patients. Arch Orthop Trauma Surg. 1999;119(7-8):401–4. PMID:10613228
**1655.** de Andrea CE, San-Julian M, Bovée JVMG. Integrating morphology and genetics in the diagnosis of cartilage tumors. Surg Pathol Clin. 2017 Sep;10(3):537–52. PMID:28797501
**1656.** Deavers MT, Malpica A, Liu J, et al. Ovarian sex cord-stromal tumors: an immunohistochemical study including a comparison of calretinin and inhibin. Mod Pathol. 2003 Jun;16(6):584–90. PMID:12808064
**1657.** Debelenko LV, Arthur DC, Pack SD, et al. Identification of CARS-ALK fusion in primary and metastatic lesions of an inflammatory myofibroblastic tumor. Lab Invest. 2003 Sep;83(9):1255–65. PMID:13679433
**1658.** Debelenko LV, Perez-Atayde AR, Dubois SG, et al. p53+/mdm2- atypical lipomatous tumor/well-differentiated liposarcoma in young children: an early expression of Li-Fraumeni syndrome. Pediatr Dev Pathol. 2010 May-Jun;13(3):218–24. PMID:20028212
**1659.** Debelenko LV, Raimondi SC, Daw N, et al. Renal cell carcinoma with novel VCL-ALK fusion: new representative of ALK-associated tumor spectrum. Mod Pathol. 2011 Mar;24(3):430–42. PMID:21076462
**1660.** Debiec-Rychter M, Van Valckenborgh I, Van den Broeck C, et al. Histologic localization of PLAG1 (pleomorphic adenoma gene 1) in pleomorphic adenoma of the salivary gland: cytogenetic evidence of common origin of phenotypically diverse cells. Lab Invest. 2001 Sep;81(9):1289–97. PMID:11555676
**1661.** Debray D, Baudouin V, Lacaille F, et al. De novo malignancy after solid organ transplantation in children. Transplant Proc. 2009 Mar;41(2):674–5. PMID:19328954
**1662.** De Bruin GP, Stefan DC. Children with Kaposi sarcoma in two southern African hospitals: clinical presentation, management, and outcome. J Trop Med. 2013;2013:213490. PMID:24396347
**1663.** Decarolis B, Simon T, Krug B, et al. Treatment and outcome of ganglioneuroma and ganglioneuroblastoma intermixed. BMC Cancer. 2016 Jul 27;16:542. PMID:27465021
**1664.** DeDavid M, Orlow SJ, Provost N, et al. Neurocutaneous melanosis: clinical features of large congenital melanocytic nevi in patients with manifest central nervous system melanosis. J Am Acad Dermatol. 1996 Oct;35(4):529–38. PMID:8859278
**1665.** Deen M, Ebrahim S, Schloff D, et al. A novel PLAG1-RAD51L1 gene fusion resulting from a t(8;14)(q12;q24) in a case of lipoblastoma. Cancer Genet. 2013 Jun;206(6):233–7. PMID:23890983
**1666.** Deenik W, Mooi WJ, Rutgers EJ, et al. Clear cell sarcoma (malignant melanoma) of soft parts: a clinicopathologic study of 30 cases. Cancer. 1999 Sep 15;86(6):969–75. PMID:10491522
**1667.** Deepak P, Sifuentes H, Sherid M, et al. T-cell non-Hodgkin's lymphomas reported to the FDA AERS with tumor necrosis factor-alpha (TNF-α) inhibitors: results of the REFURBISH study. Am J Gastroenterol. 2013 Jan;108(1):99–105. PMID:23032984
**1668.** Défachelles AS, Martin De Lassalle E, Boutard P, et al. Pancreatoblastoma in childhood: clinical course and therapeutic management of seven patients. Med Pediatr Oncol. 2001 Jul;37(1):47–52. PMID:11466723
**1669.** de Feraudy S, Fletcher CD. Fibroblastic connective tissue nevus: a rare cutaneous lesion analyzed in a series of 25 cases. Am J Surg Pathol. 2012 Oct;36(10):1509–15. PMID:22892597
**1670.** Deffenbacher KE, Iqbal J, Sanger W, et al. Molecular distinctions between pediatric and adult mature B-cell non-Hodgkin lymphomas identified through genomic profiling. Blood. 2012 Apr 19;119(16):3757–66. PMID:22374697
**1671.** Dehainault C, Garancher A, Castéra L, et al. The survival gene MED4 explains low penetrance retinoblastoma in patients with large RB1 deletion. Hum Mol Genet. 2014 Oct 1;23(19):5243–50. PMID:24858910
**1672.** Dehner LP. Gonadal and extragonadal germ cell neoplasia of childhood. Hum Pathol. 1983 Jun;14(6):493–511. PMID:6343221
**1673.** Dehner LP. Juvenile xanthogranulomas in the first two decades of life: a clinicopathologic study of 174 cases with cutaneous and extracutaneous manifestations. Am J Surg Pathol. 2003 May;27(5):579–93. PMID:12717244
**1674.** Dehner LP. The challenges of vasoformative tumors of the liver in children. Pediatr Dev Pathol. 2004 Sep-Oct;7(5):A5–7. PMID:15568213
**1675.** Dehner LP, Gru AA. Nonepithelial tumors and tumor-like lesions of the skin and subcutis in children. Pediatr Dev Pathol. 2018 Mar-Apr;21(2):150–207. PMID:29607758
**1676.** Dehner LP, Hill DA. Adrenal cortical neoplasms in children: Why so many carcinomas and yet so many survivors? Pediatr Dev Pathol. 2009 Jul-Aug;12(4):284–91. PMID:19326954
**1677.** Dehner LP, Ishak KG. Vascular tumors of the liver in infants and children. A study of 30 cases and review of the literature. Arch Pathol. 1971 Aug;92(2):101–11. PMID:5559952
**1678.** Dehner LP, Schultz KA, Hill DA. Pleuropulmonary blastoma: more than a lung neoplasm of childhood. Mo Med. 2019 May-Jun;116(3):206–10. PMID:31527943
**1679.** Dekkers OM, Karavitaki N, Pereira AM. The epidemiology of aggressive pituitary tumors

(and its challenges). Rev Endocr Metab Disord. 2020 Jun;21(2):209–12. PMID:32361816

**1680.** del Bufalo F, Carai A, Figà-Talamanca L, et al. Response of recurrent BRAFV600E mutated ganglioglioma to Vemurafenib as single agent. J Transl Med. 2014 Dec 19;12:356. PMID:25524464

**1681.** Delahunt B, Thomson KJ, Ferguson AF, et al. Familial cystic nephroma and pleuropulmonary blastoma. Cancer. 1993 Feb 15;71(4):1338–42. PMID:8382107

**1682.** de Lange J, van den Akker HP, Klip H. Incidence and disease-free survival after surgical therapy of central giant cell granulomas of the jaw in the Netherlands: 1990-1995. Head Neck. 2004 Sep;26(9):792–5. PMID:15350025

**1683.** Delattre O, Zucman J, Plougastel B, et al. Gene fusion with an ETS DNA-binding domain caused by chromosome translocation in human tumours. Nature. 1992 Sep 10;359(6391):162–5. PMID:1522903

**1684.** DeLellis RA, Mangray S. Heritable forms of primary hyperparathyroidism: a current perspective. Histopathology. 2018 Jan;72(1):117–32. PMID:29239035

**1685.** Delgado-López PD, Corrales-García EM, Alonso-García E, et al. Central nervous system ependymoma: clinical implications of the new molecular classification, treatment guidelines and controversial issues. Clin Transl Oncol. 2019 Nov;21(11):1450–63. PMID:30868390

**1686.** Delgrange E, Vasiljevic A, Wierinckx A, et al. Expression of estrogen receptor alpha is associated with prolactin pituitary tumor prognosis and supports the sex-related difference in tumor growth. Eur J Endocrinol. 2015 Jun;172(6):791–801. PMID:25792376

**1687.** Della Rocca C, Huvos AG. Osteoblastoma: varied histological presentations with a benign clinical course. An analysis of 55 cases. Am J Surg Pathol. 1996 Jul;20(7):841–50. PMID:8669532

**1688.** Delsol G, Al Saati T, Gatter KC, et al. Coexpression of epithelial membrane antigen (EMA), Ki-1, and interleukin-2 receptor by anaplastic large cell lymphomas. Diagnostic value in so-called malignant histiocytosis. Am J Pathol. 1988 Jan;130(1):59–70. PMID:2827494

**1689.** Delsol G, Lamant L, Mariamé B, et al. A new subtype of large B-cell lymphoma expressing the ALK kinase and lacking the 2; 5 translocation. Blood. 1997 Mar 1;89(5):1483–90. PMID:9057627

**1690.** DeMaioribus CA, Lally KP, Sim K, et al. Mesenchymal hamartoma of the liver. A 35-year review. Arch Surg. 1990 May;125(5):598–600. PMID:2331217

**1691.** DeMay RM, Kay S. Granular cell tumor of the breast. Pathol Annu. 1984;19(Pt 2):121–48. PMID:6095165

**1692.** Dembowska-Baginska B, Perek D, Brozyna A, et al. Non-Hodgkin lymphoma (NHL) in children with Nijmegen Breakage syndrome (NBS). Pediatr Blood Cancer. 2009 Feb;52(2):186–90. PMID:18937313

**1693.** Demehri S, Paschka P, Schultheis B, et al. e8a2 BCR-ABL: more frequent than other atypical BCR-ABL variants? Leukemia. 2005 Apr;19(4):681–4. PMID:15703785

**1694.** Demicco EG. Molecular updates in adipocytic neoplasms. Semin Diagn Pathol. 2019 Mar;36(2):85–94. PMID:30857767

**1695.** Demicco EG, Griffin AM, Gladdy RA, et al. Comparison of published risk models for prediction of outcome in patients with extrameningeal solitary fibrous tumour. Histopathology. 2019 Nov;75(5):723–37. PMID:31206727

**1696.** Demicco EG, Wagner MJ, Maki RG, et al. Risk assessment in solitary fibrous tumors: validation and refinement of a risk stratification model. Mod Pathol. 2017 Oct;30(10):1433–42. PMID:28731041

**1697.** Demir HA, Ekici F, Yazal Erdem A, et al. Everolimus: a challenging drug in the treatment of multifocal inoperable cardiac rhabdomyoma. Pediatrics. 2012 Jul;130(1):e243–7. PMID:22732179

**1698.** Demir MK, Yapıcıer Ö, Karakaya ÖF, et al. A primary third ventricle mixed germ cell tumor with leptomeningeal dissemination of immature teratoma component. Childs Nerv Syst. 2020 Mar;36(3):629–33. PMID:31418081

**1699.** den Bakker MA, Beverloo BH, van den Heuvel-Eibrink MM, et al. NUT midline carcinoma of the parotid gland with mesenchymal differentiation. Am J Surg Pathol. 2009 Aug;33(8):1253–8. PMID:19561446

**1700.** Denadai R, Bertola DR, Raposo-Amaral CE. Hyaline fibromatosis syndrome: new unifying term and surgical approach. Indian J Pathol Microbiol. 2012 Apr-Jun;55(2):262. PMID:22771664

**1701.** Denadai R, Raposo-Amaral CE, Bertola D, et al. Identification of 2 novel ANTXR2 mutations in patients with hyaline fibromatosis syndrome and proposal of a modified grading system. Am J Med Genet A. 2012 Apr;158A(4):732–42. PMID:22383261

**1702.** Deneau MR, El-Matary W, Valentino PL, et al. The natural history of primary sclerosing cholangitis in 781 children: a multicenter, international collaboration. Hepatology. 2017 Aug;66(2):518–27. PMID:28390159

**1703.** Deng MY, Sill M, Chiang J, et al. Molecularly defined diffuse leptomeningeal glioneuronal tumor (DLGNT) comprises two subgroups with distinct clinical and genetic features. Acta Neuropathol. 2018 Aug;136(2):239–53. PMID:29766299

**1704.** Deng MY, Sill M, Sturm D, et al. Diffuse glioneuronal tumour with oligodendroglioma-like features and nuclear clusters (DGONC) - a molecularly defined glioneuronal CNS tumour class displaying recurrent monosomy 14. Neuropathol Appl Neurobiol. 2020 Aug;46(5):422–30. PMID:31867747

**1705.** Denschlag D, Kontny U, Tempfer C, et al. Low-grade myxofibrosarcoma of the vulva in a 15-year-old adolescent: a case report. Int J Surg Pathol. 2005 Jan;13(1):117–9. PMID:15735866

**1706.** DeParis SW, Bloomer M, Han Y, et al. Uveal Ganglioneuroma due to Germline PTEN Mutation (Cowden Syndrome) Presenting as Unilateral Infantile Glaucoma. Ocul Oncol Pathol. 2017 Jul;3(2):122–8. PMID:28868283

**1707.** Depowski PL, Setzen G, Chui A, et al. Familial occurrence of acinic cell carcinoma of the parotid gland. Arch Pathol Lab Med. 1999 Nov;123(11):1118–20. PMID:10539921

**1708.** Depuydt P, Boeva V, Hocking TD, et al. Genomic amplifications and distal 6q Loss: novel Markers for Poor Survival in High-risk Neuroblastoma Patients. J Natl Cancer Inst. 2018 Oct 1;110(10):1084–93. PMID:29514301

**1709.** D'Ercole C, Cravello L, Boubli L, et al. Large chorioangioma associated with hydrops fetalis: prenatal diagnosis and management. Fetal Diagn Ther. 1996 Sep-Oct;11(5):357–60. PMID:8894632

**1710.** Derkay CS, Wiatrak B. Recurrent respiratory papillomatosis: a review. Laryngoscope. 2008 Jul;118(7):1236–47. PMID:18496162

**1711.** Derlin T, Tornquist K, Münster S, et al. Comparative effectiveness of 18F-FDG PET/CT versus whole-body MRI for detection of malignant peripheral nerve sheath tumors in neurofibromatosis type 1. Clin Nucl Med. 2013 Jan;38(1):e19–25. PMID:23242059

**1712.** Dermawan JK, Mukhopadhyay S, Shah AA. Frequency and extent of cytokeratin expression in paraganglioma: an immunohistochemical study of 60 cases from 5 anatomic sites and review of the literature. Hum Pathol. 2019 Nov;93:16–22. PMID:31442521

**1713.** Dermody S, Walls A, Harley EH Jr. Pediatric thyroid cancer: an update from the SEER database 2007-2012. Int J Pediatr Otorhinolaryngol. 2016 Oct;89:121–6. PMID:27619041

**1714.** Desai DC, Lockman JC, Chadwick RB, et al. Recurrent germline mutation in MSH2 arises frequently de novo. J Med Genet. 2000 Sep;37(9):646–52. PMID:10978353

**1715.** Desch AK, Hartung K, Botzen A, et al. Genotyping circulating tumor DNA of pediatric Hodgkin lymphoma. Leukemia. 2020 Jan;34(1):151–66. PMID:31431735

**1716.** Deshmukh H, Yu J, Shaik J, et al. Identification of transcriptional regulatory networks specific to pilocytic astrocytoma. BMC Med Genomics. 2011 Jul 11;4:57. PMID:21745356

**1717.** Deshpande V, Oliva E, Young RH. Solid pseudopapillary neoplasm of the ovary: a report of 3 primary ovarian tumors resembling those of the pancreas. Am J Surg Pathol. 2010 Oct;34(10):1514–20. PMID:20871224

**1718.** de Silva MV, Reid R. Chondroblastoma: varied histologic appearance, potential diagnostic pitfalls, and clinicopathologic features associated with local recurrence. Ann Diagn Pathol. 2003 Aug;7(4):205–13. PMID:12913842

**1719.** Dessars B, De Raeve LE, Morandini R, et al. Genotypic and gene expression studies in congenital melanocytic nevi: insight into initial steps of melanotumorigenesis. J Invest Dermatol. 2009 Jan;129(1):139–47. PMID:18633438

**1719A.** Deuquet J, Lausch E, Superti-Furga A, et al. The dark sides of capillary morphogenesis gene 2. EMBO J. 2012 Jan 4;31(1):3–13. PMID:22215446

**1720.** Devaney K, Snyder R, Norris HJ, et al. Proliferative and histologically malignant struma ovarii: a clinicopathologic study of 54 cases. Int J Gynecol Pathol. 1993 Oct;12(4):333–43. PMID:8253550

**1721.** Dewaele B, Libbrecht L, Levy G, et al. A novel EWS-CREB3L3 gene fusion in a mesenteric sclerosing epithelioid fibrosarcoma. Genes Chromosomes Cancer. 2017 Sep;56(9):695–9. PMID:28569045

**1722.** Dewald GW, Smyrk TC, Thorland EC, et al. Fluorescence in situ hybridization to visualize genetic abnormalities in interphase cells of acinar cell carcinoma, ductal adenocarcinoma, and islet cell carcinoma of the pancreas. Mayo Clin Proc. 2009 Sep;84(9):801–10. PMID:19720778

**1723.** Dewan R, Pemov A, Kim HJ, et al. Evidence of polyclonality in neurofibromatosis type 2-associated multilobulated vestibular schwannomas. Neuro Oncol. 2015 Apr;17(4):566–73. PMID:25452392

**1724.** Dexeus FH, Logothetis CJ, Chong C, et al. Genetic abnormalities in men with germ cell tumors. J Urol. 1988 Jul;140(1):80–4. PMID:2837589

**1725.** Deyrup AT, Lee VK, Hill CE, et al. Epstein-Barr virus-associated smooth muscle tumors are distinctive mesenchymal tumors reflecting multiple infection events: a clinicopathologic and molecular analysis of 29 tumors from 19 patients. Am J Surg Pathol. 2006 Jan;30(1):75–82. PMID:16330945

**1726.** Deyrup AT, Miettinen M, North PE, et al. Angiosarcomas arising in the viscera and soft tissue of children and young adults: a clinicopathologic study of 15 cases. Am J Surg Pathol. 2009 Feb;33(2):264–9. PMID:18987547

**1727.** Deyrup AT, Miettinen M, North PE, et al. Pediatric cutaneous angiosarcomas: a clinicopathologic study of 10 cases. Am J Surg Pathol. 2011 Jan;35(1):70–5. PMID:21164289

**1728.** Deyrup AT, Tighiouart M, Montag AG, et al. Epithelioid hemangioendothelioma of soft tissue: a proposal for risk stratification based on 49 cases. Am J Surg Pathol. 2008 Jun;32(6):924–7. PMID:18551749

**1729.** Dharnidharka VR, Ho PL, Stablein DM, et al. Mycophenolate, tacrolimus and post-transplant lymphoproliferative disorder: a report of the North American Pediatric Renal Transplant Cooperative Study. Pediatr Transplant. 2002 Oct;6(5):396–9. PMID:12390426

**1730.** Dharnidharka VR, Lamb KE, Gregg JA, et al. Associations between EBV serostatus and organ transplant type in PTLD risk: an analysis of the SRTR National Registry Data in the United States. Am J Transplant. 2012 Apr;12(4):976–83. PMID:22226225

**1731.** Dharnidharka VR, Tejani AH, Ho PL, et al. Post-transplant lymphoproliferative disorder in the United States: young Caucasian males are at highest risk. Am J Transplant. 2002 Nov;2(10):993–8. PMID:12482154

**1732.** Dhebri AR, Connor S, Campbell F, et al. Diagnosis, treatment and outcome of pancreatoblastoma. Pancreatology. 2004;4(5):441–51. PMID:15256806

**1733.** D'Hooghe E, Mifsud W, Vujanić GM. "Teratoid" Wilms tumor: the extreme end of heterologous element differentiation, not a separate entity. Am J Surg Pathol. 2019 Nov;43(11):1583–90. PMID:31600178

**1734.** Di Ieva A, Davidson JM, Syro LV, et al. Crooke's cell tumors of the pituitary. Neurosurgery. 2015 May;76(5):616–22. PMID:25635886

**1735.** Di Ieva A, Rotondo F, Syro LV, et al. Aggressive pituitary adenomas–diagnosis and emerging treatments. Nat Rev Endocrinol. 2014 Jul;10(7):423–35. PMID:24821329

**1736.** Di Micco R, Prüfer F, Bruder E, et al. Sialoblastoma of the submandibular gland: a distinct entity? Eur J Pediatr. 2019 Aug;178(8):1301–4. PMID:31257547

**1737.** Dias-Santagata D, Lam Q, Vernovsky K, et al. BRAF V600E mutations are common in pleomorphic xanthoastrocytoma: diagnostic and therapeutic implications. PLoS One. 2011 Mar 29;6(3):e17948. PMID:21479234

**1738.** Diaz-Cascajo C, Borghi S, Weyers W. Angiomatoid Spitz nevus: a distinct variant of desmoplastic Spitz nevus with prominent vasculature. Am J Dermatopathol. 2000 Apr;22(2):135–9. PMID:10770433

**1739.** Diaz-Perez JA, Nielsen GP, Antonescu C, et al. EWSR1/FUS-NFATc2 rearranged round cell sarcoma: clinicopathological series of 4 cases and literature review. Hum Pathol. 2019 Aug;90:45–53. PMID:31078563

**1740.** Dickersin GR, Kline IW, Scully RE. Small cell carcinoma of the ovary with hypercalcemia: a report of eleven cases. Cancer. 1982 Jan 1;49(1):188–97. PMID:6274502

**1741.** Dickie B, Dasgupta R, Nair R, et al. Spectrum of hepatic hemangiomas: management and outcome. J Pediatr Surg. 2009 Jan;44(1):125–33. PMID:19159729

**1742.** Dickson BC, Gortzak Y, Bell RS, et al. p63 expression in adamantinoma. Virchows Arch. 2011 Jul;459(1):109–13. PMID:21674157

**1743.** Dickson BC, Sung YS, Rosenblum MK, et al. NUTM1 gene fusions characterize a subset of undifferentiated soft tissue and visceral tumors. Am J Surg Pathol. 2018 May;42(5):636–45. PMID:29356724

**1744.** Dictor M, Ek S, Sundberg M, et al. Strong lymphoid nuclear expression of SOX11 transcription factor defines lymphoblastic neoplasms, mantle cell lymphoma and Burkitt's lymphoma. Haematologica. 2009 Nov;94(11):1563–8. PMID:19880779

**1745.** Dieckmann KP, Anheuser P, Sattler F, et al. Sequential bilateral testicular tumours presenting with intervals of 20 years and more. BMC Urol. 2013 Dec 9;13:71. PMID:24321309

1746. Dieckmann KP, Kulejewski M, Pichlmeier U, et al. Diagnosis of contralateral testicular intraepithelial neoplasia (TIN) in patients with testicular germ cell cancer: systematic two-site biopsies are more sensitive than a single random biopsy. Eur Urol. 2007 Jan;51(1):175–83. PMID:16814456
1747. Diepstra A, Niens M, Vellenga E, et al. Association with HLA class I in Epstein-Barr-virus-positive and with HLA class III in Epstein-Barr-virus-negative Hodgkin's lymphoma. Lancet. 2005 Jun 25;365(9478):2216–24. PMID:15978930
1748. Dierickx D, Habermann TM. Post-transplantation lymphoproliferative disorders in adults. N Engl J Med. 2018 Feb 8;378(6):549–62. PMID:29414277
1749. Dietl J, Horny HP, Ruck P, et al. Dysgerminoma of the ovary. An immunohistochemical study of tumor-infiltrating lymphoreticular cells and tumor cells. Cancer. 1993 Apr 15;71(8):2562–8. PMID:8453580
1750. DiGiovanna JJ, Kraemer KH. Shining a light on xeroderma pigmentosum. J Invest Dermatol. 2012 Mar;132(3 Pt 2):785–96. PMID:22217736
1751. DiGiovanna JJ, Patronas N, Katz D, et al. Xeroderma pigmentosum: spinal cord astrocytoma with 9-year survival after radiation and isotretinoin therapy. J Cutan Med Surg. 1998 Jan;2(3):153–8. PMID:9479081
1752. Dilek FH, Akpolat N, Metin A, et al. Atypical fibroxanthoma of the skin and the lower lip in xeroderma pigmentosum. Br J Dermatol. 2000 Sep;143(3):618–20. PMID:10971340
1753. Dillon JL, Gonzalez JL, DeMars L, et al. Universal screening for Lynch syndrome in endometrial cancers: frequency of germline mutations and identification of patients with Lynch-like syndrome. Hum Pathol. 2017 Dec;70:121–8. PMID:29107668
1754. Dimaras H, Khetan V, Halliday W, et al. Loss of RB1 induces non-proliferative retinoma: increasing genomic instability correlates with progression to retinoblastoma. Hum Mol Genet. 2008 May 15;17(10):1363–72. PMID:18211953
1755. Dimaras H, Khetan V, Halliday W, et al. Retinoma underlying retinoblastoma revealed after tumor response to 1 cycle of chemotherapy. Arch Ophthalmol. 2009 Aug;127(8):1066–8. PMID:19667353
1756. Dimashkieh HH, Mo JQ, Wyatt-Ashmead J, et al. Pediatric hepatic angiosarcoma: case report and review of the literature. Pediatr Dev Pathol. 2004 Sep-Oct;7(5):527–32. PMID:15547777
1757. Dimitriades VR, Devlin V, Pittaluga S, et al. DOCK 8 deficiency, EBV+ lymphomatoid granulomatosis, and intrafamilial variation in presentation. Front Pediatr. 2017 Feb 28;5:38. PMID:28293550
1758. Dimitrijevic MV, Sopta J, Ivisevic TB, et al. Chondroma of the tongue. J Craniofac Surg. 2019 Jun;30(4):e315–7. PMID:30845089
1759. Dinarvand P, Lai J. Solid pseudopapillary neoplasm of the pancreas: a rare entity with unique features. Arch Pathol Lab Med. 2017 Jul;141(7):990–5. PMID:28661210
1760. Dinauer CA, Breuer C, Rivkees SA. Differentiated thyroid cancer in children: diagnosis and management. Curr Opin Oncol. 2008 Jan;20(1):59–65. PMID:18043257
1761. Diociaiuti A, Castiglia D, Corbeddu M, et al. First case of KRT2 epidermolytic nevus and novel clinical and genetic findings in 26 Italian patients with keratinopathic ichthyoses. Int J Mol Sci. 2020 Oct 18;21(20):E7707. PMID:33081034
1762. Diotallevi F, Simonetti O, Radi G, et al. Buschke-Ollendorff syndrome in a 6-year-old patient: clinical and histopathological aspects of a rare disease. Acta Dermatovenerol Alp Pannonica Adriat. 2020 Mar;29(1):31–3. PMID:32206820
1763. Dirks MS, Butman JA, Kim HJ, et al. Long-term natural history of neurofibromatosis type 2-associated intracranial tumors. J Neurosurg. 2012 Jul;117(1):109–17. PMID:22503123
1764. Di Rocco C, Iannelli A. Bilateral thalamic tumors in children. Childs Nerv Syst. 2002 Aug;18(8):440–4. PMID:12192503
1765. Dishop MK, McKay EM, Kreiger PA, et al. Fetal lung interstitial tumor (FLIT): a proposed newly recognized lung tumor of infancy to be differentiated from cystic pleuropulmonary blastoma and other developmental pulmonary lesions. Am J Surg Pathol. 2010 Dec;34(12):1762–72. PMID:21107081
1766. Dishop MK, O'Connor WN, Abraham S, et al. Primary cardiac lipoblastoma. Pediatr Dev Pathol. 2001 May-Jun;4(3):276–80. PMID:11370265
1767. Djordjevic B, Euscher ED, Malpica A. Growing teratoma syndrome of the ovary: review of literature and first report of a carcinoid tumor arising in a growing teratoma of the ovary. Am J Surg Pathol. 2007 Dec;31(12):1913–8. PMID:18043048
1768. Do JE, Noh S, Jee HJ, et al. Familial multiple pilomatricomas showing clinical features of a giant mass without associated diseases. Int J Dermatol. 2013 Feb;52(2):250–2. PMID:23347315
1769. Dobbs SP, Shaw PA, Brown LJ, et al. Borderline malignant change in recurrent müllerian papilloma of the vagina. J Clin Pathol. 1998 Nov;51(11):875–7. PMID:10193336
1770. Dodgshun AJ, Maixner WJ, Hansford JR, et al. Low rates of recurrence and slow progression of pediatric pilocytic astrocytoma after gross-total resection: justification for reducing surveillance imaging. J Neurosurg Pediatr. 2016 May;17(5):569–72. PMID:26722760
1771. Dodgshun AJ, SantaCruz N, Hwang J, et al. Disseminated glioneuronal tumors occurring in childhood: treatment outcomes and BRAF alterations including V600E mutation. J Neurooncol. 2016 Jun;128(2):293–302. PMID:26994902
1772. Doede T, Foss HD, Waldschmidt J. Carcinoid tumors of the appendix in children–epidemiology, clinical aspects and procedure. Eur J Pediatr Surg. 2000 Dec;10(6):372–7. PMID:11215778
1773. Doeden K, Molina-Kirsch H, Perez E, et al. Hydroa-like lymphoma with CD56 expression. J Cutan Pathol. 2008 May;35(5):488–94. PMID:17976208
1774. Doğanşen SÇ, Bilgiç B, Yalin GY, et al. Clinical significance of granulation pattern in corticotroph pituitary adenomas. Turk Patoloji Derg. 2019;35(1):9–14. PMID:30035294
1775. Dogansen SC, Yalin GY, Tanrikulu S, et al. Clinicopathological significance of baseline T2-weighted signal intensity in functional pituitary adenomas. Pituitary. 2018 Aug;21(4):347–54. PMID:29460202
1776. Doglioni C, Dell'Orto P, Coggi G, et al. Choroid plexus tumors. An immunocytochemical study with particular reference to the coexpression of intermediate filament proteins. Am J Pathol. 1987 Jun;127(3):519–29. PMID:2438940
1777. Dojcinov SD, Fend F, Quintanilla-Martinez L. EBV-positive lymphoproliferations of B- T- and NK-cell derivation in non-immunocompromised hosts. Pathogens. 2018 Mar 7;7(1):E28. PMID:29518976
1778. Dojcinov SD, Venkataraman G, Raffeld M, et al. EBV positive mucocutaneous ulcer–a study of 26 cases associated with various sources of immunosuppression. Am J Surg Pathol. 2010 Mar;34(3):405–17. PMID:20154586
1779. Dolcetti R, Gloghini A, Caruso A, et al. A lymphomagenic role for HIV beyond immune suppression? Blood. 2016 Mar 17;127(11):1403–9. PMID:26773045
1779A. Dombrowski ND, Wolter NE, Irace AL, et al. Mucoepidermoid carcinoma of the head and neck in children. Int J Pediatr Otorhinolaryngol. 2019 May;120:93–9. PMID:30772619
1780. Dombrowski ND, Wolter NE, Irace AL, et al. Pleomorphic adenoma of the head and neck in children: presentation and management. Laryngoscope. 2019 Nov;129(11):2603–9. PMID:30431646
1781. Dome JS, Cotton CA, Perlman EJ, et al. Treatment of anaplastic histology Wilms' tumor: results from the fifth National Wilms' Tumor Study. J Clin Oncol. 2006 May 20;24(15):2352–8. PMID:16710034
1782. Dome JS, Graf N, Geller JI, et al. Advances in Wilms Tumor treatment and biology: progress through international collaboration. J Clin Oncol. 2015 Sep 20;33(27):2999–3007. PMID:26304882
1783. Dome JS, Perlman EJ, Graf N. Risk stratification for Wilms tumor: current approach and future directions. Am Soc Clin Oncol Educ Book. 2014:215–23. PMID:24857079
1784. Domingo RP, Ogden LL, Been LC, et al. Identification of parathyroid tissue in thyroid fine-needle aspiration: a combined approach using cytology, immunohistochemical, and molecular methods. Diagn Cytopathol. 2017 Jun;45(6):526–32. PMID:28371486
1785. Domm JA, Thompson M, Kuttesch JF, et al. Allogeneic bone marrow transplantation for chemotherapy-refractory hepatosplenic gammadelta T-cell lymphoma: case report and review of the literature. J Pediatr Hematol Oncol. 2005 Nov;27(11):607–10. PMID:16282893
1786. Dômont J, Salas S, Lacroix L, et al. High frequency of beta-catenin heterozygous mutations in extra-abdominal fibromatosis: a potential molecular tool for disease management. Br J Cancer. 2010 Mar 16;102(6):1032–6. PMID:20197769
1787. Domovitov SV, Healey JH. Primary malignant giant-cell tumor of bone has high survival rate. Ann Surg Oncol. 2010 Mar;17(3):694–701. PMID:19902306
1788. Donahoo JS, Miller JA, Lal B, et al. Chest wall hamartoma in an adult: an unusual chest wall tumor. Thorac Cardiovasc Surg. 1996 Apr;44(2):110–1. PMID:8782339
1789. Dong Y, Wang WP, Mao F, et al. Imaging features of fibrolamellar hepatocellular carcinoma with contrast-enhanced ultrasound. Ultraschall Med. 2021 Jun;42(3):306–13. PMID:32102105
1790. Donovan DT, Conley JJ. Capsular significance in parotid tumor surgery: reality and myths of lateral lobectomy. Laryngoscope. 1984 Mar;94(3):324–9. PMID:6321863
1791. Donovan MJ, Yunis EJ, DeGirolami U, et al. Chromosome aberrations in choroid plexus papillomas. Genes Chromosomes Cancer. 1994 Dec;11(4):267–70. PMID:7533531
1792. Donson AM, Kleinschmidt-DeMasters BK, Aisner DL, et al. Pediatric brainstem gangliogliomas show BRAF(V600E) mutation in a high percentage of cases. Brain Pathol. 2014 Mar;24(2):173–83. PMID:24238153
1793. Dorfman DM, Shahsafaei A, Alonso MA. Utility of CD200 immunostaining in the diagnosis of primary mediastinal large B cell lymphoma: comparison with MAL, CD23, and other markers. Mod Pathol. 2012 Dec;25(12):1637–43. PMID:22899296
1794. Dorfman HD. Proceedings: Malignant transformation of benign bone lesions. Proc Natl Cancer Conf. 1972;7:901–13. PMID:4764948
1795. Dorfman HD, Czerniak B. Bone cancers. Cancer. 1995 Jan 1;75(1 Suppl):203–10. PMID:8000997
1796. Dorfman HD, Weiss SW. Borderline osteoblastic tumors: problems in the differential diagnosis of aggressive osteoblastoma and low-grade osteosarcoma. Semin Diagn Pathol. 1984 Aug;1(3):215–34. PMID:6600112
1797. Dornbos D 3rd, Kim HJ, Butman JA, et al. Review of the neurological implications of von Hippel-Lindau disease. JAMA Neurol. 2018 May 1;75(5):620–7. PMID:29379961
1798. Doros L, Schultz KA, Stewart DR, et al. DICER1-related disorders. In: Adam MP, Ardinger HH, Pagon RA, et al., editors. GeneReviews. Seattle (WA): University of Washington, Seattle; 2014 Apr 24. PMID:24761742
1799. Doros LA, Rossi CT, Yang J, et al. DICER1 mutations in childhood cystic nephroma and its relationship to DICER1-renal sarcoma. Mod Pathol. 2014 Sep;27(9):1267–80. PMID:24481001
1800. Dorssers LCJ, Gillis AJM, Stoop H, et al. Molecular heterogeneity and early metastatic clone selection in testicular germ cell cancer development. Br J Cancer. 2019 Feb;120(4):444–52. PMID:30739914
1801. Dos Santos L, Mok E, Iasonos A, et al. Squamous cell carcinoma arising in mature cystic teratoma of the ovary: a case series and review of the literature. Gynecol Oncol. 2007 May;105(2):321–4. PMID:17240432
1802. dos Santos NR, de Bruijn DR, van Kessel AG. Molecular mechanisms underlying human synovial sarcoma development. Genes Chromosomes Cancer. 2001 Jan;30(1):1–14. PMID:11107170
1803. Dotti G, Garattini E, Borleri G, et al. Leucocyte alkaline phosphatase identifies terminally differentiated normal neutrophils and its lack in chronic myelogenous leukaemia is not dependent on p210 tyrosine kinase activity. Br J Haematol. 1999 Apr;105(1):163–72. PMID:10233380
1804. Dougherty MJ, Santi M, Brose MS, et al. Activating mutations in BRAF characterize a spectrum of pediatric low-grade gliomas. Neuro Oncol. 2010 Jul;12(7):621–30. PMID:20156809
1805. Douis H, Saifuddin A. The imaging of cartilaginous bone tumours. I. Benign lesions. Skeletal Radiol. 2012 Sep;41(10):1195–212. PMID:22707094
1806. Dounies R, Chwals WJ, Lally KP, et al. Hamartomas of the chest wall in infants. Ann Thorac Surg. 1994 Apr;57(4):868–75. PMID:8166533
1807. Dourthe ME, Bolle S, Temam S, et al. Childhood nasopharyngeal carcinoma: state-of-the-art, and questions for the future. J Pediatr Hematol Oncol. 2018 Mar;40(2):85–92. PMID:29300240
1808. Dow DE, Cunningham CK, Buchanan AM. A review of human herpesvirus 8, the Kaposi's sarcoma-associated herpesvirus, in the pediatric population. J Pediatric Infect Dis Soc. 2014 Mar;3(1):66–76. PMID:24567845
1809. Doyle LA, Fletcher CD. Peripheral hemangioblastoma: clinicopathologic characterization in a series of 22 cases. Am J Surg Pathol. 2014 Jan;38(1):119–27. PMID:24145646
1810. Doyle LA, Fletcher CD, Hornick JL. Nuclear expression of CAMTA1 distinguishes epithelioid hemangioendothelioma from histologic mimics. Am J Surg Pathol. 2016 Jan;40(1):94–102. PMID:26414223
1811. Doyle LA, Hornick JL. EWSR1 rearrangements in sclerosing epithelioid fibrosarcoma. Am J Surg Pathol. 2013 Oct;37(10):1630–1. PMID:24025527
1812. Doyle LA, Hornick JL. Pathology of extramedullary mastocytosis. Immunol Allergy

Clin North Am. 2014 May;34(2):323–39. PMID:24745677
1813. Doyle LA, Mariño-Enriquez A, Fletcher CD, et al. ALK rearrangement and overexpression in epithelioid fibrous histiocytoma. Mod Pathol. 2015 Jul;28(7):904–12. PMID:25857825
1814. Doyle LA, Möller E, Dal Cin P, et al. MUC4 is a highly sensitive and specific marker for low-grade fibromyxoid sarcoma. Am J Surg Pathol. 2011 May;35(5):733–41. PMID:21415703
1815. Doyle LA, Nelson D, Heinrich MC, et al. Loss of succinate dehydrogenase subunit B (SDHB) expression is limited to a distinctive subset of gastric wild-type gastrointestinal stromal tumours: a comprehensive genotype-phenotype correlation study. Histopathology. 2012 Nov;61(5):801–9. PMID:22804613
1816. Doyle LA, Sepehr GJ, Hamilton MJ, et al. A clinicopathologic study of 24 cases of systemic mastocytosis involving the gastrointestinal tract and assessment of mucosal mast cell density in irritable bowel syndrome and asymptomatic patients. Am J Surg Pathol. 2014 Jun;38(6):832–43. PMID:24618605
1817. Doyle LA, Wang WL, Dal Cin P, et al. MUC4 is a sensitive and extremely useful marker for sclerosing epithelioid fibrosarcoma: association with FUS gene rearrangement. Am J Surg Pathol. 2012 Oct;36(10):1444–51. PMID:22982887
1818. Draper GJ, Sanders BM, Brownbill PA, et al. Patterns of risk of hereditary retinoblastoma and applications to genetic counselling. Br J Cancer. 1992 Jul;66(1):211–9. PMID:1637670
1819. Dray MS, McCarthy SW, Palmer AA, et al. Myopericytoma: a unifying term for a spectrum of tumours that show overlapping features with myofibroma. A review of 14 cases. J Clin Pathol. 2006 Jan;59(1):67–73. PMID:16394283
1820. Drilon A, Siena S, Ou SI, et al. Safety and antitumor activity of the multitargeted pan-TRK, ROS1, and ALK inhibitor entrectinib: combined results from two phase I trials (ALKA-372-001 and STARTRK-1). Cancer Discov. 2017 Apr;7(4):400–9. PMID:28183697
1821. Drolet BA, Esterly NB, Frieden IJ. Hemangiomas in children. N Engl J Med. 1999 Jul 15;341(3):173–81. PMID:10403856
1822. Drolet BA, Frieden IJ. Characteristics of infantile hemangiomas as clues to pathogenesis: Does hypoxia connect the dots? Arch Dermatol. 2010 Nov;146(11):1295–9. PMID:21079070
1823. Drolet BA, Trenor CC 3rd, Brandão LR, et al. Consensus-derived practice standards plan for complicated Kaposiform hemangioendothelioma. J Pediatr. 2013 Jul;163(1):285–91. PMID:23796341
1824. Drut R, Jones MC. Congenital pancreatoblastoma in Beckwith-Wiedemann syndrome: an emerging association. Pediatr Pathol. 1988;8(3):331–9. PMID:2845376
1825. Dryja TP, Cavenee W, White R, et al. Homozygosity of chromosome 13 in retinoblastoma. N Engl J Med. 1984 Mar 1;310(9):550–3. PMID:6694706
1826. Dryja TP, Rapaport J, McGee TL, et al. Molecular etiology of low-penetrance retinoblastoma in two pedigrees. Am J Hum Genet. 1993 Jun;52(6):1122–8. PMID:8099255
1827. D'Souza AM, Shah R, Gupta A, et al. Surgical management of children and adolescents with upfront completely resected hepatocellular carcinoma. Pediatr Blood Cancer. 2018 Nov;65(11):e27293. PMID:29968976
1828. Du J, Wang J, Cui Y, et al. Clinicopathologic study of endolymphatic sac tumor (ELST) and differential diagnosis of papillary tumors located at the cerebellopontine angle. Neuropathology. 2015 Oct;35(5):410–20. PMID:25944396
1829. Du S, Scuderi R, Malicki DM, et al. Hodgkin's and non-Hodgkin's lymphomas occurring in two brothers with Wiskott-Aldrich syndrome and review of the literature. Pediatr Dev Pathol. 2011 Jan-Feb;14(1):64–70. PMID:20429642
1830. Duan F, Smith LM, Gustafson DM, et al. Genomic and clinical analysis of fusion gene amplification in rhabdomyosarcoma: a report from the Children's Oncology Group. Genes Chromosomes Cancer. 2012 Jul;51(7):662–74. PMID:22447499
1831. Duan K, Asa SL, Winer D, et al. Xanthomatous hypophysitis is associated with ruptured Rathke's cleft cyst. Endocr Pathol. 2017 Mar;28(1):83–90. PMID:28120170
1832. Duan K, Mete O. Algorithmic approach to neuroendocrine tumors in targeted biopsies: practical applications of immunohistochemical markers. Cancer Cytopathol. 2016 Dec;124(12):871–84. PMID:27529763
1833. Duan K, Mete O. Hereditary endocrine tumor syndromes: the clinical and predictive role of molecular histopathology. AJSP rev reports. 2017;22(5):246–68. doi:10.1097/PCR.0000000000000206.
1834. Dubois S, Viailly PJ, Mareschal S, et al. Next-generation sequencing in diffuse large B-cell lymphoma highlights molecular divergence and therapeutic opportunities: a LYSA study. Clin Cancer Res. 2016 Jun 15;22(12):2919–28. PMID:26819451
1835. Dubuc AM, Remke M, Korshunov A, et al. Aberrant patterns of H3K4 and H3K27 histone lysine methylation occur across subgroups in medulloblastoma. Acta Neuropathol. 2013 Mar;125(3):373–84. PMID:23184418
1836. Ducatman BS, Scheithauer BW. Malignant peripheral nerve sheath tumors with divergent differentiation. Cancer. 1984 Sep 15;54(6):1049–57. PMID:6432304
1837. Dudič R, Dudičová V, Urdzík P. The rare cause of childhood bleeding - recurrent Müllerian papilloma. J Obstet Gynaecol. 2019 Apr;39(3):432–3. PMID:30406704
1838. Dudley RW, Torok MR, Gallegos DR, et al. Pediatric low-grade ganglioglioma: epidemiology, treatments, and outcome analysis on 348 children from the Surveillance, Epidemiology, and End Results database. Neurosurgery. 2015 Mar;76(3):313–9. PMID:25603107
1839. Duff J, Meyer FB, Ilstrup DM, et al. Long-term outcomes for surgically resected craniopharyngiomas. Neurosurgery. 2000 Feb;46(2):291–302. PMID:10690718
1840. Duffner PK, Horowitz ME, Krischer JP, et al. The treatment of malignant brain tumors in infants and very young children: an update of the Pediatric Oncology Group experience. Neuro Oncol. 1999 Apr;1(2):152–61. PMID:11554387
1841. Dufva O, Kankainen M, Kelkka T, et al. Aggressive natural killer-cell leukemia mutational landscape and drug profiling highlight JAK-STAT signaling as therapeutic target. Nat Commun. 2018 Apr 19;9(1):1567. PMID:29674644
1842. Duhil de Bénazé G, Pacquement H, Faure-Conter C, et al. Paediatric dysgerminoma: results of three consecutive French germ cell tumours clinical studies (TGM-85/90/95) with late effects study. Eur J Cancer. 2018 Mar;91:30–7. PMID:29331749
1843. Dujardin F, Binh MB, Bouvier C, et al. MDM2 and CDK4 immunohistochemistry is a valuable tool in the differential diagnosis of low-grade osteosarcomas and other primary fibro-osseous lesions of the bone. Mod Pathol. 2011 May;24(5):624–37. PMID:21336260
1844. Duke DS, Yoo EY, Newton C, et al. A rare cause of vaginal bleeding in a 7-month-old female infant. J Pediatr Surg. 2008 Mar;43(3):E1–4. PMID:18358265
1845. Dulon M, Weichenthal M, Blettner M, et al. Sun exposure and number of nevi in 5- to 6-year-old European children. J Clin Epidemiol. 2002 Nov;55(11):1075–81. PMID:12507670
1846. Dumitriu D, Dudea SM, Botar-Jid C, et al. Ultrasonographic and sonoelastographic features of pleomorphic adenomas of the salivary glands. Med Ultrason. 2010 Sep;12(3):175–83. PMID:21203593
1847. Duncan JL, Golabi M, Fredrick DR, et al. Complex limbal choristomas in linear nevus sebaceous syndrome. Ophthalmology. 1998 Aug;105(8):1459–65. PMID:9709758
1848. Đunđerović D, Lipkovski JM, Boričic I, et al. Defining the value of CD56, CK19, Galectin 3 and HBME-1 in diagnosis of follicular cell derived lesions of thyroid with systematic review of literature. Diagn Pathol. 2015 Oct 26;10:196. PMID:26503236
1849. Dunham C, Hussong J, Seiff M, et al. Primary intracerebral angiomatoid fibrous histiocytoma: report of a case with a t(12;22)(q13;q12) causing type 1 fusion of the EWS and ATF-1 genes. Am J Surg Pathol. 2008 Mar;32(3):478–84. PMID:18300800
1850. Dunham C, Sugo E, Tobias V, et al. Embryonal tumor with abundant neuropil and true rosettes (ETANTR): report of a case with prominent neurocytic differentiation. J Neurooncol. 2007 Aug;84(1):91–8. PMID:17332950
1851. Dunkel IJ, Chan HS, Jubran R, et al. High-dose chemotherapy with autologous hematopoietic stem cell rescue for stage 4B retinoblastoma. Pediatr Blood Cancer. 2010 Jul 15;55(1):149–52. PMID:20486181
1852. Dunkel IJ, Khakoo Y, Kernan NA, et al. Intensive multimodality therapy for patients with stage 4a metastatic retinoblastoma. Pediatr Blood Cancer. 2010 Jul 15;55(1):55–9. PMID:20486171
1853. Dunphy CH, Gardner LJ, Grosso LE, et al. Flow cytometric immunophenotyping in posttransplant lymphoproliferative disorders. Am J Clin Pathol. 2002 Jan;117(1):24–8. PMID:11789726
1854. Dunzendorfer-Matt T, Mercado EL, Maly K, et al. The neurofibromin recruitment factor Spred1 binds to the GAP related domain without affecting Ras inactivation. Proc Natl Acad Sci U S A. 2016 Jul 5;113(27):7497–502. PMID:27313208
1855. Duò D, Gasverde S, Benech F, et al. MIB-1 immunoreactivity in craniopharyngiomas: a clinico-pathological analysis. Clin Neuropathol. 2003 Sep-Oct;22(5):229–34. PMID:14531547
1856. Dupree WB, Langloss JM, Weiss SW. Pigmented dermatofibrosarcoma protuberans (Bednar tumor). A pathologic, ultrastructural, and immunohistochemical study. Am J Surg Pathol. 1985 Sep;9(9):630–9. PMID:3901787
1857. Dupuy A, Sarasin A. DNA damage and gene therapy of xeroderma pigmentosum, a human DNA repair-deficient disease. Mutat Res. 2015 Jun;776:2–8. PMID:26255934
1858. Dupuy A, Valton J, Leduc S, et al. Targeted gene therapy of xeroderma pigmentosum cells using meganuclease and TALEN™. PLoS One. 2013 Nov 13;8(11):e78678. PMID:24236034
1859. Durakbaşa ÇU, Erkoç G, Çağlar Oskaylı M, et al. A retrospective evaluation of pediatric breast fibroadenomas with mid-term follow-up results. Breast J. 2020 Sep;26(9):1898–9. PMID:32281202
1860. Durandy A, Kracker S. Increased activation of PI3 kinase-δ predisposes to B-cell lymphoma. Blood. 2020 Feb 27;135(9):638–43. PMID:31942637
1861. Durell J, Dagash H, Eradi B, et al. Pediatric benign cystic peritoneal mesothelioma. J Pediatr Adolesc Gynecol. 2016 Apr;29(2):e33–4. PMID:26524665
1862. Durham BH, Lopez Rodrigo E, Picarsic J, et al. Activating mutations in CSF1R and additional receptor tyrosine kinases in histiocytic neoplasms. Nat Med. 2019 Dec;25(12):1839–42. PMID:31768065
1863. Durham BH, Roos-Weil D, Baillou C, et al. Functional evidence for derivation of systemic histiocytic neoplasms from hematopoietic stem/progenitor cells. Blood. 2017 Jul 13;130(2):176–80. PMID:28566492
1864. Durieux E, Descotes F, Nguyen AM, et al. Somatic DICER1 gene mutation in sporadic intraocular medulloepithelioma without pleuropulmonary blastoma syndrome. Hum Pathol. 2015 May;46(5):783–7. PMID:25791583
1865. Durno C, Boland CR, Cohen S, et al. Recommendations on surveillance and management of biallelic mismatch repair deficiency (BMMRD) syndrome: a consensus statement by the US multi-society task force on colorectal cancer. gastroenterology. 2017 May;152(6):1605–14. PMID:28363489
1866. Durno CA, Aronson M, Tabori U, et al. Oncologic surveillance for subjects with biallelic mismatch repair gene mutations: 10 year follow-up of a kindred. Pediatr Blood Cancer. 2012 Oct;59(4):652–6. PMID:22180144
1867. Durno CA, Sherman PM, Aronson M, et al. Phenotypic and genotypic characterisation of biallelic mismatch repair deficiency (BMMR-D) syndrome. Eur J Cancer. 2015 May;51(8):977–83. PMID:25883011
1868. Dursun H, Bayazit AK, Büyükçelik M, et al. Aggressive angiomyxoma in a child with chronic renal failure. Pediatr Surg Int. 2005 Jul;21(7):563–5. PMID:15776247
1869. Dwight T, Benn DE, Clarkson A, et al. Loss of SDHA expression identifies SDHA mutations in succinate dehydrogenase-deficient gastrointestinal stromal tumors. Am J Surg Pathol. 2013 Feb;37(2):226–33. PMID:23060355
1870. Dymerska D, Gołębiewska K, Kuświk M, et al. New EPCAM founder deletion in Polish population. Clin Genet. 2017 Dec;92(6):649–53. PMID:28369810
1871. Dymock RB, Allen PW, Stirling JW, et al. Giant cell fibroblastoma. A distinctive, recurrent tumor of childhood. Am J Surg Pathol. 1987 Apr;11(4):263–71. PMID:3565673
1872. Dyson K, Rivera-Zengotita M, Kresak J, et al. FGFR1 N546K and H3F3A K27M mutations in a diffuse leptomeningeal tumour with glial and neuronal markers. Histopathology. 2016 Oct;69(4):704–7. PMID:27061725
1873. Dyson NJ. RB1: a prototype tumor suppressor and an enigma. Genes Dev. 2016 Jul 1;30(13):1492–502. PMID:27401552
1874. Eagle RC Jr. High-risk features and tumor differentiation in retinoblastoma: a retrospective histopathologic study. Arch Pathol Lab Med. 2009 Aug;133(8):1203–9. PMID:19653710
1875. Eagle RC Jr, Font RL, Swerczek TW. Malignant medulloepithelioma of the optic nerve in a horse. Vet Pathol. 1978 Jul;15(4):488–94. PMID:695223
1876. Eagle RC Jr, Shields JA, Donoso L, et al. Malignant transformation of spontaneously regressed retinoblastoma, retinoma/retinocytoma variant. Ophthalmology. 1989 Sep;96(9):1389–95. PMID:2780006
1877. Easton JA, Donnelly S, Kamps MA, et al. Porokeratotic eccrine nevus may be caused by somatic connexin26 mutations. J Invest Dermatol. 2012 Sep;132(9):2184–91. PMID:22592158
1878. Eaton KW, Tooke LS, Wainwright LM, et al. Spectrum of SMARCB1/INI1 mutations in familial and sporadic rhabdoid tumors. Pediatr Blood Cancer. 2011 Jan;56(1):7–15. PMID:21108436

**1879.** Ebeid WA, Hasan BZ, Badr IT, et al. Functional and oncological outcome after treatment of chondroblastoma with intralesional curettage. J Pediatr Orthop. 2019 Apr;39(4):e312–7. PMID:30839485

**1880.** Eberhart CG, Brat DJ, Cohen KJ, et al. Pediatric neuroblastic brain tumors containing abundant neuropil and true rosettes. Pediatr Dev Pathol. 2000 Jul-Aug;3(4):346–52. PMID:10890250

**1881.** Eberhart CG, Kepner JL, Goldthwaite PT, et al. Histopathologic grading of medulloblastomas: a Pediatric Oncology Group study. Cancer. 2002 Jan 15;94(2):552–60. PMID:11900240

**1882.** Eberhart CG, Kratz J, Wang Y, et al. Histopathological and molecular prognostic markers in medulloblastoma: c-myc, N-myc, TrkC, and anaplasia. J Neuropathol Exp Neurol. 2004 May;63(5):441–9. PMID:15198123

**1883.** Eberle FC, Rodriguez-Canales J, Wei L, et al. Methylation profiling of mediastinal gray zone lymphoma reveals a distinctive signature with elements shared by classical Hodgkin's lymphoma and primary mediastinal large B-cell lymphoma. Haematologica. 2011 Apr;96(4):558–66. PMID:21454882

**1884.** Eberle FC, Salaverria I, Steidl C, et al. Gray zone lymphoma: chromosomal aberrations with immunophenotypic and clinical correlations. Mod Pathol. 2011 Dec;24(12):1586–97. PMID:21822207

**1884A.** Ebert C, von Haken M, Meyer-Puttlitz B, et al. Molecular genetic analysis of ependymal tumors. NF2 mutations and chromosome 22q loss occur preferentially in intramedullary spinal ependymomas. Am J Pathol. 1999 Aug;155(2):627–32. PMID:10433955

**1885.** Echegaray JJ, Al-Zahrani YA, Singh A. Episcleral brachytherapy for retinoblastoma. Br J Ophthalmol. 2020 Feb;104(2):208–13. PMID:31122912

**1886.** Eckardt JJ, Grogan TJ. Giant cell tumor of bone. Clin Orthop Relat Res. 1986 Mar;(204):45–58. PMID:3514036

**1887.** Eckardt JJ, Pritchard DJ, Soule EH. Clear cell sarcoma. A clinicopathologic study of 27 cases. Cancer. 1983 Oct 15;52(8):1482–8. PMID:6616410

**1888.** Eckelt F, Vogel M, Geserick M, et al. Calcitonin measurement in pediatrics: reference ranges are gender-dependent, validation in medullary thyroid cancer and thyroid diseases. Clin Chem Lab Med. 2019 Jul 26;57(8):1242–50. PMID:30794525

**1889.** Eder N, Roncaroli F, Domart MC, et al. YAP1/TAZ drives ependymoma-like tumour formation in mice. Nat Commun. 2020 May 13;11(1):2380. PMID:32404936

**1890.** Edis AJ. Surgical anatomy and technique of neck exploration for primary hyperparathyroidism. Surg Clin North Am. 1977 Jun;57(3):495–504. PMID:867217

**1891.** Edward DP, Alkatan H, Rafiq Q, et al. MicroRNA profiling in intraocular medulloepitheliomas. PLoS One. 2015 Mar 25;10(3):e0121706. PMID:25807141

**1892.** Edward DP, Morales J, Bouhenni RA, et al. Congenital ectropion uvea and mechanisms of glaucoma in neurofibromatosis type 1: new insights. Ophthalmology. 2012 Jul;119(7):1485–94. PMID:22480745

**1893.** Eefting D, Schrage YM, Geirnaerdt MJ, et al. Assessment of interobserver variability and histologic parameters to improve reliability in classification and grading of central cartilaginous tumors. Am J Surg Pathol. 2009 Jan;33(1):50–7. PMID:18852676

**1894.** Eerola I, Boon LM, Mulliken JB, et al. Capillary malformation-arteriovenous malformation, a new clinical and genetic disorder caused by RASA1 mutations. Am J Hum Genet. 2003 Dec;73(6):1240–9. PMID:14639529

**1895.** Efanov AA, Brenner AV, Bogdanova TI, et al. Investigation of the relationship between radiation dose and gene mutations and fusions in post-Chernobyl thyroid cancer. J Natl Cancer Inst. 2018 Apr 1;110(4):371–8. PMID:29165687

**1896.** Egan D, Radich J. Making the diagnosis, the tools, and risk stratification: more than just BCR-ABL. Best Pract Res Clin Haematol. 2016 Sep;29(3):252–63. PMID:27839566

**1897.** Egg D, Schwab C, Gabrysch A, et al. Increased risk for malignancies in 131 affected CTLA4 mutation carriers. Front Immunol. 2018 Sep 10;9:2012. PMID:30250467

**1898.** Eggermann T, Perez de Nanclares G, Maher ER, et al. Imprinting disorders: a group of congenital disorders with overlapping patterns of molecular changes affecting imprinted loci. Clin Epigenetics. 2015 Nov 14;7:123. PMID:26583054

**1899.** Eichenmüller M, Trippel F, Kreuder M, et al. The genomic landscape of hepatoblastoma and their progenies with HCC-like features. J Hepatol. 2014 Dec;61(6):1312–20. PMID:25135868

**1900.** Eidenschink Brodersen L, Alonzo TA, Menssen AJ, et al. A recurrent immunophenotype at diagnosis independently identifies high-risk pediatric acute myeloid leukemia: a report from Children's Oncology Group. Leukemia. 2016 Oct;30(10):2077–80. PMID:27133823

**1901.** Eiger-Moscovich M, Eagle RC Jr, Lally SE, et al. Conjunctival melanocytic nevi with granular cell change. Arch Pathol Lab Med. 2020 Apr;144(4):457–65. PMID:31469587

**1902.** Einhorn LH, Brames MJ, Heinrich MC, et al. Phase II study of imatinib mesylate in chemotherapy refractory germ cell tumors expressing KIT. Am J Clin Oncol. 2006 Feb;29(1):12–3. PMID:16462496

**1903.** Eisenhofer G, Klink B, Richter S, et al. Metabologenomics of phaeochromocytoma and paraganglioma: an integrated approach for personalised biochemical and genetic testing. Clin Biochem Rev. 2017 Apr;38(2):69–100. PMID:29332973

**1904.** Eisenhofer G, Lenders JW, Timmers H, et al. Measurements of plasma methoxytyramine, normetanephrine, and metanephrine as discriminators of different hereditary forms of pheochromocytoma. Clin Chem. 2011 Mar;57(3):411–20. PMID:21262951

**1905.** Eisenhofer G, Tischler AS, de Krijger RR. Diagnostic tests and biomarkers for pheochromocytoma and extra-adrenal paraganglioma: from routine laboratory methods to disease stratification. Endocr Pathol. 2012 Mar;23(1):4–14. PMID:22180288

**1906.** Eisenhut CC, King DE, Nelson WA, et al. Fine-needle biopsy of pediatric lesions: a three-year study in an outpatient biopsy clinic. Diagn Cytopathol. 1996 Feb;14(1):43–50. PMID:8834076

**1907.** Ekfors TO, Kulju T, Aaltonen M, et al. Ossifying fibromyxoid tumour of soft parts: report of four cases including one mediastinal and one infantile. APMIS. 1998 Dec;106(12):1124–30. PMID:10052720

**1908.** El Demellawy D, Cundiff CA, Nasr A, et al. Congenital mesoblastic nephroma: a study of 19 cases using immunohistochemistry and ETV6-NTRK3 fusion gene rearrangement. Pathology. 2016 Jan;48(1):47–50. PMID:27020209

**1909.** El Demellawy D, Nasr AL, Babay S, et al. Diagnostic utility of CD56 immunohistochemistry in papillary carcinoma of the thyroid. Pathol Res Pract. 2009;205(5):303–9. PMID:19153015

**1910.** El Hussein S, Patel KP, Fang H, et al. Genomic and immunophenotypic landscape of aggressive NK-cell leukemia. Am J Surg Pathol. 2020 Sep;44(9):1235–43. PMID:32590457

**1911.** El Wakil A, Doghman M, Latre De Late P, et al. Genetics and genomics of childhood adrenocortical tumors. Mol Cell Endocrinol. 2011 Apr 10;336(1-2):169–73. PMID:21094206

**1912.** El Zein S, Boccara O, Soupre V, et al. The histopathology of congenital haemangioma and its clinical correlations: a long-term follow-up study of 55 cases. Histopathology. 2020 Aug;77(2):275–83. PMID:32281140

**1913.** Elder DE, Bastian BC, Cree IA, et al. The 2018 World Health Organization classification of cutaneous, mucosal, and uveal melanoma: detailed analysis of 9 distinct subtypes defined by their evolutionary pathway. Arch Pathol Lab Med. 2020 Apr;144(4):500–22. PMID:32057276

**1914.** Elder DE, Massi D, Scolyer RA, et al., editors. WHO classification of skin tumours. Lyon (France): International Agency for Research on Cancer; 2018. (WHO classification of tumours series, 4th ed.; vol. 11). https://publications.iarc.fr/560.

**1915.** Elenitoba-Johnson KS, Kumar S, Lim MS, et al. Marginal zone B-cell lymphoma with monocytoid B-cell lymphocytes in pediatric patients without immunodeficiency. A report of two cases. Am J Clin Pathol. 1997 Jan;107(1):92–8. PMID:8980374

**1916.** Elezaby M, Lees B, Maturen KE, et al. BRCA mutation carriers: breast and ovarian cancer screening guidelines and imaging considerations. Radiology. 2019 Jun;291(3):554–69. PMID:31038410

**1917.** El-Fattah AM, Naguib A, El-Sisi H, et al. Midline nasofrontal dermoids in children: a review of 29 cases managed at Mansoura University Hospitals. Int J Pediatr Otorhinolaryngol. 2016 Apr;83:88–92. PMID:26968060

**1918.** El Hussein S, Vincentelli C. Pituicytoma: review of commonalities and distinguishing features among TTF-1 positive tumors of the central nervous system. Ann Diagn Pathol. 2017 Aug;29:57–61. PMID:28807344

**1919.** Elkaim E, Neven B, Bruneau J, et al. Clinical and immunologic phenotype associated with activated phosphoinositide 3-kinase δ syndrome 2: a cohort study. J Allergy Clin Immunol. 2016 Jul;138(1):210–218.e9. PMID:27221134

**1919A.** El-Kamah GY, Fong K, El-Ruby M, et al. Spectrum of mutations in the ANTXR2 (CMG2) gene in infantile systemic hyalinosis and juvenile hyaline fibromatosis. Br J Dermatol. 2010 Jul;163(1):213–5. PMID:20331448

**1920.** Ellerkamp V, Warmann SW, Vorwerk P, et al. Exocrine pancreatic tumors in childhood in Germany. Pediatr Blood Cancer. 2012 Mar;58(3):366–71. PMID:21681931

**1921.** Elliott P, Kleinschmidt I. Angiosarcoma of the liver in Great Britain in proximity to vinyl chloride sites. Occup Environ Med. 1997 Jan;54(1):14–8. PMID:9072028

**1922.** Ellis CL, Eble JN, Subhawong AP, et al. Clinical heterogeneity of Xp11 translocation renal cell carcinoma: impact of fusion subtype, age, and stage. Mod Pathol. 2014 Jun;27(6):875–86. PMID:24309327

**1923.** Ellis D, Fitzgerald TN. Invited commentary: Clinical assessment of pediatric patients with differentiated thyroid carcinoma: a 30-year experience at the single institution. World J Surg. 2020 Oct;44(10):3393–4. PMID:32535641

**1924.** Ellis MB, Gridley D, Lal S, et al. Phosphaturic mesenchymal tumor of the brain without tumor-induced osteomalacia in an 8-year-old girl: case report. J Neurosurg Pediatr. 2016 May;17(5):573–7. PMID:26722864

**1925.** Ellis RJ, Patel D, Prodanov T, et al. The presence of SDHB mutations should modify surgical indications for carotid body paragangliomas. Ann Surg. 2014 Jul;260(1):158–62. PMID:24169168

**1926.** Ellison DA, Adada B, Qualman SJ, et al. Melanotic neuroectodermal tumor of infancy: report of a case with myogenic differentiation. Pediatr Dev Pathol. 2007 Mar-Apr;10(2):157–60. PMID:17378694

**1927.** Ellison DA, Parham DM, Bridge J, et al. Immunohistochemistry of primary malignant neuroepithelial tumors of the kidney: a potential source of confusion? A study of 30 cases from the National Wilms Tumor Study Pathology Center. Hum Pathol. 2007 Feb;38(2):205–11. PMID:17134738

**1928.** Ellison DW. Childhood medulloblastoma: novel approaches to the classification of a heterogeneous disease. Acta Neuropathol. 2010 Sep;120(3):305–16. PMID:20652577

**1929.** Ellison DW. Mini-symposium in medulloblastoma genomics in the modern molecular era. Brain Pathol. 2020 May;30(3):661–3. PMID:32243002

**1930.** Ellison DW, Aldape KD, Capper D, et al. cIMPACT-NOW update 7: advancing the molecular classification of ependymal tumors. Brain Pathol. 2020 Sep;30(5):863–6. PMID:32502305

**1931.** Ellison DW, Dalton J, Kocak M, et al. Medulloblastoma: clinicopathological correlates of SHH, WNT, and non-SHH/WNT molecular subgroups. Acta Neuropathol. 2011 Mar;121(3):381–96. PMID:21267586

**1932.** Ellison DW, Hawkins C, Jones DTW, et al. cIMPACT-NOW update 4: diffuse gliomas characterized by MYB, MYBL1, or FGFR1 alterations or BRAFV600E mutation. Acta Neuropathol. 2019 Apr;137(4):683–7. PMID:30848347

**1933.** Ellison DW, Kocak M, Dalton J, et al. Definition of disease-risk stratification groups in childhood medulloblastoma using combined clinical, pathologic, and molecular variables. J Clin Oncol. 2011 Apr 10;29(11):1400–7. PMID:20921458

**1934.** Ellison DW, Kocak M, Figarella-Branger D, et al. Histopathological grading of pediatric ependymoma: reproducibility and clinical relevance in European trial cohorts. J Negat Results Biomed. 2011 May 31;10:7. PMID:21627842

**1935.** Ellison DW, Onilude OE, Lindsey JC, et al. Beta-catenin status predicts a favorable outcome in childhood medulloblastoma: the United Kingdom Children's Cancer Study Group Brain Tumour Committee. J Clin Oncol. 2005 Nov 1;23(31):7951–7. PMID:16258095

**1936.** El-Mallawany NK, Kamiyango W, Slone JS, et al. Clinical factors associated with long-term complete remission versus poor response to chemotherapy in HIV-infected children and adolescents with Kaposi sarcoma receiving bleomycin and vincristine: a retrospective observational study. PLoS One. 2016 Apr 15;11(4):e0153335. PMID:27082863

**1937.** El-Mallawany NK, McAtee CL, Campbell LR, et al. Pediatric Kaposi sarcoma in context of the HIV epidemic in sub-Saharan Africa: current perspectives. Pediatric Health Med Ther. 2018 Apr 19;9:35–46. PMID:29722363

**1938.** El-Mallawany NK, Villiera J, Kamiyango W, et al. Endemic Kaposi sarcoma in HIV-negative children and adolescents: an evaluation of overlapping and distinct clinical features in comparison with HIV-related disease. Infect Agent Cancer. 2018 Nov 9;13:33. PMID:30455728

**1939.** El-Maouche D, Sadowski SM, Papadakis GZ, et al. 68Ga-DOTATATE for tumor localization in tumor-induced osteomalacia. J Clin Endocrinol Metab. 2016 Oct;101(10):3575–81. PMID:27533306

**1940.** El-Mofty S. Psammomatoid and trabecular juvenile ossifying fibroma of the craniofacial skeleton: two distinct clinicopathologic entities. Oral Surg Oral Med Oral Pathol Oral

Radiol Endod. 2002 Mar;93(3):296–304. PMID:11925539

**1941.** El-Mofty SK. Fibro-osseous lesions of the craniofacial skeleton: an update. Head Neck Pathol. 2014 Dec;8(4):432–44. PMID:25409851

**1942.** el-Naggar AK, Ro JY, McLemore D, et al. DNA ploidy in testicular germ cell neoplasms. Histogenetic and clinical implications. Am J Surg Pathol. 1992 Jun;16(6):611–8. PMID:1318004

**1943.** Elowe-Gruau E, Beltrand J, Brauner R, et al. Childhood craniopharyngioma: hypothalamus-sparing surgery decreases the risk of obesity. J Clin Endocrinol Metab. 2013 Jun;98(6):2376–82. PMID:23633208

**1944.** Elsahy NI, Lorimer A. Congenital fibrolipomata in both heels. Case report. Plast Reconstr Surg. 1977 Mar;59(3):434–5. PMID:840946

**1945.** Elsamadicy AA, Koo AB, David WB, et al. Comparison of epidemiology, treatments, and outcomes in pediatric versus adult ependymoma. Neurooncol Adv. 2020 Feb 21;2(1):vdaa019. PMID:32642681

**1946.** Elsamna ST, Amer K, Elkattawy O, et al. Epithelioid sarcoma: half a century later. Acta Oncol. 2020 Jan;59(1):48–54. PMID:31478778

**1947.** Elsas FJ, Green WR. Epibulbar tumors in childhood. Am J Ophthalmol. 1975 Jun;79(6):1001–7. PMID:166560

**1948.** Else T. Association of adrenocortical carcinoma with familial cancer susceptibility syndromes. Mol Cell Endocrinol. 2012 Mar 31;351(1):66–70. PMID:22209747

**1949.** Else T, Kim AC, Sabolch A, et al. Adrenocortical carcinoma. Endocr Rev. 2014 Apr;35(2):282–326. PMID:24423978

**1950.** El-Shabrawi-Caelen L, Cerroni L, Medeiros LJ, et al. Hypopigmented mycosis fungoides: frequent expression of a CD8+ T-cell phenotype. Am J Surg Pathol. 2002 Apr;26(4):450–7. PMID:11914622

**1951.** Elsheikh TM, Bernacki EG. Fine needle aspiration cytology of cellular pleomorphic adenoma. Acta Cytol. 1996 Nov-Dec;40(6):1165–75. PMID:8960024

**1951A.** Elston MS, Sehgal S, Dray M, et al. A duodenal SDH-deficient gastrointestinal stromal tumor in a patient with a germline SDHB mutation. J Clin Endocrinol Metab. 2017 May 1;102(5):1447–50. PMID:28324028

**1952.** Elzinga-Tinke JE, Sirre ME, Looijenga LH, et al. The predictive value of testicular ultrasound abnormalities for carcinoma in situ of the testis in men at risk for testicular cancer. Int J Androl. 2010 Aug 1;33(4):597–603. PMID:19845800

**1953.** Emberger M, Laimer M, Steiner H, et al. Retiform hemangioendothelioma: presentation of a case expressing D2-40. J Cutan Pathol. 2009 Sep;36(9):987–90. PMID:19674202

**1954.** Emile JF, Abla O, Fraitag S, et al. Revised classification of histiocytoses and neoplasms of the macrophage-dendritic cell lineages. Blood. 2016 Jun 2;127(22):2672–81. PMID:26966089

**1955.** Emmerich D, Zemojtel T, Hecht J, et al. Somatic neurofibromatosis type 1 (NF1) inactivation events in cutaneous neurofibromas of a single NF1 patient. Eur J Hum Genet. 2015 Jun;23(6):870–3. PMID:25293717

**1956.** Emory TS, Scheithauer BW, Hirose T, et al. Intraneural perineurioma. A clonal neoplasm associated with abnormalities of chromosome 22. Am J Clin Pathol. 1995 Jun;103(6):696–704. PMID:7785653

**1957.** Endo M, Hasegawa T, Tashiro T, et al. Bizarre parosteal osteochondromatous proliferation with a t(1;17) translocation. Virchows Arch. 2005 Jul;447(1):99–102. PMID:15926071

**1957A.** Engelhard HH, Villano JL, Porter KR, et al. Clinical presentation, histology, and treatment in 430 patients with primary tumors of the spinal cord, spinal meninges, or cauda equina. J Neurosurg Spine. 2010 Jul;13(1):67–77. PMID:20594020

**1958.** Engelholm LH, Riaz A, Serra D, et al. CRISPR/Cas9 engineering of adult mouse liver demonstrates that the Dnajb1-Prkaca gene fusion is sufficient to induce tumors resembling fibrolamellar hepatocellular carcinoma. Gastroenterology. 2017 Dec;153(6):1662–1673.e10. PMID:28923495

**1959.** Engels EA, Clarke CA, Pfeiffer RM, et al. Plasma cell neoplasms in US solid organ transplant recipients. Am J Transplant. 2013 Jun;13(6):1523–32. PMID:23635036

**1960.** Englund A, Glimelius I, Rostgaard K, et al. Hodgkin lymphoma in children, adolescents and young adults - a comparative study of clinical presentation and treatment outcome. Acta Oncol. 2018 Feb;57(2):276–82. PMID:28760045

**1961.** Enjolras O, Mulliken JB, Boon LM, et al. Noninvoluting congenital hemangioma: a rare cutaneous vascular anomaly. Plast Reconstr Surg. 2001 Jun;107(7):1647–54. PMID:11391180

**1962.** Enjolras O, Mulliken JB, Wassef M, et al. Residual lesions after Kasabach-Merritt phenomenon in 41 patients. J Am Acad Dermatol. 2000 Feb;42(2 Pt 1):225–35. PMID:10642677

**1963.** Enneking WF. A system of staging musculoskeletal neoplasms. Clin Orthop Relat Res. 1986 Mar; (204):9–24. PMID:3456859

**1964.** Enomoto Y, Enomoto K, Uchino S, et al. Clinical features, treatment, and long-term outcome of papillary thyroid cancer in children and adolescents without radiation exposure. World J Surg. 2012 Jun;36(6):1241–6. PMID:22411092

**1965.** Enríquez-Vega ME, Muñoz-Paredes JG, Cossío-Zazueta A, et al. SDHD gene mutation in Mexican population whit carotid body tumor. Cir Cir. 2018;86(1):38–42. PMID:29681642

**1966.** Enzinger FM. Angiomatoid malignant fibrous histiocytoma: a distinct fibrohistiocytic tumor of children and young adults simulating a vascular neoplasm. Cancer. 1979 Dec;44(6):2147–57. PMID:228836

**1967.** Enzinger FM. Clear-cell sarcoma of tendons and aponeuroses. An analysis of 21 cases. Cancer. 1965 Sep;18:1163–74. PMID:14332545

**1968.** Enzinger FM, Dulcey F. Proliferative myositis. Report of thirty-three cases. Cancer. 1967 Dec;20(12):2213–23. PMID:6073898

**1969.** Enzinger FM, Zhang RY. Plexiform fibrohistiocytic tumor presenting in children and young adults. An analysis of 65 cases. Am J Surg Pathol. 1988 Nov;12(11):818–26. PMID:2847569

**1970.** Epifanio M, Baldissera M, Esteban FG, et al. Mature testicular teratoma in children: multifaceted tumors on ultrasound. Urology. 2014 Jan;83(1):195–7. PMID:24080220

**1971.** Epstein BE, Pajak TF, Haulk TL, et al. Metastatic nonresectable fibrolamellar hepatoma: prognostic features and natural history. Am J Clin Oncol. 1999 Feb;22(1):22–8. PMID:10025374

**1972.** Epstein DS, Pashaei S, Hunt E Jr, et al. Pustulo-ovoid bodies of Milian in granular cell tumors. J Cutan Pathol. 2007 May;34(5):405–9. PMID:17448196

**1973.** Erickson D, Kudva YC, Ebersold MJ, et al. Benign paragangliomas: clinical presentation and treatment outcomes in 236 patients. J Clin Endocrinol Metab. 2001 Nov;86(11):5210–6. PMID:11701678

**1974.** Erickson D, Scheithauer B, Atkinson J, et al. Silent subtype 3 pituitary adenoma: a clinicopathologic analysis of the Mayo Clinic experience. Clin Endocrinol (Oxf). 2009 Jul;71(1):92–9. PMID:19170710

**1975.** Erickson LA, Mete O. Immunohistochemistry in diagnostic parathyroid pathology. Endocr Pathol. 2018 Jun;29(2):113–29. PMID:29626276

**1976.** Erickson-Johnson MR, Chou MM, Evers BR, et al. Nodular fasciitis: a novel model of transient neoplasia induced by MYH9-USP6 gene fusion. Lab Invest. 2011 Oct;91(10):1427–33. PMID:21826056

**1977.** Erkek S, Johann PD, Finetti MA, et al. Comprehensive analysis of chromatin states in atypical teratoid/rhabdoid tumor identifies diverging roles for SWI/SNF and polycomb in gene regulation. Cancer Cell. 2019 Jan 14;35(1):95–110.e8. PMID:30595504

**1978.** Ernst T, Busch M, Rinke J, et al. Frequent ASXL1 mutations in children and young adults with chronic myeloid leukemia. Leukemia. 2018 Sep;32(9):2046–9. PMID:29899367

**1979.** Errani C, Zhang L, Panicek DM, et al. Epithelioid hemangioma of bone and soft tissue: a reappraisal of a controversial entity. Clin Orthop Relat Res. 2012 May;470(5):1498–506. PMID:21948309

**1980.** Errani C, Zhang L, Sung YS, et al. A novel WWTR1-CAMTA1 gene fusion is a consistent abnormality in epithelioid hemangioendothelioma of different anatomic sites. Genes Chromosomes Cancer. 2011 Aug;50(8):644–53. PMID:21584898

**1981.** Escribano L, Orfao A, Díaz-Agustin B, et al. Indolent systemic mast cell disease in adults: immunophenotypic characterization of bone marrow mast cells and its diagnostic implications. Blood. 1998 Apr 15;91(8):2731–6. PMID:9531582

**1982.** Espersen ADL, Noren-Nyström U, Abrahamsson J, et al. Acute myeloid leukemia (AML) with t(7;12)(q36;p13) is associated with infancy and trisomy 19: data from Nordic Society for Pediatric Hematology and Oncology (NOPHO-AML) and review of the literature. Genes Chromosomes Cancer. 2018 Jul;57(7):359–65. PMID:29569294

**1983.** Estrella JS, Li L, Rashid A, et al. Solid pseudopapillary neoplasm of the pancreas: clinicopathologic and survival analyses of 64 cases from a single institution. Am J Surg Pathol. 2014 Feb;38(2):147–57. PMID:24418850

**1984.** Etchevers HC, Dupin E, Le Douarin NM. The diverse neural crest: from embryology to human pathology. Development. 2019 Mar 11;146(5):dev169821. PMID:30858200

**1985.** Ethunandan M, Pratt CA, Macpherson DW. Changing frequency of parotid gland neoplasms–analysis of 560 tumours treated in a district general hospital. Ann R Coll Surg Engl. 2002 Jan;84(1):1–6. PMID:11890618

**1986.** Etoz M, Asantogrol F, Akyol R. Central giant cell granulomas of the jaws: retrospective radiographic analysis of 13 patients. Oral Radiol. 2020 Jan;36(1):60–8. PMID:30825099

**1987.** European Association for the Study of the Liver. EASL Clinical Practice Guidelines: management of hepatocellular carcinoma. J Hepatol. 2018 Jul;69(1):182–236. PMID:29628281

**1988.** Evans AG, French CA, Cameron MJ, et al. Pathologic characteristics of NUT midline carcinoma arising in the mediastinum. Am J Surg Pathol. 2012 Aug;36(8):1222–7. PMID:22790861

**1989.** Evans DG. Neurofibromatosis type 2 (NF2): a clinical and molecular review. Orphanet J Rare Dis. 2009 Jun 19;4:16. PMID:19545378

**1990.** Evans DG, Baser ME, O'Reilly B, et al. Management of the patient and family with neurofibromatosis 2: a consensus conference statement. Br J Neurosurg. 2005 Feb;19(1):5–12. PMID:16147576

**1991.** Evans DG, Birch JM, Ramsden RT. Paediatric presentation of type 2 neurofibromatosis. Arch Dis Child. 1999 Dec;81(6):496–9. PMID:10569966

**1992.** Evans DG, Farndon PA. Nevoid basal cell carcinoma syndrome. In: Adam MP, Ardinger HH, Pagon RA, et al., editors. GeneReviews. Seattle (WA): University of Washington, Seattle; 2002 Jun 20. PMID:20301330

**1993.** Evans DG, Hartley CL, Smith PT, et al. Incidence of mosaicism in 1055 de novo NF2 cases: much higher than previous estimates with high utility of next-generation sequencing. Genet Med. 2020 Jan;22(1):53–9. PMID:31273341

**1994.** Evans DG, Howard E, Giblin C, et al. Birth incidence and prevalence of tumor-prone syndromes: estimates from a UK family genetic register service. Am J Med Genet A. 2010 Feb;152A(2):327–32. PMID:20082463

**1995.** Evans DG, Huson SM, Birch JM. Malignant peripheral nerve sheath tumours in inherited disease. Clin Sarcoma Res. 2012 Oct 4;2(1):17. PMID:23036231

**1996.** Evans DG, Huson SM, Donnai D, et al. A clinical study of type 2 neurofibromatosis. Q J Med. 1992 Aug;84(304):603–18. PMID:1484939

**1996A.** Evans DG, King AT, Bowers NL, et al. Identifying the deficiencies of current diagnostic criteria for neurofibromatosis 2 using databases of 2777 individuals with molecular testing. Genet Med. 2019 Jul;21(7):1525–33. PMID:30523344

**1997.** Evans DG, Ladusans EJ, Rimmer S, et al. Complications of the naevoid basal cell carcinoma syndrome: results of a population based study. J Med Genet. 1993 Jun;30(6):460–4. PMID:8326488

**1998.** Evans DG, Moran A, King A, et al. Incidence of vestibular schwannoma and neurofibromatosis 2 in the North West of England over a 10-year period: higher incidence than previously thought. Otol Neurotol. 2005 Jan;26(1):93–7. PMID:15699726

**1999.** Evans DG, O'Hara C, Wilding A, et al. Mortality in neurofibromatosis 1: in North West England: an assessment of actuarial survival in a region of the UK since 1989. Eur J Hum Genet. 2011 Nov;19(11):1187–91. PMID:21694737

**2000.** Evans DG, Oudit D, Smith MJ, et al. First evidence of genotype-phenotype correlations in Gorlin syndrome. J Med Genet. 2017 Aug;54(8):530–6. PMID:28596197

**2001.** Evans DG, Ramsden RT, Shenton A, et al. Mosaicism in neurofibromatosis type 2: an update of risk based on uni/bilaterality of vestibular schwannoma at presentation and sensitive mutation analysis including multiple ligation-dependent probe amplification. J Med Genet. 2007 Jul;44(7):424–8. PMID:17307835

**2002.** Evans DG, Wallace AJ, Wu CL, et al. Somatic mosaicism: a common cause of classic disease in tumor-prone syndromes? Lessons from type 2 neurofibromatosis. Am J Hum Genet. 1998 Sep;63(3):727–36. PMID:9718334

**2003.** Evans HL. Low-grade fibromyxoid sarcoma. A report of 12 cases. Am J Surg Pathol. 1993 Jun;17(6):595–600. PMID:8333558

**2004.** Evans HL. Low-grade fibromyxoid sarcoma. A report of two metastasizing neoplasms having a deceptively benign appearance. Am J Clin Pathol. 1987 Nov;88(5):615–9. PMID:3673943

**2005.** Evans HL. Synovial sarcoma. A study of 23 biphasic and 17 probable monophasic examples. Pathol Annu. 1980;15(Pt 2):309–31. PMID:6256705

**2006.** Evans RW. Developmental stages of embryo-like bodies in teratoma testis. J Clin Pathol. 1957 Feb;10(1):31–9. PMID:13406071

**2007.** Eveslage M, Calaminus G, Warmuth-Metz M, et al. The postoperative

quality of life in children and adolescents with craniopharyngioma. Dtsch Arztebl Int. 2019 May 3;116(18):321–8. PMID:31219033
**2008.** Eveson JW, Cawson RA. Salivary gland tumours. A review of 2410 cases with particular reference to histological types, site, age and sex distribution. J Pathol. 1985 May;146(1):51–8. PMID:4009321
**2009.** Eveson JW, Cawson RA. Tumours of the minor (oropharyngeal) salivary glands: a demographic study of 336 cases. J Oral Pathol. 1985 Jul;14(6):500–9. PMID:2991488
**2010.** Ewens KG, Bhatti TR, Moran KA, et al. Phosphorylation of pRb: mechanism for RB pathway inactivation in MYCN-amplified retinoblastoma. Cancer Med. 2017 Mar;6(3):619–30. PMID:28211617
**2011.** Eyden B, Banerjee SS, Shenjere P, et al. The myofibroblast and its tumours. J Clin Pathol. 2009 Mar;62(3):236–49. PMID:18930983
**2012.** Eyden BP, Manson C, Banerjee SS, et al. Sclerosing epithelioid fibrosarcoma: a study of five cases emphasizing diagnostic criteria. Histopathology. 1998 Oct;33(4):354–60. PMID:9822926
**2013.** Eyssartier E, Villemagne T, Maurin L, et al. Intrascrotal lipoblastoma: a report of two cases and a review of the literature. J Pediatr Urol. 2013 Dec;9 6 Pt B:e151–4. PMID:23664430
**2014.** Ezekian B, Englum B, Gilmore BF, et al. Renal medullary carcinoma: a national analysis of 159 patients. Pediatr Blood Cancer. 2017 Nov;64(11). PMID:28485059
**2015.** Ezekian B, Mulvihill MS, Schroder PM, et al. Improved contemporary outcomes of liver transplantation for pediatric hepatoblastoma and hepatocellular carcinoma. Pediatr Transplant. 2018 Dec;22(8):e13305. PMID:30341782
**2016.** Ezon I, Zilbert N, Pinkney L, et al. A large struma ovarii tumor removed via laparoscopy in a 16-year-old adolescent. J Pediatr Surg. 2007 Aug;42(8):E19–22. PMID:17706482
**2017.** Ezzat S, Asa SL, Couldwell WT, et al. The prevalence of pituitary adenomas: a systematic review. Cancer. 2004 Aug 1;101(3):613–9. PMID:15274075
**2018.** Ezzat S, Cheng S, Asa SL. Epigenetics of pituitary tumors: pathogenetic and therapeutic implications. Mol Cell Endocrinol. 2018 Jul 5;469:70–6. PMID:28711607
**2019.** Ezzat S, Zhu X, Loeper S, et al. Tumor-derived Ikaros 6 acetylates the Bcl-XL promoter to up-regulate a survival signal in pituitary cells. Mol Endocrinol. 2006 Nov;20(11):2976–86. PMID:16873443
**2020.** Fabian ID, Johnson KP, Stacey AW, et al. Focal laser treatment in addition to chemotherapy for retinoblastoma. Cochrane Database Syst Rev. 2017 Jun 7;6:CD012366. PMID:28589646
**2021.** Fabian ID, Stacey AW, Chowdhury T, et al. High-risk histopathology features in primary and secondary enucleated international intraocular retinoblastoma classification group D eyes. Ophthalmology. 2017 Jun;124(6):851–8. PMID:28302322
**2022.** Fabian ID, Stacey AW, Johnson KC, et al. Primary enucleation for group D retinoblastoma in the era of systemic and targeted chemotherapy: the price of retaining an eye. Br J Ophthalmol. 2018 Feb;102(2):265–71. PMID:28659391
**2023.** Fabien-Dupuis C, Niver B, Shillingford N, et al. Melanotic neuroectodermal tumor of infancy presenting with fast-growing scrotal swelling: a case report and literature review. Pediatr Dev Pathol. 2017 Sep-Oct;20(5):411–5. PMID:28812465
**2024.** Fabrizi G, Massi G. Polypoid Spitz naevus: the benign counterpart of polypoid malignant melanoma. Br J Dermatol. 2000 Jan;142(1):128–32. PMID:10651708
**2025.** Faderl S, Talpaz M, Estrov Z, et al. The biology of chronic myeloid leukemia. N Engl J Med. 1999 Jul 15;341(3):164–72. PMID:10403855
**2026.** Faham M, Zheng J, Moorhead M, et al. Deep-sequencing approach for minimal residual disease detection in acute lymphoblastic leukemia. Blood. 2012 Dec 20;120(26):5173–80. PMID:23074282
**2027.** Falco NA, Upton J. Infantile digital fibromas. J Hand Surg Am. 1995 Nov;20(6):1014–20. PMID:8583050
**2028.** Falini B, Bigerna B, Fizzotti M, et al. ALK expression defines a distinct group of T/null lymphomas ("ALK lymphomas") with a wide morphological spectrum. Am J Pathol. 1998 Sep;153(3):875–86. PMID:9736036
**2029.** Falini B, Mason DY. Proteins encoded by genes involved in chromosomal alterations in lymphoma and leukemia: clinical value of their detection by immunocytochemistry. Blood. 2002 Jan 15;99(2):409–26. PMID:11781220
**2030.** Falk H, Thomas LB, Popper H, et al. Hepatic angiosarcoma associated with androgenic-anabolic steroids. Lancet. 1979 Nov 24;2(8152):1120–3. PMID:91848
**2031.** Fallon SC, Brandt ML, Rodriguez JR, et al. Cytogenetic analysis in the diagnosis and management of lipoblastomas: results from a single institution. J Surg Res. 2013 Sep;184(1):341–6. PMID:23751806
**2032.** Fan LD, Zang HY, Zhang XS. Ovarian epidermoid cyst: report of eight cases. Int J Gynecol Pathol. 1996 Jan;15(1):69–71. PMID:8852449
**2033.** Fan XL, Han ZJ, Gong XY, et al. Morphological classification for prediction of malignant transformation in multiple exostoses. Eur Rev Med Pharmacol Sci. 2014;18(6):840–5. PMID:24706308
**2034.** Fan Z, Li J, Du J, et al. A missense mutation in PTCH2 underlies dominantly inherited NBCCS in a Chinese family. J Med Genet. 2008 May;45(5):303–8. PMID:18285427
**2035.** Fan Z, Natkunam Y, Bair E, et al. Characterization of variant patterns of nodular lymphocyte predominant hodgkin lymphoma with immunohistologic and clinical correlation. Am J Surg Pathol. 2003 Oct;27(10):1346–56. PMID:14508396
**2036.** Fanaian NK, Cohen C, Waldrop S, et al. Epstein-Barr virus (EBV)-encoded RNA: automated in-situ hybridization (ISH) compared with manual ISH and immunohistochemistry for detection of EBV in pediatric lymphoproliferative disorders. Pediatr Dev Pathol. 2009 May-Jun;12(3):195–9. PMID:18442302
**2037.** Fanburg JC, Meis-Kindblom JM, Rosenberg AE. Multiple enchondromas associated with spindle-cell hemangioendotheliomas. An overlooked variant of Maffucci's syndrome. Am J Surg Pathol. 1995 Sep;19(9):1029–38. PMID:7661276
**2038.** Fanburg-Smith JC, Hengge M, Hengge UR, et al. Extrarenal rhabdoid tumors of soft tissue: a clinicopathologic and immunohistochemical study of 18 cases. Ann Diagn Pathol. 1998 Dec;2(6):351–62. PMID:9930572
**2039.** Fanburg-Smith JC, Majidi M, Miettinen M. Keratin expression in schwannoma; a study of 115 retroperitoneal and 22 peripheral schwannomas. Mod Pathol. 2006 Jan;19(1):115–21. PMID:16357842
**2040.** Fanburg-Smith JC, Meis-Kindblom JM, Fante R, et al. Malignant granular cell tumor of soft tissue: diagnostic criteria and clinicopathologic correlation. Am J Surg Pathol. 1998 Jul;22(7):779–94. PMID:9669341
**2041.** Fanburg-Smith JC, Michal M, Partanen TA, et al. Papillary intralymphatic angioendothelioma (PILA): a report of twelve cases of a distinctive vascular tumor with phenotypic features of lymphatic vessels. Am J Surg Pathol. 1999 Sep;23(9):1004–10. PMID:10478659
**2042.** Fanburg-Smith JC, Miettinen M. Angiomatoid "malignant" fibrous histiocytoma: a clinicopathologic study of 158 cases and further exploration of the myoid phenotype. Hum Pathol. 1999 Nov;30(11):1336–43. PMID:10571514
**2043.** Fanburg-Smith JC, Miettinen M, Folpe AL, et al. Lingual alveolar soft part sarcoma; 14 cases: novel clinical and morphological observations. Histopathology. 2004 Nov;45(5):526–37. PMID:15500657
**2044.** Fang D, Gan H, Lee JH, et al. The histone H3.3K36M mutation reprograms the epigenome of chondroblastomas. Science. 2016 Jun 10;352(6291):1344–8. PMID:27229140
**2045.** Fang H, Langstraat CL, Visscher DW, et al. Epithelioid inflammatory myofibroblastic sarcoma of the ovary with RANB2-ALK fusion: report of a case. Int J Gynecol Pathol. 2018 Sep;37(5):468–72. PMID:28787324
**2046.** Fang J, Huang Y, Mao G, et al. Cancer-driving H3G34V/R/D mutations block H3K36 methylation and H3K36me3-MutSα interaction. Proc Natl Acad Sci U S A. 2018 Sep 18;115(38):9598–603. PMID:30181289
**2047.** Fang QG, Shi S, Sun CF. Odontogenic lesions in pediatric patients. J Craniofac Surg. 2014 May;25(3):e248–51. PMID:24785745
**2048.** Fankhauser CD, Grogg JB, Hayoz S, et al. Risk factors and treatment outcomes of 1,375 patients with testicular leydig cell tumors: analysis of published case series data. J Urol. 2020 May;203(5):949–56. PMID:31845841
**2049.** Fanna M, Rougemont AL, Arni D, et al. Giant intrahepatic lipoblastoma in a child. J Pediatr. 2019 Jul;210:235–236.e1. PMID:30955788
**2050.** Faquin WC, Wong LQ, Afrogheh AH, et al. Impact of reclassifying noninvasive follicular variant of papillary thyroid carcinoma on the risk of malignancy in The Bethesda System for Reporting Thyroid Cytopathology. Cancer Cytopathol. 2016 Mar;124(3):181–7. PMID:26457584
**2051.** Farah N, Kirkwood AA, Rahman S, et al. Prognostic impact of the absence of biallelic deletion at the TRG locus for pediatric patients with T-cell acute lymphoblastic leukemia treated on the Medical Research Council UK Acute Lymphoblastic Leukemia 2003 trial. Haematologica. 2018 Jul;103(7):e288–92. PMID:29519867
**2052.** Fardet L, Blanche S, Brousse N, et al. Cutaneous EBV-related lymphoproliferative disorder in a 15-year-old boy with AIDS: an unusual clinical presentation. J Pediatr Hematol Oncol. 2002 Nov;24(8):666–9. PMID:12439041
**2053.** Farhi DC, Shikes RH, Murari PJ, et al. Hepatocellular carcinoma in young people. Cancer. 1983 Oct 15;52(8):1516–25. PMID:6311397
**2054.** Farhi DC, Shikes RH, Silverberg SG. Ultrastructure of fibrolamellar oncocytic hepatoma. Cancer. 1982 Aug 15;50(4):702–9. PMID:6284337
**2055.** Faria P, Beckwith JB, Mishra K, et al. Focal versus diffuse anaplasia in Wilms tumor–new definitions with prognostic significance: a report from the National Wilms Tumor Study Group. Am J Surg Pathol. 1996 Aug;20(8):909–20. PMID:8712292
**2056.** Farmer JR, Ong MS, Barmettler S, et al. Common variable immunodeficiency non-infectious disease endotypes redefined using unbiased network clustering in large electronic datasets. Front Immunol. 2018 Jan 9;8:1740. PMID:29375540
**2057.** Farnia B, Allen PK, Brown PD, et al. Clinical outcomes and patterns of failure in pineoblastoma: a 30-year, single-institution retrospective review. World Neurosurg. 2014 Dec;82(6):1232–41. PMID:25045788
**2058.** Farrow JH, Ashikari H. Breast lesions in young girls. Surg Clin North Am. 1969 Apr;49(2):261–9. PMID:5813207
**2059.** Fassnacht M, Kroiss M, Allolio B. Update in adrenocortical carcinoma. J Clin Endocrinol Metab. 2013 Dec;98(12):4551–64. PMID:24081734
**2060.** Fatobene G, Haroche J, Hélias-Rodzwicz Z, et al. BRAF V600E mutation detected in a case of Rosai-Dorfman disease. Haematologica. 2018 Aug;103(8):e377–9. PMID:29748446
**2061.** Fattizzo B, Rosa J, Giannotta JA, et al. The physiopathology of T- cell acute lymphoblastic leukemia: focus on molecular aspects. Front Oncol. 2020 Feb 28;10:273. PMID:32185137
**2062.** Fauchon F, Jouvet A, Paquis P, et al. Parenchymal pineal tumors: a clinicopathological study of 76 cases. Int J Radiat Oncol Biol Phys. 2000 Mar 1;46(4):959–68. PMID:10705018
**2063.** Faucz FR, Tirosh A, Tatsi C, et al. Somatic USP8 gene mutations are a common cause of pediatric cushing disease. J Clin Endocrinol Metab. 2017 Aug 1;102(8):2836–43. PMID:28505279
**2064.** Favara BE, Jaffe R, Egeler RM. Macrophage activation and hemophagocytic syndrome in langerhans cell histiocytosis: report of 30 cases. Pediatr Dev Pathol. 2002 Mar-Apr;5(2):130–40. PMID:11910507
**2065.** Favier J, Meatchi T, Robidel E, et al. Carbonic anhydrase 9 immunohistochemistry as a tool to predict or validate germline and somatic VHL mutations in pheochromocytoma and paraganglioma-a retrospective and prospective study. Mod Pathol. 2020 Jan;33(1):57–64. PMID:31383958
**2066.** Faye A, Vilmer E. Post-transplant lymphoproliferative disorder in children: incidence, prognosis, and treatment options. Paediatr Drugs. 2005;7(1):55–65. PMID:15777111
**2067.** Fazlollahi L, Hsiao SJ, Kochhar M, et al. Malignant rhabdoid tumor, an aggressive tumor often misclassified as small cell variant of hepatoblastoma. Cancers (Basel). 2019 Dec 11;11(12):E1992. PMID:31835848
**2068.** Feany MB, Anthony DC, Fletcher CD. Nerve sheath tumours with hybrid features of neurofibroma and schwannoma: a conceptual challenge. Histopathology. 1998 May;32(5):405–10. PMID:9639114
**2069.** Feasel P, Al-Ibraheemi A, Fritchie K, et al. Superficial solitary fibrous tumor: a series of 26 cases. Am J Surg Pathol. 2018 Jun;42(6):778–85. PMID:29438169
**2070.** Feasel PC, Cheah AL, Fritchie K, et al. Primary clear cell sarcoma of the head and neck: a case series with review of the literature. J Cutan Pathol. 2016 Oct;43(10):838–46. PMID:27264732
**2071.** Fedele M, Crescenzi E, Cerchia L. The POZ/BTB and AT-hook containing zinc finger 1 (PATZ1) transcription regulator: physiological functions and disease involvement. Int J Mol Sci. 2017 Nov 24;18(12):E2524. PMID:29186807
**2072.** Fehr A, Röser K, Heidorn K, et al. A new type of MAML2 fusion in mucoepidermoid carcinoma. Genes Chromosomes Cancer. 2008 Mar;47(3):203–6. PMID:18050304
**2073.** Feldman AL, Vasmatzis G, Asmann YW, et al. Novel TRAF1-ALK fusion identified by deep RNA sequencing of anaplastic large cell lymphoma. Genes Chromosomes Cancer. 2013 Nov;52(11):1097–102. PMID:23999969
**2074.** Feliciano DM, Quon JL, Su T, et al. Postnatal neurogenesis generates heterotopias, olfactory micronodules and cortical infiltration following single-cell Tsc1 deletion.

Hum Mol Genet. 2012 Feb 15;21(4):799–810. PMID:22068588
**2075.** Felix IA, Horvath E, Kovacs K, et al. Mammosomatotroph adenoma of the pituitary associated with gigantism and hyperprolactinemia. A morphological study including immunoelectron microscopy. Acta Neuropathol. 1986;71(1-2):76–82. PMID:3776476
**2076.** Feng J, Polychronidis G, Heger U, et al. Incidence trends and survival prediction of hepatoblastoma in children: a population-based study. Cancer Commun (Lond). 2019 Oct 24;39(1):62. PMID:31651371
**2077.** Feng J, Sethi A, Reyes-Múgica M, et al. Life-threatening blood loss from scratching provoked by pruritus in the bulky perineal nevocytoma variant of giant congenital melanocytic nevus in a child. J Am Acad Dermatol. 2005 Aug;53(2 Suppl 1):S139–42. PMID:16021164
**2078.** Fenoglio JJ Jr, MCAllister HA Jr, Ferrans VJ. Cardiac rhabdomyoma: a clinicopathologic and electron microscopic study. Am J Cardiol. 1976 Aug;38(2):241–51. PMID:952267
**2079.** Fenton CL, Lukes Y, Nicholson D, et al. The ret/PTC mutations are common in sporadic papillary thyroid carcinoma of children and young adults. J Clin Endocrinol Metab. 2000 Mar;85(3):1170–5. PMID:10720057
**2080.** Feoli-Fonseca JC, Oligny LL, Filion M, et al. Direct human papillomavirus (HPV) sequencing method yields a novel HPV in a human immunodeficiency virus-positive Quebec woman and distinguishes a new HPV clade. J Infect Dis. 1998 Nov;178(5):1492–6. PMID:9780273
**2081.** Ferguson L, Agoulnik AI. Testicular cancer and cryptorchidism. Front Endocrinol (Lausanne). 2013 Mar 20;4:32. PMID:23519268
**2082.** Ferla V, Rossi FG, Goldaniga MC, et al. Biological difference between Epstein-Barr virus positive and negative post-transplant lymphoproliferative disorders and their clinical impact. Front Oncol. 2020 May 8;10:506. PMID:32457824
**2083.** Ferlay J, Ervik M, Lam F, et al. Global Cancer Observatory: Cancer Today [Internet]. Lyon (France): International Agency for Research on Cancer; 2020. Available from: https://gco.iarc.fr/today.
**2084.** Fernanda Amary M, Ye H, Berisha F, et al. Fibroblastic growth factor receptor 1 amplification in osteosarcoma is associated with poor response to neo-adjuvant chemotherapy. Cancer Med. 2014 Aug;3(4):980–7. PMID:24861215
**2085.** Fernandes T, Silva R, Devesa V, et al. AIRP best cases in radiologic-pathologic correlation: gastroblastoma: a rare biphasic gastric tumor. Radiographics. 2014 Nov-Dec;34(7):1929–33. PMID:25384293
**2086.** Fernandez A, Karavitaki N, Wass JA. Prevalence of pituitary adenomas: a community-based, cross-sectional study in Banbury (Oxfordshire, UK). Clin Endocrinol (Oxf). 2010 Mar;72(3):377–82. PMID:19650784
**2087.** Fernandez AP, Billings SD, Bergfeld WF, et al. Pagetoid Spitz nevi: clinicopathologic characterization of a series of 12 cases. J Cutan Pathol. 2016 Nov;43(11):932–9. PMID:27442449
**2088.** Fernandez AP, Sun Y, Tubbs RR, et al. FISH for MYC amplification and anti-MYC immunohistochemistry: useful diagnostic tools in the assessment of secondary angiosarcoma and atypical vascular proliferations. J Cutan Pathol. 2012 Feb;39(2):234–42. PMID:22121953
**2089.** Fernandez C, Figarella-Branger D, Girard N, et al. Pilocytic astrocytomas in children: prognostic factors–a retrospective study of 80 cases. Neurosurgery. 2003 Sep;53(3):544–53. PMID:12943571
**2090.** Fernandez C, Girard N, Paz Paredes A, et al. The usefulness of MR imaging in the diagnosis of dysembryoplastic neuroepithelial tumor in children: a study of 14 cases. AJNR Am J Neuroradiol. 2003 May;24(5):829–34. PMID:12748079
**2091.** Ferrando AA, Neuberg DS, Staunton J, et al. Gene expression signatures define novel oncogenic pathways in T cell acute lymphoblastic leukemia. Cancer Cell. 2002 Feb;1(1):75–87. PMID:12086890
**2092.** Ferraresi S, Garozzo D, Bianchini E, et al. Perineurioma of the sciatic nerve: a possible cause of idiopathic foot drop in children: report of 4 cases. J Neurosurg Pediatr. 2010 Nov;6(5):506–10. PMID:21039177
**2093.** Ferrari A, Bisogno G, Cecchetto G, et al. Cutaneous melanoma in children and adolescents: the Italian Rare Tumors in Pediatric Age Project experience. J Pediatr. 2014 Feb;164(2):376–82.e1, 2. PMID:24252782
**2094.** Ferrari A, Bleyer A. Participation of adolescents with cancer in clinical trials. Cancer Treat Rev. 2007 Nov;33(7):603–8. PMID:17250970
**2095.** Ferrari A, Casanova M. Current chemotherapeutic strategies for rhabdomyosarcoma. Expert Rev Anticancer Ther. 2005 Apr;5(2):283–94. PMID:15877525
**2096.** Ferrari A, Casanova M. New concepts for the treatment of pediatric nonrhabdomyosarcoma soft tissue sarcomas. Expert Rev Anticancer Ther. 2005 Apr;5(2):307–18. PMID:15877527
**2097.** Ferrari A, Casanova M, Bisogno G, et al. Clear cell sarcoma of tendons and aponeuroses in pediatric patients: a report from the Italian and German Soft Tissue Sarcoma Cooperative Group. Cancer. 2002 Jun 15;94(12):3269–76. PMID:12115360
**2098.** Ferrari A, Casanova M, Collini P, et al. Adult-type soft tissue sarcomas in pediatric-age patients: experience at the Istituto Nazionale Tumori in Milan. J Clin Oncol. 2005 Jun 20;23(18):4021–30. PMID:15767645
**2099.** Ferrari A, Chi YY, De Salvo GL, et al. Surgery alone is sufficient therapy for children and adolescents with low-risk synovial sarcoma: a joint analysis from the European paediatric soft tissue sarcoma Study Group and the Children's Oncology Group. Eur J Cancer. 2017 Jun;78:1–6. PMID:28391003
**2100.** Ferrari A, De Salvo GL, Brennan B, et al. Synovial sarcoma in children and adolescents: the European Pediatric Soft Tissue Sarcoma Study Group prospective trial (EpSSG NRSTS 2005). Ann Oncol. 2015 Mar;26(3):567–72. PMID:25488687
**2101.** Ferrari A, Miceli R, Rey A, et al. Non-metastatic unresected paediatric non-rhabdomyosarcoma soft tissue sarcomas: results of a pooled analysis from United States and European groups. Eur J Cancer. 2011 Mar;47(5):724–31. PMID:21145727
**2102.** Ferrari B, Taliercio V, Restrepo P, et al. Nevus comedonicus: a case series. Pediatr Dermatol. 2015 Mar-Apr;32(2):216–9. PMID:25557057
**2103.** Ferreira AM, Brondani VB, Helena VP, et al. Clinical spectrum of Li-Fraumeni syndrome/Li-Fraumeni-like syndrome in Brazilian individuals with the TP53 p.R337H mutation. J Steroid Biochem Mol Biol. 2019 Jun;190:250–5. PMID:30974190
**2104.** Ferreira J, Esteves G, Fonseca R, et al. Fine-needle aspiration of lipoblastoma: cytological, molecular, and clinical features. Cancer Cytopathol. 2017 Dec;125(12):934–9. PMID:28902468
**2105.** Ferreiro JA, Nascimento AG. Hyaline-cell rich chondroid syringoma. A tumor mimicking malignancy. Am J Surg Pathol. 1995 Aug;19(8):912–7. PMID:7541966
**2106.** Ferreiro JF, Morscio J, Dierickx D, et al. EBV-positive and EBV-negative posttransplant diffuse large B cell lymphomas have distinct genomic and transcriptomic features. Am J Transplant. 2016 Feb;16(2):414–25. PMID:26780579
**2107.** Ferreiro JF, Morscio J, Dierickx D, et al. Post-transplant molecularly defined Burkitt lymphomas are frequently MYC-negative and characterized by the 11q-gain/loss pattern. Haematologica. 2015 Jul;100(7):e275–9. PMID:25795716
**2108.** Ferringer T. Syringocystadenoma papilliferum. Cutis. 2011 Dec;88(6):268, 273–4. PMID:22372162
**2109.** Ferris SP, Velazquez Vega J, Aboian M, et al. High-grade neuroepithelial tumor with BCOR exon 15 internal tandem duplication-a comprehensive clinical, radiographic, pathologic, and genomic analysis. Brain Pathol. 2020 Jan;30(1):46–62. PMID:31104347
**2110.** Ferry JA, Scully RE. Mesonephric remnants, hyperplasia, and neoplasia in the uterine cervix. A study of 49 cases. Am J Surg Pathol. 1990 Dec;14(12):1100–11. PMID:2252101
**2111.** Festen C, Otten BJ, van de Kaa CA. Follicular adenoma of the thyroid gland in children. Eur J Pediatr Surg. 1995 Oct;5(5):262–4. PMID:8555125
**2112.** Fetsch JF, Laskin WB, Miettinen M. Nerve sheath myxoma: a clinicopathologic and immunohistochemical analysis of 57 morphologically distinctive, S-100 protein- and GFAP-positive, myxoid peripheral nerve sheath tumors with a predilection for the extremities and a high local recurrence rate. Am J Surg Pathol. 2005 Dec;29(12):1615–24. PMID:16327434
**2113.** Fetsch JF, Laskin WB, Miettinen M. Palmar-plantar fibromatosis in children and preadolescents: a clinicopathologic study of 56 cases with newly recognized demographics and extended follow-up information. Am J Surg Pathol. 2005 Aug;29(8):1095–105. PMID:16006806
**2114.** Fetsch JF, Laskin WB, Miettinen M. Superficial acral fibromyxoma: a clinicopathologic and immunohistochemical analysis of 37 cases of a distinctive soft tissue tumor with a predilection for the fingers and toes. Hum Pathol. 2001 Jul;32(7):704–14. PMID:11486169
**2115.** Fetsch JF, Miettinen M. Calcifying aponeurotic fibroma: a clinicopathologic study of 22 cases arising in uncommon sites. Hum Pathol. 1998 Dec;29(12):1504–10. PMID:9865839
**2116.** Fetsch JF, Miettinen M. Sclerosing perineurioma: a clinicopathologic study of 19 cases of a distinctive soft tissue lesion with a predilection for the fingers and palms of young adults. Am J Surg Pathol. 1997 Dec;21(12):1433–42. PMID:9414186
**2117.** Fetsch JF, Miettinen M, Laskin WB, et al. A clinicopathologic study of 45 pediatric soft tissue tumors with an admixture of adipose tissue and fibroblastic elements, and a proposal for classification as lipofibromatosis. Am J Surg Pathol. 2000 Nov;24(11):1491–500. PMID:11075850
**2118.** Fetsch JF, Sesterhenn IA, Miettinen M, et al. Epithelioid hemangioma of the penis: a clinicopathologic and immunohistochemical analysis of 19 cases, with special reference to exuberant examples often confused with epithelioid hemangioendothelioma and epithelioid angiosarcoma. Am J Surg Pathol. 2004 Apr;28(4):523–33. PMID:15087672
**2119.** Fetsch JF, Weiss SW. Observations concerning the pathogenesis of epithelioid hemangioma (angiolymphoid hyperplasia). Mod Pathol. 1991 Jul;4(4):449–55. PMID:1924276
**2120.** Feurstein S, Adegunsoye A, Mojsilovic D, et al. Telomere biology disorder prevalence and phenotypes in adults with familial hematologic and/or pulmonary presentations. Blood Adv. 2020 Oct 13;4(19):4873–86. PMID:33035329
**2121.** Fèvre-Montange M, Vasiljevic A, Frappaz D, et al. Utility of Ki67 immunostaining in the grading of pineal parenchymal tumours: a multicentre study. Neuropathol Appl Neurobiol. 2012 Feb;38(1):87–94. PMID:21696422
**2122.** Figarella-Branger D, Lechapt-Zalcman E, Tabouret E, et al. Supratentorial clear cell ependymomas with branching capillaries demonstrate characteristic clinicopathological features and pathological activation of nuclear factor-kappaB signaling. Neuro Oncol. 2016 Jul;18(7):919–27. PMID:26984744
**2123.** Filbin MG, Tirosh I, Hovestadt V, et al. Developmental and oncogenic programs in H3K27M gliomas dissected by single-cell RNA-seq. Science. 2018 Apr 20;360(6386):331–5. PMID:29674595
**2124.** Filho FB, Alves AO. Penile eruptive syringoma. Pan Afr Med J. 2017 Nov 28;28:268. PMID:29881510
**2125.** Filie AC, Lage JM, Azumi N. Immunoreactivity of S100 protein, alpha-1-antitrypsin, and CD68 in adult and congenital granular cell tumors. Mod Pathol. 1996 Sep;9(9):888–92. PMID:8878020
**2126.** Fina F, Barets D, Colin C, et al. Droplet digital PCR is a powerful technique to demonstrate frequent FGFR1 duplication in dysembryoplastic neuroepithelial tumors. Oncotarget. 2017 Jan 10;8(2):2104–13. PMID:27791984
**2127.** Finalet Ferreiro J, Rouhigharabaei L, Urbankova H, et al. Integrative genomic and transcriptomic analysis identified candidate genes implicated in the pathogenesis of hepatosplenic T-cell lymphoma. PLoS One. 2014 Jul 24;9(7):e102977. PMID:25057852
**2128.** Finch SC, Linet MS. Chronic leukaemias. Baillieres Clin Haematol. 1992 Jan;5(1):27–56. PMID:1350742
**2129.** Finck C, Moront M, Newton C, et al. Pediatric granular cell tumor of the tracheobronchial tree. J Pediatr Surg. 2008 Mar;43(3):568–70. PMID:18358305
**2130.** Finzi G, Cerati M, Marando A, et al. Mixed pituitary adenoma/craniopharyngioma: clinical, morphological, immunohistochemical and ultrastructural study of a case, review of the literature, and pathogenetic and nosological considerations. Pituitary. 2014 Feb;17(1):53–9. PMID:23344977
**2131.** Fischbach BV, Trout KL, Lewis J, et al. WAGR syndrome: a clinical review of 54 cases. Pediatrics. 2005 Oct;116(4):984–8. PMID:16199712
**2132.** Fischer U, Forster M, Rinaldi A, et al. Genomics and drug profiling of fatal TCF3-HLF-positive acute lymphoblastic leukemia identifies recurrent mutation patterns and therapeutic options. Nat Genet. 2015 Sep;47(9):1020–9. PMID:26214592
**2133.** Fishbein L, Leshchiner I, Walter V, et al. Comprehensive molecular characterization of pheochromocytoma and paraganglioma. Cancer Cell. 2017 Feb 13;31(2):181–93. PMID:28162975
**2134.** Fishbein L, Nathanson KL. Pheochromocytoma and paraganglioma susceptibility genes: estimating the associated risk of disease. JAMA Oncol. 2017 Sep 1;3(9):1212–3. PMID:28384677
**2135.** Fisher C. Myofibroblastic malignancies. Adv Anat Pathol. 2004 Jul;11(4):190–201. PMID:15220822
**2136.** Fisher C. Myofibrosarcoma. Virchows Arch. 2004 Sep;445(3):215–23. PMID:15173943
**2137.** Fisher C, Folpe AL, Hashimoto H, et al. Intra-abdominal synovial sarcoma: a

clinicopathological study. Histopathology. 2004 Sep;45(3):245–53. PMID:15330802

2138. Fisher C, Hedges M, Weiss SW. Ossifying fibromyxoid tumor of soft parts with stromal cyst formation and ribosome-lamella complexes. Ultrastruct Pathol. 1994 Nov-Dec;18(6):593–600. PMID:7855933

2139. Fishman SJ, Burrows PE. Chapter 7: Treatment of visceral vascular tumors. In: Mulliken JB, Burrows PE, Fishman SJ, editors. Mulliken and Young's vascular anomalies: hemangiomas and malformations. 2nd ed. New York (NY): Oxford University Press; 2013. pp. 242–9.

2140. Fite JJ, Maleki Z. Paraganglioma: cytomorphologic features, radiologic and clinical findings in 12 cases. Diagn Cytopathol. 2018 Jun;46(6):473–81. PMID:29575826

2141. Fittall MW, Mifsud W, Pillay N, et al. Recurrent rearrangements of FOS and FOSB define osteoblastoma. Nat Commun. 2018 Jun 1;9(1):2150. PMID:29858576

2142. Fjalldal S, Holmer H, Rylander L, et al. Hypothalamic involvement predicts cognitive performance and psychosocial health in long-term survivors of childhood craniopharyngioma. J Clin Endocrinol Metab. 2013 Aug;98(8):3253–62. PMID:23771923

2143. Flaig MJ, Cerroni L, Schuhmann K, et al. Follicular mycosis fungoides. A histopathologic analysis of nine cases. J Cutan Pathol. 2001 Nov;28(10):525–30. PMID:11737522

2144. Flamme I, Krieg M, Plate KH. Up-regulation of vascular endothelial growth factor in stromal cells of hemangioblastomas is correlated with up-regulation of the transcription factor HRF/HIF-2alpha. Am J Pathol. 1998 Jul;153(1):25–9. PMID:9665461

2144A. Flasinski M, Scheibke K, Zimmermann M, et al. Low-dose cytarabine to prevent myeloid leukemia in children with Down syndrome: TMD Prevention 2007 study. Blood Adv. 2018 Jul 10;2(13):1532–40. PMID:29959152

2145. Flavahan WA, Drier Y, Johnstone SE, et al. Altered chromosomal topology drives oncogenic programs in SDH-deficient GISTs. Nature. 2019 Nov;575(7781):229–33. PMID:31666694

2146. Flemming DJ, Murphey MD. Enchondroma and chondrosarcoma. Semin Musculoskelet Radiol. 2000;4(1):59–71. PMID:11061692

2147. Fletcher CD. Solitary circumscribed neuroma of the skin (so-called palisaded, encapsulated neuroma). A clinicopathologic and immunohistochemical study. Am J Surg Pathol. 1989 Jul;13(7):574–80. PMID:2660609

2148. Fletcher CD, Beham A, Bekir S, et al. Epithelioid angiosarcoma of deep soft tissue: a distinctive tumor readily mistaken for an epithelial neoplasm. Am J Surg Pathol. 1991 Oct;15(10):915–24. PMID:1718176

2149. Fletcher CD, Dal Cin P, de Wever I, et al. Correlation between clinicopathological features and karyotype in spindle cell sarcomas. A report of 130 cases from the CHAMP study group. Am J Pathol. 1999 Jun;154(6):1841–7. PMID:10362810

2150. Fletcher CD, Davies SE. Benign plexiform (multinodular) schwannoma: a rare tumour unassociated with neurofibromatosis. Histopathology. 1986 Sep;10(9):971–80. PMID:3096870

2151. Fletcher JS, Wu J, Jessen WJ, et al. Cxcr3-expressing leukocytes are necessary for neurofibroma formation in mice. JCI Insight. 2019 Feb 7;4(3):98601. PMID:30728335

2152. Flex E, Jaiswal M, Pantaleoni F, et al. Activating mutations in RRAS underlie a phenotype within the RASopathy spectrum and contribute to leukaemogenesis. Hum Mol Genet. 2014 Aug 15;23(16):4315–27. PMID:24705357

2153. Flieder DB, Moran CA, Suster S. Primary alveolar soft-part sarcoma of the mediastinum:

a clinicopathological and immunohistochemical study of two cases. Histopathology. 1997 Nov;31(5):469–73. PMID:9416489

2154. Flores RJ, Harrison DJ, Federman NC, et al. Alveolar soft part sarcoma in children and young adults: a report of 69 cases. Pediatr Blood Cancer. 2018 May;65(5):e26953. PMID:29350467

2155. Flucke U, Hulsebos TJ, van Krieken JH, et al. Myxoid epithelioid sarcoma: a diagnostic challenge. A report on six cases. Histopathology. 2010 Nov;57(5):753–9. PMID:21083605

2156. Flucke U, Mentzel T, Verdijk MA, et al. EWSR1-ATF1 chimeric transcript in a myoepithelial tumor of soft tissue: a case report. Hum Pathol. 2012 May;43(5):764–8. PMID:22154050

2157. Flucke U, Palmedo G, Blankenhorn N, et al. EWSR1 gene rearrangement occurs in a subset of cutaneous myoepithelial tumors: a study of 18 cases. Mod Pathol. 2011 Nov;24(11):1444–50. PMID:21725291

2158. Flucke U, Shepard SJ, Bekers EM, et al. Fibro-osseous pseudotumor of digits - Expanding the spectrum of clonal transient neoplasms harboring USP6 rearrangement. Ann Diagn Pathol. 2018 Aug;35:53–5. PMID:29787930

2159. Flucke U, Tops BB, van Diest PJ, et al. Desmoid-type fibromatosis of the head and neck region in the paediatric population: a clinicopathological and genetic study of seven cases. Histopathology. 2014 May;64(6):769–76. PMID:24206198

2160. Flucke U, van Noesel MM, Wijnen M, et al. TFG-MET fusion in an infantile spindle cell sarcoma with neural features. Genes Chromosomes Cancer. 2017 Sep;56(9):663–7. PMID:28510278

2161. Flucke U, Vogels RJ, de Saint Aubain Somerhausen N, et al. Epithelioid hemangioendothelioma: clinicopathologic, immunhistochemical, and molecular genetic analysis of 39 cases. Diagn Pathol. 2014 Jul 1;9:131. PMID:24986479

2162. Fluhr S, Krombholz CF, Meier A, et al. Epigenetic dysregulation of the erythropoietic transcription factor KLF1 and the β-like globin locus in juvenile myelomonocytic leukemia. Epigenetics. 2017 Aug;12(8):715–23. PMID:28749240

2163. Fluri S, Ammann R, Lüthy AR, et al. High-dose therapy and autologous stem cell transplantation for children with HIV-associated non-Hodgkin lymphoma. Pediatr Blood Cancer. 2007 Dec;49(7):984–7. PMID:16685736

2164. Flynt KA, Dillman JR, Davenport MS, et al. Pediatric adrenocortical neoplasms: Can imaging reliably discriminate adenomas from carcinomas? Pediatr Radiol. 2015 Jul;45(8):1160–8. PMID:25794486

2165. Fogt F, Vortmeyer AO, Ahn G, et al. Neural cyst of the ovary with central nervous system microvasculature. Histopathology. 1994 May;24(5):477–80. PMID:8088721

2166. Folberg R, Jakobiec FA, Bernardino VB, et al. Benign conjunctival melanocytic lesions. Clinicopathologic features. Ophthalmology. 1989 Apr;96(4):436–61. PMID:2657539

2167. Folk GS, Williams SB, Foss RB, et al. Oral and maxillofacial sclerosing epithelioid fibrosarcoma: report of five cases. Head Neck Pathol. 2007 Sep;1(1):13–20. PMID:20614275

2168. Folpe AL, Agoff SN, Willis J, et al. Parachordoma is immunohistochemically and cytogenetically distinct from axial chordoma and extraskeletal myxoid chondrosarcoma. Am J Surg Pathol. 1999 Sep;23(9):1059–67. PMID:10478665

2169. Folpe AL, Billings SD, McKenney JK, et al. Expression of claudin-1, a recently described tight junction-associated protein, distinguishes soft tissue perineurioma from potential mimics.

Am J Surg Pathol. 2002 Dec;26(12):1620–6. PMID:12459629

2170. Folpe AL, Fanburg-Smith JC, Billings SD, et al. Most osteomalacia-associated mesenchymal tumors are a single histopathologic entity: an analysis of 32 cases and a comprehensive review of the literature. Am J Surg Pathol. 2004 Jan;28(1):1–30. PMID:14707860

2171. Folpe AL, Fanburg-Smith JC, Miettinen M, et al. Atypical and malignant glomus tumors: analysis of 52 cases, with a proposal for the reclassification of glomus tumors. Am J Surg Pathol. 2001 Jan;25(1):1–12. PMID:11145243

2172. Folpe AL, Goldblum JR, Rubin BP, et al. Morphologic and immunophenotypic diversity in Ewing family tumors: a study of 66 genetically confirmed cases. Am J Surg Pathol. 2005 Aug;29(8):1025–33. PMID:16006796

2173. Folpe AL, Hill CE, Parham DM, et al. Immunohistochemical detection of FLI-1 protein expression: a study of 132 round cell tumors with emphasis on CD99-positive mimics of Ewing's sarcoma/primitive neuroectodermal tumor. Am J Surg Pathol. 2000 Dec;24(12):1657–62. PMID:11117787

2174. Folpe AL, Lane KL, Paull G, et al. Low-grade fibromyxoid sarcoma and hyalinizing spindle cell tumor with giant rosettes: a clinicopathologic study of 73 cases supporting their identity and assessing the impact of high-grade areas. Am J Surg Pathol. 2000 Oct;24(10):1353–60. PMID:11023096

2175. Folpe AL, Lloyd RV, Bacchi CE, et al. Spindle epithelial tumor with thymus-like differentiation: a morphologic, immunohistochemical, and molecular genetic study of 11 cases. Am J Surg Pathol. 2009 Aug;33(8):1179–86. PMID:19417583

2176. Folpe AL, Mentzel T, Lehr HA, et al. Perivascular epithelioid cell neoplasms of soft tissue and gynecologic origin: a clinicopathologic study of 26 cases and review of the literature. Am J Surg Pathol. 2005 Dec;29(12):1558–75. PMID:16327428

2177. Folpe AL, Morris RJ, Weiss SW. Soft tissue giant cell tumor of low malignant potential: a proposal for the reclassification of malignant giant cell tumor of soft parts. Mod Pathol. 1999 Sep;12(9):894–902. PMID:10496598

2178. Folpe AL, Weiss SW. Pleomorphic hyalinizing angiectatic tumor: analysis of 41 cases supporting evolution from a distinctive precursor lesion. Am J Surg Pathol. 2004 Nov;28(11):1417–25. PMID:15489645

2179. Fonseca EKUN, Ponte MPTR, Yamauchi FI, et al. The light bulb sign in pheochromocytoma. Abdom Radiol (NY). 2017 Nov;42(11):2779. PMID:28580539

2180. Fonseca FP, Carvalho MdeV, de Almeida OP, et al. Clinicopathologic analysis of 493 cases of salivary gland tumors in a Southern Brazilian population. Oral Surg Oral Med Oral Pathol Oral Radiol. 2012 Aug;114(2):230–9. PMID:22769409

2181. Font RL, Jurco S 3rd, Zimmerman LE. Alveolar soft-part sarcoma of the orbit: a clinicopathologic analysis of seventeen cases and a review of the literature. Hum Pathol. 1982 Jun;13(6):569–79. PMID:7076238

2182. Fontana E, Gaillard R. [Epidemiology of pituitary adenoma: results of the first Swiss study]. Rev Med Suisse. 2009 Oct 28;5(223):2172–4. French. PMID:19968031

2183. Fontebasso AM, Papillon-Cavanagh S, Schwartzentruber J, et al. Recurrent somatic mutations in ACVR1 in pediatric midline high-grade astrocytoma. Nat Genet. 2014 May;46(5):462–6. PMID:24705250

2184. Foo WC, Cruise MW, Wick MR, et al. Immunohistochemical staining for TLE1 distinguishes synovial sarcoma from histologic

mimics. Am J Clin Pathol. 2011 Jun;135(6):839–44. PMID:21571956

2185. Foote FW Jr, Frazell EL. Tumors of the major salivary glands. Cancer. 1953 Nov;6(6):1065–133. PMID:13106826

2186. Forbes JA, Ordóñez-Rubiano EG, Tomasiewicz HC, et al. Endonasal endoscopic transsphenoidal resection of intrinsic third ventricular craniopharyngioma: surgical results. J Neurosurg. 2018 Nov 1:1–11. PMID:30497140

2187. Forero Molina MA, Garcia E, Gonzalez-Devia D, et al. A 17-year-old male with a small bowel neuroendocrine tumor: flushing differential diagnosis. World Allergy Organ J. 2017 Sep 4;10(1):30. PMID:28904734

2188. Forest F, David A, Arrufat S, et al. Conventional chondrosarcoma in a survivor of rhabdoid tumor: enlarging the spectrum of tumors associated with SMARCB1 germline mutations. Am J Surg Pathol. 2012 Dec;36(12):1892–6. PMID:23154773

2189. Forshew T, Tatevossian RG, Lawson AR, et al. Activation of the ERK/MAPK pathway: a signature genetic defect in posterior fossa pilocytic astrocytomas. J Pathol. 2009 Jun;218(2):172–81. PMID:19373855

2190. Fortna RR, Junkins-Hopkins JM. A case of lobular capillary hemangioma (pyogenic granuloma), localized to the subcutaneous tissue, and a review of the literature. Am J Dermatopathol. 2007 Aug;29(4):408–11. PMID:17667179

2191. Fortunati N, Guaraldi F, Zunino V, et al. Effects of environmental pollutants on signaling pathways in rat pituitary GH3 adenoma cells. Environ Res. 2017 Oct;158:660–8. PMID:28732322

2192. Foss HD, Anagnostopoulos I, Araujo I, et al. Anaplastic large-cell lymphomas of T-cell and null-cell phenotype express cytotoxic molecules. Blood. 1996 Nov 15;88(10):4005–11. PMID:8916967

2193. Fosså A, Fosså SD. Serum lactate dehydrogenase and human choriogonadotrophin in seminoma. Br J Urol. 1989 Apr;63(4):408–15. PMID:2653557

2194. Fosså SD, Aass N, Heilo A, et al. Testicular carcinoma in situ in patients with extragonadal germ-cell tumours: the clinical role of pretreatment biopsy. Ann Oncol. 2003 Sep;14(9):1412–8. PMID:12954581

2195. Fosså SD, Cvancarova M, Chen L, et al. Adverse prognostic factors for testicular cancer-specific survival: a population-based study of 27,948 patients. J Clin Oncol. 2011 Mar 10;29(8):963–70. PMID:21300926

2196. Fossey M, Li H, Afzal S, et al. Atypical teratoid rhabdoid tumor in the first year of life: the Canadian ATRT registry experience and review of the literature. J Neurooncol. 2017 Mar;132(1):155–62. PMID:28102486

2197. Foster RD, Williams ML, Barkovich AJ, et al. Giant congenital melanocytic nevi: the significance of neurocutaneous melanosis in neurologically asymptomatic children. Plast Reconstr Surg. 2001 Apr 1;107(4):933–41. PMID:11252085

2198. Foster RS, Hermans B, Bihrle R, et al. Clinical stage I pure yolk sac tumor of the testis in adults has different clinical behavior than juvenile yolk sac tumor. J Urol. 2000 Dec;164(6):1943–4. PMID:11061887

2199. Foulkes WD, Bahubeshi A, Hamel N, et al. Extending the phenotypes associated with DICER1 mutations. Hum Mutat. 2011 Dec;32(12):1381–4. PMID:21882293

2200. Foulkes WD, Clarke BA, Hasselblatt M, et al. No small surprise - small cell carcinoma of the ovary, hypercalcaemic type, is a malignant rhabdoid tumour. J Pathol. 2014 Jul;233(3):209–14. PMID:24752781

2201. Foulkes WD, Kamihara J, Evans DGR, et al. Cancer surveillance in Gorlin syndrome and rhabdoid tumor predisposition syndrome. Clin Cancer Res. 2017 Jun 15;23(12):e62–7. PMID:28620006
2202. Foulkes WD, Priest JR, Duchaine TF. DICER1: mutations, microRNAs and mechanisms. Nat Rev Cancer. 2014 Oct;14(10):662–72. PMID:25176334
2203. Fournier B, Balducci E, Duployez N, et al. B-ALL with t(5;14)(q31;q32); IGH-IL3 rearrangement and eosinophilia: a comprehensive analysis of a peculiar IGH-rearranged B-ALL. Front Oncol. 2019 Dec 10;9:1374. PMID:31921638
2204. Fowler M, Simpson DA. A malignant melanin-forming tumour of the cerebellum. J Pathol Bacteriol. 1962 Oct;84:307–11. PMID:13958991
2205. Fox MD, Billings SD, Gleason BC, et al. Cutaneous meningioma: a potential diagnostic pitfall in p63 positive cutaneous neoplasms. J Cutan Pathol. 2013 Oct;40(10):891–5. PMID:23924346
2206. França JA, Gayden T, Bareke E, et al. Whole-exome sequencing reveals novel vacuolar ATPase genes' variants and variants in genes involved in lysosomal biology and autophagosomal formation in oral granular cell tumors. J Oral Pathol Med. 2021 Apr;50(4):410–7. PMID:33289181
2207. Franceschi E, Hofer S, Brandes AA, et al. EANO-EURACAN clinical practice guideline for diagnosis, treatment, and follow-up of post-pubertal and adult patients with medulloblastoma. Lancet Oncol. 2019 Dec;20(12):e715–28. PMID:31797797
2208. Francis GL, Waguespack SG, Bauer AJ, et al. Management guidelines for children with thyroid nodules and differentiated thyroid cancer. Thyroid. 2015 Jul;25(7):716–59. PMID:25900731
2209. Francis JH, Abramson DH, Gaillard MC, et al. The classification of vitreous seeds in retinoblastoma and response to intravitreal melphalan. Ophthalmology. 2015 Jun;122(6):1173–9. PMID:25795478
2210. Francis JH, Grossniklaus HE, Habib LA, et al. BRAF, NRAS, and GNAQ mutations in conjunctival melanocytic nevi. Invest Ophthalmol Vis Sci. 2018 Jan 1;59(1):117–21. PMID:29332123
2211. Francis JH, Levin AM, Zabor EC, et al. Ten-year experience with ophthalmic artery chemosurgery: ocular and recurrence-free survival. PLoS One. 2018 May 23;13(5):e0197081. PMID:29791475
2212. Francis R, Bower M, Brunström G, et al. Surveillance for stage I testicular germ cell tumours: results and cost benefit analysis of management options. Eur J Cancer. 2000 Oct;36(15):1925–32. PMID:11000572
2213. Franco AT, Labourier E, Ablordeppey KK, et al. miRNA expression can classify pediatric thyroid lesions and increases the diagnostic yield of mutation testing. Pediatr Blood Cancer. 2020 Jun;67(6):e28276. PMID:32196952
2214. Francom CR, Leoniak SM, Lovell MA, et al. Head and neck pleomorphic myxoid liposarcoma in a child with Li-Fraumeni syndrome. Int J Pediatr Otorhinolaryngol. 2019 Aug;123:191–4. PMID:31129458
2215. Franz DN, Belousova E, Sparagana S, et al. Efficacy and safety of everolimus for subependymal giant cell astrocytomas associated with tuberous sclerosis complex (EXIST-1): a multicentre, randomised, placebo-controlled phase 3 trial. Lancet. 2013 Jan 12;381(9861):125–32. PMID:23158522
2216. Franz DN, Belousova E, Sparagana S, et al. Everolimus for subependymal giant cell astrocytoma in patients with tuberous sclerosis complex: 2-year open-label extension of the randomised EXIST-1 study. Lancet Oncol. 2014 Dec;15(13):1513–20. PMID:25456370
2217. Franz DN, Belousova E, Sparagana S, et al. Long-term use of everolimus in patients with tuberous sclerosis complex: final results from the EXIST-1 study. PLoS One. 2016 Jun 28;11(6):e0158476. PMID:27351628
2218. Frayling IM. Microsatellite instability. Gut. 1999 Jul;45(1):1–4. PMID:10369691
2219. Frayling IM, Arends M. Adenomatous polyposis coli. In: Maloy S, Hughes K, editors. Brenner's encyclopedia of genetics. Volume 1. 2nd ed. San Diego (CA): Academic Press; 2013. pp. 27–9.
2220. Frayling IM. Familial adenomatous polyposis (FAP) and adenomatous polyposis (due to MUTYH, NTHL1, POLE & POLD1). In: Firth HV, Hurst JA, editors. Oxford Desk Reference: clinical genetics & genomics. 2nd ed. Oxford (UK): Oxford University Press; 2017.
2221. Frazier AL, Rumcheva P, Olson T, et al. Application of the adult international germ cell classification system to pediatric malignant non-seminomatous germ cell tumors: a report from the Children's Oncology Group. Pediatr Blood Cancer. 2008 Apr;50(4):746–51. PMID:18085675
2222. Frebourg T, Bajalica Lagercrantz S, Oliveira C, et al. Guidelines for the Li-Fraumeni and heritable TP53-related cancer syndromes. Eur J Hum Genet. 2020 Oct;28(10):1379–86. PMID:32457520
2223. Freeburn AM, McAloon J. Infantile chest hamartoma–case outcome aged 11. Arch Dis Child. 2001 Sep;85(3):244–5. PMID:11517112
2224. Freedom RM, Lee KJ, MacDonald C, et al. Selected aspects of cardiac tumors in infancy and childhood. Pediatr Cardiol. 2000 Jul-Aug;21(4):299–316. PMID:10865003
2225. Freilich RJ, Thompson SJ, Walker RW, et al. Adenocarcinomatous transformation of intracranial germ cell tumors. Am J Surg Pathol. 1995 May;19(5):537–44. PMID:7726363
2226. French CA. Pathogenesis of NUT midline carcinoma. Annu Rev Pathol. 2012;7:247–65. PMID:22017582
2227. French CA, Kutok JL, Faquin WC, et al. Midline carcinoma of children and young adults with NUT rearrangement. J Clin Oncol. 2004 Oct 15;22(20):4135–9. PMID:15483023
2228. French CA, Ramirez CL, Kolmakova J, et al. BRD-NUT oncoproteins: a family of closely related nuclear proteins that block epithelial differentiation and maintain the growth of carcinoma cells. Oncogene. 2008 Apr 3;27(15):2237–42. PMID:17934517
2229. Freudenstein D, Wagner A, Bornemann A, et al. Primary melanocytic lesions of the CNS: report of five cases. Zentralbl Neurochir. 2004;65(3):146–53. PMID:15306980
2230. Frezza AM, Cesari M, Baumhoer D, et al. Mesenchymal chondrosarcoma: prognostic factors and outcome in 113 patients. A European Musculoskeletal Oncology Society study. Eur J Cancer. 2015 Feb;51(3):374–81. PMID:25529371
2231. Frezza AM, Sbaraglia M, Lo Vullo S, et al. The natural history of epithelioid sarcoma. A retrospective multicentre case-series within the Italian Sarcoma Group. Eur J Surg Oncol. 2020 Jul;46(7):1320–6. PMID:32307188
2232. Fridman M, Lam AK, Krasko O, et al. Morphological and clinical presentation of papillary thyroid carcinoma in children and adolescents of Belarus: the influence of radiation exposure and the source of irradiation. Exp Mol Pathol. 2015 Jun;98(3):527–31. PMID:25841866
2233. Fridman MV, Savva NN, Krasko OV, et al. Clinical and pathologic features of "sporadic" papillary thyroid carcinoma registered in the years 2005 to 2008 in children and adolescents of Belarus. Thyroid. 2012 Oct;22(10):1016–24. PMID:22947350
2234. Friedman AC, Lichtenstein JE, Goodman Z, et al. Fibrolamellar hepatocellular carcinoma. Radiology. 1985 Dec;157(3):583–7. PMID:2997835
2235. Friedman DL, Whitton J, Leisenring W, et al. Subsequent neoplasms in 5-year survivors of childhood cancer: the Childhood Cancer Survivor Study. J Natl Cancer Inst. 2010 Jul 21;102(14):1083–95. PMID:20634481
2236. Friedman SM, Margo CE. Choroidal melanoma and neurofibromatosis type 1. Arch Ophthalmol. 1998 May;116(5):694–5. PMID:9596516
2237. Friend KE, Chiou YK, Laws ER Jr, et al. Pit-1 messenger ribonucleic acid is differentially expressed in human pituitary adenomas. J Clin Endocrinol Metab. 1993 Nov;77(5):1281–6. PMID:8077322
2238. Friend KE, Chiou YK, Lopes MB, et al. Estrogen receptor expression in human pituitary: correlation with immunohistochemistry in normal tissue, and immunohistochemistry and morphology in macroadenomas. J Clin Endocrinol Metab. 1994 Jun;78(6):1497–504. PMID:7515390
2239. Friend SH, Bernards R, Rogelj S, et al. A human DNA segment with properties of the gene that predisposes to retinoblastoma and osteosarcoma. Nature. 1986 Oct 16-22;323(6089):643–6. PMID:2877398
2240. Frigerio M, Martinelli-Kläy CP, Lombardi T. Clinical, histopathological and immunohistochemical study of oral squamous papillomas. Acta Odontol Scand. 2015;73(7):508–15. PMID:25598510
2241. Frismantas V, Dobay MP, Rinaldi A, et al. Ex vivo drug response profiling detects recurrent sensitivity patterns in drug-resistant acute lymphoblastic leukemia. Blood. 2017 Mar 16;129(11):e26–37. PMID:28122742
2242. Fritchie K, Wang L, Yin Z, et al. Lipoblastomas presenting in older children and adults: analysis of 22 cases with identification of novel PLAG1 fusion partners. Mod Pathol. 2021 Mar;34(3):584–91. PMID:33097826
2243. Fritz A, Percy C, Jack A, et al., editors. International classification of diseases for oncology (ICD-O). 3rd ed. 1st rev. Geneva (Switzerland): World Health Organization; 2013.
2244. Fröstad B, Tani E, Brosjö O, et al. Fine needle aspiration cytology in the diagnosis and management of children and adolescents with Ewing sarcoma and peripheral primitive neuroectodermal tumor. Med Pediatr Oncol. 2002 Jan;38(1):33–40. PMID:11835234
2245. Fruehwald-Pallamar J, Puchner SB, Rossi A, et al. Magnetic resonance imaging spectrum of medulloblastoma. Neuroradiology. 2011 Jun;53(6):387–96. PMID:21279509
2246. Frühwald MC, Hasselblatt M, Nemes K, et al. Age and DNA methylation subgroup as potential independent risk factors for treatment stratification in children with atypical teratoid/rhabdoid tumors. Neuro Oncol. 2020 Jul 7;22(7):1006–17. PMID:31883020
2247. Fujii K, Miyashita T. Gorlin syndrome (nevoid basal cell carcinoma syndrome): update and literature review. Pediatr Int. 2014 Oct;56(5):667–74. PMID:25131638
2248. Fujii K, Ohashi H, Suzuki M, et al. Frameshift mutation in the PTCH2 gene can cause nevoid basal cell carcinoma syndrome. Fam Cancer. 2013 Dec;12(4):611–4. PMID:23479190
2249. Fujii S, Nagata K, Matsumoto S, et al. Wnt/β-catenin signaling, which is activated in odontomas, reduces Sema3A expression to regulate odontogenic epithelial cell proliferation and tooth germ development. Sci Rep. 2019 Mar 12;9(1):4257. PMID:30862786
2250. Fujisawa K, Suzuki N, Hoshino M, et al. [Congenital dermal sinus of the nose complicated with a brain abscess – a case report (author's transl)]. Neurol Med Chir (Tokyo). 1981 May;21(5):521–4. Japanese. PMID:6168964
2251. Fujiwara K, Ginzan S, Silverberg SG. Mature cystic teratomas of the ovary with intestinal wall structures harboring intestinal- type epithelial neoplasms. Gynecol Oncol. 1995 Jan;56(1):97–101. PMID:7821857
2252. Fukuda M, Horibe K, Miyajima Y, et al. Spontaneous remission of juvenile chronic myelomonocytic leukemia in an infant with Noonan syndrome. J Pediatr Hematol Oncol. 1997 Mar-Apr;19(2):177–9. PMID:9149755
2253. Fukuda T, Akiyama N, Ikegami M, et al. Expression of hydroxyindole-O-methyltransferase enzyme in the human central nervous system and in pineal parenchymal cell tumors. J Neuropathol Exp Neurol. 2010 May;69(5):498–510. PMID:20418777
2254. Fukuda T, Igarashi T, Hiraki H, et al. Abnormal pigmentation of schwannoma attributed to excess production of neuromelanin-like pigment. Pathol Int. 2000 Mar;50(3):230–7. PMID:10792787
2255. Fukunaga M, Endo Y, Masui F, et al. Retiform haemangioendothelioma. Virchows Arch. 1996 Jul;428(4-5):301–4. PMID:8764941
2256. Fukunaga M, Ishibashi T, Koyama T, et al. Malignant struma ovarii with a predominant component of anaplastic carcinoma. Int J Gynecol Pathol. 2016 Jul;35(4):357–61. PMID:26630220
2257. Fukuoka K, Kanemura Y, Shofuda T, et al. Significance of molecular classification of ependymomas: C11orf95-RELA fusion-negative supratentorial ependymomas are a heterogeneous group of tumors. Acta Neuropathol Commun. 2018 Dec 4;6(1):134. PMID:30514397
2258. Fukuoka K, Mamatjan Y, Ryall S, et al. BRAF V600E mutant oligodendroglioma-like tumors with chromosomal instability in adolescents and young adults. Brain Pathol. 2020 May;30(3):515–23. PMID:31630459
2259. Fukuoka K, Mamatjan Y, Tatevossian R, et al. Clinical impact of combined epigenetic and molecular analysis of pediatric low-grade gliomas. Neuro Oncol. 2020 Oct 14;22(10):1474–83. PMID:32242226
2260. Fukushima S, Otsuka A, Suzuki T, et al. Mutually exclusive mutations of KIT and RAS are associated with KIT mRNA expression and chromosomal instability in primary intracranial pure germinomas. Acta Neuropathol. 2014;127(6):911–25. PMID:24452629
2261. Fukushima S, Yamashita S, Kobayashi H, et al. Genome-wide methylation profiles in primary intracranial germ cell tumors indicate a primordial germ cell origin for germinomas. Acta Neuropathol. 2017 Mar;133(3):445–62. PMID:28078450
2262. Fuld AD, Speck ME, Harris BT, et al. Primary melanoma of the spinal cord: a case report, molecular footprint, and review of the literature. J Clin Oncol. 2011 Jun 10;29(17):e499–502. PMID:21444862
2263. Funato K, Major T, Lewis PW, et al. Use of human embryonic stem cells to model pediatric gliomas with H3.3K27M histone mutation. Science. 2014 Dec 19;346(6216):1529–33. PMID:25525250
2264. Funch DP, Brady J, Ko HH, et al. Methods and objectives of a large US multicenter case-control study of post-transplant lymphoproliferative disorder in renal transplant patients. Recent Results Cancer Res. 2002;159:81–8. PMID:11785847
2265. Funkhouser AW, Katzman PJ, Sickel JZ, et al. CD30-positive anaplastic large cell lymphoma (ALCL) of T-cell lineage in a

14-month-old infant with perinatally acquired HIV-1 infection. J Pediatr Hematol Oncol. 1998 Nov-Dec;20(6):556–9. PMID:9856678
**2266.** Furey C, Antwi P, Duran D, et al. 9p24 triplication in syndromic hydrocephalus with diffuse villous hyperplasia of the choroid plexus. Cold Spring Harb Mol Case Stud. 2018 Oct 1;4(5):a003145. PMID:29895553
**2267.** Furlan A, Adameyko I. Schwann cell precursor: a neural crest cell in disguise? Dev Biol. 2018 Dec 1;444 Suppl 1:S25–35. PMID:29454705
**2268.** Furlan A, Dyachuk V, Kastriti ME, et al. Multipotent peripheral glial cells generate neuroendocrine cells of the adrenal medulla. Science. 2017 Jul 7;357(6346):eaal3753. PMID:28684471
**2269.** Furlan D, Sahnane N, Bernasconi B, et al. APC alterations are frequently involved in the pathogenesis of acinar cell carcinoma of the pancreas, mainly through gene loss and promoter hypermethylation. Virchows Arch. 2014 May;464(5):553–64. PMID:24590585
**2270.** Furlong MA, Fanburg-Smith JC, Miettinen M. The morphologic spectrum of hibernoma: a clinicopathologic study of 170 cases. Am J Surg Pathol. 2001 Jun;25(6):809–14. PMID:11395560
**2271.** Furtwängler R, Schmolze M, Gräber S, et al. Pretreatment for bilateral nephroblastomatosis is an independent risk factor for progressive disease in patients with stage V nephroblastoma. Klin Padiatr. 2014 May;226(3):175–81. PMID:24819388
**2272.** Furuta T, Moritsubo M, Muta H, et al. Central nervous system neuroblastic tumor with FOXR2 activation presenting both neuronal and glial differentiation: a case report. Brain Tumor Pathol. 2020 Jul;37(3):100–4. PMID:32535663
**2273.** Futani H, Fukunaga S, Tsukamoto Y, et al. Small cell osteosarcoma successfully treated by high-dose ifosfamide and methotrexate, combined with carboplatin and pirarubicin. Anticancer Res. 2012 Mar;32(3):965–71. PMID:22399618
**2274.** Gaal J, Stratakis CA, Carney JA, et al. SDHB immunohistochemistry: a useful tool in the diagnosis of Carney-Stratakis and Carney triad gastrointestinal stromal tumors. Mod Pathol. 2011 Jan;24(1):147–51. PMID:20890271
**2275.** Gabel BC, Cleary DR, Martin JR, et al. Unusual and rare locations for craniopharyngiomas: clinical significance and review of the literature. World Neurosurg. 2017 Feb;98:381–7. PMID:27908738
**2276.** Gadd S, Beezhold P, Jennings L, et al. Mediators of receptor tyrosine kinase activation in infantile fibrosarcoma: a Children's Oncology Group study. J Pathol. 2012 Sep;228(1):119–30. PMID:22374738
**2277.** Gadd S, Huff V, Walz AL, et al. A Children's Oncology Group and TARGET initiative exploring the genetic landscape of Wilms tumor. Nat Genet. 2017 Oct;49(10):1487–94. PMID:28825729
**2278.** Gadducci A, Giuliani D, Cosio S, et al. Clinical outcome of patients with malignant tumors associated with mature cystic teratomas of the ovary: a retrospective multicenter Italian study. Anticancer Res. 2019 May;39(5):2513–7. PMID:31092447
**2278A.** Gadgeel M, AlQanber B, Buck S, et al. Aberrant myelomonocytic CD56 expression in Down syndrome is frequent and not associated with leukemogenesis. Ann Hematol. 2021 Jul;100(7):1695–700. PMID:33890142
**2279.** Gadish T, Tulchinsky H, Deutsch AA, et al. Pinealoblastoma in a patient with familial adenomatous polyposis: variant of Turcot syndrome type 2? Report of a case and review of the literature. Dis Colon Rectum. 2005 Dec;48(12):2343–6. PMID:16400511
**2280.** Gadner H, Minkov M, Grois N, et al. Therapy prolongation improves outcome in multisystem Langerhans cell histiocytosis. Blood. 2013 Jun 20;121(25):5006–14. PMID:23589673
**2281.** Gadwal SR, Fanburg-Smith JC, Gannon FH, et al. Primary chondrosarcoma of the head and neck in pediatric patients: a clinicopathologic study of 14 cases with a review of the literature. Cancer. 2000 May 1;88(9):2181–8. PMID:10813732
**2282.** Gaertner EM, Steinberg DM, Huber M, et al. Pulmonary and mediastinal glomus tumors–report of five cases including a pulmonary glomangiosarcoma: a clinicopathologic study with literature review. Am J Surg Pathol. 2000 Aug;24(8):1105–14. PMID:10935651
**2283.** Gaffey MJ, Mills SE, Boyd JC. Aggressive papillary tumor of middle ear/temporal bone and adnexal papillary cystadenoma. Manifestations of von Hippel-Lindau disease. Am J Surg Pathol. 1994 Dec;18(12):1254–60. PMID:7977949
**2284.** Gahr N, Darge K, Hahn G, et al. Diffusion-weighted MRI for differentiation of neuroblastoma and ganglioneuroblastoma/ganglioneuroma. Eur J Radiol. 2011 Sep;79(3):443–6. PMID:20462716
**2285.** Gaiani F, de'Angelis N, Minelli R, et al. Pediatric gastroenteropancreatic neuroendocrine tumor: a case report and review of the literature. Medicine (Baltimore). 2019 Sep;98(37):e17154. PMID:31517859
**2286.** Gajjar A, Pfister SM, Taylor MD, et al. Molecular insights into pediatric brain tumors have the potential to transform therapy. Clin Cancer Res. 2014 Nov 15;20(22):5630–40. PMID:25398846
**2287.** Galgano MA, Goulart CR, Iwenofu H, et al. Osteoblastomas of the spine: a comprehensive review. Neurosurg Focus. 2016 Aug;41(2):E4. PMID:27476846
**2288.** Galili N, Davis RJ, Fredericks WJ, et al. Fusion of a fork head domain gene to PAX3 in the solid tumour alveolar rhabdomyosarcoma. Nat Genet. 1993 Nov;5(3):230–5. PMID:8275086
**2289.** Galimberti S, Devidas M, Lucenti A, et al. Validation of minimal residual disease as surrogate endpoint for event-free survival in childhood acute lymphoblastic leukemia. JNCI Cancer Spectr. 2018 Dec 19;2(4):pky069. PMID:31360884
**2290.** Galle TS, Juel K, Bülow S. Causes of death in familial adenomatous polyposis. Scand J Gastroenterol. 1999 Aug;34(8):808–12. PMID:10499482
**2291.** Gallie BL, Campbell C, Devlin H, et al. Developmental basis of retinal-specific induction of cancer by RB mutation. Cancer Res. 1999 Apr 1;59(7 Suppl):1731s–5s. PMID:10197588
**2292.** Gallon R, Mühlegger B, Wenzel SS, et al. A sensitive and scalable microsatellite instability assay to diagnose constitutional mismatch repair deficiency by sequencing of peripheral blood leukocytes. Hum Mutat. 2019 May;40(5):649–55. PMID:30740824
**2293.** Galluzzo ML, Garcia de Davila MT, Vujanić GM. A composite renal tumor: metanephric adenofibroma, Wilms tumor, and renal cell carcinoma: a missing link? Pediatr Dev Pathol. 2012 Jan-Feb;15(1):65–70. PMID:21711207
**2294.** Galluzzo Mutti L, Álvarez M, Siminovich M, et al. Disseminated visceral Kaposi's sarcoma in a pediatric bilateral lung transplant recipient. Pediatr Transplant. 2019 Feb;23(1):e13311. PMID:30362299
**2295.** Gambarotti M, Benini S, Gamberi G, et al. CIC-DUX4 fusion-positive round-cell sarcomas of soft tissue and bone: a single-institution morphological and molecular analysis of seven cases. Histopathology. 2016 Oct;69(4):624–34. PMID:27079694
**2296.** Gambarotti M, Dei Tos AP, Vanel D, et al. Osteoblastoma-like osteosarcoma: high-grade or low-grade osteosarcoma? Histopathology. 2019 Feb;74(3):494–503. PMID:30152881
**2297.** Gambarotti M, Righi A, Picci P, et al. Paediatric chondrosarcomas: a retrospective review of 17 cases. Histopathology. 2016 Jun;68(7):1073–8. PMID:26408960
**2298.** Gambarotti M, Righi A, Sbaraglia M, et al. Intraosseous papillary intralymphatic angioendothelioma (PILA): one new case and review of the literature. Clin Sarcoma Res. 2018 Jan 30;8:1. PMID:29423171
**2299.** Gamberi G, Cocchi S, Benini S, et al. Molecular diagnosis in Ewing family tumors: the Rizzoli experience–222 consecutive cases in four years. J Mol Diagn. 2011 May;13(3):313–24. PMID:21458383
**2300.** Gambichler T, Al-Muhammadi R, Boms S. Immunologically mediated photodermatoses: diagnosis and treatment. Am J Clin Dermatol. 2009;10(3):169–80. PMID:19354331
**2301.** Gamboa NT, Karsy M, Gamboa JT, et al. Preoperative and intraoperative perfusion magnetic resonance imaging in a RELA fusion-positive anaplastic ependymoma: a case report. Surg Neurol Int. 2018 Jul 24;9:144. PMID:30105138
**2302.** Gamborino E, Carrilho C, Ferro J, et al. Fine-needle aspiration diagnosis of Kaposi's sarcoma in a developing country. Diagn Cytopathol. 2000 Nov;23(5):322–5. PMID:11074626
**2303.** Gamis AS, Alonzo TA, Gerbing RB, et al. Natural history of transient myeloproliferative disorder clinically diagnosed in Down syndrome neonates: a report from the Children's Oncology Group Study A2971. Blood. 2011 Dec 22;118(26):6752–9. PMID:21849481
**2304.** Gamis AS, Alonzo TA, Meshinchi S, et al. Gemtuzumab ozogamicin in children and adolescents with de novo acute myeloid leukemia improves event-free survival by reducing relapse risk: results from the randomized phase III Children's Oncology Group trial AAML0531. J Clin Oncol. 2014 Sep 20;32(27):3021–32. PMID:25092781
**2305.** Gan S, Xie D, Dai H, et al. Proliferative myositis and nodular fasciitis: a retrospective study with clinicopathologic and radiologic correlation. Int J Clin Exp Pathol. 2019 Dec 1;12(12):4319–28. PMID:31933833
**2306.** Gandhi JS, Malik F, Amin MB, et al. MiT family translocation renal cell carcinomas: a 15th anniversary update. Histol Histopathol. 2020 Feb;35(2):125–36. PMID:31489603
**2307.** Ganeshan D, Szklaruk J, Kundra V, et al. Imaging features of fibrolamellar hepatocellular carcinoma. AJR Am J Roentgenol. 2014 Mar;202(3):544–52. PMID:24555590
**2308.** Ganmore I, Smooha G, Izraeli S. Constitutional aneuploidy and cancer predisposition. Hum Mol Genet. 2009 Apr 15;18 R1:R84–93. PMID:19297405
**2309.** Gannon FH, Glaser D, Caron R, et al. Mast cell involvement in fibrodysplasia ossificans progressiva. Hum Pathol. 2001 Aug;32(8):842–8. PMID:11521229
**2310.** Gantner S, Rütten A, Requena L, et al. CHILD syndrome with mild skin lesions: histopathologic clues for the diagnosis. J Cutan Pathol. 2014 Oct;41(10):787–90. PMID:25093865
**2311.** Gao J, Gauerke SJ, Martinez-Escala ME, et al. Bone marrow involvement by subcutaneous panniculitis-like T-cell lymphoma: a report of three cases. Mod Pathol. 2014 Jun;27(6):800–7. PMID:24201122
**2312.** Gao M, Hao Y, Huang MX, et al. Salivary gland tumours in a northern Chinese population: a 50-year retrospective study of 7190 cases. Int J Oral Maxillofac Surg. 2017 Mar;46(3):343–9. PMID:27769738
**2313.** Gao X, Zhang Y, Arrazola P, et al. Tsc tumour suppressor proteins antagonize amino-acid-TOR signalling. Nat Cell Biol. 2002 Sep;4(9):699–704. PMID:12172555
**2314.** Gao Y, Jiang J, Liu Q. Clinicopathological and immunohistochemical features of primary central nervous system germ cell tumors: a 24-years experience. Int J Clin Exp Pathol. 2014 Sep 15;7(10):6965–72. PMID:25400782
**2315.** Gao Y, Saksena MA, Brachtel EF, et al. How to approach breast lesions in children and adolescents. Eur J Radiol. 2015 Jul;84(7):1350–64. PMID:25958188
**2315A.** Garcia C, Gutmann DH. Nf2/Merlin controls spinal cord neural progenitor function in a Rac1/ErbB2-dependent manner. PLoS One. 2014 May 9;9(5):e97320. PMID:24817309
**2316.** Garcia CA, Spencer RP. Bone and In-111 octreotide imaging in oncogenic osteomalacia: a case report. Clin Nucl Med. 2002 Aug;27(8):582–3. PMID:12170004
**2317.** Garcia RA, Inwards CY, Unni KK. Benign bone tumors–recent developments. Semin Diagn Pathol. 2011 Feb;28(1):73–85. PMID:21675379
**2318.** Garcia-Lavandeira M, Saez C, Diaz-Rodriguez E, et al. Craniopharyngiomas express embryonic stem cell markers (SOX2, OCT4, KLF4, and SOX9) as pituitary stem cells but do not coexpress RET/GFRA3 receptors. J Clin Endocrinol Metab. 2012 Jan;97(1):E80–7. PMID:22031517
**2319.** Garcia-Montero AC, Jara-Acevedo M, Teodosio C, et al. KIT mutation in mast cells and other bone marrow hematopoietic cell lineages in systemic mast cell disorders: a prospective study of the Spanish Network on Mastocytosis (REMA) in a series of 113 patients. Blood. 2006 Oct 1;108(7):2366–72. PMID:16741248
**2320.** García-Morales I, Requena-Caballero L, Happle R, et al. Segmental Hailey-Hailey disease of the vulva. Pediatr Dermatol. 2018 Nov;35(6):e398–9. PMID:30168169
**2321.** Garcia-Reyero J, Martinez Magunacelaya N, Gonzalez de Villambrosia S, et al. Genetic lesions in MYC and STAT3 drive oncogenic transcription factor overexpression in plasmablastic lymphoma. Haematologica. 2021 Apr 1;106(4):1120–8. PMID:32273478
**2322.** Garcias-Ladaria J, Cuadrado Rosón M, Pascual-López M. Epidermal nevi and related syndromes – Part 1: keratinocytic nevi. Actas Dermosifiliogr (Engl Ed). 2018 Oct;109(8):677–86. PMID:29983155
**2323.** Garcias-Ladaria J, Cuadrado Rosón M, Pascual-López M. Epidermal nevi and related syndromes - Part 2: nevi derived from adnexal structures. Actas Dermosifiliogr (Engl Ed). 2018 Oct;109(8):687–98. PMID:30041869
**2324.** Gardiman MP, Fassan M, Orvieto E, et al. Diffuse leptomeningeal glioneuronal tumors: a new entity? Brain Pathol. 2010 Mar;20(2):361–6. PMID:19486008
**2325.** Gareton A, Tauziède-Espariat A, Dangouloff-Ros V, et al. The histomolecular criteria established for adult anaplastic pilocytic astrocytoma are not applicable to the pediatric population. Acta Neuropathol. 2020 Feb;139(2):287–303. PMID:31677015
**2326.** Garfield EM, Walton KE, Quan VL, et al. Histomorphologic spectrum of germline-related and sporadic BAP1-inactivated melanocytic tumors. J Am Acad Dermatol. 2018 Sep;79(3):525–34. PMID:29753057
**2327.** Garg K, Soslow RA, Rivera M, et al. Histologically bland "extremely well differentiated" thyroid carcinomas arising in struma ovarii can

recur and metastasize. Int J Gynecol Pathol. 2009 May;28(3):222–30. PMID:19620939

**2328.** Garland SM, Pitisuttithum P, Ngan HYS, et al. Efficacy, immunogenicity, and safety of a 9-valent human papillomavirus vaccine: subgroup analysis of participants from Asian countries. J Infect Dis. 2018 Jun 5;218(1):95–108. PMID:29767739

**2329.** Garnier L, Ducray F, Verlut C, et al. Prolonged response induced by single agent vemurafenib in a BRAF V600E spinal ganglioglioma: a case report and review of the literature. Front Oncol. 2019 Mar 26;9:177. PMID:30984614

**2330.** Garrè ML, Cama A, Bagnasco F, et al. Medulloblastoma variants: age-dependent occurrence and relation to Gorlin syndrome–a new clinical perspective. Clin Cancer Res. 2009 Apr 1;15(7):2463–71. PMID:19276247

**2331.** Garrido A, Humphrey G, Squire RS, et al. Sialoblastoma. Br J Plast Surg. 2000 Dec;53(8):697–9. PMID:11090328

**2332.** Garriga MM, Friedman MM, Metcalfe DD. A survey of the number and distribution of mast cells in the skin of patients with mast cell disorders. J Allergy Clin Immunol. 1988 Sep;82(3 Pt 1):425–32. PMID:3170991

**2333.** Garvin JH Jr, Selch MT, Holmes E, et al. Phase II study of pre-irradiation chemotherapy for childhood intracranial ependymoma. Children's Cancer Group protocol 9942: a report from the Children's Oncology Group. Pediatr Blood Cancer. 2012 Dec 15;59(7):1183–9. PMID:22949057

**2334.** Garzia L, Kijima N, Morrissy AS, et al. A hematogenous route for medulloblastoma leptomeningeal metastases. Cell. 2018 Feb 22;172(5):1050–1062.e14. PMID:29474906

**2335.** Gascoyne RD, Lamant L, Martin-Subero JI, et al. ALK-positive diffuse large B-cell lymphoma is associated with Clathrin-ALK rearrangements: report of 6 cases. Blood. 2003 Oct 1;102(7):2568–73. PMID:12763927

**2336.** Gaspard M, Lamant L, Tournier E, et al. Evaluation of eight melanocytic and neural crest-associated markers in a well-characterised series of 124 malignant peripheral nerve sheath tumours (MPNST): useful to distinguish MPNST from melanoma? Histopathology. 2018 Dec;73(6):969–82. PMID:30137667

**2337.** Gaston-Massuet C, Andoniadou CL, Signore M, et al. Increased Wingless (Wnt) signaling in pituitary progenitor/stem cells gives rise to pituitary tumors in mice and humans. Proc Natl Acad Sci U S A. 2011 Jul 12;108(28):11482–7. PMID:21636786

**2338.** Sohn JH, Cho MY, Park Y, et al. Prognostic significance of defining L-cell type on the biologic behavior of rectal neuroendocrine tumors in relation with pathological parameters. Cancer Res Treat. 2015 Oct;47(4):813–22. PMID:25715764

**2339.** Gates GA, Rice DH, Koopmann CF Jr, et al. Flutamide-induced regression of angiofibroma. Laryngoscope. 1992 Jun;102(6):641–4. PMID:1318484

**2340.** Gatta G, Botta L, Rossi S, et al. Childhood cancer survival in Europe 1999-2007: results of EUROCARE-5–a population-based study. Lancet Oncol. 2014 Jan;15(1):35–47. PMID:24314616

**2341.** Gattuso P, Castelli MJ, Peng Y, et al. Posttransplant lymphoproliferative disorders: a fine-needle aspiration biopsy study. Diagn Cytopathol. 1997 May;16(5):392–5. PMID:9143839

**2342.** Gaujoux S, Tissier F, Ragazzon B, et al. Pancreatic ductal and acinar cell neoplasms in Carney complex: a possible new association. J Clin Endocrinol Metab. 2011 Nov;96(11):E1888–95. PMID:21900385

**2343.** Gayden T, Sepulveda FE, Khuong-Quang DA, et al. Germline HAVCR2 mutations altering TIM-3 characterize subcutaneous panniculitis-like T cell lymphomas with hemophagocytic lymphohistiocytic syndrome. Nat Genet. 2018 Dec;50(12):1650–7. PMID:30374066

**2344.** Gayre GS, Proia AD, Dutton JJ. Epibulbar osseous choristoma: case report and review of the literature. Ophthalmic Surg Lasers. 2002 Sep-Oct;33(5):410–5. PMID:12358295

**2345.** Gearhart MD, Corcoran CM, Wamstad JA, et al. Polycomb group and SCF ubiquitin ligases are found in a novel BCOR complex that is recruited to BCL6 targets. Mol Cell Biol. 2006 Sep;26(18):6880–9. PMID:16943429

**2346.** Geirnaerdt MJ, Hogendoorn PC, Bloem JL, et al. Cartilaginous tumors: fast contrast-enhanced MR imaging. Radiology. 2000 Feb;214(2):539–46. PMID:10671608

**2347.** Gélinas JF, Manoukian J, Côté A. Lung involvement in juvenile onset recurrent respiratory papillomatosis: a systematic review of the literature. Int J Pediatr Otorhinolaryngol. 2008 Apr;72(4):433–52. PMID:18281102

**2348.** Geller JI, Dome JS. Local lymph node involvement does not predict poor outcome in pediatric renal cell carcinoma. Cancer. 2004 Oct 1;101(7):1575–83. PMID:15378495

**2349.** Geller JI, Ehrlich PF, Cost NG, et al. Characterization of adolescent and pediatric renal cell carcinoma: a report from the Children's Oncology Group study AREN03B2. Cancer. 2015 Jul 15;121(14):2457–64. PMID:25845370

**2350.** Geller JI, Roth JJ, Biegel JA. Biology and treatment of rhabdoid tumor. Crit Rev Oncog. 2015;20(3-4):199–216. PMID:26349416

**2351.** Gentry M, Bodo J, Durkin L, et al. Performance of a commercially available MAL antibody in the diagnosis of primary mediastinal large B-cell lymphoma. Am J Surg Pathol. 2017 Feb;41(2):189–94. PMID:27879516

**2352.** Geoerger B, Hero B, Harms D, et al. Metabolic activity and clinical features of primary ganglioneuromas. Cancer. 2001 May 15;91(10):1905–13. PMID:11346873

**2353.** George DH, Scheithauer BW, Kovacs K, et al. Crooke's cell adenoma of the pituitary: an aggressive variant of corticotroph adenoma. Am J Surg Pathol. 2003 Oct;27(10):1330–6. PMID:14508394

**2354.** George RE, London WB, Cohn SL, et al. Hyperdiploidy plus nonamplified MYCN confers a favorable prognosis in children 12 to 18 months old with disseminated neuroblastoma: a Pediatric Oncology Group study. J Clin Oncol. 2005 Sep 20;23(27):6466–73. PMID:16116152

**2355.** Georgesen C, Magro C. Lymphomatoid papulosis in children and adolescents: a clinical and histopathologic retrospective cohort. Ann Diagn Pathol. 2020 Jun;46:151486. PMID:32172217

**2356.** Gerald WL, Haber DA. The EWS-WT1 gene fusion in desmoplastic small round cell tumor. Semin Cancer Biol. 2005 Jun;15(3):197–205. PMID:15826834

**2357.** Gerald WL, Ladanyi M, de Alava E, et al. Clinical, pathologic, and molecular spectrum of tumors associated with t(11;22)(p13;q12): desmoplastic small round-cell tumor and its variants. J Clin Oncol. 1998 Sep;16(9):3028–36. PMID:9738572

**2358.** Gerald WL, Miller HK, Battifora H, et al. Intra-abdominal desmoplastic small round-cell tumor. Report of 19 cases of a distinctive type of high-grade polyphenotypic malignancy affecting young individuals. Am J Surg Pathol. 1991 Jun;15(6):499–513. PMID:1709557

**2359.** Gerald WL, Rosai J. Case 2. Desmoplastic small cell tumor with divergent differentiation. Pediatr Pathol. 1989;9(2):177–83. PMID:2473463

**2360.** Gerald WL, Rosai J, Ladanyi M. Characterization of the genomic breakpoint and chimeric transcripts in the EWS-WT1 gene fusion of desmoplastic small round cell tumor. Proc Natl Acad Sci U S A. 1995 Feb 14;92(4):1028–32. PMID:7862627

**2361.** Gerami P, Scolyer RA, Xu X, et al. Risk assessment for atypical spitzoid melanocytic neoplasms using FISH to identify chromosomal copy number aberrations. Am J Surg Pathol. 2013 May;37(5):676–84. PMID:23388126

**2361A.** Geramizadeh B. Nested stromal-epithelial tumor of the liver: a review. Gastrointest Tumors. 2019 Aug;6(1-2):1–10. PMID:31602372

**2362.** Gerber NU, von Hoff K, von Bueren AO, et al. Outcome of 11 children with ependymoblastoma treated within the prospective HIT-trials between 1991 and 2006. J Neurooncol. 2011 May;102(3):459–69. PMID:21308398

**2363.** Germain M, Smith KJ. Hair follicle nevus in a distribution following Blaskho's lines. J Am Acad Dermatol. 2002 May;46(5 Suppl):S125–7. PMID:12004289

**2364.** German J. Bloom's syndrome. XX. The first 100 cancers. Cancer Genet Cytogenet. 1997 Jan;93(1):100–6. PMID:9062585

**2365.** Gerner N, Nørregaard JC, Jensen OA, et al. Conjunctival naevi in Denmark 1960-1980. A 21-year follow-up study. Acta Ophthalmol Scand. 1996 Aug;74(4):334–7. PMID:8883545

**2366.** Gerrand C, Athanasou N, Brennan B, et al. UK guidelines for the management of bone sarcomas. Clin Sarcoma Res. 2016 May 4;6:7. PMID:27148438

**2367.** Gerrard DJ, Donaldson DR. Salivary pleomorphic adenoma in familial adenomatous polyposis. J R Soc Med. 1998 Feb;91(2):86–7. PMID:9602747

**2368.** Gerrard M, Cairo MS, Weston C, et al. Excellent survival following two courses of COPAD chemotherapy in children and adolescents with resected localized B-cell non-Hodgkin's lymphoma: results of the FAB/LMB 96 international study. Br J Haematol. 2008 Jun;141(6):840–7. PMID:18371107

**2369.** Gersell DJ, King TC. Papillary cystadenoma of the mesosalpinx in von Hippel-Lindau disease. Am J Surg Pathol. 1988 Feb;12(2):145–9. PMID:3341511

**2370.** Gershenson DM, Okamoto A, Ray-Coquard I. Management of rare ovarian cancer histologies. J Clin Oncol. 2019 Sep 20;37(27):2406–15. PMID:31403866

**2371.** Gesk S, Gascoyne RD, Schnitzer B, et al. ALK-positive diffuse large B-cell lymphoma with ALK-Clathrin fusion belongs to the spectrum of pediatric lymphomas. Leukemia. 2005 Oct;19(10):1839–40. PMID:16107887

**2372.** Gessi M, Capper D, Sahm F, et al. Evidence of H3 K27M mutations in posterior fossa ependymomas. Acta Neuropathol. 2016 Oct;132(4):635–7. PMID:27539613

**2373.** Gessi M, Dörner E, Dreschmann V, et al. Intramedullary gangliogliomas: histopathologic and molecular features of 25 cases. Hum Pathol. 2016 Mar;49:107–13. PMID:26826417

**2374.** Gessi M, Giagnacovo M, Modena P, et al. Role of immunohistochemistry in the identification of supratentorial C11ORF95-RELA fused ependymoma in routine neuropathology. Am J Surg Pathol. 2019 Jan;43(1):56–63. PMID:29266023

**2375.** Gessi M, Giangaspero F, Lauriola L, et al. Embryonal tumors with abundant neuropil and true rosettes: a distinctive CNS primitive neuroectodermal tumor. Am J Surg Pathol. 2009 Feb;33(2):211–7. PMID:18987548

**2376.** Gessi M, Giangaspero F, Pietsch T. Atypical teratoid/rhabdoid tumors and choroid plexus tumors: when genetics "surprise" pathology. Brain Pathol. 2003 Jul;13(3):409–14. PMID:12946029

**2377.** Gessi M, Gielen GH, Dreschmann V, et al. High frequency of H3F3A (K27M) mutations characterizes pediatric and adult high-grade gliomas of the spinal cord. Acta Neuropathol. 2015 Sep;130(3):435–7. PMID:26231952

**2378.** Gessi M, Hattingen E, Dörner E, et al. Dysembryoplastic neuroepithelial tumor of the septum pellucidum and the supratentorial midline: histopathologic, neuroradiologic, and molecular features of 7 cases. Am J Surg Pathol. 2016 Jun;40(6):806–11. PMID:26796505

**2379.** Gessi M, Japp AS, Dreschmann V, et al. High-resolution genomic analysis of cribriform neuroepithelial tumors of the central nervous system. J Neuropathol Exp Neurol. 2015 Oct;74(10):970–4. PMID:26352987

**2380.** Gessi M, von Bueren A, Treszl A, et al. MYCN amplification predicts poor outcome for patients with supratentorial primitive neuroectodermal tumors of the central nervous system. Neuro Oncol. 2014 Jul;16(7):924–32. PMID:24470553

**2381.** Gessi M, Zur Mühlen A, Hammes J, et al. Genome-wide DNA copy number analysis of desmoplastic infantile astrocytomas and desmoplastic infantile gangliogliomas. J Neuropathol Exp Neurol. 2013 Sep;72(9):807–15. PMID:23965740

**2382.** Geurts van Kessel A, van Drunen E, de Jong B, et al. Chromosome 12q heterozygosity is retained in i(12p)-positive testicular germ cell tumor cells. Cancer Genet Cytogenet. 1989 Jul 1;40(1):129–34. PMID:2569358

**2383.** Gezginç K, Karataylı R, Yazıcı F, et al. Ovarian cancer during pregnancy. Int J Gynaecol Obstet. 2011 Nov;115(2):140–3. PMID:21872237

**2384.** Ghasemi DR, Sill M, Okonechnikov K, et al. MYCN amplification drives an aggressive form of spinal ependymoma. Acta Neuropathol. 2019 Dec;138(6):1075–89. PMID:31414211

**2385.** Gherlinzoni F, Rock M, Picci P. Chondromyxoid fibroma. The experience at the Istituto Ortopedico Rizzoli. J Bone Joint Surg Am. 1983 Feb;65(2):198–204. PMID:6337162

**2386.** Ghobrial IM, Habermann TM, Macon WR, et al. Differences between early and late posttransplant lymphoproliferative disorders in solid organ transplant patients: Are they two different diseases? Transplantation. 2005 Jan 27;79(2):244–7. PMID:15665775

**2387.** Gholam D, Fizazi K, Terrier-Lacombe MJ, et al. Advanced seminoma–treatment results and prognostic factors for survival after first-line, cisplatin-based chemotherapy and for patients with recurrent disease: a single-institution experience in 145 patients. Cancer. 2003 Aug 15;98(4):745–52. PMID:12910518

**2388.** Gholve PA, Hosalkar HS, Kreiger PA, et al. Giant cell tumor of tendon sheath: largest single series in children. J Pediatr Orthop. 2007 Jan-Feb;27(1):67–74. PMID:17195801

**2389.** Ghosal N, Rudrappa S, Tandon AS, et al. Atypical ossifying fibromyxoid tumor in left maxillo-ethmoid sinus with intracranial extension in a child. Clin Neuropathol. 2016 Sep-Oct;35(5):329–32. PMID:27345437

**2390.** Ghosh S, Sinha R, Bandyopadhyay R, et al. Oncogenous osteomalacia. J Cancer Res Ther. 2009 Jul-Sep;5(3):210–2. PMID:19841566

**2391.** Ghossein R, Barletta J, Bullock M, et al., editors. Carcinoma of the thyroid histopathology reporting guide. 2nd ed. Sydney (Australia): International Collaboration on Cancer Reporting; 2020.

**2392.** Ghossein RA, Katabi N, Fagin JA. Immunohistochemical detection of mutated BRAF V600E supports the clonal origin of BRAF-induced thyroid cancers along the spectrum of disease progression. J Clin Endocrinol Metab. 2013 Aug;98(8):E1414–21. PMID:23775351

**2393.** Ghuman M, Hwang S, Antonescu CR, et al. Plexiform fibrohistiocytic tumor: imaging features and clinical findings. Skeletal Radiol. 2019 Mar;48(3):437–43. PMID:30145610
**2394.** Giacchero D, Maire G, Nuin PA, et al. No correlation between the molecular subtype of COL1A1-PDGFB fusion gene and the clinico-histopathological features of dermatofibrosarcoma protuberans. J Invest Dermatol. 2010 Mar;130(3):904–7. PMID:19890351
**2395.** Giacomazzi J, Graudenz MS, Osorio CA, et al. Prevalence of the TP53 p.R337H mutation in breast cancer patients in Brazil. PLoS One. 2014 Jun 17;9(6):e99893. PMID:24936644
**2396.** Giagnacovo M, Antonelli M, Biassoni V, et al. Retrospective analysis on the consistency of MRI features with histological and molecular markers in diffuse intrinsic pontine glioma (DIPG). Childs Nerv Syst. 2020 Apr;36(4):697–704. PMID:31848724
**2397.** Giagulli C, Marsico S, Magiera AK, et al. Opposite effects of HIV-1 p17 variants on PTEN activation and cell growth in B cells. PLoS One. 2011 Mar 14;6(3):e17831. PMID:21423810
**2398.** Giancane G, Tanturri de Horatio L, Buonuomo PS, et al. Swollen knee due to primary synovial chondromatosis in pediatrics: a rare and possibly misdiagnosed condition. Rheumatol Int. 2013 Aug;33(8):2183–5. PMID:22457006
**2399.** Giangaspero F, Chieco P, Ceccarelli C, et al. "Desmoplastic" versus "classic" medulloblastoma: comparison of DNA content, histopathology and differentiation. Virchows Arch A Pathol Anat Histopathol. 1991;418(3):207–14. PMID:1900966
**2400.** Giangaspero F, Perilongo G, Fondelli MP, et al. Medulloblastoma with extensive nodularity: a variant with favorable prognosis. J Neurosurg. 1999 Dec;91(6):971–7. PMID:10584843
**2401.** Giangaspero F, Rigobello L, Badiali M, et al. Large-cell medulloblastomas. A distinct variant with highly aggressive behavior. Am J Surg Pathol. 1992 Jul;16(7):687–93. PMID:1530108
**2401A.** Giannelli SM, McPhaul L, Nakamoto J, et al. Familial adenomatous polyposis-associated, cribriform morular variant of papillary thyroid carcinoma harboring a K-RAS mutation: case presentation and review of molecular mechanisms. Thyroid. 2014 Jul;24(7):1184–9. PMID:24702198
**2402.** Giannini C, Hebrink D, Scheithauer BW, et al. Analysis of p53 mutation and expression in pleomorphic xanthoastrocytoma. Neurogenetics. 2001 Jul;3(3):159–62. PMID:11523567
**2403.** Giannini C, Scheithauer BW, Burger PC, et al. Cellular proliferation in pilocytic and diffuse astrocytomas. J Neuropathol Exp Neurol. 1999 Jan;58(1):46–53. PMID:10068313
**2404.** Giannini C, Scheithauer BW, Burger PC, et al. Pleomorphic xanthoastrocytoma: What do we really know about it? Cancer. 1999 May 1;85(9):2033–45. PMID:10223246
**2405.** Giannini C, Scheithauer BW, Lopes MB, et al. Immunophenotype of pleomorphic xanthoastrocytoma. Am J Surg Pathol. 2002 Apr;26(4):479–85. PMID:11914626
**2406.** Gianno F, Antonelli M, Ferretti E, et al. Pediatric high-grade glioma: a heterogeneous group of neoplasms with different molecular drivers. Glioma. 2018;1:117–24. doi:10.4103/glioma.glioma_27_18.
**2407.** Giardiello FM, Offerhaus GJ, Krush AJ, et al. Risk of hepatoblastoma in familial adenomatous polyposis. J Pediatr. 1991 Nov;119(5):766–8. PMID:1658283
**2408.** Giarola M, Stagi L, Presciuttini S, et al. Screening for mutations of the APC gene in 66 Italian familial adenomatous polyposis patients: evidence for phenotypic differences in cases with and without identified mutation. Hum Mutat. 1999;13(2):116–23. PMID:10094547
**2409.** Gibault L, Pérot G, Chibon F, et al. New insights in sarcoma oncogenesis: a comprehensive analysis of a large series of 160 soft tissue sarcomas with complex genomics. J Pathol. 2011 Jan;223(1):64–71. PMID:21125665
**2410.** Gibbons D, Leitch M, Coscia J, et al. Fine needle aspiration cytology and histologic findings of granular cell tumor of the breast: review of 19 cases with clinical/radiologic correlation. Breast J. 2000 Jan;6(1):27–30. PMID:11348331
**2411.** Gibson BE, Webb DK, Howman AJ, et al. Results of a randomized trial in children with acute myeloid leukaemia: Medical Research Council AML12 trial. Br J Haematol. 2011 Nov;155(3):366–76. PMID:21902686
**2412.** Gibson P, Tong Y, Robinson G, et al. Subtypes of medulloblastoma have distinct developmental origins. Nature. 2010 Dec 23;468(7327):1095–9. PMID:21150899
**2413.** Gilbert AR, Zaky W, Gokden M, et al. Extending the neuroanatomic territory of diffuse midline glioma, K27M mutant: pineal region origin. Pediatr Neurosurg. 2018;53(1):59–63. PMID:29131126
**2414.** Gil-Gouveia R, Cristino N, Farias JP, et al. Pleomorphic xanthoastrocytoma of the cerebellum: illustrated review. Acta Neurochir (Wien). 2004 Nov;146(11):1241–4. PMID:15455217
**2415.** Gill AJ. Succinate dehydrogenase (SDH)-deficient neoplasia. Histopathology. 2018 Jan;72(1):106–16. PMID:29239034
**2416.** Gill AJ. Understanding the genetic basis of parathyroid carcinoma. Endocr Pathol. 2014 Mar;25(1):30–4. PMID:24402736
**2417.** Gill AJ, Benn DE, Chou A, et al. Immunohistochemistry for SDHB triages genetic testing of SDHB, SDHC, and SDHD in paraganglioma-pheochromocytoma syndromes. Hum Pathol. 2010 Jun;41(6):805–14. PMID:20236688
**2418.** Gill AJ, Chou A, Vilain R, et al. Immunohistochemistry for SDHB divides gastrointestinal stromal tumors (GISTs) into 2 distinct types. Am J Surg Pathol. 2010 May;34(5):636–44. PMID:20305538
**2419.** Gill AJ, Clarkson A, Gimm O, et al. Loss of nuclear expression of parafibromin distinguishes parathyroid carcinomas and hyperparathyroidism-jaw tumor (HPT-JT) syndrome-related adenomas from sporadic parathyroid adenomas and hyperplasias. Am J Surg Pathol. 2006 Sep;30(9):1140–9. PMID:16931959
**2420.** Gill AJ, Lim G, Cheung VKY, et al. Parafibromin-deficient (HPT-JT type, CDC73 mutated) parathyroid tumors demonstrate distinctive morphologic features. Am J Surg Pathol. 2019 Jan;43(1):35–46. PMID:29324469
**2421.** Gill JR, Reyes-Múgica M, Iyengar S, et al. Early presentation of metastatic medullary carcinoma in multiple endocrine neoplasia, type IIA: implications for therapy. J Pediatr. 1996 Sep;129(3):459–64. PMID:8804341
**2422.** Gill RM, Buelow B, Mather C, et al. Hepatic small vessel neoplasm, a rare infiltrative vascular neoplasm of uncertain malignant potential. Hum Pathol. 2016 Aug;54:143–51. PMID:27090685
**2423.** Gilligan TD, Seidenfeld J, Basch EM, et al. American Society of Clinical Oncology Clinical Practice Guideline on uses of serum tumor markers in adult males with germ cell tumors. J Clin Oncol. 2010 Jul 10;28(20):3388–404. PMID:20530278
**2424.** Gillis AJ, Rijlaarsdam MA, Eini R, et al. Targeted serum miRNA (TSmiR) test for diagnosis and follow-up of (testicular) germ cell cancer patients: a proof of principle. Mol Oncol. 2013 Dec;7(6):1083–92. PMID:24012110
**2425.** Gillis AJ, Stoop H, Biermann K, et al. Expression and interdependencies of pluripotency factors LIN28, OCT3/4, NANOG and SOX2 in human testicular germ cells and tumours of the testis. Int J Androl. 2011 Aug;34(4 Pt 2):e160–74. PMID:21631526
**2426.** Giona F, Putti MC, Micalizzi C, et al. Long-term results of high-dose imatinib in children and adolescents with chronic myeloid leukaemia in chronic phase: the Italian experience. Br J Haematol. 2015 Aug;170(3):398–407. PMID:25891192
**2427.** Girardi T, Vicente C, Cools J, et al. The genetics and molecular biology of T-ALL. Blood. 2017 Mar 2;129(9):1113–23. PMID:28115373
**2428.** Giridhar P, Mallick S, Kashyap L, et al. Patterns of care and impact of prognostic factors in the outcome of NUT midline carcinoma: a systematic review and individual patient data analysis of 119 cases. Eur Arch Otorhinolaryngol. 2018 Mar;275(3):815–21. PMID:29356890
**2429.** Girolami I, Mancini I, Simoni A, et al. Denosumab treated giant cell tumour of bone: a morphological, immunohistochemical and molecular analysis of a series. J Clin Pathol. 2016 Mar;69(3):240–7. PMID:26338802
**2430.** Gisselsson D, Hibbard MK, Dal Cin P, et al. PLAG1 alterations in lipoblastoma: involvement in varied mesenchymal cell types and evidence for alternative oncogenic mechanisms. Am J Pathol. 2001 Sep;159(3):955–62. PMID:11549588
**2431.** Gitelson E, Al-Saleem T, Robu V, et al. Pediatric nodal marginal zone lymphoma may develop in the adult population. Leuk Lymphoma. 2010 Jan;51(1):89–94. PMID:19863176
**2432.** Gittleman H, Cioffi G, Vecchione-Koval T, et al. Descriptive epidemiology of germ cell tumors of the central nervous system diagnosed in the United States from 2006 to 2015. J Neurooncol. 2019 Jun;143(2):251–60. PMID:31025275
**2433.** Giulino-Roth L, O'Donohue T, Chen Z, et al. Outcomes of adults and children with primary mediastinal B-cell lymphoma treated with dose-adjusted EPOCH-R. Br J Haematol. 2017 Dec;179(5):739–47. PMID:29082519
**2434.** Giussani C, Isimbaldi G, Massimino M, et al. Ganglioglioma of the spinal cord in neurofibromatosis type 1. Pediatr Neurosurg. 2013;49(1):50–4. PMID:24192615
**2435.** Givon U, Ganel A, Heim M. Pigmented villonodular synovitis. Arch Dis Child. 1991 Dec;66(12):1449–50. PMID:1776897
**2436.** Giza A, Gałązka K, Jońca M, et al. Subcutaneous panniculitis-like T-cell lymphoma (SPTCL) with probable mesentery involvement with associated hemophagocytic syndrome (HPS) - how to treat it? J Dermatolog Treat. 2022 Aug;33(5):2674–6. PMID:32924664
**2437.** Gkourogianni A, Lodish MB, Zilbermint M, et al. Death in pediatric Cushing syndrome is uncommon but still occurs. Eur J Pediatr. 2015 Apr;174(4):501–7. PMID:25241829
**2438.** Glad H, Vainer B, Buchwald C, et al. Juvenile nasopharyngeal angiofibromas in Denmark 1981-2003: diagnosis, incidence, and treatment. Acta Otolaryngol. 2007 Mar;127(3):292–9. PMID:17364367
**2439.** Gładkowska-Dura M, Dzierzanowska-Fangrat K, Dura WT, et al. Unique morphological spectrum of lymphomas in Nijmegen breakage syndrome (NBS) patients with high frequency of consecutive lymphoma formation. J Pathol. 2008 Nov;216(3):337–44. PMID:18788073
**2440.** Gläsker S, Lonser RR, Tran MG, et al. Effects of VHL deficiency on endolymphatic duct and sac. Cancer Res. 2005 Dec 1;65(23):10847–53. PMID:16322231
**2441.** Gleason BC, Fletcher CD. Deep "benign" fibrous histiocytoma: clinicopathologic analysis of 69 cases of a rare tumor indicating occasional metastatic potential. Am J Surg Pathol. 2008 Mar;32(3):354–62. PMID:18300816
**2442.** Gleason BC, Fletcher CD. Myoepithelial carcinoma of soft tissue in children: an aggressive neoplasm analyzed in a series of 29 cases. Am J Surg Pathol. 2007 Dec;31(12):1813–24. PMID:18043035
**2443.** Gleason BC, Hornick JL. Inflammatory myofibroblastic tumours: Where are we now? J Clin Pathol. 2008 Apr;61(4):428–37. PMID:17938159
**2444.** Gleason BC, Liegl-Atzwanger B, Kozakewich HP, et al. Osteofibrous dysplasia and adamantinoma in children and adolescents: a clinicopathologic reappraisal. Am J Surg Pathol. 2008 Mar;32(3):363–76. PMID:18300815
**2445.** Gleason BC, Nascimento AF. HMB-45 and Melan-A are useful in the differential diagnosis between granular cell tumor and malignant melanoma. Am J Dermatopathol. 2007 Feb;29(1):22–7. PMID:17284958
**2446.** Glick RD, Pashankar FD, Pappo A, et al. Management of pancreatoblastoma in children and young adults. J Pediatr Hematol Oncol. 2012 May;34 Suppl 2:S47–50. PMID:22525406
**2447.** Global Health Observatory [Internet]. Geneva (Switzerland): World Health Organization; 2021. Distribution of causes of death among children aged < 5 years (%). Available from: https://www.who.int/data/gho/data/indicators/indicator-details/GHO/distribution-of-causes-of-death-among-children-aged-5-years-(-).
**2448.** Fabian ID, Abdallah E, Abdullahi SU, et al. Global retinoblastoma presentation and analysis by national income level. JAMA Oncol. 2020 May 1;6(5):685–95. PMID:32105305
**2449.** Glover MT, Malone M, Atherton DJ. Michelin-tire baby syndrome resulting from diffuse smooth muscle hamartoma. Pediatr Dermatol. 1989 Dec;6(4):329–31. PMID:2694131
**2450.** Gnekow AK, Walker DA, Kandels D, et al. A European randomised controlled trial of the addition of etoposide to standard vincristine and carboplatin induction as part of an 18-month treatment programme for childhood (≤16 years) low grade glioma - a final report. Eur J Cancer. 2017 Aug;81:206–25. PMID:28649001
**2451.** Gnepp DR, Schroeder W, Heffner D. Synchronous tumors arising in a single major salivary gland. Cancer. 1989 Mar 15;63(6):1219–24. PMID:2917323
**2452.** Gnepp DR, Wang LJ, Brandwein-Gensler M, et al. Sclerosing polycystic adenosis of the salivary gland: a report of 16 cases. Am J Surg Pathol. 2006 Feb;30(2):154–64. PMID:16434888
**2453.** Göbel U, Schneider DT, Calaminus G, et al. Multimodal treatment of malignant sacrococcygeal germ cell tumors: a prospective analysis of 66 patients of the German cooperative protocols MAKEI 83/86 and 89. J Clin Oncol. 2001 Apr 1;19(7):1943–50. PMID:11283126
**2454.** Gochhait D, Dey P, Mitra S, et al. Fine-needle aspiration cytology of melanotic neuroectodermal tumor of infancy. Diagn Cytopathol. 2015 Sep;43(9):770–2. PMID:26173836
**2455.** Göckeritz W, Borchert HH. [The effect of chlorpromazine and carbamazepine on diagnostically relevant liver enzymes]. Pharmazie. 1990 Jul;45(8):579–81. German. PMID:2080202
**2456.** Goddard DS, Rogers M, Frieden IJ, et al. Widespread porokeratotic adnexal ostial nevus: clinical features and proposal of a new name unifying porokeratotic eccrine ostial and dermal duct nevus and porokeratotic eccrine and hair follicle nevus. J Am Acad Dermatol. 2009 Dec;61(6):1060.e1–14. PMID:19664847
**2457.** Goddard MJ, Lonsdale RN. The histogenesis of appendiceal carcinoid tumours. Histopathology. 1992 Apr;20(4):345–9. PMID:1577412

**2458.** Godette GA, O'Sullivan M, Menelaus MB. Plantar fibromatosis of the heel in children: a report of 14 cases. J Pediatr Orthop. 1997 Jan-Feb;17(1):16–7. PMID:8989694
**2459.** Godfraind C, Calicchio ML, Kozakewich H. Pyogenic granuloma, an impaired wound healing process, linked to vascular growth driven by FLT4 and the nitric oxide pathway. Mod Pathol. 2013 Feb;26(2):247–55. PMID:22955520
**2460.** Godfraind C, Kaczmarska JM, Kocak M, et al. Distinct disease-risk groups in pediatric supratentorial and posterior fossa ependymomas. Acta Neuropathol. 2012 Aug;124(2):247–57. PMID:22526017
**2461.** Godot C, Patte C, Blanche S, et al. Characteristics and prognosis of B-cell lymphoma in HIV-infected children in the HAART era. J Pediatr Hematol Oncol. 2012 Oct;34(7):e282–8. PMID:22935659
**2462.** Goebel EA, McCluggage WG, Walsh JC. Mitotically active sclerosing stromal tumor of the ovary: report of a case series with parallels to mitotically active cellular fibroma. Int J Gynecol Pathol. 2016 Nov;35(6):549–53. PMID:27149006
**2463.** Goebel HH, Cravioto H. Ultrastructure of human and experimental ependymomas. A comparative study. J Neuropathol Exp Neurol. 1972 Jan;31(1):54–71. PMID:5060130
**2464.** Goel A, Nguyen TP, Leung HC, et al. De novo constitutional MLH1 epimutations confer early-onset colorectal cancer in two new sporadic Lynch syndrome cases, with derivation of the epimutation on the paternal allele in one. Int J Cancer. 2011 Feb 15;128(4):869–78. PMID:20473912
**2465.** Gogia A, Bakhshi S. Plasmablastic lymphoma of oral cavity in a HIV-negative child. Pediatr Blood Cancer. 2010 Aug;55(2):390–1. PMID:20582963
**2466.** Gogia A, Sharma MC, Bakhshi S. Subcutaneous nodules as initial presentation of Burkitt lymphoma in HIV-negative child. J Pediatr Hematol Oncol. 2013 Nov;35(8):e326–8. PMID:23426001
**2467.** Goh S, Butler W, Thiele EA. Subependymal giant cell tumors in tuberous sclerosis complex. Neurology. 2004 Oct 26;63(8):1457–61. PMID:15505165
**2468.** Gokden M, Mrak RE. Pituitary adenoma with craniopharyngioma component. Hum Pathol. 2009 Aug;40(8):1189–93. PMID:19427020
**2469.** Göktay F, Atış G, Güneş P, et al. Subungual exostosis and subungual osteochondromas: a description of 25 cases. Int J Dermatol. 2018 Jul;57(7):872–81. PMID:29704255
**2470.** Goldblum JR, Folpe AL, Weiss SW, editors. Enzinger and Weiss's soft tissue tumors. 7th ed. Philadelphia (PA): Elsevier; 2019.
**2471.** Goldenberg-Cohen N, Cohen Y, Rosenbaum E, et al. T1799A BRAF mutations in conjunctival melanocytic lesions. Invest Ophthalmol Vis Sci. 2005 Sep;46(9):3027–30. PMID:16123397
**2472.** Goldfisher R, Awal D, Amodio J. Peritoneal inclusion cysts in female children: pathogenesis, treatment, and multimodality imaging review. Case Rep Radiol. 2014;2014:427427. PMID:25143853
**2473.** Goldman S, Smith L, Anderson JR, et al. Rituximab and FAB/LMB 96 chemotherapy in children with Stage III/IV B-cell non-Hodgkin lymphoma: a Children's Oncology Group report. Leukemia. 2013 Apr;27(5):1174–7. PMID:22940833
**2474.** Goldstein AM, Stidd KC, Yang XR, et al. Pediatric melanoma in melanoma-prone families. Cancer. 2018 Sep 15;124(18):3715–23. PMID:30207590
**2475.** Gomes CC, Diniz MG, de Menezes GH, et al. BRAFV600E mutation in melanotic neuroectodermal tumor of infancy: toward personalized medicine? Pediatrics. 2015 Jul;136(1):e267–9. PMID:26122804
**2475A.** Gomez DR, Missett BT, Wara WM, et al. High failure rate in spinal ependymomas with long-term follow-up. Neuro Oncol. 2005 Jul;7(3):254–9. PMID:16053700
**2476.** Gomez LM, Bagazgotia L, Requena L. A Rare presentation and histopathologic findings of woolly hair nevus. Int J Trichology. 2015 Jul-Sep;7(3):131–2. PMID:26622159
**2477.** Gomez MR. Phenotypes of the tuberous sclerosis complex with a revision of diagnostic criteria. Ann N Y Acad Sci. 1991;615:1–7. PMID:2039135
**2478.** Gómez García EB, Knoers NV. Gardner's syndrome (familial adenomatous polyposis): a cilia-related disorder. Lancet Oncol. 2009 Jul;10(7):727–35. PMID:19573802
**2479.** Gomez-Hernandez K, Ezzat S, Asa SL, et al. Clinical implications of accurate subtyping of pituitary adenomas: perspectives from the treating physician. Turk Patoloji Derg. 2015;31 Suppl 1:4–17. PMID:26177314
**2480.** Gompels MM, Hodges E, Lock RJ, et al. Lymphoproliferative disease in antibody deficiency: a multi-centre study. Clin Exp Immunol. 2003 Nov;134(2):314–20. PMID:14616793
**2481.** Gonen R, Fong K, Chiasson DA. Prenatal sonographic diagnosis of hepatic hemangioendothelioma with secondary nonimmune hydrops fetalis. Obstet Gynecol. 1989 Mar;73(3 Pt 2):485–7. PMID:2644601
**2482.** Gonzalez CL, Medeiros LJ, Braziel RM, et al. T-cell lymphoma involving subcutaneous tissue. A clinicopathologic entity commonly associated with hemophagocytic syndrome. Am J Surg Pathol. 1991 Jan;15(1):17–27. PMID:1985499
**2483.** Gonzalez KD, Noltner KA, Buzin CH, et al. Beyond Li Fraumeni syndrome: clinical characteristics of families with p53 germline mutations. J Clin Oncol. 2009 Mar 10;27(8):1250–6. PMID:19204208
**2484.** Gonzalez S, Duarte I. Benign fibrous histiocytoma of the skin. A morphologic study of 290 cases. Pathol Res Pract. 1982 Oct;174(4):379–91. PMID:6296802
**2485.** González-Acosta M, Marín F, Puliafito B, et al. High-sensitivity microsatellite instability assessment for the detection of mismatch repair defects in normal tissue of biallelic germline mismatch repair mutation carriers. J Med Genet. 2020 Apr;57(4):269–73. PMID:31494577
**2486.** Gonzalez-Crussi F, Winkler RF, Mirkin DL. Sacrococcygeal teratomas in infants and children: relationship of histology and prognosis in 40 cases. Arch Pathol Lab Med. 1978 Aug;102(8):420–5. PMID:580884
**2487.** Gonzalez-Farre B, Ramis-Zaldivar JE, Salmeron-Villalobos J, et al. Burkitt-like lymphoma with 11q aberration: a germinal center-derived lymphoma genetically unrelated to Burkitt lymphoma. Haematologica. 2019 Sep;104(9):1822–9. PMID:30733272
**2488.** González-Lois C, Cuevas C, Abdullah O, et al. Intracranial extraskeletal myxoid chondrosarcoma: case report and review of the literature. Acta Neurochir (Wien). 2002 Jul;144(7):735–40. PMID:12181708
**2489.** Gonzalez-Meljem JM, Haston S, Carreno G, et al. Stem cell senescence drives age-attenuated induction of pituitary tumours in mouse models of paediatric craniopharyngioma. Nat Commun. 2017 Nov 28;8(1):1819. PMID:29180744
**2490.** Goodlad JR, Mentzel T, Fletcher CD. Low grade fibromyxoid sarcoma: clinicopathological analysis of eleven new cases in support of a distinct entity. Histopathology. 1995 Mar;26(3):229–37. PMID:7797200
**2491.** Goodrich LV, Scott MP. Hedgehog and patched in neural development and disease. Neuron. 1998 Dec;21(6):1243–57. PMID:9883719
**2492.** Goodwin ML, Jin H, Straessler K, et al. Modeling alveolar soft part sarcomagenesis in the mouse: a role for lactate in the tumor microenvironment. Cancer Cell. 2014 Dec 8;26(6):851–62. PMID:25453902
**2493.** Gooskens SL, Furtwängler R, Spreafico F, et al. Treatment and outcome of patients with relapsed clear cell sarcoma of the kidney: a combined SIOP and AIEOP study. Br J Cancer. 2014 Jul 15;111(2):227–33. PMID:24937667
**2494.** Gooskens SL, Furtwängler R, Vujanic GM, et al. Clear cell sarcoma of the kidney: a review. Eur J Cancer. 2012 Sep;48(14):2219–26. PMID:22579455
**2495.** Gooskens SL, Houwing ME, Vujanic GM, et al. Congenital mesoblastic nephroma 50 years after its recognition: a narrative review. Pediatr Blood Cancer. 2017 Jul;64(7). PMID:28124468
**2496.** Gooskens SL, Oranje AP, van Adrichem LN, et al. Imatinib mesylate for children with dermatofibrosarcoma protuberans (DFSP). Pediatr Blood Cancer. 2010 Aug;55(2):369–73. PMID:20582941
**2497.** Gopal S, Gross TG. How I treat Burkitt lymphoma in children, adolescents, and young adults in sub-Saharan Africa. Blood. 2018 Jul 19;132(3):254–63. PMID:29769263
**2498.** Gopalan A, Dhall D, Olgac S, et al. Testicular mixed germ cell tumors: a morphological and immunohistochemical study using stem cell markers, OCT3/4, SOX2 and GDF3, with emphasis on morphologically difficult-to-classify areas. Mod Pathol. 2009 Aug;22(8):1066–74. PMID:19396148
**2499.** Gordon A, Lipton D, Woodruff JD. Dysgerminoma: a review of 158 cases from the Emil Novak Ovarian Tumor Registry. Obstet Gynecol. 1981 Oct;58(4):497–504. PMID:7279343
**2500.** Gordon K, Varney R, Keeley V, et al. Update and audit of the St George's classification algorithm of primary lymphatic anomalies: a clinical and molecular approach to diagnosis. J Med Genet. 2020 Oct;57(10):653–9. PMID:32409509
**2501.** Gore AC. Neuroendocrine targets of endocrine disruptors. Hormones (Athens). 2010 Jan-Mar;9(1):16–27. PMID:20363718
**2502.** Gorelyshev A, Mazerkina N, Medvedeva O, et al. Second-hit APC mutation in a familial adamantinomatous craniopharyngioma. Neuro Oncol. 2020 Jun 9;22(6):889–91. PMID:32170310
**2503.** Gorlin RJ. Nevoid basal-cell carcinoma syndrome. Medicine (Baltimore). 1987 Mar;66(2):98–113. PMID:3547011
**2504.** Goschzik T, Gessi M, Dreschmann V, et al. Genomic alterations of adamantinomatous and papillary craniopharyngioma. J Neuropathol Exp Neurol. 2017 Feb 1;76(2):126–34. PMID:28069929
**2505.** Goschzik T, Schwalbe EC, Hicks D, et al. Prognostic effect of whole chromosomal aberration signatures in standard-risk, non-WNT/non-SHH medulloblastoma: a retrospective, molecular analysis of the HIT-SIOP PNET 4 trial. Lancet Oncol. 2018 Dec;19(12):1602–16. PMID:30392813
**2506.** Goss JA, Konczyk DJ, Smits PJ, et al. Intramuscular fast-flow vascular anomaly contains somatic MAP2K1 and KRAS mutations. Angiogenesis. 2019 Nov;22(4):547–52. PMID:31486960
**2507.** Gossage L, Eisen T, Maher ER. VHL, the story of a tumour suppressor gene. Nat Rev Cancer. 2015 Jan;15(1):55–64. PMID:25533676
**2508.** Goto H, Hirano N, Kadowaki H, et al. Clinical features of infantile subcutaneous panniculitis-like T-cell lymphoma. Pediatr Int. 2019 Dec;61(12):1261–2. PMID:31808238
**2509.** Goto S, Umehara S, Gerbing RB, et al. Histopathology (International Neuroblastoma Pathology Classification) and MYCN status in patients with peripheral neuroblastic tumors: a report from the Children's Cancer Group. Cancer. 2001 Nov 15;92(10):2699–708. PMID:11745206
**2510.** Goucha S, Khaled A, Zéglaoui F, et al. Nevus lipomatosus cutaneous superficialis: report of eight cases. Dermatol Ther (Heidelb). 2011 Dec;1(2):25–30. PMID:22984661
**2511.** Goulvent T, Ray-Coquard I, Borel S, et al. DICER1 and FOXL2 mutations in ovarian sex cord-stromal tumours: a GINECO Group study. Histopathology. 2016 Jan;68(2):279–85. PMID:26033501
**2512.** Gouveia MH, Otim I, Ogwang MD, et al. Endemic Burkitt Lymphoma in second-degree relatives in Northern Uganda: in-depth genome-wide analysis suggests clues about genetic susceptibility. Leukemia. 2021 Apr;35(4):1209–13. PMID:33051549
**2513.** Goyal A, Yang B. Differential patterns of PAX8, p16, and ER immunostains in mesonephric lesions and adenocarcinomas of the cervix. Int J Gynecol Pathol. 2014 Nov;33(6):613–9. PMID:25272301
**2514.** Goyal G, Heaney ML, Collin M, et al. Erdheim-Chester disease: consensus recommendations for evaluation, diagnosis, and treatment in the molecular era. Blood. 2020 May 28;135(22):1929–45. PMID:32187362
**2515.** Gozali AE, Britt B, Shane L, et al. Choroid plexus tumors; management, outcome, and association with the Li-Fraumeni syndrome: the Children's Hospital Los Angeles (CHLA) experience, 1991-2010. Pediatr Blood Cancer. 2012 Jun;58(6):905–9. PMID:21990040
**2516.** Graadt van Roggen JF, McMenamin ME, Belchis DA, et al. Reticular perineurioma: a distinctive variant of soft tissue perineurioma. Am J Surg Pathol. 2001 Apr;25(4):485–93. PMID:11257623
**2517.** Graetz D, Crews KR, Azzato EM, et al. Leukemic presentation of ALK-positive anaplastic large cell lymphoma with a novel partner, poly(A) binding protein cytoplasmic 1 (PABPC1), responding to single-agent crizotinib. Haematologica. 2019 May;104(5):e218–21. PMID:30819904
**2518.** Graham C, Chilton-MacNeill S, Zielenska M, et al. The CIC-DUX4 fusion transcript is present in a subgroup of pediatric primitive round cell sarcomas. Hum Pathol. 2012 Feb;43(2):180–9. PMID:21813156
**2519.** Graham R, Krishnamurthy S, Oliveira A, et al. Frequent expression of fibroblast growth factor-23 (FGF23) mRNA in aneurysmal bone cysts and chondromyxoid fibromas. J Clin Pathol. 2012 Oct;65(10):907–9. PMID:22933546
**2520.** Graham RP, Jin L, Knutson DL, et al. DNAJB1-PRKACA is specific for fibrolamellar carcinoma. Mod Pathol. 2015 Jun;28(6):822–9. PMID:25698061
**2521.** Graham RP, Kerr SE, Butz ML, et al. Heterogenous MSH6 loss is a result of microsatellite instability within MSH6 and occurs in sporadic and hereditary colorectal and endometrial carcinomas. Am J Surg Pathol. 2015 Oct;39(10):1370–6. PMID:26099011
**2522.** Graham RP, Lackner C, Terracciano L, et al. Fibrolamellar carcinoma in the Carney complex: PRKAR1A loss instead of the classic DNAJB1-PRKACA fusion. Hepatology. 2018 Oct;68(4):1441–7. PMID:29222914
**2523.** Graham RP, Nair AA, Davila JI, et al. Gastroblastoma harbors a recurrent somatic

MALAT1-GLI1 fusion gene. Mod Pathol. 2017 Oct;30(10):1443–52. PMID:28731043
**2524.** Graham RP, Terracciano LM, Meves A, et al. Hepatic adenomas with synchronous or metachronous fibrolamellar carcinomas: both are characterized by LFABP loss. Mod Pathol. 2016 Jun;29(6):607–15. PMID:27015136
**2525.** Graham RP, Torbenson MS. Fibrolamellar carcinoma: a histologically unique tumor with unique molecular findings. Semin Diagn Pathol. 2017 Mar;34(2):146–52. PMID:28110996
**2526.** Graham RP, Yeh MM, Lam-Himlin D, et al. Molecular testing for the clinical diagnosis of fibrolamellar carcinoma. Mod Pathol. 2018 Jan;31(1):141–9. PMID:28862261
**2527.** Grajkowska W, Kotulska K, Jurkiewicz E, et al. Subependymal giant cell astrocytomas with atypical histological features mimicking malignant gliomas. Folia Neuropathol. 2011;49(1):39–46. PMID:21455842
**2528.** Grajo JR, Paspulati RM, Sahani DV, et al. Multiple endocrine neoplasia syndromes: a comprehensive imaging review. Radiol Clin North Am. 2016 May;54(3):441–51. PMID:27153782
**2529.** Granai M, Amato T, Di Napoli A, et al. IGHV mutational status of nodal marginal zone lymphoma by NGS reveals distinct pathogenic pathways with different prognostic implications. Virchows Arch. 2020 Jul;477(1):143–50. PMID:31802229
**2530.** Grande BM, Gerhard DS, Jiang A, et al. Genome-wide discovery of somatic coding and noncoding mutations in pediatric endemic and sporadic Burkitt lymphoma. Blood. 2019 Mar 21;133(12):1313–24. PMID:30617194
**2531.** Grani G, Lamartina L, Ascoli V, et al. Reducing the number of unnecessary thyroid biopsies while improving diagnostic accuracy: toward the "Right" TIRADS. J Clin Endocrinol Metab. 2019 Jan 1;104(1):95–102. PMID:30299457
**2532.** Grapsa D, Kairi-Vassilatou E, Kleanthis C, et al. Epithelial ovarian tumors in adolescents: a retrospective pathologic study and a critical review of the literature. J Pediatr Adolesc Gynecol. 2011 Dec;24(6):386–8. PMID:21945630
**2533.** Grass B, Wachtel M, Behnke S, et al. Immunohistochemical detection of EGFR, fibrillin-2, P-cadherin and AP2beta as biomarkers for rhabdomyosarcoma diagnostics. Histopathology. 2009 Jun;54(7):873–9. PMID:19469909
**2534.** Grassia KL, Peterman CM, Iacobas I, et al. Clinical case series of pediatric hepatic angiosarcoma. Pediatr Blood Cancer. 2017 Nov;64(11). PMID:28521077
**2535.** Gratzinger D, de Jong D, Jaffe ES, et al. T- and NK-cell lymphomas and systemic lymphoproliferative disorders and the immunodeficiency setting: 2015 SH/EAHP workshop report-part 4. Am J Clin Pathol. 2017 Feb 1;147(2):188–203. PMID:28395105
**2536.** Gray MJ, Kannu P, Sharma S, et al. Mutations preventing regulated exon skipping in MET cause osteofibrous dysplasia. Am J Hum Genet. 2015 Dec 3;97(6):837–47. PMID:26637977
**2537.** Green M, Cacciarelli TV, Mazariegos GV, et al. Serial measurement of Epstein-Barr viral load in peripheral blood in pediatric liver transplant recipients during treatment for posttransplant lymphoproliferative disease. Transplantation. 1998 Dec 27;66(12):1641–4. PMID:9884252
**2538.** Green MR, Monti S, Rodig SJ, et al. Integrative analysis reveals selective 9p24.1 amplification, increased PD-1 ligand expression, and further induction via JAK2 in nodular sclerosing Hodgkin lymphoma and primary mediastinal large B-cell lymphoma. Blood. 2010 Oct 28;116(17):3268–77. PMID:20628145
**2539.** Green NM, Pagkalos J, Jeys LM, et al. Humeral simple bone cysts: observational versus interventional management. J Pediatr Orthop. 2019 Jul;39(6):e472–7. PMID:30702640
**2540.** Green RC, Green JS, Buehler SK, et al. Very high incidence of familial colorectal cancer in Newfoundland: a comparison with Ontario and 13 other population-based studies. Fam Cancer. 2007;6(1):53–62. PMID:17039269
**2541.** Green RS, Tunkel DE, Small D, et al. Sialoblastoma: association with cutaneous hamartoma (organoid nevus)? Pediatr Dev Pathol. 2000 Sep-Oct;3(5):504–5. PMID:10890938
**2542.** Green WM, Yonescu R, Morsberger L, et al. Utilization of a TFE3 break-apart FISH assay in a renal tumor consultation service. Am J Surg Pathol. 2013 Aug;37(8):1150–63. PMID:23715164
**2543.** Green WR, Iliff WJ, Trotter RR. Malignant teratoid medulloepithelioma of the optic nerve. Arch Ophthalmol. 1974 Jun;91(6):451–4. PMID:4827430
**2544.** Greene AK, Karnes J, Padua HM, et al. Diffuse lipofibromatosis of the lower extremity masquerading as a vascular anomaly. Ann Plast Surg. 2009 Jun;62(6):703–6. PMID:19461290
**2545.** Greenspan A. Benign bone-forming lesions: osteoma, osteoid osteoma, and osteoblastoma. Clinical, imaging, pathologic, and differential considerations. Skeletal Radiol. 1993 Oct;22(7):485–500. PMID:8272884
**2546.** Greer A, Foreman NK, Donson A, et al. Desmoplastic infantile astrocytoma/ganglioglioma with rare BRAF V600D mutation. Pediatr Blood Cancer. 2017 Jun;64(6):10.1002/pbc.26350. PMID:27860162
**2547.** Greiner G, Gurbisz M, Ratzinger F, et al. Digital PCR: a sensitive and precise method for KIT D816V quantification in mastocytosis. Clin Chem. 2018 Mar;64(3):547–55. PMID:29237714
**2548.** Grenga TE. Intratendinous fibroma of flexor tendon. J Hand Surg Am. 1990 Jan;15(1):92–3. PMID:2299175
**2549.** Gressel GM, Buza N, Pal L. Ovarian Sertoli-Leydig cell tumors: a single institution experience and review of the literature. Eur J Gynaecol Oncol. 2017;38(2):214–20. PMID:29953783
**2550.** Griewank KG, Koelsche C, van de Nes JAP, et al. Integrated genomic classification of melanocytic tumors of the central nervous system using mutation analysis, copy number alterations, and DNA methylation profiling. Clin Cancer Res. 2018 Sep 15;24(18):4494–504. PMID:29891723
**2551.** Griewank KG, Müller H, Jackett LA, et al. SF3B1 and BAP1 mutations in blue nevus-like melanoma. Mod Pathol. 2017 Jul;30(7):928–39. PMID:28409567
**2552.** Griffin CA, Hawkins AL, Dvorak C, et al. Recurrent involvement of 2p23 in inflammatory myofibroblastic tumors. Cancer Res. 1999 Jun 15;59(12):2776–80. PMID:10383129
**2553.** Griffith CC, Thompson LD, Assaad A, et al. Salivary duct carcinoma and the concept of early carcinoma ex pleomorphic adenoma. Histopathology. 2014 Dec;65(6):854–60. PMID:24804831
**2554.** Griffith JL, Morris SM, Mahdi J, et al. Increased prevalence of brain tumors classified as T2 hyperintensities in neurofibromatosis 1. Neurol Clin Pract. 2018 Aug;8(4):283–91. PMID:30140579
**2555.** Grignon DJ, Eble JN. Papillary and metanephric adenomas of the kidney. Semin Diagn Pathol. 1998 Feb;15(1):41–53. PMID:9503505
**2556.** Grimer RJ, Bielack S, Flege S, et al. Periosteal osteosarcoma–a European review of outcome. Eur J Cancer. 2005 Dec;41(18):2806–11. PMID:16290134
**2557.** Grimm F, Maurus R, Beschorner R, et al. Ki-67 labeling index and expression of p53 are non-predictive for invasiveness and tumor size in functional and nonfunctional pituitary adenomas. Acta Neurochir (Wien). 2019 Jun;161(6):1149–56. PMID:31037500
**2558.** Gröbner SN, Worst BC, Weischenfeldt J, et al. Author correction: The landscape of genomic alterations across childhood cancers. Nature. 2018 Jul;559(7714):E10. PMID:29875405
**2559.** Gröbner SN, Worst BC, Weischenfeldt J, et al. The landscape of genomic alterations across childhood cancers. Nature. 2018 Mar 15;555(7696):321–7. PMID:29489754
**2560.** Groesser L, Herschberger E, Ruetten A, et al. Postzygotic HRAS and KRAS mutations cause nevus sebaceous and Schimmelpenning syndrome. Nat Genet. 2012 Jun 10;44(7):783–7. PMID:22683711
**2561.** Groesser L, Herschberger E, Sagrera A, et al. Phacomatosis pigmentokeratotica is caused by a postzygotic HRAS mutation in a multipotent progenitor cell. J Invest Dermatol. 2013 Aug;133(8):1998–2003. PMID:23337891
**2562.** Groesser L, Peterhof E, Evert M, et al. BRAF and RAS mutations in sporadic and secondary pyogenic granuloma. J Invest Dermatol. 2016 Feb;136(2):481–6. PMID:26802240
**2563.** Grogan RH, Pacak K, Pasche L, et al. Bilateral adrenal medullary hyperplasia associated with an SDHB mutation. J Clin Oncol. 2011 Mar 10;29(8):e200–2. PMID:21172883
**2564.** Grogg J, Schneider K, Bode PK, et al. Sertoli cell tumors of the testes: systematic literature review and meta-analysis of outcomes in 435 patients. Oncologist. 2020 Jul;25(7):585–90. PMID:32043680
**2565.** Grogg JB, Schneider K, Bode PK, et al. Risk factors and treatment outcomes of 239 patients with testicular granulosa cell tumors: a systematic review of published case series data. J Cancer Res Clin Oncol. 2020 Nov;146(11):2829–41. PMID:32719989
**2566.** Groom KR, Murphey MD, Howard LM, et al. Mesenchymal hamartoma of the chest wall: radiologic manifestations with emphasis on cross-sectional imaging and histopathologic comparison. Radiology. 2002 Jan;222(1):205–11. PMID:11756727
**2567.** Gross AM, Wolters PL, Dombi E, et al. Selumetinib in children with inoperable plexiform neurofibromas. N Engl J Med. 2020 Apr 9;382(15):1430–42. PMID:32187457
**2568.** Groves C, Lamlum H, Crabtree M, et al. Mutation cluster region, association between germline and somatic mutations and genotype-phenotype correlation in upper gastrointestinal familial adenomatous polyposis. Am J Pathol. 2002 Jun;160(6):2055–61. PMID:12057910
**2569.** Gru AA, Jaffe ES. Cutaneous EBV-related lymphoproliferative disorders. Semin Diagn Pathol. 2017 Jan;34(1):60–75. PMID:27988064
**2570.** Gruber TA, Larson Gedman A, Zhang J, et al. An Inv(16)(p13.3q24.3)-encoded CBFA2T3-GLIS2 fusion protein defines an aggressive subtype of pediatric acute megakaryoblastic leukemia. Cancer Cell. 2012 Nov 13;22(5):683–97. PMID:23153540
**2571.** Grünewald TGP, Cidre-Aranaz F, Surdez D, et al. Ewing sarcoma. Nat Rev Dis Primers. 2018 Jul 5;4(1):5. PMID:29977059
**2572.** Grygalewicz B, Woroniecka R, Rymkiewicz G, et al. The 11q-gain/loss aberration occurs recurrently in MYC-negative Burkitt-like lymphoma with 11q aberration, as well as MYC-positive Burkitt lymphoma and MYC-positive high-grade B-cell lymphoma, NOS. Am J Clin Pathol. 2017 Dec 20;149(1):17–28. PMID:29272887
**2573.** Gu Z, Churchman ML, Roberts KG, et al. PAX5-driven subtypes of B-progenitor acute lymphoblastic leukemia. Nat Genet. 2019 Feb;51(2):296–307. PMID:30643249
**2574.** Guan W, Yan Y, He W, et al. Ossifying renal tumor of infancy (ORIT): the clinicopathological and cytogenetic feature of two cases and literature review. Pathol Res Pract. 2016 Nov;212(11):1004–9. PMID:27633911
**2575.** Guan XQ, Xu L, Ke ZY, et al. Five Chinese pediatric patients with leukemias possibly arising from immature natural killer cells: clinical features and courses. Pediatr Hematol Oncol. 2011 Apr;28(3):187–93. PMID:21271777
**2576.** Gudowius S, Engelbrecht V, Messing-Jünger M, et al. Diagnostic difficulties in childhood bilateral thalamic astrocytomas. Neuropediatrics. 2002 Dec;33(6):331–5. PMID:12571791
**2577.** Guermazi A, De Kerviler E, Zagdanski AM, et al. Diagnostic imaging of choroid plexus disease. Clin Radiol. 2000 Jul;55(7):503–16. PMID:10924373
**2578.** Guerreiro Stucklin AS, Ryall S, Fukuoka K, et al. Alterations in ALK/ROS1/NTRK/MET drive a group of infantile hemispheric gliomas. Nat Commun. 2019 Sep 25;10(1):4343. PMID:31554817
**2579.** Guerrini-Rousseau L, Dufour C, Varlet P, et al. Germline SUFU mutation carriers and medulloblastoma: clinical characteristics, cancer risk, and prognosis. Neuro Oncol. 2018 Jul 5;20(8):1122–32. PMID:29186568
**2579A.** Guerrini-Rousseau L, Smith MJ, Kratz CP, et al. Current recommendations for cancer surveillance in Gorlin syndrome: a report from the SIOPE host genome working group (SIOPE HGWG). Fam Cancer. 2021 Oct;20(4):317–25. PMID:33860896
**2580.** Guerrini-Rousseau L, Varlet P, Colas C, et al. Constitutional mismatch repair deficiency-associated brain tumors: report from the European C4CMMRD consortium. Neurooncol Adv. 2019 Dec 2;1(1):vdz033. PMID:32642664
**2581.** Guerrisi M, Piloni MJ, Keszler A. Odontogenic tumors in children and adolescents. A 15-year retrospective study in Argentina. Med Oral Patol Oral Cir Bucal. 2007 May 1;12(3):E180–5. PMID:17468710
**2582.** Gugel I, Grimm F, Teuber C, et al. Presenting symptoms in children with neurofibromatosis type 2. Childs Nerv Syst. 2020 Oct;36(10):2463–70. PMID:32537663
**2583.** Gui T, Cao D, Shen K, et al. A clinicopathological analysis of 40 cases of ovarian Sertoli-Leydig cell tumors. Gynecol Oncol. 2012 Nov;127(2):384–9. PMID:22850410
**2584.** Guidry CA, McGahren ED, Rodgers BM, et al. Pediatric cervicomediastinal hibernoma: a case report. J Pediatr Surg. 2013 Jan;48(1):258–61. PMID:23331827
**2585.** Guilhamon P, Eskandarpour M, Halai D, et al. Meta-analysis of IDH-mutant cancers identifies EBF1 as an interaction partner for TET2. Nat Commun. 2013;4:2166. PMID:23863747
**2586.** Guillerman RP, Foulkes WD, Priest JR. Imaging of DICER1 syndrome. Pediatr Radiol. 2019 Oct;49(11):1488–505. PMID:31620849
**2587.** Guillet C, Rechsteiner M, Bellini E, et al. Juvenile papillomatosis of the breast (Swiss cheese disease) has frequent associations with PIK3CA and/or AKT1 mutations. Hum Pathol. 2020 Apr;98:64–73. PMID:32088208
**2588.** Guillou L, Aurias A. Soft tissue sarcomas with complex genomic profiles. Virchows Arch. 2010 Feb;456(2):201–17. PMID:20217954
**2589.** Guillou L, Benhattar J, Bonichon F, et al. Histologic grade, but not SYT-SSX fusion type, is an important prognostic factor in patients with synovial sarcoma: a multicenter,

retrospective analysis. J Clin Oncol. 2004 Oct 15;22(20):4040–50. PMID:15364967
**2590.** Guillou L, Benhattar J, Gengler C, et al. Translocation-positive low-grade fibromyxoid sarcoma: clinicopathologic and molecular analysis of a series expanding the morphologic spectrum and suggesting potential relationship to sclerosing epithelioid fibrosarcoma: a study from the French Sarcoma Group. Am J Surg Pathol. 2007 Sep;31(9):1387–402. PMID:17721195
**2591.** Guillou L, Coindre JM, Bonichon F, et al. Comparative study of the National Cancer Institute and French Federation of Cancer Centers Sarcoma Group grading systems in a population of 410 adult patients with soft tissue sarcoma. J Clin Oncol. 1997 Jan;15(1):350–62. PMID:8996162
**2592.** Guillou L, Gebhard S, Salmeron M, et al. Metastasizing fibrous histiocytoma of the skin: a clinicopathologic and immunohistochemical analysis of three cases. Mod Pathol. 2000 Jun;13(6):654–60. PMID:10874670
**2593.** Guillou L, Wadden C, Coindre JM, et al. "Proximal-type" epithelioid sarcoma, a distinctive aggressive neoplasm showing rhabdoid features. Clinicopathologic, immunohistochemical, and ultrastructural study of a series. Am J Surg Pathol. 1997 Feb;21(2):130–46. PMID:9042279
**2593A.** Guilmette J, Nosé V. Hereditary and familial thyroid tumours. Histopathology. 2018 Jan;72(1):70–81. PMID:29239041
**2594.** Guinand S, Hedinger C. [Atypical intratubular germ cells and testicular germ cell tumors in children (author's transl)]. Ann Pathol. 1981;1(4):251–7. French. PMID:6119099
**2595.** Guinot-Moya R, Valmaseda-Castellon E, Berini-Aytes L, et al. Pilomatrixoma. Review of 205 cases. Med Oral Patol Oral Cir Bucal. 2011 Jul 1;16(4):e552–5. PMID:20711110
**2596.** Gül D, Oğur G, Tunca Y, et al. Third case of WAGR syndrome with severe obesity and constitutional deletion of chromosome (11)(p12p14). Am J Med Genet. 2002 Jan 1;107(1):70–1. PMID:11807873
**2597.** Gulack BC, Rialon KL, Englum BR, et al. Factors associated with survival in pediatric adrenocortical carcinoma: an analysis of the National Cancer Data Base (NCDB). J Pediatr Surg. 2016 Jan;51(1):172–7. PMID:26572849
**2598.** Gulluoglu S, Turksoy O, Kuskucu A, et al. The molecular aspects of chordoma. Neurosurg Rev. 2016 Apr;39(2):185–96. PMID:26363792
**2599.** Gunes D, Uysal KM, Cecen E, et al. Stromal-predominant mesenchymal hamartoma of the liver with elevated serum alpha-fetoprotein level. Pediatr Hematol Oncol. 2008 Sep;25(7):685–92. PMID:18850482
**2600.** Güngör Ş, Şişman S, Kocaturk E, et al. Benign nerve sheath myxoma in an infant misdiagnosed as infantile digital fibromatosis. Pediatr Dermatol. 2016 Jul;33(4):e252–3. PMID:27196676
**2601.** Gunsilius E, Duba HC, Petzer AL, et al. Evidence from a leukaemia model for maintenance of vascular endothelium by bone-marrow-derived endothelial cells. Lancet. 2000 May 13;355(9216):1688–91. PMID:10905245
**2602.** Guo H, Garcia RA, Perle MA, et al. Giant cell tumor of soft tissue with pulmonary metastases: pathologic and cytogenetic study. Pediatr Dev Pathol. 2005 Nov-Dec;8(6):718–24. PMID:16328671
**2603.** Guo H, Keefe KA, Kohler MF, et al. Juvenile granulosa cell tumor of the ovary associated with tuberous sclerosis. Gynecol Oncol. 2006 Jul;102(1):118–20. PMID:16516278
**2604.** Guo J, Tretiakova MS, Troxell ML, et al. Tuberous sclerosis-associated renal cell carcinoma: a clinicopathologic study of 57 separate carcinomas in 18 patients. Am J Surg Pathol. 2014 Nov;38(11):1457–67. PMID:25093518
**2604A.** Guo N, Chen Y, Wang Y, et al. Clinicopathological categorization of hydroa vacciniforme-like lymphoproliferative disorder: an analysis of prognostic implications and treatment based on 19 cases. Diagn Pathol. 2019 Jul 17;14(1):82. PMID:31315684
**2605.** Guo R, Wang X, Chou MM, et al. PPP6R3-USP6 amplification: novel oncogenic mechanism in malignant nodular fasciitis. Genes Chromosomes Cancer. 2016 Aug;55(8):640–9. PMID:27113271
**2606.** Guo T, Zhang L, Chang NE, et al. Consistent MYC and FLT4 gene amplification in radiation-induced angiosarcoma but not in other radiation-associated atypical vascular lesions. Genes Chromosomes Cancer. 2011 Jan;50(1):25–33. PMID:20949568
**2607.** Guo Y, Yuan F, Deng H, et al. Paranuclear dot-like immunostaining for CD99: a unique staining pattern for diagnosing solid-pseudopapillary neoplasm of the pancreas. Am J Surg Pathol. 2011 Jun;35(6):799–806. PMID:21566515
**2608.** Gupta A, Kozakewich H. Histopathology of vascular anomalies. Clin Plast Surg. 2011 Jan;38(1):31–44. PMID:21095470
**2609.** Gupta A, Ly S, Castroneves LA, et al. A standardized assessment of thyroid nodules in children confirms higher cancer prevalence than in adults. J Clin Endocrinol Metab. 2013 Aug;98(8):3238–45. PMID:23737541
**2610.** Gupta A, Sheridan RM, Towbin A, et al. Multifocal hepatic neoplasia in 3 children with APC gene mutation. Am J Surg Pathol. 2013 Jul;37(7):1058–66. PMID:23715166
**2611.** Gupta AK, Gupta MK, Gupta K. Dermoid cyst of the testis (a case report). Indian J Cancer. 1986 Mar;23(1):21–3. PMID:3817858
**2612.** Gupta C, Iyer VK, Kaushal S, et al. Fine needle aspiration cytology of undifferentiated embryonal sarcoma of the liver. Cytopathology. 2010 Dec;21(6):414–6. PMID:20105209
**2613.** Gupta D, Deavers MT, Silva EG, et al. Malignant melanoma involving the ovary: a clinicopathologic and immunohistochemical study of 23 cases. Am J Surg Pathol. 2004 Jun;28(6):771–80. PMID:15166669
**2614.** Gupta G, Garg R, Wadhwa C, et al. A rare primary dumbbell lipoblastoma. Asian J Neurosurg. 2018 Jan-Mar;13(1):83–5. PMID:29492129
**2615.** Gupta G, Man I, Kemmett D. Hydroa vacciniforme: a clinical and follow-up study of 17 cases. J Am Acad Dermatol. 2000 Feb;42(2 Pt 1):208–13. PMID:10642674
**2616.** Gupta K, Harreld JH, Sabin ND, et al. Massively calcified low-grade glioma - a rare and distinctive entity. Neuropathol Appl Neurobiol. 2014 Feb;40(2):221–4. PMID:23927783
**2617.** Gupta K, Orisme W, Harreld JH, et al. Posterior fossa and spinal gangliogliomas form two distinct clinicopathologic and molecular subgroups. Acta Neuropathol Commun. 2014 Feb 14;2:18. PMID:24529209
**2618.** Gupta MP, Lane AM, DeAngelis MM, et al. Clinical characteristics of uveal melanoma in patients with germline BAP1 mutations. JAMA Ophthalmol. 2015 Aug;133(8):881–7. PMID:25974357
**2619.** Gupta N, Gupta R, Bakhshi S. Transient myeloproliferation mimicking JMML associated with parvovirus infection of infancy. Pediatr Blood Cancer. 2009 Mar;52(3):411–3. PMID:18989883
**2620.** Gupta R, Billis A, Shah RB, et al. Carcinoma of the collecting ducts of Bellini and renal medullary carcinoma: clinicopathologic analysis of 52 cases of rare aggressive subtypes of renal cell carcinoma with a focus on their interrelationship. Am J Surg Pathol. 2012 Sep;36(9):1265–78. PMID:22895263
**2621.** Gupta S, Argani P, Jungbluth AA, et al. TFEB expression profiling in renal cell carcinomas: clinicopathologic correlations. Am J Surg Pathol. 2019 Nov;43(11):1445–61. PMID:31600176
**2622.** Gupta S, Johnson SH, Vasmatzis G, et al. TFEB-VEGFA (6p21.1) co-amplified renal cell carcinoma: a distinct entity with potential implications for clinical management. Mod Pathol. 2017 Jul;30(7):998–1012. PMID:28338654
**2623.** Gupta S, Yeh S, Chami R, et al. The prognostic impact of tumour-associated macrophages and Reed-Sternberg cells in paediatric Hodgkin lymphoma. Eur J Cancer. 2013 Oct;49(15):3255–61. PMID:23791542
**2624.** Gupta S, Zhang J, Erickson LA. Composite pheochromocytoma/paraganglioma-ganglioneuroma: a clinicopathologic study of eight cases with analysis of succinate dehydrogenase. Endocr Pathol. 2017 Sep;28(3):269–75. PMID:28752484
**2625.** Gupta VR, Giller C, Kolhe R, et al. Polymorphous low-grade neuroepithelial tumor of the young: a case report with genomic findings. World Neurosurg. 2019 Dec;132:347–55. PMID:31520766
**2626.** Gurbuz AK, Giardiello FM, Petersen GM, et al. Desmoid tumours in familial adenomatous polyposis. Gut. 1994 Mar;35(3):377–81. PMID:8150351
**2627.** Gurda GT, VandenBussche CJ, Yonescu R, et al. Sacrococcygeal teratomas: clinico-pathological characteristics and isochromosome 12p status. Mod Pathol. 2014 Apr;27(4):562–8. PMID:24051698
**2628.** Guschmann M, Henrich W, Entezami M, et al. Chorioangioma–new insights into a well-known problem. I. Results of a clinical and morphological study of 136 cases. J Perinat Med. 2003;31(2):163–9. PMID:12747233
**2629.** Gusella JF, Ramesh V, MacCollin M, et al. Merlin: the neurofibromatosis 2 tumor suppressor. Biochim Biophys Acta. 1999 Mar 25;1423(2):M29–36. PMID:10214350
**2630.** Gusella JF, Ramesh V, MacCollin M, et al. Neurofibromatosis 2: loss of merlin's protective spell. Curr Opin Genet Dev. 1996 Feb;6(1):87–92. PMID:8791482
**2631.** Guseva NV, Jaber O, Tanas MR, et al. Anchored multiplex PCR for targeted next-generation sequencing reveals recurrent and novel USP6 fusions and upregulation of USP6 expression in aneurysmal bone cyst. Genes Chromosomes Cancer. 2017 Apr;56(4):266–77. PMID:27910166
**2632.** Gustavson KH, Gamstorp I, Meurling S. Bilateral teratoma of testis in two brothers with 47,XXY Klinefelter's syndrome. Clin Genet. 1975 Jul;8(1):5–10. PMID:1149322
**2633.** Guthery SL, Heubi JE, Bucuvalas JC, et al. Determination of risk factors for Epstein-Barr virus-associated posttransplant lymphoproliferative disorder in pediatric liver transplant recipients using objective case ascertainment. Transplantation. 2003 Apr 15;75(7):987–93. PMID:12698085
**2634.** Gutmann DH, Aylsworth A, Carey JC, et al. The diagnostic evaluation and multidisciplinary management of neurofibromatosis 1 and neurofibromatosis 2. JAMA. 1997 Jul 2;278(1):51–7. PMID:9207339
**2635.** Gutmann DH, Donahoe J, Brown T, et al. Loss of neurofibromatosis 1 (NF1) gene expression in NF1-associated pilocytic astrocytomas. Neuropathol Appl Neurobiol. 2000 Aug;26(4):361–7. PMID:10931370
**2636.** Gutmann DH, Ferner RE, Listernick RH, et al. Neurofibromatosis type 1. Nat Rev Dis Primers. 2017 Feb 23;3:17004. PMID:28230061
**2637.** Gutmann DH, McLellan MD, Hussain I, et al. Somatic neurofibromatosis type 1 (NF1) inactivation characterizes NF1-associated pilocytic astrocytoma. Genome Res. 2013 Mar;23(3):431–9. PMID:23222849
**2638.** Guyot-Goubin A, Donadieu J, Barkaoui M, et al. Descriptive epidemiology of childhood Langerhans cell histiocytosis in France, 2000-2004. Pediatr Blood Cancer. 2008 Jul;51(1):71–5. PMID:18260117
**2639.** Guzzo M, Ferrari A, Marcon I, et al. Salivary gland neoplasms in children: the experience of the Istituto Nazionale Tumori of Milan. Pediatr Blood Cancer. 2006 Nov;47(6):806–10. PMID:16425245
**2640.** Gwin K, Cajaiba MM, Caminoa-Lizarralde A, et al. Expanding the clinical spectrum of Frasier syndrome. Pediatr Dev Pathol. 2008 Mar-Apr;11(2):122–7. PMID:17378674
**2641.** Gwin K, Mariño-Enriquez A, Martel M, et al. Sclerosing stromal tumor: an important differential diagnosis of ovarian neoplasms in childhood and adolescence. Pediatr Dev Pathol. 2009 Sep-Oct;12(5):366–70. PMID:19071970
**2642.** Gylling A, Abdel-Rahman WM, Juhola M, et al. Is gastric cancer part of the tumour spectrum of hereditary non-polyposis colorectal cancer? A molecular genetic study. Gut. 2007 Jul;56(7):926–33. PMID:17267619
**2643.** Gyure KA, Morrison AL. Cytokeratin 7 and 20 expression in choroid plexus tumors: utility in differentiating these neoplasms from metastatic carcinomas. Mod Pathol. 2000 Jun;13(6):638–43. PMID:10874668
**2644.** Gyure KA, Prayson RA. Subependymal giant cell astrocytoma: a clinicopathologic study with HMB45 and MIB-1 immunohistochemical analysis. Mod Pathol. 1997 Apr;10(4):313–7. PMID:9110292
**2645.** Haack H, Johnson LA, Fry CJ, et al. Diagnosis of NUT midline carcinoma using a NUT-specific monoclonal antibody. Am J Surg Pathol. 2009 Jul;33(7):984–91. PMID:19363441
**2646.** Haase GM, O'Leary MC, Stram DO, et al. Pelvic neuroblastoma–implications for a new favorable subgroup: a Children's Cancer Group experience. Ann Surg Oncol. 1995 Nov;2(6):516–23. PMID:8591082
**2647.** Habek M, Brinar VV, Mubrin Z, et al. Bilateral thalamic astrocytoma. J Neurooncol. 2007 Sep;84(2):175–7. PMID:17522784
**2648.** Haberler C, Laggner U, Slavc I, et al. Immunohistochemical analysis of INI1 protein in malignant pediatric CNS tumors: lack of INI1 in atypical teratoid/rhabdoid tumors and in a fraction of primitive neuroectodermal tumors without rhabdoid phenotype. Am J Surg Pathol. 2006 Nov;30(11):1462–8. PMID:17063089
**2649.** Haberler C, Reiniger L, Rajnai H, et al. Case of the month 1-2019: CNS high-grade neuroepithelial tumor with BCOR alteration. Clin Neuropathol. 2019 Jan/Feb;38(1):4–7. PMID:30526817
**2650.** Häcker U, Nybakken K, Perrimon N. Heparan sulphate proteoglycans: the sweet side of development. Nat Rev Mol Cell Biol. 2005 Jul;6(7):530–41. PMID:16072037
**2651.** Hackethal A, Brueggmann D, Bohlmann MK, et al. Squamous-cell carcinoma in mature cystic teratoma of the ovary: systematic review and analysis of published data. Lancet Oncol. 2008 Dec;9(12):1173–80. PMID:19038764
**2651A.** Hadar T, Rahima M, Kahan E, et al. Significance of specific Epstein-Barr virus IgA and elevated IgG antibodies to viral capsid antigens in nasopharyngeal carcinoma patients. J Med Virol. 1986 Dec;20(4):329–39. PMID:3025351
**2652.** Haddad AF, Young JS, Oh T, et al. Clinical characteristics and outcomes of null-cell versus silent gonadotroph adenomas in a series of 1166 pituitary adenomas from

a single institution. Neurosurg Focus. 2020 Jun;48(6):E13. PMID:32480370
**2653.** Hadi HA, Finley J, Strickland D. Placental chorioangioma: prenatal diagnosis and clinical significance. Am J Perinatol. 1993 Mar;10(2):146–9. PMID:8476479
**2654.** Hadj-Rabia S, Oriot D, Soufir N, et al. Unexpected extradermatological findings in 31 patients with xeroderma pigmentosum type C. Br J Dermatol. 2013 May;168(5):1109–13. PMID:23278166
**2655.** Hadzic N, Quaglia A, Mieli-Vergani G. Hepatocellular carcinoma in a 12-year-old child with PiZZ alpha1-antitrypsin deficiency. Hepatology. 2006 Jan;43(1):194. PMID:16374862
**2656.** Hadžić N, Quaglia A, Portmann B, et al. Hepatocellular carcinoma in biliary atresia: King's College Hospital experience. J Pediatr. 2011 Oct;159(4):617–22.e1. PMID:21489554
**2657.** Hafeez S, Balarezo F, Ricci A Jr. Benign phyllodes tumor in children: a study of 8 cases and review of the literature. J Pediatr Hematol Oncol. 2020 Jul;42(5):e388–91. PMID:31107366
**2658.** Hafner C, Hafner H, Groesser L. [Genetic basis of seborrheic keratosis and epidermal nevi]. Pathologe. 2014 Sep;35(5):413–23. German. PMID:25187080
**2659.** Hafner C, Toll A, Gantner S, et al. Keratinocytic epidermal nevi are associated with mosaic RAS mutations. J Med Genet. 2012 Apr;49(4):249–53. PMID:22499344
**2660.** Hafner C, van Oers JM, Vogt T, et al. Mosaicism of activating FGFR3 mutations in human skin causes epidermal nevi. J Clin Invest. 2006 Aug;116(8):2201–7. PMID:16841094
**2661.** Hagel C, Stemmer-Rachamimov AO, Bornemann A, et al. Clinical presentation, immunohistochemistry and electron microscopy indicate neurofibromatosis type 2-associated gliomas to be spinal ependymomas. Neuropathology. 2012 Dec;32(6):611–6. PMID:22394059
**2662.** Hahn H, Wicking C, Zaphiropoulous PG, et al. Mutations of the human homolog of Drosophila patched in the nevoid basal cell carcinoma syndrome. Cell. 1996 Jun 14;85(6):841–51. PMID:8681379
**2663.** Haimes JD, Stewart CJR, Kudlow BA, et al. Uterine inflammatory myofibroblastic tumors frequently harbor ALK fusions with IGFBP5 and THBS1. Am J Surg Pathol. 2017 Jun;41(6):773–80. PMID:28490045
**2664.** Haines K, Sarabia SF, Alvarez KR, et al. Characterization of pediatric hepatocellular carcinoma reveals genomic heterogeneity and diverse signaling pathway activation. Pediatr Blood Cancer. 2019 Jul;66(7):e27745. PMID:30977242
**2665.** Hajiran A, Jessop M, Werner Z, et al. Ossifying renal tumor of infancy: laparoscopic treatment and literature review. Case Rep Urol. 2018 Oct 23;2018:1935657. PMID:30425880
**2666.** Hajnsek S, Paladino J, Gadze ZP, et al. Clinical and neurophysiological changes in patients with pineal region expansions. Coll Antropol. 2013 Mar;37(1):35–40. PMID:23697248
**2667.** Halabi M, Oliva E, Mazal PR, et al. Prostatic tissue in mature cystic teratomas of the ovary: a report of four cases, including one with features of prostatic adenocarcinoma, and cytogenetic studies. Int J Gynecol Pathol. 2002 Jul;21(3):261–7. PMID:12068172
**2668.** Halac I, Zimmerman D. Thyroid nodules and cancers in children. Endocrinol Metab Clin North Am. 2005 Sep;34(3):725–44, x. PMID:16085168
**2669.** Hall OR, Pascasio JM, Morrissette JJ, et al. Study of an ovarian sclerosing stromal tumor presenting as vaginal bleeding in a 7-month-old. Pediatr Dev Pathol. 2008 Jul-Aug;11(4):300–4. PMID:17990931
**2670.** Hall RK. Solitary median maxillary central incisor (SMMCI) syndrome. Orphanet J Rare Dis. 2006 Apr 9;1:12. PMID:16722608
**2671.** Haller F, Bieg M, Will R, et al. Enhancer hijacking activates oncogenic transcription factor NR4A3 in acinic cell carcinomas of the salivary glands. Nat Commun. 2019 Jan 21;10(1):368. PMID:30664630
**2672.** Haller F, Knopf J, Ackermann A, et al. Paediatric and adult soft tissue sarcomas with NTRK1 gene fusions: a subset of spindle cell sarcomas unified by a prominent myopericytic/haemangiopericytic pattern. J Pathol. 2016 Apr;238(5):700–10. PMID:26863915
**2673.** Haller F, Moskalev EA, Kuck S, et al. Nuclear NR4A2 (Nurr1) Immunostaining is a novel marker for acinic cell carcinoma of the salivary glands lacking the classic NR4A3 (NOR-1) upregulation. Am J Surg Pathol. 2020 Sep;44(9):1290–2. PMID:32341238
**2674.** Haller F, Skálová A, Ihrler S, et al. Nuclear NR4A3 immunostaining is a specific and sensitive novel marker for acinic cell carcinoma of the salivary glands. Am J Surg Pathol. 2019 Sep;43(9):1264–72. PMID:31094928
**2675.** Hallor KH, Micci F, Meis-Kindblom JM, et al. Fusion genes in angiomatoid fibrous histiocytoma. Cancer Lett. 2007 Jun 18;251(1):158–63. PMID:17188428
**2676.** Halme A, Kellokumpu-Lehtinen P, Lehtonen T, et al. Morphology of testicular germ cell tumours in treated and untreated cryptorchidism. Br J Urol. 1989 Jul;64(1):78–83. PMID:2569902
**2677.** Hama A, Takahashi Y, Muramatsu H, et al. Comparison of long-term outcomes between children with aplastic anemia and refractory cytopenia of childhood who received immunosuppressive therapy with antithymocyte globulin and cyclosporine. Haematologica. 2015 Nov;100(11):1426–33. PMID:26273061
**2678.** Hambraeus M, Arnbjörnsson E, Börjesson A, et al. Sacrococcygeal teratoma: a population-based study of incidence and prenatal prognostic factors. J Pediatr Surg. 2016 Mar;51(3):481–5. PMID:26454470
**2679.** Hameetman L, Szuhai K, Yavas A, et al. The role of EXT1 in nonhereditary osteochondroma: identification of homozygous deletions. J Natl Cancer Inst. 2007 Mar 7;99(5):396–406. PMID:17341731
**2680.** Hamidi O, Young WF Jr, Gruber L, et al. Outcomes of patients with metastatic phaeochromocytoma and paraganglioma: a systematic review and meta-analysis. Clin Endocrinol (Oxf). 2017 Nov;87(5):440–50. PMID:28746746
**2681.** Hamilton SR, Liu B, Parsons RE, et al. The molecular basis of Turcot's syndrome. N Engl J Med. 1995 Mar 30;332(13):839–47. PMID:7661930
**2682.** Han HJ, Lim GY, You CY. A large infiltrating fibrous hamartoma of infancy in the abdominal wall with rare associated tuberous sclerosis. Pediatr Radiol. 2009 Jul;39(7):743–6. PMID:19319513
**2683.** Han JC, Liu QR, Jones M, et al. Brain-derived neurotrophic factor and obesity in the WAGR syndrome. N Engl J Med. 2008 Aug 28;359(9):918–27. PMID:18753648
**2684.** Han JW, Kim H, Youn JK, et al. Analysis of clinical features of lipoblastoma in children. Pediatr Hematol Oncol. 2017 May;34(4):212–20. PMID:29035641
**2685.** Han JY, Yum MS, Kim EH, et al. A rare case of dysembryoplastic neuroepithelial tumor combined with encephalocraniocutaneous lipomatosis and intractable seizures. Korean J Pediatr. 2016 Nov;59 Suppl 1:S139–44. PMID:28018467
**2686.** Han Y, Qiu XS, Li QC, et al. Epididymis rhabdomyoma: a case report and literature review. Diagn Pathol. 2012 Apr 20;7:47. PMID:22520028
**2687.** Han Z, Kang P, Zhang H, et al. Prognostic value of H3K27me3 in children with ependymoma. Pediatr Blood Cancer. 2020 Mar;67(3):e28121. PMID:31850684
**2688.** Hanafy AK, Mujtaba B, Roman-Colon AM, et al. Imaging features of adrenal gland masses in the pediatric population. Abdom Radiol (NY). 2020 Apr;45(4):964–81. PMID:31538225
**2689.** Hanahan D, Weinberg RA. Hallmarks of cancer: the next generation. Cell. 2011 Mar 4;144(5):646–74. PMID:21376230
**2690.** Handa U, Palta A, Mohan H, et al. Aspiration cytology of glomus tumor: a case report. Acta Cytol. 2001 Nov-Dec;45(6):1073–6. PMID:11726106
**2691.** Hang JF, Hsu CY, Lin SC, et al. Thyroid transcription factor-1 distinguishes subependymal giant cell astrocytoma from its mimics and supports its cell origin from the progenitor cells in the medial ganglionic eminence. Mod Pathol. 2017 Mar;30(3):318–28. PMID:27910945
**2692.** Hanna SA, Tirabosco R, Amin A, et al. Dedifferentiated chordoma: a report of four cases arising 'de novo'. J Bone Joint Surg Br. 2008 May;90(5):652–6. PMID:18450635
**2692A.** Hansen MF, Johansen J, Sylvander AE, et al. Use of multigene-panel identifies pathogenic variants in several CRC-predisposing genes in patients previously tested for Lynch syndrome. Clin Genet. 2017 Oct;92(4):405–14. PMID:28195393
**2693.** Hansen MF, Koufos A, Gallie BL, et al. Osteosarcoma and retinoblastoma: a shared chromosomal mechanism revealing recessive predisposition. Proc Natl Acad Sci U S A. 1985 Sep;82(18):6216–20. PMID:2994066
**2694.** Hansen TH, Myers NB, Lee DR. Studies of two antigenic forms of Ld with disparate beta 2-microglobulin (beta 2m) associations suggest that beta 2m facilitate the folding of the alpha 1 and alpha 2 domains during de novo synthesis. J Immunol. 1988 May 15;140(10):3522–7. PMID:2452190
**2695.** Happle R. [Syndromes with vascular skin anomalies]. Hautarzt. 2019 Jul;70(7):474–80. German. PMID:31111168
**2696.** Happle R. Capillary malformations: a classification using specific names for specific skin disorders. J Eur Acad Dermatol Venereol. 2015 Dec;29(12):2295–305. PMID:25864701
**2697.** Happle R. Linear Cowden nevus: a new distinct epidermal nevus. Eur J Dermatol. 2007 Mar-Apr;17(2):133–6. PMID:17337396
**2698.** Happle R. Molecular corroboration of type 2 segmental mosaicism in various types of porokeratosis. JAMA Dermatol. 2019 May 1;155(5):531–2. PMID:30942834
**2699.** Happle R. Nevus sebaceus is a mosaic RASopathy. J Invest Dermatol. 2013 Mar;133(3):597–600. PMID:23399824
**2700.** Happle R. The group of epidermal nevus syndromes Part I. Well defined phenotypes. J Am Acad Dermatol. 2010 Jul;63(1):1–22. PMID:20542174
**2701.** Happle R. The group of epidermal nevus syndromes Part II. Less well defined phenotypes. J Am Acad Dermatol. 2010 Jul;63(1):25–30. PMID:20542175
**2702.** Happle R, Koopman RJ. Becker nevus syndrome. Am J Med Genet. 1997 Jan 31;68(3):357–61. PMID:9024572
**2703.** Happle R, Küster W. Nevus psiloliparus: a distinct fatty tissue nevus. Dermatology. 1998;197(1):6–10. PMID:9693178
**2704.** Happle R, Torrelo A. Superimposed mosaicism in tuberous sclerosis complex: a key to understanding all of the manifold manifestations? J Eur Acad Dermatol Venereol. 2020 Nov;34(11):2511–7. PMID:32396651
**2705.** Haque AK, Myers JL, Hudnall SD, et al. Pulmonary lymphomatoid granulomatosis in acquired immunodeficiency syndrome: lesions with Epstein-Barr virus infection. Mod Pathol. 1998 Apr;11(4):347–56. PMID:9578085
**2706.** Hara T, Akutsu H, Takano S, et al. Clinical and biological significance of adamantinomatous craniopharyngioma with CTNNB1 mutation. J Neurosurg. 2018 Aug 3;131(1):217–26. PMID:30074466
**2707.** Harach HR, Williams ED. Childhood thyroid cancer in England and Wales. Br J Cancer. 1995 Sep;72(3):777–83. PMID:7669594
**2707A.** Harach HR, Williams GT, Williams ED. Familial adenomatous polyposis associated thyroid carcinoma: a distinct type of follicular cell neoplasm. Histopathology. 1994 Dec;25(6):549–61. PMID:7698732
**2708.** Haralambieva E, Rosati S, van Noesel C, et al. Florid granulomatous reaction in Epstein-Barr virus-positive nonendemic Burkitt lymphomas: report of four cases. Am J Surg Pathol. 2004 Mar;28(3):379–83. PMID:15104301
**2709.** Haraldsdottir S, Rafnar T, Frankel WL, et al. Comprehensive population-wide analysis of Lynch syndrome in Iceland reveals founder mutations in MSH6 and PMS2. Nat Commun. 2017 May 3;8:14755. PMID:28466842
**2710.** Harbour JW. Molecular basis of low-penetrance retinoblastoma. Arch Ophthalmol. 2001 Nov;119(11):1699–704. PMID:11709023
**2711.** Harbour JW, Dean DC. Rb function in cell-cycle regulation and apoptosis. Nat Cell Biol. 2000 Apr;2(4):E65–7. PMID:10783254
**2712.** Harbour JW, Onken MD, Roberson ED, et al. Frequent mutation of BAP1 in metastasizing uveal melanomas. Science. 2010 Dec 3;330(6009):1410–3. PMID:21051595
**2713.** Harder A, Wesemann M, Hagel C, et al. Hybrid neurofibroma/schwannoma is overrepresented among schwannomatosis and neurofibromatosis patients. Am J Surg Pathol. 2012 May;36(5):702–9. PMID:22446939
**2714.** Harding CO, Pagon RA. Incidence of tuberous sclerosis in patients with cardiac rhabdomyoma. Am J Med Genet. 1990 Dec;37(4):443–6. PMID:2260584
**2715.** Haresh KP, Prabhakar R, Anand Rajan KD, et al. A rare case of paraganglioma of the sella with bone metastases. Pituitary. 2009;12(3):276–9. PMID:18320326
**2716.** Hargrave DR, Bouffet E, Tabori U, et al. Efficacy and safety of dabrafenib in pediatric patients with BRAF V600 mutation-positive relapsed or refractory low-grade glioma: results from a phase I/IIa study. Clin Cancer Res. 2019 Dec 15;25(24):7303–11. PMID:31811016
**2717.** Harland SJ, Cook PA, Fossa SD, et al. Intratubular germ cell neoplasia of the contralateral testis in testicular cancer: defining a high risk group. J Urol. 1998 Oct;160(4):1353–7. PMID:9751353
**2718.** Harms D. Alveolar rhabdomyosarcoma: a prognostically unfavorable rhabdomyosarcoma type and its necessary distinction from embryonal rhabdomyosarcoma. Curr Top Pathol. 1995;89:273–96. PMID:7882714
**2719.** Harms D, Jänig U. Germ cell tumours of childhood. Report of 170 cases including 59 pure and partial yolk-sac tumours. Virchows Arch A Pathol Anat Histopathol. 1986;409(2):223–39. PMID:2424170
**2720.** Harms D, Kock LR. Testicular juvenile granulosa cell and Sertoli cell tumours: a clinicopathological study of 29 cases from the Kiel Paediatric Tumour Registry. Virchows Arch. 1997 Apr;430(4):301–9. PMID:9134041
**2721.** Harms D, Schmidt D, Leuschner I. Abdominal, retroperitoneal and sacrococcygeal tumours of the newborn and the very young

infant. Report from the Kiel Paediatric Tumour Registry. Eur J Pediatr. 1989 Aug;148(8):720–8. PMID:2551691
2722. Harms D, Zahn S, Göbel U, et al. Pathology and molecular biology of teratomas in childhood and adolescence. Klin Padiatr. 2006 Nov-Dec;218(6):296–302. PMID:17080330
2723. Haroche J, Charlotte F, Arnaud L, et al. High prevalence of BRAF V600E mutations in Erdheim-Chester disease but not in other non-Langerhans cell histiocytoses. Blood. 2012 Sep 27;120(13):2700–3. PMID:22879539
2724. Haroon S, Idrees R, Zia A, et al. Ovarian sex cord stromal tumours in children and young girls - a more than two decade clinicopathological experience in a developing country, Pakistan. Asian Pac J Cancer Prev. 2014;15(3):1351–5. PMID:24606464
2725. Harrington DS, Weisenburger DD, Purtilo DT. Malignant lymphoma in the X-linked lymphoproliferative syndrome. Cancer. 1987 Apr 15;59(8):1419–29. PMID:3815312
2726. Harris BF, Harris JP, Ducey TJ, et al. Phakomatous choristoma of the orbit with involvement of the inferior oblique muscle. Ophthalmic Plast Reconstr Surg. 2019 Jan/Feb;35(1):e10–9. PMID:30407999
2727. Harris MH, Czuchlewski DR, Arber DA, et al. Genetic testing in the diagnosis and biology of acute leukemia. Am J Clin Pathol. 2019 Aug 1;152(3):322–46. PMID:31367767
2728. Harris NL, Jaffe ES, Diebold J, et al. World Health Organization classification of neoplastic diseases of the hematopoietic and lymphoid tissues: report of the Clinical Advisory Committee meeting-Airlie House, Virginia, November 1997. J Clin Oncol. 1999 Dec;17(12):3835–49. PMID:10577857
2729. Harrison CJ, Moorman AV, Schwab C, et al. An international study of intrachromosomal amplification of chromosome 21 (iAMP21): cytogenetic characterization and outcome. Leukemia. 2014 May;28(5):1015–21. PMID:24166298
2730. Harrison G, Hemmerich A, Guy C, et al. Overexpression of SOX11 and TFE3 in solid-pseudopapillary neoplasms of the pancreas. Am J Clin Pathol. 2017 Dec 20;149(1):67–75. PMID:29272888
2731. Hart AH, Hartley L, Parker K, et al. The pluripotency homeobox gene NANOG is expressed in human germ cell tumors. Cancer. 2005 Nov 15;104(10):2092–8. PMID:16206293
2732. Hart DN, Baker BW, Inglis MJ, et al. Epstein-Barr viral DNA in acute large granular lymphocyte (natural killer) leukemic cells. Blood. 1992 Apr 15;79(8):2116–23. PMID:1314113
2733. Hart J, Gardner JM, Edgar M, et al. Epithelioid schwannomas: an analysis of 58 cases including atypical variants. Am J Surg Pathol. 2016 May;40(5):704–13. PMID:26752543
2734. Hartley BE, Eze N, Trozzi M, et al. Nasal dermoids in children: a proposal for a new classification based on 103 cases at Great Ormond Street Hospital. Int J Pediatr Otorhinolaryngol. 2015 Jan;79(1):18–22. PMID:25481331
2735. Hartmann K, Escribano L, Grattan C, et al. Cutaneous manifestations in patients with mastocytosis: consensus report of the European Competence Network on Mastocytosis; the American Academy of Allergy, Asthma & Immunology; and the European Academy of Allergology and Clinical Immunology. J Allergy Clin Immunol. 2016 Jan;137(1):35–45. PMID:26476479
2736. Hartmann S, Eichenauer DA. Nodular lymphocyte predominant Hodgkin lymphoma: pathology, clinical course and relation to T-cell/histiocyte rich large B-cell lymphoma. Pathology. 2020 Jan;52(1):142–53. PMID:31785822
2737. Hartmann S, Schuhmacher B, Rausch T, et al. Highly recurrent mutations of SGK1, DUSP2 and JUNB in nodular lymphocyte predominant Hodgkin lymphoma. Leukemia. 2016 Apr;30(4):844–53. PMID:26658840
2738. Hartmann S, Winkelmann R, Metcalf RA, et al. Immunoarchitectural patterns of progressive transformation of germinal centers with and without nodular lymphocyte-predominant Hodgkin lymphoma. Hum Pathol. 2015 Nov;46(11):1655–61. PMID:26410017
2739. Harutyunyan AS, Krug B, Chen H, et al. H3K27M induces defective chromatin spread of PRC2-mediated repressive H3K27me2/me3 and is essential for glioma tumorigenesis. Nat Commun. 2019 Mar 19;10(1):1262. PMID:30890717
2740. Harvell JD, Bastian BC, LeBoit PE. Persistent (recurrent) Spitz nevi: a histopathologic, immunohistochemical, and molecular pathologic study of 22 cases. Am J Surg Pathol. 2002 May;26(5):654–61. PMID:11979096
2741. Harvell JD, Meehan SA, LeBoit PE. Spitz's nevi with halo reaction: a histopathologic study of 17 cases. J Cutan Pathol. 1997 Nov;24(10):611–9. PMID:9449488
2742. Hasegawa D. The current perspective of low-grade myelodysplastic syndrome in children. Int J Hematol. 2016 Apr;103(4):360–4. PMID:26939774
2743. Hasegawa D, Chen X, Hirabayashi S, et al. Clinical characteristics and treatment outcome in 65 cases with refractory cytopenia of childhood defined according to the WHO 2008 classification. Br J Haematol. 2014 Sep;166(5):758–66. PMID:24894311
2744. Hasegawa T, Hirose T, Sakamoto R, et al. Mechanism of pain in osteoid osteomas: an immunohistochemical study. Histopathology. 1993 May;22(5):487–91. PMID:8344659
2745. Hasegawa T, Matsuno Y, Shimoda T, et al. Proximal-type epithelioid sarcoma: a clinicopathologic study of 20 cases. Mod Pathol. 2001 Jul;14(7):655–63. PMID:11454997
2746. Hasegawa T, Seki K, Ono K, et al. Angiomatoid (malignant) fibrous histiocytoma: a peculiar low-grade tumor showing immunophenotypic heterogeneity and ultrastructural variations. Pathol Int. 2000 Sep;50(9):731–8. PMID:11012987
2747. Hashii Y, Okuda T, Ohta H, et al. Pediatric myeloid/NK cell precursor lymphoma/leukemia expressing T/NK immunophenotype markers. Int J Hematol. 2010 Apr;91(3):525–9. PMID:20146030
2748. Hashimoto M, Yamashita Y, Mori N. Immunohistochemical detection of CD79a expression in precursor T cell lymphoblastic lymphoma/leukaemias. J Pathol. 2002 Jul;197(3):341–7. PMID:12115880
2749. Hashimoto N, Handa H, Nishi S. Intracranial and intraspinal dissemination from a growth hormone-secreting pituitary tumor. Case report. J Neurosurg. 1986 Jan;64(1):140–4. PMID:3941337
2750. Hashimoto T, Fujimoto M, Nishikori M, et al. Plasmacytic ALK-positive large B-cell lymphoma: a potential mimic of extramedullary plasmacytoma. Pathol Int. 2014 Jun;64(6):292–4. PMID:24965113
2751. Hasle H. Myelodysplastic and myeloproliferative disorders of childhood. Hematology Am Soc Hematol Educ Program. 2016 Dec 2;2016(1):598–604. PMID:27913534
2752. Hasle H. Myelodysplastic syndromes in childhood–classification, epidemiology, and treatment. Leuk Lymphoma. 1994 Mar;13(1-2):11–26. PMID:8025513
2753. Hasle H, Abrahamsson J, Arola M, et al. Myeloid leukemia in children 4 years or older with Down syndrome often lacks GATA1 mutation and cytogenetics and risk of relapse are more akin to sporadic AML. Leukemia. 2008 Jul;22(7):1428–30. PMID:18059480
2754. Hasle H, Clemmensen IH, Mikkelsen M. Risks of leukaemia and solid tumours in individuals with Down's syndrome. Lancet. 2000 Jan 15;355(9199):165–9. PMID:10675114
2754A. Hasle H, Kerndrup G, Jacobsen BB. Childhood myelodysplastic syndrome in Denmark: incidence and predisposing conditions. Leukemia. 1995 Sep;9(9):1569–72. PMID:7658725
2755. Hasle H, Niemeyer CM. Advances in the prognostication and management of advanced MDS in children. Br J Haematol. 2011 Jul;154(2):185–95. PMID:21554264
2756. Hasle H, Niemeyer CM, Chessells JM, et al. A pediatric approach to the WHO classification of myelodysplastic and myeloproliferative diseases. Leukemia. 2003 Feb;17(2):277–82. PMID:12592323
2757. Hasle H, Wadsworth LD, Massing BG, et al. A population-based study of childhood myelodysplastic syndrome in British Columbia, Canada. Br J Haematol. 1999 Sep;106(4):1027–32. PMID:10520007
2758. Hassan M, Butler E, Wilson R, et al. Novel PDGFRB rearrangement in multifocal infantile myofibromatosis is tumorigenic and sensitive to imatinib. Cold Spring Harb Mol Case Stud. 2019 Oct 23;5(5):a004440. PMID:31645346
2759. Hassan SF, Stephens E, Fallon SC, et al. Characterizing pilomatricomas in children: a single institution experience. J Pediatr Surg. 2013 Jul;48(7):1551–6. PMID:23895971
2760. Hasselblatt M, Böhm C, Tatenhorst L, et al. Identification of novel diagnostic markers for choroid plexus tumors: a microarray-based approach. Am J Surg Pathol. 2006 Jan;30(1):66–74. PMID:16330944
2761. Hasselblatt M, Gesk S, Oyen F, et al. Nonsense mutation and inactivation of SMARCA4 (BRG1) in an atypical teratoid/rhabdoid tumor showing retained SMARCB1 (INI1) expression. Am J Surg Pathol. 2011 Jun;35(6):933–5. PMID:21566516
2762. Hasselblatt M, Isken S, Linge A, et al. High-resolution genomic analysis suggests the absence of recurrent genomic alterations other than SMARCB1 aberrations in atypical teratoid/rhabdoid tumors. Genes Chromosomes Cancer. 2013 Feb;52(2):185–90. PMID:23074045
2763. Hasselblatt M, Jeibmann A, Guerry M, et al. Choroid plexus papilloma with neuropil-like islands. Am J Surg Pathol. 2008 Jan;32(1):162–6. PMID:18162784
2764. Hasselblatt M, Nagel I, Oyen F, et al. SMARCA4-mutated atypical teratoid/rhabdoid tumors are associated with inherited germline alterations and poor prognosis. Acta Neuropathol. 2014 Sep;128(3):453–6. PMID:25060813
2765. Hasselblatt M, Oyen F, Gesk S, et al. Cribriform neuroepithelial tumor (CRINET): a nonrhabdoid ventricular tumor with INI1 loss and relatively favorable prognosis. J Neuropathol Exp Neurol. 2009 Dec;68(12):1249–55. PMID:19915490
2766. Hasselblatt M, Paulus W. Sensitivity and specificity of epithelial membrane antigen staining patterns in ependymomas. Acta Neuropathol. 2003 Oct;106(4):385–8. PMID:12898159
2767. Hasselblatt M, Thomas C, Hovestadt V, et al. Poorly differentiated chordoma with SMARCB1/INI1 loss: a distinct molecular entity with dismal prognosis. Acta Neuropathol. 2016 Jul;132(1):149–51. PMID:27067307
2768. Hasselblatt M, Thomas C, Nemes K, et al. Tyrosinase immunohistochemistry can be employed for the diagnosis of atypical teratoid/rhabdoid tumours of the tyrosinase subgroup (ATRT-TYR). Neuropathol Appl Neurobiol. 2020 Feb;46(2):186–9. PMID:31077608
2769. Hasserjian RP, Harris NL. NK-cell lymphomas and leukemias: a spectrum of tumors with variable manifestations and immunophenotype. Am J Clin Pathol. 2007 Jun;127(6):860–8. PMID:17509983
2770. Haston S, Pozzi S, Carreno G, et al. MAPK pathway control of stem cell proliferation and differentiation in the embryonic pituitary provides insights into the pathogenesis of papillary craniopharyngioma. Development. 2017 Jun 15;144(12):2141–52. PMID:28506993
2771. Hata JL, Correa H, Krishnan C, et al. Diagnostic utility of PHOX2B in primary and treated neuroblastoma and in neuroblastoma metastatic to the bone marrow. Arch Pathol Lab Med. 2015 Apr;139(4):543–6. PMID:25822764
2772. Hatakeyama S, Satoh M, Yoshimura N, et al. Immunocytochemical localization of bone morphogenetic proteins (BMPs) in salivary gland pleomorphic adenoma. J Oral Pathol Med. 1994 May;23(5):232–6. PMID:7519267
2773. Hattab EM, Tu PH, Wilson JD, et al. OCT4 immunohistochemistry is superior to placental alkaline phosphatase (PLAP) in the diagnosis of central nervous system germinoma. Am J Surg Pathol. 2005 Mar;29(3):368–71. PMID:15725806
2774. Hatzipantelis E, Panagopoulou P, Sidi-Fragandrea V, et al. Carcinoid tumors of the appendix in children: experience from a tertiary center in northern Greece. J Pediatr Gastroenterol Nutr. 2010 Nov;51(5):622–5. PMID:20948448
2775. Hauben EI, Weeden S, Pringle J, et al. Does the histological subtype of high-grade central osteosarcoma influence the response to treatment with chemotherapy and does it affect overall survival? A study on 570 patients of two consecutive trials of the European Osteosarcoma Intergroup. Eur J Cancer. 2002 Jun;38(9):1218–25. PMID:12044509
2776. Hauck F, Voss R, Urban C, et al. Intrinsic and extrinsic causes of malignancies in patients with primary immunodeficiency disorders. J Allergy Clin Immunol. 2018 Jan;141(1):59–68.e4. PMID:28669558
2777. Haugen BR, Alexander EK, Bible KC, et al. 2015 American Thyroid Association management guidelines for adult patients with thyroid nodules and differentiated thyroid cancer: the American Thyroid Association guidelines task force on thyroid nodules and differentiated thyroid cancer. Thyroid. 2016 Jan;26(1):1–133. PMID:26462967
2778. Haugh AM, Njauw CN, Bubley JA, et al. Genotypic and phenotypic features of BAP1 cancer syndrome: a report of 8 new families and review of cases in the literature. JAMA Dermatol. 2017 Oct 1;153(10):999–1006. PMID:28793149
2779. Haupt R, Minkov M, Astigarraga I, et al. Langerhans cell histiocytosis (LCH): guidelines for diagnosis, clinical work-up, and treatment for patients till the age of 18 years. Pediatr Blood Cancer. 2013 Feb;60(2):175–84. PMID:23109216
2780. Hauser BM, Lau A, Gupta S, et al. The epigenomics of pituitary adenoma. Front Endocrinol (Lausanne). 2019 May 14;10:290. PMID:31139150
2781. Havelange V, Ameye G, Théate I, et al. The peculiar 11q-gain/loss aberration reported in a subset of MYC-negative high-grade B-cell lymphomas can also occur in a MYC-rearranged lymphoma. Cancer Genet. 2016 Mar;209(3):117–8. PMID:26776268
2782. Håvik AL, Bruland O, Myrseth E, et al. Genetic landscape of sporadic vestibular schwannoma. J Neurosurg. 2018 Mar;128(3):911–22. PMID:28409725

**2783.** Hawkins DS, Chi YY, Anderson JR, et al. Addition of vincristine and irinotecan to vincristine, dactinomycin, and cyclophosphamide does not improve outcome for intermediate-risk rhabdomyosarcoma: a report from the Children's Oncology Group. J Clin Oncol. 2018 Sep 20;36(27):2770–7. PMID:30091945

**2784.** Hawkins E, Heifetz SA, Giller R, et al. The prepubertal testis (prenatal and postnatal): its relationship to intratubular germ cell neoplasia: a combined Pediatric Oncology Group and Children's Cancer Study Group. Hum Pathol. 1997 Apr;28(4):404–10. PMID:9104938

**2785.** Hawkins EP, Finegold MJ, Hawkins HK, et al. Nongerminomatous malignant germ cell tumors in children. A review of 89 cases from the Pediatric Oncology Group, 1971-1984. Cancer. 1986 Dec 15;58(12):2579–84. PMID:3022907

**2786.** Hay ID, Johnson TR, Kaggal S, et al. Papillary Thyroid Carcinoma (PTC) in children and adults: comparison of initial presentation and long-term postoperative outcome in 4432 patients consecutively treated at the Mayo Clinic during eight decades (1936-2015). World J Surg. 2018 Feb;42(2):329–42. PMID:29030676

**2787.** Hayashi K, Inoshita N, Kawaguchi K, et al. The USP8 mutational status may predict drug susceptibility in corticotroph adenomas of Cushing's disease. Eur J Endocrinol. 2016 Feb;174(2):213–26. PMID:26578638

**2788.** Hayashi RJ, Winter SS, Dunsmore KP, et al. Successful outcomes of newly diagnosed T lymphoblastic lymphoma: results from Children's Oncology Group AALL0434. J Clin Oncol. 2020 Sep 10;38(26):3062–70. PMID:32552472

**2789.** Haybittle JL, Hayhoe FG, Easterling MJ, et al. Review of British National Lymphoma Investigation studies of Hodgkin's disease and development of prognostic index. Lancet. 1985 Apr 27;1(8435):967–72. PMID:2859421

**2790.** Hays DM, Newton W Jr, Soule EH, et al. Mortality among children with rhabdomyosarcomas of the alveolar histologic subtype. J Pediatr Surg. 1983 Aug;18(4):412–7. PMID:6620082

**2791.** Hayter JP, Robertson JM. Familial occurrence of pleomorphic adenoma of the parotid gland. Br J Oral Maxillofac Surg. 1990 Oct;28(5):333–4. PMID:2174255

**2792.** Hazelbag HM, Fleuren GJ, Cornelisse CJ, et al. DNA aberrations in the epithelial cell component of adamantinoma of long bones. Am J Pathol. 1995 Dec;147(6):1770–9. PMID:7495301

**2793.** Hazelbag HM, Fleuren GJ, vd Broek LJ, et al. Adamantinoma of the long bones: keratin subclass immunoreactivity pattern with reference to its histogenesis. Am J Surg Pathol. 1993 Dec;17(12):1225–33. PMID:7694513

**2794.** Hazelbag HM, Laforga JB, Roels HJ, et al. Dedifferentiated adamantinoma with revertant mesenchymal phenotype. Am J Surg Pathol. 2003 Dec;27(12):1530–7. PMID:14657712

**2795.** Hazelbag HM, Wessels JW, Mollevangers P, et al. Cytogenetic analysis of adamantinoma of long bones: further indications for a common histogenesis with osteofibrous dysplasia. Cancer Genet Cytogenet. 1997 Aug;97(1):5–11. PMID:9242211

**2796.** He H, Trpkov K, Martinek P, et al. "High-grade oncocytic renal tumor": morphologic, immunohistochemical, and molecular genetic study of 14 cases. Virchows Arch. 2018 Dec;473(6):725–38. PMID:30232607

**2797.** He WG, Yan Y, Tang W, et al. Clinical and biological features of neuroblastic tumors: a comparison of neuroblastoma and ganglioneuroblastoma. Oncotarget. 2017 Jun 6;8(23):37730–9. PMID:28465480

**2798.** He X, Pang Z, Zhang X, et al. Consistent Amplification of FRS2 and MDM2 in Low-grade Osteosarcoma: a Genetic Study of 22 Cases With Clinicopathologic Analysis. Am J Surg Pathol. 2018 Sep;42(9):1143–55. PMID:30001240

**2799.** He Y, Yang KX, Jiang W, et al. Sclerosing stromal tumor of the ovary in a 4-year-old girl with characteristics of an ovarian signet-ring stromal tumor. Pathol Res Pract. 2010 May 15;206(5):338–41. PMID:19604650

**2800.** Healey JH, Ghelman B. Osteoid osteoma and osteoblastoma. Current concepts and recent advances. Clin Orthop Relat Res. 1986 Mar; (204):76–85. PMID:3956019

**2801.** Heaney AP. Clinical review: pituitary carcinoma: difficult diagnosis and treatment. J Clin Endocrinol Metab. 2011 Dec;96(12):3649–60. PMID:21956419

**2802.** Hébert-Blouin MN, Scheithauer BW, Amrami KK, et al. Fibromatosis: a potential sequela of neuromuscular choristoma. J Neurosurg. 2012 Feb;116(2):399–408. PMID:21819193

**2803.** Heck A, Emblem KE, Casar-Borota O, et al. Quantitative analyses of T2-weighted MRI as a potential marker for response to somatostatin analogs in newly diagnosed acromegaly. Endocrine. 2016 May;52(2):333–43. PMID:26475495

**2804.** Heck JE, Lee PC, Wu CK, et al. Gestational risk factors and childhood cancers: a cohort study in Taiwan. Int J Cancer. 2020 Sep 1;147(5):1343–53. PMID:32020595

**2805.** Hedrick HL, Flake AW, Crombleholme TM, et al. Sacrococcygeal teratoma: prenatal assessment, fetal intervention, and outcome. J Pediatr Surg. 2004 Mar;39(3):430–8. PMID:15017565

**2806.** Heenan PJ, Quirk CJ, Papadimitriou JM. Epithelioid sarcoma. A diagnostic problem. Am J Dermatopathol. 1986 Apr;8(2):95–104. PMID:3717528

**2807.** Heerema NA, Carroll AJ, Devidas M, et al. Intrachromosomal amplification of chromosome 21 is associated with inferior outcomes in children with acute lymphoblastic leukemia treated in contemporary standard-risk children's oncology group studies: a report from the children's oncology group. J Clin Oncol. 2013 Sep 20;31(27):3397–402. PMID:23940221

**2808.** Heerema-McKenney A, Harrison MR, Bratton B, et al. Congenital teratoma: a clinicopathologic study of 22 fetal and neonatal tumors. Am J Surg Pathol. 2005 Jan;29(1):29–38. PMID:15613854

**2809.** Heerema-McKenney A, Leuschner I, Smith N, et al. Nested stromal epithelial tumor of the liver: six cases of a distinctive pediatric neoplasm with frequent calcifications and association with cushing syndrome. Am J Surg Pathol. 2005 Jan;29(1):10–20. PMID:15613852

**2810.** Heerema-McKenney A, Popek EJ, De Paepe ME, et al. Diagnostic pathology: placenta. 1st ed. Philadelphia (PA): Elsevier; 2015. Section II-8, pp. 6–7.

**2811.** Heffner DK. Problems in pediatric otorhinolaryngic pathology, III. Teratoid and neural tumors of the nose, sinonasal tract, and nasopharynx. Int J Pediatr Otorhinolaryngol. 1983 Sep;6(1):1–21. PMID:6668102

**2812.** Heffner DK. Problems in pediatric otorhinolaryngic pathology. I. Sinonasal and nasopharyngeal tumors and masses with myxoid features. Int J Pediatr Otorhinolaryngol. 1983 Jan;5(1):77–91. PMID:6302014

**2813.** Heffner DK. Sinonasal myxomas and fibromyxomas in children. Ear Nose Throat J. 1993 May;72(5):365–8. PMID:8334970

**2814.** Heffner DK, Thompson LD, Schall DG, et al. Pharyngeal dermoids ("hairy polyps") as accessory auricles. Ann Otol Rhinol Laryngol. 1996 Oct;105(10):819–24. PMID:8865778

**2815.** Hehlmann R. How I treat CML blast crisis. Blood. 2012 Jul 26;120(4):737–47. PMID:22653972

**2816.** Heide S, Masliah-Planchon J, Isidor B, et al. Oncologic phenotype of peripheral neuroblastic tumors associated with PHOX2B non-polyalanine repeat expansion mutations. Pediatr Blood Cancer. 2016 Jan;63(1):71–7. PMID:26375764

**2817.** Heider A, Arnold S, Jing X. Bethesda system for reporting thyroid cytopathology in pediatric thyroid nodules: experience of a tertiary care referral center. Arch Pathol Lab Med. 2020 Apr;144(4):473–7. PMID:31403334

**2818.** Heifetz SA, Cushing B, Giller R, et al. Immature teratomas in children: pathologic considerations: a report from the combined Pediatric Oncology Group/Children's Cancer Group. Am J Surg Pathol. 1998 Sep;22(9):1115–24. PMID:9737245

**2819.** Heikinheimo K, Huhtala JM, Thiel A, et al. The mutational profile of unicystic ameloblastoma. J Dent Res. 2019 Jan;98(1):54–60. PMID:30216733

**2820.** Heiland DH, Staszewski O, Hirsch M, et al. Malignant transformation of a dysembryoplastic neuroepithelial tumor (DNET) characterized by genome-wide methylation analysis. J Neuropathol Exp Neurol. 2016 Apr;75(4):358–65. PMID:26921879

**2821.** Heimbach JK, Kulik LM, Finn RS, et al. AASLD guidelines for the treatment of hepatocellular carcinoma. Hepatology. 2018 Jan;67(1):358–80. PMID:28130846

**2822.** Heimdal K, Evensen SA, Fosså SD, et al. Karyotyping of a hematologic neoplasia developing shortly after treatment for cerebral extragonadal germ cell tumor. Cancer Genet Cytogenet. 1991 Nov;57(1):41–6. PMID:1756483

**2823.** Hein K, Dell R, Cohen MI. Self-detection of a breast mass in adolescent females. J Adolesc Health Care. 1982 Aug;3(1):15–7. PMID:7118680

**2824.** Hein KD, Mulliken JB, Kozakewich HP, et al. Venous malformations of skeletal muscle. Plast Reconstr Surg. 2002 Dec;110(7):1625–35. PMID:12447041

**2825.** Heinze A, Kuemmet TJ, Chiu YE, et al. Longitudinal study of pediatric urticaria pigmentosa. Pediatr Dermatol. 2017 Mar;34(2):144–9. PMID:28133781

**2826.** Heiss NS, Knight SW, Vulliamy TJ, et al. X-linked dyskeratosis congenita is caused by mutations in a highly conserved gene with putative nucleolar functions. Nat Genet. 1998 May;19(1):32–8. PMID:9590285

**2827.** Hejmadi RK, Gearty JC, Waddell C, et al. Mesonephric hyperplasia can cause abnormal cervical smears: report of three cases with review of literature. Cytopathology. 2005 Oct;16(5):240–3. PMID:16181310

**2828.** Helgager J, Lidov HG, Mahadevan NR, et al. A novel GIT2-BRAF fusion in pilocytic astrocytoma. Diagn Pathol. 2017 Nov 15;12(1):82. PMID:29141672

**2829.** Hellemans J, Preobrazhenska O, Willaert A, et al. Loss-of-function mutations in LEMD3 result in osteopoikilosis, Buschke-Ollendorff syndrome and melorheostosis. Nat Genet. 2004 Nov;36(11):1213–8. PMID:15489854

**2830.** Helming KC, Wang X, Roberts CWM. Vulnerabilities of mutant SWI/SNF complexes in cancer. Cancer Cell. 2014 Sep 8;26(3):309–17. PMID:25203320

**2831.** Haggstrom AN, Drolet BA, Baselga E, et al. Prospective study of infantile hemangiomas: demographic, prenatal, and perinatal characteristics. J Pediatr. 2007 Mar;150(3):291–4. PMID:17307549

**2832.** Hempenstall LE, Siriwardana AR, Desai DJ. Investigation of a renal mass: diagnosing renal paraganglioma. Urol Case Rep. 2018 Aug 9;21:8–9. PMID:30116720

**2833.** Hemsrichart V, Charoenkwan P. Fatal bilateral congenital mesenchymal hamartoma of the chest wall. J Med Assoc Thai. 2007 Nov;90(11):2519–23. PMID:18181344

**2834.** Henderson H, Peng YJ, Salter DM. Anti-calponin 1 antibodies highlight intracytoplasmic inclusions of infantile digital fibromatosis. Histopathology. 2014 Apr;64(5):752–5. PMID:24117680

**2835.** Henderson L, Fehily C, Folaranmi S, et al. Management and outcome of neuroendocrine tumours of the appendix-a two centre UK experience. J Pediatr Surg. 2014 Oct;49(10):1513–7. PMID:25280658

**2836.** Hendrick SJ, Sanchez RL, Blackwell SJ, et al. Striated muscle hamartoma: description of two cases. Pediatr Dermatol. 1986 Feb;3(2):153–7. PMID:3952032

**2837.** Hendy GN, Cole DE. Genetic defects associated with familial and sporadic hyperparathyroidism. Front Horm Res. 2013;41:149–65. PMID:23652676

**2838.** Heng YK, Koh MJ, Giam YC, et al. Pediatric mycosis fungoides in Singapore: a series of 46 children. Pediatr Dermatol. 2014 Jul-Aug;31(4):477–82. PMID:24890628

**2839.** Henke AC, Kelley CM, Jensen CS, et al. Fine-needle aspiration cytology of pancreatoblastoma. Diagn Cytopathol. 2001 Aug;25(2):118–21. PMID:11477717

**2840.** Henley JD, Young RH, Wade CL, et al. Seminomas with exclusive intertubular growth: a report of 12 clinically and grossly inconspicuous tumors. Am J Surg Pathol. 2004 Sep;28(9):1163–8. PMID:15316315

**2841.** Hennessy MJ, Elwes RD, Rabe-Hesketh S, et al. Prognostic factors in the surgical treatment of medically intractable epilepsy associated with mesial temporal sclerosis. Acta Neurol Scand. 2001 Jun;103(6):344–50. PMID:11421846

**2842.** Hennigar RA, Beckwith JB. Nephrogenic adenofibroma. A novel kidney tumor of young people. Am J Surg Pathol. 1992 Apr;16(4):325–34. PMID:1373578

**2843.** Henrickson SE, Dolan JG, Forbes LR, et al. Gain-of-function STAT1 mutation with familial lymphadenopathy and Hodgkin lymphoma. Front Pediatr. 2019 Apr 30;7:160. PMID:31114772

**2844.** Henriksson G, Westrin KM, Carlsöö B, et al. Recurrent primary pleomorphic adenomas of salivary gland origin: intrasurgical rupture, histopathologic features, and pseudopodia. Cancer. 1998 Feb 15;82(4):617–20. PMID:9477091

**2845.** Henry SC, Walsh PC, Rotner MB. Choriocarcinoma of the testis. J Urol. 1974 Jul;112(1):105–8. PMID:4134907

**2846.** Henske EP, Wessner LL, Golden J, et al. Loss of tuberin in both subependymal giant cell astrocytomas and angiomyolipomas supports a two-hit model for the pathogenesis of tuberous sclerosis tumors. Am J Pathol. 1997 Dec;151(6):1639–47. PMID:9403714

**2847.** Henter JI, Horne A, Aricó M, et al. HLH-2004: diagnostic and therapeutic guidelines for hemophagocytic lymphohistiocytosis. Pediatr Blood Cancer. 2007 Feb;48(2):124–31. PMID:16937360

**2848.** Herath M, Parameswaran V, Thompson M, et al. Paediatric and young adult manifestations and outcomes of multiple endocrine neoplasia type 1. Clin Endocrinol (Oxf). 2019 Nov;91(5):633–8. PMID:31348545

**2849.** Heravi-Moussavi A, Anglesio MS, Cheng SW, et al. Recurrent somatic DICER1 mutations in nonepithelial ovarian cancers. N Engl J Med. 2012 Jan 19;366(3):234–42. PMID:22187960

**2850.** Herber M, Mertz P, Dieudonné Y, et al. Primary immunodeficiencies and lymphoma: a

systematic review of literature. Leuk Lymphoma. 2020 Feb;61(2):274–84. PMID:31580160
**2851.** Herbrueggen H, Mueller S, Rohde J, et al. Treatment and outcome of IG-MYC+ neoplasms with precursor B-cell phenotype in childhood and adolescence. Leukemia. 2020 Mar;34(3):942–6. PMID:31611629
**2852.** Hered RW, Hiles DA. Epibulbar osseous choristoma and ectopic lacrimal gland underlying a dermolipoma. J Pediatr Ophthalmol Strabismus. 1987 Sep-Oct;24(5):255–8. PMID:3681614
**2853.** Héritier S, Emile JF, Barkaoui MA, et al. BRAF mutation correlates with high-risk Langerhans cell histiocytosis and increased resistance to first-line therapy. J Clin Oncol. 2016 Sep 1;34(25):3023–30. PMID:27382093
**2854.** Herman TE, McAlister WH, Dehner LP, et al. Dedifferentiated chondrosarcoma in childhood: report of a case. Pediatr Radiol. 1995 Nov;25 Suppl 1:S140–2. PMID:8577508
**2855.** Herman TE, Siegel MJ, Dehner LP. CT of pancreatoblastoma derived from the dorsal pancreatic anlage. J Comput Assist Tomogr. 1994 Jul-Aug;18(4):648–50. PMID:8040456
**2856.** Herman V, Fagin J, Gonsky R, et al. Clonal origin of pituitary adenomas. J Clin Endocrinol Metab. 1990 Dec;71(6):1427–33. PMID:1977759
**2857.** Hernandez KG, Ezzat S, Morel CF, et al. Familial pheochromocytoma and renal cell carcinoma syndrome: TMEM127 as a novel candidate gene for the association. Virchows Arch. 2015 Jun;466(6):727–32. PMID:25800244
**2858.** Hernández L, Pinyol M, Hernández S, et al. TRK-fused gene (TFG) is a new partner of ALK in anaplastic large cell lymphoma producing two structurally different TFG-ALK translocations. Blood. 1999 Nov 1;94(9):3265–8. PMID:10556217
**2859.** Hernandez RK, Maegbaek ML, Liede A, et al. Bone metastases, skeletal-related events, and survival among children with cancer in Denmark. J Pediatr Hematol Oncol. 2014 Oct;36(7):528–33. PMID:24390452
**2860.** Hernández-Monjaraz B, Santiago-Osorio E, Ledesma-Martínez E, et al. Retrieval of a periodontally compromised tooth by allogeneic grafting of mesenchymal stem cells from dental pulp: a case report. J Int Med Res. 2018 Jul;46(7):2983–93. PMID:29911458
**2861.** Hernández-Núñez A, Nájera Botello L, Romero Maté A, et al. Retrospective study of pilomatricoma: 261 tumors in 239 patients. Actas Dermosifiliogr. 2014 Sep;105(7):699–705. PMID:24838222
**2862.** Hernández-Ramírez LC, Gam R, Valdés N, et al. Loss-of-function mutations in the CABLES1 gene are a novel cause of Cushing's disease. Endocr Relat Cancer. 2017 Aug;24(8):379–92. PMID:28533356
**2863.** Herndier BG, Sanchez HC, Chang KL, et al. High prevalence of Epstein-Barr virus in the Reed-Sternberg cells of HIV-associated Hodgkin's disease. Am J Pathol. 1993 Apr;142(4):1073–9. PMID:8386441
**2864.** Herrick MK, Rubinstein LJ. The cytological differentiating potential of pineal parenchymal neoplasms (true pinealomas). A clinicopathological study of 28 tumours. Brain. 1979 Jun;102(2):289–320. PMID:88244
**2865.** Herrington H, Adil E, Moritz E, et al. Update on current evaluation and management of pediatric nasal dermoid. Laryngoscope. 2016 Sep;126(9):2151–60. PMID:26891409
**2866.** Herrmann JL, Allan A, Trapp KM, et al. Pilomatrix carcinoma: 13 new cases and review of the literature with emphasis on predictors of metastasis. J Am Acad Dermatol. 2014 Jul;71(1):38–43.e2. PMID:24739254
**2867.** Herrod HG, Dow LW, Sullivan JL. Persistent epstein-barr virus infection mimicking juvenile chronic myelogenous leukemia: immunologic and hematologic studies. Blood. 1983 Jun;61(6):1098–104. PMID:6301580
**2868.** Hershkovitz D, Amitai B, Sprecher E. Familial cutaneous collagenomas resulting from a novel mutation in LEMD3. Br J Dermatol. 2007 Feb;156(2):375–7. PMID:17223882
**2869.** Hersmus R, Kalfa N, de Leeuw B, et al. FOXL2 and SOX9 as parameters of female and male gonadal differentiation in patients with various forms of disorders of sex development (DSD). J Pathol. 2008 May;215(1):31–8. PMID:18348162
**2870.** Hersmus R, Stoop H, van de Geijn GJ, et al. Prevalence of c-KIT mutations in gonadoblastoma and dysgerminomas of patients with disorders of sex development (DSD) and ovarian dysgerminomas. PLoS One. 2012;7(8):e43952. PMID:22937135
**2871.** Hersmus R, Stoop H, White SJ, et al. Delayed recognition of Disorders of Sex Development (DSD): a missed opportunity for early diagnosis of malignant germ cell tumors. Int J Endocrinol. 2012;2012:671209. PMID:22315593
**2872.** Hersmus R, van der Zwan YG, Stoop H, et al. A 46,XY female DSD patient with bilateral gonadoblastoma, a novel SRY missense mutation combined with a WT1 KTS splice-site mutation. PLoS One. 2012;7(7):e40858. PMID:22815844
**2873.** Hertel JD, Huettner PC, Dehner LP, et al. The chromosome Y-linked testis-specific protein locus TSPY1 is characteristically present in gonadoblastoma. Hum Pathol. 2010 Nov;41(11):1544–9. PMID:20656323
**2874.** Hes FJ, Nielsen M, Bik EC, et al. Somatic APC mosaicism: an underestimated cause of polyposis coli. Gut. 2008 Jan;57(1):71–6. PMID:17604324
**2875.** Hettmer S, Archer NM, Somers GR, et al. Anaplastic rhabdomyosarcoma in TP53 germline mutation carriers. Cancer. 2014 Apr 1;120(7):1068–75. PMID:24382691
**2876.** Hettmer S, Teot LA, Kozakewich H, et al. Myogenic tumors in nevoid Basal cell carcinoma syndrome. J Pediatr Hematol Oncol. 2015 Mar;37(2):147–9. PMID:24517962
**2877.** Hettmer S, Teot LA, van Hummelen P, et al. Mutations in Hedgehog pathway genes in fetal rhabdomyomas. J Pathol. 2013 Sep;231(1):44–52. PMID:23780909
**2878.** Heukamp LC, Thor T, Schramm A, et al. Targeted expression of mutated ALK induces neuroblastoma in transgenic mice. Sci Transl Med. 2012 Jul 4;4(141):141ra91. PMID:22764207
**2879.** Hewer E, Knecht U, Ulrich CT. Two adult cases of massively calcified low-grade glioma: expanding clinical spectrum of an emerging entity. Neuropathology. 2016 Oct;36(5):508–9. PMID:26991895
**2880.** Hewer E, Vajtai I. Consistent nuclear expression of thyroid transcription factor 1 in subependymal giant cell astrocytomas suggests lineage-restricted histogenesis. Clin Neuropathol. 2015 May-Jun;34(3):128–31. PMID:25669749
**2881.** Heymann S, Delaloge S, Rahal A, et al. Radio-induced malignancies after breast cancer postoperative radiotherapy in patients with Li-Fraumeni syndrome. Radiat Oncol. 2010 Nov 8;5:104. PMID:21059199
**2882.** Hibbard MK, Kozakewich HP, Dal Cin P, et al. PLAG1 fusion oncogenes in lipoblastoma. Cancer Res. 2000 Sep 1;60(17):4869–72. PMID:10987300
**2883.** Hicks D, Rafiee G, Schwalbe EC, et al. The molecular landscape and associated clinical experience in infant medulloblastoma: prognostic significance of second-generation subtypes. Neuropathol Appl Neurobiol. 2021 Feb;47(2):236–50. PMID:32779246
**2884.** Hicks J, Flaitz C. Mucoepidermoid carcinoma of salivary glands in children and adolescents: assessment of proliferation markers. Oral Oncol. 2000 Sep;36(5):454–60. PMID:10964053
**2885.** Hicks MJ, Roth JR, Kozinetz CA, et al. Clinicopathologic features of osteosarcoma in patients with Rothmund-Thomson syndrome. J Clin Oncol. 2007 Feb 1;25(4):370–5. PMID:17264332
**2886.** Hidalgo ET, Orillac C, Kvint S, et al. Quality of life, hypothalamic obesity, and sexual function in adulthood two decades after primary gross-total resection for childhood craniopharyngioma. Childs Nerv Syst. 2020 Feb;36(2):281–9. PMID:31222446
**2887.** Higgins JP, Warnke RA. CD30 expression is common in mediastinal large B-cell lymphoma. Am J Clin Pathol. 1999 Aug;112(2):241–7. PMID:10439805
**2888.** Higham CS, Dombi E, Rogiers A, et al. The characteristics of 76 atypical neurofibromas as precursors to neurofibromatosis 1 associated malignant peripheral nerve sheath tumors. Neuro Oncol. 2018 May 18;20(6):818–25. PMID:29409029
**2889.** Hijiya N, Millot F, Suttorp M. Chronic myeloid leukemia in children: clinical findings, management, and unanswered questions. Pediatr Clin North Am. 2015 Feb;62(1):107–19. PMID:25435115
**2890.** Hildebrandt RH, Rouse RV, Longacre TA. Value of inhibin in the identification of granulosa cell tumors of the ovary. Hum Pathol. 1997 Dec;28(12):1387–95. PMID:9416696
**2891.** Hill DA, Dehner LP, White FV, et al. Gliomatosis peritonei as a complication of a ventriculoperitoneal shunt: case report and review of the literature. J Pediatr Surg. 2000 Mar;35(3):497–9. PMID:10726696
**2892.** Hill DA, Ivanovich J, Priest JR, et al. DICER1 mutations in familial pleuropulmonary blastoma. Science. 2009 Aug 21;325(5943):965. PMID:19556464
**2893.** Hill DA, Jarzembowski JA, Priest JR, et al. Type I pleuropulmonary blastoma: pathology and biology study of 51 cases from the international pleuropulmonary blastoma registry. Am J Surg Pathol. 2008 Feb;32(2):282–95. PMID:18223332
**2894.** Hill DA, Pfeifer JD, Marley EF, et al. WT1 staining reliably differentiates desmoplastic small round cell tumor from Ewing sarcoma/primitive neuroectodermal tumor. An immunohistochemical and molecular diagnostic study. Am J Clin Pathol. 2000 Sep;114(3):345–53. PMID:10989634
**2895.** Hill DA, Swanson PE, Anderson K, et al. Desmoplastic nested spindle cell tumor of liver: report of four cases of a proposed new entity. Am J Surg Pathol. 2005 Jan;29(1):1–9. PMID:15613851
**2896.** Hill RM, Richardson S, Schwalbe EC, et al. Time, pattern, and outcome of medulloblastoma relapse and their association with tumour biology at diagnosis and therapy: a multicentre cohort study. Lancet Child Adolesc Health. 2020 Dec;4(12):865–74. PMID:33222802
**2897.** Hill S, Rademaker M. A collection of rare anomalies: multiple digital glomuvenous malformations, epidermal naevus, temporal alopecia, heterochromia and abdominal lipoblastoma. Clin Exp Dermatol. 2009 Dec;34(8):e862–4. PMID:20055849
**2898.** Hingorani M, Williamson KA, Moore AT, et al. Detailed ophthalmologic evaluation of 43 individuals with PAX6 mutations. Invest Ophthalmol Vis Sci. 2009 Jun;50(6):2581–90. PMID:19218613
**2899.** Hingorani P, Dinu V, Zhang X, et al. Transcriptome analysis of desmoplastic small round cell tumors identifies actionable therapeutic targets: a report from the Children's Oncology Group. Sci Rep. 2020 Jul 23;10(1):12318. PMID:32703985
**2900.** Hinkes BG, von Hoff K, Deinlein F, et al. Childhood pineoblastoma: experiences from the prospective multicenter trials HIT-SKK87, HIT-SKK92 and HIT91. J Neurooncol. 2007 Jan;81(2):217–23. PMID:16941074
**2901.** Hinshaw M, Trowers AB, Kodish E, et al. Three children with CD30 cutaneous anaplastic large cell lymphomas bearing the t(2;5)(p23;q35) translocation. Pediatr Dermatol. 2004 May-Jun;21(3):212–7. PMID:15165197
**2902.** Hinton RB, Prakash A, Romp RL, et al. Cardiovascular manifestations of tuberous sclerosis complex and summary of the revised diagnostic criteria and surveillance and management recommendations from the International Tuberous Sclerosis Consensus Group. J Am Heart Assoc. 2014 Nov 25;3(6):e001493. PMID:25424575
**2903.** Hirabayashi S, Flotho C, Moetter J, et al. Spliceosomal gene aberrations are rare, coexist with oncogenic mutations, and are unlikely to exert a driver effect in childhood MDS and JMML. Blood. 2012 Mar 15;119(11):e96–9. PMID:22238327
**2904.** Hirai Y, Kodama Y, Moriwaki S, et al. Heterozygous individuals bearing a founder mutation in the XPA DNA repair gene comprise nearly 1% of the Japanese population. Mutat Res. 2006 Oct 10;601(1-2):171–8. PMID:16905156
**2905.** Hirai Y, Yamamoto T, Kimura H, et al. Hydroa vacciniforme is associated with increased numbers of Epstein-Barr virus-infected γδT cells. J Invest Dermatol. 2012 May;132(5):1401–8. PMID:22297643
**2906.** Hirakawa T, Tsuneyoshi M, Enjoji M. Squamous cell carcinoma arising in mature cystic teratoma of the ovary. Clinicopathologic and topographic analysis. Am J Surg Pathol. 1989 May;13(5):397–405. PMID:2712191
**2907.** Hirata Y, Brems H, Suzuki M, et al. Interaction between a domain of the negative regulator of the Ras-ERK pathway, SPRED1 protein, and the GTPase-activating protein-related domain of neurofibromin is implicated in legius syndrome and neurofibromatosis type 1. J Biol Chem. 2016 Feb 12;291(7):3124–34. PMID:26635368
**2908.** Hirokawa M, Maekawa M, Kuma S, et al. Cribriform-morular variant of papillary thyroid carcinoma–cytological and immunocytochemical findings of 18 cases. Diagn Cytopathol. 2010 Dec;38(12):890–6. PMID:20091902
**2909.** Hirose T, Giannini C, Scheithauer BW. Ultrastructural features of pleomorphic xanthoastrocytoma: a comparative study with glioblastoma multiforme. Ultrastruct Pathol. 2001 Nov-Dec;25(6):469–78. PMID:11783911
**2910.** Hirose T, Nobusawa S, Sugiyama K, et al. Astroblastoma: a distinct tumor entity characterized by alterations of the X chromosome and MN1 rearrangement. Brain Pathol. 2018 Sep;28(5):684–94. PMID:28990708
**2911.** Hirose T, Scheithauer BW, Lopes MB, et al. Ganglioglioma: an ultrastructural and immunohistochemical study. Cancer. 1997 Mar 1;79(5):989–1003. PMID:9041162
**2912.** Hirose T, Scheithauer BW, Lopes MB, et al. Tuber and subependymal giant cell astrocytoma associated with tuberous sclerosis: an immunohistochemical, ultrastructural, and immunoelectron and microscopic study. Acta Neuropathol. 1995;90(4):387–99. PMID:8546029
**2913.** Hirose T, Scheithauer BW, Sano T. Perineurial malignant peripheral nerve sheath tumor (MPNST): a clinicopathologic, immunohistochemical, and ultrastructural study of seven cases. Am J Surg Pathol. 1998 Nov;22(11):1368–78. PMID:9808129

2914. Hirschowitz L, Ansari A, Cahill DJ, et al. Central neurocytoma arising within a mature cystic teratoma of the ovary. Int J Gynecol Pathol. 1997 Apr;16(2):176–9. PMID:9100074
2915. Hisaoka M, Ishida T, Kuo TT, et al. Clear cell sarcoma of soft tissue: a clinicopathologic, immunohistochemical, and molecular analysis of 33 cases. Am J Surg Pathol. 2008 Mar;32(3):452–60. PMID:18300804
2916. Hitchins MP, Ward RL. Constitutional (germline) MLH1 epimutation as an aetiological mechanism for hereditary non-polyposis colorectal cancer. J Med Genet. 2009 Dec;46(12):793–802. PMID:19564652
2917. Hitzler JK, Cheung J, Li Y, et al. GATA1 mutations in transient leukemia and acute megakaryoblastic leukemia of Down syndrome. Blood. 2003 Jun 1;101(11):4301–4. PMID:12586620
2918. Hmada YA, Bernieh A, Morris RW, et al. Chondroblastoma-like osteosarcoma. Arch Pathol Lab Med. 2020 Jan;144(1):15–7. PMID:31389716
2919. Ho B, Johann PD, Grabovska Y, et al. Molecular subgrouping of atypical teratoid/rhabdoid tumors-a reinvestigation and current consensus. Neuro Oncol. 2020 May 15;22(5):613–24. PMID:31889194
2920. Ho DM, Liu HC. Primary intracranial germ cell tumor. Pathologic study of 51 patients. Cancer. 1992 Sep 15;70(6):1577–84. PMID:1325276
2921. Ho HE, Cunningham-Rundles C. Non-infectious complications of common variable immunodeficiency: updated clinical spectrum, sequelae, and insights to pathogenesis. Front Immunol. 2020 Feb 7;11:149. PMID:32117289
2922. Hoang JK, Lee WK, Lee M, et al. US features of thyroid malignancy: pearls and pitfalls. Radiographics. 2007 May-Jun;27(3):847–60. PMID:17495296
2923. Hoang MP. Myxoid Spitz nevus. J Cutan Pathol. 2003 Oct;30(9):566–8. PMID:14507405
2924. Hoch BL, Nielsen GP, Liebsch NJ, et al. Base of skull chordomas in children and adolescents: a clinicopathologic study of 73 cases. Am J Surg Pathol. 2006 Jul;30(7):811–8. PMID:16819322
2925. Hochberg J, Waxman IM, Kelly KM, et al. Adolescent non-Hodgkin lymphoma and Hodgkin lymphoma: state of the science. Br J Haematol. 2009 Jan;144(1):24–40. PMID:19087093
2926. Hochhaus A, Baccarani M, Silver RT, et al. European LeukemiaNet 2020 recommendations for treating chronic myeloid leukemia. Leukemia. 2020 Apr;34(4):966–84. PMID:32127639
2927. Hochhaus A, Reiter A, Skladny H, et al. A novel BCR-ABL fusion gene (e6a2) in a patient with Philadelphia chromosome-negative chronic myelogenous leukemia. Blood. 1996 Sep 15;88(6):2236–40. PMID:8822944
2928. Hockman D, Adameyko I, Kaucka M, et al. Striking parallels between carotid body glomus cell and adrenal chromaffin cell development. Dev Biol. 2018 Dec 1;444 Suppl 1:S308–24. PMID:29807017
2929. Hoda SA, Brogi E, Koerner FC, et al., editors. Rosen's breast pathology. 4th ed. Philadelphia (PA): Lippincott Williams & Wilkins; 2014.
2930. Hoei-Hansen CE, Almstrup K, Nielsen JE, et al. Stem cell pluripotency factor NANOG is expressed in human fetal gonocytes, testicular carcinoma in situ and germ cell tumours. Histopathology. 2005 Jul;47(1):48–56. PMID:15982323
2931. Hoei-Hansen CE, Carlsen E, Jorgensen N, et al. Towards a non-invasive method for early detection of testicular neoplasia in semen samples by identification of fetal germ cell-specific markers. Hum Reprod. 2007 Jan;22(1):167–73. PMID:16920726
2932. Hoei-Hansen CE, Holm M, Rajpert-De Meyts E, et al. Histological evidence of testicular dysgenesis in contralateral biopsies from 218 patients with testicular germ cell cancer. J Pathol. 2003 Jul;200(3):370–4. PMID:12845633
2933. Hoei-Hansen CE, Kraggerud SM, Abeler VM, et al. Ovarian dysgerminomas are characterised by frequent KIT mutations and abundant expression of pluripotency markers. Mol Cancer. 2007 Feb 2;6:12. PMID:17274819
2934. Hoei-Hansen CE, Nielsen JE, Almstrup K, et al. Transcription factor AP-2gamma is a developmentally regulated marker of testicular carcinoma in situ and germ cell tumors. Clin Cancer Res. 2004 Dec 15;10(24):8521–30. PMID:15623634
2935. Hoesly PM, Lowe GC, Lohse CM, et al. Prognostic impact of fibrosarcomatous transformation in dermatofibrosarcoma protuberans: a cohort study. J Am Acad Dermatol. 2015 Mar;72(3):419–25. PMID:25582537
2936. Hoffman LM, DeWire M, Ryall S, et al. Spatial genomic heterogeneity in diffuse intrinsic pontine and midline high-grade glioma: implications for diagnostic biopsy and targeted therapeutics. Acta Neuropathol Commun. 2016 Jan 4;4:1. PMID:26727948
2937. Hoffman LM, Richardson EA, Ho B, et al. Advancing biology-based therapeutic approaches for atypical teratoid rhabdoid tumors. Neuro Oncol. 2020 Jul 7;22(7):944–54. PMID:32129445
2938. Hoffman LM, Veldhuijzen van Zanten SEM, Colditz N, et al. Clinical, radiologic, pathologic, and molecular characteristics of long-term survivors of Diffuse Intrinsic Pontine Glioma (DIPG): a collaborative report from the International and European Society for Pediatric Oncology DIPG registries. J Clin Oncol. 2018 Jul 1;36(19):1963–72. PMID:29746225
2939. Hoffmann A, Boekhoff S, Gebhardt U, et al. History before diagnosis in childhood craniopharyngioma: associations with initial presentation and long-term prognosis. Eur J Endocrinol. 2015 Dec;173(6):853–62. PMID:26392473
2940. Hoffmann A, Brentrup A, Müller HL. First report on spinal metastasis in childhood-onset craniopharyngioma. J Neurooncol. 2016 Aug;129(1):193–4. PMID:27278607
2941. Hoffmann C, Hentrich M, Gillor D, et al. Hodgkin lymphoma is as common as non-Hodgkin lymphoma in HIV-positive patients with sustained viral suppression and limited immune deficiency: a prospective cohort study. HIV Med. 2015 Apr;16(4):261–4. PMID:25252101
2942. Hoffmann VS, Baccarani M, Hasford J, et al. The EUTOS population-based registry: incidence and clinical characteristics of 2904 CML patients in 20 European Countries. Leukemia. 2015 Jun;29(6):1336–43. PMID:25783795
2943. Hofmann M, Schlegel PG, Hippert F, et al. Testicular sex cord stromal tumors: analysis of patients from the MAKEI study. Pediatr Blood Cancer. 2013 Oct;60(10):1651–5. PMID:23733594
2944. Hofvander J, Jo VY, Ghanei I, et al. Comprehensive genetic analysis of a paediatric pleomorphic myxoid liposarcoma reveals near-haploidization and loss of the RB1 gene. Histopathology. 2016 Jul;69(1):141–7. PMID:26647907
2945. Hofvander J, Tayebwa J, Nilsson J, et al. Recurrent PRDM10 gene fusions in undifferentiated pleomorphic sarcoma. Clin Cancer Res. 2015 Feb 15;21(4):864–9. PMID:25516889
2946. Hogan AR, Zhuge Y, Perez EA, et al. Pediatric thyroid carcinoma: incidence and outcomes in 1753 patients. J Surg Res. 2009 Sep;156(1):167–72. PMID:19631341
2947. Hogstad B, Berres ML, Chakraborty R, et al. RAF/MEK/extracellular signal-related kinase pathway suppresses dendritic cell migration and traps dendritic cells in Langerhans cell histiocytosis lesions. J Exp Med. 2018 Jan 2;215(1):319–36. PMID:29263218
2948. Hollanda LM, Lima CS, Cunha AF, et al. An inherited mutation leading to production of only the short isoform of GATA-1 is associated with impaired erythropoiesis. Nat Genet. 2006 Jul;38(7):807–12. PMID:16783379
2949. Holley DG, Martin GR, Brenner JI, et al. Diagnosis and management of fetal cardiac tumors: a multicenter experience and review of published reports. J Am Coll Cardiol. 1995 Aug;26(2):516–20. PMID:7608458
2950. Hollmann TJ, Bovée JV, Fletcher CD. Digital fibromyxoma (superficial acral fibromyxoma): a detailed characterization of 124 cases. Am J Surg Pathol. 2012 Jun;36(6):789–98. PMID:22367301
2951. Hollmann TJ, Brenn T, Hornick JL. CD25 expression on cutaneous mast cells from adult patients presenting with urticaria pigmentosa is predictive of systemic mastocytosis. Am J Surg Pathol. 2008 Jan;32(1):139–45. PMID:18162781
2952. Hollmann TJ, Hornick JL. INI1-deficient tumors: diagnostic features and molecular genetics. Am J Surg Pathol. 2011 Oct;35(10):e47–63. PMID:21934399
2953. Hollowell ML, Goulart RA, Gang DL, et al. Cytologic features of müllerian papilloma of the cervix: mimic of malignancy. Diagn Cytopathol. 2007 Sep;35(9):607–11. PMID:17703455
2954. Hollowood K, Holley MP, Fletcher CD. Plexiform fibrohistiocytic tumour: clinicopathological, immunohistochemical and ultrastructural analysis in favour of a myofibroblastic lesion. Histopathology. 1991 Dec;19(6):503–13. PMID:1723956
2955. Hollstein M, Marion MJ, Lehman T, et al. p53 mutations at A:T base pairs in angiosarcomas of vinyl chloride-exposed factory workers. Carcinogenesis. 1994 Jan;15(1):1–3. PMID:8293534
2956. Holm M, Hoei-Hansen CE, Rajpert-De Meyts E, et al. Increased risk of carcinoma in situ in patients with testicular germ cell cancer with ultrasonic microlithiasis in the contralateral testicle. J Urol. 2003 Oct;170(4 Pt 1):1163–7. PMID:14501716
2957. Holmfeldt L, Wei L, Diaz-Flores E, et al. The genomic landscape of hypodiploid acute lymphoblastic leukemia. Nat Genet. 2013 Mar;45(3):242–52. PMID:23334668
2958. Hölsken A, Kreutzer J, Hofmann BM, et al. Target gene activation of the Wnt signaling pathway in nuclear beta-catenin accumulating cells of adamantinomatous craniopharyngiomas. Brain Pathol. 2009 Jul;19(3):357–64. PMID:18540944
2959. Hölsken A, Sill M, Merkle J, et al. Adamantinomatous and papillary craniopharyngiomas are characterized by distinct epigenomic as well as mutational and transcriptomic profiles. Acta Neuropathol Commun. 2016 Feb 29;4:20. PMID:26927026
2960. Holsten T, Bens S, Oyen F, et al. Germline variants in SMARCB1 and other members of the BAF chromatin-remodeling complex across human disease entities: a meta-analysis. Eur J Hum Genet. 2018 Aug;26(8):1083–93. PMID:29706634
2961. Holsten T, Lubieniecki F, Spohn M, et al. Detailed clinical and histopathological description of 8 cases of molecularly defined CNS neuroblastomas. J Neuropathol Exp Neurol. 2021 Jan 1;80(1):52–9. PMID:33270865
2962. Holyoake TL, Vetrie D. The chronic myeloid leukemia stem cell: stemming the tide of persistence. Blood. 2017 Mar 23;129(12):1595–606. PMID:28159740
2963. Hommann M, Kaemmerer D, Daffner W, et al. Nested stromal epithelial tumor of the liver–liver transplantation and follow-up. J Gastrointest Cancer. 2011 Dec;42(4):292–5. PMID:21221846
2964. Honavar M, Janota I, Polkey CE. Histological heterogeneity of dysembryoplastic neuroepithelial tumour: identification and differential diagnosis in a series of 74 cases. Histopathology. 1999 Apr;34(4):342–56. PMID:10231402
2965. Honecker F, Aparicio J, Berney D, et al. ESMO Consensus Conference on testicular germ cell cancer: diagnosis, treatment and follow-up. Ann Oncol. 2018 Aug 1;29(8):1658–86. PMID:30113631
2966. Honecker F, Stoop H, de Krijger RR, et al. Pathobiological implications of the expression of markers of testicular carcinoma in situ by fetal germ cells. J Pathol. 2004 Jul;203(3):849–57. PMID:15221945
2967. Honeyman JN, Simon EP, Robine N, et al. Detection of a recurrent DNAJB1-PRKACA chimeric transcript in fibrolamellar hepatocellular carcinoma. Science. 2014 Feb 28;343(6174):1010–4. PMID:24578576
2968. Hong JY, Yoon DH, Suh C, et al. EBV-positive diffuse large B-cell lymphoma in young adults: Is this a distinct disease entity? Ann Oncol. 2015 Mar;26(3):548–55. PMID:25475080
2969. Hong Kong Cancer Registry [Internet]. Hong Kong SAR (China): Hong Kong Cancer Registry, Hospital Authority; cited 2020 Aug. Available from: https://www3.ha.org.hk/cancereg/.
2970. Hong YH, Kim DG, Lee JH, et al. The unusual case of fibroma of tendon sheath in a young girl with turner syndrome undergoing growth hormone treatment. J Clin Res Pediatr Endocrinol. 2021 Feb 26;13(1):104–8. PMID:32349463
2971. Honig GR, Suarez CR, Vida LN, et al. Juvenile myelomonocytic leukemia (JMML) with the hematologic phenotype of severe beta thalassemia. Am J Hematol. 1998 May;58(1):67–71. PMID:9590152
2972. Hoorens A, Lemoine NR, McLellan E, et al. Pancreatic acinar cell carcinoma. An analysis of cell lineage markers, p53 expression, and Ki-ras mutation. Am J Pathol. 1993 Sep;143(3):685–98. PMID:8362971
2973. Hoot AC, Russo P, Judkins AR, et al. Immunohistochemical analysis of hSNF5/INI1 distinguishes renal and extra-renal malignant rhabdoid tumors from other pediatric soft tissue tumors. Am J Surg Pathol. 2004 Nov;28(11):1485–91. PMID:15489652
2974. Hopkins KL, Dickson PK, Ball TI, et al. Fetus-in-fetu with malignant recurrence. J Pediatr Surg. 1997 Oct;32(10):1476–9. PMID:9349774
2975. Hopp RN, de Siqueira DC, Sena-Filho M, et al. Oral vascular malformation in a patient with hereditary hemorrhagic telangiectasia: a case report. Spec Care Dentist. 2013 May-Jun;33(3):150–3. PMID:23600987
2976. Horbinski C, Kofler J, Yeaney G, et al. Isocitrate dehydrogenase 1 analysis differentiates gangliogliomas from infiltrative gliomas. Brain Pathol. 2011 Sep;21(5):564–74. PMID:21314850
2977. Horie A, Haratake J, Jimi A, et al. Pancreatoblastoma in Japan, with differential diagnosis from papillary cystic tumor (ductuloacinar adenoma) of the pancreas. Acta Pathol Jpn. 1987 Jan;37(1):47–63. PMID:3554891
2978. Horie A, Yano Y, Kotoo Y, et al. Morphogenesis of pancreatoblastoma, infantile carcinoma of the pancreas: report of two cases. Cancer. 1977 Jan;39(1):247–54. PMID:188539

2979. Horikawa H, Sato T, Gomi H, et al. Medallion-like dermal dendrocyte hamartoma: a rare congenital CD34-positive dermal lesion clinically and pathologically overlapping with fibroblastic connective tissue nevus. Pediatr Dermatol. 2019 May;36(3):397–9. PMID:30811625
2980. Horiuchi A, Muraji T, Tsugawa C, et al. Thoracic neuroblastoma: outcome of incomplete resection. Pediatr Surg Int. 2004 Sep;20(9):714–8. PMID:15278374
2981. Hornick JL, Bosenberg MW, Mentzel T, et al. Pleomorphic liposarcoma: clinicopathologic analysis of 57 cases. Am J Surg Pathol. 2004 Oct;28(10):1257–67. PMID:15371941
2982. Hornick JL, Bundock EA, Fletcher CD. Hybrid schwannoma/perineurioma: clinicopathologic analysis of 42 distinctive benign nerve sheath tumors. Am J Surg Pathol. 2009 Oct;33(10):1554–61. PMID:19623031
2983. Hornick JL, Dal Cin P, Fletcher CD. Loss of INI1 expression is characteristic of both conventional and proximal-type epithelioid sarcoma. Am J Surg Pathol. 2009 Apr;33(4):542–50. PMID:19033866
2984. Hornick JL, Fletcher CD. Cutaneous myoepithelioma: a clinicopathologic and immunohistochemical study of 14 cases. Hum Pathol. 2004 Jan;35(1):14–24. PMID:14745720
2985. Hornick JL, Fletcher CD. Intraarticular nodular fasciitis–a rare lesion: clinicopathologic analysis of a series. Am J Surg Pathol. 2006 Feb;30(2):237–41. PMID:16434899
2986. Hornick JL, Fletcher CD. Myoepithelial tumors of soft tissue: a clinicopathologic and immunohistochemical study of 101 cases with evaluation of prognostic parameters. Am J Surg Pathol. 2003 Sep;27(9):1183–96. PMID:12960802
2987. Hornick JL, Fletcher CD. Pseudomyogenic hemangioendothelioma: a distinctive, often multicentric tumor with indolent behavior. Am J Surg Pathol. 2011 Feb;35(2):190–201. PMID:21263239
2988. Hornick JL, Fletcher CD. Soft tissue perineurioma: clinicopathologic analysis of 81 cases including those with atypical histologic features. Am J Surg Pathol. 2005 Jul;29(7):845–58. PMID:15958848
2989. Hornick JL, Nielsen GP. Beyond "triton": malignant peripheral nerve sheath tumors with complete heterologous rhabdomyoblastic differentiation mimicking spindle cell rhabdomyosarcoma. Am J Surg Pathol. 2019 Oct;43(10):1323–30. PMID:31107719
2990. Hornick JL, Sholl LM, Dal Cin P, et al. Expression of ROS1 predicts ROS1 gene rearrangement in inflammatory myofibroblastic tumors. Mod Pathol. 2015 May;28(5):732–9. PMID:25612511
2991. Horny HP, Sotlar K, Stellmacher F, et al. The tryptase positive compact round cell infiltrate of the bone marrow (TROCI-BM): a novel histopathological finding requiring the application of lineage specific markers. J Clin Pathol. 2006 Mar;59(3):298–302. PMID:16505282
2992. Horten BC, Rubinstein LJ. Primary cerebral neuroblastoma. A clinicopathological study of 35 cases. Brain. 1976 Dec;99(4):735–56. PMID:1030655
2993. Horvath E, Kovacs K, Killinger DW, et al. Mammosomatotroph cell adenoma of the human pituitary: a morphologic entity. Virchows Arch A Pathol Anat Histopathol. 1983;398(3):277–89. PMID:6402839
2994. Horvath E, Kovacs K, Singer W, et al. Acidophil stem cell adenoma of the human pituitary. Arch Pathol Lab Med. 1977 Nov;101(11):594–9. PMID:199135
2995. Horvath E, Kovacs K, Singer W, et al. Acidophil stem cell adenoma of the human pituitary: clinicopathologic analysis of 15 cases. Cancer. 1981 Feb 15;47(4):761–71. PMID:6261917
2996. Horvath E, Kovacs K, Smyth HS, et al. Silent adenoma subtype 3 of the pituitary–immunohistochemical and ultrastructural classification: a review of 29 cases. Ultrastruct Pathol. 2005 Nov-Dec;29(6):511–24. PMID:16316952
2997. Horwitz M, Dufour C, Leblond P, et al. Embryonal tumors with multilayered rosettes in children: the SFCE experience. Childs Nerv Syst. 2016 Feb;32(2):299–305. PMID:26438544
2998. Hosono J, Nitta M, Masui K, et al. Role of a Promoter Mutation in TERT in Malignant Transformation of Pleomorphic Xanthoastrocytoma. World Neurosurg. 2019 Jun;126:624–30. PMID:30599247
2999. Hotokebuchi Y, Kohashi K, Toyoshima S, et al. Congenital peribronchial myofibroblastic tumor. Pathol Int. 2014 Apr;64(4):189–91. PMID:24750190
3000. Houk CP, Hughes IA, Ahmed SF, et al. Summary of consensus statement on intersex disorders and their management. Pediatrics. 2006 Aug;118(2):753–7. PMID:16882833
3001. Hovestadt V, Ayrault O, Swartling FJ, et al. Medulloblastomics revisited: biological and clinical insights from thousands of patients. Nat Rev Cancer. 2020 Jan;20(1):42–56. PMID:31819232
3002. Hovestadt V, Remke M, Kool M, et al. Robust molecular subgrouping and copy-number profiling of medulloblastoma from small amounts of archival tumour material using high-density DNA methylation arrays. Acta Neuropathol. 2013 Jun;125(6):913–6. PMID:23670100
3003. Hovestadt V, Smith KS, Bihannic L, et al. Resolving medulloblastoma cellular architecture by single-cell genomics. Nature. 2019 Aug;572(7767):74–9. PMID:31341285
3004. Howell SM, Bray DW. Amelanotic melanoma in a patient with Rothmund-Thomson syndrome. Arch Dermatol. 2008 Mar;144(3):416–7. PMID:18347307
3005. Howitt BE, Berney DM. Tumors of the testis: morphologic features and molecular alterations. Surg Pathol Clin. 2015 Dec;8(4):687–716. PMID:26612222
3006. Howitt BE, Emori MM, Drapkin R, et al. GATA3 is a sensitive and specific marker of benign and malignant mesonephric lesions in the lower female genital tract. Am J Surg Pathol. 2015 Oct;39(10):1411–9. PMID:26135559
3007. Howitt BE, Fletcher CD. Mammary-type myofibroblastoma: clinicopathologic characterization in a series of 143 cases. Am J Surg Pathol. 2016 Mar;40(3):361–7. PMID:26523539
3008. Howitt BE, Nucci MR. Mesonephric proliferations of the female genital tract. Pathology. 2018 Feb;50(2):141–50. PMID:29269124
3009. Howley S, Stack D, Morris T, et al. Ectomesenchymoma with t(1;12)(p32;p13) evolving from embryonal rhabdomyosarcoma shows no rearrangement of ETV6. Hum Pathol. 2012 Feb;43(2):299–302. PMID:21803398
3010. Howman-Giles R, Shaw HM, Scolyer RA, et al. Sentinel lymph node biopsy in pediatric and adolescent cutaneous melanoma patients. Ann Surg Oncol. 2010 Jan;17(1):138–43. PMID:19672660
3011. Hoyoux C, Dresse MF, Forget P, et al. Osteopetrosis mimicking juvenile myelomonocytic leukemia. Pediatr Int. 2014 Oct;56(5):779–82. PMID:25335998
3012. Hoyt WF, Baghdassarian SA. Optic glioma of childhood. Natural history and rationale for conservative management. Br J Ophthalmol. 1969 Dec;53(12):793–8. PMID:5386369
3013. Hrusák O, Porwit-MacDonald A. Antigen expression patterns reflecting genotype of acute leukemias. Leukemia. 2002 Jul;16(7):1233–58. PMID:12094248
3014. Hsiao SJ, Karajannis MA, Diolaiti D, et al. A novel, potentially targetable TMEM106B-BRAF fusion in pleomorphic xanthoastrocytoma. Cold Spring Harb Mol Case Stud. 2017 Mar;3(2):a001396. PMID:28299358
3015. Hsi Dickie B, Fishman SJ, Azizkhan RG. Hepatic vascular tumors. Semin Pediatr Surg. 2014 Aug;23(4):168–72. PMID:25241093
3016. Hsieh MS, Jeng YM, Lee YH. Mist1: a novel nuclear marker for acinic cell carcinoma of the salivary gland. Virchows Arch. 2019 Nov;475(5):617–24. PMID:31187185
3017. Hsieh MS, Lee YH, Chang YL. SOX10-positive salivary gland tumors: a growing list, including mammary analogue secretory carcinoma of the salivary gland, sialoblastoma, low-grade salivary duct carcinoma, basal cell adenoma/adenocarcinoma, and a subgroup of mucoepidermoid carcinoma. Hum Pathol. 2016 Oct;56:134–42. PMID:27327192
3018. Hsieh MS, Wang H, Lee YH, et al. Reevaluation of MAML2 fusion-negative mucoepidermoid carcinoma: a subgroup being actually hyalinizing clear cell carcinoma of the salivary gland with EWSR1 translocation. Hum Pathol. 2017 Mar;61:9–18. PMID:27769871
3019. Hsu AP, Sampaio EP, Khan J, et al. Mutations in GATA2 are associated with the autosomal dominant and sporadic monocytopenia and mycobacterial infection (MonoMAC) syndrome. Blood. 2011 Sep 8;118(10):2653–5. PMID:21670465
3020. Hsueh C, Hsueh S, Gonzalez-Crussi F, et al. Nasal chondromesenchymal hamartoma in children: report of 2 cases with review of the literature. Arch Pathol Lab Med. 2001 Mar;125(3):400–3. PMID:11231491
3021. Hu S, Xu X, Xu J, et al. Prognostic factors and long-term outcomes of nasopharyngeal carcinoma in children and adolescents. Pediatr Blood Cancer. 2013 Jul;60(7):1122–7. PMID:23303571
3022. Hu W, Huang J, Zhang Y, et al. A rare and easily misdiagnosed tumor of the urinary bladder: primary composite pheochromocytoma. Int J Clin Exp Pathol. 2017 Oct 1;10(10):10522–30. PMID:31966391
3023. Hu ZL, Sang H, Deng L, et al. Subcutaneous panniculitis-like T-cell lymphoma in children: a review of the literature. Pediatr Dermatol. 2015 Jul-Aug;32(4):526–32. PMID:25727090
3024. Huang FL, Liao EC, Li CL, et al. Pathogenesis of pediatric B-cell acute lymphoblastic leukemia: molecular pathways and disease treatments. Oncol Lett. 2020 Jul;20(1):448–54. PMID:32565969
3025. Huang H, Reis R, Yonekawa Y, et al. Identification in human brain tumors of DNA sequences specific for SV40 large T antigen. Brain Pathol. 1999 Jan;9(1):33–42. PMID:9989448
3026. Huang H, Wang C, Tian Q. Gonadal tumour risk in 292 phenotypic female patients with disorders of sex development containing Y chromosome or Y-derived sequence. Clin Endocrinol (Oxf). 2017 Apr;86(4):621–7. PMID:27862157
3027. Huang IH, Wu YY, Huang TC, et al. Statistics and outlook of primary hepatic angiosarcoma based on clinical stage. Oncol Lett. 2016 May;11(5):3218–22. PMID:27123094
3028. Huang J, Grotzer MA, Watanabe T, et al. Mutations in the Nijmegen breakage syndrome gene in medulloblastomas. Clin Cancer Res. 2008 Jul 1;14(13):4053–8. PMID:18593981
3029. Huang J, Luo RK, Du M, et al. Clear cell sarcoma of the pancreas: a case report and review of literature. Int J Clin Exp Pathol. 2015 Feb 1;8(2):2171–5. PMID:25973121
3030. Huang JG, Tan MYQ, Quak SH, et al. Risk factors and clinical outcomes of pediatric liver transplant recipients with post-transplant lymphoproliferative disease in a multi-ethnic Asian cohort. Transpl Infect Dis. 2018 Feb;20(1). PMID:29071779
3031. Huang L, Liu D, Wang N, et al. Integrated genomic analysis identifies deregulated JAK/STAT-MYC-biosynthesis axis in aggressive NK-cell leukemia. Cell Res. 2018 Feb;28(2):172–86. PMID:29148541
3032. Huang L, Wang SA, Konoplev S, et al. Well-differentiated systemic mastocytosis showed excellent clinical response to imatinib in the absence of known molecular genetic abnormalities: a case report. Medicine (Baltimore). 2016 Oct;95(41):e4934. PMID:27741105
3033. Huang R, Jaffer S. Imprint cytology of metastatic sialoblastoma. A case report. Acta Cytol. 2003 Nov-Dec;47(6):1123–6. PMID:14674095
3034. Huang SA, Tu HM, Harney JW, et al. Severe hypothyroidism caused by type 3 iodothyronine deiodinase in infantile hemangiomas. N Engl J Med. 2000 Jul 20;343(3):185–9. PMID:10900278
3035. Huang SC, Alaggio R, Sung YS, et al. Frequent HRAS mutations in malignant ectomesenchymoma: overlapping genetic abnormalities with embryonal rhabdomyosarcoma. Am J Surg Pathol. 2016 Jul;40(7):876–85. PMID:26872011
3036. Huang SC, Chen HW, Zhang L, et al. Novel FUS-KLF17 and EWSR1-KLF17 fusions in myoepithelial tumors. Genes Chromosomes Cancer. 2015 May;54(5):267–75. PMID:25706482
3037. Huang SC, Durno CA, Erdman SH. Lynch syndrome: a pediatric perspective. J Pediatr Gastroenterol Nutr. 2014 Feb;58(2):144–52. PMID:24051481
3038. Huang SC, Zhang L, Sung YS, et al. Frequent FOS gene rearrangements in epithelioid hemangioma: a molecular study of 58 cases with morphologic reappraisal. Am J Surg Pathol. 2015 Oct;39(10):1313–21. PMID:26135557
3039. Huang SC, Zhang L, Sung YS, et al. Recurrent CIC gene abnormalities in angiosarcomas: a molecular study of 120 cases with concurrent investigation of PLCG1, KDR, MYC, and FLT4 gene alterations. Am J Surg Pathol. 2016 May;40(5):645–55. PMID:26735859
3040. Huang SC, Zhang L, Sung YS, et al. Secondary EWSR1 gene abnormalities in SMARCB1-deficient tumors with 22q11-12 regional deletions: potential pitfalls in interpreting EWSR1 FISH results. Genes Chromosomes Cancer. 2016 Oct;55(10):767–76. PMID:27218413
3041. Huang T, Garcia R, Qi J, et al. Detection of histone H3 K27M mutation and post-translational modifications in pediatric diffuse midline glioma via tissue immunohistochemistry informs diagnosis and clinical outcomes. Oncotarget. 2018 Dec 14;9(98):37112–24. PMID:30647848
3042. Huang TB. Cancer of the nasopharynx in childhood. Cancer. 1990 Sep 1;66(5):968–71. PMID:2386925
3043. Huang Y, Cao YF, Lin JL, et al. Acinar cell cystadenocarcinoma of the pancreas in a 4-year-old child. Pancreas. 2006 Oct;33(3):311–2. PMID:17003655
3044. Huang Y, Yang W, Hu J, et al. Diagnosis and treatment of pancreatoblastoma in children: a retrospective study in a single pediatric center. Pediatr Surg Int. 2019 Nov;35(11):1231–8. PMID:31338582
3045. Hubbard AK, Spector LG, Fortuna G, et al. Trends in international incidence of pediatric cancers in children under 5 years of

age: 1988-2012. JNCI Cancer Spectr. 2019 Mar;3(1):pkz007. PMID:30984908
3046. Huber K, Janoueix-Lerosey I, Kummer W, et al. The sympathetic nervous system: malignancy, disease, and novel functions. Cell Tissue Res. 2018 May;372(2):163–70. PMID:29623426
3047. Hübner JM, Müller T, Papageorgiou DN, et al. EZHIP/CXorf67 mimics K27M mutated oncohistones and functions as an intrinsic inhibitor of PRC2 function in aggressive posterior fossa ependymoma. Neuro Oncol. 2019 Jul 11;21(7):878–89. PMID:30923826
3048. Huddart SN, Mann JR, Robinson K, et al. Sacrococcygeal teratomas: the UK Children's Cancer Study Group's experience. I. Neonatal. Pediatr Surg Int. 2003 Apr;19(1-2):47–51. PMID:12721723
3049. Huegel J, Mundy C, Sgariglia F, et al. Perichondrium phenotype and border function are regulated by Ext1 and heparan sulfate in developing long bones: a mechanism likely deranged in Hereditary Multiple Exostoses. Dev Biol. 2013 May 1;377(1):100–12. PMID:23458899
3050. Hueso L, Hernández A, Torrelo A, et al. [Agminated Spitz nevi on a hyperpigmented macule]. Actas Dermosifiliogr. 2008 Jan-Feb;99(1):69–72. Spanish. PMID:18206090
3051. Huh WW, Yuen C, Munsell M, et al. Liposarcoma in children and young adults: a multi-institutional experience. Pediatr Blood Cancer. 2011 Dec 15;57(7):1142–6. PMID:21394894
3052. Huizenga NA, de Lange P, Koper JW, et al. Human adrenocorticotropin-secreting pituitary adenomas show frequent loss of heterozygosity at the glucocorticoid receptor gene locus. J Clin Endocrinol Metab. 1998 Mar;83(3):917–21. PMID:9506748
3053. Hulsebos TJ, Plomp AS, Wolterman RA, et al. Germline mutation of INI1/SMARCB1 in familial schwannomatosis. Am J Hum Genet. 2007 Apr;80(4):805–10. PMID:17357086
3054. Humke EW, Dorn KV, Milenkovic L, et al. The output of Hedgehog signaling is controlled by the dynamic association between Suppressor of Fused and the Gli proteins. Genes Dev. 2010 Apr 1;24(7):670–82. PMID:20360384
3055. Hummel M, Bentink S, Berger H, et al. A biologic definition of Burkitt's lymphoma from transcriptional and genomic profiling. N Engl J Med. 2006 Jun 8;354(23):2419–30. PMID:16760442
3056. Humphrey GM, Brown I, Squire R, et al. Extraosseous osteogenic sarcoma–a rare pediatric malignancy: case report and review of the literature. J Pediatr Surg. 1999 Jun;34(6):1025–8. PMID:10392928
3057. Hung GY, Horng JL, Yen HJ, et al. Changing incidence patterns of hepatocellular carcinoma among age groups in Taiwan. J Hepatol. 2015 Dec;63(6):1390–6. PMID:26256438
3058. Hung GY, Horng JL, Yen HJ, et al. Pre-pubertal and adolescent germ cell neoplasms in Taiwan: time trends and geographic variation. Andrology. 2015 Sep;3(5):895–901. PMID:26227297
3059. Hung NA, Silver MM, Chitayat D, et al. Gonadoblastoid testicular dysplasia in Walker-Warburg syndrome. Pediatr Dev Pathol. 1998 Sep-Oct;1(5):393–404. PMID:9688764
3060. Hung T, Argenyi Z, Erickson L, et al. Cellular blue nevomelanocytic lesions: analysis of clinical, histological, and outcome data in 37 cases. Am J Dermatopathol. 2016 Jul;38(7):499–503. PMID:26909585
3061. Hung T, Piris A, Lobo A, et al. Sentinel lymph node metastasis is not predictive of poor outcome in patients with problematic spitzoid melanocytic tumors. Hum Pathol. 2013 Jan;44(1):87–94. PMID:22939951
3062. Hung T, Yang A, Mihm MC, et al. The plexiform spindle cell nevus nevi and atypical variants: report of 128 cases. Hum Pathol. 2014 Dec;45(12):2369–78. PMID:25300464
3063. Hung W. Solitary thyroid nodules in 93 children and adolescents. a 35-years experience. Horm Res. 1999;52(1):15–8. PMID:10640894
3064. Hung YP, Diaz-Perez JA, Cote GM, et al. Dedifferentiated chordoma: clinicopathologic and molecular characteristics with integrative analysis. Am J Surg Pathol. 2020 Sep;44(9):1213–23. PMID:32427623
3065. Hung YP, Fletcher CD, Hornick JL. Evaluation of ETV4 and WT1 expression in CIC-rearranged sarcomas and histologic mimics. Mod Pathol. 2016 Nov;29(11):1324–34. PMID:27443513
3066. Hung YP, Fletcher CD, Hornick JL. Evaluation of NKX2-2 expression in round cell sarcomas and other tumors with EWSR1 rearrangement: imperfect specificity for Ewing sarcoma. Mod Pathol. 2016 Apr;29(4):370–80. PMID:26847175
3067. Hung YP, Fletcher CD, Hornick JL. FOSB is a useful diagnostic marker for pseudomyogenic Hemangioendothelioma. Am J Surg Pathol. 2017 May;41(5):596–606. PMID:28009608
3068. Hung YP, Fletcher CDM. Myopericytomatosis: clinicopathologic analysis of 11 cases with molecular identification of recurrent PDGFRB alterations in myopericytomatosis and myopericytoma. Am J Surg Pathol. 2017 Aug;41(8):1034–44. PMID:28505006
3069. Hung YP, Fletcher CDM, Hornick JL. Evaluation of pan-TRK immunohistochemistry in infantile fibrosarcoma, lipofibromatosis-like neural tumour and histological mimics. Histopathology. 2018 Oct;73(4):634–44. PMID:29863809
3070. Huppmann AR, Coffin CM, Hoot AC, et al. Congenital peribronchial myofibroblastic tumor: comparison of fetal and postnatal morphology. Pediatr Dev Pathol. 2011 Mar-Apr;14(2):124–9. PMID:20367454
3071. Huppmann AR, Nicolae A, Slack GW, et al. EBV may be expressed in the LP cells of nodular lymphocyte-predominant Hodgkin lymphoma (NLPHL) in both children and adults. Am J Surg Pathol. 2014 Mar;38(3):316–24. PMID:24525501
3072. Huppmann AR, Xi L, Raffeld M, et al. Subcutaneous panniculitis-like T-cell lymphoma in the pediatric age group: a lymphoma of low malignant potential. Pediatr Blood Cancer. 2013 Jul;60(7):1165–70. PMID:23382035
3073. Huq AJ, Walsh M, Rajagopalan B, et al. Mutations in SUFU and PTCH1 genes may cause different cutaneous cancer predisposition syndromes: similar, but not the same. Fam Cancer. 2018 Oct;17(4):601–6. PMID:29356994
3074. Hurwitz JL, Fenton A, McCluggage WG, et al. Squamous cell carcinoma arising in a dermoid cyst of the ovary: a case series. BJOG. 2007 Oct;114(10):1283–7. PMID:17877681
3075. Huryn LA, Turriff A, Harney LA, et al. DICER1 Syndrome: characterization of the ocular phenotype in a family-based cohort study. Ophthalmology. 2019 Feb;126(2):296–304. PMID:30339877
3076. Huse JT, Edgar M, Halliday J, et al. Multinodular and vacuolating neuronal tumors of the cerebrum: 10 cases of a distinctive seizure-associated lesion. Brain Pathol. 2013 Sep;23(5):515–24. PMID:23324039
3077. Huse JT, Snuderl M, Jones DT, et al. Polymorphous low-grade neuroepithelial tumor of the young (PLNTY): an epileptogenic neoplasm with oligodendroglioma-like components, aberrant CD34 expression, and genetic alterations involving the MAP kinase pathway. Acta Neuropathol. 2017 Mar;133(3):417–29. PMID:27812792
3078. Hussain N, Curran A, Pilling D, et al. Congenital subependymal giant cell astrocytoma diagnosed on fetal MRI. Arch Dis Child. 2006 Jun;91(6):520. PMID:16714726
3079. Hussein K, Rath B, Ludewig B, et al. Clinico-pathological characteristics of different types of immunodeficiency-associated smooth muscle tumours. Eur J Cancer. 2014 Sep;50(14):2417–24. PMID:25027306
3080. Hussein K, Stucki-Koch A, Göhring G, et al. Increased megakaryocytic proliferation, pro-platelet deposition and expression of fibrosis-associated factors in children with chronic myeloid leukaemia with bone marrow fibrosis. Leukemia. 2017 Jul;31(7):1540–6. PMID:28239144
3081. Hussein K, Suttorp M, Stucki-Koch A, et al. Molecular profile of inflammatory and megakaryocytic factors in pediatric myelodysplastic syndrome with acute myelofibrosis. Pediatr Blood Cancer. 2018 Jul;65(7):e27048. PMID:29667765
3082. Hutchison RE, Laver JH, Chang M, et al. Non-anaplastic peripheral T-cell lymphoma in childhood and adolescence: a Children's Oncology Group study. Pediatr Blood Cancer. 2008 Jul;51(1):29–33. PMID:18300314
3083. Huttenlocher PR, Heydemann PT. Fine structure of cortical tubers in tuberous sclerosis: a Golgi study. Ann Neurol. 1984 Nov;16(5):595–602. PMID:6508241
3084. Huvos AG, Rosen G, Dabska M, et al. Mesenchymal chondrosarcoma. A clinicopathologic analysis of 35 patients with emphasis on treatment. Cancer. 1983 Apr 1;51(7):1230–7. PMID:6825046
3085. Hvarness T, Nielsen JE, Almstrup K, et al. Phenotypic characterisation of immune cell infiltrates in testicular germ cell neoplasia. J Reprod Immunol. 2013 Dec;100(2):135–45. PMID:24290033
3086. Hwang EI, Kool M, Burger PC, et al. Extensive molecular and clinical heterogeneity in patients with histologically diagnosed CNS-PNET treated as a single entity: a report from the Children's Oncology Group randomized ACNS0332 trial. J Clin Oncol. 2018 Oct 17; (Oct):JCO2017764720. PMID:30332335
3087. Hwang HC, Mills SE, Patterson K, et al. Expression of androgen receptors in nasopharyngeal angiofibroma: an immunohistochemical study of 24 cases. Mod Pathol. 1998 Nov;11(11):1122–6. PMID:9831211
3088. Hwang J, Kim DY, Kim SC, et al. Solid-pseudopapillary neoplasm of the pancreas in children: Can we predict malignancy? J Pediatr Surg. 2014 Dec;49(12):1730–3. PMID:25487471
3089. Hyjek E, Isaacson PG. Primary B cell lymphoma of the thyroid and its relationship to Hashimoto's thyroiditis. Hum Pathol. 1988 Nov;19(11):1315–26. PMID:3141260
3090. Hyjek E, Smith WJ, Isaacson PG. Primary B-cell lymphoma of salivary glands and its relationship to myoepithelial sialadenitis. Hum Pathol. 1988 Jul;19(7):766–76. PMID:3136072
3091. Hyrcza MD, Ezzat S, Mete O, et al. Pituitary adenomas presenting as sinonasal or nasopharyngeal masses: a case series illustrating potential diagnostic pitfalls. Am J Surg Pathol. 2017 Apr;41(4):525–34. PMID:28009611
3092. Iacobas I, Phung TL, Adams DM, et al. Guidance document for hepatic hemangioma (infantile and congenital) evaluation and monitoring. J Pediatr. 2018 Dec;203:294–300.e2. PMID:30244993
3093. Iacobucci I, Kimura S, Mullighan CG. Biologic and therapeutic implications of genomic alterations in acute lymphoblastic leukemia. J Clin Med. 2021 Aug 25;10(17):3792. PMID:34501239
3094. Iacobucci I, Mullighan CG. Genetic basis of acute lymphoblastic leukemia. J Clin Oncol. 2017 Mar 20;35(9):975–83. PMID:28297628
3095. Iacobucci I, Wen J, Meggendorfer M, et al. Genomic subtyping and therapeutic targeting of acute erythroleukemia. Nat Genet. 2019 Apr;51(4):694–704. PMID:30926971
3096. Iacovazzo D, Carlsen E, Lugli F, et al. Factors predicting pasireotide responsiveness in somatotroph pituitary adenomas resistant to first-generation somatostatin analogues: an immunohistochemical study. Eur J Endocrinol. 2016 Feb;174(2):241–50. PMID:26586796
3097. Iacovazzo D, Caswell R, Bunce B, et al. Germline or somatic GPR101 duplication leads to X-linked acrogigantism: a clinico-pathological and genetic study. Acta Neuropathol Commun. 2016 Jun 1;4(1):56. PMID:27245663
3098. Iacovelli R, Modica D, Palazzo A, et al. Clinical outcome and prognostic factors in renal medullary carcinoma: a pooled analysis from 18 years of medical literature. Can Urol Assoc J. 2015 Mar-Apr;9(3-4):E172–7. PMID:26085875
3099. Iannelli F, Collino A, Sinha S, et al. Massive gene amplification drives paediatric hepatocellular carcinoma caused by bile salt export pump deficiency. Nat Commun. 2014 May 13;5:3850. PMID:24819516
3100. IARC TP53 Database [Internet]. Lyon (France): International Agency for Research on Cancer; 2018. Version R19, August 2018. Available from: http://p53.iarc.fr/.
3101. Iaria G, Pisani F, De Luca L, et al. Prospective study of switch from cyclosporine to tacrolimus for fibroadenomas of the breast in kidney transplantation. Transplant Proc. 2010 May;42(4):1169–70. PMID:20534252
3102. Ibrahim GM, Huang A, Halliday W, et al. Cribriform neuroepithelial tumour: novel clinicopathological, ultrastructural and cytogenetic findings. Acta Neuropathol. 2011 Oct;122(4):511–4. PMID:21918902
3103. Ibrahim ZA, Chan WH, Wong SL, et al. Extraskeletal myxoid chondrosarcoma of the thigh in a child: a case report. J Orthop Surg (Hong Kong). 2014 Dec;22(3):423–6. PMID:25550031
3104. Ichikawa T, Federle MP, Grazioli L, et al. Fibrolamellar hepatocellular carcinoma: imaging and pathologic findings in 31 recent cases. Radiology. 1999 Nov;213(2):352–61. PMID:10551212
3105. Ichikawa T, Federle MP, Grazioli L, et al. Fibrolamellar hepatocellular carcinoma: pre- and posttherapy evaluation with CT and MR imaging. Radiology. 2000 Oct;217(1):145–51. PMID:11012437
3106. Ichimura K, Fukushima S, Totoki Y, et al. Recurrent neomorphic mutations of MTOR in central nervous system and testicular germ cell tumors may be targeted for therapy. Acta Neuropathol. 2016 Jun;131(6):889–901. PMID:26956871
3107. Iczkowski KA, Butler SL, Shanks JH, et al. Trials of new germ cell immunohistochemical stains in 93 extragonadal and metastatic germ cell tumors. Hum Pathol. 2008 Feb;39(2):275–81. PMID:18045648
3108. Ida CM, Rodriguez FJ, Burger PC, et al. Pleomorphic xanthoastrocytoma: natural history and long-term follow-up. Brain Pathol. 2015 Sep;25(5):575–86. PMID:25318587
3109. Ida CM, Vrana JA, Rodriguez FJ, et al. Immunohistochemistry is highly sensitive and specific for detection of BRAF V600E mutation in pleomorphic xanthoastrocytoma. Acta Neuropathol Commun. 2013 May 30;1:20. PMID:24252190
3110. Ide F. Oral endovascular

papillary angioendothelioma (Dabska tumor). J Oral Pathol Med. 2004 Apr;33(4):249. PMID:15061715
3111. Ide T, Miyoshi T, Katsuragi S, et al. Prediction of postnatal arrhythmia in fetuses with cardiac rhabdomyoma. J Matern Fetal Neonatal Med. 2019 Aug;32(15):2463–8. PMID:29415597
3112. Idowu BD, Thomas G, Frow R, et al. Mutations in SH3BP2, the cherubism gene, were not detected in central or peripheral giant cell tumours of the jaw. Br J Oral Maxillofac Surg. 2008 Apr;46(3):229–30. PMID:17544554
3113. Ijiri R, Tanaka Y, Misugi K, et al. Ossifying fibromyxoid tumor of soft parts in a child: a case report. J Pediatr Surg. 1999 Aug;34(8):1294–6. PMID:10466619
3114. Ikeda J, Sawamura Y, van Meir EG. Pineoblastoma presenting in familial adenomatous polyposis (FAP): random association, FAP variant or Turcot syndrome? Br J Neurosurg. 1998 Dec;12(6):576–8. PMID:10070471
3115. Ikeda R, Tateda M, Okoshi A, et al. Extraosseous chondroma of anterior neck in pediatric patient. Int J Pediatr Otorhinolaryngol. 2015 Aug;79(8):1374–6. PMID:26104481
3116. Ikegaki N, Shimada H, Fox AM, et al. Transient treatment with epigenetic modifiers yields stable neuroblastoma stem cells resembling aggressive large-cell neuroblastomas. Proc Natl Acad Sci U S A. 2013 Apr 9;110(15):6097–102. PMID:23479628
3117. Ikegaki N, Shimada H, International Neuroblastoma Pathology Committee. Subgrouping of unfavorable histology neuroblastomas with immunohistochemistry toward precision prognosis and therapy stratification. JCO Precis Oncol. 2019;3:PO.18.00312. PMID:31840131
3118. Ilica AT, Mossa-Basha M, Zan E, et al. Cranial intraosseous meningioma: spectrum of neuroimaging findings with respect to histopathological grades in 65 patients. Clin Imaging. 2014 Sep-Oct;38(5):599–604. PMID:24997535
3119. Illyés G, Luczay A, Benyó G, et al. Cushing's syndrome in a child with pancreatic acinar cell carcinoma. Endocr Pathol. 2007 Summer;18(2):95–102. PMID:17917000
3120. Imperial R, Helwig EB. Angiokeratoma. A clinicopathological study. Arch Dermatol. 1967 Feb;95(2):166–75. PMID:6018992
3121. Inaba H, Greaves M, Mullighan CG. Acute lymphoblastic leukaemia. Lancet. 2013 Jun 1;381(9881):1943–55. PMID:23523389
3122. Inagaki J, Fukano R, Kurauchi K, et al. Hematopoietic stem cell transplantation in children with refractory cytopenia of childhood: single-center experience using high-dose cytarabine containing myeloablative and aplastic anemia oriented reduced-intensity conditioning regimens. Biol Blood Marrow Transplant. 2015 Mar;21(3):565–9. PMID:25498905
3123. Inamura K, Kobayashi M, Nagano H, et al. A novel fusion of HNRNPA1-ALK in inflammatory myofibroblastic tumor of urinary bladder. Hum Pathol. 2017 Nov;69:96–100. PMID:28504207
3124. Inano S, Sato K, Katsuki Y, et al. RFWD3-mediated ubiquitination promotes timely removal of both RPA and RAD51 from DNA damage sites to facilitate homologous recombination. Mol Cell. 2017 Jun 1;66(5):622–634.e8. PMID:28575658
3125. Inatomi Y, Ito T, Nagae K, et al. Hybrid perineurioma-neurofibroma in a patient with neurofibromatosis type 1, clinically mimicking malignant peripheral nerve sheath tumor. Eur J Dermatol. 2014 May-Jun;24(3):412–3. PMID:24751814
3126. Ingham PW. The patched gene in development and cancer. Curr Opin Genet Dev. 1998 Feb;8(1):88–94. PMID:9529611
3127. Inoue T, Nishi Y, Okumura F, et al. Solid pseudopapillary neoplasm of the pancreas associated with familial adenomatous polyposis. Intern Med. 2015;54(11):1349–55. PMID:26027985
3128. Inoue Y, Nemoto Y, Murata R, et al. CT and MR imaging of cerebral tuberous sclerosis. Brain Dev. 1998 Jun;20(4):209–21. PMID:9661965
3129. International Association of Cancer Registries (IACR) [Internet]. Lyon (France): International Agency for Research on Cancer; 2021. International Classification of Diseases for Oncology (ICD-O) – ICD-O-3.2; updated 2021 Jan 25. Available from: http://www.iacr.com.fr/index.php?option=com_content&view=category&layout=blog&id=100&Itemid=577.
3130. International Germ Cell Cancer Collaborative Group. International Germ Cell Consensus Classification: a prognostic factor-based staging system for metastatic germ cell cancers. J Clin Oncol. 1997 Feb;15(2):594–603. PMID:9053482
3131. International Society for Gastrointestinal Hereditary Tumours [Internet]. Middlesex (UK): International Society for Gastrointestinal Hereditary Tumours; 2018. MMR gene variant classification criteria. Available from: https://www.insight-group.org/criteria/.
3132. Inyang A, Mertens F, Puls F, et al. Primary pseudomyogenic hemangioendothelioma of bone. Am J Surg Pathol. 2016 May;40(5):587–98. PMID:26872012
3133. Ippolito E, Bray EW, Corsi A, et al. Natural history and treatment of fibrous dysplasia of bone: a multicenter clinicopathologic study promoted by the European Pediatric Orthopaedic Society. J Pediatr Orthop B. 2003 May;12(3):155–77. PMID:12703030
3134. Ippolito S, Bellevicine C, Arpaia D, et al. Spindle epithelial tumor with thymus-like differentiation (SETTLE): clinical-pathological features, differential pathological diagnosis and therapy. Endocrine. 2016 Mar;51(3):402–12. PMID:26289127
3135. Iqbal CW, St Peter S, Ishitani MB. Pediatric dermatofibrosarcoma protuberans: multi-institutional outcomes. J Surg Res. 2011 Sep;170(1):69–72. PMID:21429521
3136. Irace AL, Adil EA, Archer NM, et al. Pediatric sialoblastoma: evaluation and management. Int J Pediatr Otorhinolaryngol. 2016 Aug;87:44–9. PMID:27368441
3137. Ireland DC, Soule EH, Ivins JC. Myxoma of somatic soft tissues. A report of 58 patients, 3 with multiple tumors and fibrous dysplasia of bone. Mayo Clin Proc. 1973 Jun;48(6):401–10. PMID:4709710
3138. Irie N, Weinberger L, Tang WW, et al. SOX17 is a critical specifier of human primordial germ cell fate. Cell. 2015 Jan 15;160(1-2):253–68. PMID:25543152
3139. Ironside JW, Jefferson AA, Royds JA, et al. Carcinoid tumour arising in a recurrent intradural spinal teratoma. Neuropathol Appl Neurobiol. 1984 Nov-Dec;10(6):479–89. PMID:6084821
3140. Irving JA, Alkushi A, Young RH, et al. Cellular fibromas of the ovary: a study of 75 cases including 40 mitotically active tumors emphasizing their distinction from fibrosarcoma. Am J Surg Pathol. 2006 Aug;30(8):929–38. PMID:16861962
3141. Irving JA, Young RH. Granulosa cell tumors of the ovary with a pseudopapillary pattern: a study of 14 cases of an unusual morphologic variant emphasizing their distinction from transitional cell neoplasms and other papillary ovarian tumors. Am J Surg Pathol. 2008 Apr;32(4):581–6. PMID:18301054
3142. Isaacs H Jr. Fetal intracranial teratoma. A review. Fetal Pediatr Pathol. 2014 Oct-Dec;33(5-6):289–92. PMID:25353702
3143. Isacsson G, Shear M. Intraoral salivary gland tumors: a retrospective study of 201 cases. J Oral Pathol. 1983 Feb;12(1):57–62. PMID:6300361
3144. Isakoff MS, Bielack SS, Meltzer P, et al. Osteosarcoma: current treatment and a collaborative pathway to success. J Clin Oncol. 2015 Sep 20;33(27):3029–35. PMID:26304877
3145. Isaza-Guzmán DM, Teller-Carrero CB, Laberry-Bermúdez MP, et al. Assessment of clinicopathological characteristics and immunoexpression of COX-2 and IL-10 in oral pyogenic granuloma. Arch Oral Biol. 2012 May;57(5):503–12. PMID:22153609
3145A. Ishibashi K, Ito Y, Masaki A, et al. Warthin-like mucoepidermoid carcinoma: a combined study of fluorescence in situ hybridization and whole-slide imaging. Am J Surg Pathol. 2015 Nov;39(11):1479–87. PMID:26457352
3146. Ishibashi T, Nishio J, Kobayashi S, et al. Chondrolipoma of the ankle in a child: a case report. J Foot Ankle Surg. 2017 Nov-Dec;56(6):1284–7. PMID:28606791
3147. Ishida M, Yoshida K, Kagotani A, et al. Anaplastic lymphoma kinase-positive large B-cell lymphoma: a case report with emphasis on the cytological features of the pleural effusion. Int J Clin Exp Pathol. 2013 Oct 15;6(11):2631–5. PMID:24228132
3148. Ishida S, Yoshida K, Kaneko Y, et al. The genomic breakpoint and chimeric transcripts in the EWSR1-ETV4/E1AF gene fusion in Ewing sarcoma. Cytogenet Cell Genet. 1998;82(3-4):278–83. PMID:9858836
3149. Ishida T, Tagatz GE, Okagaki T. Gonadoblastoma: ultrastructural evidence for testicular origin. Cancer. 1976 Apr;37(4):1770–81. PMID:1260688
3150. Ishige T, Kikuchi K, Miyazaki Y, et al. Differentiation and apoptosis in pilomatrixoma. Am J Dermatopathol. 2011 Feb;33(1):60–4. PMID:21239898
3151. Ishihara S, Ohshima K, Tokura Y, et al. Hypersensitivity to mosquito bites conceals clonal lymphoproliferation of Epstein-Barr viral DNA-positive natural killer cells. Jpn J Cancer Res. 1997 Jan;88(1):82–7. PMID:9045900
3152. Ishihara S, Okada S, Wakiguchi H, et al. Clonal lymphoproliferation following chronic active Epstein-Barr virus infection and hypersensitivity to mosquito bites. Am J Hematol. 1997 Apr;54(4):276–81. PMID:9092681
3153. Ishijima K, Kase S, Noda M, et al. Intraocular neovascularization associated with choroidal ganglioneuroma in neurofibromatosis type 1. Eur J Ophthalmol. 2011 Nov-Dec;21(6):837–40. PMID:21574161
3154. Ishikawa K, Hatano Y, Ichikawa H, et al. The spontaneous regression of tufted angioma. A case of regression after two recurrences and a review of 27 cases reported in the literature. Dermatology. 2005;210(4):346–8. PMID:15942226
3155. Ishikawa O, Ishiguro S, Ohhigashi H, et al. Solid and papillary neoplasm arising from an ectopic pancreas in the mesocolon. Am J Gastroenterol. 1990 May;85(5):597–601. PMID:2337064
3156. Ishizawa K, Komori T, Shimada S, et al. Olig2 and CD99 are useful negative markers for the diagnosis of brain tumors. Clin Neuropathol. 2008 May-Jun;27(3):118–28. PMID:18552083
3157. Ishoo E. Intramuscular myxoma presenting as a rare posterior neck mass in a young child: case report and literature review. Arch Otolaryngol Head Neck Surg. 2007 Apr;133(4):398–401. PMID:17438256
3158. Isidor B, Capito C, Paris F, et al. Familial frameshift SRY mutation inherited from a mosaic father with testicular dysgenesis syndrome. J Clin Endocrinol Metab. 2009 Sep;94(9):3467–71. PMID:19531589
3159. Isimbaldi G, Bandiera L, d'Amore ES, et al. ALK-positive plasmablastic B-cell lymphoma with the clathrin-ALK gene rearrangement. Pediatr Blood Cancer. 2006 Mar;46(3):390–1. PMID:16086416
3160. Isler C, Erturk Cetin O, Ugurlar D, et al. Dysembryoplastic neuroepithelial tumours: clinical, radiological, pathological features and outcome. Br J Neurosurg. 2018 Aug;32(4):436–41. PMID:29792345
3161. Ismail H, Broniszczak D, Kaliciński P, et al. Liver transplantation in children with hepatocellular carcinoma. Do Milan criteria apply to pediatric patients? Pediatr Transplant. 2009 Sep;13(6):682–92. PMID:19496985
3162. Isobe T, Seki M, Yoshida K, et al. Integrated molecular characterization of the lethal pediatric cancer pancreatoblastoma. Cancer Res. 2018 Feb 15;78(4):865–76. PMID:29233928
3163. Itakura E, Yamamoto H, Oda Y, et al. Detection and characterization of vascular endothelial growth factors and their receptors in a series of angiosarcomas. J Surg Oncol. 2008 Jan 1;97(1):74–81. PMID:18041747
3164. Italiano A, Bianchini L, Gjernes E, et al. Clinical and biological significance of CDK4 amplification in well-differentiated and dedifferentiated liposarcomas. Clin Cancer Res. 2009 Sep 15;15(18):5696–703. PMID:19737942
3165. Italiano A, Chen CL, Thomas R, et al. Alterations of the p53 and PIK3CA/AKT/mTOR pathways in angiosarcomas: a pattern distinct from other sarcomas with complex genomics. Cancer. 2012 Dec 1;118(23):5878–87. PMID:22648906
3166. Italiano A, Di Mauro I, Rapp J, et al. Clinical effect of molecular methods in sarcoma diagnosis (GENSARC): a prospective, multicentre, observational study. Lancet Oncol. 2016 Apr;17(4):532–8. PMID:26970672
3167. Italiano A, Sung YS, Zhang L, et al. High prevalence of CIC fusion with double-homeobox (DUX4) transcription factors in EWSR1-negative undifferentiated small blue round cell sarcomas. Genes Chromosomes Cancer. 2012 Mar;51(3):207–18. PMID:22072439
3168. Itin PH, Lautenschlager S. Lower and upper extremity atrophy associated with a giant congenital melanocytic nevus. Pediatr Dermatol. 1998 Jul-Aug;15(4):287–9. PMID:9720694
3169. Ito J, Nakano Y, Shima H, et al. Central nervous system ganglioneuroblastoma harboring MYO5A-NTRK3 fusion. Brain Tumor Pathol. 2020 Jul;37(3):105–10. PMID:32556925
3170. Iwafuchi H, Ito M. Differences in the bone marrow histology between childhood myelodysplastic syndrome with multilineage dysplasia and refractory cytopenia of childhood without multilineage dysplasia. Histopathology. 2019 Jan;74(2):239–47. PMID:30062702
3171. Iwafuchi H, Nakazawa A, Sekimizu M, et al. Clinicopathological features and prognostic significance of programmed death ligand 1 in pediatric ALK-positive anaplastic large cell lymphoma: results of the ALCL99 treatment in Japan. Hum Pathol. 2021 Oct;116:112–21. PMID:34363798
3172. Iwasaki H, Kikuchi M, Mori R, et al. Infantile digital fibromatosis. Ultrastructural, histochemical, and tissue culture observations. Cancer. 1980 Nov 15;46(10):2238–47. PMID:6253042
3173. Iwasaki T, Murakami M, Sugisaki C, et al. Characterization of myelodysplastic syndrome and aplastic anemia by immunostaining of p53 and hemoglobin F and karyotype analysis: differential diagnosis between refractory anemia and aplastic anemia. Pathol Int. 2008 Jun;58(6):353–60. PMID:18477214

**3173A.** Iwatsuki K, Miyake T, Hirai Y, et al. Hydroa vacciniforme: a distinctive form of Epstein-Barr virus-associated T-cell lymphoproliferative disorders. Eur J Dermatol. 2019 Feb 1;29(1):21–8. PMID:30998212

**3174.** Iyer RS, Chapman T, Chew FS. Pediatric bone imaging: diagnostic imaging of osteoid osteoma. AJR Am J Roentgenol. 2012 May;198(5):1039–52. PMID:22528893

**3175.** Izadpanah A, Viezel-Mathieu A, Izadpanah A, et al. Dupuytren contracture in the pediatric population: a systematic review. Eur J Pediatr Surg. 2015 Apr;25(2):151–4. PMID:24163199

**3176.** Izquierdo FM, Ramos LR, Sánchez-Herráez S, et al. Dedifferentiated classic adamantinoma of the tibia: a report of a case with eventual complete revertant mesenchymal phenotype. Am J Surg Pathol. 2010 Sep;34(9):1388–92. PMID:20717000

**3177.** Izquierdo MA, Van der Valk P, Van Ark-Otte J, et al. Differential expression of the c-kit proto-oncogene in germ cell tumours. J Pathol. 1995 Nov;177(3):253–8. PMID:8551387

**3178.** Jaafar R, Tang IP, Jong DE, et al. Cervical lipoblastoma: an uncommon presentation. Ear Nose Throat J. 2015 Jul;94(7):E8–10. PMID:26214680

**3179.** Jääskeläinen J, Paetau A, Pyykkö I, et al. Interface between the facial nerve and large acoustic neurinomas. Immunohistochemical study of the cleavage plane in NF2 and non-NF2 cases. J Neurosurg. 1994 Mar;80(3):541–7. PMID:8113868

**3180.** Jabarin B, Solomon A, Amer R. Interleukin-17 and its correlation with vascular endothelial growth factor expression in ocular surface pathologies: a histologic study. Eur J Ophthalmol. 2016 Jun 10;26(4):283–6. PMID:26615952

**3181.** Jablenska L, Trinidade A, Meranagri V, et al. Salivary gland pathology in the paediatric population: implications for management and presentation of a rare case. J Laryngol Otol. 2014 Jan;128(1):104–6. PMID:24507800

**3182.** Jacknow G, Frizzera G, Gajl-Peczalska K, et al. Extramedullary presentation of the blast crisis of chronic myelogenous leukaemia. Br J Haematol. 1985 Oct;61(2):225–36. PMID:3862425

**3183.** Jacks SK, Witman PM. Tuberous sclerosis complex: an update for dermatologists. Pediatr Dermatol. 2015 Sep-Oct;32(5):563–70. PMID:25776100

**3184.** Jackson CC, Dickson MA, Sadjadi M, et al. Kaposi sarcoma of childhood: inborn or acquired immunodeficiency to oncogenic HHV-8. Pediatr Blood Cancer. 2016 Mar;63(3):392–7. PMID:26469702

**3185.** Jackson TJ, Williams RD, Brok J, et al. The diagnostic accuracy and clinical utility of pediatric renal tumor biopsy: report of the UK experience in the SIOP UK WT 2001 trial. Pediatr Blood Cancer. 2019 Jun;66(6):e27627. PMID:30761727

**3186.** Jacobs JJ, Rosenberg AE. Extracranial skeletal metastasis from a pinealoblastoma. A case report and review of the literature. Clin Orthop Relat Res. 1989 Oct; (247):256–60. PMID:2676297

**3187.** Jacobsen GK, Henriksen OB, von der Maase H. Carcinoma in situ of testicular tissue adjacent to malignant germ-cell tumors: a study of 105 cases. Cancer. 1981 Jun 1;47(11):2660–2. PMID:7260858

**3188.** Jacobsen GK, Nørgaard-Pedersen B. Placental alkaline phosphatase in testicular germ cell tumours and in carcinoma-in-situ of the testis. An immunohistochemical study. Acta Pathol Microbiol Immunol Scand A. 1984 Sep;92(5):323–9. PMID:6209917

**3189.** Jacobsen GK, Rørth M, Osterlind K, et al. Histopathological features in stage I non-seminomatous testicular germ cell tumours correlated to relapse. APMIS. 1990 Apr;98(4):377–82. PMID:2162186

**3190.** Jacoby LB, MacCollin M, Barone R, et al. Frequency and distribution of NF2 mutations in schwannomas. Genes Chromosomes Cancer. 1996 Sep;17(1):45–55. PMID:8889506

**3191.** Jafarian F, McCuaig C, Kokta V, et al. Dermatofibrosarcoma protuberans in childhood and adolescence: report of eight patients. Pediatr Dermatol. 2008 May-Jun;25(3):317–25. PMID:18577035

**3192.** Jaffe ES, Diebold J, Harris NL, et al. Burkitt's lymphoma: a single disease with multiple variants. The World Health Organization classification of neoplastic diseases of the hematopoietic and lymphoid tissues. Blood. 1999 Feb 1;93(3):1124. PMID:10025990

**3193.** Jaffe HL. Osteoid-osteoma. Proc R Soc Med. 1953 Dec;46(12):1007–12. PMID:13120827

**3194.** Jaffe HL, Lichtenstein L. Non-osteogenic fibroma of bone. Am J Pathol. 1942 Mar;18(2):205–21. PMID:19970624

**3195.** Jaffe JD, Wang Y, Chan HM, et al. Global chromatin profiling reveals NSD2 mutations in pediatric acute lymphoblastic leukemia. Nat Genet. 2013 Nov;45(11):1386–91. PMID:24076604

**3196.** Jaffe N, Spears R, Eftekhari F, et al. Pathologic fracture in osteosarcoma. Impact of chemotherapy on primary tumor and survival. Cancer. 1987 Feb 15;59(4):701–9. PMID:3492261

**3197.** Jager B, Schuhmann MU, Schober R, et al. Induction of gliosarcoma and atypical meningioma 13 years after radiotherapy of residual pilocytic astrocytoma in childhood. Pediatr Neurosurg. 2008;44(2):153–8. PMID:18230932

**3198.** Jager MJ, Shields CL, Cebulla CM, et al. Uveal melanoma. Nat Rev Dis Primers. 2020 Apr 9;6(1):24. PMID:32273508

**3199.** Jaiman S, Fernandez E, Gundabattula SR. Chorangioendothelioma of the placenta: a myth or reality? Pediatr Dev Pathol. 2015 Sep-Oct;18(5):410–5. PMID:25906437

**3200.** Jain P, Mohamed A, Sigamani E, et al. Bilateral thalamic lesions in a child. Eur Neurol. 2013;70(1-2):33–4. PMID:23689275

**3201.** Jain SU, Do TJ, Lund PJ, et al. PFA ependymoma-associated protein EZHIP inhibits PRC2 activity through a H3 K27M-like mechanism. Nat Commun. 2019 May 13;10(1):2146. PMID:31086175

**3202.** Jaiswal S, Vij M, Jaiswal AK, et al. Squash cytology of subependymal giant cell astrocytoma: report of four cases with brief review of literature. Diagn Cytopathol. 2012 Apr;40(4):333–6. PMID:22431322

**3203.** Jaju A, Hwang EI, Kool M, et al. MRI Features of histologically diagnosed supratentorial primitive neuroectodermal tumors and pineoblastomas in correlation with molecular diagnoses and outcomes: a report from the Children's Oncology Group ACNS0332 Trial. AJNR Am J Neuroradiol. 2019 Nov;40(11):1796–803. PMID:31601576

**3204.** Jaju PD, Ransohoff KJ, Tang JY, et al. Familial skin cancer syndromes: increased risk of nonmelanotic skin cancers and extracutaneous tumors. J Am Acad Dermatol. 2016 Mar;74(3):437–51. PMID:26892653

**3205.** Jakacki RI, Burger PC, Kocak M, et al. Outcome and prognostic factors for children with supratentorial primitive neuroectodermal tumors treated with carboplatin during radiotherapy: a report from the Children's Oncology Group. Pediatr Blood Cancer. 2015 May;62(5):776–83. PMID:25704363

**3206.** Jakchairoongruang K, Khakoo Y, Beckwith M, et al. New insights into neurocutaneous melanosis. Pediatr Radiol. 2018 Nov;48(12):1786–96. PMID:30074086

**3207.** Jakobiec FA, Bhat P, Colby KA. Immunohistochemical studies of conjunctival nevi and melanomas. Arch Ophthalmol. 2010 Feb;128(2):174–83. PMID:20142539

**3208.** Jakobiec FA, Colby K, Bajart AM, et al. Immunohistochemical studies of atypical conjunctival melanocytic nevi. Arch Ophthalmol. 2009 Aug;127(8):970–80. PMID:19667333

**3209.** Jakobiec FA, Folberg R, Iwamoto T. Clinicopathologic characteristics of premalignant and malignant melanocytic lesions of the conjunctiva. Ophthalmology. 1989 Feb;96(2):147–66. PMID:2649838

**3210.** Jakobiec FA, Kool M, Stagner AM, et al. Intraocular medulloepitheliomas and embryonal tumors with multilayered rosettes of the brain: comparative roles of LIN28A and C19MC. Am J Ophthalmol. 2015 Jun;159(6):1065–1074.e1. PMID:25748578

**3211.** Jakobiec FA, Rose MF, Trief D, et al. Immunohistochemical investigations of adult intraocular medulloepitheliomas. Clin Exp Ophthalmol. 2015 May-Jun;43(4):379–85. PMID:25251824

**3212.** Jakobiec FA, Trief D, Rashid A, et al. New insights into the development of infantile intraocular medulloepithelioma. Am J Ophthalmol. 2014 Dec;158(6):1275–1296.e1. PMID:25174896

**3213.** Jakowski JD, Wakely PE Jr. Primary intrathoracic low-grade fibromyxoid sarcoma. Hum Pathol. 2008 Apr;39(4):623–8. PMID:18275982

**3214.** Jalali M, Netscher DT, Connelly JH. Glomangiomatosis. Ann Diagn Pathol. 2002 Oct;6(5):326–8. PMID:12376927

**3215.** Jamilloux Y, Favier J, Pertuit M, et al. A MEN1 syndrome with a paraganglioma. Eur J Hum Genet. 2014 Feb;22(2):283–5. PMID:23778871

**3216.** Jamshidi F, Bashashati A, Shumansky K, et al. The genomic landscape of epithelioid sarcoma cell lines and tumours. J Pathol. 2016 Jan;238(1):63–73. PMID:26365879

**3217.** Janeway KA, Kim SY, Lodish M, et al. Defects in succinate dehydrogenase in gastrointestinal stromal tumors lacking KIT and PDGFRA mutations. Proc Natl Acad Sci U S A. 2011 Jan 4;108(1):314–8. PMID:21173220

**3218.** Janeway KA, Weldon CB. Pediatric gastrointestinal stromal tumor. Semin Pediatr Surg. 2012 Feb;21(1):31–43. PMID:22248968

**3219.** Jänisch W, Staneczek W. [Primary tumors of the choroid plexus. Frequency, localization and age]. Zentralbl Allg Pathol. 1989;135(3):235–40. German. PMID:2773602

**3220.** Janoueix-Lerosey I, Lopez-Delisle L, Delattre O, et al. The ALK receptor in sympathetic neuron development and neuroblastoma. Cell Tissue Res. 2018 May;372(2):325–37. PMID:29374774

**3221.** Janson K, Nedzi LA, David O, et al. Predisposition to atypical teratoid/rhabdoid tumor due to an inherited INI1 mutation. Pediatr Blood Cancer. 2006 Sep;47(3):279–84. PMID:16261613

**3222.** Janssen D, Harms D. Juvenile xanthogranuloma in childhood and adolescence: a clinicopathologic study of 129 patients from the kiel pediatric tumor registry. Am J Surg Pathol. 2005 Jan;29(1):21–8. PMID:15613853

**3223.** Janz TA, Lentsch EJ, Nguyen SA, et al. Are demographics associated with mucoepidermoid or acinic cell carcinoma parotid malignancies in children? World J Otorhinolaryngol Head Neck Surg. 2020 Jan 14;5(4):222–7. PMID:32083250

**3224.** Janzarik WG, Kratz CP, Loges NT, et al. Further evidence for a somatic KRAS mutation in a pilocytic astrocytoma. Neuropediatrics. 2007 Apr;38(2):61–3. PMID:17712732

**3225.** Japp AS, Gessi M, Messing-Jünger M, et al. High-resolution genomic analysis does not qualify atypical plexus papilloma as a separate entity among choroid plexus tumors. J Neuropathol Exp Neurol. 2015 Feb;74(2):110–20. PMID:25575132

**3226.** Jaquemus J, Perron E, Buisson A, et al. Compound blue nevus: a reappraisal of the concept in the genomic era. Virchows Arch. 2020 Mar;476(3):439–43. PMID:31754815

**3227.** Jaqueti G, Requena L, Sánchez Yus E. Trichoblastoma is the most common neoplasm developed in nevus sebaceus of Jadassohn: a clinicopathologic study of a series of 155 cases. Am J Dermatopathol. 2000 Apr;22(2):108–18. PMID:10770429

**3228.** Jaramillo S, Grosshans DR, Philip N, et al. Radiation for ETMR: literature review and case series of patients treated with proton therapy. Clin Transl Radiat Oncol. 2018 Nov 7;15:31–7. PMID:30582019

**3229.** Jardin F, Pujals A, Pelletier L, et al. Recurrent mutations of the exportin 1 gene (XPO1) and their impact on selective inhibitor of nuclear export compounds sensitivity in primary mediastinal B-cell lymphoma. Am J Hematol. 2016 Sep;91(9):923–30. PMID:27312795

**3230.** Järvinen HJ, Peltomäki P. The complex genotype-phenotype relationship in familial adenomatous polyposis. Eur J Gastroenterol Hepatol. 2004 Jan;16(1):5–8. PMID:15095846

**3231.** Jarzembowski JA. New prognostic indicators in pediatric adrenal tumors: Neuroblastoma and adrenal cortical tumors, can we predict when these will behave badly? Surg Pathol Clin. 2020 Dec;13(4):625–41. PMID:33183724

**3232.** Jaunmuktane Z, Capper D, Jones DTW, et al. Methylation array profiling of adult brain tumours: diagnostic outcomes in a large, single centre. Acta Neuropathol Commun. 2019 Feb 20;7(1):24. PMID:30786920

**3233.** Javadpour N. Significance of elevated serum alphafetoprotein (AFP) in seminoma. Cancer. 1980 Apr 15;45(8):2166–8. PMID:6154525

**3234.** Javadpour N. The role of biologic tumor markers in testicular cancer. Cancer. 1980 Apr;45 Suppl 7:1755–61. PMID:29603174

**3235.** Javanmardi N, Fransson S, Djos A, et al. Low frequency ALK hotspots mutations in neuroblastoma tumours detected by ultradeep sequencing: implications for ALK inhibitor treatment. Sci Rep. 2019 Feb 18;9(1):2199. PMID:30778092

**3236.** Jawad MU, Cheung MC, Min ES, et al. Ewing sarcoma demonstrates racial disparities in incidence-related and sex-related differences in outcome: an analysis of 1631 cases from the SEER database, 1973-2005. Cancer. 2009 Aug 1;115(15):3526–36. PMID:19548262

**3237.** Jay V, Squire J, Becker LE, et al. Malignant transformation in a ganglioglioma with anaplastic neuronal and astrocytic components. Report of a case with flow cytometric and cytogenetic analysis. Cancer. 1994 Jun 1;73(11):2862–8. PMID:8194028

**3238.** Jee KJ, Persson M, Heikinheimo K, et al. Genomic profiles and CRTC1-MAML2 fusion distinguish different subtypes of mucoepidermoid carcinoma. Mod Pathol. 2013 Feb;26(2):213–22. PMID:23018873

**3239.** Jeha S, Choi J, Roberts KG, et al. Clinical significance of novel subtypes of acute lymphoblastic leukemia in the context of minimal residual disease-directed therapy. Blood Cancer Discov. 2021 Jul;2(4):326–37. PMID:34250504

**3240.** Jeha S, Pei D, Raimondi SC, et al. Increased risk for CNS relapse in pre-B cell leukemia with the t(1;19)/TCF3-PBX1. Leukemia. 2009 Aug;23(8):1406–9. PMID:19282835

**3241.** Jehangir S, Kurian JJ, Selvarajah D, et al. Recurrent and metastatic congenital mesoblastic nephroma: Where does the evidence stand? Pediatr Surg Int. 2017 Nov;33(11):1183–8. PMID:28850451
**3242.** Jeibmann A, Eikmeier K, Linge A, et al. Identification of genes involved in the biology of atypical teratoid/rhabdoid tumours using Drosophila melanogaster. Nat Commun. 2014 Jun 3;5:4005. PMID:24892285
**3243.** Jeibmann A, Hasselblatt M, Gerss J, et al. Prognostic implications of atypical histologic features in choroid plexus papilloma. J Neuropathol Exp Neurol. 2006 Nov;65(11):1069–73. PMID:17086103
**3244.** Jeibmann A, Wrede B, Peters O, et al. Malignant progression in choroid plexus papillomas. J Neurosurg. 2007 Sep;107(3 Suppl):199–202. PMID:17918524
**3245.** Jelinic P, Mueller JJ, Olvera N, et al. Recurrent SMARCA4 mutations in small cell carcinoma of the ovary. Nat Genet. 2014 May;46(5):424–6. PMID:24658004
**3246.** Jelinic P, Schlappe BA, Conlon N, et al. Concomitant loss of SMARCA2 and SMARCA4 expression in small cell carcinoma of the ovary, hypercalcemic type. Mod Pathol. 2016 Jan;29(1):60–6. PMID:26564006
**3247.** Jeng MR, Fuh B, Blatt J, et al. Malignant transformation of infantile hemangioma to angiosarcoma: response to chemotherapy with bevacizumab. Pediatr Blood Cancer. 2014 Nov;61(11):2115–7. PMID:24740626
**3248.** Jennes I, de Jong D, Mees K, et al. Breakpoint characterization of large deletions in EXT1 or EXT2 in 10 multiple osteochondromas families. BMC Med Genet. 2011 Jun 26;12:85. PMID:21703028
**3249.** Jennes I, Pedrini E, Zuntini M, et al. Multiple osteochondromas: mutation update and description of the multiple osteochondromas mutation database (MOdb). Hum Mutat. 2009 Dec;30(12):1620–7. PMID:19810120
**3250.** Jennings MT, Gelman R, Hochberg F. Intracranial germ-cell tumors: natural history and pathogenesis. J Neurosurg. 1985 Aug;63(2):155–67. PMID:2991485
**3251.** Jensen DE, Proctor M, Marquis ST, et al. BAP1: a novel ubiquitin hydrolase which binds to the BRCA1 RING finger and enhances BRCA1-mediated cell growth suppression. Oncogene. 1998 Mar 5;16(9):1097–112. PMID:9528852
**3252.** Jensen JL, Venner PM. Predictive factors for outcome in treatment of metastatic nonseminomatous germ cell tumors. Urology. 1992 Mar;39(3):237–42. PMID:1372134
**3253.** Jensen LH, Bojesen A, Byriel L, et al. Implementing population-based screening for Lynch syndrome [abstract]. J Clin Oncol. 2013 May 20;31(15 Suppl). Abstract no. 6600. doi:10.1200/jco.2013.31.15_suppl.6600.
**3254.** Jensen RL, Caamano E, Jensen EM, et al. Development of contrast enhancement after long-term observation of a dysembryoplastic neuroepithelial tumor. J Neurooncol. 2006 May;78(1):59–62. PMID:16314940
**3255.** Jeon YK, Cheon JE, Kim SK, et al. Clinicopathological features and global genomic copy number alterations of pilomyxoid astrocytoma in the hypothalamus/optic pathway: comparative analysis with pilocytic astrocytoma using array-based comparative genomic hybridization. Mod Pathol. 2008 Nov;21(11):1345–56. PMID:18622384
**3256.** Jeong D, Lee DS, Kim N, et al. Prevalence of germline predisposition gene mutations in pediatric acute myeloid leukemia: genetic background of pediatric AML. Leuk Res. 2019 Oct;85:106210. PMID:31470354
**3257.** Jeong HJ, Ahn YH, Park E, et al. Post-transplantation lymphoproliferative disorder after pediatric solid organ transplantation: experiences of 20 years in a single center. Korean J Pediatr. 2017 Mar;60(3):86–93. PMID:28392824
**3258.** Jessa S, Blanchet-Cohen A, Krug B, et al. Stalled developmental programs at the root of pediatric brain tumors. Nat Genet. 2019 Dec;51(12):1702–13. PMID:31768071
**3259.** Jet Aw S, Hong Kuick C, Hwee Yong M, et al. Novel karyotypes and cyclin D1 immunoreactivity in clear cell sarcoma of the kidney. Pediatr Dev Pathol. 2015 Jul-Aug;18(4):297–304. PMID:25751590
**3260.** Jett K, Friedman JM. Clinical and genetic aspects of neurofibromatosis 1. Genet Med. 2010 Jan;12(1):1–11. PMID:20027112
**3261.** Jha A, Ling A, Millo C, et al. Superiority of 68Ga-DOTATATE over 18F-FDG and anatomic imaging in the detection of succinate dehydrogenase mutation (SDHx )-related pheochromocytoma and paraganglioma in the pediatric population. Eur J Nucl Med Mol Imaging. 2018 May;45(5):787–97. PMID:29204718
**3262.** Jha P, Moosavi C, Fanburg-Smith JC. Giant cell fibroblastoma: an update and addition of 86 new cases from the Armed Forces Institute of Pathology, in honor of Dr. Franz M. Enzinger. Ann Diagn Pathol. 2007 Apr;11(2):81–8. PMID:17349565
**3263.** Jhala DN, Eltoum I, Carroll AJ, et al. Osteosarcoma in a patient with McCune-Albright syndrome and Mazabraud's syndrome: a case report emphasizing the cytological and cytogenetic findings. Hum Pathol. 2003 Dec;34(12):1354–7. PMID:14691924
**3264.** Ji Y, Yang K, Peng S, et al. Kaposiform haemangioendothelioma: clinical features, complications and risk factors for Kasabach-Merritt phenomenon. Br J Dermatol. 2018 Aug;179(2):457–63. PMID:29603128
**3265.** Jia L, Carlo MI, Khan H, et al. Distinctive mechanisms underlie the loss of SMARCB1 protein expression in renal medullary carcinoma: morphologic and molecular analysis of 20 cases. Mod Pathol. 2019 Sep;32(9):1329–43. PMID:30980040
**3266.** Jia WH, Qin HD. Non-viral environmental risk factors for nasopharyngeal carcinoma: a systematic review. Semin Cancer Biol. 2012 Apr;22(2):117–26. PMID:22311401
**3267.** Jiang JF, Xue W, Deng Y, et al. Gonadal malignancy in 202 female patients with disorders of sex development containing Y-chromosome material. Gynecol Endocrinol. 2016;32(4):338–41. PMID:26608236
**3268.** Jiang L, Gu ZH, Yan ZX, et al. Exome sequencing identifies somatic mutations of DDX3X in natural killer/T-cell lymphoma. Nat Genet. 2015 Sep;47(9):1061–6. PMID:26192917
**3269.** Jiang T, Raynald, Yang H, et al. Predictive factors of overall survival in primary intracranial pure choriocarcinoma. J Clin Neurosci. 2019 Mar;61:93–101. PMID:30442453
**3270.** Jiang T, Raynald, Yang H, et al. Primary intracranial embryonal carcinoma in children: report of two cases with review of the literature. Int J Clin Exp Pathol. 2017 Nov 1;10(11):10700–10. PMID:31966414
**3271.** Jiang XN, Yu BH, Wang WG, et al. Anaplastic lymphoma kinase-positive large B-cell lymphoma: clinico-pathological study of 17 cases with review of literature. PLoS One. 2017 Jun 30;12(6):e0178416. PMID:28665943
**3272.** Jiang Z, Zhang T, Liu X, et al. Multimodal imaging features of bilateral choroidal ganglioneuroma. J Ophthalmol. 2020 May 11;2020:6231269. PMID:32454990
**3273.** Jiao Y, Yonescu R, Offerhaus GJ, et al. Whole-exome sequencing of pancreatic neoplasms with acinar differentiation. J Pathol. 2014 Mar;232(4):428–35. PMID:24293293
**3274.** Jiménez I, Chicard M, Colmet-Daage L, et al. Circulating tumor DNA analysis enables molecular characterization of pediatric renal tumors at diagnosis. Int J Cancer. 2019 Jan 1;144(1):68–79. PMID:29923174
**3275.** Jiménez I, Laé M, Tanguy ML, et al. Craniofacial second primary tumors in patients with germline retinoblastoma previously treated with external beam radiotherapy: a retrospective institutional analysis. Pediatr Blood Cancer. 2020 Apr;67(4):e28158. PMID:31904159
**3276.** Jiménez-Heffernan JA, Freih Fraih A, Álvarez F, et al. Cytologic features of pleomorphic xanthoastrocytoma, WHO grade II. A comparative study with glioblastoma. Diagn Cytopathol. 2017 Apr;45(4):339–44. PMID:28084690
**3277.** Jin L, Sui Y, Zhu H, et al. Primary mediastinal clear cell sarcoma: a case report and review of the literature. Diagn Pathol. 2017 Jan 13;12(1):5. PMID:28086809
**3278.** Jin Y, Elalaf H, Watanabe M, et al. Mutant IDH1 dysregulates the differentiation of mesenchymal stem cells in association with gene-specific histone modifications to cartilage- and bone-related genes. PLoS One. 2015 Jul 10;10(7):e0131998. PMID:26161668
**3279.** Jin Y, Möller E, Nord KH, et al. Fusion of the AHRR and NCOA2 genes through a recurrent translocation t(5;8)(p15;q13) in soft tissue angiofibroma results in upregulation of aryl hydrocarbon receptor target genes. Genes Chromosomes Cancer. 2012 May;51(5):510–20. PMID:22337624
**3280.** Jinkala SR, Muthalagan E, Badhe BA. Granulomatous response in intracranial germinomas: diagnostic problems. Int J Appl Basic Med Res. 2018 Jan-Mar;8(1):51–3. PMID:29552538
**3281.** Jinnin M, Medici D, Park L, et al. Suppressed NFAT-dependent VEGFR1 expression and constitutive VEGFR2 signaling in infantile hemangioma. Nat Med. 2008 Nov;14(11):1236–46. PMID:18931684
**3282.** Jo VY, Antonescu CR, Dickson BC, et al. Cutaneous syncytial myoepithelioma is characterized by recurrent EWSR1-PBX3 fusions. Am J Surg Pathol. 2019 Oct;43(10):1349–54. PMID:31135487
**3283.** Jo VY, Antonescu CR, Zhang L, et al. Cutaneous syncytial myoepithelioma: clinicopathologic characterization in a series of 38 cases. Am J Surg Pathol. 2013 May;37(5):710–8. PMID:23588365
**3284.** Jo VY, Fletcher CD. Epithelioid malignant peripheral nerve sheath tumor: clinicopathologic analysis of 63 cases. Am J Surg Pathol. 2015 May;39(5):673–82. PMID:25602794
**3285.** Jo VY, Fletcher CD. p63 immunohistochemical staining is limited in soft tissue tumors. Am J Clin Pathol. 2011 Nov;136(5):762–6. PMID:22031315
**3286.** Jo VY, Fletcher CDM. SMARCB1/INI1 Loss in epithelioid schwannoma: a clinicopathologic and immunohistochemical study of 65 cases. Am J Surg Pathol. 2017 Aug;41(8):1013–22. PMID:28368924
**3287.** Jo VY, Sholl LM, Krane JF. Distinctive patterns of CTNNB1 (β-Catenin) alterations in salivary gland basal cell adenoma and basal cell adenocarcinoma. Am J Surg Pathol. 2016 Aug;40(8):1143–50. PMID:27259009
**3288.** Job S, Draskovic I, Burnichon N, et al. Telomerase activation and ATRX mutations are independent risk factors for metastatic pheochromocytoma and paraganglioma. Clin Cancer Res. 2019 Jan 15;25(2):760–70. PMID:30301828
**3289.** Jochmanova I, Abcede AMT, Guerrero RJS, et al. Clinical characteristics and outcomes of SDHB-related pheochromocytoma and paraganglioma in children and adolescents. J Cancer Res Clin Oncol. 2020 Apr;146(4):1051–63. PMID:32062700
**3290.** Johann PD, Bens S, Oyen F, et al. Sellar region atypical teratoid/rhabdoid tumors (ATRT) in adults display DNA methylation profiles of the ATRT-MYC subgroup. Am J Surg Pathol. 2018 Apr;42(4):506–11. PMID:29324471
**3291.** Johann PD, Erkek S, Zapatka M, et al. Atypical teratoid/rhabdoid tumors are comprised of three epigenetic subgroups with distinct enhancer landscapes. Cancer Cell. 2016 Mar 14;29(3):379–93. PMID:26923874
**3292.** Johann PD, Hovestadt V, Thomas C, et al. Cribriform neuroepithelial tumor: molecular characterization of a SMARCB1-deficient non-rhabdoid tumor with favorable long-term outcome. Brain Pathol. 2017 Jul;27(4):411–8. PMID:27380723
**3293.** Johnson A, Severson E, Gay L, et al. Comprehensive genomic profiling of 282 pediatric low- and high-grade gliomas reveals genomic drivers, tumor mutational burden, and hypermutation signatures. Oncologist. 2017 Dec;22(12):1478–90. PMID:28912153
**3294.** Johnson DR, Giannini C, Jenkins RB, et al. Plenty of calcification: imaging characterization of polymorphous low-grade neuroepithelial tumor of the young. Neuroradiology. 2019 Nov;61(11):1327–32. PMID:31396664
**3295.** Johnson LC, Yousefi M, Vinh TN, et al. Juvenile active ossifying fibroma. Its nature, dynamics and origin. Acta Otolaryngol Suppl. 1991;488:1–40. PMID:1843064
**3296.** Johnson LN, Hepler RS, Yee RD, et al. Magnetic resonance imaging of craniopharyngioma. Am J Ophthalmol. 1986 Aug 15;102(2):242–4. PMID:3740186
**3297.** Johnson LR, Nalesnik MA, Swerdlow SH. Impact of Epstein-Barr virus in monomorphic B-cell posttransplant lymphoproliferative disorders: a histogenetic study. Am J Surg Pathol. 2006 Dec;30(12):1604–12. PMID:17122518
**3298.** Johnson MW, Eberhart CG, Perry A, et al. Spectrum of pilomyxoid astrocytomas: intermediate pilomyxoid tumors. Am J Surg Pathol. 2010 Dec;34(12):1783–91. PMID:21107083
**3299.** Johnson MW, Emelin JK, Park SH, et al. Co-localization of TSC1 and TSC2 gene products in tubers of patients with tuberous sclerosis. Brain Pathol. 1999 Jan;9(1):45–54. PMID:9989450
**3300.** Johnson MW, Kerfoot C, Bushnell T, et al. Hamartin and tuberin expression in human tissues. Mod Pathol. 2001 Mar;14(3):202–10. PMID:11266527
**3301.** Johnson NR, Gannon OM, Savage NW, et al. Frequency of odontogenic cysts and tumors: a systematic review. J Investig Clin Dent. 2014 Feb;5(1):9–14. PMID:23766099
**3302.** Johnson PR. Gastroenteropancreatic neuroendocrine (carcinoid) tumors in children. Semin Pediatr Surg. 2014 Apr;23(2):91–5. PMID:24931354
**3302A.** Johnson RA, Wright KD, Poppleton H, et al. Cross-species genomics matches driver mutations and cell compartments to model ependymoma. Nature. 2010 Jul 29;466(7306):632–6. PMID:20639864
**3303.** Johnson RL, Rothman AL, Xie J, et al. Human homolog of patched, a candidate gene for the basal cell nevus syndrome. Science. 1996 Jun 14;272(5268):1668–71. PMID:8658145
**3304.** Johnson S, Têtu B, Ayala AG, et al. Chondrosarcoma with additional mesenchymal component (dedifferentiated chondrosarcoma). I. A clinicopathologic study of 26 cases. Cancer. 1986 Jul 15;58(2):278–86. PMID:3719521
**3305.** Johnson TL, Lloyd RV, Thompson NW, et al. Prognostic implications of the tall cell variant of papillary thyroid carcinoma. Am J Surg Pathol. 1988 Jan;12(1):22–7. PMID:3337337

3306. Johnston EE, LeBlanc RE, Kim J, et al. Subcutaneous panniculitis-like T-cell lymphoma: pediatric case series demonstrating heterogeneous presentation and option for watchful waiting. Pediatr Blood Cancer. 2015 Nov;62(11):2025–8. PMID:26146844
3307. Jokinen CH, Ragsdale BD, Argenyi ZB. Expanding the clinicopathologic spectrum of palisaded encapsulated neuroma. J Cutan Pathol. 2010 Jan;37(1):43–8. PMID:19614730
3308. Jones AC, Prihoda TJ, Kacher JE, et al. Osteoblastoma of the maxilla and mandible: a report of 24 cases, review of the literature, and discussion of its relationship to osteoid osteoma of the jaws. Oral Surg Oral Med Oral Pathol Oral Radiol Endod. 2006 Nov;102(5):639–50. PMID:17052641
3309. Jones AC, Shyamsundar MM, Thomas MW, et al. Comprehensive mutation analysis of TSC1 and TSC2-and phenotypic correlations in 150 families with tuberous sclerosis. Am J Hum Genet. 1999 May;64(5):1305–15. PMID:10205261
3310. Jones AV, Craig GT, Speight PM, et al. The range and demographics of salivary gland tumours diagnosed in a UK population. Oral Oncol. 2008 Apr;44(4):407–17. PMID:17825603
3311. Jones AV, Franklin CD. An analysis of oral and maxillofacial pathology found in children over a 30-year period. Int J Paediatr Dent. 2006 Jan;16(1):19–30. PMID:16364089
3312. Jones DC, Reyes-Múgica M, Gallagher PG, et al. Three-dimensional sonographic imaging of a highly developed fetus in fetu with spontaneous movement of the extremities. J Ultrasound Med. 2001 Dec;20(12):1357–63. PMID:11762548
3313. Jones DT, Hutter B, Jäger N, et al. Recurrent somatic alterations of FGFR1 and NTRK2 in pilocytic astrocytoma. Nat Genet. 2013 Aug;45(8):927–32. PMID:23817572
3314. Jones DT, Ichimura K, Liu L, et al. Genomic analysis of pilocytic astrocytomas at 0.97 Mb resolution shows an increasing tendency toward chromosomal copy number change with age. J Neuropathol Exp Neurol. 2006 Nov;65(11):1049–58. PMID:17086101
3315. Jones DT, Kocialkowski S, Liu L, et al. Oncogenic RAF1 rearrangement and a novel BRAF mutation as alternatives to KIAA1549:BRAF fusion in activating the MAPK pathway in pilocytic astrocytoma. Oncogene. 2009 May 21;28(20):2119–23. PMID:19363522
3316. Jones DT, Kocialkowski S, Liu L, et al. Tandem duplication producing a novel oncogenic BRAF fusion gene defines the majority of pilocytic astrocytomas. Cancer Res. 2008 Nov 1;68(21):8673–7. PMID:18974108
3317. Jones DT, Northcott PA, Kool M, et al. The role of chromatin remodeling in medulloblastoma. Brain Pathol. 2013 Mar;23(2):193–9. PMID:23432644
3318. Jones EC, Pins M, Dickersin GR, et al. Metanephric adenoma of the kidney. A clinicopathological, immunohistochemical, flow cytometric, cytogenetic, and electron microscopic study of seven cases. Am J Surg Pathol. 1995 Jun;19(6):615–26. PMID:7755148
3319. Jones EW, Marks R, Pongsehirun D. Naevus superficialis lipomatosus. A clinicopathological report of twenty cases. Br J Dermatol. 1975 Aug;93(2):121–33. PMID:1235780
3320. Jones G, Arthurs B, Kaya H, et al. Overall survival analysis of adjuvant radiation versus observation in stage I testicular seminoma: a Surveillance, Epidemiology, and End Results (SEER) analysis. Am J Clin Oncol. 2013 Oct;36(5):500–4. PMID:22781383
3321. Jones JF, Shurin S, Abramowsky C, et al. T-cell lymphomas containing Epstein-Barr viral DNA in patients with chronic Epstein-Barr virus infections. N Engl J Med. 1988 Mar 24;318(12):733–41. PMID:2831453
3322. Jones KB, Barrott JJ, Xie M, et al. The impact of chromosomal translocation locus and fusion oncogene coding sequence in synovial sarcomagenesis. Oncogene. 2016 Sep 22;35(38):5021–32. PMID:26947017
3323. Jones KB, Piombo V, Searby C, et al. A mouse model of osteochondromagenesis from clonal inactivation of Ext1 in chondrocytes. Proc Natl Acad Sci U S A. 2010 Feb 2;107(5):2054–9. PMID:20080592
3324. Jones TD, Ulbright TM, Eble JN, et al. OCT4 staining in testicular tumors: a sensitive and specific marker for seminoma and embryonal carcinoma. Am J Surg Pathol. 2004 Jul;28(7):935–40. PMID:15223965
3325. Jones TD, Ulbright TM, Eble JN, et al. OCT4: a sensitive and specific biomarker for intratubular germ cell neoplasia of the testis. Clin Cancer Res. 2004 Dec 15;10(24):8544–7. PMID:15623637
3326. Jong B, Shahabpour M, Spruyt D, et al. Imaging and differential diagnosis of synovial sarcoma. J Belge Radiol. 1992 Aug;75(4):335–9. PMID:1334066
3327. Jonigk D, Laenger F, Maegel L, et al. Molecular and clinicopathological analysis of Epstein-Barr virus-associated posttransplant smooth muscle tumors. Am J Transplant. 2012 Jul;12(7):1908–17. PMID:22420456
3328. Jonkman-Berk BM, van den Berg JM, Ten Berge IJ, et al. Primary immunodeficiencies in the Netherlands: national patient data demonstrate the increased risk of malignancy. Clin Immunol. 2015 Feb;156(2):154–62. PMID:25451158
3329. Joos S, Otaño-Joos MI, Ziegler S, et al. Primary mediastinal (thymic) B-cell lymphoma is characterized by gains of chromosomal material including 9p and amplification of the REL gene. Blood. 1996 Feb 15;87(4):1571–8. PMID:8608249
3330. Joosse ME, Aardoom MA, Kemos P, et al. Malignancy and mortality in paediatric-onset inflammatory bowel disease: a 3-year prospective, multinational study from the paediatric IBD Porto group of ESPGHAN. Aliment Pharmacol Ther. 2018 Sep;48(5):523–37. PMID:29984520
3331. Jordan MB, Allen CE, Greenberg J, et al. Challenges in the diagnosis of hemophagocytic lymphohistiocytosis: recommendations from the North American Consortium for Histiocytosis (NACHO). Pediatr Blood Cancer. 2019 Nov;66(11):e27929. PMID:31339233
3332. Jordan MB, Allen CE, Weitzman S, et al. How I treat hemophagocytic lymphohistiocytosis. Blood. 2011 Oct 13;118(15):4041–52. PMID:21828139
3333. Jorge S, Jones NL, Chen L, et al. Characteristics, treatment and outcomes of women with immature ovarian teratoma, 1998-2012. Gynecol Oncol. 2016 Aug;142(2):261–6. PMID:27222024
3334. Jørgensen A, Nielsen JE, Almstrup K, et al. Dysregulation of the mitosis-meiosis switch in testicular carcinoma in situ. J Pathol. 2013 Mar;229(4):588–98. PMID:23303528
3335. Jørgensen N, Müller J, Giwercman A, et al. DNA content and expression of tumour markers in germ cells adjacent to germ cell tumours in childhood: probably a different origin for infantile and adolescent germ cell tumours. J Pathol. 1995 Jul;176(3):269–78. PMID:7674089
3336. Joseph J, Ritchie D, MacDuff E, et al. Bizarre parosteal osteochondromatous proliferation: a locally aggressive benign tumor. Clin Orthop Relat Res. 2011 Jul;469(7):2019–27. PMID:21533526
3337. Joshi VV, Gagnon GA, Chadwick EG, et al. The spectrum of mucosa-associated lymphoid tissue lesions in pediatric patients infected with HIV: a clinicopathologic study of six cases. Am J Clin Pathol. 1997 May;107(5):592–600. PMID:9128273
3338. Jouvet A, Fauchon F, Liberski P, et al. Papillary tumor of the pineal region. Am J Surg Pathol. 2003 Apr;27(4):505–12. PMID:12657936
3339. Jouvet A, Saint-Pierre G, Fauchon F, et al. Pineal parenchymal tumors: a correlation of histological features with prognosis in 66 cases. Brain Pathol. 2000 Jan;10(1):49–60. PMID:10668895
3340. Joyce MJ, Harmon DC, Mankin HJ, et al. Ewing's sarcoma in female siblings. A clinical report and review of the literature. Cancer. 1984 May 1;53(9):1959–62. PMID:6704922
3341. Jozwiak J, Jozwiak S, Skopinski P. Immunohistochemical and microscopic studies on giant cells in tuberous sclerosis. Histol Histopathol. 2005 Oct;20(4):1321–6. PMID:16136513
3342. Jóźwiak S, Kwiatkowski D, Kotulska K, et al. Tuberin and hamartin expression is reduced in the majority of subependymal giant cell astrocytomas in tuberous sclerosis complex consistent with a two-hit model of pathogenesis. J Child Neurol. 2004 Feb;19(2):102–6. PMID:15072102
3343. Jóźwiak S, Schwartz RA, Janniger CK, et al. Skin lesions in children with tuberous sclerosis complex: their prevalence, natural course, and diagnostic significance. Int J Dermatol. 1998 Dec;37(12):911–7. PMID:9888331
3344. Ju WT, Zhao TC, Liu Y, et al. Clinical and pathologic analysis of myopericytoma in the oral and maxillofacial region. Oral Surg Oral Med Oral Pathol Oral Radiol. 2019 Oct;128(4):393–9. PMID:31350225
3345. Judkins AR. Immunohistochemistry of INI1 expression: a new tool for old challenges in CNS and soft tissue pathology. Adv Anat Pathol. 2007 Sep;14(5):335–9. PMID:17717433
3346. Judkins AR, Burger PC, Hamilton RL, et al. INI1 protein expression distinguishes atypical teratoid/rhabdoid tumor from choroid plexus carcinoma. J Neuropathol Exp Neurol. 2005 May;64(5):391–7. PMID:15892296
3347. Judkins AR, Ellison DW. Ependymoblastoma: dear, damned, distracting diagnosis, farewell!. Brain Pathol. 2010 Jan;20(1):133–9. PMID:19120373
3348. Judkins AR, Mauger J, Ht A, et al. Immunohistochemical analysis of hSNF5/INI1 in pediatric CNS neoplasms. Am J Surg Pathol. 2004 May;28(5):644–50. PMID:15105654
3349. Juhlin CC, Stenman A, Haglund F, et al. Whole-exome sequencing defines the mutational landscape of pheochromocytoma and identifies KMT2D as a recurrently mutated gene. Genes Chromosomes Cancer. 2015 Sep;54(9):542–54. PMID:26032282
3349A. Jung CK, Choi YJ, Lee KY, et al. The cytological, clinical, and pathological features of the cribriform-morular variant of papillary thyroid carcinoma and mutation analysis of CTNNB1 and BRAF genes. Thyroid. 2009 Aug;19(8):905–13. PMID:19534622
3350. Jung H, Kim HN, Jang Y, et al. CAMTA-1 expression in 24 cases of hepatic epithelioid hemangioendothelioma in a single institute: diagnostic utility for differential diagnosis from hepatic angiosarcoma. In Vivo. 2019 Nov-Dec;33(6):2293–7. PMID:31662570
3351. Jung H, Kim HN, Jang Y, et al. Hepatic angiosarcoma: clinicopathologic study with an investigation of ROS1 gene rearrangements. In Vivo. 2020 May-Jun;34(3):1463–7. PMID:32354947
3352. Jung SM, Chang PY, Luo CC, et al. Lipoblastoma/lipoblastomatosis: a clinicopathologic study of 16 cases in Taiwan. Pediatr Surg Int. 2005 Oct;21(10):809–12. PMID:16180007
3353. Jünger ST, Andreiuolo F, Mynarek M, et al. CDKN2A deletion in supratentorial ependymoma with RELA alteration indicates a dismal prognosis: a retrospective analysis of the HIT ependymoma trial cohort. Acta Neuropathol. 2020 Sep;140(3):405–7. PMID:32514758
3354. Jünger ST, Mynarek M, Wohlers I, et al. Improved risk-stratification for posterior fossa ependymoma of childhood considering clinical, histological and genetic features - a retrospective analysis of the HIT ependymoma trial cohort. Acta Neuropathol Commun. 2019 Nov 14;7(1):181. PMID:31727173
3355. Justin N, Zhang Y, Tarricone C, et al. Structural basis of oncogenic histone H3K27M inhibition of human polycomb repressive complex 2. Nat Commun. 2016 Apr 28;7:11316. PMID:27121947
3356. Jutric Z, Rozenfeld Y, Grendar J, et al. Analysis of 340 patients with solid pseudopapillary tumors of the pancreas: a closer look at patients with metastatic disease. Ann Surg Oncol. 2017 Jul;24(7):2015–22. PMID:28299507
3357. Kaatsch P. Epidemiology of childhood cancer. Cancer Treat Rev. 2010 Jun;36(4):277–85. PMID:20231056
3358. Kaatsch P, Rickert CH, Kühl J, et al. Population-based epidemiologic data on brain tumors in German children. Cancer. 2001 Dec 15;92(12):3155–64. PMID:11753995
3359. Kacerovska D, Michal M, Kuroda N, et al. Hybrid peripheral nerve sheath tumors, including a malignant variant in type 1 neurofibromatosis. Am J Dermatopathol. 2013 Aug;35(6):641–9. PMID:23676318
3360. Kadar A, Kleinstern G, Morsy M, et al. Multiple enchondromas of the hand in children: long-term follow-up of mean 15.4 years. J Pediatr Orthop. 2018 Nov/Dec;38(10):543–8. PMID:27603196
3361. Kaddu S, McMenamin ME, Fletcher CD. Atypical fibrous histiocytoma of the skin: clinicopathologic analysis of 59 cases with evidence of infrequent metastasis. Am J Surg Pathol. 2002 Jan;26(1):35–46. PMID:11756767
3362. Kadin ME, Hamilton RG, Vonderheid EC. Evidence linking atopy and staphylococcal superantigens to the pathogenesis of lymphomatoid papulosis, a recurrent CD30+ cutaneous lymphoproliferative disorder. PLoS One. 2020 Feb 12;15(2):e0228751. PMID:32049976
3363. Kadlub N, Mbou VB, Leboulanger N, et al. Infant odontogenic myxoma: a specific entity. J Craniomaxillofac Surg. 2014 Dec;42(8):2082–6. PMID:24429059
3364. Kadoch C, Crabtree GR. Reversible disruption of mSWI/SNF (BAF) complexes by the SS18-SSX oncogenic fusion in synovial sarcoma. Cell. 2013 Mar 28;153(1):71–85. PMID:23540691
3365. Kadoch C, Williams RT, Calarco JP, et al. Dynamics of BAF-Polycomb complex opposition on heterochromatin in normal and oncogenic states. Nat Genet. 2017 Feb;49(2):213–22. PMID:27941796
3366. Kadonaga JN, Frieden IJ. Neurocutaneous melanosis: definition and review of the literature. J Am Acad Dermatol. 1991 May;24(5 Pt 1):747–55. PMID:1869648
3367. Käfer G, Willer A, Ludwig W, et al. Intracellular expression of CD61 precedes surface expression. Ann Hematol. 1999 Oct;78(10):472–4. PMID:10550559
3368. Kageji T, Miyamoto T, Kotani Y, et al. Congenital craniopharyngioma treated by radical surgery: case report and review of the literature. Childs Nerv Syst. 2017 Feb;33(2):357–62. PMID:27669698

**3369.** Kager L, Zoubek A, Pötschger U, et al. Primary metastatic osteosarcoma: presentation and outcome of patients treated on neoadjuvant Cooperative Osteosarcoma Study Group protocols. J Clin Oncol. 2003 May 15;21(10):2011–8. PMID:12743156

**3370.** Kaido T, Sasaoka Y, Hashimoto H, et al. De novo germinoma in the brain in association with Klinefelter's syndrome: case report and review of the literature. Surg Neurol. 2003 Dec;60(6):553–8. PMID:14670679

**3371.** Kaito K, Otsubo H, Usui N, et al. Secondary polycythemia as a paraneoplastic syndrome of testicular seminoma. Ann Hematol. 2004 Jan;83(1):55–7. PMID:12923663

**3372.** Kakar S, Chen X, Ho C, et al. Chromosomal changes in fibrolamellar hepatocellular carcinoma detected by array comparative genomic hybridization. Mod Pathol. 2009 Jan;22(1):134–41. PMID:18997738

**3373.** Kakkar A, Majumdar A, Kumar A, et al. Alterations in BRAF gene, and enhanced mTOR and MAPK signaling in dysembryoplastic neuroepithelial tumors (DNTs). Epilepsy Res. 2016 Nov;127:141–51. PMID:27599148

**3374.** Kalani N, Guidry JA, Farahi JM, et al. Pediatric melanoma: characterizing 256 cases from the Colorado Central Cancer Registry. Pediatr Dermatol. 2019 Mar;36(2):219–22. PMID:30793788

**3375.** Kalfa N, Ecochard A, Patte C, et al. Activating mutations of the stimulatory G protein in juvenile ovarian granulosa cell tumors: a new prognostic factor? J Clin Endocrinol Metab. 2006 May;91(5):1842–7. PMID:16507630

**3376.** Kalfa N, Fellous M, Boizet-Bonhoure B, et al. Aberrant expression of ovary determining gene FOXL2 in the testis and juvenile granulosa cell tumor in children. J Urol. 2008 Oct;180(4 Suppl):1810–3. PMID:18721930

**3377.** Kalifa G, Adamsbaum C, Job-Deslande C, et al. Fibrodysplasia ossificans progressiva and synovial chondromatosis. Pediatr Radiol. 1993;23(2):91–3. PMID:8516051

**3378.** Kaliki S, Eagle RC, Grossniklaus HE, et al. Inadvertent implantation of aqueous tube shunts in glaucomatous eyes with unrecognized intraocular neoplasms: report of 5 cases. JAMA Ophthalmol. 2013 Jul;131(7):925–8. PMID:23699787

**3379.** Kaliki S, Shields CL, Eagle RC Jr, et al. Ciliary body medulloepithelioma: analysis of 41 cases. Ophthalmology. 2013 Dec;120(12):2552–9. PMID:23796765

**3380.** Kaliki S, Shields CL, Shah SU, et al. Postenucleation adjuvant chemotherapy with vincristine, etoposide, and carboplatin for the treatment of high-risk retinoblastoma. Arch Ophthalmol. 2011 Nov;129(11):1422–7. PMID:22084213

**3381.** Kaliki S, Srinivasan V, Gupta A, et al. Clinical features predictive of high-risk retinoblastoma in 403 Asian Indian patients: a case-control study. Ophthalmology. 2015 Jun;122(6):1165–72. PMID:25841975

**3382.** Kalina PH, Bartley GB, Campbell RJ, et al. Isolated neurofibromas of the conjunctiva. Am J Ophthalmol. 1991 Jun 15;111(6):694–8. PMID:2039037

**3383.** Kalish JM, Conlin LK, Mostoufi-Moab S, et al. Bilateral pheochromocytomas, hemihyperplasia, and subtle somatic mosaicism: the importance of detecting low-level uniparental disomy. Am J Med Genet A. 2013 May;161A(5):993–1001. PMID:23532898

**3384.** Kalish JM, Doros L, Helman LJ, et al. Surveillance recommendations for children with overgrowth syndromes and predisposition to Wilms tumors and hepatoblastoma. Clin Cancer Res. 2017 Jul 1;23(13):e115–22. PMID:28674120

**3385.** Kaliya-Perumal AK, Carney TJ, Ingham PW. Fibrodysplasia ossificans progressiva:

current concepts from bench to bedside. Dis Model Mech. 2020 Sep 21;13(9):dmm046441. PMID:32988985

**3386.** Kalkan E, Waguespack SG. Endocrine tumors associated with neurofibromatosis type 1, Peutz-Jeghers syndrome and other familial neoplasia syndromes. Front Horm Res. 2013;41:166–81. PMID:23652677

**3387.** Kallen ME, Dulau-Florea A, Wang W, et al. Acquired and germline predisposition to bone marrow failure: diagnostic features and clinical implications. Semin Hematol. 2019 Jan;56(1):69–82. PMID:30573048

**3388.** Kalmanti L, Saussele S, Lauseker M, et al. Younger patients with chronic myeloid leukemia do well in spite of poor prognostic indicators: results from the randomized CML study IV. Ann Hematol. 2014 Jan;93(1):71–80. PMID:24162333

**3389.** Kamal D, Breton P, Bouletreau P. Congenital infiltrating lipomatosis of the face: report of three cases and review of the literature. J Craniomaxillofac Surg. 2010 Dec;38(8):610–4. PMID:20338773

**3390.** Kamei K, Funabiki T, Ochiai M, et al. Three cases of solid and cystic tumor of the pancreas. Analysis comparing the histopathological findings and DNA histograms. Int J Pancreatol. 1991 Nov-Dec;10(3-4):269–78. PMID:1787338

**3391.** Kamihara J, Bourdeaut F, Foulkes WD, et al. Retinoblastoma and neuroblastoma predisposition and surveillance. Clin Cancer Res. 2017 Jul 1;23(13):e98–106. PMID:28674118

**3392.** Kamino H, Flotte TJ, Misheloff E, et al. Eosinophilic globules in Spitz's nevi. New findings and a diagnostic sign. Am J Dermatopathol. 1979 Winter;1(4):319–24. PMID:94511

**3393.** Kanamori M, Antonescu CR, Scott M, et al. Extra copies of chromosomes 7, 8, 12, 19, and 21 are recurrent in adamantinoma. J Mol Diagn. 2001 Feb;3(1):16–21. PMID:11227067

**3394.** Kanavaros P, Gaulard P, Charlotte F, et al. Discordant expression of immunoglobulin and its associated molecule mb-1/CD79a is frequently found in mediastinal large B cell lymphomas. Am J Pathol. 1995 Mar;146(3):735–41. PMID:7887454

**3395.** Kanayama T, Imamura T, Kawabe Y, et al. KMT2A-rearranged infantile acute myeloid leukemia masquerading as juvenile myelomonocytic leukemia. Int J Hematol. 2018 Dec;108(6):665–9. PMID:30143999

**3396.** Kanazawa T, Fukushima N, Imayoshi S, et al. Rare case of malignant transformation of recurrent respiratory papillomatosis associated with human papillomavirus type 6 infection and p53 overexpression. Springerplus. 2013 Apr 10;2(1):153. PMID:23641321

**3397.** Kandt RS, Haines JL, Smith M, et al. Linkage of an important gene locus for tuberous sclerosis to a chromosome 16 marker for polycystic kidney disease. Nat Genet. 1992 Sep;2(1):37–41. PMID:1303246

**3398.** Kane LA, Leinung MC, Scheithauer BW, et al. Pituitary adenomas in childhood and adolescence. J Clin Endocrinol Metab. 1994 Oct;79(4):1135–40. PMID:7525627

**3399.** Kane PJ, Phipps KP, Harkness WF, et al. Intracranial neoplasms in the first year of life: results of a second cohort of patients from a single institution. Br J Neurosurg. 1999 Jun;13(3):294–8. PMID:10562841

**3400.** Kaneda HJ, Mack J, Kasales CJ, et al. Pediatric and adolescent breast masses: a review of pathophysiology, imaging, diagnosis, and treatment. AJR Am J Roentgenol. 2013 Feb;200(2):W204-12. PMID:23345385

**3401.** Kanegane H, Bhatia K, Gutierrez M, et al. A syndrome of peripheral blood T-cell

infection with Epstein-Barr virus (EBV) followed by EBV-positive T-cell lymphoma. Blood. 1998 Mar 15;91(6):2085–91. PMID:9490694

**3402.** Kaneko M, Fukaya M, Nakayama K, et al. Holoprosencephaly: report of a case. Aichi Gakuin Dent Sci. 1989;2:29–37. PMID:2641432

**3403.** Kanetsky PA, Mitra N, Vardhanabhuti S, et al. Common variation in KITLG and at 5q31.3 predisposes to testicular germ cell cancer. Nat Genet. 2009 Jul;41(7):811–5. PMID:19483682

**3404.** Kang H, Tan M, Bishop JA, et al. Whole-exome sequencing of salivary gland mucoepidermoid carcinoma. Clin Cancer Res. 2017 Jan 1;23(1):283–8. PMID:27340278

**3405.** Kang HJ, Park JH, Chen W, et al. EWS-WT1 oncoprotein activates neuronal reprogramming factor ASCL1 and promotes neural differentiation. Cancer Res. 2014 Aug 15;74(16):4526–35. PMID:24934812

**3406.** Kang JH, Buckley AF, Nagpal S, et al. A diffuse leptomeningeal glioneuronal tumor without diffuse leptomeningeal involvement: detailed molecular and clinical characterization. J Neuropathol Exp Neurol. 2018 Sep 1;77(9):751–6. PMID:29931222

**3407.** Kang JM, Ha J, Hong EK, et al. A nationwide, population-based epidemiologic study of childhood brain tumors in Korea, 2005-2014: a comparison with United States data. Cancer Epidemiol Biomarkers Prev. 2019 Feb;28(2):409–16. PMID:30348678

**3407A.** Kang SY, Park CK, Chang DK, et al. Lynch-like syndrome: characterization and comparison with EPCAM deletion carriers. Int J Cancer. 2015 Apr 1;136(7):1568–78. PMID:25110875

**3408.** Kang Y, Pekmezci M, Folpe AL, et al. Diagnostic utility of SOX10 to distinguish malignant peripheral nerve sheath tumor from synovial sarcoma, including intraneural synovial sarcoma. Mod Pathol. 2014 Jan;27(1):55–61. PMID:23929265

**3409.** Kanitakis J, Kyamidis K, Toussinas A, et al. Pure apocrine nevus: immunohistochemical study of a new case and literature review. Dermatology. 2011;222(2):97–101. PMID:21212656

**3410.** Kanjilal B, Ghosh M, Mitra A, et al. Cytological diagnosis of adrenocortical carcinoma: a report of 2 cases in children. Diagn Cytopathol. 2018 Dec;46(12):1064–7. PMID:30354004

**3411.** Kansara M, Teng MW, Smyth MJ, et al. Translational biology of osteosarcoma. Nat Rev Cancer. 2014 Nov;14(11):722–35. PMID:25319867

**3412.** Kansy K, Juergens P, Krol Z, et al. Odontogenic myxoma: diagnostic and therapeutic challenges in paediatric and adult patients—a case series and review of the literature. J Craniomaxillofac Surg. 2012 Apr;40(3):271–6. PMID:21624835

**3413.** Kanu A, Oermann CM, Malicki D, et al. Pulmonary lipoblastoma in an 18-month-old child: a unique tumor in children. Pediatr Pulmonol. 2002 Aug;34(2):150–4. PMID:12112785

**3414.** Kao CS, Cornejo KM, Ulbright TM, et al. Juvenile granulosa cell tumors of the testis: a clinicopathologic study of 70 cases with emphasis on its wide morphologic spectrum. Am J Surg Pathol. 2015 Sep;39(9):1159–69. PMID:26076062

**3415.** Kao CS, Idrees MT, Young RH, et al. "Dissecting gonadoblastoma" of Scully: a morphologic variant that often mimics germinoma. Am J Surg Pathol. 2016 Oct;40(10):1417–23. PMID:27454939

**3416.** Kao CS, Idrees MT, Young RH, et al. Solid pattern yolk sac tumor: a morphologic and immunohistochemical study of 52 cases. Am J Surg Pathol. 2012 Mar;36(3):360–7. PMID:22261704

**3417.** Kao CS, Ulbright TM, Idrees MT. Gonadoblastoma: an immunohistochemical study and comparison to Sertoli cell nodule with intratubular germ cell neoplasia, with pathogenetic implications. Histopathology. 2014 Dec;65(6):861–7. PMID:24766183

**3418.** Kao CS, Ulbright TM, Young RH, et al. Testicular embryonal carcinoma: a morphologic study of 180 cases highlighting unusual and unemphasized aspects. Am J Surg Pathol. 2014 May;38(5):689–97. PMID:24503753

**3419.** Kao JL, Tsung SH, Shiao CC. Rare anaplastic sarcoma of the kidney: a case report. World J Clin Cases. 2020 Apr 26;8(8):1495–501. PMID:32368542

**3420.** Kao YC, Fletcher CDM, Alaggio R, et al. Recurrent BRAF gene fusions in a subset of pediatric spindle cell sarcomas: expanding the genetic spectrum of tumors with overlapping features with infantile fibrosarcoma. Am J Surg Pathol. 2018 Jan;42(1):28–38. PMID:28877062

**3421.** Kao YC, Flucke U, Eijkelenboom A, et al. Novel EWSR1-SMAD3 gene fusions in a group of acral fibroblastic spindle cell neoplasms. Am J Surg Pathol. 2018 Apr;42(4):522–8. PMID:29309308

**3422.** Kao YC, Lan J, Tai HC, et al. Angiomatoid fibrous histiocytoma: clinicopathological and molecular characterisation with emphasis on variant histomorphology. J Clin Pathol. 2014 Mar;67(3):210–5. PMID:24043718

**3423.** Kao YC, Lee JC, Zhang L, et al. Recurrent YAP1 and KMT2A gene rearrangements in a subset of MUC4-negative sclerosing epithelioid fibrosarcoma. Am J Surg Pathol. 2020 Mar;44(3):368–77. PMID:31592798

**3424.** Kao YC, Owosho AA, Sung YS, et al. BCOR-CCNB3 fusion positive sarcomas: a clinicopathologic and molecular analysis of 36 cases with comparison to morphologic spectrum and clinical behavior of other round cell sarcomas. Am J Surg Pathol. 2018 May;42(5):604–15. PMID:29300189

**3425.** Kao YC, Sung YS, Chen CL, et al. ETV transcriptional upregulation is more reliable than RNA sequencing algorithms and FISH in diagnosing round cell sarcomas with CIC gene rearrangements. Genes Chromosomes Cancer. 2017 Jun;56(6):501–10. PMID:28233365

**3426.** Kao YC, Sung YS, Zhang L, et al. BCOR overexpression is a highly sensitive marker in round cell sarcomas with BCOR genetic abnormalities. Am J Surg Pathol. 2016 Dec;40(12):1670–8. PMID:27428733

**3427.** Kao YC, Sung YS, Zhang L, et al. EWSR1 fusions with CREB family transcription factors define a novel myxoid mesenchymal tumor with predilection for intracranial location. Am J Surg Pathol. 2017 Apr;41(4):482–90. PMID:28009602

**3428.** Kao YC, Sung YS, Zhang L, et al. Recurrent BCOR internal tandem duplication and YWHAE-NUTM2B fusions in soft tissue undifferentiated round cell sarcoma of infancy: overlapping genetic features with clear cell sarcoma of kidney. Am J Surg Pathol. 2016 Aug;40(8):1009–20. PMID:26945340

**3429.** Kao YC, Suurmeijer AJH, Argani P, et al. Soft tissue tumors characterized by a wide spectrum of kinase fusions share a lipofibromatosis-like neural tumor pattern. Genes Chromosomes Cancer. 2020 Oct;59(10):575–83. PMID:32506523

**3430.** Kapadia SB, Meis JM, Frisman DM, et al. Fetal rhabdomyoma of the head and neck: a clinicopathologic and immunophenotypic study of 24 cases. Hum Pathol. 1993 Jul;24(7):754–65. PMID:8319954

**3431.** Kapatai G, Brundler MA, Jenkinson H, et al. Gene expression profiling identifies different sub-types of retinoblastoma. Br J Cancer. 2013 Jul 23;109(2):512–25. PMID:23756868

**3432.** Kaplan FS, Al Mukaddam M, Stanley A, et al. Fibrodysplasia ossificans progressiva (FOP): a disorder of osteochondrogenesis. Bone. 2020 Nov;140:115539. PMID:32730934

**3433.** Kaplan FS, Fiori J, DE LA Peña LS, et al. Dysregulation of the BMP-4 signaling pathway in fibrodysplasia ossificans progressiva. Ann N Y Acad Sci. 2006 Apr;1068:54–65. PMID:16831905

**3434.** Kaplan FS, Zasloff MA, Kitterman JA, et al. Early mortality and cardiorespiratory failure in patients with fibrodysplasia ossificans progressiva. J Bone Joint Surg Am. 2010 Mar;92(3):686–91. PMID:20194327

**3435.** Kaprova-Pleskacova J, Stoop H, Brüggenwirth H, et al. Complete androgen insensitivity syndrome: factors influencing gonadal histology including germ cell pathology. Mod Pathol. 2014 May;27(5):721–30. PMID:24186138

**3436.** Kapur RP, Berry JE, Tsuchiya KD, et al. Activation of the chromosome 19q microRNA cluster in sporadic and androgenetic-biparental mosaicism-associated hepatic mesenchymal hamartoma. Pediatr Dev Pathol. 2014 Mar-Apr;17(2):75–84. PMID:24555441

**3437.** Karai LJ, Kadin ME, Hsi ED, et al. Chromosomal rearrangements of 6p25.3 define a new subtype of lymphomatoid papulosis. Am J Surg Pathol. 2013 Aug;37(8):1173–81. PMID:23648461

**3438.** Karamchandani JR, Nielsen TO, van de Rijn M, et al. Sox10 and S100 in the diagnosis of soft-tissue neoplasms. Appl Immunohistochem Mol Morphol. 2012 Oct;20(5):445–50. PMID:22495377

**3439.** Karamurzin Y, Zeng Z, Stadler ZK, et al. Unusual DNA mismatch repair-deficient tumors in Lynch syndrome: a report of new cases and review of the literature. Hum Pathol. 2012 Oct;43(10):1677–87. PMID:22516243

**3440.** Karamzadeh Dashti N, Bahrami A, Lee SJ, et al. BRAF V600E mutations occur in a subset of glomus tumors, and are associated with malignant histologic characteristics. Am J Surg Pathol. 2017 Nov;41(11):1532–41. PMID:28834810

**3441.** Karanian M, Kelsey A, Paindavoine S, et al. SRF fusions other than with RELA expand the molecular definition of SRF-fused perivascular tumors. Am J Surg Pathol. 2020 Dec;44(12):1725–35. PMID:33021523

**3442.** Karanian M, Pérot G, Coindre JM, et al. Fluorescence in situ hybridization analysis is a helpful test for the diagnosis of dermatofibrosarcoma protuberans. Mod Pathol. 2015 Feb;28(2):230–7. PMID:25081750

**3443.** Karanian M, Pissaloux D, Gomez-Brouchet A, et al. SRF-FOXO1 and SRF-NCOA1 fusion genes delineate a distinctive subset of well-differentiated rhabdomyosarcoma. Am J Surg Pathol. 2020 May;44(5):607–16. PMID:32187044

**3444.** Karanian-Philippe M, Velasco V, Longy M, et al. SMARCA4 (BRG1) loss of expression is a useful marker for the diagnosis of ovarian small cell carcinoma of the hypercalcemic type (ovarian rhabdoid tumor): a comprehensive analysis of 116 rare gynecologic tumors, 9 soft tissue tumors, and 9 melanomas. Am J Surg Pathol. 2015 Sep;39(9):1197–205. PMID:26135561

**3445.** Karavitaki N, Brufani C, Warner JT, et al. Craniopharyngiomas in children and adults: systematic analysis of 121 cases with long-term follow-up. Clin Endocrinol (Oxf). 2005 Apr;62(4):397–409. PMID:15807869

**3446.** Kardos G, Baumann I, Passmore SJ, et al. Refractory anemia in childhood: a retrospective analysis of 67 patients with particular reference to monosomy 7. Blood. 2003 Sep 15;102(6):1997–2003. PMID:12763938

**3447.** Karl SR, Ballantine TV, Zaino R. Juvenile secretory carcinoma of the breast. J Pediatr Surg. 1985 Aug;20(4):368–71. PMID:4045662

**3448.** Karlberg S, Lipsanen-Nyman M, Lassus H, et al. Gynecological tumors in Mulibrey nanism and role for RING finger protein TRIM37 in the pathogenesis of ovarian fibrothecomas. Mod Pathol. 2009 Apr;22(4):570–8. PMID:19329943

**3449.** Karmakar S, Reilly KM. The role of the immune system in neurofibromatosis type 1-associated nervous system tumors. CNS Oncol. 2017 Jan;6(1):45–60. PMID:28001089

**3450.** Karnak I, Senocak ME, Ciftci AO, et al. Inflammatory myofibroblastic tumor in children: diagnosis and treatment. J Pediatr Surg. 2001 Jun;36(6):908–12. PMID:11381424

**3451.** Karnezis AN, Wang Y, Keul J, et al. DICER1 and FOXL2 mutation status correlates with clinicopathologic features in ovarian Sertoli-Leydig cell tumors. Am J Surg Pathol. 2019 May;43(5):628–38. PMID:30986800

**3452.** Karnezis AN, Wang Y, Ramos P, et al. Dual loss of the SWI/SNF complex ATPases SMARCA4/BRG1 and SMARCA2/BRM is highly sensitive and specific for small cell carcinoma of the ovary, hypercalcaemic type. J Pathol. 2016 Feb;238(3):389–400. PMID:26356327

**3453.** Karow A, Baumann I, Niemeyer CM. Morphologic differential diagnosis of juvenile myelomonocytic leukemia–pitfalls apart from viral infection. J Pediatr Hematol Oncol. 2009 May;31(5):380. PMID:19415027

**3454.** Karow A, Flotho C, Schneider M, et al. Mutations of the Shwachman-Bodian-Diamond syndrome gene in patients presenting with refractory cytopenia–Do we have to screen? Haematologica. 2010 Apr;95(4):689–90. PMID:19951977

**3455.** Karpelowsky JS, Pansini A, Lazarus C, et al. Difficulties in the management of mesenchymal hamartomas. Pediatr Surg Int. 2008 Oct;24(10):1171–5. PMID:18751987

**3456.** Karremann M, Pietsch T, Janssen G, et al. Anaplastic ganglioglioma in children. J Neurooncol. 2009 Apr;92(2):157–63. PMID:19043777

**3457.** Karsy M, Guan J, Ravindra VM, et al. Diagnostic quality of magnetic resonance imaging interpretation for peripheral nerve sheath tumors: Can malignancy be determined? J Neurol Surg A Cent Eur Neurosurg. 2016 Nov;77(6):495–504. PMID:27276118

**3458.** Karube K, Ohshima K, Tsuchiya T, et al. A "floral" variant of nodal marginal zone lymphoma. Hum Pathol. 2005 Feb;36(2):202–6. PMID:15754298

**3459.** Kas K, Voz ML, Röijer E, et al. Promoter swapping between the genes for a novel zinc finger protein and beta-catenin in pleiomorphic adenomas with t(3;8)(p21;q12) translocations. Nat Genet. 1997 Feb;15(2):170–4. PMID:9020842

**3460.** Kasahara Y, Yachie A, Takei K, et al. Differential cellular targets of Epstein-Barr virus (EBV) infection between acute EBV-associated hemophagocytic lymphohistiocytosis and chronic active EBV infection. Blood. 2001 Sep 15;98(6):1882–8. PMID:11535525

**3461.** Kasaliwal R, Sarathi V, Pandit R, et al. Pheochromocytoma and tetralogy of Fallot: a rare but potentially dangerous combination. Endocr Pract. 2014 May;20(5):e80–5. PMID:24449673

**3462.** Kaseb AO, Shama M, Sahin IH, et al. Prognostic indicators and treatment outcome in 94 cases of fibrolamellar hepatocellular carcinoma. Oncology. 2013;85(4):197–203. PMID:24051705

**3463.** Kashima HK, Shah F, Lyles A, et al. A comparison of risk factors in juvenile-onset and adult-onset recurrent respiratory papillomatosis. Laryngoscope. 1992 Jan;102(1):9–13. PMID:1309932

**3464.** Kasper B, Baumgarten C, Garcia J, et al. An update on the management of sporadic desmoid-type fibromatosis: a European Consensus Initiative between Sarcoma PAtients EuroNet (SPAEN) and European Organization for Research and Treatment of Cancer (EORTC)/ Soft Tissue and Bone Sarcoma Group (STBSG). Ann Oncol. 2017 Oct 1;28(10):2399–408. PMID:28961825

**3465.** Kasper LH, Baker SJ. Invited review: Emerging functions of histone H3 mutations in paediatric diffuse high-grade gliomas. Neuropathol Appl Neurobiol. 2020 Feb;46(1):73–85. PMID:31859390

**3466.** Kaste SC, Fuller CE, Saharia A, et al. Pediatric surface osteosarcoma: clinical, pathologic, and radiologic features. Pediatr Blood Cancer. 2006 Aug;47(2):152–62. PMID:16123997

**3467.** Kastenhuber ER, Lowe SW. Putting p53 in Context. Cell. 2017 Sep 7;170(6):1062–78. PMID:28886379

**3468.** Kastriti ME, Kameneva P, Kamenev D, et al. Schwann cell precursors generate the majority of chromaffin cells in Zuckerkandl organ and some sympathetic neurons in paraganglia. Front Mol Neurosci. 2019 Jan 25;12:6. PMID:30740044

**3469.** Katabi N, Ghossein R, Ho A, et al. Consistent PLAG1 and HMGA2 abnormalities distinguish carcinoma ex-pleomorphic adenoma from its de novo counterparts. Hum Pathol. 2015 Jan;46(1):26–33. PMID:25439740

**3470.** Katabi N, Lewis JS. Update from the 4th edition of the World Health Organization classification of head and neck tumours: What is new in the 2017 WHO Blue Book for tumors and tumor-like lesions of the neck and lymph nodes. Head Neck Pathol. 2017 Mar;11(1):48–54. PMID:28247228

**3471.** Katabi N, Xu B, Jungbluth AA, et al. PLAG1 immunohistochemistry is a sensitive marker for pleomorphic adenoma: a comparative study with PLAG1 genetic abnormalities. Histopathology. 2018 Jan;72(2):285–93. PMID:28796899

**3472.** Kataria SP, Kumar S, Singh G, et al. Sialoblastoma. diagnosis by FNAC: a case report. Diagn Cytopathol. 2015 Nov;43(11):924–7. PMID:26214398

**3473.** Kato I, Furuya M, Matsuo K, et al. Giant cell tumours of bone treated with denosumab: histological, immunohistochemical and H3F3A mutation analyses. Histopathology. 2018 May;72(6):914–22. PMID:29206281

**3474.** Kato K, Nakatani Y, Kanno H, et al. Possible linkage between specific histological structures and aberrant reactivation of the Wnt pathway in adamantinomatous craniopharyngioma. J Pathol. 2004 Jul;203(3):814–21. PMID:15221941

**3475.** Kato K, Ohshima K, Ishihara S, et al. Elevated serum soluble Fas ligand in natural killer cell proliferative disorders. Br J Haematol. 1998 Dec;103(4):1164–6. PMID:9886336

**3476.** Kato K, Takeuchi M, Yonekawa Y, et al. Management of inflamed conjunctival nevus with topical antiallergic medications: case series. Clin Ophthalmol. 2021 Feb 12;15:559–64. PMID:33603334

**3477.** Kato N, Motoyama T, Kameda N, et al. Primary carcinoid tumor of the testis: immunohistochemical, ultrastructural and FISH analysis with review of the literature. Pathol Int. 2003 Oct;53(10):680–5. PMID:14516318

**3478.** Kato N, Romero M, Catasus L, et al. The STK11/LKB1 Peutz-Jegher gene is not involved in the pathogenesis of sporadic sex cord-stromal tumors, although loss of heterozygosity at 19p13.3 indicates other gene alteration in these tumors. Hum Pathol. 2004 Sep;35(9):1101–4. PMID:15343512

**3479.** Katsenos S, Becker HD. Recurrent respiratory papillomatosis: a rare chronic disease, difficult to treat, with potential to lung cancer transformation: apropos of two cases and a brief literature review. Case Rep Oncol. 2011 Mar 23;4(1):162–71. PMID:21526134

**3480.** Katzenstein AL, Doxtader E, Narendra S. Lymphomatoid granulomatosis: insights gained over 4 decades. Am J Surg Pathol. 2010 Dec;34(12):e35–48. PMID:21107080

**3481.** Katzenstein HM, Krailo MD, Malogolowkin MH, et al. Fibrolamellar hepatocellular carcinoma in children and adolescents. Cancer. 2003 Apr 15;97(8):2006–12. PMID:12673731

**3482.** Katzenstein HM, Krailo MD, Malogolowkin MH, et al. Hepatocellular carcinoma in children and adolescents: results from the Pediatric Oncology Group and the Children's Cancer Group intergroup study. J Clin Oncol. 2002 Jun 15;20(12):2789–97. PMID:12065555

**3483.** Katzenstein HM, López-Terrada DH, Tiao G, et al. Chapter 31: Liver tumors. In: Blaney SM, Adamson PC, Helman LJ, editors. Pizzo and Poplack's Pediatric Oncology. 8th ed. Philadelphia (PA): Wolters Kluwer Health; 2020. pp. 842–67.

**3484.** Katzenstein HM, Langham MR, Malogolowkin MH, et al. Minimal adjuvant chemotherapy for children with hepatoblastoma resected at diagnosis (AHEP0731): a Children's Oncology Group, multicentre, phase 3 trial. Lancet Oncol. 2019 May;20(5):719–27. PMID:30975630

**3485.** Kaulich K, Blaschke B, Nümann A, et al. Genetic alterations commonly found in diffusely infiltrating cerebral gliomas are rare or absent in pleomorphic xanthoastrocytomas. J Neuropathol Exp Neurol. 2002 Dec;61(12):1092–9. PMID:12484572

**3486.** Kaur K, Agarwal S, Rajeshwari M, et al. Melanotic neuroectodermal tumour of infancy: an enigmatic tumour with unique cytomorphological features. Cytopathology. 2018 Feb;29(1):104–8. PMID:29027726

**3487.** Kaur K, Jha P, Pathak P, et al. Approach to molecular subgrouping of medulloblastomas: comparison of NanoString nCounter assay versus combination of immunohistochemistry and fluorescence in-situ hybridization in resource constrained centres. J Neurooncol. 2019 Jul;143(3):393–403. PMID:31104222

**3488.** Kaur K, Kakkar A, Kumar A, et al. Integrating molecular subclassification of medulloblastomas into routine clinical practice: a simplified approach. Brain Pathol. 2016 May;26(3):334–43. PMID:26222673

**3489.** Kausar A, Zafar SN, Altaf S, et al. Ophthalmic manifestations of linear nevus sebaceous/organoid nevus syndrome. J Coll Physicians Surg Pak. 2015 Mar;25(3):220–2. PMID:25772967

**3490.** Kawaguchi T, Kumabe T, Kanamori M, et al. Logarithmic decrease of serum alpha-fetoprotein or human chorionic gonadotropin in response to chemotherapy can distinguish a subgroup with better prognosis among highly malignant intracranial non-germinomatous germ cell tumors. J Neurooncol. 2011 Sep;104(3):779–87. PMID:21359564

**3491.** Kawa-Ha K, Ishihara S, Ninomiya T, et al. CD3-negative lymphoproliferative disease of granular lymphocytes containing Epstein-Barr viral DNA. J Clin Invest. 1989 Jul;84(1):51–5. PMID:2544630

**3492.** Kawamoto EH, Weidner N, Agostini RM Jr, et al. Malignant ectomesenchymoma of soft tissue. Report of two cases and review of the literature. Cancer. 1987 May 15;59(10):1791–802. PMID:2950992

**3493.** Kawamura M, Matsumoto F, Matsui F, et al. Aggressive angiomyxoma of the vulva mimicking clitoromegaly in a young child. Urology. 2017 Mar;101:142–4. PMID:27984053
**3494.** Kawamura-Saito M, Yamazaki Y, Kaneko K, et al. Fusion between CIC and DUX4 up-regulates PEA3 family genes in Ewing-like sarcomas with t(4;19)(q35;q13) translocation. Hum Mol Genet. 2006 Jul 1;15(13):2125–37. PMID:16717057
**3495.** Kawano N, Yasui Y, Utsuki S, et al. Light microscopic demonstration of the microlumen of ependymoma: a study of the usefulness of antigen retrieval for epithelial membrane antigen (EMA) immunostaining. Brain Tumor Pathol. 2004;21(1):17–21. PMID:15696964
**3496.** Kawaoka JC, Gray J, Schappell D, et al. Eccrine nevus. J Am Acad Dermatol. 2004 Aug;51(2):301–4. PMID:15280853
**3497.** Kawata R, Lee K, Yoshimura K, et al. [Review of 300 cases of parotidectomy for benign parotid tumors]. Nihon Jibiinkoka Gakkai Kaiho. 2012 Jun;115(6):618–24. Japanese. PMID:22844822
**3498.** Kawauchi D, Ogg RJ, Liu L, et al. Novel MYC-driven medulloblastoma models from multiple embryonic cerebellar cells. Oncogene. 2017 Sep 14;36(37):5231–42. PMID:28504719
**3499.** Kawauchi S, Fukuda T, Miyamoto S, et al. Peripheral primitive neuroectodermal tumor of the ovary confirmed by CD99 immunostaining, karyotypic analysis, and RT-PCR for EWS/FLI-1 chimeric mRNA. Am J Surg Pathol. 1998 Nov;22(11):1417–22. PMID:9808135
**3500.** Kay M, Eng K, Wyllie R. Colonic polyps and polyposis syndromes in pediatric patients. Curr Opin Pediatr. 2015 Oct;27(5):634–41. PMID:26208235
**3501.** Kayembe MK, Kalengayi MM. Salivary gland tumours in Congo (Zaire). Odontostomatol Trop. 2002 Sep;25(99):19–22. PMID:12430350
**3502.** Kaymaz Y, Oduor CI, Yu H, et al. Comprehensive transcriptome and mutational profiling of endemic Burkitt lymphoma reveals EBV type-specific differences. Mol Cancer Res. 2017 May;15(5):563–76. PMID:28465297
**3503.** Kazakov DV, Requena L, Kutzner H, et al. Morphologic diversity of syringocystadenocarcinoma papilliferum based on a clinicopathologic study of 6 cases and review of the literature. Am J Dermatopathol. 2010 Jun;32(4):340–7. PMID:20216201
**3504.** Keating S, Taylor GP. Undifferentiated (embryonal) sarcoma of the liver: ultrastructural and immunohistochemical similarities with malignant fibrous histiocytoma. Hum Pathol. 1985 Jul;16(7):693–9. PMID:2989150
**3505.** Keene D, Johnston D, Strother D, et al. Epidemiological survey of central nervous system germ cell tumors in Canadian children. J Neurooncol. 2007 May;82(3):289–95. PMID:17120159
**3506.** Keeney GL, Unni KK, Beabout JW, et al. Adamantinoma of long bones. A clinicopathologic study of 85 cases. Cancer. 1989 Aug 1;64(3):730–7. PMID:2743266
**3507.** Kehrer-Sawatzki H, Farschtschi S, Mautner VF, et al. The molecular pathogenesis of schwannomatosis, a paradigm for the co-involvement of multiple tumour suppressor genes in tumorigenesis. Hum Genet. 2017 Feb;136(2):129–48. PMID:27921248
**3508.** Kehrer-Sawatzki H, Kordes U, Seiffert S, et al. Co-occurrence of schwannomatosis and rhabdoid tumor predisposition syndrome 1. Mol Genet Genomic Med. 2018 May 20;6(4):627–37. PMID:29779243
**3509.** Keiler SA, Honda K, Bordeaux JS. Retiform hemangioendothelioma treated with Mohs micrographic surgery. J Am Acad Dermatol. 2011 Jul;65(1):233–5. PMID:21679834
**3510.** Kelley MJ, Shi J, Ballew B, et al. Characterization of T gene sequence variants and germline duplications in familial and sporadic chordoma. Hum Genet. 2014 Oct;133(10):1289–97. PMID:24990759
**3511.** Kelley RR, Scully RE. Cancer developing in dermoid cysts of the ovary. A report of 8 cases, including a carcinoid and a leiomyosarcoma. Cancer. 1961 Sep-Oct;14:989–1000. PMID:13752348
**3512.** Kelly D, Sharif K, Brown RM, et al. Hepatocellular carcinoma in children. Clin Liver Dis. 2015 May;19(2):433–47. PMID:25921672
**3513.** Kelly TG, Hong S, Jarzembowski J, et al. Infant with nasolacrimal sinonasal myxoma: diffusion MRI features. Radiol Case Rep. 2016 Feb 17;10(2):1104. PMID:27398121
**3514.** Kempers MJ, Kuiper RP, Ockeloen CW, et al. Risk of colorectal and endometrial cancers in EPCAM deletion-positive Lynch syndrome: a cohort study. Lancet Oncol. 2011 Jan;12(1):49–55. PMID:21145788
**3515.** Kempf W. A new era for cutaneous CD30-positive T-cell lymphoproliferative disorders. Semin Diagn Pathol. 2017 Jan;34(1):22–35. PMID:27993440
**3516.** Kempf W, Kazakov DV, Paredes BE, et al. Primary cutaneous anaplastic large cell lymphoma with angioinvasive features and cytotoxic phenotype: a rare lymphoma variant within the spectrum of CD30+ lymphoproliferative disorders. Dermatology. 2013;227(4):346–52. PMID:24246691
**3517.** Kempf W, Kazakov DV, Schärer L, et al. Angioinvasive lymphomatoid papulosis: a new variant simulating aggressive lymphomas. Am J Surg Pathol. 2013 Jan;37(1):1–13. PMID:23026936
**3518.** Kempf W, Pfaltz K, Vermeer MH, et al. EORTC, ISCL, and USCLC consensus recommendations for the treatment of primary cutaneous CD30-positive lymphoproliferative disorders: lymphomatoid papulosis and primary cutaneous anaplastic large-cell lymphoma. Blood. 2011 Oct 13;118(15):4024–35. PMID:21841159
**3519.** Kenawy N, Kalirai H, Sacco JJ, et al. Conjunctival melanoma copy number alterations and correlation with mutation status, tumor features, and clinical outcome. Pigment Cell Melanoma Res. 2019 Jul;32(4):564–75. PMID:30672666
**3520.** Kennedy AL, Shimamura A. Genetic predisposition to MDS: clinical features and clonal evolution. Blood. 2019 Mar 7;133(10):1071–85. PMID:30670445
**3521.** Kennedy RD, Boughey JC. Management of pediatric and adolescent breast masses. Semin Plast Surg. 2013 Feb;27(1):19–22. PMID:24872734
**3522.** Kenney B, Richkind KE, Friedlaender G, et al. Chromosomal rearrangements in lipofibromatosis. Cancer Genet Cytogenet. 2007 Dec;179(2):136–9. PMID:18036401
**3523.** Kenny C, Grehan D, Ulas M, et al. Immunophenotype-genotype correlations in clear cell sarcoma of kidney-an evaluation of diagnostic ancillary studies. Pediatr Dev Pathol. 2020 Sep-Oct;23(5):345–51. PMID:32364435
**3524.** Kenny SL, McBride HA, Jamison J, et al. Mesonephric adenocarcinomas of the uterine cervix and corpus: HPV-negative neoplasms that are commonly PAX8, CA125, and HMGA2 positive and that may be immunoreactive with TTF1 and hepatocyte nuclear factor 1-β. Am J Surg Pathol. 2012 Jun;36(6):799–807. PMID:22456609
**3525.** Kenny SL, Patel K, Humphries A, et al. Ovarian cellular fibroma harbouring an isocitrate dehydrogenase 1 (1DH1) mutation in a patient with Ollier disease: evidence for a causal relationship. Histopathology. 2013 Mar;62(4):667–70. PMID:23347143
**3526.** Kepes JJ, Rubinstein LJ, Eng LF. Pleomorphic xanthoastrocytoma: a distinctive meningocerebral glioma of young subjects with relatively favorable prognosis. A study of 12 cases. Cancer. 1979 Nov;44(5):1839–52. PMID:498051
**3527.** Keppler-Noreuil KM, Rios JJ, Parker VE, et al. PIK3CA-related overgrowth spectrum (PROS): diagnostic and testing eligibility criteria, differential diagnosis, and evaluation. Am J Med Genet A. 2015 Feb;167A(2):287–95. PMID:25557259
**3528.** Keppler-Noreuil KM, Sapp JC, Lindhurst MJ, et al. Clinical delineation and natural history of the PIK3CA-related overgrowth spectrum. Am J Med Genet A. 2014 Jul;164A(7):1713–33. PMID:24782230
**3529.** Kerfoot C, Wienecke R, Menchine M, et al. Localization of tuberous sclerosis 2 mRNA and its protein product tuberin in normal human brain and in cerebral lesions of patients with tuberous sclerosis. Brain Pathol. 1996 Oct;6(4):367–75. PMID:8944308
**3530.** Kern WH. Proliferative myositis; a pseudosarcomatous reaction to injury: a report of seven cases. Arch Pathol. 1960 Feb;69:209–16. PMID:14408614
**3531.** Kerr DA, Lopez HU, Deshpande V, et al. Molecular distinction of chondrosarcoma from chondroblastic osteosarcoma through IDH1/2 mutations. Am J Surg Pathol. 2013 Jun;37(6):787–95. PMID:23598960
**3532.** Kerr NJ, Chun YH, Yun K, et al. Pancreatoblastoma is associated with chromosome 11p loss of heterozygosity and IGF2 overexpression. Med Pediatr Oncol. 2002 Jul;39(1):52–4. PMID:12116082
**3533.** Kerr NJ, Fukuzawa R, Reeve AE, et al. Beckwith-Wiedemann syndrome, pancreatoblastoma, and the WNT signaling pathway. Am J Pathol. 2002 Apr;160(4):1541–2. PMID:11943738
**3534.** Kersemaekers AM, Honecker F, Stoop H, et al. Identification of germ cells at risk for neoplastic transformation in gonadoblastoma: an immunohistochemical study for OCT3/4 and TSPY. Hum Pathol. 2005 May;36(5):512–21. PMID:15948118
**3535.** Kervarrec T, Collin C, Larousserie F, et al. H3F3 mutation status of giant cell tumors of the bone, chondroblastomas and their mimics: a combined high resolution melting and pyrosequencing approach. Mod Pathol. 2017 Mar;30(3):393–406. PMID:28059095
**3536.** Kesserwan C, Sokolic R, Cowen EW, et al. Multicentric dermatofibrosarcoma protuberans in patients with adenosine deaminase-deficient severe combined immune deficiency. J Allergy Clin Immunol. 2012 Mar;129(3):762–769.e1. PMID:22153773
**3537.** Ketteler P, Hülsenbeck I, Frank M, et al. The impact of RB1 genotype on incidence of second tumours in heritable retinoblastoma. Eur J Cancer. 2020 Jul;133:47–55. PMID:32434110
**3538.** Kezlarian B, Alhyari M, Venkataraman G, et al. GATA3 immunohistochemical staining in Hodgkin lymphoma: diagnostic utility in differentiating classic Hodgkin lymphoma from nodular lymphocyte predominant Hodgkin lymphoma and other mimicking entities. Appl Immunohistochem Mol Morphol. 2019 Mar;27(3):180–4. PMID:28877074
**3539.** Khalidi HS, Brynes RK, Medeiros LJ, et al. The immunophenotype of blast transformation of chronic myelogenous leukemia: a high frequency of mixed lineage phenotype in "lymphoid" blasts and A comparison of morphologic, immunophenotypic, and molecular findings. Mod Pathol. 1998 Dec;11(12):1211–21. PMID:9872654
**3540.** Khalidi HS, Chang KL, Medeiros LJ, et al. Acute lymphoblastic leukemia. Survey of immunophenotype, French-American-British classification, frequency of myeloid antigen expression, and karyotypic abnormalities in 210 pediatric and adult cases. Am J Clin Pathol. 1999 Apr;111(4):467–76. PMID:10191766
**3541.** Khan NE, Bauer AJ, Schultz KAP, et al. Quantification of thyroid cancer and multinodular goiter risk in the DICER1 syndrome: a family-based cohort study. J Clin Endocrinol Metab. 2017 May 1;102(5):1614–22. PMID:28323992
**3542.** Khan S, Jetley S, Jairajpuri Z, et al. Fibromatosis colli - a rare cytological diagnosis in infantile neck swellings. J Clin Diagn Res. 2014 Nov;8(11):FD08–09. PMID:25584233
**3543.** Khan ZA, Boscolo E, Picard A, et al. Multipotential stem cells recapitulate human infantile hemangioma in immunodeficient mice. J Clin Invest. 2008 Jul;118(7):2592–9. PMID:18535669
**3544.** Khanna R, Verma SK. Pediatric hepatocellular carcinoma. World J Gastroenterol. 2018 Sep 21;24(35):3980–99. PMID:30254403
**3545.** Khanna V, Achey RL, Ostrom QT, et al. Incidence and survival trends for medulloblastomas in the United States from 2001 to 2013. J Neurooncol. 2017 Dec;135(3):433–41. PMID:28828582
**3546.** Khater F, Langlois S, Cassart P, et al. Recurrent somatic BRAF insertion (p.V504_R506dup): a tumor marker and a potential therapeutic target in pilocytic astrocytoma. Oncogene. 2019 Apr;38(16):2994–3002. PMID:30575814
**3547.** Khedmati F, Chirolas C, Seidman JD. Ovarian and paraovarian squamous-lined cysts (epidermoid cysts): a clinicopathologic study of 18 cases with comparison to mature cystic teratomas. Int J Gynecol Pathol. 2009 Mar;28(2):193–6. PMID:19188813
**3548.** Kholaki O, Metter D, Tandon R, et al. Tumorigenic potential of granulocyte colony-stimulating factor therapy-a case report and review of literature. J Oral Maxillofac Surg. 2020 Dec;78(12):2219–25. PMID:32628932
**3549.** Khoshnam N, Robinson H, Clay MR, et al. Calcifying nested stromal-epithelial tumor (CNSET) of the liver in Beckwith-Wiedemann syndrome. Eur J Med Genet. 2017 Feb;60(2):136–9. PMID:27965001
**3550.** Khoueir N, Nicolas N, Rohayem Z, et al. Exclusive endoscopic resection of juvenile nasopharyngeal angiofibroma: a systematic review of the literature. Otolaryngol Head Neck Surg. 2014 Mar;150(3):350–8. PMID:24381014
**3551.** Khoury JD, Solary E, Abla O, et al. The 5th edition of the World Health Organization Classification of Haematolymphoid Tumours: myeloid and histiocytic/dendritic neoplasms. Leukemia. 2022 Jul;36(7):1703–19. PMID:35732831
**3552.** Khurana KK, Truong LD, LiVolsi VA, et al. Cytokeratin 19 immunolocalization in cell block preparation of thyroid aspirates. An adjunct to fine-needle aspiration diagnosis of papillary thyroid carcinoma. Arch Pathol Lab Med. 2003 May;127(5):579–83. PMID:12708901
**3553.** Kiani B, Ferrell LD, Qualman S, et al. Immunohistochemical analysis of embryonal sarcoma of the liver. Appl Immunohistochem Mol Morphol. 2006 Jun;14(2):193–7. PMID:16785789
**3554.** Kiessling P, Dowling E, Huang Y, et al. Identification of aggressive Gardner syndrome phenotype associated with a de novo APC variant, c.4666dup. Cold Spring Harb Mol Case Stud. 2019 Apr 1;5(2):a003640. PMID:30696621
**3555.** Kiil K, Bein J, Schuhmacher B, et al. A high number of IgG4-positive plasma cells rules out nodular lymphocyte predominant Hodgkin lymphoma. Virchows Arch. 2018 Dec;473(6):759–64. PMID:30259184

**3556.** Kikuchi A, Hasegawa D, Ohtsuka Y, et al. Outcome of children with refractory anaemia with excess of blast (RAEB) and RAEB in transformation (RAEB-T) in the Japanese MDS99 study. Br J Haematol. 2012 Sep;158(5):657–61. PMID:22734597
**3557.** Kikuchi Y, Wada R, Sakihara S, et al. Pheochromocytoma with histologic transformation to composite type, complicated by watery diarrhea, hypokalemia, and achlorhydria syndrome. Endocr Pract. 2012 Jul-Aug;18(4):e91–6. PMID:22440998
**3558.** Kikuta H, Sakiyama Y, Matsumoto S, et al. Fatal Epstein-Barr virus-associated hemophagocytic syndrome. Blood. 1993 Dec 1;82(11):3259–64. PMID:8241498
**3559.** Kilcline C, Frieden IJ. Infantile hemangiomas: How common are they? A systematic review of the medical literature. Pediatr Dermatol. 2008 Mar-Apr;25(2):168–73. PMID:18429772
**3560.** Kilday JP, Mitra B, Domerg C, et al. Copy number gain of 1q25 predicts poor progression-free survival for pediatric intracranial ependymomas and enables patient risk stratification: a prospective European clinical trial cohort analysis on behalf of the Children's Cancer Leukaemia Group (CCLG), Societe Francaise d'Oncologie Pediatrique (SFOP), and International Society for Pediatric Oncology (SIOP). Clin Cancer Res. 2012 Apr 1;18(7):2001–11. PMID:22338015
**3561.** Kilian A, Latino GA, White AJ, et al. Genotype-phenotype correlations in children with HHT. J Clin Med. 2020 Aug 22;9(9):E2714. PMID:32842615
**3562.** Kilickesmez O, Sanal HT, Haholu A, et al. Coexistence of pleomorphic xanthoastrocytoma with Sturge-Weber syndrome: MRI features. Pediatr Radiol. 2005 Sep;35(9):910–3. PMID:15883827
**3563.** Killian JK, Kim SY, Miettinen M, et al. Succinate dehydrogenase mutation underlies global epigenomic divergence in gastrointestinal stromal tumor. Cancer Discov. 2013 Jun;3(6):648–57. PMID:23550148
**3564.** Killian JK, Miettinen M, Walker RL, et al. Recurrent epimutation of SDHC in gastrointestinal stromal tumors. Sci Transl Med. 2014 Dec 24;6(268):268ra177. PMID:25540324
**3565.** Kilpatrick SE, Hitchcock MG, Kraus MD, et al. Mixed tumors and myoepitheliomas of soft tissue: a clinicopathologic study of 19 cases with a unifying concept. Am J Surg Pathol. 1997 Jan;21(1):13–22. PMID:8990137
**3566.** Kilpatrick SE, Teot LA, Stanley MW, et al. Fine-needle aspiration biopsy of synovial sarcoma. A cytomorphologic analysis of primary, recurrent, and metastatic tumors. Am J Clin Pathol. 1996 Dec;106(6):769–75. PMID:8980353
**3567.** Kilpatrick SE, Ward WG, Bos GD, et al. The role of fine needle aspiration biopsy in the diagnosis and management of osteosarcoma. Pediatr Pathol Mol Med. 2001 May-Jun;20(3):175–87. PMID:11486348
**3568.** Kilpatrick SE, Ward WG, Chauvenet AR, et al. The role of fine-needle aspiration biopsy in the initial diagnosis of pediatric bone and soft tissue tumors: an institutional experience. Mod Pathol. 1998 Oct;11(10):923–8. PMID:9796716
**3569.** Kim B, Giardiello FM. Chemoprevention in familial adenomatous polyposis. Best Pract Res Clin Gastroenterol. 2011 Aug;25(4-5):607–22. PMID:22122775
**3570.** Kim B, Park SH, Yang HR, et al. Hepatocellular carcinoma occurring in alagille syndrome. Pathol Res Pract. 2005;201(1):55–60. PMID:15807312
**3571.** Kim B, Tabori U, Hawkins C. An update on the CNS manifestations of brain tumor polyposis syndromes. Acta Neuropathol. 2020 Apr;139(4):703–15. PMID:31970492
**3572.** Kim CA, Konig A, Bertola DR, et al. CHILD syndrome caused by a deletion of exons 6-8 of the NSDHL gene. Dermatology. 2005;211(2):155–8. PMID:16088165
**3573.** Kim CY, Choi JW, Lee JY, et al. Intracranial growing teratoma syndrome: clinical characteristics and treatment strategy. J Neurooncol. 2011 Jan;101(1):109–15. PMID:20532955
**3574.** Kim DG, Lee DY, Paek SH, et al. Supratentorial primitive neuroectodermal tumors in adults. J Neurooncol. 2002 Oct;60(1):43–52. PMID:12416545
**3575.** Kim ES, Kwon MJ, Song JH, et al. Adenocarcinoma arising from intracranial recurrent mature teratoma and featuring mutated KRAS and wild-type BRAF genes. Neuropathology. 2015 Feb;35(1):44–9. PMID:25039399
**3576.** Kim HJ, McCormick SA, Nath S, et al. Melanocytic nevi of the tarsal conjunctiva: clinicopathologic case series with review of literature. Ophthalmic Plast Reconstr Surg. 2010 Nov-Dec;26(6):438–42. PMID:20683369
**3577.** Kim HS, Park SH, Chi JG. Aggressive angiomyxoma of childhood: two unusual cases developed in the scrotum. Pediatr Dev Pathol. 2003 Mar-Apr;6(2):187–91. PMID:12548375
**3578.** Kim J, Ellis GL. Dental follicular tissue: misinterpretation as odontogenic tumors. J Oral Maxillofac Surg. 1993 Jul;51(7):762–7. PMID:8509916
**3579.** Kim J, Field A, Schultz KAP, et al. The prevalence of DICER1 pathogenic variation in population databases. Int J Cancer. 2017 Nov 15;141(10):2030–6. PMID:28748527
**3580.** Kim J, Horowitz G, Hong M, et al. The dangers of parathyroid biopsy. J Otolaryngol Head Neck Surg. 2017 Jan 7;46(1):4. PMID:28061891
**3581.** Kim J, Kumar R, Raymond AK, et al. Non-epiphyseal chondroblastoma arising in the iliac bone, and complicated by an aneurysmal bone cyst: a case report and review of the literature. Skeletal Radiol. 2010 Jun;39(6):583–7. PMID:19936740
**3582.** Kim JH, Moon H, Noh J, et al. Epidemiology and prognosis of pheochromocytoma/paraganglioma in Korea: a nationwide study based on the National Health Insurance Service. Endocrinol Metab (Seoul). 2020 Mar;35(1):157–64. PMID:32207276
**3583.** Kim JW, Park SH, Park SS, et al. Fetus-in-fetu in the cranium of a 4-month-old boy: histopathology and short tandem repeat polymorphism-based genotyping. Case report. J Neurosurg Pediatr. 2008 May;1(5):410–4. PMID:18447681
**3584.** Kim JY, Jung WH, Yoon CS, et al. Mesenchymal hamartomas of the chest wall in infancy: radiologic and pathologic correlation. Yonsei Med J. 2000 Oct;41(5):615–22. PMID:11079622
**3585.** Kim JY, Kim KS, Kim KJ, et al. Non-L-cell immunophenotype and large tumor size in rectal neuroendocrine tumors are associated with aggressive clinical behavior and worse prognosis. Am J Surg Pathol. 2015 May;39(5):632–43. PMID:25724002
**3586.** Kim KH, Roberts CW. Mechanisms by which SMARCB1 loss drives rhabdoid tumor growth. Cancer Genet. 2014 Sep;207(9):365–72. PMID:24853101
**3587.** Kim KH, Roberts CW. Targeting EZH2 in cancer. Nat Med. 2016 Feb;22(2):128–34. PMID:26845405
**3588.** Kim MS, Lee SH, Yoo NJ, et al. DICER1 exons 25 and 26 mutations are rare in common human tumours besides Sertoli-Leydig cell tumour. Histopathology. 2013 Sep;63(3):436–8. PMID:23763383
**3589.** Kim SH, Da Cruz Paula A, Basili T, et al. Identification of recurrent FHL2-GLI2 oncogenic fusion in sclerosing stromal tumors of the ovary. Nat Commun. 2020 Jan 2;11(1):44. PMID:31896750
**3590.** Kim SI, Lee Y, Kim SK, et al. Aggressive Supratentorial Ependymoma, RELA Fusion-Positive with Extracranial Metastasis: a Case Report. J Pathol Transl Med. 2017 Nov;51(6):588–93. PMID:29161788
**3591.** Kim SJ, Park YM, Jung SJ, et al. Sonographic appearances of juvenile fibroadenoma of the breast. J Ultrasound Med. 2014 Nov;33(11):1879–84. PMID:25336474
**3592.** Kim SS, Kays DW, Larson SD, et al. Appendiceal carcinoids in children–management and outcomes. J Surg Res. 2014 Dec;192(2):250–3. PMID:25039014
**3593.** Kim Y, Wen X, Bae JM, et al. The distribution of intratumoral macrophages correlates with molecular phenotypes and impacts prognosis in colorectal carcinoma. Histopathology. 2018 Oct;73(4):663–71. PMID:29906313
**3594.** Kim YD, Goldberg RA. Orbital fat prolapse and dermolipoma: two distinct entities. Korean J Ophthalmol. 1994 Jun;8(1):42–3. PMID:7933633
**3595.** Kimonis VE, Goldstein AM, Pastakia B, et al. Clinical manifestations in 105 persons with nevoid basal cell carcinoma syndrome. Am J Med Genet. 1997 Mar 31;69(3):299–308. PMID:9096761
**3596.** Kimura H, Hoshino Y, Kanegane H, et al. Clinical and virologic characteristics of chronic active Epstein-Barr virus infection. Blood. 2001 Jul 15;98(2):280–6. PMID:11435294
**3597.** Kimura N, Pilichowska M, Okamoto H, et al. Immunohistochemical expression of chromogranins A and B, prohormone convertases 2 and 3, and amidating enzyme in carcinoid tumors and pancreatic endocrine tumors. Mod Pathol. 2000 Feb;13(2):140–6. PMID:10697270
**3598.** Kimura N, Shiga K, Kaneko K, et al. The diagnostic dilemma of GATA3 immunohistochemistry in pheochromocytoma and paraganglioma. Endocr Pathol. 2020 Jun;31(2):95–100. PMID:32303954
**3599.** Kimura N, Takayanagi R, Takizawa N, et al. Pathological grading for predicting metastasis in phaeochromocytoma and paraganglioma. Endocr Relat Cancer. 2014 May 6;21(3):405–14. PMID:24521857
**3600.** Kimura N, Takekoshi K, Horii A, et al. Clinicopathological study of SDHB mutation-related pheochromocytoma and sympathetic paraganglioma. Endocr Relat Cancer. 2014 May 6;21(3):L13–6. PMID:24659481
**3601.** Kimura T, Budka H, Soler-Federsppiel S. An immunocytochemical comparison of the glia-associated proteins glial fibrillary acidic protein (GFAP) and S-100 protein (S100P) in human brain tumors. Clin Neuropathol. 1986 Jan-Feb;5(1):21–7. PMID:3512139
**3602.** King KS, Prodanov T, Kantorovich V, et al. Metastatic pheochromocytoma/paraganglioma related to primary tumor development in childhood or adolescence: significant link to SDHB mutations. J Clin Oncol. 2011 Nov 1;29(31):4137–42. PMID:21969497
**3603.** King RL, Howard MT, Bagg A. Hodgkin lymphoma: pathology, pathogenesis, and a plethora of potential prognostic predictors. Adv Anat Pathol. 2014 Jan;21(1):12–25. PMID:24316907
**3604.** Kingma DW, Mueller BU, Frekko K, et al. Low-grade monoclonal Epstein-Barr virus-associated lymphoproliferative disorder of the brain presenting as human immunodeficiency virus-associated encephalopathy in a child with acquired immunodeficiency syndrome. Arch Pathol Lab Med. 1999 Jan;123(1):83–7. PMID:9923843
**3605.** Kinkor Z, Vaneček T, Svajdler M Jr, et al. [Where does Ewing sarcoma end and begin - two cases of unusual bone tumors with t(20;22)(EWSR1-NFATc2) alteration]. Cesk Patol. 2014 Apr;50(2):87–91. Czech. PMID:24758504
**3606.** Kinmonth JB, Eustace PW. Lymph nodes and vessels in primary lymphoedema. Their relative importance in aetiology. Ann R Coll Surg Engl. 1976 Jul;58(4):278–84. PMID:182058
**3607.** Kinney MC, Collins RD, Greer JP, et al. A small-cell-predominant variant of primary Ki-1 (CD30)+ T-cell lymphoma. Am J Surg Pathol. 1993 Sep;17(9):859–68. PMID:8394652
**3608.** Kinney SN, Eble JN, Hes O, et al. Metanephric adenoma: the utility of immunohistochemical and cytogenetic analyses in differential diagnosis, including solid variant papillary renal cell carcinoma and epithelial-predominant nephroblastoma. Mod Pathol. 2015 Sep;28(9):1236–48. PMID:26248896
**3609.** Kinsler VA, O'Hare P, Bulstrode N, et al. Melanoma in congenital melanocytic naevi. Br J Dermatol. 2017 May;176(5):1131–43. PMID:28078671
**3610.** Kinsler VA, O'Hare P, Jacques T, et al. MEK inhibition appears to improve symptom control in primary NRAS-driven CNS melanoma in children. Br J Cancer. 2017 Apr 11;116(8):990–3. PMID:28253523
**3611.** Kinsler VA, Polubothu S, Calonje JE, et al. Copy number abnormalities in new or progressive 'neurocutaneous melanosis' confirm it to be primary CNS melanoma. Acta Neuropathol. 2017 Feb;133(2):329–31. PMID:27933403
**3612.** Kinsler VA, Thomas AC, Ishida M, et al. Multiple congenital melanocytic nevi and neurocutaneous melanosis are caused by postzygotic mutations in codon 61 of NRAS. J Invest Dermatol. 2013 Sep;133(9):2229–36. PMID:23392294
**3613.** Kinzler KW, Vogelstein B. Lessons from hereditary colorectal cancer. Cell. 1996 Oct 18;87(2):159–70. PMID:8861899
**3614.** Kirby PA, Ellison WA, Thomas PA. Spindle epithelial tumor with thymus-like differentiation (SETTLE) of the thyroid with prominent mitotic activity and focal necrosis. Am J Surg Pathol. 1999 Jun;23(6):712–6. PMID:10366154
**3615.** Kirchhoff C, Buhmann S, Braunstein V, et al. Synovial chondromatosis of the long biceps tendon sheath in a child: a case report and review of the literature. J Shoulder Elbow Surg. 2008 May-Jun;17(3):e6–10. PMID:18178490
**3616.** Kirk CW, Donnelly DE, Hardy R, et al. Natural history of a fibrous cephalic plaque and sustained eight decade follow-up in an 80 year old with tuberous sclerosis complex type 2. Ulster Med J. 2020 Jan;89(1):14–6. PMID:32218621
**3617.** Kirkman MA, Pickles JC, Fairchild AR, et al. Early wound site seeding in a patient with central nervous system high-grade neuroepithelial tumor with BCOR alteration. World Neurosurg. 2018 Aug;116:279–84. PMID:29859355
**3618.** Kirschner LS, Sandrini F, Monbo J, et al. Genetic heterogeneity and spectrum of mutations of the PRKAR1A gene in patients with the carney complex. Hum Mol Genet. 2000 Dec 12;9(20):3037–46. PMID:11115848
**3619.** Kirwan EO, Hutton PA, Pozo JL, et al. Osteoid osteoma and benign osteoblastoma of the spine. Clinical presentation and treatment. J Bone Joint Surg Br. 1984 Jan;66(1):21–6. PMID:6693472
**3620.** Kiseljak-Vassiliades K, Xu M, Mills TS, et al. Differential somatostatin receptor (SSTR) 1-5 expression and downstream effectors in histologic subtypes of growth hormone pituitary tumors. Mol Cell Endocrinol. 2015 Dec 5;417:73–83. PMID:26391562
**3621.** Kishore M, Gupta P, Bhardwaj M. Cerebrospinal fluid cytology of choroid plexus tumor:

a report of two cases. Cytojournal. 2019 Apr 22;16:9. PMID:31080487
**3622.** Kissil JL, Wilker EW, Johnson KC, et al. Merlin, the product of the Nf2 tumor suppressor gene, is an inhibitor of the p21-activated kinase, Pak1. Mol Cell. 2003 Oct;12(4):841–9. PMID:14580336
**3623.** Kitayama T, Akaki S, Hisazumi K, et al. An adult case of nasal chondromesenchymal hamartoma: imaging characteristics including diffusion-weighted images. Acta Med Okayama. 2019 Dec;73(6):529–32. PMID:31871336
**3624.** Kittah NE, Gruber LM, Bancos I, et al. Bilateral pheochromocytoma: clinical characteristics, treatment and longitudinal follow-up. Clin Endocrinol (Oxf). 2020 Sep;93(3):288–95. PMID:32410303
**3625.** Klairmont MM, Hoskoppal D, Yadak N, et al. The comparative sensitivity of immunohistochemical markers of megakaryocytic differentiation in acute megakaryoblastic leukemia. Am J Clin Pathol. 2018 Oct 1;150(5):461–7. PMID:30052718
**3626.** Klapper W, Kreuz M, Kohler CW, et al. Patient age at diagnosis is associated with the molecular characteristics of diffuse large B-cell lymphoma. Blood. 2012 Feb 23;119(8):1882–7. PMID:22238326
**3627.** Klapper W, Szczepanowski M, Burkhardt B, et al. Molecular profiling of pediatric mature B-cell lymphoma treated in population-based prospective clinical trials. Blood. 2008 Aug 15;112(4):1374–81. PMID:18509088
**3628.** Klapsinou E, Despoina P, Dimitra D. Cytologic findings and potential pitfalls in proliferative myositis and myositis ossificans diagnosed by fine needle aspiration cytology: report of four cases and review of the literature. Diagn Cytopathol. 2012 Mar;40(3):239–44. PMID:20890998
**3629.** Klausner RD, Handler SD. Familial occurrence of pleomorphic adenoma. Int J Pediatr Otorhinolaryngol. 1994 Nov;30(3):205–10. PMID:7836033
**3630.** Klco JM, Miller CA, Griffith M, et al. Association between mutation clearance after induction therapy and outcomes in acute myeloid leukemia. JAMA. 2015 Aug 25;314(8):811–22. PMID:26305651
**3631.** Klco JM, Welch JS, Nguyen TT, et al. State of the art in myeloid sarcoma. Int J Lab Hematol. 2011 Dec;33(6):555–65. PMID:21883967
**3632.** Kleer CG, Unni KK, McLeod RA. Epithelioid hemangioendothelioma of bone. Am J Surg Pathol. 1996 Nov;20(11):1301–11. PMID:8898834
**3633.** Kleijer WJ, Laugel V, Berneburg M, et al. Incidence of DNA repair deficiency disorders in western Europe: xeroderma pigmentosum, Cockayne syndrome and trichothiodystrophy. DNA Repair (Amst). 2008 May 3;7(5):744–50. PMID:18329345
**3634.** Klein CJ, Wu Y, Jentoft ME, et al. Genomic analysis reveals frequent TRAF7 mutations in intraneural perineuriomas. Ann Neurol. 2017 Feb;81(2):316–21. PMID:28019650
**3635.** Klein JA, Barr RJ. Diffuse lipomatosis and tuberous sclerosis. Arch Dermatol. 1986 Nov;122(11):1298–302. PMID:3777976
**3636.** Klein K, de Haas V, Kaspers GJL. Clinical challenges in de novo pediatric acute myeloid leukemia. Expert Rev Anticancer Ther. 2018 Mar;18(3):277–93. PMID:29338495
**3637.** Klein MH, Shankman S. Osteoid osteoma: radiologic and pathologic correlation. Skeletal Radiol. 1992;21(1):23–31. PMID:1546333
**3638.** Klein S, Lee H, Ghahremani S, et al. Expanding the phenotype of mutations in DICER1: mosaic missense mutations in the RNase IIIb domain of DICER1 cause GLOW syndrome. J Med Genet. 2014 May;51(5):294–302. PMID:24676357
**3639.** Kleinerman RA, Schonfeld SJ, Sigel BS, et al. Bone and soft-tissue sarcoma risk in long-term survivors of hereditary retinoblastoma treated with radiation. J Clin Oncol. 2019 Dec 10;37(35):3436–45. PMID:31622129
**3640.** Kleinerman RA, Tucker MA, Tarone RE, et al. Risk of new cancers after radiotherapy in long-term survivors of retinoblastoma: an extended follow-up. J Clin Oncol. 2005 Apr 1;23(10):2272–9. PMID:15800318
**3641.** Kleinman CL, Gerges N, Papillon-Cavanagh S, et al. Fusion of TTYH1 with the C19MC microRNA cluster drives expression of a brain-specific DNMT3B isoform in the embryonal brain tumor ETMR. Nat Genet. 2014 Jan;46(1):39–44. PMID:24316981
**3642.** Kleinman GM, Young RH, Scully RE. Ependymoma of the ovary: report of three cases. Hum Pathol. 1984 Jul;15(7):632–8. PMID:6204919
**3643.** Kleinman GM, Young RH, Scully RE. Primary neuroectodermal tumors of the ovary. A report of 25 cases. Am J Surg Pathol. 1993 Aug;17(8):764–78. PMID:8393302
**3644.** Kleinschmidt-DeMasters BK, Donson A, Foreman NK, et al. H3 K27M Mutation in Gangliogliomas can be Associated with Poor Prognosis. Brain Pathol. 2017 Nov;27(6):846–50. PMID:28378357
**3645.** Kleinschmidt-DeMasters BK, Donson AM, Richmond AM, et al. SOX10 distinguishes pilocytic and pilomyxoid astrocytomas from ependymomas but shows no differences in expression level in ependymomas from infants versus older children or among molecular subgroups. J Neuropathol Exp Neurol. 2016 Apr;75(4):295–8. PMID:26945037
**3646.** Kleinschmidt-DeMasters BK, Donson AM, Vogel H, et al. Pilomyxoid astrocytoma (PMA) shows significant differences in gene expression vs. pilocytic astrocytoma (PA) and variable tendency toward maturation to PA. Brain Pathol. 2015 Jul;25(4):429–40. PMID:25521223
**3647.** Kleinschmidt-DeMasters BK, Lillehei KO, Hankinson TC. Review of xanthomatous lesions of the sella. Brain Pathol. 2017 May;27(3):377–95. PMID:28236350
**3648.** Kleinschmidt-DeMasters BK, Lopes MB. Update on hypophysitis and TTF-1 expressing sellar region masses. Brain Pathol. 2013 Sep;23(5):495–514. PMID:23701182
**3649.** Klesse LJ, Jordan JT, Radtke HB, et al. The use of MEK inhibitors in neurofibromatosis type 1-associated tumors and management of toxicities. Oncologist. 2020 Jul;25(7):e1109–16. PMID:32272491
**3650.** Kletter GB, Sweetser DA, Wallace SF, et al. Adrenocorticotropin-secreting pancreatoblastoma. J Pediatr Endocrinol Metab. 2007 May;20(5):639–42. PMID:17642425
**3651.** Klijanienko J, Vielh P. Fine-needle sampling of salivary gland lesions. I. Cytology and histology correlation of 412 cases of pleomorphic adenoma. Diagn Cytopathol. 1996 May;14(3):195–200. PMID:8732648
**3652.** Klimstra DS. Nonductal neoplasms of the pancreas. Mod Pathol. 2007 Feb;20 Suppl 1:S94–112. PMID:17486055
**3653.** Klimstra DS, Heffess CS, Oertel JE, et al. Acinar cell carcinoma of the pancreas. A clinicopathologic study of 28 cases. Am J Surg Pathol. 1992 Sep;16(9):815–37. PMID:1384374
**3654.** Klimstra DS, Wenig BM, Adair CF, et al. Pancreatoblastoma. A clinicopathologic study and review of the literature. Am J Surg Pathol. 1995 Dec;19(12):1371–89. PMID:7503360
**3655.** Kline CN, Joseph NM, Grenert JP, et al. Targeted next-generation sequencing of pediatric neuro-oncology patients improves diagnosis, identifies pathogenic germline mutations, and directs targeted therapy. Neuro Oncol. 2017 May 1;19(5):699–709. PMID:28453743
**3656.** Klöppel G, Anlauf M, Perren A, et al. Hyperplasia to neoplasia sequence of duodenal and pancreatic neuroendocrine diseases and pseudohyperplasia of the PP-cells in the pancreas. Endocr Pathol. 2014 Jun;25(2):181–5. PMID:24718881
**3657.** Kluckova K, Tennant DA. Metabolic implications of hypoxia and pseudohypoxia in pheochromocytoma and paraganglioma. Cell Tissue Res. 2018 May;372(2):367–78. PMID:29450727
**3658.** Kluijfhout WP, Pasternak JD, van der Kaay D, et al. Is it time to reconsider lobectomy in low-risk paediatric thyroid cancer? Clin Endocrinol (Oxf). 2017 Apr;86(4):591–6. PMID:27896825
**3659.** Kluin PM, Langerak AW, Beverdam-Vincent J, et al. Paediatric nodal marginal zone B-cell lymphadenopathy of the neck: a Haemophilus influenzae-driven immune disorder? J Pathol. 2015 Jul;236(3):302–14. PMID:25722108
**3660.** Klusmann JH, Creutzig U, Zimmermann M, et al. Treatment and prognostic impact of transient leukemia in neonates with Down syndrome. Blood. 2008 Mar 15;111(6):2991–8. PMID:18182574
**3661.** Kluwe L, MacCollin M, Tatagiba M, et al. Phenotypic variability associated with 14 splice-site mutations in the NF2 gene. Am J Med Genet. 1998 May 18;77(3):228–33. PMID:9605590
**3662.** Kluwe L, Mautner V, Heinrich B, et al. Molecular study of frequency of mosaicism in neurofibromatosis 2 patients with bilateral vestibular schwannomas. J Med Genet. 2003 Feb;40(2):109–14. PMID:12566519
**3663.** Kluwe L, Mautner VF. Mosaicism in sporadic neurofibromatosis 2 patients. Hum Mol Genet. 1998 Dec;7(13):2051–5. PMID:9817921
**3664.** Knezevich SR, Garnett MJ, Pysher TJ, et al. ETV6-NTRK3 gene fusions and trisomy 11 establish a histogenetic link between mesoblastic nephroma and congenital fibrosarcoma. Cancer Res. 1998 Nov 15;58(22):5046–8. PMID:9823307
**3665.** Knisely AS, Strautnieks SS, Meier Y, et al. Hepatocellular carcinoma in ten children under five years of age with bile salt export pump deficiency. Hepatology. 2006 Aug;44(2):478–86. PMID:16871584
**3666.** Knöpfel N, Colmenero I, Matito A, et al. Cutaneous mastocytosis with predominant infiltration of promastocytes. Am J Dermatopathol. 2019 Apr;41(4):296–9. PMID:30252695
**3667.** Knosp E, Steiner E, Kitz K, et al. Pituitary adenomas with invasion of the cavernous sinus space: a magnetic resonance imaging classification compared with surgical findings. Neurosurgery. 1993 Oct;33(4):610–7. PMID:8232800
**3668.** Knowles DM, Cesarman E, Chadburn A, et al. Correlative morphologic and molecular genetic analysis demonstrates three distinct categories of posttransplantation lymphoproliferative disorders. Blood. 1995 Jan 15;85(2):552–65. PMID:7812011
**3669.** Knudsen AL, Bülow S, Tomlinson I, et al. Attenuated familial adenomatous polyposis: results from an international collaborative study. Colorectal Dis. 2010 Oct;12 10 Online:e243–9. PMID:20105204
**3670.** Knudson AG Jr. Mutation and cancer: statistical study of retinoblastoma. Proc Natl Acad Sci U S A. 1971 Apr;68(4):820–3. PMID:5279523
**3671.** Ko CJ, McNiff JM, Glusac EJ. Melanocytic nevi with features of Spitz nevi and Clark's/dysplastic nevi ("Spark's" nevi). J Cutan Pathol. 2009 Oct;36(10):1063–8. PMID:19187111
**3672.** Ko E, Mortimer E, Fraire AE. Extraarticular synovial chondromatosis: review of epidemiology, imaging studies, microscopy and pathogenesis, with a report of an additional case in a child. Int J Surg Pathol. 2004 Jul;12(3):273–80. PMID:15306942
**3673.** Ko JS, Marusic Z, Azzato EM, et al. Superficial sarcomas with CIC rearrangement are aggressive neoplasms: a series of eight cases. J Cutan Pathol. 2020 Jun;47(6):509–16. PMID:32026485
**3674.** Kobayashi C, Monforte-Munoz HL, Gerbing RB, et al. Enlarged and prominent nucleoli may be indicative of MYCN amplification: a study of neuroblastoma (Schwannian stroma-poor), undifferentiated/poorly differentiated subtype with high mitosis-karyorrhexis index. Cancer. 2005 Jan 1;103(1):174–80. PMID:15549714
**3675.** Kobayashi R, Yamato K, Tanaka F, et al. Retrospective analysis of non-anaplastic peripheral T-cell lymphoma in pediatric patients in Japan. Pediatr Blood Cancer. 2010 Feb;54(2):212–5. PMID:19856396
**3676.** Kobayashi T, Kimura T, Takabayashi N, et al. Two synchronous solid and cystic tumors of the pancreas. J Gastroenterol. 1998 Jun;33(3):439–42. PMID:9658328
**3677.** Kobos R, Nagai M, Tsuda M, et al. Combining integrated genomics and functional genomics to dissect the biology of a cancer-associated, aberrant transcription factor, the ASPSCR1-TFE3 fusion oncoprotein. J Pathol. 2013 Apr;229(5):743–54. PMID:23288701
**3678.** Kobos R, Steinherz PG, Kernan NA, et al. Allogeneic hematopoietic stem cell transplantation for pediatric patients with treatment-related myelodysplastic syndrome or acute myelogenous leukemia. Biol Blood Marrow Transplant. 2012 Mar;18(3):473–80. PMID:22079789
**3679.** Koch CA, Mauro D, Walther MM, et al. Pheochromocytoma in von hippel-lindau disease: distinct histopathologic phenotype compared to pheochromocytoma in multiple endocrine neoplasia type 2. Endocr Pathol. 2002 Spring;13(1):17–27. PMID:12114747
**3680.** Kochummen E, Tong S, Umpaichitra V, et al. A unique case of bilateral Hürthle cell adenoma in an adolescent. Horm Res Paediatr. 2017;87(2):136–42. PMID:27467101
**3681.** Kocjan BJ, Gale N, Hočevar Boltežar I, et al. Identical human papillomavirus (HPV) genomic variants persist in recurrent respiratory papillomatosis for up to 22 years. J Infect Dis. 2013 Feb 15;207(4):583–7. PMID:23204170
**3682.** Koczkowska M, Callens T, Gomes A, et al. Expanding the clinical phenotype of individuals with a 3-bp in-frame deletion of the NF1 gene (c.2970_2972del): an update of genotype-phenotype correlation. Genet Med. 2019 Apr;21(4):867–76. PMID:30190611
**3683.** Koczkowska M, Chen Y, Callens T, et al. Genotype-phenotype correlation in NF1: evidence for a more severe phenotype associated with missense mutations affecting NF1 codons 844-848. Am J Hum Genet. 2018 Jan 4;102(1):69–87. PMID:29290338
**3684.** Kodet R, Newton WA Jr, Sachs N, et al. Rhabdoid tumors of soft tissues: a clinicopathologic study of 26 cases enrolled on the Intergroup Rhabdomyosarcoma Study. Hum Pathol. 1991 Jul;22(7):674–84. PMID:1712749
**3684A.** Koeller KK, Rosenblum RS, Morrison AL. Neoplasms of the spinal cord and filum terminale: radiologic-pathologic correlation. Radiographics. 2000 Nov-Dec;20(6):1721–49. PMID:11112826
**3685.** Koelsche C, Hartmann W, Schrimpf D, et al. Array-based DNA-methylation profiling in sarcomas with small blue round cell histology provides valuable diagnostic information. Mod Pathol. 2018 Aug;31(8):1246–56. PMID:29572501

**3686.** Koelsche C, Hovestadt V, Jones DT, et al. Melanotic tumors of the nervous system are characterized by distinct mutational, chromosomal and epigenomic profiles. Brain Pathol. 2015 Mar;25(2):202–8. PMID:25399693

**3687.** Koelsche C, Kriegsmann M, Kommoss FKF, et al. DNA methylation profiling distinguishes Ewing-like sarcoma with EWSR1-NFATc2 fusion from Ewing sarcoma. J Cancer Res Clin Oncol. 2019 May;145(5):1273–81. PMID:30895378

**3688.** Koelsche C, Sahm F, Capper D, et al. Distribution of TERT promoter mutations in pediatric and adult tumors of the nervous system. Acta Neuropathol. 2013 Dec;126(6):907–15. PMID:24154961

**3689.** Koelsche C, Sahm F, Paulus W, et al. BRAF V600E expression and distribution in desmoplastic infantile astrocytoma/ganglioglioma. Neuropathol Appl Neurobiol. 2014 Apr;40(3):337–44. PMID:23822828

**3690.** Koelsche C, Sahm F, Wöhrer A, et al. BRAF-mutated pleomorphic xanthoastrocytoma is associated with temporal location, reticulin fiber deposition and CD34 expression. Brain Pathol. 2014 Apr;24(3):221–9. PMID:24345274

**3691.** Koelsche C, Wöhrer A, Jeibmann A, et al. Mutant BRAF V600E protein in ganglioglioma is predominantly expressed by neuronal tumor cells. Acta Neuropathol. 2013 Jun;125(6):891–900. PMID:23435618

**3692.** Koga M, Koga K, Kiryu H, et al. Congenital Spitz nevus on the foot. J Dermatol. 2014 Mar;41(3):282–3. PMID:24506180

**3693.** Koh CM, Khattar E, Leow SC, et al. Telomerase regulates MYC-driven oncogenesis independent of its reverse transcriptase activity. J Clin Invest. 2015 May;125(5):2109–22. PMID:25893605

**3694.** Koh HY, Kim SH, Jang J, et al. BRAF somatic mutation contributes to intrinsic epileptogenicity in pediatric brain tumors. Nat Med. 2018 Nov;24(11):1662–8. PMID:30224756

**3695.** Koh JM, Ahn SH, Kim H, et al. Validation of pathological grading systems for predicting metastatic potential in pheochromocytoma and paraganglioma. PLoS One. 2017 Nov 8;12(11):e0187398. PMID:29117221

**3696.** Koh TH, Cooper JE, Newman CL, et al. Pancreatoblastoma in a neonate with Wiedemann-Beckwith syndrome. Eur J Pediatr. 1986 Oct;145(5):435–8. PMID:3792392

**3697.** Kohashi K, Izumi T, Oda Y, et al. Infrequent SMARCB1/INI1 gene alteration in epithelioid sarcoma: a useful tool in distinguishing epithelioid sarcoma from malignant rhabdoid tumor. Hum Pathol. 2009 Mar;40(3):349–55. PMID:18973917

**3698.** Kohashi K, Nakatsura T, Kinoshita Y, et al. Glypican 3 expression in tumors with loss of SMARCB1/INI1 protein expression. Hum Pathol. 2013 Apr;44(4):526–33. PMID:23084579

**3699.** Kohashi K, Oda Y, Yamamoto H, et al. Reduced expression of SMARCB1/INI1 protein in synovial sarcoma. Mod Pathol. 2010 Jul;23(7):981–90. PMID:20305614

**3700.** Kohashi K, Tanaka Y, Kishimoto H, et al. Reclassification of rhabdoid tumor and pediatric undifferentiated/unclassified sarcoma with complete loss of SMARCB1/INI1 protein expression: three subtypes of rhabdoid tumor according to their histological features. Mod Pathol. 2016 Oct;29(10):1232–42. PMID:27338635

**3701.** Kohashi K, Yamada Y, Hotokebuchi Y, et al. ERG and SALL4 expressions in SMARCB1/INI1-deficient tumors: a useful tool for distinguishing epithelioid sarcoma from malignant rhabdoid tumor. Hum Pathol. 2015 Feb;46(2):225–30. PMID:25479928

**3702.** Kohashi K, Yamamoto H, Kumagai R, et al. Differential microRNA expression profiles between malignant rhabdoid tumor and epithelioid sarcoma: miR193a-5p is suggested to downregulate SMARCB1 mRNA expression. Mod Pathol. 2014 Jun;27(6):832–9. PMID:24287458

**3703.** Kohda E, Iseki M, Ikawa H, et al. Pancreatoblastoma. Three original cases and review of the literature. Acta Radiol. 2000 Jul;41(4):334–7. PMID:10937753

**3704.** Kohout MP, Hansen M, Pribaz JJ, et al. Arteriovenous malformations of the head and neck: natural history and management. Plast Reconstr Surg. 1998 Sep;102(3):643–54. PMID:9727427

**3705.** Kohsaka S, Shukla N, Ameur N, et al. A recurrent neomorphic mutation in MYOD1 defines a clinically aggressive subset of embryonal rhabdomyosarcoma associated with PI3K-AKT pathway mutations. Nat Genet. 2014 Jun;46(6):595–600. PMID:24793135

**3706.** Kojima Y, Sasaki K, Yokobayashi S, et al. Evolutionarily distinctive transcriptional and signaling programs drive human germ cell lineage specification from pluripotent stem cells. Cell Stem Cell. 2017 Oct 5;21(4):517–532.e5. PMID:28985527

**3707.** Kokubun K, Matsuzaka K, Akashi Y, et al. Congenital epulis: a case and review of the literature. Bull Tokyo Dent Coll. 2018;59(2):127–32. PMID:29962420

**3708.** Kolin DL, Duan K, Ngan B, et al. Expanding the spectrum of colonic manifestations in tuberous sclerosis: L-cell neuroendocrine tumor arising in the background of rectal PEComa. Endocr Pathol. 2018 Mar;29(1):21–6. PMID:28733877

**3709.** Kolin DL, Geddie WR, Ko HM. CSF cytology diagnosis of NRAS-mutated primary leptomeningeal melanomatosis with neurocutaneous melanosis. Cytopathology. 2017 Jun;28(3):235–8. PMID:27696542

**3710.** Kollars J, Zarroug AE, van Heerden J, et al. Primary hyperparathyroidism in pediatric patients. Pediatrics. 2005 Apr;115(4):974–80. PMID:15805373

**3711.** Kollipara R, Odhav A, Rentas KE, et al. Vascular anomalies in pediatric patients: updated classification, imaging, and therapy. Radiol Clin North Am. 2013 Jul;51(4):659–72. PMID:23830791

**3712.** Kollur SM, El Hag IA. Fine-needle aspiration cytology of metastatic nasopharyngeal carcinoma in cervical lymph nodes: comparison with metastatic squamous-cell carcinoma, and Hodgkin's and non-Hodgkin's lymphoma. Diagn Cytopathol. 2003 Jan;28(1):18–22. PMID:12508177

**3713.** Komai Y, Fujiwara M, Fujii Y, et al. Adult Xp11 translocation renal cell carcinoma diagnosed by cytogenetics and immunohistochemistry. Clin Cancer Res. 2009 Feb 15;15(4):1170–6. PMID:19228722

**3714.** Komatsu H, Inui A, Kishiki K, et al. Liver disease secondary to congenital heart disease in children. Expert Rev Gastroenterol Hepatol. 2019 Jul;13(7):651–66. PMID:31131680

**3715.** Kominami A, Fujino M, Murakami H, et al. β-catenin mutation in ovarian solid pseudopapillary neoplasm. Pathol Int. 2014 Sep;64(9):460–4. PMID:25186079

**3716.** Kommoss F, Oliva E, Bhan AK, et al. Inhibin expression in ovarian tumors and tumor-like lesions: an immunohistochemical study. Mod Pathol. 1998 Jul;11(7):656–64. PMID:9688187

**3717.** Komori K, Hoshino K, Shirai J, et al. Mesothelial cyst of the liver in a neonate. Pediatr Surg Int. 2008 Apr;24(4):463–5. PMID:17598115

**3718.** Komotar RJ, Burger PC, Carson BS, et al. Pilocytic and pilomyxoid hypothalamic/chiasmatic astrocytomas. Neurosurgery. 2004 Jan;54(1):72–9. PMID:14683543

**3719.** Konczyk DJ, Goss JA, Smits PJ, et al. Arteriovenous malformation associated with a HRAS mutation. Hum Genet. 2019 Dec;138(11-12):1419–21. PMID:31637524

**3720.** Kong G, Grozinsky-Glasberg S, Hofman MS, et al. Efficacy of peptide receptor radionuclide therapy for functional metastatic paraganglioma and pheochromocytoma. J Clin Endocrinol Metab. 2017 Sep 1;102(9):3278–87. PMID:28605448

**3721.** Kong YY, Dai B, Kong JC, et al. Neutrophil/eosinophil-rich type of primary cutaneous anaplastic large cell lymphoma: a clinicopathological, immunophenotypic and molecular study of nine cases. Histopathology. 2009 Aug;55(2):189–96. PMID:19694826

**3722.** Koni A, Ozseker HS, Arpali E, et al. Histopathological evaluation of orchiectomy specimens in 51 late postpubertal men with unilateral cryptorchidism. J Urol. 2014 Oct;192(4):1183–8. PMID:24840535

**3723.** Konishi E, Nakashima Y, Iwasa Y, et al. Immunohistochemical analysis for Sox9 reveals the cartilaginous character of chondroblastoma and chondromyxoid fibroma of the bone. Hum Pathol. 2010 Feb;41(2):208–13. PMID:19801163

**3724.** Konishi E, Nakashima Y, Mano M, et al. Chondroblastoma of extra-craniofacial bones: clinicopathological analyses of 103 cases. Pathol Int. 2017 Oct;67(10):495–502. PMID:28971570

**3725.** Konno S, Oka H, Utsuki S, et al. Germinoma with a granulomatous reaction. Problems of differential diagnosis. Clin Neuropathol. 2002 Nov-Dec;21(6):248–51. PMID:12489672

**3726.** Kontny U, Oschlies I, Woessmann W, et al. Non-anaplastic peripheral T-cell lymphoma in children and adolescents–a retrospective analysis of the NHL-BFM study group. Br J Haematol. 2015 Mar;168(6):835–44. PMID:25395120

**3727.** Koo M, Ohgami RS. Pediatric-type follicular lymphoma and pediatric nodal marginal zone lymphoma: recent clinical, morphologic, immunophenotypic, and genetic insights. Adv Anat Pathol. 2017 May;24(3):128–35. PMID:28277421

**3728.** Kooi IE, Mol BM, Massink MP, et al. Somatic genomic alterations in retinoblastoma beyond RB1 are rare and limited to copy number changes. Sci Rep. 2016 Apr 29;6:25264. PMID:27126562

**3729.** Kool M, Jones DT, Jäger N, et al. Genome sequencing of SHH medulloblastoma predicts genotype-related response to smoothened inhibition. Cancer Cell. 2014 Mar 17;25(3):393–405. PMID:24651015

**3730.** Kool M, Korshunov A, Remke M, et al. Molecular subgroups of medulloblastoma: an international meta-analysis of transcriptome, genetic aberrations, and clinical data of WNT, SHH, Group 3, and Group 4 medulloblastomas. Acta Neuropathol. 2012 Apr;123(4):473–84. PMID:22358457

**3731.** Koopmans AE, Verdijk RM, Brouwer RW, et al. Clinical significance of immunohistochemistry for detection of BAP1 mutations in uveal melanoma. Mod Pathol. 2014 Oct;27(10):1321–30. PMID:24633195

**3732.** Koperek O, Kornauth C, Capper D, et al. Immunohistochemical detection of the BRAF V600E-mutated protein in papillary thyroid carcinoma. Am J Surg Pathol. 2012 Jun;36(6):844–50. PMID:22592144

**3733.** Köpf S, Tönshoff B. Adenotonsillar hypertrophy and post-transplant lymphoproliferative disorder in pediatric renal transplant recipients. Pediatr Nephrol. 2004 Apr;19(4):471–2. PMID:14963764

**3734.** Koral K, Koral KM, Sklar F. Angiocentric glioma in a 4-year-old boy: imaging characteristics and review of the literature. Clin Imaging. 2012 Jan-Feb;36(1):61–4. PMID:22226445

**3735.** Koral K, Sayre J, Bhuta S, et al. Recurrent pleomorphic adenoma of the parotid gland in pediatric and adult patients: value of multiple lesions as a diagnostic indicator. AJR Am J Roentgenol. 2003 Apr;180(4):1171–4. PMID:12646477

**3736.** Kordek R, Biernat W, Sapieja W, et al. Pleomorphic xanthoastrocytoma with a gangliomatous component: an immunohistochemical and ultrastructural study. Acta Neuropathol. 1995;89(2):194–7. PMID:7732793

**3737.** Kordes U, Flitsch J, Hagel C, et al. Ectopic craniopharyngioma. Klin Padiatr. 2011 May;223(3):176–7. PMID:21462099

**3738.** Koren R, Bernheim J, Schachter P, et al. Black thyroid adenoma. Clinical, histochemical, and ultrastructural features. Appl Immunohistochem Mol Morphol. 2000 Mar;8(1):80–4. PMID:10937053

**3739.** Korfhage J, Lombard DB. Malignant peripheral nerve sheath tumors: from epigenome to bedside. Mol Cancer Res. 2019 Jul;17(7):1417–28. PMID:31023785

**3740.** Korinek V, Barker N, Morin PJ, et al. Constitutive transcriptional activation by a beta-catenin-Tcf complex in APC-/- colon carcinoma. Science. 1997 Mar 21;275(5307):1784–7. PMID:9065401

**3741.** Korn WT, Schatzki SC, DiSciullo AJ, et al. Papillary cystadenoma of the broad ligament in von Hippel-Lindau disease. Am J Obstet Gynecol. 1990 Aug;163(2):596–8. PMID:2386149

**3742.** Kornreich L, Blaser S, Schwarz M, et al. Optic pathway glioma: correlation of imaging findings with the presence of neurofibromatosis. AJNR Am J Neuroradiol. 2001 Nov-Dec;22(10):1963–9. PMID:11733333

**3743.** Korpershoek E, Favier J, Gaal J, et al. SDHA immunohistochemistry detects germline SDHA gene mutations in apparently sporadic paragangliomas and pheochromocytomas. J Clin Endocrinol Metab. 2011 Sep;96(9):E1472–6. PMID:21752896

**3744.** Korshunov A, Capper D, Reuss D, et al. Histologically distinct neuroepithelial tumors with histone 3 G34 mutation are molecularly similar and comprise a single nosologic entity. Acta Neuropathol. 2016 Jan;131(1):137–46. PMID:26482474

**3745.** Korshunov A, Chavez L, Northcott PA, et al. DNA-methylation profiling discloses significant advantages over NanoString method for molecular classification of medulloblastoma. Acta Neuropathol. 2017 Dec;134(6):965–7. PMID:29027579

**3746.** Korshunov A, Chavez L, Sharma T, et al. Epithelioid glioblastomas stratify into established diagnostic subsets upon integrated molecular analysis. Brain Pathol. 2018 Sep;28(5):656–62. PMID:28990704

**3747.** Korshunov A, Jakobiec FA, Eberhart CG, et al. Comparative integrated molecular analysis of intraocular medulloepitheliomas and central nervous system embryonal tumors with multilayered rosettes confirms that they are distinct nosologic entities. Neuropathology. 2015 Dec;35(6):538–44. PMID:26183384

**3748.** Korshunov A, Okonechnikov K, Sahm F, et al. Molecular progression of SHH-activated medulloblastomas. Acta Neuropathol. 2019 Aug;138(2):327–30. PMID:31030238

**3749.** Korshunov A, Okonechnikov K, Sahm F, et al. Transcriptional profiling of medulloblastoma with extensive nodularity (MBEN) reveals two clinically relevant tumor subsets with VSNL1 as potent prognostic marker. Acta Neuropathol. 2020 Mar;139(3):583–96. PMID:31781912

3750. Korshunov A, Remke M, Werft W, et al. Adult and pediatric medulloblastomas are genetically distinct and require different algorithms for molecular risk stratification. J Clin Oncol. 2010 Jun 20;28(18):3054–60. PMID:20479417
3751. Korshunov A, Ryzhova M, Hovestadt V, et al. Integrated analysis of pediatric glioblastoma reveals a subset of biologically favorable tumors with associated molecular prognostic markers. Acta Neuropathol. 2015 May;129(5):669–78. PMID:25752754
3752. Korshunov A, Sahm F, Okonechnikov K, et al. Desmoplastic/nodular medulloblastomas (DNMB) and medulloblastomas with extensive nodularity (MBEN) disclose similar epigenetic signatures but different transcriptional profiles. Acta Neuropathol. 2019 Jun;137(6):1003–15. PMID:30826918
3753. Korshunov A, Schrimpf D, Ryzhova M, et al. H3-/IDH-wild type pediatric glioblastoma is comprised of molecularly and prognostically distinct subtypes with associated oncogenic drivers. Acta Neuropathol. 2017 Sep;134(3):507–16. PMID:28401334
3754. Korshunov A, Sturm D, Ryzhova M, et al. Embryonal tumor with abundant neuropil and true rosettes (ETANTR), ependymoblastoma, and medulloepithelioma share molecular similarity and comprise a single clinicopathological entity. Acta Neuropathol. 2014 Aug;128(2):279–89. PMID:24337497
3755. Körver RJ, Theunissen PH, van de Kreeke WT, et al. Juxta-articular myxoma of the knee in a 5-year-old boy: a case report and review of the literature (2009: 12b). Eur Radiol. 2010 Mar;20(3):764–8. PMID:20157818
3756. Koshida K, Wahren B. Placental-like alkaline phosphatase in seminoma. Urol Res. 1990;18(2):87–92. PMID:2187297
3757. Kosmahl M, Seada LS, Jänig U, et al. Solid-pseudopapillary tumor of the pancreas: its origin revisited. Virchows Arch. 2000 May;436(5):473–80. PMID:10881741
3758. Koss MN, Hochholzer L, Langloss JM, et al. Lymphomatoid granulomatosis: a clinicopathologic study of 42 patients. Pathology. 1986 Jul;18(3):283–8. PMID:3785978
3759. Koster R, Mitra N, D'Andrea K, et al. Pathway-based analysis of GWAs data identifies association of sex determination genes with susceptibility to testicular germ cell tumors. Hum Mol Genet. 2014 Nov 15;23(22):6061–8. PMID:24943593
3760. Kotiligam D, Lazar AJ, Pollock RE, et al. Desmoid tumor: a disease opportune for molecular insights. Histol Histopathol. 2008 Jan;23(1):117–26. PMID:17952864
3761. Kotler E, Segal E, Oren M. Functional characterization of the p53 "mutome". Mol Cell Oncol. 2018 Sep 25;5(6):e1511207. PMID:30525089
3762. Koubaa Mahjoub W, Jouini R, Khanchel F, et al. Neuroblastoma-like schwannoma with giant rosette: a potential diagnostic pitfall for hyalinizing spindle cell tumor. J Cutan Pathol. 2019 Mar;46(3):234–7. PMID:30582192
3763. Koutlas IG, Scheithauer BW. Palisaded encapsulated ("solitary circumscribed") neuroma of the oral cavity: a review of 55 cases. Head Neck Pathol. 2010 Mar;4(1):15–26. PMID:20237984
3764. Kovac M, Blattmann C, Ribi S, et al. Exome sequencing of osteosarcoma reveals mutation signatures reminiscent of BRCA deficiency. Nat Commun. 2015 Dec 3;6:8940. PMID:26632267
3765. Kovalchuk AL, Ansarah-Sobrinho C, Hakim O, et al. Mouse model of endemic Burkitt translocations reveals the long-range boundaries of Ig-mediated oncogene deregulation. Proc Natl Acad Sci U S A. 2012 Jul 3;109(27):10972–7. PMID:22711821
3766. Kox C, Zimmermann M, Stanulla M, et al. The favorable effect of activating NOTCH1 receptor mutations on long-term outcome in T-ALL patients treated on the ALL-BFM 2000 protocol can be separated from FBXW7 loss of function. Leukemia. 2010 Dec;24(12):2005–13. PMID:20944675
3767. Kozakewich HPW, Mulliken JB. Chapter 12: Histopathology of vascular malformations. In: Mulliken JB, Burrows PE, Fishman SJ, editors. Mulliken and Young's vascular anomalies: hemangiomas and malformations. 2nd ed. New York (NY): Oxford University Press; 2013.
3768. Koziel L, Kunath M, Kelly OG, et al. Ext1-dependent heparan sulfate regulates the range of Ihh signaling during endochondral ossification. Dev Cell. 2004 Jun;6(6):801–13. PMID:15177029
3769. Kraemer KH, DiGiovanna JJ. Xeroderma pigmentosum. In: Adam MP, Ardinger HH, Pagon RA, et al., editors. GeneReviews. Seattle (WA): University of Washington, Seattle; 2003 Jun 20. PMID:20301571
3770. Kraemer KH, Lee MM, Scotto J. Xeroderma pigmentosum. Cutaneous, ocular, and neurologic abnormalities in 830 published cases. Arch Dermatol. 1987 Feb;123(2):241–50. PMID:3545087
3771. Kraft S, Granter SR. Molecular pathology of skin neoplasms of the head and neck. Arch Pathol Lab Med. 2014 Jun;138(6):759–87. PMID:24878016
3772. Krag Jacobsen G, Barlebo H, Olsen J, et al. Testicular germ cell tumours in Denmark 1976-1980. Pathology of 1058 consecutive cases. Acta Radiol Oncol. 1984;23(4):239–47. PMID:6093440
3773. Kraggerud SM, Szymanska J, Abeler VM, et al. DNA copy number changes in malignant ovarian germ cell tumors. Cancer Res. 2000 Jun 1;60(11):3025–30. PMID:10850452
3774. Kramer GD, Arepalli S, Shields CL, et al. Ciliary body medulloepithelioma association with pleuropulmonary blastoma in a familial tumor predisposition syndrome. J Pediatr Ophthalmol Strabismus. 2014 Jul 16;51 Online:e48–50. PMID:25032694
3775. Kramer K, Hicks DG, Palis J, et al. Epithelioid osteosarcoma of bone. Immunocytochemical evidence suggesting divergent epithelial and mesenchymal differentiation in a primary osseous neoplasm. Cancer. 1993 May 15;71(10):2977–82. PMID:7683966
3776. Krane JF, Alexander EK, Cibas ES, et al. Coming to terms with NIFTP: a provisional approach for cytologists. Cancer Cytopathol. 2016 Nov;124(11):767–72. PMID:27564464
3777. Kransdorf MJ, Sweet DE. Aneurysmal bone cyst: concept, controversy, clinical presentation, and imaging. AJR Am J Roentgenol. 1995 Mar;164(3):573–80. PMID:7863874
3778. Kratz CP, Achatz MI, Brugières L, et al. Cancer screening recommendations for individuals with Li-Fraumeni syndrome. Clin Cancer Res. 2017 Jun 1;23(11):e38–45. PMID:28572266
3779. Kratz CP, Niemeyer CM, Castleberry RP, et al. The mutational spectrum of PTPN11 in juvenile myelomonocytic leukemia and Noonan syndrome/myeloproliferative disease. Blood. 2005 Sep 15;106(6):2183–5. PMID:15928039
3780. Kratz CP, Stanulla M, Cavé H. Genetic predisposition to acute lymphoblastic leukemia: overview on behalf of the I-BFM ALL Host Genetic Variation Working Group. Eur J Med Genet. 2016 Mar;59(3):111–5. PMID:26699264
3781. Krauss T, Ferrara AM, Links TP, et al. Preventive medicine of von Hippel-Lindau disease-associated pancreatic neuroendocrine tumors. Endocr Relat Cancer. 2018 Sep;25(9):783–93. PMID:29748190
3782. Krengel S, Reyes-Múgica M. Melanoma risk in congenital melanocytic naevi. Br J Dermatol. 2017 May;176(5):1114. PMID:28504374
3783. Krengel S, Scope A, Dusza SW, et al. New recommendations for the categorization of cutaneous features of congenital melanocytic nevi. J Am Acad Dermatol. 2013 Mar;68(3):441–51. PMID:22982004
3784. Kresse SH, Ohnstad HO, Bjerkehagen B, et al. DNA copy number changes in human malignant fibrous histiocytomas by array comparative genomic hybridisation. PLoS One. 2010 Nov 9;5(11):e15378. PMID:21085701
3785. Kreutzer J, Vance ML, Lopes MB, et al. Surgical management of GH-secreting pituitary adenomas: an outcome study using modern remission criteria. J Clin Endocrinol Metab. 2001 Sep;86(9):4072–7. PMID:11549628
3786. Krewer J, Rolle U, Koscielniak E, et al. Dermatofibrosarcoma protuberans in children and adolescents: primary and relapsed disease-experience of the Cooperative Weichteilsarkomstudiengruppe (CWS). J Surg Oncol. 2020 Aug;122(2):263–72. PMID:32430916
3787. Krieg AH, Hefti F, Speth BM, et al. Synovial sarcomas usually metastasize after >5 years: a multicenter retrospective analysis with minimum follow-up of 10 years for survivors. Ann Oncol. 2011 Feb;22(2):458–67. PMID:20716627
3788. Krieg M, Marti HH, Plate KH. Coexpression of erythropoietin and vascular endothelial growth factor in nervous system tumors associated with von Hippel-Lindau tumor suppressor gene loss of function. Blood. 1998 Nov 1;92(9):3388–93. PMID:9787178
3789. Kriegsmann K, Zgorzelski C, Kazdal D, et al. Insulinoma-associated protein 1 (INSM1) in thoracic tumors is less sensitive but more specific compared with synaptophysin, chromogranin A, and CD56. Appl Immunohistochem Mol Morphol. 2020 Mar;28(3):237–42. PMID:30358615
3790. Krishnan S, Brown PD, Scheithauer BW, et al. Choroid plexus papillomas: a single institutional experience. J Neurooncol. 2004 May;68(1):49–55. PMID:15174521
3791. Krishnatry R, Zhukova N, Guerreiro Stucklin AS, et al. Clinical and treatment factors determining long-term outcomes for adult survivors of childhood low-grade glioma: a population-based study. Cancer. 2016 Apr 15;122(8):1261–9. PMID:26970559
3792. Kristensen DG, Nielsen JE, Jørgensen A, et al. Evidence that active demethylation mechanisms maintain the genome of carcinoma in situ cells hypomethylated in the adult testis. Br J Cancer. 2014 Feb 4;110(3):668–78. PMID:24292451
3793. Kristensen DG, Skakkebæk NE, Rajpert-De Meyts E, et al. Epigenetic features of testicular germ cell tumours in relation to epigenetic characteristics of foetal germ cells. Int J Dev Biol. 2013;57(2-4):309–17. PMID:23784842
3794. Kristensen T, Vestergaard H, Møller MB. Improved detection of the KIT D816V mutation in patients with systemic mastocytosis using a quantitative and highly sensitive real-time qPCR assay. J Mol Diagn. 2011 Mar;13(2):180–8. PMID:21354053
3795. Kroeze E, Loeffen JLC, Poort VM, et al. T-cell lymphoblastic lymphoma and leukemia: different diseases from a common premalignant progenitor? Blood Adv. 2020 Jul 28;4(14):3466–73. PMID:32722786
3796. Kros JM, Delwel EJ, de Jong TH, et al. Desmoplastic infantile astrocytoma and ganglioglioma: a search for genomic characteristics. Acta Neuropathol. 2002 Aug;104(2):144–8. PMID:12111357
3797. Krown SE, Moser CB, MacPhail P, et al. Treatment of advanced AIDS-associated Kaposi sarcoma in resource-limited settings: a three-arm, open-label, randomised, non-inferiority trial. Lancet. 2020 Apr 11;395(10231):1195–207. PMID:32145827
3798. Krueger DA, Northrup H, International Tuberous Sclerosis Complex Consensus Group. Tuberous sclerosis complex surveillance and management: recommendations of the 2012 International Tuberous Sclerosis Complex Consensus Conference. Pediatr Neurol. 2013 Oct;49(4):255–65. PMID:24053983
3799. Krueger EM, Invergo DL, Lin JJ. Germinoma with diffuse subependymal spread: a case report. Cureus. 2016 Jun 15;8(6):e643. PMID:27433421
3800. Krumbholz M, Karl M, Tauer JT, et al. Genomic BCR-ABL1 breakpoints in pediatric chronic myeloid leukemia. Genes Chromosomes Cancer. 2012 Nov;51(11):1045–53. PMID:22887688
3801. Krutilkova V, Trkova M, Fleitz J, et al. Identification of five new families strengthens the link between childhood choroid plexus carcinoma and germline TP53 mutations. Eur J Cancer. 2005 Jul;41(11):1597–603. PMID:15925506
3802. Kuan JW, Su AT, Leong CF, et al. Systematic review of normal subjects harbouring BCR-ABL1 fusion gene. Acta Haematol. 2020;143(2):96–111. PMID:31401626
3803. Kubo O, Sasahara A, Tajika Y, et al. Pleomorphic xanthoastrocytoma with neurofibromatosis type 1: case report. Noshuyo Byori. 1996 Apr;13(1):79–83. PMID:8916131
3804. Kubota T, Sato K, Arishima H, et al. Astroblastoma: immunohistochemical and ultrastructural study of distinctive epithelial and probable tanycytic differentiation. Neuropathology. 2006 Feb;26(1):72–81. PMID:16521483
3805. Kuentz P, Fraitag S, Gonzales M, et al. Mosaic-activating FGFR2 mutation in two fetuses with papillomatous pedunculated sebaceous naevus. Br J Dermatol. 2017 Jan;176(1):204–8. PMID:27095246
3806. Kuhlen M, Taeubner J, Brozou T, et al. Family-based germline sequencing in children with cancer. Oncogene. 2019 Feb;38(9):1367–80. PMID:30305723
3807. Kuijjer ML, Hogendoorn PC, Cleton-Jansen AM. Genome-wide analyses on high-grade osteosarcoma: making sense of a genomically most unstable tumor. Int J Cancer. 2013 Dec 1;133(11):2512–21. PMID:23436697
3808. Kuimov AN, Konareva NV, Kochetov GA. Morphological differences in crystals of multiple forms of yeast transketolase. Biochem Int. 1992 Mar;26(3):451–5. PMID:1627155
3809. Kuiper RP, Schepens M, Thijssen J, et al. Upregulation of the transcription factor TFEB in t(6;11)(p21;q13)-positive renal cell carcinomas due to promoter substitution. Hum Mol Genet. 2003 Jul 15;12(14):1661–9. PMID:12837690
3810. Kuiper RP, Vissers LE, Venkatachalam R, et al. Recurrence and variability of germline EPCAM deletions in Lynch syndrome. Hum Mutat. 2011 Apr;32(4):407–14. PMID:21309036
3811. Kujas M, Faillot T, Lalam T, et al. Astroblastomas revisited. Report of two cases with immunocytochemical and electron microscopic study. Histogenetic considerations. Neuropathol Appl Neurobiol. 2000 Jun;26(3):295–8. PMID:10886687
3812. Kulac I, Tihan T. Pilomyxoid astrocytomas: a short review. Brain Tumor Pathol. 2019 Apr;36(2):52–5. PMID:30945015
3813. Kulkarni K, Desai S, Grundy P, et al. Infantile myofibromatosis: report on a family with autosomal dominant inheritance and

variable penetrance. J Pediatr Surg. 2012 Dec;47(12):2312–5. PMID:23217896
3814. Kumar A, Paswan SS, Kumar B, et al. Fetus in fetu in an adult woman. BMJ Case Rep. 2019 Aug 12;12(8):e230835. PMID:31409619
3815. Kumar B, Pradhan A. Diagnosis of sternomastoid tumor of infancy by fine-needle aspiration cytology. Diagn Cytopathol. 2011 Jan;39(1):13–7. PMID:20091898
3816. Kumar M, Kumar V, Talukdar B, et al. Cushing syndrome in an infant due to cortisol secreting adrenal pheochromocytoma: a rare association. J Pediatr Endocrinol Metab. 2010 Jun;23(6):621–5. PMID:20662337
3817. Kumar R. New insights into phosphate homeostasis: fibroblast growth factor 23 and frizzled-related protein-4 are phosphaturic factors derived from tumors associated with osteomalacia. Curr Opin Nephrol Hypertens. 2002 Sep;11(5):547–53. PMID:12187320
3818. Kumar R, Galardy PJ, Dogan A, et al. Rituximab in combination with multiagent chemotherapy for pediatric follicular lymphoma. Pediatr Blood Cancer. 2011 Aug;57(2):317–20. PMID:21462303
3819. Kumar R, Liu APY, Northcott PA. Medulloblastoma genomics in the modern molecular era. Brain Pathol. 2020 May;30(3):679–90. PMID:31799776
3820. Kumar S, Krenacs L, Medeiros J, et al. Subcutaneous panniculitic T-cell lymphoma is a tumor of cytotoxic T lymphocytes. Hum Pathol. 1998 Apr;29(4):397–403. PMID:9563791
3821. Kumar S, Pittaluga S, Raffeld M, et al. Primary cutaneous CD30-positive anaplastic large cell lymphoma in childhood: report of 4 cases and review of the literature. Pediatr Dev Pathol. 2005 Jan-Feb;8(1):52–60. PMID:15719203
3822. Kunz G Jr, Chung J, Ali SZ. Hepatocellular carcinoma-fibrolamellar variant: cytopathology of an unusual case. Diagn Cytopathol. 2002 Apr;26(4):257–61. PMID:11933273
3823. Kunze E, Enderle A, Radig K, et al. Aggressive osteoblastoma with focal malignant transformation and development of pulmonary metastases. A case report with a review of literature. Gen Diagn Pathol. 1996 May;141(5-6):377–92. PMID:8780939
3824. Küpers AM, Andriessen P, van Kempen MJ, et al. Congenital epulis of the jaw: a series of five cases and review of literature. Pediatr Surg Int. 2009 Feb;25(2):207–10. PMID:19082830
3825. Küppers R. B cells under influence: transformation of B cells by Epstein-Barr virus. Nat Rev Immunol. 2003 Oct;3(10):801–12. PMID:14523386
3826. Kupryjańczyk J, Dansonka-Mieszkowska A, Moes-Sosnowska J, et al. Ovarian small cell carcinoma of hypercalcemic type - evidence of germline origin and SMARCA4 gene inactivation. a pilot study. Pol J Pathol. 2013 Dec;64(4):238–46. PMID:24375037
3827. Kurek KC, Howard E, Tennant LB, et al. PTEN harnartoma of soft tissue: a distinctive lesion in PTEN syndromes. Am J Surg Pathol. 2012 May;36(5):671–87. PMID:22446940
3828. Kurihara S, Hiyama E, Onitake Y, et al. Clinical features of ATRX or DAXX mutated neuroblastoma. J Pediatr Surg. 2014 Dec;49(12):1835–8. PMID:25487495
3829. Kurisaka M, Moriki A, Mori K, et al. Primary yolk sac tumor in the spinal cord. Childs Nerv Syst. 1998 Nov;14(11):653–7. PMID:9840366
3830. Kurita T, Iwasa K, Yano H. [Primary extragenital choriocarcinoma in spinal cord: report of a case]. Hinyokika Kiyo. 1966 May;12(5):466–70. Japanese. PMID:6006788
3831. Kuroda N, Hirano K, Inui Y, et al. Compound melanocytic nevus arising in a mature cystic teratoma of the ovary. Pathol Int. 2001 Nov;51(11):902–4. PMID:11844060
3832. Kuroda N, Trpkov K, Gao Y, et al. ALK rearranged renal cell carcinoma (ALK-RCC): a multi-institutional study of twelve cases with identification of novel partner genes CLIP1, KIF5B and KIAA1217. Mod Pathol. 2020 Dec;33(12):2564–79. PMID:32467651
3833. Kuroda T, Kumagai M, Nosaka S, et al. Critical infantile hepatic hemangioma: results of a nationwide survey by the Japanese Infantile Hepatic Hemangioma Study Group. J Pediatr Surg. 2011 Dec;46(12):2239–43. PMID:22152857
3834. Kuroki S, Akiyoshi M, Tokura M, et al. JMJD1C, a JmjC domain-containing protein, is required for long-term maintenance of male germ cells in mice. Biol Reprod. 2013 Oct 17;89(4):93. PMID:24006281
3835. Kurosaki M, Saeger W, Lüdecke DK. Immunohistochemical localisation of cytokeratins in craniopharyngioma. Acta Neurochir (Wien). 2001;143(2):147–51. PMID:11459086
3836. Kurosawa A, Kurosawa H. Ovoid bodies in choroidal neurofibromatosis. Arch Ophthalmol. 1982 Dec;100(12):1939–41. PMID:6816197
3837. Kurt AM, Unni KK, McLeod RA, et al. Low-grade intraosseous osteosarcoma. Cancer. 1990 Mar 15;65(6):1418–28. PMID:2306687
3838. Kurt AM, Unni KK, Sim FH, et al. Chondroblastoma of bone. Hum Pathol. 1989 Oct;20(10):965–76. PMID:2793161
3839. Kurtkaya-Yapicier O, Scheithauer BW, Woodruff JM, et al. Schwannoma with rhabdomyoblastic differentiation: a unique variant of malignant triton tumor. Am J Surg Pathol. 2003 Jun;27(6):848–53. PMID:12766593
3840. Kurtycz DF, Logroño R, Hoerl HD, et al. Diagnosis of fibromatosis colli by fine-needle aspiration. Diagn Cytopathol. 2000 Nov;23(5):338–42. PMID:11074630
3841. Kuruvilla S, Marco R, Raymond AK, et al. Bizarre parosteal osteochondromatous proliferation (Nora's lesion) with translocation t(1;17)(q32;q21): a case report and role of cytogenetic studies on diagnosis. Ann Clin Lab Sci. 2011 Summer;41(3):285–7. PMID:22075515
3842. Kurzawa P, Kattapuram S, Hornicek FJ, et al. Primary myoepithelioma of bone: a report of 8 cases. Am J Surg Pathol. 2013 Jul;37(7):960–8. PMID:23681076
3843. Kurzrock EA, Busby JE, Gandour-Edwards R. Paratesticular rhabdomyoma. J Pediatr Surg. 2003 Oct;38(10):1546–7. PMID:14577086
3844. Kusafuka K, Yamaguchi A, Kayano T, et al. Immunohistochemical localization of members of the transforming growth factor (TGF)-beta superfamily in normal human salivary glands and pleomorphic adenomas. J Oral Pathol Med. 2001 Aug;30(7):413–20. PMID:11488419
3845. Kusano H, Togashi Y, Akiba J, et al. Two cases of renal cell carcinoma harboring a novel STRN-ALK fusion gene. Am J Surg Pathol. 2016 Jun;40(6):761–9. PMID:26848800
3846. Kushner BH. Neuroblastoma: a disease requiring a multitude of imaging studies. J Nucl Med. 2004 Jul;45(7):1172–88. PMID:15235064
3847. Kussick SJ, Kalnoski M, Braziel RM, et al. Prominent clonal B-cell populations identified by flow cytometry in histologically reactive lymphoid proliferations. Am J Clin Pathol. 2004 Apr;121(4):464–72. PMID:15080297
3848. Küsters-Vandevelde HV, Küsters B, van Engen-van Grunsven AC, et al. Primary melanocytic tumors of the central nervous system: a review with focus on molecular aspects. Brain Pathol. 2015 Mar;25(2):209–26. PMID:25534128
3849. Küsters-Vandevelde HV, van Engen-van Grunsven IA, Küsters B, et al. Improved discrimination of melanotic schwannoma from melanocytic lesions by combined morphological and GNAQ mutational analysis. Acta Neuropathol. 2010 Dec;120(6):755–64. PMID:20865267
3850. Kutzner H, Mentzel T, Palmedo G, et al. Plaque-like CD34-positive dermal fibroma ("medallion-like dermal dendrocyte hamartoma"): clinicopathologic, immunohistochemical, and molecular analysis of 5 cases emphasizing its distinction from superficial, plaque-like dermatofibrosarcoma protuberans. Am J Surg Pathol. 2010 Feb;34(2):190–201. PMID:20061935
3851. Kuznetsov JN, Aguero TH, Owens DA, et al. BAP1 regulates epigenetic switch from pluripotency to differentiation in developmental lineages giving rise to BAP1-mutant cancers. Sci Adv. 2019 Sep 18;5(9):eaax1738. PMID:31555735
3852. Kwiatkowski JL, Rutkowski JL, Yamashiro DJ, et al. Schwann cell-conditioned medium promotes neuroblastoma survival and differentiation. Cancer Res. 1998 Oct 15;58(20):4602–6. PMID:9788610
3853. Kwon CH, Zhu X, Zhang J, et al. Pten regulates neuronal soma size: a mouse model of Lhermitte-Duclos disease. Nat Genet. 2001 Dec;29(4):404–11. PMID:11726927
3853A. Kwon MJ, Rho YS, Jeong JC, et al. Cribriform-morular variant of papillary thyroid carcinoma: a study of 3 cases featuring the PIK3CA mutation. Hum Pathol. 2015 Aug;46(8):1180–8. PMID:26054797
3854. Kyrgiou M, Mitra A, Moscicki AB. Does the vaginal microbiota play a role in the development of cervical cancer? Transl Res. 2017 Jan;179:168–82. PMID:27477083
3855. Kyritsis AP. Management of primary intracranial germ cell tumors. J Neurooncol. 2010 Jan;96(2):143–9. PMID:19588227
3856. La Quaglia MP, Spiro SA, Ghavimi F, et al. Liposarcoma in patients younger than or equal to 22 years of age. Cancer. 1993 Nov 15;72(10):3114–9. PMID:8221578
3857. La Rosa S, Adsay V, Albarello L, et al. Clinicopathologic study of 62 acinar cell carcinomas of the pancreas: insights into the morphology and immunophenotype and search for prognostic markers. Am J Surg Pathol. 2012 Dec;36(12):1782–95. PMID:23026929
3858. La Rosa S, Bernasconi B, Frattini M, et al. TP53 alterations in pancreatic acinar cell carcinoma: new insights into the molecular pathology of this rare cancer. Virchows Arch. 2016 Mar;468(3):289–96. PMID:26586531
3859. La Rosa S, Bernasconi B, Vanoli A, et al. c-MYC amplification and c-myc protein expression in pancreatic acinar cell carcinomas. New insights into the molecular signature of these rare cancers. Virchows Arch. 2018 Oct;473(4):435–41. PMID:29721608
3860. La Rosa S, Franzi F, Marchet S, et al. The monoclonal anti-BCL10 antibody (clone 331.1) is a sensitive and specific marker of pancreatic acinar cell carcinoma and pancreatic metaplasia. Virchows Arch. 2009 Feb;454(2):133–42. PMID:19066953
3861. Labuhn M, Perkins K, Matzk S, et al. Mechanisms of progression of myeloid preleukemia to transformed myeloid leukemia in children with Down syndrome. Cancer Cell. 2019 Aug 12;36(2):123–138.e10. PMID:31303423
3862. Lacaria M, El Demellawy D, McGowan-Jordan J. A rare case of pediatric lipoma with t(9;12)(p22;q14) and evidence of HMGA2-NFIB gene fusion. Cancer Genet. 2017 Oct;216-217:100–4. PMID:29025583
3863. Lack EE, Schloo BL, Azumi N, et al. Undifferentiated (embryonal) sarcoma of the liver. Clinical and pathologic study of 16 cases with emphasis on immunohistochemical features. Am J Surg Pathol. 1991 Jan;15(1):1–16. PMID:1702267
3864. Lack EE, Worsham GF, Callihan MD, et al. Granular cell tumor: a clinicopathologic study of 110 patients. J Surg Oncol. 1980;13(4):301–16. PMID:6246310
3865. Lacoste C, Avril MF, Frassati-Biaggi A, et al. Malignant melanoma arising in patients with a large congenital melanocytic naevus: retrospective study of 10 cases with cytogenetic analysis. Acta Derm Venereol. 2015 Jul;95(6):686–90. PMID:25594732
3866. LaCour DE, Trimble C. Human papillomavirus in infants: transmission, prevalence, and persistence. J Pediatr Adolesc Gynecol. 2012 Apr;25(2):93–7. PMID:21600804
3867. Lad S, Seely J, Elmaadawi M, et al. Juvenile papillomatosis: a case report and literature review. Clin Breast Cancer. 2014 Oct;14(5):e103–5. PMID:24997851
3868. Ladanyi M, Antonescu CR, Drobnjak M, et al. The precrystalline cytoplasmic granules of alveolar soft part sarcoma contain monocarboxylate transporter 1 and CD147. Am J Pathol. 2002 Apr;160(4):1215–21. PMID:11943706
3869. Ladanyi M, Antonescu CR, Leung DH, et al. Impact of SYT-SSX fusion type on the clinical behavior of synovial sarcoma: a multi-institutional retrospective study of 243 patients. Cancer Res. 2002 Jan 1;62(1):135–40. PMID:11782370
3870. Ladanyi M, Gerald W. Fusion of the EWS and WT1 genes in the desmoplastic small round cell tumor. Cancer Res. 1994 Jun 1;54(11):2837–40. PMID:8187063
3871. Ladanyi M, Lui MY, Antonescu CR, et al. The der(17)t(X;17)(p11;q25) of human alveolar soft part sarcoma fuses the TFE3 transcription factor gene to ASPL, a novel gene at 17q25. Oncogene. 2001 Jan 4;20(1):48–57. PMID:11244503
3872. Ladd AP, Grosfeld JL. Gastrointestinal tumors in children and adolescents. Semin Pediatr Surg. 2006 Feb;15(1):37–47. PMID:16458845
3873. Lafay-Cousin L, Bouffet E, Strother D, et al. Phase II study of nonmetastatic desmoplastic medulloblastoma in children younger than 4 years of age: a report of the Children's Oncology Group (ACNS1221). J Clin Oncol. 2020 Jan 20;38(3):223–31. PMID:31774708
3874. Lafay-Cousin L, Hader W, Wei XC, et al. Post-chemotherapy maturation in supratentorial primitive neuroectodermal tumors. Brain Pathol. 2014 Mar;24(2):166–72. PMID:24033491
3875. Lafay-Cousin L, Hawkins C, Carret AS, et al. Central nervous system atypical teratoid rhabdoid tumours: the Canadian Paediatric Brain Tumour Consortium experience. Eur J Cancer. 2012 Feb;48(3):353–9. PMID:22023887
3876. Lafay-Cousin L, Keene D, Carret AS, et al. Choroid plexus tumors in children less than 36 months: the Canadian Pediatric Brain Tumor Consortium (CPBTC) experience. Childs Nerv Syst. 2011 Feb;27(2):259–64. PMID:20809071
3877. Lafferty AR, Batch JA. Thyroid nodules in childhood and adolescence–thirty years of experience. J Pediatr Endocrinol Metab. 1997 Sep-Oct;10(5):479–86. PMID:9401903
3878. Lagarde P, Przybyl J, Brulard C, et al. Chromosome instability accounts for reverse metastatic outcomes of pediatric and adult synovial sarcomas. J Clin Oncol. 2013 Feb 10;31(5):608–15. PMID:23319690
3879. Lai JP, Liu YC, Alimchandani M, et al. The influence of DNA repair on neurological degeneration, cachexia, skin cancer and internal neoplasms: autopsy report of four xeroderma pigmentosum patients (XP-A, XP-C and XP-D). Acta Neuropathol Commun. 2013 May 8;1:4. PMID:24252196
3880. Lai R, Juco J, Lee SF, et al. Flow cytometric detection of CD79a expression

in T-cell acute lymphoblastic leukemias. Am J Clin Pathol. 2000 Jun;113(6):823–30. PMID:10874883

**3881.** Lai R, Weiss LM, Chang KL, et al. Frequency of CD43 expression in non-Hodgkin lymphoma. A survey of 742 cases and further characterization of rare CD43+ follicular lymphomas. Am J Clin Pathol. 1999 Apr;111(4):488–94. PMID:10191768

**3882.** Laird PW, Grossniklaus HE, Hubbard GB. Ciliary body medulloepithelioma associated with pleuropulmonary blastoma. Br J Ophthalmol. 2013 Aug;97(8):1079, 1086–7. PMID:23613510

**3883.** Laje P, Palladino AA, Bhatti TR, et al. Pancreatic surgery in infants with Beckwith-Wiedemann syndrome and hyperinsulinism. J Pediatr Surg. 2013 Dec;48(12):2511–6. PMID:24314195

**3884.** Lake JA, Donson AM, Prince E, et al. Targeted fusion analysis can aid in the classification and treatment of pediatric glioma, ependymoma, and glioneuronal tumors. Pediatr Blood Cancer. 2020 Jan;67(1):e28028. PMID:31595628

**3885.** Lal DR, Su WT, Wolden SL, et al. Results of multimodal treatment for desmoplastic small round cell tumors. J Pediatr Surg. 2005 Jan;40(1):251–5. PMID:15868593

**3886.** Lal G, Leavitt JA, Lindor NM, et al. Unilateral Lisch nodules in the absence of other features of neurofibromatosis 1. Am J Ophthalmol. 2003 Apr;135(4):567–8. PMID:12654389

**3887.** Lallas A, Kyrgidis A, Ferrara G, et al. Atypical Spitz tumours and sentinel lymph node biopsy: a systematic review. Lancet Oncol. 2014 Apr;15(4):e178–83. PMID:24694641

**3888.** Lalli E, Figueiredo BC. Pediatric adrenocortical tumors: what they can tell us on adrenal development and comparison with adult adrenal tumors. Front Endocrinol (Lausanne). 2015 Feb 18;6:23. PMID:25741319

**3889.** Lalloo F, Varley J, Ellis D, et al. Prediction of pathogenic mutations in patients with early-onset breast cancer by family history. Lancet. 2003 Mar 29;361(9363):1101–2. PMID:12672316

**3890.** Lam AK, Fridman M. Characteristics of cribriform morular variant of papillary thyroid carcinoma in post-Chernobyl affected region. Hum Pathol. 2018 Apr;74:170–7. PMID:29320754

**3891.** Lam AK, Lo CY. Diffuse sclerosing variant of papillary carcinoma of the thyroid: a 35-year comparative study at a single institution. Ann Surg Oncol. 2006 Feb;13(2):176–81. PMID:16411146

**3892.** Lam AK, Lo CY, Lam KS. Papillary carcinoma of thyroid: a 30-yr clinicopathological review of the histological variants. Endocr Pathol. 2005 Winter;16(4):323–30. PMID:16627919

**3893.** Lam AK, Saremi N. Cribriform-morular variant of papillary thyroid carcinoma: a distinctive type of thyroid cancer. Endocr Relat Cancer. 2017 Apr;24(4):R109–21. PMID:28314770

**3894.** Lam KH, Wei WI, Ho HC, et al. Whole organ sectioning of mixed parotid tumors. Am J Surg. 1990 Oct;160(4):377–81. PMID:2171368

**3895.** Lam KY, Lo CY. Composite pheochromocytoma-ganglioneuroma of the adrenal gland: an uncommon entity with distinctive clinicopathologic features. Endocr Pathol. 1999 Winter;10(4):343–52. PMID:12114771

**3896.** Lam KY, Lo CY, Wat NM, et al. The clinicopathological features and importance of p53, Rb, and mdm2 expression in phaeochromocytomas and paragangliomas. J Clin Pathol. 2001 Jun;54(6):443–8. PMID:11376017

**3897.** Lam KY, Loong F, Shek TW, et al. Composite paraganglioma-ganglioneuroma of the urinary bladder: a clinicopathologic,

immunohistochemical, and ultrastructural study of a case and review of the literature. Endocr Pathol. 1998 Winter;9(1):353–61. PMID:12114785

**3898.** Lam SW, Cleton Jansen AM, Cleven AHG, et al. Molecular analysis of gene fusions in bone and soft tissue tumors by anchored multiplex PCR-based targeted next-generation sequencing. J Mol Diagn. 2018 Sep;20(5):653–63. PMID:30139549

**3899.** Lam SW, Cleven AHG, Kroon HM, et al. Utility of FOS as diagnostic marker for osteoid osteoma and osteoblastoma. Virchows Arch. 2020 Mar;476(3):455–63. PMID:31768625

**3900.** Lamant L, Dastugue N, Pulford K, et al. A new fusion gene TPM3-ALK in anaplastic large cell lymphoma created by a (1;2)(q25;p23) translocation. Blood. 1999 May 1;93(9):3088–95. PMID:10216106

**3901.** Lamant L, Gascoyne RD, Duplantier MM, et al. Non-muscle myosin heavy chain (MYH9): a new partner fused to ALK in anaplastic large cell lymphoma. Genes Chromosomes Cancer. 2003 Aug;37(4):427–32. PMID:12800156

**3902.** Lamant L, McCarthy K, d'Amore E, et al. Prognostic impact of morphologic and phenotypic features of childhood ALK-positive anaplastic large-cell lymphoma: results of the ALCL99 study. J Clin Oncol. 2011 Dec 10;29(35):4669–76. PMID:22084369

**3903.** Lamant L, Meggetto F, al Saati T, et al. High incidence of the t(2;5)(p23;q35) translocation in anaplastic large cell lymphoma and its lack of detection in Hodgkin's disease. Comparison of cytogenetic analysis, reverse transcriptase-polymerase chain reaction, and P-80 immunostaining. Blood. 1996 Jan 1;87(1):284–91. PMID:8547653

**3904.** Lamant L, Pulford K, Bischof D, et al. Expression of the ALK tyrosine kinase gene in neuroblastoma. Am J Pathol. 2000 May;156(5):1711–21. PMID:10793082

**3905.** Lambert SR, Witt H, Hovestadt V, et al. Differential expression and methylation of brain developmental genes define location-specific subsets of pilocytic astrocytoma. Acta Neuropathol. 2013 Aug;126(2):291–301. PMID:23660940

**3906.** Lambert WA, DiGiuseppe JA, Lara-Ospina T, et al. Juvenile myelomonocytic leukemia presenting in an infant with a subdural hematoma. Childs Nerv Syst. 2021 Jun;37(6):2075–9. PMID:33404720

**3907.** Lamberts R, Nitsche R, de Vivie RE, et al. Budd-Chiari syndrome as the primary manifestation of a fibrolamellar hepatocellular carcinoma. Digestion. 1992;53(3-4):200–9. PMID:1337896

**3908.** Lambo S, Gröbner SN, Rausch T, et al. The molecular landscape of ETMR at diagnosis and relapse. Nature. 2019 Dec;576(7786):274–80. PMID:31802000

**3909.** Lambo S, von Hoff K, Korshunov A, et al. ETMR: a tumor entity in its infancy. Acta Neuropathol. 2020 Sep;140(3):249–66. PMID:32601913

**3910.** Lamlum H, Ilyas M, Rowan A, et al. The type of somatic mutation at APC in familial adenomatous polyposis is determined by the site of the germline mutation: a new facet to Knudson's 'two-hit' hypothesis. Nat Med. 1999 Sep;5(9):1071–5. PMID:10470088

**3911.** Lamzabi I, Arvanitis LD, Reddy VB, et al. Immunophenotype of myxopapillary ependymomas. Appl Immunohistochem Mol Morphol. 2013 Dec;21(6):485–9. PMID:23455181

**3912.** Lan F, Shi Y. Histone H3.3 and cancer: a potential reader connection. Proc Natl Acad Sci U S A. 2015 Jun 2;112(22):6814–9. PMID:25453099

**3913.** Landa I, Ibrahimpasic T, Boucai L, et al. Genomic and transcriptomic hallmarks of poorly

differentiated and anaplastic thyroid cancers. J Clin Invest. 2016 Mar 1;126(3):1052–66. PMID:26878173

**3914.** Landberg A, Fält A, Montgomery S, et al. Overweight and obesity during adolescence increases the risk of renal cell carcinoma. Int J Cancer. 2019 Sep 1;145(5):1232–7. PMID:30790271

**3915.** Landis CA, Masters SB, Spada A, et al. GTPase inhibiting mutations activate the alpha chain of Gs and stimulate adenylyl cyclase in human pituitary tumours. Nature. 1989 Aug 31;340(6236):692–6. PMID:2549426

**3916.** Landmann A, Calisto JL, Reyes-Múgica M, et al. Fetus-in-fetu presenting as a cryptorchid testis and abdominal mass: a report of a case and review of the literature. J Pediatr Surg Case Rep. 2016 Oct;13:38–40. doi:10.1016/j.epsc.2016.07.010.

**3917.** Landmann E, Oschlies I, Zimmermann M, et al. Secondary non-Hodgkin lymphoma (NHL) in children and adolescents after childhood cancer other than NHL. Br J Haematol. 2008 Nov;143(3):387–94. PMID:18729852

**3918.** Landon GC, Johnson KA, Dahlin DC. Subungual exostoses. J Bone Joint Surg Am. 1979 Mar;61(2):256–9. PMID:422611

**3919.** Lane BR, Ross JH, Hart WR, et al. Müllerian papilloma of the cervix in a child with multiple renal cysts. Urology. 2005 Feb;65(2):388. PMID:15708065

**3920.** Lane KL, Shannon RJ, Weiss SW. Hyalinizing spindle cell tumor with giant rosettes: a distinctive tumor closely resembling low-grade fibromyxoid sarcoma. Am J Surg Pathol. 1997 Dec;21(12):1481–8. PMID:9414192

**3921.** Lang FF, Epstein FJ, Ransohoff J, et al. Central nervous system gangliogliomas. Part 2: clinical outcome. J Neurosurg. 1993 Dec;79(6):867–73. PMID:8246055

**3922.** Lang FF, Macdonald OK, Fuller GN, et al. Primary extradural meningiomas: a report on nine cases and review of the literature from the era of computerized tomography scanning. J Neurosurg. 2000 Dec;93(6):940–50. PMID:11117866

**3923.** Lang SS, Beslow LA, Gabel B, et al. Surgical treatment of brain tumors in infants younger than six months of age and review of the literature. World Neurosurg. 2012 Jul;78(1-2):137–44. PMID:22120270

**3924.** Lange M, Niedoszytko M, Nedoszytko B, et al. Diffuse cutaneous mastocytosis: analysis of 10 cases and a brief review of the literature. J Eur Acad Dermatol Venereol. 2012 Dec;26(12):1565–71. PMID:22092511

**3925.** Lange M, Żawrocki A, Nedoszytko B, et al. Does the aberrant expression of CD2 and CD25 by skin mast cells truly correlate with systemic involvement in patients presenting with mastocytosis in the skin? Int Arch Allergy Immunol. 2014;165(2):104–10. PMID:25402852

**3926.** Langebrake C, Creutzig U, Reinhardt D. Immunophenotype of Down syndrome acute myeloid leukemia and transient myeloproliferative disease differs significantly from other diseases with morphologically identical or similar blasts. Klin Padiatr. 2005 May-Jun;217(3):126–34. PMID:15858703

**3927.** Langebrake C, Klusmann JH, Wortmann K, et al. Concomitant aberrant overexpression of RUNX1 and NCAM in regenerating bone marrow of myeloid leukemia of Down's syndrome. Haematologica. 2006 Nov;91(11):1473–80. PMID:17043020

**3928.** Langman G, Andrews CL, Weissferdt A. WT1 expression in salivary gland pleomorphic adenomas: a reliable marker of the neoplastic myoepithelium. Mod Pathol. 2011 Feb;24(2):168–74. PMID:21057459

**3929.** Lanzafame S, Caltabiano R, Puzzo L, et al. Expression of thyroid transcription factor 1

(TTF-1) in extra thyroidal sites: papillary thyroid carcinoma of branchial cleft cysts and thyroglossal duct cysts and struma ovarii. Pathologica. 2006 Dec;98(6):640–4. PMID:17285841

**3930.** Lapunzina P. Risk of tumorigenesis in overgrowth syndromes: a comprehensive review. Am J Med Genet C Semin Med Genet. 2005 Aug 15;137C(1):53–71. PMID:16010678

**3931.** LaQuaglia MJ, Grijalva JL, Mueller KA, et al. YAP subcellular localization and hippo pathway transcriptome analysis in pediatric hepatocellular carcinoma. Sci Rep. 2016 Sep 8;6:30238. PMID:27605415

**3932.** Larizza L, Magnani I, Roversi G. Rothmund-Thomson syndrome and RECQL4 defect: splitting and lumping. Cancer Lett. 2006 Jan 28;232(1):107–20. PMID:16271439

**3933.** Larizza L, Roversi G, Volpi L. Rothmund-Thomson syndrome. Orphanet J Rare Dis. 2010 Jan 29;5:2. PMID:20113479

**3934.** La Rosa S, Sessa F, Capella C. Acinar cell carcinoma of the pancreas: overview of clinicopathologic features and insights into the molecular pathology. Front Med (Lausanne). 2015 Jun 15;2:41. PMID:26137463

**3935.** Larralde M, Boggio P, Abad ME, et al. Nevus trichilemmocysticus: report of a new case of a recently recognized entity. Pediatr Dermatol. 2011 May-Jun;28(3):286–9. PMID:20825570

**3936.** Larsen AC, Dahl C, Dahmcke CM, et al. BRAF mutations in conjunctival melanoma: investigation of incidence, clinicopathological features, prognosis and paired premalignant lesions. Acta Ophthalmol. 2016 Aug;94(5):463–70. PMID:27009410

**3937.** Larson JD, Kasper LH, Paugh BS, et al. Histone H3.3 K27M accelerates spontaneous brainstem glioma and drives restricted changes in bivalent gene expression. Cancer Cell. 2019 Jan 14;35(1):140–155.e7. PMID:30595505

**3938.** Larson KN, O'Shea P, Zedek DC, et al. Hair follicle nevus located on the chin of an infant: case report and review of literature. Pediatr Dermatol. 2016 Mar-Apr;33(2):e106–8. PMID:27001331

**3939.** Laskar S, Sanghavi V, Muckaden MA, et al. Nasopharyngeal carcinoma in children: ten years' experience at the Tata Memorial Hospital, Mumbai. Int J Radiat Oncol Biol Phys. 2004 Jan 1;58(1):189–95. PMID:14697438

**3940.** Laskin WB, Fetsch JF, Miettinen M. Myxoinflammatory fibroblastic sarcoma: a clinicopathologic analysis of 104 cases, with emphasis on predictors of outcome. Am J Surg Pathol. 2014 Jan;38(1):1–12. PMID:24121178

**3941.** Laskin WB, Fetsch JF, Miettinen M. The "neurothekeoma": immunohistochemical analysis distinguishes the true nerve sheath myxoma from its mimics. Hum Pathol. 2000 Oct;31(10):1230–41. PMID:11070116

**3942.** Laskin WB, Miettinen M. Epithelioid sarcoma: new insights based on an extended immunohistochemical analysis. Arch Pathol Lab Med. 2003 Sep;127(9):1161–8. PMID:12946229

**3943.** Laskin WB, Miettinen M, Fetsch JF. Infantile digital fibroma/fibromatosis: a clinicopathologic and immunohistochemical study of 69 tumors from 57 patients with long-term follow-up. Am J Surg Pathol. 2009 Jan;33(1):1–13. PMID:18830128

**3944.** Laskin WB, Weiss SW, Bratthauer GL. Epithelioid variant of malignant peripheral nerve sheath tumor (malignant epithelioid schwannoma). Am J Surg Pathol. 1991 Dec;15(12):1136–45. PMID:1746681

**3945.** Lassaletta A, Zapotocky M, Mistry M, et al. Therapeutic and prognostic implications of BRAF V600E in pediatric low-grade gliomas. J Clin Oncol. 2017 Sep 1;35(25):2934–41. PMID:28727518

**3946.** Lassaletta L, Torres-Martín M, Peña-Granero C, et al. NF2 genetic alterations in sporadic vestibular schwannomas: clinical implications. Otol Neurotol. 2013 Sep;34(7):1355–61. PMID:23921927

**3947.** Łastowska M, Trubicka J, Sobocińska A, et al. Molecular identification of CNS NB-FOXR2, CNS EFT-CIC, CNS HGNET-MN1 and CNS HGNET-BCOR pediatric brain tumors using tumor-specific signature genes. Acta Neuropathol Commun. 2020 Jul 10;8(1):105. PMID:32650833

**3948.** Latour S, Winter S. Inherited immunodeficiencies with high predisposition to Epstein-Barr virus-driven lymphoproliferative diseases. Front Immunol. 2018 Jun 4;9:1103. PMID:29942301

**3949.** Lau AH, Soltys K, Sindhi RK, et al. Chronic high Epstein-Barr viral load carriage in pediatric small bowel transplant recipients. Pediatr Transplant. 2010 Jun;14(4):549–53. PMID:20102529

**3950.** Lau CS, Mahendraraj K, Chamberlain RS. Hepatocellular carcinoma in the pediatric population: a population based clinical outcomes study involving 257 patients from the Surveillance, Epidemiology, and End Result (SEER) database (1973-2011). HPB Surg. 2015;2015:670728. PMID:26663981

**3951.** Lau K, Massad M, Pollak C, et al. Clinical patterns and outcome in epithelioid hemangioendothelioma with or without pulmonary involvement: insights from an internet registry in the study of a rare cancer. Chest. 2011 Nov;140(5):1312–8. PMID:21546438

**3952.** Lau PP, Lui PC, Lau GT, et al. EWSR1-CREB3L1 gene fusion: a novel alternative molecular aberration of low-grade fibromyxoid sarcoma. Am J Surg Pathol. 2013 May;37(5):734–8. PMID:23588368

**3953.** Lau PP, Wong OK, Lui PC, et al. Myopericytoma in patients with AIDS: a new class of Epstein-Barr virus-associated tumor. Am J Surg Pathol. 2009 Nov;33(11):1666–72. PMID:19675451

**3954.** Lau SK, Luthringer DJ, Eisen RN. Thyroid transcription factor-1: a review. Appl Immunohistochem Mol Morphol. 2002 Jun;10(2):97–102. PMID:12051643

**3955.** Lau SK, Weiss LM, Chu PG. Association of intratubular seminoma and intratubular embryonal carcinoma with invasive testicular germ cell tumors. Am J Surg Pathol. 2007 Jul;31(7):1045–9. PMID:17592271

**3956.** Lau SK, Weiss LM, Chu PG. D2-40 immunohistochemistry in the differential diagnosis of seminoma and embryonal carcinoma: a comparative immunohistochemical study with KIT (CD117) and CD30. Mod Pathol. 2007 Mar;20(3):320–5. PMID:17277761

**3957.** Lau YC, Li Y, Kido T. Battle of the sexes: contrasting roles of testis-specific protein Y-encoded (TSPY) and TSPX in human oncogenesis. Asian J Androl. 2019 May-Jun;21(3):260–9. PMID:29974883

**3958.** Lau YF, Li Y, Kido T. Gonadoblastoma locus and the TSPY gene on the human Y chromosome. Birth Defects Res C Embryo Today. 2009 Mar;87(1):114–22. PMID:19306348

**3959.** Lauer DH, Enzinger FM. Cranial fasciitis of childhood. Cancer. 1980 Jan 15;45(2):401–6. PMID:7351023

**3960.** Lauer SR, Edgar MA, Gardner JM, et al. Soft tissue chordomas: a clinicopathologic analysis of 11 cases. Am J Surg Pathol. 2013 May;37(5):719–26. PMID:23588366

**3961.** Launbjerg K, Bache I, Galanakis M, et al. von Hippel-Lindau development in children and adolescents. Am J Med Genet A. 2017 Sep;173(9):2381–94. PMID:28650583

**3962.** Lauper JM, Krause A, Vaughan TL, et al. Spectrum and risk of neoplasia in Werner

syndrome: a systematic review. PLoS One. 2013;8(4):e59709. PMID:23573208

**3963.** Laurent C, Do C, Gascoyne RD, et al. Anaplastic lymphoma kinase-positive diffuse large B-cell lymphoma: a rare clinicopathologic entity with poor prognosis. J Clin Oncol. 2009 Sep 1;27(25):4211–6. PMID:19636007

**3964.** Laurent C, Fabiani B, Do C, et al. Immune-checkpoint expression in Epstein-Barr virus positive and negative plasmablastic lymphoma: a clinical and pathological study in 82 patients. Haematologica. 2016 Aug;101(8):976–84. PMID:27175027

**3965.** Lauretta R, Sansone A, Sansone M, et al. Endocrine disrupting chemicals: effects on endocrine glands. Front Endocrinol (Lausanne). 2019 Mar 21;10:178. PMID:30984107

**3966.** Laurini JA, Zhang L, Goldblum JR, et al. Low-grade fibromyxoid sarcoma of the small intestine: report of 4 cases with molecular cytogenetic confirmation. Am J Surg Pathol. 2011 Jul;35(7):1069–73. PMID:21677541

**3967.** Laury AR, Bongiovanni M, Tille JC, et al. Thyroid pathology in PTEN-hamartoma tumor syndrome: characteristic findings of a distinct entity. Thyroid. 2011 Feb;21(2):135–44. PMID:21190448

**3968.** Lauwers GY, Grant LD, Donnelly WH, et al. Hepatic undifferentiated (embryonal) sarcoma arising in a mesenchymal hamartoma. Am J Surg Pathol. 1997 Oct;21(10):1248–54. PMID:9331300

**3969.** La Vecchia C, Morris HB, Draper GJ. Malignant ovarian tumours in childhood in Britain, 1962-78. Br J Cancer. 1983 Sep;48(3):363–74. PMID:6311234

**3970.** Lawrence B, Perez-Atayde A, Hibbard MK, et al. TPM3-ALK and TPM4-ALK oncogenes in inflammatory myofibroblastic tumors. Am J Pathol. 2000 Aug;157(2):377–84. PMID:10934142

**3971.** Lawrence W Jr, Gehan EA, Hays DM, et al. Prognostic significance of staging factors of the UICC staging system in childhood rhabdomyosarcoma: a report from the Intergroup Rhabdomyosarcoma Study (IRS-II). J Clin Oncol. 1987 Jan;5(1):46–54. PMID:3543238

**3972.** Lawrence WD, Young RH, Scully RE. Juvenile granulosa cell tumor of the infantile testis. A report of 14 cases. Am J Surg Pathol. 1985 Feb;9(2):87–94. PMID:3976984

**3973.** Lawson ML, Miller SF, Ellis G, et al. Primary hyperparathyroidism in a paediatric hospital. QJM. 1996 Dec;89(12):921–32. PMID:9015486

**3974.** Layfield LJ. Fine-needle aspiration of the head and neck. Pathology (Phila). 1996;4(2):409–38. PMID:9238365

**3975.** Layfield LJ, Emerson L, Crim JR, et al. Squamous differentiation and cytokeratin expression in an osteosarcoma: a case report and review of the literature. Clin Med Pathol. 2008;1:55–9. PMID:21876652

**3976.** Layfield LJ, Reznicek M, Lowe M, et al. Spontaneous infarction of a parotid gland pleomorphic adenoma. Report of a case with cytologic and radiographic overlap with a primary salivary gland malignancy. Acta Cytol. 1992 May-Jun;36(3):381–6. PMID:1316031

**3977.** Lazar AJ, Hajibashi S, Lev D. Desmoid tumor: from surgical extirpation to molecular dissection. Curr Opin Oncol. 2009 Jul;21(4):352–9. PMID:19436199

**3978.** Lazar AJ, Tuvin D, Hajibashi S, et al. Specific mutations in the beta-catenin gene (CTNNB1) correlate with local recurrence in sporadic desmoid tumors. Am J Pathol. 2008 Nov;173(5):1518–27. PMID:18832571

**3979.** Lazar DA, Cass DL, Dishop MK, et al. Fetal lung interstitial tumor: a cause of late gestation fetal hydrops. J Pediatr Surg. 2011 Jun;46(6):1263–6. PMID:21683234

**3980.** Lazar RH, Younis RT, Kluka EA, et al. Granular cell tumor of the larynx: report of two pediatric cases. Ear Nose Throat J. 1992 Sep;71(9):440–3. PMID:1425384

**3981.** Le BH, Towfighi J, Kapadia SB, et al. Comparative immunohistochemical assessment of craniopharyngioma and related lesions. Endocr Pathol. 2007 Spring;18(1):23–30. PMID:17652797

**3982.** Le Deley MC, Reiter A, Williams D, et al. Prognostic factors in childhood anaplastic large cell lymphoma: results of a large European intergroup study. Blood. 2008 Feb 1;111(3):1560–6. PMID:17957029

**3983.** Le DT, Uram JN, Wang H, et al. PD-1 blockade in tumors with mismatch-repair deficiency. N Engl J Med. 2015 Jun 25;372(26):2509–20. PMID:26028255

**3984.** Le Guellec S, Soubeyran I, Rochaix P, et al. CTNNB1 mutation analysis is a useful tool for the diagnosis of desmoid tumors: a study of 260 desmoid tumors and 191 potential morphologic mimics. Mod Pathol. 2012 Dec;25(12):1551–8. PMID:22766794

**3985.** Le Guellec S, Velasco V, Pérot G, et al. ETV4 is a useful marker for the diagnosis of CIC-rearranged undifferentiated round-cell sarcomas: a study of 127 cases including mimicking lesions. Mod Pathol. 2016 Dec;29(12):1523–31. PMID:27562494

**3986.** Le Huu AR, Jokinen CH, Rubin BP, et al. Expression of prox1, lymphatic endothelial nuclear transcription factor, in Kaposiform hemangioendothelioma and tufted angioma. Am J Surg Pathol. 2010 Nov;34(11):1563–73. PMID:20975337

**3987.** Le Loarer F, Cleven AHG, Bouvier C, et al. A subset of epithelioid and spindle cell rhabdomyosarcomas is associated with TFCP2 fusions and common ALK upregulation. Mod Pathol. 2020 Mar;33(3):404–19. PMID:31383960

**3988.** Le Loarer F, Pissaloux D, Watson S, et al. Clinicopathologic features of CIC-NUTM1 sarcomas, a new molecular variant of the family of CIC-fused sarcomas. Am J Surg Pathol. 2019 Feb;43(2):268–76. PMID:30407212

**3989.** Le Loarer F, Watson S, Pierron G, et al. SMARCA4 inactivation defines a group of undifferentiated thoracic malignancies transcriptionally related to BAF-deficient sarcomas. Nat Genet. 2015 Oct;47(10):1200–5. PMID:26343384

**3990.** Le Loarer F, Zhang L, Fletcher CD, et al. Consistent SMARCB1 homozygous deletions in epithelioid sarcoma and in a subset of myoepithelial carcinomas can be reliably detected by FISH in archival material. Genes Chromosomes Cancer. 2014 Jun;53(6):475–86. PMID:24585572

**3991.** Le LQ, Shipman T, Burns DK, et al. Cell of origin and microenvironment contribution for NF1-associated dermal neurofibromas. Cell Stem Cell. 2009 May 8;4(5):453–63. PMID:19427294

**3992.** Leão RR, Ahmad AE, Richard PO. Should small renal masses be biopsied? Curr Urol Rep. 2017 Jan;18(1):7. PMID:28188595

**3993.** LeBlanc RE, Tavallaee M, Kim YH, et al. Useful parameters for distinguishing subcutaneous panniculitis-like T-cell lymphoma from lupus erythematosus panniculitis. Am J Surg Pathol. 2016 Jun;40(6):745–54. PMID:26796503

**3994.** Lee AF, Hayes MM, Lebrun D, et al. FLI-1 distinguishes Ewing sarcoma from small cell osteosarcoma and mesenchymal chondrosarcoma. Appl Immunohistochem Mol Morphol. 2011 May;19(3):233–8. PMID:21084965

**3995.** Lee B, Chiu M, Soriano T, et al. Adult-onset tufted angioma: a case report and review of the literature. Cutis. 2006 Nov;78(5):341–5. PMID:17186794

**3996.** Lee CH, Su SY, Sittampalam K, et al. Frequent overexpression of klotho in fusion-negative phosphaturic mesenchymal tumors with tumorigenic implications. Mod Pathol. 2020 May;33(5):858–70. PMID:31792355

**3997.** Lee CH, Yu JR, Granat J, et al. Automethylation of PRC2 promotes H3K27 methylation and is impaired in H3K27M pediatric glioma. Genes Dev. 2019 Oct 1;33(19-20):1428–40. PMID:31488577

**3998.** Lee CT, Tung YC, Hwu WL, et al. Mosaic paternal haploidy in a patient with pancreatoblastoma and Beckwith-Wiedemann spectrum. Am J Med Genet A. 2019 Sep;179(9):1878–83. PMID:31231953

**3999.** Lee D, Cho YH, Kang SY, et al. BRAF V600E mutations are frequent in dysembryoplastic neuroepithelial tumors and subependymal giant cell astrocytomas. J Surg Oncol. 2015 Mar;111(3):359–64. PMID:25346165

**4000.** Lee DW, Yang JH, Lee SM, et al. Subcutaneous panniculitis-like T-cell lymphoma: a clinical and pathologic study of 14 korean patients. Ann Dermatol. 2011 Aug;23(3):329–37. PMID:21909203

**4001.** Lee EB, Tihan T, Scheithauer BW, et al. Thyroid transcription factor 1 expression in sellar tumors: a histogenetic marker? J Neuropathol Exp Neurol. 2009 May;68(5):482–8. PMID:19525896

**4002.** Lee EJ, Chang YW, Oh JH, et al. Breast lesions in children and adolescents: diagnosis and management. Korean J Radiol. 2018 Sep-Oct;19(5):978–91. PMID:30174488

**4003.** Lee H, Roh JL, Choi YJ, et al. High grade transformation in mucoepidermoid carcinoma of the minor salivary gland with polyploidy of the rearranged MAML2 gene. Head Neck Pathol. 2020 Sep;14(3):822–7. PMID:31535311

**4004.** Lee HY, Yoon CS, Sevenet N, et al. Rhabdoid tumor of the kidney is a component of the rhabdoid predisposition syndrome. Pediatr Dev Pathol. 2002 Jul-Aug;5(4):395–9. PMID:12016529

**4005.** Lee JC, Huang HY. Soft tissue special issue: giant cell-rich lesions of the head and neck region. Head Neck Pathol. 2020 Mar;14(1):97–108. PMID:31950466

**4006.** Lee JC, Jeng YM, Su SY, et al. Identification of a novel FN1-FGFR1 genetic fusion as a frequent event in phosphaturic mesenchymal tumour. J Pathol. 2015 Mar;235(4):539–45. PMID:25319834

**4007.** Lee JC, Li CF, Huang HY, et al. ALK oncoproteins in atypical inflammatory myofibroblastic tumours: novel RRBP1-ALK fusions in epithelioid inflammatory myofibroblastic sarcoma. J Pathol. 2017 Feb;241(3):316–23. PMID:27874193

**4008.** Lee JC, Liang CW, Fletcher CD. Giant cell tumor of soft tissue is genetically distinct from its bone counterpart. Mod Pathol. 2017 May;30(5):728–33. PMID:28084336

**4009.** Lee JC, Mazor T, Lao R, et al. Recurrent KBTBD4 small in-frame insertions and absence of DROSHA deletion or DICER1 mutation differentiate pineal parenchymal tumor of intermediate differentiation (PPTID) from pineoblastoma. Acta Neuropathol. 2019 May;137(5):851–4. PMID:30877433

**4010.** Lee JC, Sharifai N, Dahiya S, et al. Clinicopathologic features of anaplastic myxopapillary ependymomas. Brain Pathol. 2019 Jan;29(1):75–84. PMID:30417460

**4011.** Lee JC, Su SY, Changou CA, et al. Characterization of FN1-FGFR1 and novel FN1-FGF1 fusion genes in a large series of phosphaturic mesenchymal tumors. Mod Pathol. 2016 Nov;29(11):1335–46. PMID:27443518

**4012.** Lee JY, Wakabayashi T, Yoshida J. Management and survival of pineoblastoma: an analysis of 34 adults from the brain tumor

registry of Japan. Neurol Med Chir (Tokyo). 2005 Mar;45(3):132–41. PMID:15782004
4013. Lee LH, Bos GD, Marsh WL Jr, et al. Fine-needle aspiration cytology of sclerosing perineurioma. Ann Diagn Pathol. 2004 Apr;8(2):80–6. PMID:15060885
4014. Lee MJ, Sallomi DF, Munk PL, et al. Pictorial review: giant cell tumours of bone. Clin Radiol. 1998 Jul;53(7):481–9. PMID:9714386
4015. Lee RS, Stewart C, Carter SL, et al. A remarkably simple genome underlies highly malignant pediatric rhabdoid cancers. J Clin Invest. 2012 Aug;122(8):2983–8. PMID:22797305
4016. Lee S, Barnhill RL, Dummer R, et al. TERT Promoter mutations are predictive of aggressive clinical behavior in patients with spitzoid melanocytic neoplasms. Sci Rep. 2015 Jun 10;5:11200. PMID:26061100
4017. Lee S, Borah S, Bahrami A. Detection of aberrant TERT promoter methylation by combined bisulfite restriction enzyme analysis for cancer diagnosis. J Mol Diagn. 2017 May;19(3):378–86. PMID:28284778
4018. Lee SC, Kim KH, Kim SH, et al. Mixed testicular germ cell tumor presenting as metastatic pure choriocarcinoma involving multiple lung metastases that was effectively treated with high-dose chemotherapy. Cancer Res Treat. 2009 Dec;41(4):229–32. PMID:20057969
4019. Lee SD, Korean Society of Pediatric Urology. Epidemiological and clinical behavior of prepubertal testicular tumors in Korea. J Urol. 2004 Aug;172(2):674–8. PMID:15247758
4020. Lee SE, Jang JY, Hwang DW, et al. Clinical features and outcome of solid pseudopapillary neoplasm: differences between adults and children. Arch Surg. 2008 Dec;143(12):1218–21. PMID:19075175
4021. Lee SE, Kang SY, Takeuchi K, et al. Identification of RANBP2-ALK fusion in ALK positive diffuse large B-cell lymphoma. Hematol Oncol. 2014 Dec;32(4):221–4. PMID:24470379
4022. Lee SE, Lee EH, Park H, et al. The diagnostic utility of the GNAS mutation in patients with fibrous dysplasia: meta-analysis of 168 sporadic cases. Hum Pathol. 2012 Aug;43(8):1234–42. PMID:22245114
4023. Lee SH, Kim BC, Chang HJ, et al. Rectal neuroendocrine and L-cell tumors: diagnostic dilemma and therapeutic strategy. Am J Surg Pathol. 2013 Jul;37(7):1044–52. PMID:23648459
4024. Lee W, Teckie S, Wiesner T, et al. PRC2 is recurrently inactivated through EED or SUZ12 loss in malignant peripheral nerve sheath tumors. Nat Genet. 2014 Nov;46(11):1227–32. PMID:25240281
4025. Lee YA, Im SW, Jung KC, et al. Predominant DICER1 pathogenic variants in pediatric follicular thyroid carcinomas. Thyroid. 2020 Aug;30(8):1120–31. PMID:32228164
4026. Lee YH, Park EK, Park YS, et al. Treatment and outcomes of primary intracranial teratoma. Childs Nerv Syst. 2009 Dec;25(12):1581–7. PMID:19693515
4027. Lee-Jones L, Aligianis I, Davies PA, et al. Sacrococcygeal chordomas in patients with tuberous sclerosis complex show somatic loss of TSC1 or TSC2. Genes Chromosomes Cancer. 2004 Sep;41(1):80–5. PMID:15236319
4028. Legeai-Mallet L, Munnich A, Maroteaux P, et al. Incomplete penetrance and expressivity skewing in hereditary multiple exostoses. Clin Genet. 1997 Jul;52(1):12–6. PMID:9272707
4029. Legius E, Marchuk DA, Collins FS, et al. Somatic deletion of the neurofibromatosis type 1 gene in a neurofibrosarcoma supports a tumour suppressor gene hypothesis. Nat Genet. 1993 Feb;3(2):122–6. PMID:8499945
4030. Leguit RJ, van den Tweel JG. The pathology of bone marrow failure. Histopathology. 2010 Nov;57(5):655–70. PMID:20727024
4031. Lehman NL, Usubalieva A, Lin T, et al. Genomic analysis demonstrates that histologically-defined astroblastomas are molecularly heterogeneous and that tumors with MN1 rearrangement exhibit the most favorable prognosis. Acta Neuropathol Commun. 2019 Mar 15;7(1):42. PMID:30876455
4032. Leibovitch I, Baniel J, Rowland RG, et al. Malignant testicular neoplasms in immunosuppressed patients. J Urol. 1996 Jun;155(6):1938–42. PMID:8618292
4033. Leibovitch I, Foster RS, Ulbright TM, et al. Adult primary pure teratoma of the testis. The Indiana experience. Cancer. 1995 May 1;75(9):2244–50. PMID:7712432
4033A. Leiden University Medical Center. LOVD v.3.0 - Leiden Open Variation Database [Internet]. Leiden (Netherlands): Leiden University Medical Center; 2021. The TSC1 gene homepage; updated 2021 Mar 9. Available from: https://databases.lovd.nl/shared/genes/TSC1.
4033B. Leiden University Medical Center. LOVD v.3.0 - Leiden Open Variation Database [Internet]. Leiden (Netherlands): Leiden University Medical Center; 2021. The TSC2 gene homepage; updated 2021 Mar 9. Available from: https://databases.lovd.nl/shared/genes/TSC2.
4034. Leithner A, Windhager R, Lang S, et al. Aneurysmal bone cyst. A population based epidemiologic study and literature review. Clin Orthop Relat Res. 1999 Jun; (363):176–9. PMID:10379320
4035. Lellouch-Tubiana A, Boddaert N, Bourgeois M, et al. Angiocentric neuroepithelial tumor (ANET): a new epilepsy-related clinicopathological entity with distinctive MRI. Brain Pathol. 2005 Oct;15(4):281–6. PMID:16389940
4036. Lellouch-Tubiana A, Bourgeois M, Vekemans M, et al. Dysembryoplastic neuroepithelial tumors in two children with neurofibromatosis type 1. Acta Neuropathol. 1995;90(3):319–22. PMID:8525807
4037. Lelotte J, Mourin A, Fomekong E, et al. Both invasiveness and proliferation criteria predict recurrence of non-functioning pituitary macroadenomas after surgery: a retrospective analysis of a monocentric cohort of 120 patients. Eur J Endocrinol. 2018 Mar;178(3):237–46. PMID:29259039
4038. Lenherr-Taube N, Lam CK, Vali R, et al. Severe primary hyperparathyroidism caused by parathyroid carcinoma in a 13-year-old child; novel findings from HRpQCT. JBMR Plus. 2020 Jan 2;4(3):e10324. PMID:32161840
4039. Lennert K, Kaiserling E, Mazzanti T. Diagnosis and differential diagnosis of lymphoepithelial carcinoma in lymph nodes: histological, cytological and electron-microscopic findings. IARC Sci Publ (1971). 1978;(20):51–64. PMID:83286
4040. Leoncini L. Epstein-Barr virus positivity as a defining pathogenetic feature of Burkitt lymphoma subtypes. Br J Haematol. 2022 Feb;196(3):468–70. PMID:34725813
4041. Leong SC. A systematic review of surgical outcomes for advanced juvenile nasopharyngeal angiofibroma with intracranial involvement. Laryngoscope. 2013 May;123(5):1125–31. PMID:23553370
4042. Lepreux S, Rebouissou S, Le Bail B, et al. Mutation of TP53 gene is involved in carcinogenesis of hepatic undifferentiated (embryonal) sarcoma of the adult, in contrast with Wnt or telomerase pathways: an immunohistochemical study of three cases with genomic relation in two cases. J Hepatol. 2005 Mar;42(3):424–9. PMID:15710230
4043. Leraas HJ, Rosenberger LH, Ren Y, et al. Pediatric phyllodes tumors: a review of the National Cancer Data Base and adherence to NCCN guidelines for phyllodes tumor treatment. J Pediatr Surg. 2018 Jun;53(6):1123–8. PMID:29605260
4044. Lerner J, Goldfarb M. Follicular variant papillary thyroid carcinoma in a pediatric population. Pediatr Blood Cancer. 2015 Nov;62(11):1942–6. PMID:26131690
4045. Leroy B, Ballinger ML, Baran-Marszak F, et al. Recommended guidelines for validation, quality control, and reporting of TP53 variants in clinical practice. Cancer Res. 2017 Mar 15;77(6):1250–60. PMID:28254861
4046. Leroy B, Fournier JL, Ishioka C, et al. The TP53 website: an integrative resource centre for the TP53 mutation database and TP53 mutant analysis. Nucleic Acids Res. 2013 Jan;41(Database issue):D962–9. PMID:23161690
4047. Leroy X, Augusto D, Leteurtre E, et al. CD30 and CD117 (c-kit) used in combination are useful for distinguishing embryonal carcinoma from seminoma. J Histochem Cytochem. 2002 Feb;50(2):283–5. PMID:11799147
4048. Leruste A, Tosello J, Ramos RN, et al. Clonally expanded T cells reveal immunogenicity of rhabdoid tumors. Cancer Cell. 2019 Dec 9;36(6):597–612.e8. PMID:31708437
4049. Leske H, Dalgleish R, Lazar AJ, et al. A common classification framework for histone sequence alterations in tumours: an expert consensus proposal. J Pathol. 2021 Jun;254(2):109–20. PMID:33779999
4050. Leske H, Rushing E, Budka H, et al. K27/G34 versus K28/G35 in histone H3-mutant gliomas: a note of caution. Acta Neuropathol. 2018 Jul;136(1):175–6. PMID:29766298
4051. Lesluyes T, Delespaul L, Coindre JM, et al. The CINSARC signature as a prognostic marker for clinical outcome in multiple neoplasms. Sci Rep. 2017 Jul 14;7(1):5480. PMID:28710396
4052. Leucci E, Cocco M, Onnis A, et al. MYC translocation-negative classical Burkitt lymphoma cases: an alternative pathogenetic mechanism involving miRNA deregulation. J Pathol. 2008 Dec;216(4):440–50. PMID:18802929
4053. Leung AKC, Lam JM, Leong KF, et al. Infantile hemangioma: an updated review. Curr Pediatr Rev. 2021;17(1):55–69. PMID:32384034
4054. Leuschner I, Newton WA Jr, Schmidt D, et al. Spindle cell variants of embryonal rhabdomyosarcoma in the paratesticular region. A report of the Intergroup Rhabdomyosarcoma Study. Am J Surg Pathol. 1993 Mar;17(3):221–30. PMID:8434703
4055. Leventaki V, Bhattacharyya S, Lim MS. Pathology and genetics of anaplastic large cell lymphoma. Semin Diagn Pathol. 2020 Jan;37(1):57–71. PMID:31882178
4056. Leventaki V, Drakos E, Medeiros LJ, et al. NPM-ALK oncogenic kinase promotes cell-cycle progression through activation of JNK/cJun signaling in anaplastic large-cell lymphoma. Blood. 2007 Sep 1;110(5):1621–30. PMID:17416736
4057. Leverstein H, van der Wal JE, Tiwari RM, et al. Surgical management of 246 previously untreated pleomorphic adenomas of the parotid gland. Br J Surg. 1997 Mar;84(3):399–403. PMID:9117322
4058. Levine E, Fréneaux P, Schleiermacher G, et al. Risk-adapted therapy for infantile myofibromatosis in children. Pediatr Blood Cancer. 2012 Jul 15;59(1):115–20. PMID:22038698
4059. Levinsohn JL, Sugarman JL, McNiff JM, et al. Somatic mutations in NEK9 cause nevus comedonicus. Am J Hum Genet. 2016 May 5;98(5):1030–7. PMID:27153399
4060. Levinsohn JL, Tian LC, Boyden LM, et al. Whole-exome sequencing reveals somatic mutations in HRAS and KRAS, which cause nevus sebaceus. J Invest Dermatol. 2013 Mar;133(3):827–30. PMID:23096712
4061. Levi-Schaffer F, Micera A, Zamir E, et al. Nerve growth factor and eosinophils in inflamed juvenile conjunctival nevus. Invest Ophthalmol Vis Sci. 2002 Jun;43(6):1850–6. PMID:12036989
4062. Levy A, Le Péchoux C, Terrier P, et al. Epithelioid sarcoma: need for a multimodal approach to maximize the chances of curative conservative treatment. Ann Surg Oncol. 2014 Jan;21(1):269–76. PMID:24046109
4063. Levy M, Trivedi A, Zhang J, et al. Expression of glypican-3 in undifferentiated embryonal sarcoma and mesenchymal hamartoma of the liver. Hum Pathol. 2012 May;43(5):695–701. PMID:21937079
4064. Levy MT, Braun JT, Pennant M, et al. Primary paraganglioma of the parathyroid: a case report and clinicopathologic review. Head Neck Pathol. 2010 Mar;4(1):37–43. PMID:20237987
4065. Levy RM, Ming ME, Shapiro M, et al. Eruptive disseminated Spitz nevi. J Am Acad Dermatol. 2007 Sep;57(3):519–23. PMID:17467853
4066. Lewis JE, Olsen KD, Sebo TJ. Carcinoma ex pleomorphic adenoma: pathologic analysis of 73 cases. Hum Pathol. 2001 Jun;32(6):596–604. PMID:11431714
4067. Lewis PW, Müller MM, Koletsky MS, et al. Inhibition of PRC2 activity by a gain-of-function H3 mutation found in pediatric glioblastoma. Science. 2013 May 17;340(6134):857–61. PMID:23539183
4068. Lewis RH. Foetus in foetu and the retroperitoneal teratoma. Arch Dis Child. 1961 Apr;36:220–6. PMID:13761753
4069. Li B, Jie W, He H. Myb immunohistochemical staining and fluorescence in situ hybridization in salivary rare basaloid lesions. Front Oncol. 2020 Jun 30;10:870. PMID:32695659
4070. Li BK, Vasiljevic A, Dufour C, et al. Pineoblastoma segregates into molecular subgroups with distinct clinico-pathologic features: a Rare Brain Tumor Consortium registry study. Acta Neuropathol. 2020 Feb;139(2):223–41. PMID:31820118
4071. Li C, Tian Y, Wang J, et al. Abnormal immunophenotype provides a key diagnostic marker: a report of 29 cases of de novo aggressive natural killer cell leukemia. Transl Res. 2014 Jun;163(6):565–77. PMID:24524877
4072. Li D, Wenger TL, Seiler C, et al. Pathogenic variant in EPHB4 results in central conducting lymphatic anomaly. Hum Mol Genet. 2018 Sep 15;27(18):3233–45. PMID:29905864
4073. Li GM. Mechanisms and functions of DNA mismatch repair. Cell Res. 2008 Jan;18(1):85–98. PMID:18157157
4074. Li GY, Fan B, Jiao YY. Endonasal endoscopy for removing nasal chondromesenchymal hamartoma extending from the lacrimal sac region. Can J Ophthalmol. 2013 Apr;48(2):e22–3. PMID:23561613
4075. Li J, Woods SL, Healey S, et al. Point mutations in exon 1B of APC reveal gastric adenocarcinoma and proximal polyposis of the stomach as a familial adenomatous polyposis variant. Am J Hum Genet. 2016 May 5;98(5):830–42. PMID:27087319
4076. Li JF, Dai YT, Lilljebjörn H, et al. Transcriptional landscape of B cell precursor acute lymphoblastic leukemia based on an international study of 1,223 cases. Proc Natl Acad Sci U S A. 2018 Dec 11;115(50):E11711–20. PMID:30487223
4077. Li JY, Langford LA, Adesina A, et al. The high mitotic count detected by phospho-histone H3 immunostain does not alter the benign

behavior of angiocentric glioma. Brain Tumor Pathol. 2012 Jan;29(1):68–72. PMID:21892765
**4078.** Li JY, Lopez JI, Powell SZ, et al. Giant cell ependymoma-report of three cases and review of the literature. Int J Clin Exp Pathol. 2012;5(5):458–62. PMID:22808300
**4079.** Li L, Grausam KB, Wang J, et al. Sonic Hedgehog promotes proliferation of Notch-dependent monociliated choroid plexus tumour cells. Nat Cell Biol. 2016 Apr;18(4):418–30. PMID:26999738
**4080.** Li L, Othman M, Rashid A, et al. Solid pseudopapillary neoplasm of the pancreas with prominent atypical multinucleated giant tumour cells. Histopathology. 2013 Feb;62(3):465–71. PMID:23134473
**4081.** Li L, Zeng Y, Fang K, et al. Anetodermic pilomatricoma: molecular characteristics and trauma in the development of its bullous appearance. Am J Dermatopathol. 2012 Jun;34(4):e41–5. PMID:22307232
**4082.** Li LJ, Li Y, Wen YM, et al. Clinical analysis of salivary gland tumor cases in West China in past 50 years. Oral Oncol. 2008 Feb;44(2):187–92. PMID:17418612
**4083.** Li M, Wang C, Liu P, et al. Clinical and genetic features of pediatric PCCs/PGLs patients: a single-center experience in China. Transl Androl Urol. 2020 Apr;9(2):267–75. PMID:32420132
**4084.** Li MM, Datto M, Duncavage EJ, et al. Standards and guidelines for the interpretation and reporting of sequence variants in cancer: a joint consensus recommendation of the Association for Molecular Pathology, American Society of Clinical Oncology, and College of American Pathologists. J Mol Diagn. 2017 Jan;19(1):4–23. PMID:27993330
**4085.** Li N, Gao X, Xu Z, et al. Prevalence of developmental odontogenic cysts in children and adolescents with emphasis on dentigerous cyst and odontogenic keratocyst (keratocystic odontogenic tumor). Acta Odontol Scand. 2014 Nov;72(8):795–800. PMID:24832690
**4086.** Li S. Anaplastic lymphoma kinase-positive large B-cell lymphoma: a distinct clinicopathological entity. Int J Clin Exp Pathol. 2009 Mar 13;2(6):508–18. PMID:19636398
**4087.** Li S, Baloch ZW, Tomaszewski JE, et al. Worrisome histologic alterations following fine-needle aspiration of benign parotid lesions. Arch Pathol Lab Med. 2000 Jan;124(1):87–91. PMID:10629137
**4088.** Li W, Cooley LD. Unusual infant eosinophilia: myeloid neoplasm with FGFR1 abnormality. Blood. 2016 Sep 8;128(10):1440. PMID:27769039
**4089.** Li W, Cooley LD, August K. Juvenile myelomonocytic leukemia with t(3;5)(q25;q35), Auer rods and marked myelodysplasia. Pathol Res Pract. 2018 Jun;214(6):919–23. PMID:29496305
**4090.** Li W, Cooper J, Zhou L, et al. Merlin/NF2 loss-driven tumorigenesis linked to CRL4(DCAF1)-mediated inhibition of the hippo pathway kinases Lats1 and 2 in the nucleus. Cancer Cell. 2014 Jul 14;26(1):48–60. PMID:25026211
**4091.** Li WS, Liao IC, Wen MC, et al. BCOR-CCNB3-positive soft tissue sarcoma with round-cell and spindle-cell histology: a series of four cases highlighting the pitfall of mimicking poorly differentiated synovial sarcoma. Histopathology. 2016 Nov;69(5):792–801. PMID:27228320
**4092.** Li Y, Reuter VE, Matoso A, et al. Re-evaluation of 33 'unclassified' eosinophilic renal cell carcinomas in young patients. Histopathology. 2018 Mar;72(4):588–600. PMID:28898443
**4093.** Li Y, Schwab C, Ryan S, et al. Constitutional and somatic rearrangement of chromosome 21 in acute lymphoblastic leukaemia. Nature. 2014 Apr 3;508(7494):98–102. PMID:24670643
**4094.** Li Y, Vilain E, Conte F, et al. Testis-specific protein Y-encoded gene is expressed in early and late stages of gonadoblastoma and testicular carcinoma in situ. Urol Oncol. 2007 Mar-Apr;25(2):141–6. PMID:17349529
**4095.** Li Y, Yang QX, Tian XT, et al. Malignant transformation of nasal chondromesenchymal hamartoma in adult: a case report and review of the literature. Histol Histopathol. 2013 Mar;28(3):337–44. PMID:23348387
**4096.** Li Y, Zheng D, Zuo M, et al. Chondromesenchymal hamartomas in a 24-year-old male mimicking a posterior mediastinal tumor and a 5-month-old boy with postoperative disseminated intravascular coagulation: two case reports. Diagn Pathol. 2020 May 12;15(1):53. PMID:32398154
**4097.** Li YP, Chang K, Chen TW, et al. Primary Ewing family of tumor arising in the ovary: a case report. Int J Gynecol Pathol. 2019 Sep;38(5):470–3. PMID:30085939
**4098.** Li YY, Chung GT, Lui VW, et al. Exome and genome sequencing of nasopharynx cancer identifies NF-κB pathway activating mutations. Nat Commun. 2017 Jan 18;8:14121. PMID:28098136
**4099.** Li Z, Lu L, Zhou Z, et al. Recurrent mutations in epigenetic modifiers and the PI3K/AKT/mTOR pathway in subcutaneous panniculitis-like T-cell lymphoma. Br J Haematol. 2018 May;181(3):406–10. PMID:28294301
**4100.** Lian F, Wang LM, Qi XL, et al. MYB-QKI rearrangement in angiocentric glioma. Clin Neuropathol. 2020 Nov/Dec;39(6):263–70. PMID:32589128
**4101.** Liang L, Korogi Y, Sugahara T, et al. MRI of intracranial germ-cell tumours. Neuroradiology. 2002 May;44(5):382–8. PMID:12012121
**4102.** Liang L, Olar A, Niu N, et al. Primary glial and neuronal tumors of the ovary or peritoneum: a clinicopathologic study of 11 cases. Am J Surg Pathol. 2016 Jun;40(6):847–56. PMID:26990854
**4103.** Liang L, Zhang Y, Malpica A, et al. Gliomatosis peritonei: a clinicopathologic and immunohistochemical study of 21 cases. Mod Pathol. 2015 Dec;28(12):1613–20. PMID:26564007
**4104.** Liang Y, Yang YS, Zhang Y. Multiple congenital granular cell epulis in a female newborn: a case report. J Med Case Rep. 2014 Dec 8;8:413. PMID:25482350
**4105.** Lianjia Y, Yan J, Hitoshi N, et al. An immunohistochemical study of bone morphogenetic protein in pleomorphic adenoma of the salivary gland. Virchows Arch A Pathol Anat Histopathol. 1993;422(6):439–43. PMID:8333147
**4106.** Liao CP, Booker RC, Brosseau JP, et al. Contributions of inflammation and tumor microenvironment to neurofibroma tumorigenesis. J Clin Invest. 2018 Jul 2;128(7):2848–61. PMID:29596064
**4107.** Liao CP, Pradhan S, Chen Z, et al. The role of nerve microenvironment for neurofibroma development. Oncotarget. 2016 Sep 20;7(38):61500–8. PMID:27517146
**4108.** Liberman L, Bonaccio E, Hamele-Bena D, et al. Benign and malignant phyllodes tumors: mammographic and sonographic findings. Radiology. 1996 Jan;198(1):121–4. PMID:8539362
**4109.** Licis AK, Vallorani A, Gao F, et al. Prevalence of sleep disturbances in children with neurofibromatosis type 1. J Child Neurol. 2013 Nov;28(11):1400–5. PMID:24065580
**4110.** Lieber MR, Lack EE, Roberts JR Jr, et al. Solid and papillary epithelial neoplasm of the pancreas. An ultrastructural and immunocytochemical study of six cases. Am J Surg Pathol. 1987 Feb;11(2):85–93. PMID:3812876
**4111.** Lieberman PH, Brennan MF, Kimmel M, et al. Alveolar soft-part sarcoma. A clinico-pathologic study of half a century. Cancer. 1989 Jan 1;63(1):1–13. PMID:2642727
**4112.** Liede A, Hernandez RK, Tang ET, et al. Epidemiology of benign giant cell tumor of bone in the Chinese population. J Bone Oncol. 2018 Jul 26;12:96–100. PMID:30148063
**4113.** Lietman SA, Germain-Lee EL, Levine MA. Hypercalcemia in children and adolescents. Curr Opin Pediatr. 2010 Aug;22(4):508–15. PMID:20601885
**4114.** Ligtenberg MJ, Kuiper RP, Geurts van Kessel A, et al. EPCAM deletion carriers constitute a unique subgroup of Lynch syndrome patients. Fam Cancer. 2013 Jun;12(2):169–74. PMID:23264089
**4115.** Lillard JC, Venable GT, Khan NR, et al. Pediatric supratentorial ependymoma: surgical, clinical, and molecular analysis. Neurosurgery. 2019 Jul 1;85(1):41–9. PMID:29917116
**4116.** Lilljebjörn H, Henningsson R, Hyrenius-Wittsten A, et al. Identification of ETV6-RUNX1-like and DUX4-rearranged subtypes in paediatric B-cell precursor acute lymphoblastic leukaemia. Nat Commun. 2016 Jun 6;7:11790. PMID:27265895
**4117.** Lim D, Oliva E. Gynecological neoplasms associated with paraneoplastic hypercalcemia. Semin Diagn Pathol. 2019 Jul;36(4):246–59. PMID:30772079
**4118.** Lim D, Oliva E. Ovarian sex cord-stromal tumours: an update in recent molecular advances. Pathology. 2018 Feb;50(2):178–89. PMID:29275930
**4119.** Lim II, Farber BA, LaQuaglia MP. Advances in fibrolamellar hepatocellular carcinoma: a review. Eur J Pediatr Surg. 2014 Dec;24(6):461–6. PMID:25486412
**4120.** Lim JS, Gopalappa R, Kim SH, et al. Somatic Mutations in TSC1 and TSC2 Cause Focal Cortical Dysplasia. Am J Hum Genet. 2017 Mar 2;100(3):454–72. PMID:28215400
**4121.** Lim MS, Straus SE, Dale JK, et al. Pathological findings in human autoimmune lymphoproliferative syndrome. Am J Pathol. 1998 Nov;153(5):1541–50. PMID:9811346
**4121A.** Lim S, Lim KY, Koh J, et al. Pediatric-type indolent B-cell lymphomas with overlapping clinical, pathologic, and genetic features. Am J Surg Pathol. 2022 Oct 1;46(10):1397–406. PMID:35834399
**4122.** Lim YH, Bacchiocchi A, Qiu J, et al. GNA14 somatic mutation causes congenital and sporadic vascular tumors by MAPK activation. Am J Hum Genet. 2016 Aug 4;99(2):443–50. PMID:27476652
**4123.** Lima JF, Jin L, de Araujo AR, et al. FOXL2 mutations in granulosa cell tumors occurring in males. Arch Pathol Lab Med. 2012 Jul;136(7):825–8. PMID:22742556
**4124.** Lin CN, Chou SC, Li CF, et al. Prognostic factors of myxofibrosarcomas: implications of margin status, tumor necrosis, and mitotic rate on survival. J Surg Oncol. 2006 Mar 15;93(4):294–303. PMID:16496357
**4125.** Lin CW, Liu TY, Chen SU, et al. CD94 1A transcripts characterize lymphoblastic lymphoma/leukemia of immature natural killer cell origin with distinct clinical features. Blood. 2005 Nov 15;106(10):3567–74. PMID:16046525
**4126.** Lin DC, Meng X, Hazawa M, et al. The genomic landscape of nasopharyngeal carcinoma. Nat Genet. 2014 Aug;46(8):866–71. PMID:24952746
**4127.** Lin HC, Chu PH, Jung SM, et al. MUC5AC in juvenile conjunctival nevus. Jpn J Ophthalmol. 2012 Mar;56(2):107–12. PMID:22139382
**4128.** Lin LL, El Naqa I, Leonard JR, et al. Long-term outcome in children treated for craniopharyngioma with and without radiotherapy. J Neurosurg Pediatr. 2008 Feb;1(2):126–30. PMID:18352781
**4129.** Lin O, Koreishi A, Brandt SM, et al. ALK+ large B-cell lymphoma: a rare variant of aggressive large B-cell lymphoma mimicking carcinoma on cytology specimens. Diagn Cytopathol. 2013 May;41(5):404–7. PMID:22351377
**4130.** Linder D. Gene loss in human teratomas. Proc Natl Acad Sci U S A. 1969 Jul;63(3):699–704. PMID:5259759
**4131.** Linder D, McCaw BK, Hecht F. Parthenogenic origin of benign ovarian teratomas. N Engl J Med. 1975 Jan 9;292(2):63–6. PMID:162806
**4132.** Linder D, Power J. Further evidence for post-meiotic origin of teratomas in the human female. Ann Hum Genet. 1970 Jul;34(1):21–30. PMID:5476662
**4133.** Lindhurst MJ, Sapp JC, Teer JK, et al. A mosaic activating mutation in AKT1 associated with the Proteus syndrome. N Engl J Med. 2011 Aug 18;365(7):611–9. PMID:21793738
**4134.** Lindhurst MJ, Wang JA, Bloomhardt HM, et al. AKT1 gene mutation levels are correlated with the type of dermatologic lesions in patients with Proteus syndrome. J Invest Dermatol. 2014 Feb;134(2):543–6. PMID:23884311
**4135.** Lindner S, Bachmann HS, Odersky A, et al. Absence of telomerase reverse transcriptase promoter mutations in neuroblastoma. Biomed Rep. 2015 Jul;3(4):443–6. PMID:26171145
**4136.** Lindsey JC, Schwalbe EC, Potluri S, et al. TERT promoter mutation and aberrant hypermethylation are associated with elevated expression in medulloblastoma and characterise the majority of non-infant SHH subgroup tumours. Acta Neuropathol. 2014 Feb;127(2):307–9. PMID:24337442
**4137.** Lindsley RC, Saber W, Mar BG, et al. Prognostic mutations in myelodysplastic syndrome after stem-cell transplantation. N Engl J Med. 2017 Feb 9;376(6):536–47. PMID:28177873
**4138.** Lindström E, Shimokawa T, Toftgård R, et al. PTCH mutations: distribution and analyses. Hum Mutat. 2006 Mar;27(3):215–9. PMID:16419085
**4139.** Linhares ND, Freire MC, Cardenas RG, et al. Exome sequencing identifies a novel homozygous variant in NDRG4 in a family with infantile myofibromatosis. Eur J Med Genet. 2014 Nov-Dec;57(11-12):643–8. PMID:25241110
**4140.** Linhares ND, Freire MC, Cardenas RG, et al. Modulation of expressivity in PDGFRB-related infantile myofibromatosis: a role for PTPRG? Genet Mol Res. 2014 Aug 15;13(3):6287–92. PMID:25158255
**4141.** Link MP, Goorin AM, Miser AW, et al. The effect of adjuvant chemotherapy on relapse-free survival in patients with osteosarcoma of the extremity. N Engl J Med. 1986 Jun 19;314(25):1600–6. PMID:3520317
**4142.** Linn Murphree A. Intraocular retinoblastoma: the case for a new group classification. Ophthalmol Clin North Am. 2005 Mar;18(1):41–53, viii. PMID:15763190
**4143.** Linos K, Carter JM, Gardner JM, et al. Myofibromas with atypical features: expanding the morphologic spectrum of a benign entity. Am J Surg Pathol. 2014 Dec;38(12):1649–54. PMID:24921644
**4144.** Lipka DB, Witte T, Toth R, et al. RAS-pathway mutation patterns define epigenetic subclasses in juvenile myelomonocytic leukemia. Nat Commun. 2017 Dec 19;8(1):2126. PMID:29259247
**4145.** Lips DJ, Barker N, Clevers H, et al. The role of APC and beta-catenin in the aetiology of aggressive fibromatosis (desmoid tumors). Eur J Surg Oncol. 2009 Jan;35(1):3–10. PMID:18722078

4146. Liso A, Capello D, Marafioti T, et al. Aberrant somatic hypermutation in tumor cells of nodular-lymphocyte-predominant and classic Hodgkin lymphoma. Blood. 2006 Aug 1;108(3):1013–20. PMID:16614247

4147. Listernick R, Charrow J. Neurofibromatosis type 1 in childhood. J Pediatr. 1990 Jun;116(6):845–53. PMID:2112186

4148. Listernick R, Charrow J, Greenwald M, et al. Natural history of optic pathway tumors in children with neurofibromatosis type 1: a longitudinal study. J Pediatr. 1994 Jul;125(1):63–6. PMID:8021787

4149. Listernick R, Ferner RE, Liu GT, et al. Optic pathway gliomas in neurofibromatosis-1: controversies and recommendations. Ann Neurol. 2007 Mar;61(3):189–98. PMID:17387725

4150. Litchfield K, Summersgill B, Yost S, et al. Whole-exome sequencing reveals the mutational spectrum of testicular germ cell tumours. Nat Commun. 2015 Jan 22;6:5973. PMID:25609015

4151. Liu APY, Gudenas B, Lin T, et al. Risk-adapted therapy and biological heterogeneity in pineoblastoma: integrated clinico-pathological analysis from the prospective, multi-center SJMB03 and SJYC07 trials. Acta Neuropathol. 2020 Feb;139(2):259–71. PMID:31802236

4152. Liu APY, Li BK, Pfaff E, et al. Clinical and molecular heterogeneity of pineal parenchymal tumors: a consensus study. Acta Neuropathol. 2021 May;141(5):771–85. PMID:33619588

4153. Liu APY, Priesterbach-Ackley LP, Orr BA, et al. WNT-activated embryonal tumors of the pineal region: ectopic medulloblastomas or a novel pineoblastoma subgroup? Acta Neuropathol. 2020 Oct;140(4):595–7. PMID:32772175

4154. Liu GY, Song H, Xu XL. Multiple palisaded encapsulated neuromas in siblings: a case report and review of the published work. J Dermatol. 2016 May;43(5):560–3. PMID:26460241

4155. Liu H, Lin F. Application of immunohistochemistry in thyroid pathology. Arch Pathol Lab Med. 2015 Jan;139(1):67–82. PMID:25549145

4156. Liu H, Wang X, Lu D, et al. Ovarian masses in children and adolescents in China: analysis of 203 cases. J Ovarian Res. 2013 Jul 4;6:47. PMID:23826706

4157. Liu J, Guzman MA, Pawel BR, et al. Clonal trisomy 4 cells detected in the ossifying renal tumor of infancy: study of 3 cases. Mod Pathol. 2013 Feb;26(2):275–81. PMID:22976287

4158. Liu J, Guzman MA, Pezanowski D, et al. FOXO1-FGFR1 fusion and amplification in a solid variant of alveolar rhabdomyosarcoma. Mod Pathol. 2011 Oct;24(10):1327–35. PMID:21666686

4159. Liu J, Hudkins PG, Swee RG, et al. Bone sarcomas associated with Ollier's disease. Cancer. 1987 Apr 1;59(7):1376–85. PMID:3815310

4160. Liu KX, Duggan EM, Al-Ibraheemi A, et al. Characterization of long-term outcomes for pediatric patients with epithelioid hemangioma. Pediatr Blood Cancer. 2019 Jan;66(1):e27451. PMID:30207085

4161. Liu PT, Kujak JL, Roberts CC, et al. The vascular groove sign: a new CT finding associated with osteoid osteomas. AJR Am J Roentgenol. 2011 Jan;196(1):168–73. PMID:21178063

4162. Liu Q, Galli S, Srinivasan R, et al. Renal medullary carcinoma: molecular, immunohistochemistry, and morphologic correlation. Am J Surg Pathol. 2013 Mar;37(3):368–74. PMID:23348212

4163. Liu Q, Salaverria I, Pittaluga S, et al. Follicular lymphomas in children and young adults: a comparison of the pediatric variant with usual follicular lymphoma. Am J Surg Pathol. 2013 Mar;37(3):333–43. PMID:23108024

4164. Liu Q, Wang Y, Tong D, et al. A Somatic HIF2α mutation-induced multiple and recurrent pheochromocytoma/paraganglioma with polycythemia: clinical study with literature review. Endocr Pathol. 2017 Mar;28(1):75–82. PMID:28116635

4165. Liu S, Tian Y, Chlenski A, et al. Cross-talk between Schwann cells and neuroblasts influences the biology of neuroblastoma xenografts. Am J Pathol. 2005 Mar;166(3):891–900. PMID:15743800

4166. Liu W, Shia J, Gönen M, et al. DNA mismatch repair abnormalities in acinar cell carcinoma of the pancreas: frequency and clinical significance. Pancreas. 2014 Nov;43(8):1264–70. PMID:25058881

4167. Liu W, Tang Y, Gao L, et al. Nasopharyngeal carcinoma in children and adolescents - a single institution experience of 158 patients. Radiat Oncol. 2014 Dec 5;9:274. PMID:25477058

4168. Liu Y, Bian T, Zhang Y, et al. A combination of LMO2 negative and CD38 positive is useful for the diagnosis of Burkitt lymphoma. Diagn Pathol. 2019 Sep 4;14(1):100. PMID:31484540

4169. Liu Y, Ma C, Wang G, et al. Hydroa vacciniforme-like lymphoproliferative disorder: clinicopathologic study of 41 cases. J Am Acad Dermatol. 2019 Aug;81(2):534–40. PMID:30654082

4170. Liu Y, Sattarzadeh A, Diepstra A, et al. The microenvironment in classical Hodgkin lymphoma: an actively shaped and essential tumor component. Semin Cancer Biol. 2014 Feb;24:15–22. PMID:23867303

4171. Liu Z, Zeng W, Chen T, et al. Correction: A comparison of the clinicopathological features and prognoses of the classical and the tall cell variant of papillary thyroid cancer: a meta-analysis. Oncotarget. 2018 Mar 23;9(22):16271. PMID:29662643

4172. LiVolsi VA. Papillary carcinoma tall cell variant (TCV): a review. Endocr Pathol. 2010 Mar;21(1):12–5. PMID:20174895

4173. LiVolsi VA, Abrosimov AA, Bogdanova T, et al. The Chernobyl thyroid cancer experience: pathology. Clin Oncol (R Coll Radiol). 2011 May;23(4):261–7. PMID:21333507

4174. Llamas-Velasco M, Hilty N, Kempf W. Porokeratotic adnexal ostial naevus: review on the entity and therapeutic approach. J Eur Acad Dermatol Venereol. 2015 Oct;29(10):2032–7. PMID:25255914

4175. Llamas-Velasco M, Kempf W, Cota C, et al. Multiple eruptive epithelioid hemangiomas: a subset of cutaneous cellular epithelioid hemangioma with expression of FOS-B. Am J Surg Pathol. 2019 Jan;43(1):26–34. PMID:29266025

4176. Llamas-Velasco M, Pérez-Gónzalez YC, Requena L, et al. Histopathologic clues for the diagnosis of Wiesner nevus. J Am Acad Dermatol. 2014 Mar;70(3):549–54. PMID:24373783

4177. Llombart B, Monteagudo C, Sanmartín O, et al. Dermatofibrosarcoma protuberans: a clinicopathological, immunohistochemical, genetic (COL1A1-PDGFB), and therapeutic study of low-grade versus high-grade (fibrosarcomatous) tumors. J Am Acad Dermatol. 2011 Sep;65(3):564–75. PMID:21570152

4178. Llombart B, Sanmartín O, López-Guerrero JA, et al. Dermatofibrosarcoma protuberans: clinical, pathological, and genetic (COL1A1-PDGFB ) study with therapeutic implications. Histopathology. 2009 Jun;54(7):860–72. PMID:19635106

4179. Llombart-Bosch A, Machado I, Navarro S, et al. Histological heterogeneity of Ewing's sarcoma/PNET: an immunohistochemical analysis of 415 genetically confirmed cases with clinical support. Virchows Arch. 2009 Nov;455(5):397–411. PMID:19841938

4180. Lloyd RV, Osamura RY, Klöppel G, et al., editors. WHO classification of tumours of endocrine organs. Lyon (France): International Agency for Research on Cancer; 2017. (WHO classification of tumours series, 4th ed.; vol. 10). https://publications.iarc.fr/554.

4181. Lobeck IN, Jeste N, Geller J, et al. Surgical management and surveillance of pediatric appendiceal carcinoid tumor. J Pediatr Surg. 2017 Jun;52(6):925–7. PMID:28363472

4182. Lobo J, Gillis AJM, Jerónimo C, et al. Human germ cell tumors are developmental cancers: impact of epigenetics on pathobiology and clinic. Int J Mol Sci. 2019 Jan 10;20(2):E258. PMID:30634670

4183. Locatelli F, Niemeyer CM. How I treat juvenile myelomonocytic leukemia. Blood. 2015 Feb 12;125(7):1083–90. PMID:25564399

4184. Locatelli F, Strahm B. How I treat myelodysplastic syndromes of childhood. Blood. 2018 Mar 29;131(13):1406–14. PMID:29438960

4185. Locati LD, Collini P, Imbimbo M, et al. Immunohistochemical and molecular profile of salivary gland cancer in children. Pediatr Blood Cancer. 2017 Sep;64(9). PMID:28139061

4186. Loconte DC, Grossi V, Bozzao C, et al. Molecular and functional characterization of three different postzygotic mutations in PIK-3CA-related overgrowth spectrum (PROS) patients: effects on PI3K/AKT/mTOR signaling and sensitivity to PIK3 inhibitors. PLoS One. 2015 Apr 27;10(4):e0123092. PMID:25915946

4187. Loddenkemper C, Anagnostopoulos I, Hummel M, et al. Differential Emu enhancer activity and expression of BOB.1/OBF.1, Oct2, PU.1, and immunoglobulin in reactive B-cell populations, B-cell non-Hodgkin lymphomas, and Hodgkin lymphomas. J Pathol. 2004 Jan;202(1):60–9. PMID:14694522

4188. Loeffler KU, McMenamin PG. An ultrastructural study of DNA precipitation in the anterior segment of eyes with retinoblastoma. Ophthalmology. 1987 Sep;94(9):1160–8. PMID:3684233

4189. Logothetis CJ, Samuels ML, Selig DE, et al. Cyclic chemotherapy with cyclophosphamide, doxorubicin, and cisplatin plus vinblastine and bleomycin in advanced germinal tumors. Results with 100 patients. Am J Med. 1986 Aug;81(2):219–28. PMID:2426944

4190. Loh JK, Lieu AS, Chai CY, et al. Malignant transformation of a desmoplastic infantile ganglioglioma. Pediatr Neurol. 2011 Aug;45(2):135–7. PMID:21763958

4191. Loh ML. Childhood myelodysplastic syndrome: focus on the approach to diagnosis and treatment of juvenile myelomonocytic leukemia. Hematology Am Soc Hematol Educ Program. 2010;2010:357–62. PMID:21239819

4192. Lohmann DR, Gallie BL. Retinoblastoma: revisiting the model prototype of inherited cancer. Am J Med Genet C Semin Med Genet. 2004 Aug 15;129C(1):23–8. PMID:15264269

4193. Lohmann DR, Gillessen-Kaesbach G. Multiple subcutaneous granular-cell tumours in a patient with Noonan syndrome. Clin Dysmorphol. 2000 Oct;9(4):301–2. PMID:11045593

4194. Lones MA, Mishalani S, Shintaku IP, et al. Changes in tonsils and adenoids in children with posttransplant lymphoproliferative disorder: report of three cases with early involvement of Waldeyer's ring. Hum Pathol. 1995 May;26(5):525–30. PMID:7750936

4195. Longhi A, Bielack SS, Grimer R, et al. Extraskeletal osteosarcoma: a European Musculoskeletal Oncology Society study on 266 patients. Eur J Cancer. 2017 Mar;74:9–16. PMID:28167373

4196. Longhi A, Fabbri N, Donati D, et al. Neoadjuvant chemotherapy for patients with synchronous multifocal osteosarcoma: results in eleven cases. J Chemother. 2001 Jun;13(3):324–30. PMID:11450892

4197. Longley BJ Jr, Metcalfe DD, Tharp M, et al. Activating and dominant inactivating c-KIT catalytic domain mutations in distinct clinical forms of human mastocytosis. Proc Natl Acad Sci U S A. 1999 Feb 16;96(4):1609–14. PMID:9990072

4198. Longo JF, Weber SM, Turner-Ivey BP, et al. Recent advances in the diagnosis and pathogenesis of neurofibromatosis type 1 (NF1)-associated peripheral nervous system neoplasms. Adv Anat Pathol. 2018 Sep;25(5):353–68. PMID:29762158

4199. Longworth MS, Laimins LA. Pathogenesis of human papillomaviruses in differentiating epithelia. Microbiol Mol Biol Rev. 2004 Jun;68(2):362–72. PMID:15187189

4200. Lo Nigro L. Biology of childhood acute lymphoblastic leukemia. J Pediatr Hematol Oncol. 2013 May;35(4):245–52. PMID:23612374

4201. Looi LM. Tumor-associated tissue eosinophilia in nasopharyngeal carcinoma. A pathologic study of 422 primary and 138 metastatic tumors. Cancer. 1987 Feb 1;59(3):466–70. PMID:3791157

4202. Looi LM, Cheah PL. An immunohistochemical study comparing clear cell sarcoma of the kidney and Wilms' tumor. Pathology. 1993 Apr;25(2):106–9. PMID:8396229

4203. Looijenga LH, Hersmus R, de Leeuw BH, et al. Gonadal tumours and DSD. Best Pract Res Clin Endocrinol Metab. 2010 Apr;24(2):291–310. PMID:20541153

4204. Looijenga LH, Oosterhuis JW. Pathogenesis of testicular germ cell tumours. Rev Reprod. 1999 May;4(2):90–100. PMID:10357096

4205. Looijenga LH, Rosenberg C, van Gurp RJ, et al. Comparative genomic hybridization of microdissected samples from different stages in the development of a seminoma and a non-seminoma. J Pathol. 2000 Jun;191(2):187–92. PMID:10861580

4206. Looijenga LH, Stoop H, de Leeuw HP, et al. POU5F1 (OCT3/4) identifies cells with pluripotent potential in human germ cell tumors. Cancer Res. 2003 May 1;63(9):2244–50. PMID:12727846

4207. Looijenga LH, Zafarana G, Grygalewicz B, et al. Role of gain of 12p in germ cell tumour development. APMIS. 2003 Jan;111(1):161–71. PMID:12752258

4208. Looijenga LHJ, Kao CS, Idrees MT. Predicting gonadal germ cell cancer in people with disorders of sex development; insights from developmental biology. Int J Mol Sci. 2019 Oct 10;20(20):E5017. PMID:31658757

4209. Look AT, Hayes FA, Nitschke R, et al. Cellular DNA content as a predictor of response to chemotherapy in infants with unresectable neuroblastoma. N Engl J Med. 1984 Jul 26;311(4):231–5. PMID:6738617

4210. Lopes MB, Altermatt HJ, Scheithauer BW, et al. Immunohistochemical characterization of subependymal giant cell astrocytomas. Acta Neuropathol. 1996;91(4):368–75. PMID:8928613

4211. Lopes MLDS, Barroso KMA, Henriques ÁCG, et al. Pleomorphic adenomas of the salivary glands: retrospective multicentric study of 130 cases with emphasis on histopathological features. Eur Arch Otorhinolaryngol. 2017 Jan;274(1):543–51. PMID:27520570

4212. López G, Oberheim Bush NA, Berger MS, et al. Diffuse non-midline glioma with H3F3A K27M mutation: a prognostic and treatment dilemma. Acta Neuropathol Commun. 2017 May 15;5(1):38. PMID:28506301

4213. López GY, Van Ziffle J, Onodera C, et al. The genetic landscape of gliomas arising after

therapeutic radiation. Acta Neuropathol. 2019 Jan;137(1):139–50. PMID:30196423
4214. López V, Martín JM, Monteagudo C, et al. [Epidemiology of pediatric dermatologic surgery: a retrospective study of 996 children]. Actas Dermosifiliogr. 2010 Nov;101(9):771–7. Spanish. PMID:21034707
4215. Lopez-Ben R, Pitt MJ, Jaffe KA, et al. Osteosarcoma in a patient with McCune-Albright syndrome and Mazabraud's syndrome. Skeletal Radiol. 1999 Sep;28(9):522–6. PMID:10525796
4216. López-Lerma I, Peñate Y, Gallardo F, et al. Subcutaneous panniculitis-like T-cell lymphoma: clinical features, therapeutic approach, and outcome in a case series of 16 patients. J Am Acad Dermatol. 2018 Nov;79(5):892–8. PMID:30126736
4217. Lopez-Nunez O, Alaggio R, Ranganathan S, et al. New molecular insights into the pathogenesis of lipoblastomas: clinicopathologic, immunohistochemical, and molecular analysis in pediatric cases. Hum Pathol. 2020 Oct;104:30–41. PMID:32692992
4218. Lopez-Nunez O, John I, Panasiti RN, et al. Infantile inflammatory myofibroblastic tumors: clinicopathological and molecular characterization of 12 cases. Mod Pathol. 2020 Apr;33(4):576–90. PMID:31690781
4219. López-Terrada D, Alaggio R, de Dávila MT, et al. Towards an international pediatric liver tumor consensus classification: proceedings of the Los Angeles COG Liver Tumors Symposium. Mod Pathol. 2014 Mar;27(3):472–91. PMID:24008558
4220. López-Terrada D, Gunaratne PH, Adesina AM, et al. Histologic subtypes of hepatoblastoma are characterized by differential canonical Wnt and Notch pathway activation in DLK+ precursors. Hum Pathol. 2009 Jun;40(6):783–94. PMID:19200579
4221. Lorenzana A, Lyons H, Sawaf H, et al. Human herpesvirus 6 infection mimicking juvenile myelomonocytic leukemia in an infant. J Pediatr Hematol Oncol. 2002 Feb;24(2):136–41. PMID:11990701
4222. Lorenzi L, Tabellini G, Vermi W, et al. Occurrence of nodular lymphocyte-predominant hodgkin lymphoma in hermansky-pudlak type 2 syndrome is associated to natural killer and natural killer T cell defects. PLoS One. 2013 Nov 26;8(11):e80131. PMID:24302998
4223. Lorenzo FR, Yang C, Ng Tang Fui M, et al. A novel EPAS1/HIF2A germline mutation in a congenital polycythemia with paraganglioma. J Mol Med (Berl). 2013 Apr;91(4):507–12. PMID:23090011
4224. Lorsbach RB, Shay-Seymore D, Moore J, et al. Clinicopathologic analysis of follicular lymphoma occurring in children. Blood. 2002 Mar 15;99(6):1959–64. PMID:11877266
4225. Losa M, Vimercati A, Acerno S, et al. Correlation between clinical characteristics and proliferative activity in patients with craniopharyngioma. J Neurol Neurosurg Psychiatry. 2004 Jun;75(6):889–92. PMID:15146007
4226. Lott JP, Wititsuwannakul J, Lee JJ, et al. Clinical characteristics associated with Spitz nevi and Spitzoid malignant melanomas: the Yale University Spitzoid Neoplasm Repository experience, 1991 to 2008. J Am Acad Dermatol. 2014 Dec;71(6):1077–82. PMID:25308882
4227. Louis DN, Ellison DW, Brat DJ, et al. cIMPACT-NOW: a practical summary of diagnostic points from Round 1 updates. Brain Pathol. 2019 Jul;29(4):469–72. PMID:31038238
4228. Louis DN, Giannini C, Capper D, et al. cIMPACT-NOW update 2: diagnostic clarifications for diffuse midline glioma, H3 K27M-mutant and diffuse astrocytoma/anaplastic astrocytoma, IDH-mutant. Acta Neuropathol. 2018 Apr;135(4):639–42. PMID:29497819
4229. Louis DN, Perry A, Burger P, et al. International Society of Neuropathology–Haarlem consensus guidelines for nervous system tumor classification and grading. Brain Pathol. 2014 Sep;24(5):429–35. PMID:24990071
4230. Louis DN, Ramesh V, Gusella JF. Neuropathology and molecular genetics of neurofibromatosis 2 and related tumors. Brain Pathol. 1995 Apr;5(2):163–72. PMID:7670657
4231. Louis DN, von Deimling A, Dickersin GR, et al. Desmoplastic cerebral astrocytomas of infancy: a histopathologic, immunohistochemical, ultrastructural, and molecular genetic study. Hum Pathol. 1992 Dec;23(12):1402–9. PMID:1468778
4232. Louis DN, Wesseling P, Aldape K, et al. cIMPACT-NOW update 6: new entity and diagnostic principle recommendations of the cIMPACT-Utrecht meeting on future CNS tumor classification and grading. Brain Pathol. 2020 Jul;30(4):844–56. PMID:32307792
4233. Louis DN, Wesseling P, Brandner S, et al. Data sets for the reporting of tumors of the central nervous system: recommendations from the International Collaboration on Cancer Reporting. Arch Pathol Lab Med. 2020 Feb;144(2):196–206. PMID:31219344
4234. Louis DN, Wesseling P, Paulus W, et al. cIMPACT-NOW update 1: not otherwise specified (NOS) and not elsewhere classified (NEC). Acta Neuropathol. 2018 Mar;135(3):481–4. PMID:29372318
4235. Louissaint A Jr, Ackerman AM, Dias-Santagata D, et al. Pediatric-type nodal follicular lymphoma: an indolent clonal proliferation in children and adults with high proliferation index and no BCL2 rearrangement. Blood. 2012 Sep 20;120(12):2395–404. PMID:22855608
4236. Louissaint A Jr, Schafernak KT, Geyer JT, et al. Pediatric-type nodal follicular lymphoma: a biologically distinct lymphoma with frequent MAPK pathway mutations. Blood. 2016 Aug 25;128(8):1093–100. PMID:27325104
4237. Louka E, Povinelli B, Rodriguez-Meira A, et al. Heterogeneous disease-propagating stem cells in juvenile myelomonocytic leukemia. J Exp Med. 2021 Feb 1;218(2):e20180853. PMID:33416891
4238. Loukola A, Salovaara R, Kristo P, et al. Microsatellite instability in adenomas as a marker for hereditary nonpolyposis colorectal cancer. Am J Pathol. 1999 Dec;155(6):1849–53. PMID:10595914
4239. Love C, Sun Z, Jima D, et al. The genetic landscape of mutations in Burkitt lymphoma. Nat Genet. 2012 Dec;44(12):1321–5. PMID:23143597
4240. Lovly CM, Gupta A, Lipson D, et al. Inflammatory myofibroblastic tumors harbor multiple potentially actionable kinase fusions. Cancer Discov. 2014 Aug;4(8):889–95. PMID:24875859
4241. Lowe EJ, Sposto R, Perkins SL, et al. Intensive chemotherapy for systemic anaplastic large cell lymphoma in children and adolescents: final results of Children's Cancer Group Study 5941. Pediatr Blood Cancer. 2009 Mar;52(3):335–9. PMID:18985718
4242. Lowry KC, Estroff JA, Rahbar R. The presentation and management of fibromatosis colli. Ear Nose Throat J. 2010 Sep;89(9):E4–8. PMID:20859860
4243. Loyola AM, Gatti AF, Pinto DS Jr, et al. Alveolar and extra-alveolar granular cell lesions of the newborn: report of case and review of literature. Oral Surg Oral Med Oral Pathol Oral Radiol Endod. 1997 Dec;84(6):668–71. PMID:9431537
4244. Lu C, Ramirez D, Hwang S, et al. Histone H3K36M mutation and trimethylation patterns in chondroblastoma. Histopathology. 2019 Jan;74(2):291–9. PMID:30098026
4245. Lu C, Zhang J, Nagahawatte P, et al. The genomic landscape of childhood and adolescent melanoma. J Invest Dermatol. 2015 Mar;135(3):816–23. PMID:25268584
4246. Lu DY, Chang S, Cook H, et al. Genital rhabdomyoma of the urethra in an infant girl. Hum Pathol. 2012 Apr;43(4):597–600. PMID:21992817
4247. Lu L, Jin W, Liu H, et al. RECQ DNA helicases and osteosarcoma. Adv Exp Med Biol. 2014;804:129–45. PMID:24924172
4248. Lubin JH, Schafer DW, Ron E, et al. A reanalysis of thyroid neoplasms in the Israeli tinea capitis study accounting for dose uncertainties. Radiat Res. 2004 Mar;161(3):359–68. PMID:14982478
4249. Lubs ML, Bauer MS, Formas ME, et al. Lisch nodules in neurofibromatosis type 1. N Engl J Med. 1991 May 2;324(18):1264–6. PMID:1901624
4250. Lucas CG, Villanueva-Meyer JE, Whipple N, et al. Myxoid glioneuronal tumor, PDGFRA p.K385-mutant: clinical, radiologic, and histopathologic features. Brain Pathol. 2020 May;30(3):479–94. PMID:31609499
4251. Lucas CL, Kuehn HS, Zhao F, et al. Dominant-activating germline mutations in the gene encoding the PI(3)K catalytic subunit p110δ result in T cell senescence and human immunodeficiency. Nat Immunol. 2014 Jan;15(1):88–97. PMID:24165795
4252. Lucas DR, Nascimento AG, Sim FH. Clear cell sarcoma of soft tissues. Mayo Clinic experience with 35 cases. Am J Surg Pathol. 1992 Dec;16(12):1197–204. PMID:1463095
4253. Lucas DR, Unni KK, McLeod RA, et al. Osteoblastoma: clinicopathologic study of 306 cases. Hum Pathol. 1994 Feb;25(2):117–34. PMID:8119712
4254. Lucas JT Jr, Huang AJ, Mott RT, et al. Anaplastic ganglioglioma: a report of three cases and review of the literature. J Neurooncol. 2015 May;123(1):171–7. PMID:25862009
4255. Lucchesi KM, Grant R, Kahle KT, et al. Primary spinal myxopapillary ependymoma in the pediatric population: a study from the Surveillance, Epidemiology, and End Results (SEER) database. J Neurooncol. 2016 Oct;130(1):133–40. PMID:27423644
4256. Luckie TM, Danzig M, Zhou S, et al. A multicenter retrospective review of pediatric Leydig cell tumor of the testis. J Pediatr Hematol Oncol. 2019 Jan;41(1):74–6. PMID:29554024
4257. Ludwig K, Alaggio R, Zin A, et al. BCOR-CCNB3 undifferentiated sarcoma-Does immunohistochemistry help in the identification? Pediatr Dev Pathol. 2017 Jul-Aug;20(4):321–9. PMID:28420319
4258. Luithle T, Szavay P, Furtwängler R, et al. Treatment of cystic nephroma and cystic partially differentiated nephroblastoma–a report from the SIOP/GPOH study group. J Urol. 2007 Jan;177(1):294–6. PMID:17162067
4259. Lukáš J, Drábek J, Lukáš D, et al. Ectopic thyroid with benign and malignant findings: a case series. Int J Surg Case Rep. 2020;66:33–8. PMID:31790949
4260. Luks VL, Kamitaki N, Vivero MP, et al. Lymphatic and other vascular malformative/overgrowth disorders are caused by somatic mutations in PIK3CA. J Pediatr. 2015 Apr;166(4):1048–54.e1, 5. PMID:25681199
4261. Luksch R, Castellani MR, Collini P, et al. Neuroblastoma (Peripheral neuroblastic tumours). Crit Rev Oncol Hematol. 2016 Nov;107:163–81. PMID:27823645
4262. Lum SH, Bonney D, Cheesman E, et al. Successful curative therapy with rituximab and allogeneic haematopoietic stem cell transplantation for MALT lymphoma associated with STK4-mutated CD4+ lymphocytopenia. Pediatr Blood Cancer. 2016 Sep;63(9):1657–9. PMID:27163767
4263. Luna PC, Panizzardi AA, Martin CI, et al. Papular epidermal nevus with skyline basal cell layer (PENS): three new cases and review of the literature. Pediatr Dermatol. 2016 May;33(3):296–300. PMID:26939784
4264. Luna-Fineman S, Shannon KM, Atwater SK, et al. Myelodysplastic and myeloproliferative disorders of childhood: a study of 167 patients. Blood. 1999 Jan 15;93(2):459–66. PMID:9885207
4265. Lundberg WB, Mitchell MS. Transient warm autoimmune hemolytic anemia and cryoglobulinemia associated with seminoma. Yale J Biol Med. 1977 Jul-Aug;50(4):419–27. PMID:906560
4266. Luo JH, Ren B, Keryanov S, et al. Transcriptomic and genomic analysis of human hepatocellular carcinomas and hepatoblastomas. Hepatology. 2006 Oct;44(4):1012–24. PMID:17006932
4267. Lüttges JE, Lübke M. Recurrent benign Müllerian papilloma of the vagina. Immunohistological findings and histogenesis. Arch Gynecol Obstet. 1994;255(3):157–60. PMID:7979569
4268. Luu MH, Press RD. BCR-ABL PCR testing in chronic myelogenous leukemia: molecular diagnosis for targeted cancer therapy and monitoring. Expert Rev Mol Diagn. 2013 Sep;13(7):749–62. PMID:24063401
4269. Luyken C, Blümcke I, Fimmers R, et al. Supratentorial gangliogliomas: histopathologic grading and tumor recurrence in 184 patients with a median follow-up of 8 years. Cancer. 2004 Jul 1;101(1):146–55. PMID:15222000
4270. Luzar B, Billings SD, de la Fouchardiere A, et al. Compound clear cell sarcoma of the skin-a potential diagnostic pitfall: report of a series of 4 new cases and a review of the literature. Am J Surg Pathol. 2020 Jan;44(1):21–9. PMID:31688004
4271. Luzar B, Ieremia E, Antonescu CR, et al. Cutaneous intravascular epithelioid hemangioma. A clinicopathological and molecular study of 21 cases. Mod Pathol. 2020 Aug;33(8):1527–36. PMID:32094426
4272. Luzar B, Shanesmith R, Ramakrishnan R, et al. Cutaneous epithelioid malignant peripheral nerve sheath tumour: a clinicopathological analysis of 11 cases. Histopathology. 2016 Jan;68(2):286–96. PMID:26096054
4273. Luzzi S, Elia A, Del Maestro M, et al. Dysembryoplastic neuroepithelial tumors: what you need to know. World Neurosurg. 2019 Jul;127:255–65. PMID:30981794
4274. Lynch HT, Cristofaro G, Rozen P, et al. History of the International Collaborative Group on Hereditary Non Polyposis Colorectal Cancer. Fam Cancer. 2003;2 Suppl 1:3–5. PMID:14574154
4275. Lynch HT, Krush AJ. Cancer family "G" revisited: 1895-1970. Cancer. 1971 Jun;27(6):1505–11. PMID:5088221
4276. Lynch HT, Lynch PM, Pester J, et al. The cancer family syndrome. Rare cutaneous phenotypic linkage of Torre's syndrome. Arch Intern Med. 1981 Apr;141(5):607–11. PMID:7224741
4277. Lynch HT, Riegert-Johnson DL, Snyder C, et al. Lynch syndrome-associated extracolonic tumors are rare in two extended families with the same EPCAM deletion. Am J Gastroenterol. 2011 Oct;106(10):1829–36. PMID:21769135
4278. Lynch HT, Smyrk T, Lynch JF. Molecular genetics and clinical-pathology features of hereditary nonpolyposis colorectal carcinoma (Lynch syndrome): historical journey from pedigree anecdote to molecular genetic confirmation. Oncology. 1998 Mar-Apr;55(2):103–8. PMID:9499183

4279. Lynskey SJ, Pianta MJ. MRI and thallium features of pigmented villonodular synovitis and giant cell tumours of tendon sheaths: a retrospective single centre study of imaging and literature review. Br J Radiol. 2015;88(1056):20150528. PMID:26440548
4280. Lyons LL, North PE, Mac-Moune Lai F, et al. Kaposiform hemangioendothelioma: a study of 33 cases emphasizing its pathologic, immunophenotypic, and biologic uniqueness from juvenile hemangioma. Am J Surg Pathol. 2004 May;28(5):559–68. PMID:15105642
4281. Lysell J, Wiegleb Edström D, Linde A, et al. Antiviral therapy in children with hydroa vacciniforme. Acta Derm Venereol. 2009;89(4):393–7. PMID:19688153
4282. Lyskjaer I, Lindsay D, Tirabosco R, et al. H3K27me3 expression and methylation status in histological variants of malignant peripheral nerve sheath tumours. J Pathol. 2020 Oct;252(2):151–64. PMID:32666581
4283. M D, S K, S R, et al. Lipoblastomatosis of the retropharyngeal space: pathogenesis, presentation, and management, with a focus on head-neck lipoblastoma(toses). B-ENT. 2016;12(1):33–9. PMID:27097392
4284. Ma C, Feng R, Chen H, et al. BRAF V600E, TERT, and IDH2 mutations in pleomorphic xanthoastrocytoma: observations from a large case-series study. World Neurosurg. 2018 Dec;120:e1225–33. PMID:30240866
4285. Ma Y, Zheng J, Zhu H, et al. Gastroblastoma in a 12-year-old Chinese boy. Int J Clin Exp Pathol. 2014 May 15;7(6):3380–4. PMID:25031764
4286. Ma ZY, Song ZJ, Chen JH, et al. Recurrent gain-of-function USP8 mutations in Cushing's disease. Cell Res. 2015 Mar;25(3):306–17. PMID:25675982
4287. Ma'aita JK, Al-Kaisi N, Al-Tamimi S, et al. Salivary gland tumors in Jordan: a retrospective study of 221 patients. Croat Med J. 1999 Dec;40(4):539–42. PMID:10554362
4288. Macarenco RS, Zamolyi R, Franco MF, et al. Genomic gains of COL1A1-PDFGB occur in the histologic evolution of giant cell fibroblastoma into dermatofibrosarcoma protuberans. Genes Chromosomes Cancer. 2008 Mar;47(3):260–5. PMID:18069662
4289. MacCarthy A, Bayne AM, Brownbill PA, et al. Second and subsequent tumours among 1927 retinoblastoma patients diagnosed in Britain 1951-2004. Br J Cancer. 2013 Jun 25;108(12):2455–63. PMID:23674091
4290. MacCarthy A, Draper GJ, Steliarova-Foucher E, et al. Retinoblastoma incidence and survival in European children (1978-1997). Report from the Automated Childhood Cancer Information System project. Eur J Cancer. 2006 Sep;42(13):2092–102. PMID:16919773
4291. Macchiaiolo M, Markowich AH, Diociaiuti A, et al. Diffuse infantile hepatic hemangiomas in a patient with Beckwith-Wiedemann syndrome: a new association? Am J Med Genet A. 2020 Aug;182(8):1972–6. PMID:32573107
4292. MacCollin M, Chiocca EA, Evans DG, et al. Diagnostic criteria for schwannomatosis. Neurology. 2005 Jun 14;64(11):1838–45. PMID:15955931
4293. MacCollin M, Ramesh V, Jacoby LB, et al. Mutational analysis of patients with neurofibromatosis 2. Am J Hum Genet. 1994 Aug;55(2):314–20. PMID:7913580
4293A. MacDonald-Jankowski DS. Keratocystic odontogenic tumour: systematic review. Dentomaxillofac Radiol. 2011 Jan;40(1):1–23. PMID:21159911
4294. MacDonald-Jankowski DS. Ossifying fibroma: a systematic review. Dentomaxillofac Radiol. 2009 Dec;38(8):495–513. PMID:20026707
4295. MacFarland SP, Zelley K, Surrey LF, et al. Pediatric somatic tumor sequencing identifies underlying cancer predisposition. JCO Precis Oncol. 2019;3:PO.19.00062. PMID:32783018
4296. Machado I, López-Soto MV, Rubio L, et al. Soft tissue myoepithelial carcinoma with rhabdoid-like features and EWSR1 rearrangement: fine needle aspiration cytology with histologic correlation. Diagn Cytopathol. 2015 May;43(5):421–6. PMID:25693574
4297. Machado I, Navarro S, Picci P, et al. The utility of SATB2 immunohistochemical expression in distinguishing between osteosarcomas and their malignant bone tumor mimickers, such as Ewing sarcomas and chondrosarcomas. Pathol Res Pract. 2016 Sep;212(9):811–6. PMID:27465835
4298. Machado I, Yoshida A, Morales MGN, et al. Review with novel markers facilitates precise categorization of 41 cases of diagnostically challenging, "undifferentiated small round cell tumors". A clinicopathologic, immunophenotypic and molecular analysis. Ann Diagn Pathol. 2018 Jun;34:1–12. PMID:29661713
4299. Machein MR, Plate KH. VEGF in brain tumors. J Neurooncol. 2000 Oct-Nov;50(1-2):109–20. PMID:11245271
4300. Machen SK, Easley KA, Goldblum JR. Synovial sarcoma of the extremities: a clinicopathologic study of 34 cases, including semi-quantitative analysis of spindled, epithelial, and poorly differentiated areas. Am J Surg Pathol. 1999 Mar;23(3):268–75. PMID:10078916
4301. Machens A, Niccoli-Sire P, Hoegel J, et al. Early malignant progression of hereditary medullary thyroid cancer. N Engl J Med. 2003 Oct 16;349(16):1517–25. PMID:14561794
4302. Maciaszek JL, Oak N, Nichols KE. Recent advances in Wilms' tumor predisposition. Hum Mol Genet. 2020 Oct 20;29 R2:R138–49. PMID:32412586
4303. Mack SC, Agnihotri S, Bertrand KC, et al. Spinal myxopapillary ependymomas demonstrate a Warburg phenotype. Clin Cancer Res. 2015 Aug 15;21(16):3750–8. PMID:25957288
4304. Mack SC, Pajtler KW, Chavez L, et al. Therapeutic targeting of ependymoma as informed by oncogenic enhancer profiling. Nature. 2018 Jan 4;553(7686):101–5. PMID:29258295
4305. Mack SC, Witt H, Piro RM, et al. Epigenomic alterations define lethal CIMP-positive ependymomas of infancy. Nature. 2014 Feb 27;506(7489):445–50. PMID:24553142
4306. Mackay A, Burford A, Carvalho D, et al. Integrated molecular meta-analysis of 1,000 pediatric high-grade and diffuse intrinsic pontine glioma. Cancer Cell. 2017 Oct 9;32(4):520–537.e5. PMID:28966033
4307. Mackay A, Burford A, Molinari V, et al. Molecular, pathological, radiological, and immune profiling of non-brainstem pediatric high-grade glioma from the HERBY phase II randomized trial. Cancer Cell. 2018 May 14;33(5):829–842.e5. PMID:29763623
4308. Mackey AC, Green L, Liang LC, et al. Hepatosplenic T cell lymphoma associated with infliximab use in young patients treated for inflammatory bowel disease. J Pediatr Gastroenterol Nutr. 2007 Feb;44(2):265–7. PMID:17255842
4309. MacLennan KA, Bennett MH, Tu A, et al. Relationship of histopathologic features to survival and relapse in nodular sclerosing Hodgkin's disease. A study of 1659 patients. Cancer. 1989 Oct 15;64(8):1686–93. PMID:2790683
4310. Macon WR, Levy NB, Kurtin PJ, et al. Hepatosplenic alphabeta T-cell lymphomas: a report of 14 cases and comparison with hepatosplenic gammadelta T-cell lymphomas. Am J Surg Pathol. 2001 Mar;25(3):285–96. PMID:11224598
4311. Madan R, Gormley R, Dulau A, et al. AIDS and non-AIDS diffuse large B-cell lymphomas express different antigen profiles. Mod Pathol. 2006 Mar;19(3):438–46. PMID:16444194
4312. Madigan CE, Armenian SH, Malogolowkin MH, et al. Extracranial malignant rhabdoid tumors in childhood: the Childrens Hospital Los Angeles experience. Cancer. 2007 Nov 1;110(9):2061–6. PMID:17828773
4313. Madsen PJ, Buch VP, Douglas JE, et al. Endoscopic endonasal resection versus open surgery for pediatric craniopharyngioma: comparison of outcomes and complications. J Neurosurg Pediatr. 2019 Jun 7:1–10. PMID:31174192
4314. Maecker B, Jack T, Zimmermann M, et al. CNS or bone marrow involvement as risk factors for poor survival in post-transplantation lymphoproliferative disorders in children after solid organ transplantation. J Clin Oncol. 2007 Nov 1;25(31):4902–8. PMID:17971586
4315. Maeyama H, Hidaka E, Ota H, et al. Familial gastrointestinal stromal tumor with hyperpigmentation: association with a germline mutation of the c-kit gene. Gastroenterology. 2001 Jan;120(1):210–5. PMID:11208730
4316. Maffeis M, Notarangelo LD, Schumacher RF, et al. Primary immunodeficiencies and oncological risk: the experience of the Children's Hospital of Brescia. Front Pediatr. 2019 Jun 19;7:232. PMID:31275905
4317. Magaki SD, Vinters HV. Tuberous sclerosis complex. In: Adle-Biassette H, Harding BN, Golden JA, editors. Developmental neuropathology. 2nd ed. Oxford (UK): John Wiley & Sons Ltd; 2018. pp. 117–31.
4318. Magaña M, Massone C, Magaña P, et al. Clinicopathologic features of hydroa vacciniforme-like lymphoma: a series of 9 patients. Am J Dermatopathol. 2016 Jan;38(1):20–5. PMID:26368647
4319. Magaña M, Sangüeza P, Gil-Beristain J, et al. Angiocentric cutaneous T-cell lymphoma of childhood (hydroa-like lymphoma): a distinctive type of cutaneous T-cell lymphoma. J Am Acad Dermatol. 1998 Apr;38(4):574–9. PMID:9580256
4320. Magdy M, Abdel Karim N, Eldessouki I, et al. Myeloid Sarcoma. Oncol Res Treat. 2019;42(4):224–9. PMID:30840960
4321. Magg T, Schober T, Walz C, et al. Epstein-barr virus+ smooth muscle tumors as manifestation of primary immunodeficiency disorders. Front Immunol. 2018 Feb 27;9:368. PMID:29535735
4322. Magri L, Cambiaghi M, Cominelli M, et al. Sustained activation of mTOR pathway in embryonic neural stem cells leads to development of tuberous sclerosis complex-associated lesions. Cell Stem Cell. 2011 Nov 4;9(5):447–62. PMID:22056141
4323. Magro G, Greco P, Alaggio R, et al. Polypoid angiomyofibroblastoma-like tumor of the oral cavity: a hitherto unreported soft tissue tumor mimicking embryonal rhabdomyosarcoma. Pathol Res Pract. 2008;204(11):837–43. PMID:18656317
4324. Maguiness S, Uihlein LC, Liang MG, et al. Rapidly involuting congenital hemangioma with fetal involution. Pediatr Dermatol. 2015 May-Jun;32(3):321–6. PMID:25492638
4325. Maguiness SM. Vascular tumors and malformations in children, Introduction. Semin Cutan Med Surg. 2016 Mar;35(3):107. PMID:27607317
4326. Mahajan P, Margolin J, Iacobas I. Kasabach-Merritt phenomenon: classic presentation and management options. Clin Med Insights Blood Disord. 2017 Mar 16;10:X17699849. PMID:28579853
4327. Mahajan S, Agarwal S, Kocheri N, et al. Cytopathology of non-invasive follicular thyroid neoplasm with papillary-like nuclear features: a comparative study with similar patterned papillary thyroid carcinoma variants. Cytopathology. 2018 Jun;29(3):233–40. PMID:29638022
4328. Mahalakshmi B, Baskaran R, Shanmugavadivu M, et al. Insulinoma-associated protein 1 (INSM1): a potential biomarker and therapeutic target for neuroendocrine tumors. Cell Oncol (Dordr). 2020 Jun;43(3):367–76. PMID:32219703
4329. Mahdi J, Goyal MS, Griffith J, et al. Nonoptic pathway tumors in children with neurofibromatosis type 1. Neurology. 2020 Aug 25;95(8):e1052–9. PMID:32300062
4330. Mahdi J, Shah AC, Sato A, et al. A multi-institutional study of brainstem gliomas in children with neurofibromatosis type 1. Neurology. 2017 Apr 18;88(16):1584–9. PMID:28330960
4331. Mahler C, Verhelst J, Klaes R, et al. Cushing's disease and hyperprolactinemia due to a mixed ACTH- and prolactin-secreting pituitary macroadenoma. Pathol Res Pract. 1991 Jun;187(5):598–602. PMID:1656408
4332. Mahoney MC, Lawvere S, Falkner KL, et al. Thyroid cancer incidence trends in Belarus: examining the impact of Chernobyl. Int J Epidemiol. 2004 Oct;33(5):1025–33. PMID:15166190
4333. Mahoney NR, Liu GT, Menacker SJ, et al. Pediatric horner syndrome: etiologies and roles of imaging and urine studies to detect neuroblastoma and other responsible mass lesions. Am J Ophthalmol. 2006 Oct;142(4):651–9. PMID:17011859
4334. Mai KT, Landry DC, Thomas J, et al. Follicular adenoma with papillary architecture: a lesion mimicking papillary thyroid carcinoma. Histopathology. 2001 Jul;39(1):25–32. PMID:11454041
4335. Maier EM, Leitner C, Löhrs U, et al. True hermaphroditism in an XY individual due to a familial point mutation of the SRY gene. J Pediatr Endocrinol Metab. 2003 Apr-May;16(4):575–80. PMID:12793612
4336. Makarova O, Oschlies I, Müller S, et al. Excellent outcome with limited treatment in paediatric patients with marginal zone lymphoma. Br J Haematol. 2018 Sep;182(5):735–9. PMID:28771659
4337. Makhlouf HR, Abdul-Al HM, Wang G, et al. Calcifying nested stromal-epithelial tumors of the liver: a clinicopathologic, immunohistochemical, and molecular genetic study of 9 cases with a long-term follow-up. Am J Surg Pathol. 2009 Jul;33(7):976–83. PMID:19363442
4338. Makino K, Nakamura H, Yano S, et al. Incidence of primary central nervous system germ cell tumors in childhood: a regional survey in Kumamoto prefecture in southern Japan. Pediatr Neurosurg. 2013;49(3):155–8. PMID:24751890
4339. Makishima H, Ito T, Momose K, et al. Chemokine system and tissue infiltration in aggressive NK-cell leukemia. Leuk Res. 2007 Sep;31(9):1237–45. PMID:17123604
4340. Makri A, Akshintala S, Derse-Anthony C, et al. Pheochromocytoma in children and adolescents with multiple endocrine neoplasia type 2B. J Clin Endocrinol Metab. 2019 Jan 1;104(1):7–12. PMID:30113649
4341. Malandrino P, Russo M, Regalbuto C, et al. Outcome of the diffuse sclerosing variant of papillary thyroid cancer: a meta-analysis. Thyroid. 2016 Sep;26(9):1285–92. PMID:27349273
4342. Malard F, Mohty M. Acute lymphoblastic leukaemia. Lancet. 2020 Apr 4;395(10230):1146–62. PMID:32247396
4343. Malempati S, Hawkins DS. Rhabdomyosarcoma: review of the Children's Oncology Group (COG) Soft-Tissue Sarcoma Committee experience and rationale for current COG studies. Pediatr Blood Cancer. 2012 Jul 15;59(1):5–10. PMID:22378628

4344. Malgulwar PB, Nambirajan A, Pathak P, et al. C11orf95-RELA fusions and upregulated NF-KB signalling characterise a subset of aggressive supratentorial ependymomas that express L1CAM and nestin. J Neurooncol. 2018 May;138(1):29–39. PMID:29354850
4345. Malgulwar PB, Nambirajan A, Pathak P, et al. Study of β-catenin and BRAF alterations in adamantinomatous and papillary craniopharyngiomas: mutation analysis with immunohistochemical correlation in 54 cases. J Neurooncol. 2017 Jul;133(3):487–95. PMID:28500561
4346. Malik F, Wang L, Yu Z, et al. Benign infiltrative myofibroblastic neoplasms of childhood with USP6 gene rearrangement. Histopathology. 2020 Nov;77(5):760–8. PMID:32583473
4347. Malinowska I, Kwiatkowski DJ, Weiss S, et al. Perivascular epithelioid cell tumors (PEComas) harboring TFE3 gene rearrangements lack the TSC2 alterations characteristic of conventional PEComas: further evidence for a biological distinction. Am J Surg Pathol. 2012 May;36(5):783–4. PMID:22456611
4348. Malkin D. Li-fraumeni syndrome. Genes Cancer. 2011 Apr;2(4):475–84. PMID:21779515
4349. Malkin D, Li FP, Strong LC, et al. Germ line p53 mutations in a familial syndrome of breast cancer, sarcomas, and other neoplasms. Science. 1990 Nov 30;250(4985):1233–8. PMID:1978757
4350. Malla I, Pérez C, Cheang Y, et al. [Human herpesvirus 8 related Kaposi's sarcoma in a pediatric liver transplant recipient: case report]. Arch Argent Pediatr. 2013 Oct;111(5):e125–8. Spanish. PMID:24092038
4351. Mallet E, Working Group on Calcium Metabolism. Primary hyperparathyroidism in neonates and childhood. The French experience (1984-2004). Horm Res. 2008;69(3):180–8. PMID:18219222
4352. Mallet JF, Rigault P, Padovani JP, et al. [Non-ossifying fibroma in children: a surgical condition?]. Chir Pediatr. 1980;21(3):179–89. French. PMID:7408072
4353. Mallory GB, Spray TL. Paediatric lung transplantation. Eur Respir J. 2004 Nov;24(5):839–45. PMID:15516681
4354. Mallory SB, Enjolras O, Boon LM, et al. Congenital plaque-type glomuvenous malformations presenting in childhood. Arch Dermatol. 2006 Jul;142(7):892–6. PMID:16847206
4355. Malogolowkin MH, Katzenstein HM, Meyers RL, et al. Complete surgical resection is curative for children with hepatoblastoma with pure fetal histology: a report from the Children's Oncology Group. J Clin Oncol. 2011 Aug 20;29(24):3301–6. PMID:21768450
4356. Malouf GG, Camparo P, Molinié V, et al. Transcription factor E3 and transcription factor EB renal cell carcinomas: clinical features, biological behavior and prognostic factors. J Urol. 2011 Jan;185(1):24–9. PMID:21074195
4357. Malowany JI, Merritt NH, Chan NG, et al. Nested stromal epithelial tumor of the liver in Beckwith-Wiedemann syndrome. Pediatr Dev Pathol. 2013 Jul-Aug;16(4):312–7. PMID:23570373
4358. Maly A, Epstein D, Meir K, et al. Histological criteria for grading of atypia in melanocytic conjunctival lesions. Pathology. 2008 Dec;40(7):676–81. PMID:18985522
4359. Mamilla D, Manukyan I, Fetsch PA, et al. Immunohistochemical distinction of paragangliomas from epithelial neuroendocrine tumors-gangliocytic duodenal and cauda equina paragangliomas align with epithelial neuroendocrine tumors. Hum Pathol. 2020 Sep;103:72–82. PMID:32668278
4360. Mamsen LS, Brøchner CB, Byskov AG, et al. The migration and loss of human primordial germ stem cells from the hind gut epithelium towards the gonadal ridge. Int J Dev Biol. 2012;56(10-12):771–8. PMID:23417399
4361. Manabe A, Yoshimasu T, Ebihara Y, et al. Viral infections in juvenile myelomonocytic leukemia: prevalence and clinical implications. J Pediatr Hematol Oncol. 2004 Oct;26(10):636-41. PMID:15454834
4362. Mancao C, Altmann M, Jungnickel B, et al. Rescue of "crippled" germinal center B cells from apoptosis by Epstein-Barr virus. Blood. 2005 Dec 15;106(13):4339–44. PMID:16076866
4363. Mancini I, Righi A, Gambarotti M, et al. Phenotypic and molecular differences between giant-cell tumour of soft tissue and its bone counterpart. Histopathology. 2017 Sep;71(3):453–60. PMID:28477388
4364. Mandal GK, Das I, Paul R, et al. Primary central nervous system teratoma with sarcomatous transformation in a young girl: report of a rare case. Asian J Neurosurg. 2016 Oct-Dec;11(4):458. PMID:27695574
4365. Mandelker DL, Dorfman DM, Li B, et al. Antigen expression patterns of MYC-rearranged versus non-MYC-rearranged B-cell lymphomas by flow cytometry. Leuk Lymphoma. 2014 Nov;55(11):2592–6. PMID:24397618
4366. Manes RP, Ryan MW, Batra PS, et al. Ossifying fibroma of the nose and paranasal sinuses. Int Forum Allergy Rhinol. 2013 Feb;3(2):161–8. PMID:22736440
4367. Mangham DC, Williams A, Lalam RK, et al. Angiomatoid fibrous histiocytoma of bone: a calcifying sclerosing variant mimicking osteosarcoma. Am J Surg Pathol. 2010 Feb;34(2):279–85. PMID:20090505
4368. Mangili G, Sigismondi C, Lorusso D, et al. Is surgical restaging indicated in apparent stage IA pure ovarian dysgerminoma? The MITO group retrospective experience. Gynecol Oncol. 2011 May 1;121(2):280–4. PMID:21277010
4369. Mangray S, Breese V, Jackson CL, et al. Application of BRAF V600E mutation analysis for the diagnosis of metanephric adenofibroma. Am J Surg Pathol. 2015 Sep;39(9):1301–4. PMID:26274032
4370. Mangray S, Kelly DR, LeGuellec S, et al. Clinicopathologic features of a series of primary renal CIC-rearranged sarcomas with comprehensive molecular analysis. Am J Surg Pathol. 2018 Oct;42(10):1360–9. PMID:29901569
4371. Manivel JC, Jessurun J, Wick MR, et al. Placental alkaline phosphatase immunoreactivity in testicular germ-cell neoplasms. Am J Surg Pathol. 1987 Jan;11(1):21–9. PMID:3538918
4372. Manivel JC, Priest JR, Watterson J, et al. Pleuropulmonary blastoma. The so-called pulmonary blastoma of childhood. Cancer. 1988 Oct 15;62(8):1516–26. PMID:3048630
4373. Manivel JC, Simonton S, Wold LE, et al. Absence of intratubular germ cell neoplasia in testicular yolk sac tumors in children. A histochemical and immunohistochemical study. Arch Pathol Lab Med. 1988 Jun;112(6):641–5. PMID:2837162
4374. Manjila S, Asmar NE, Vidalis BM, et al. Intratumoral Rathke's cleft cyst remnants within craniopharyngioma, pituitary adenoma, suprasellar dermoid, and epidermoid cysts: a ubiquitous signature of ectodermal lineage or a transitional entity? Neurosurgery. 2019 Aug 1;85(2):180–8. PMID:30010935
4375. Manjila S, Miller E, Awadallah A, et al. Ossified choroid plexus papilloma of the fourth ventricle: elucidation of the mechanism of osteogenesis in benign brain tumors. J Neurosurg Pediatr. 2013 Jul;12(1):13–20. PMID:23641963
4376. Mankuzhy NP, Anderson B, Heider A, et al. KRAS mutant tenosynovial giant cell tumor in a pediatric patient: a case report. Transl Pediatr. 2019 Dec;8(5):449–54. PMID:31993359
4377. Manlhiot C, Pollock-Barziv SM, Holmes C, et al. Post-transplant lymphoproliferative disorder in pediatric heart transplant recipients. J Heart Lung Transplant. 2010 Jun;29(6):648–57. PMID:20304682
4378. Mann AS. Bilateral exophthalmos in seminoma. J Clin Endocrinol Metab. 1967 Oct;27(10):1500–2. PMID:4168317
4379. Mann JR, Gray ES, Thornton C, et al. Mature and immature extracranial teratomas in children: the UK Children's Cancer Study Group experience. J Clin Oncol. 2008 Jul 20;26(21):3590–7. PMID:18541896
4380. Mann JR, Raafat F, Robinson K, et al. The United Kingdom Children's Cancer Study Group's second germ cell tumor study: carboplatin, etoposide, and bleomycin are effective treatment for children with malignant extracranial germ cell tumors, with acceptable toxicity. J Clin Oncol. 2000 Nov 15;18(22):3809–18. PMID:11078494
4381. Mannelli M, Castellano M, Schiavi F, et al. Clinically guided genetic screening in a large cohort of Italian patients with pheochromocytomas and/or functional or nonfunctional paragangliomas. J Clin Endocrinol Metab. 2009 May;94(5):1541–7. PMID:19223516
4382. Manner J, Radlwimmer B, Hohenberger P, et al. MYC high level gene amplification is a distinctive feature of angiosarcomas after irradiation or chronic lymphedema. Am J Pathol. 2010 Jan;176(1):34–9. PMID:20008140
4383. Manning-Geist BL, Perez-Atayde AR, Laufer MR. Pediatric granular cell tumors of the vulva: a report of 4 cases and a review of the literature. J Pediatr Adolesc Gynecol. 2018 Jun;31(3):311–4. PMID:29305965
4384. Manor E, Shubinsky G, Moser AM, et al. Conversion of childhood acute lymphocytic leukemia (L2) with a double t(12;21) to juvenile myelomonocytic leukemia with a novel t(4;11)(p12;q23): a cytogenetic, morphologic, and immunophenotypic study. Cancer Genet Cytogenet. 2003 Dec;147(2):110–4. PMID:14623459
4385. Mansour AM, Barber JC, Reinecke RD, et al. Ocular choristomas. Surv Ophthalmol. 1989 Mar-Apr;33(5):339–58. PMID:2655139
4386. Mantoan Padilha M, Billis A, Allende D, et al. Metanephric adenoma and solid variant of papillary renal cell carcinoma: common and distinctive features. Histopathology. 2013 May;62(6):941–53. PMID:23551615
4387. Manuel M, Katayama PK, Jones HW Jr. The age of occurrence of gonadal tumors in intersex patients with a Y chromosome. Am J Obstet Gynecol. 1976 Feb 1;124(3):293–300. PMID:1247071
4388. Mao C, Guvendi M, Domenico DR, et al. Papillary cystic and solid tumors of the pancreas: a pancreatic embryonic tumor? Studies of three cases and cumulative review of the world's literature. Surgery. 1995 Nov;118(5):821–8. PMID:7482268
4389. Maragliano R, Vanoli A, Albarello L, et al. ACTH-secreting pancreatic neoplasms associated with Cushing syndrome: clinicopathologic study of 11 cases and review of the literature. Am J Surg Pathol. 2015 Mar;39(3):374–82. PMID:25353285
4390. Marcel V, Dichtel-Danjoy ML, Sagne C, et al. Biological functions of p53 isoforms through evolution: lessons from animal and cellular models. Cell Death Differ. 2011 Dec;18(12):1815–24. PMID:21941372
4391. Marchese C, Montera M, Torrini M, et al. Granular cell tumor in a PHTS patient with a novel germline PTEN mutation. Am J Med Genet A. 2003 Jul 15;120A(2):286–8. PMID:12833416
4392. Marchetti AA. A consideration of certain types of benign tumors of the placenta. Surg Gynecol Obstet. 1939;68:733–74.
4393. Marcocci C, Cetani F. Clinical practice. Primary hyperparathyroidism. N Engl J Med. 2011 Dec 22;365(25):2389–97. PMID:22187986
4394. Marcon J, DiNatale RG, Sanchez A, et al. Comprehensive genomic analysis of translocation renal cell carcinoma reveals copy-number variations as drivers of disease progression. Clin Cancer Res. 2020 Jul 15;26(14):3629–40. PMID:32220885
4395. Marcotte L, Aronica E, Baybis M, et al. Cytoarchitectural alterations are widespread in cerebral cortex in tuberous sclerosis complex. Acta Neuropathol. 2012 May;123(5):685–93. PMID:22327361
4396. Marcoux D, Nadeau K, McCuaig C, et al. Pediatric anogenital warts: a 7-year review of children referred to a tertiary-care hospital in Montreal, Canada. Pediatr Dermatol. 2006 May-Jun;23(3):199–207. PMID:16780463
4397. Marghoob AA, Dusza S, Oliveria S, et al. Number of satellite nevi as a correlate for neurocutaneous melanocytosis in patients with large congenital melanocytic nevi. Arch Dermatol. 2004 Feb;140(2):171–5. PMID:14967788
4398. Margo C, Hidayat A, Kopelman J, et al. Retinocytoma. A benign variant of retinoblastoma. Arch Ophthalmol. 1983 Oct;101(10):1519–31. PMID:6626001
4399. Margraf RL, Crockett DK, Krautscheid PM, et al. Multiple endocrine neoplasia type 2 RET protooncogene database: repository of MEN2-associated RET sequence variation and reference for genotype/phenotype correlations. Hum Mutat. 2009 Apr;30(4):548–56. PMID:19177457
4400. Mariani RA, Kadakia R, Arva NC. Noninvasive encapsulated follicular variant of papillary thyroid carcinoma: Should it also be reclassified in children? Pediatr Blood Cancer. 2018 Jun;65(6):e26966. PMID:29380524
4401. Marigo V, Davey RA, Zuo Y, et al. Biochemical evidence that patched is the Hedgehog receptor. Nature. 1996 Nov 14;384(6605):176–9. PMID:8906794
4402. Marina N, London WB, Frazier AL, et al. Prognostic factors in children with extragonadal malignant germ cell tumors: a pediatric intergroup study. J Clin Oncol. 2006 Jun 1;24(16):2544–8. PMID:16735707
4403. Marina NM, Cushing B, Giller R, et al. Complete surgical excision is effective treatment for children with immature teratomas with or without malignant elements: a Pediatric Oncology Group/Children's Cancer Group Intergroup Study. J Clin Oncol. 1999 Jul;17(7):2137–43. PMID:10561269
4404. Mariño-Enríquez A, Dal Cin P. ALK as a paradigm of oncogenic promiscuity: different mechanisms of activation and different fusion partners drive tumors of different lineages. Cancer Genet. 2013 Nov;206(11):357–73. PMID:24091028
4405. Mariño-Enríquez A, Fletcher CD. Angiofibroma of soft tissue: clinicopathologic characterization of a distinctive benign fibrovascular neoplasm in a series of 37 cases. Am J Surg Pathol. 2012 Apr;36(4):500–8. PMID:22301504
4406. Mariño-Enríquez A, Ou WB, Weldon CB, et al. ALK rearrangement in sickle cell trait-associated renal medullary carcinoma. Genes Chromosomes Cancer. 2011 Mar;50(3):146–53. PMID:21213368
4407. Mariño-Enríquez A, Wang WL, Roy A, et al. Epithelioid inflammatory myofibroblastic sarcoma: an aggressive intra-abdominal variant of inflammatory myofibroblastic tumor with nuclear membrane or perinuclear ALK. Am J Surg Pathol. 2011 Jan;35(1):135–44. PMID:21164297
4408. Mark L, Delmore F, Creech JL Jr, et al. Clinical and morphologic features of hepatic

angiosarcoma in vinyl chloride workers. Cancer. 1976 Jan;37(1):149–63. PMID:942881
**4409.** Markley M. [A modern review of dental restorations]. Rev Dent (San Salv). 1968 Jun;15(43):17–31. Spanish. PMID:5247758
**4410.** Marks AM, Bindra RS, DiLuna ML, et al. Response to the BRAF/MEK inhibitors dabrafenib/trametinib in an adolescent with a BRAF V600E mutated anaplastic ganglioglioma intolerant to vemurafenib. Pediatr Blood Cancer. 2018 May;65(5):e26969. PMID:29380516
**4411.** Marks EI, Pamarthy S, Dizon D, et al. ROS1-GOPC/FIG: a novel gene fusion in hepatic angiosarcoma. Oncotarget. 2019 Jan 4;10(2):245–51. PMID:30719217
**4412.** Marque M, Bessis D, Pedeutour F, et al. Medallion-like dermal dendrocyte hamartoma: the main diagnostic pitfall is congenital atrophic dermatofibrosarcoma. Br J Dermatol. 2009 Jan;160(1):190–3. PMID:19016705
**4413.** Marques-Pereira R, Delacerda L, Lacerda HM, et al. Childhood adrenocortical tumours: a review. Hered Cancer Clin Pract. 2006 May 15;4(2):81–9. PMID:20223012
**4414.** Marsan E, Baulac S. Review: Mechanistic target of rapamycin (mTOR) pathway, focal cortical dysplasia and epilepsy. Neuropathol Appl Neurobiol. 2018 Feb;44(1):6–17. PMID:29359340
**4415.** Martelli H Jr, Pereira SM, Rocha TM, et al. White sponge nevus: report of a three-generation family. Oral Surg Oral Med Oral Pathol Oral Radiol Endod. 2007 Jan;103(1):43–7. PMID:17178493
**4416.** Martignetti JA, Tian L, Li D, et al. Mutations in PDGFRB cause autosomal-dominant infantile myofibromatosis. Am J Hum Genet. 2013 Jun 6;92(6):1001–7. PMID:23731542
**4417.** Martignoni G, Gobbo S, Camparo P, et al. Differential expression of cathepsin K in neoplasms harboring TFE3 gene fusions. Mod Pathol. 2011 Oct;24(10):1313–9. PMID:21602817
**4418.** Martignoni G, Pea M, Gobbo S, et al. Cathepsin-K immunoreactivity distinguishes MiTF/TFE family renal translocation carcinomas from other renal carcinomas. Mod Pathol. 2009 Aug;22(8):1016–22. PMID:19396149
**4419.** Martignoni G, Pea M, Zampini C, et al. PEComas of the kidney and of the genitourinary tract. Semin Diagn Pathol. 2015 Mar;32(2):140–59. PMID:25804448
**4420.** Martin C, McCarthy EF. Giant cell tumor of the sacrum and spine: series of 23 cases and a review of the literature. Iowa Orthop J. 2010;30:69–75. PMID:21045974
**4421.** Martin E, Coert JH, Flucke UE, et al. Neurofibromatosis-associated malignant peripheral nerve sheath tumors in children have a worse prognosis: a nationwide cohort study. Pediatr Blood Cancer. 2020 Apr;67(4):e28138. PMID:31889416
**4422.** Martin E, Minet N, Boschat AC, et al. Impaired lymphocyte function and differentiation in CTPS1-deficient patients result from a hypomorphic homozygous mutation. JCI Insight. 2020 Mar 12;5(5):133880. PMID:32161190
**4423.** Martin E, Muskens IS, Coert JH, et al. Treatment and survival differences across tumor sites in malignant peripheral nerve sheath tumors: a SEER database analysis and review of the literature. Neurooncol Pract. 2019 Mar;6(2):134–43. PMID:31386019
**4424.** Martin J, Chung P, Warde P. Treatment options, prognostic factors and selection of treatment in stage I seminoma. Onkologie. 2006 Dec;29(12):592–8. PMID:17202831
**4425.** Martin L, Combemale P, Dupin M, et al. The atrophic variant of dermatofibrosarcoma protuberans in childhood: a report of six cases. Br J Dermatol. 1998 Oct;139(4):719–25. PMID:10025975
**4426.** Martin SE, Dwyer A, Kissane JM, et al. Small-cell osteosarcoma. Cancer. 1982 Sep 1;50(5):990–6. PMID:6953993
**4427.** Martinelli S, Stellacci E, Pannone L, et al. Molecular diversity and associated phenotypic spectrum of germline CBL mutations. Hum Mutat. 2015 Aug;36(8):787–96. PMID:25952305
**4428.** Martinez D, Valera A, Perez NS, et al. Plasmablastic transformation of low-grade B-cell lymphomas: report on 6 cases. Am J Surg Pathol. 2013 Feb;37(2):272–81. PMID:23282972
**4429.** Martinez V, Sissons HA. Aneurysmal bone cyst. A review of 123 cases including primary lesions and those secondary to other bone pathology. Cancer. 1988 Jun 1;61(11):2291–304. PMID:2835141
**4430.** Martinez Álvarez S, Azorín Cuadrillero DL, Little KJ. Bizarre parosteal osteochondromatous proliferation (Nora lesion) in pediatric phalanges. J Hand Surg Am. 2021 Apr;46(4):344.e1–e9. PMID:32611484
**4431.** Martinez-Diaz H, Kleinschmidt-DeMasters BK, Powell SZ, et al. Giant cell glioblastoma and pleomorphic xanthoastrocytoma show different immunohistochemical profiles for neuronal antigens and p53 but share reactivity for class III beta-tubulin. Arch Pathol Lab Med. 2003 Sep;127(9):1187–91. PMID:12946225
**4432.** Martinez-Lopez A, Salvador-Rodriguez L, Montero-Vilchez T, et al. Vascular malformations syndromes: an update. Curr Opin Pediatr. 2019 Dec;31(6):747–53. PMID:31693582
**4433.** Martin-Guerrero I, Salaverria I, Burkhardt B, et al. Recurrent loss of heterozygosity in 1p36 associated with TNFRSF14 mutations in IRF4 translocation negative pediatric follicular lymphomas. Haematologica. 2013 Aug;98(8):1237–41. PMID:23445872
**4434.** Martins C, Fonseca I, Roque L, et al. PLAG1 gene alterations in salivary gland pleomorphic adenoma and carcinoma ex-pleomorphic adenoma: a combined study using chromosome banding, in situ hybridization and immunocytochemistry. Mod Pathol. 2005 Aug;18(8):1048–55. PMID:15920557
**4435.** Martins da Silva V, Martinez-Barrios E, Tell-Martí G, et al. Genetic abnormalities in large to giant congenital nevi: beyond NRAS mutations. J Invest Dermatol. 2019 Apr;139(4):900–8. PMID:30359577
**4436.** Martins R, Bugalho MJ. Paragangliomas/pheochromocytomas: clinically oriented genetic testing. Int J Endocrinol. 2014;2014:794187. PMID:24899893
**4437.** Martins-Filho SN, Almeida MQ, Soares I, et al. Clinical impact of pathological features including the Ki-67 labeling index on diagnosis and prognosis of adult and pediatric adrenocortical tumors. Endocr Pathol. 2021 Jun;32(2):288–300. PMID:33443677
**4438.** Martorell-Calatayud A, Sanz-Motilva V, Garcia-Sales MA, et al. Linear syringocystadenoma papilliferum: an uncommon event with a favorable prognosis. Dermatol Online J. 2011 Aug 15;17(8):5. PMID:21906485
**4439.** Martos-Moreno GÁ, de Prada I, Riñón C, et al. Vulvar fetal rhabdomyoma mimicking 46XX sex differentiation disorder. J Pediatr Endocrinol Metab. 2016 Feb;29(2):217–20. PMID:26352088
**4440.** Martuza RL, Eldridge R. Neurofibromatosis 2 (bilateral acoustic neurofibromatosis). N Engl J Med. 1988 Mar 17;318(11):684–8. PMID:3125435
**4441.** Marzec M, Kasprzycka M, Liu X, et al. Oncogenic tyrosine kinase NPM/ALK induces activation of the MEK/ERK signaling pathway independently of c-Raf. Oncogene. 2007 Feb 8;26(6):813–21. PMID:16909118
**4442.** Mas C, Penny DJ, Menahem S. Pre-excitation syndrome secondary to cardiac rhabdomyomas in tuberous sclerosis. J Paediatr Child Health. 2000 Feb;36(1):84–6. PMID:10723700
**4443.** Masciari S, Dillon DA, Rath M, et al. Breast cancer phenotype in women with TP53 germline mutations: a Li-Fraumeni syndrome consortium effort. Breast Cancer Res Treat. 2012 Jun;133(3):1125–30. PMID:22392042
**4444.** Masciari S, Van den Abbeele AD, Diller LR, et al. F18-fluorodeoxyglucose-positron emission tomography/computed tomography screening in Li-Fraumeni syndrome. JAMA. 2008 Mar 19;299(11):1315–9. PMID:18349092
**4445.** Masciocchi C, Zugaro L, Arrigoni F, et al. Radiofrequency ablation versus magnetic resonance guided focused ultrasound surgery for minimally invasive treatment of osteoid osteoma: a propensity score matching study. Eur Radiol. 2016 Aug;26(8):2472–81. PMID:26612546
**4446.** Masetti R, Bertuccio SN, Pession A, et al. CBFA2T3-GLIS2-positive acute myeloid leukaemia. A peculiar paediatric entity. Br J Haematol. 2019 Feb;184(3):337–47. PMID:30592296
**4447.** Mashiah J, Hadj-Rabia S, Dompmartin A, et al. Infantile myofibromatosis: a series of 28 cases. J Am Acad Dermatol. 2014 Aug;71(2):264–70. PMID:24894456
**4448.** Masliah-Planchon J, Machet MC, Fréneaux P, et al. SMARCA4-mutated atypical teratoid/rhabdoid tumor with retained BRG1 expression. Pediatr Blood Cancer. 2016 Mar;63(3):568–9. PMID:26469284
**4449.** Mas-Moya J, Dudley B, Brand RE, et al. Clinicopathological comparison of colorectal and endometrial carcinomas in patients with Lynch-like syndrome versus patients with Lynch syndrome. Hum Pathol. 2015 Nov;46(11):1616–25. PMID:26319271
**4450.** Masnari O, Neuhaus K, Aegerter T, et al. Predictors of health-related quality of life and psychological adjustment in children and adolescents with congenital melanocytic nevi: analysis of parent reports. J Pediatr Psychol. 2019 Jul 1;44(6):714–25. PMID:30916755
**4451.** Mason EF, Hornick JL. Conventional risk stratification fails to predict progression of succinate dehydrogenase-deficient gastrointestinal stromal tumors: a clinicopathologic study of 76 cases. Am J Surg Pathol. 2016 Dec;40(12):1616–21. PMID:27340750
**4452.** Mason KA, Navaratnam A, Theodorakopoulou E, et al. Nasal chondromesenchymal hamartoma (NCMH): a systematic review of the literature with a new case report. J Otolaryngol Head Neck Surg. 2015 Jul 3;44:28. PMID:26138824
**4453.** Masqué-Soler N, Szczepanowski M, Kohler CW, et al. Clinical and pathological features of Burkitt lymphoma showing expression of BCL2–an analysis including gene expression in formalin-fixed paraffin-embedded tissue. Br J Haematol. 2015 Nov;171(4):501–8. PMID:26218299
**4454.** Massei F, Laccetta G, Barrani M, et al. Osteoid osteoma mimicking monoarticular juvenile idiopathic arthritis in a girl. Pediatr Int. 2016 Aug;58(8):791–4. PMID:27325304
**4455.** Massengill JB, Sample KM, Pilarski R, et al. Analysis of the exome aggregation consortium (ExAC) database suggests that the BAP1-tumor predisposition syndrome is underreported in cancer patients. Genes Chromosomes Cancer. 2018 Sep;57(9):478–81. PMID:29761599
**4456.** Massimino M, Antonelli M, Gandola L, et al. Histological variants of medulloblastoma are the most powerful clinical prognostic indicators. Pediatr Blood Cancer. 2013 Feb;60(2):210–6. PMID:22693015
**4457.** Massimino M, Miceli R, Giangaspero F, et al. Final results of the second prospective AIEOP protocol for pediatric intracranial ependymoma. Neuro Oncol. 2016 Oct;18(10):1451–60. PMID:27194148
**4458.** Massone C, Kodama K, Salmhofer W, et al. Lupus erythematosus panniculitis (lupus profundus): clinical, histopathological, and molecular analysis of nine cases. J Cutan Pathol. 2005 Jul;32(6):396–404. PMID:15953372
**4459.** Mastboom MJL, Hoek DM, Bovée JVMG, et al. Does CSF1 overexpression or rearrangement influence biological behaviour in tenosynovial giant cell tumours of the knee? Histopathology. 2019 Jan;74(2):332–40. PMID:30152874
**4460.** Mastboom MJL, Palmerini E, Verspoor FGM, et al. Surgical outcomes of patients with diffuse-type tenosynovial giant-cell tumours: an international, retrospective, cohort study. Lancet Oncol. 2019 Jun;20(6):877–86. PMID:31029509
**4461.** Mastboom MJL, Verspoor FGM, Uittenbogaard D, et al. Tenosynovial giant cell tumors in children: a similar entity compared with adults. Clin Orthop Relat Res. 2018 Sep;476(9):1803–12. PMID:29494352
**4462.** Mastboom MJL, Verspoor FGM, Verschoor AJ, et al. Higher incidence rates than previously known in tenosynovial giant cell tumors. Acta Orthop. 2017 Dec;88(6):688–94. PMID:28787222
**4463.** Mastrangelo T, Modena P, Tornielli S, et al. A novel zinc finger gene is fused to EWS in small round cell tumor. Oncogene. 2000 Aug 3;19(33):3799–804. PMID:10949935
**4464.** Mastropolo R, Close A, Allen SW, et al. BRAF-V600E-mutated Rosai-Dorfman-Destombes disease and Langerhans cell histiocytosis with response to BRAF inhibitor. Blood Adv. 2019 Jun 25;3(12):1848–53. PMID:31213430
**4465.** Matarazzo P, Tuli G, Tessaris D, et al. Cushing syndrome due to ectopic adrenocorticotropic hormone secretion in a 3-year-old child. J Pediatr Endocrinol Metab. 2011;24(3-4):219–22. PMID:21648297
**4466.** Mathew A, Abuhammour W, Fathalla B, et al. Parvovirus B19 infection mimicking juvenile myelomonocytic leukemia in an immunocompetent child. Cureus. 2020 Jun 26;12(6):e8854. PMID:32754395
**4467.** Mathew J, Sen S, Chandi SM, et al. Pulmonary lipoblastoma: a case report. Pediatr Surg Int. 2001 Sep;17(7):543–4. PMID:11666056
**4468.** Mathew L, George R, Meeniga RS, et al. Peripheral arteriovenous malformations-a case series. Indian Dermatol Online J. 2020 May 10;11(3):367–72. PMID:32695695
**4469.** Mathew S, Ali SZ. Parotid fine-needle aspiration: a cytologic study of pediatric lesions. Diagn Cytopathol. 1997 Jul;17(1):8–13. PMID:9218896
**4470.** Mathews J, Duncavage EJ, Pfeifer JD. Characterization of translocations in mesenchymal hamartoma and undifferentiated embryonal sarcoma of the liver. Exp Mol Pathol. 2013 Dec;95(3):319–24. PMID:24120702
**4471.** Mathias MD, Ambati SR, Chou AJ, et al. A single-center experience with undifferentiated embryonal sarcoma of the liver. Pediatr Blood Cancer. 2016 Dec;63(12):2246–8. PMID:27427850
**4472.** Mathios AJ, McCausland AM. Basal cell carcinoma originating in a benign cystic teratoma of the ovary. Obstet Gynecol. 1973 Dec;42(6):892–6. PMID:4757597
**4473.** Matsumoto K, Irie F, Mackem S, et al. A mouse model of chondrocyte-specific somatic mutation reveals a role for Ext1 loss of heterozygosity in multiple hereditary

exostoses. Proc Natl Acad Sci U S A. 2010 Jun 15;107(24):10932–7. PMID:20534475
**4474.** Matsumoto K, Kakizaki H, Yagihashi N, et al. Malignant glomus tumor in the branchial muscle of a 16-year-old girl. Pathol Int. 2001 Sep;51(9):729–34. PMID:11696178
**4475.** Matsumura N, Natsume A, Maeda S, et al. Malignant transformation of a dysembryoplastic neuroepithelial tumor verified by a shared copy number gain of the tyrosine kinase domain of FGFR1. Brain Tumor Pathol. 2020 Apr;37(2):69–75. PMID:32297014
**4476.** Matsumura N, Nobusawa S, Ito J, et al. Multiplex ligation-dependent probe amplification analysis is useful for detecting a copy number gain of the FGFR1 tyrosine kinase domain in dysembryoplastic neuroepithelial tumors. J Neurooncol. 2019 May;143(1):27–33. PMID:30825062
**4477.** Matsuno R, Gifford AJ, Fang J, et al. Rare MYC-amplified neuroblastoma with large cell histology. Pediatr Dev Pathol. 2018 Sep-Oct;21(5):461–6. PMID:29426276
**4478.** Matsuno T, Unni KK, McLeod RA, et al. Telangiectatic osteogenic sarcoma. Cancer. 1976 Dec;38(6):2538–47. PMID:1069603
**4479.** Matsutani M, Japanese Pediatric Brain Tumor Study Group. Combined chemotherapy and radiation therapy for CNS germ cell tumors–the Japanese experience. J Neurooncol. 2001 Sep;54(3):311–6. PMID:11767296
**4480.** Matsutani M, Sano K, Takakura K, et al. Primary intracranial germ cell tumors: a clinical analysis of 153 histologically verified cases. J Neurosurg. 1997 Mar;86(3):446–55. PMID:9046301
**4481.** Matsuyama A, Hisaoka M, Shimajiri S, et al. Molecular detection of FUS-CREB3L2 fusion transcripts in low-grade fibromyxoid sarcoma using formalin-fixed, paraffin-embedded tissue specimens. Am J Surg Pathol. 2006 Sep;30(9):1077–84. PMID:16931951
**4482.** Matsuyama A, Shiba E, Umekita Y, et al. Clinicopathologic diversity of undifferentiated sarcoma with BCOR-CCNB3 fusion: analysis of 11 cases with a reappraisal of the utility of immunohistochemistry for BCOR and CCNB3. Am J Surg Pathol. 2017 Dec;41(12):1713–21. PMID:28877060
**4483.** Mattei TA, Nogueira GF, Ramina R. Juvenile nasopharyngeal angiofibroma with intracranial extension. Otolaryngol Head Neck Surg. 2011 Sep;145(3):498–504. PMID:21572079
**4484.** Mautner VF, Tatagiba M, Lindenau M, et al. Spinal tumors in patients with neurofibromatosis type 2: MR imaging study of frequency, multiplicity, and variety. AJR Am J Roentgenol. 1995 Oct;165(4):951–5. PMID:7676998
**4485.** Mavros MN, Mayo SC, Hyder O, et al. A systematic review: treatment and prognosis of patients with fibrolamellar hepatocellular carcinoma. J Am Coll Surg. 2012 Dec;215(6):820–30. PMID:22981432
**4486.** Maxson JE, Ries RE, Wang YC, et al. CSF3R mutations have a high degree of overlap with CEBPA mutations in pediatric AML. Blood. 2016 Jun 16;127(24):3094–8. PMID:27143256
**4487.** Mayor PC, Eng KH, Singel KL, et al. Cancer in primary immunodeficiency diseases: cancer incidence in the United States Immune Deficiency Network Registry. J Allergy Clin Immunol. 2018 Mar;141(3):1028–35. PMID:28606585
**4488.** Mayorandan S, Meyer U, Gokcay G, et al. Cross-sectional study of 168 patients with hepatorenal tyrosinaemia and implications for clinical practice. Orphanet J Rare Dis. 2014 Aug 1;9:107. PMID:25081276
**4488A.** Mayr D, Kaltz-Wittmer C, Arbogast S, et al. Characteristic pattern of genetic aberrations in ovarian granulosa cell tumors. Mod Pathol. 2002 Sep;15(9):951–7. PMID:12218213
**4489.** Mazereeuw-Hautier J, Thibaut I, Bonafé JL. Acantholytic dyskeratotic epidermal nevus: a rare histopathologic feature. J Cutan Pathol. 2002 Jan;29(1):52–4. PMID:11841519
**4490.** Mazzaferro V, Regalia E, Doci R, et al. Liver transplantation for the treatment of small hepatocellular carcinomas in patients with cirrhosis. N Engl J Med. 1996 Mar 14;334(11):693–9. PMID:8594428
**4491.** Mbagwu M, Rahmani B, Srivastava A, et al. Unsuspected ganglioneuroma of the choroid diagnosed after enucleation. Ocul Oncol Pathol. 2015 Sep;2(1):48–50. PMID:27171204
**4492.** Mbulaiteye SM, Anderson WF, Bhatia K, et al. Trimodal age-specific incidence patterns for Burkitt lymphoma in the United States, 1973-2005. Int J Cancer. 2010 Apr 1;126(7):1732–9. PMID:19810101
**4493.** Mbulaiteye SM, Anderson WF, Ferlay J, et al. Pediatric, elderly, and emerging adult-onset peaks in Burkitt's lymphoma incidence diagnosed in four continents, excluding Africa. Am J Hematol. 2012 Jun;87(6):573–8. PMID:22488262
**4494.** Mbulaiteye SM, Biggar RJ, Bhatia K, et al. Sporadic childhood Burkitt lymphoma incidence in the United States during 1992-2005. Pediatr Blood Cancer. 2009 Sep;53(3):366–70. PMID:19434731
**4495.** McAteer JP, Goldin AB, Healey PJ, et al. Surgical treatment of primary liver tumors in children: outcomes analysis of resection and transplantation in the SEER database. Pediatr Transplant. 2013 Dec;17(8):744–50. PMID:23992390
**4496.** McAteer JP, Huaco JA, Gow KW. Predictors of survival in pediatric adrenocortical carcinoma: a Surveillance, Epidemiology, and End Results (SEER) Program study. J Pediatr Surg. 2013 May;48(5):1025–31. PMID:23701777
**4497.** McCarten KM, Nadel HR, Shulkin BL, et al. Imaging for diagnosis, staging and response assessment of Hodgkin lymphoma and non-Hodgkin lymphoma. Pediatr Radiol. 2019 Oct;49(11):1545–64. PMID:31620854
**4498.** McClatchey AI, Giovannini M. Membrane organization and tumorigenesis–the NF2 tumor suppressor, Merlin. Genes Dev. 2005 Oct 1;19(19):2265–77. PMID:16204178
**4499.** McClelland S 3rd, Hentea C, Fan R, et al. Role of radiation therapy for pediatric upper extremity extraskeletal osteosarcoma: a case series. Pediatr Blood Cancer. 2020 Feb;67(2):e28018. PMID:31710168
**4500.** McCloskey JJ, Germain-Lee EL, Perman JA, et al. Gynecomastia as a presenting sign of fibrolamellar carcinoma of the liver. Pediatrics. 1988 Sep;82(3):379–82. PMID:2841641
**4501.** McCluggage WG, Ashe P, McBride H, et al. Localization of the cellular expression of inhibin in trophoblastic tissue. Histopathology. 1998 Mar;32(3):252–6. PMID:9568511
**4502.** McCluggage WG, Bissonnette JP, Young RH. Primary malignant melanoma of the ovary: a report of 9 definite or probable cases with emphasis on their morphologic diversity and mimicry of other primary and secondary ovarian neoplasms. Int J Gynecol Pathol. 2006 Oct;25(4):321–9. PMID:16990706
**4503.** McCluggage WG, Chong AL, de Kock L, et al. Somatic tumour testing establishes that bilateral DICER1-associated ovarian Sertoli-Leydig cell tumours represent independent primary neoplasms. Histopathology. 2020 Aug;77(2):223–30. PMID:32333409
**4504.** McCluggage WG, Connolly L, McBride HA. HMGA2 is a sensitive but not specific immunohistochemical marker of vulvovaginal aggressive angiomyxoma. Am J Surg Pathol. 2010 Jul;34(7):1037–42. PMID:20551826
**4505.** McCluggage WG, McKenna M, McBride HA. CD56 is a sensitive and diagnostically useful immunohistochemical marker of ovarian sex cord-stromal tumors. Int J Gynecol Pathol. 2007 Jul;26(3):322–7. PMID:17581419
**4506.** McCluggage WG, Nirmala V, Radhakumari K. Intramural müllerian papilloma of the vagina. Int J Gynecol Pathol. 1999 Jan;18(1):94–5. PMID:9891250
**4507.** McCluggage WG, Oliva E, Connolly LE, et al. An immunohistochemical analysis of ovarian small cell carcinoma of hypercalcemic type. Int J Gynecol Pathol. 2004 Oct;23(4):330–6. PMID:15381902
**4508.** McCluggage WG, Witkowski L, Clarke BA, et al. Clinical, morphological and immunohistochemical evidence that small-cell carcinoma of the ovary of hypercalcaemic type (SCCOHT) may be a primitive germ-cell neoplasm. Histopathology. 2017 Jun;70(7):1147–54. PMID:28130795
**4509.** McCluggage WG, Young RH. Immunohistochemistry as a diagnostic aid in the evaluation of ovarian tumors. Semin Diagn Pathol. 2005 Feb;22(1):3–32. PMID:16512597
**4510.** McConechy MK, Färkkilä A, Horlings HM, et al. Molecularly defined adult granulosa cell tumor of the ovary: the clinical phenotype. J Natl Cancer Inst. 2016 Jun 13;108(11):djw134. PMID:27297428
**4511.** McCormack A, Dekkers OM, Petersenn S, et al. Treatment of aggressive pituitary tumours and carcinomas: results of a European Society of Endocrinology (ESE) survey 2016. Eur J Endocrinol. 2018 Mar;178(3):265–76. PMID:29330228
**4512.** McCracken JA, Gonzales MF, Phal PM, et al. Angiocentric glioma transformed into anaplastic ependymoma: review of the evidence for malignant potential. J Clin Neurosci. 2016 Dec;34:47–52. PMID:27742374
**4513.** McCrary HC, Babajanian E, Calquin M, et al. Characterization of malignant head and neck paragangliomas at a single institution across multiple decades. JAMA Otolaryngol Head Neck Surg. 2019 Jul 1;145(7):641–6. PMID:31194233
**4514.** McCullagh M, Keen C, Dykes E. Cystic mesothelioma of the peritoneum: a rare cause of 'ascites' in children. J Pediatr Surg. 1994 Sep;29(9):1205–7. PMID:7528798
**4515.** McDermott MB, Ponder TB, Dehner LP. Nasal chondromesenchymal hamartoma: an upper respiratory tract analogue of the chest wall mesenchymal hamartoma. Am J Surg Pathol. 1998 Apr;22(4):425–33. PMID:9537469
**4516.** McDonald OG, Rodriguez R, Bergner A, et al. Metanephric stromal tumor arising in a patient with neurofibromatosis type 1 syndrome. Int J Surg Pathol. 2011 Oct;19(5):667–71. PMID:19875383
**4517.** McEvoy J, Nagahawatte P, Finkelstein D, et al. RB1 gene inactivation by chromothripsis in human retinoblastoma. Oncotarget. 2014 Jan 30;5(2):438–50. PMID:24509483
**4518.** McGinnis M, Jacobs G, el-Naggar A, et al. Congenital peribronchial myofibroblastic tumor (so-called "congenital leiomyosarcoma"). A distinct neonatal lung lesion associated with nonimmune hydrops fetalis. Mod Pathol. 1993 Jul;6(4):487–92. PMID:8415597
**4519.** McGirt LY, Jia P, Baerenwald DA, et al. Whole-genome sequencing reveals oncogenic mutations in mycosis fungoides. Blood. 2015 Jul 23;126(4):508–19. PMID:26082451
**4520.** McGuire CS, Sainani KL, Fisher PG. Incidence patterns for ependymoma: a Surveillance, Epidemiology, and End Results study. J Neurosurg. 2009 Apr;110(4):725–9. PMID:19061350
**4521.** McIntyre A, Summersgill B, Grygalewicz B, et al. Amplification and overexpression of the KIT gene is associated with progression in the seminoma subtype of testicular germ cell tumors of adolescents and adults. Cancer Res. 2005 Sep 15;65(18):8085–9. PMID:16166280
**4522.** McKay P, Fielding P, Gallop-Evans E, et al. Guidelines for the investigation and management of nodular lymphocyte predominant Hodgkin lymphoma. Br J Haematol. 2016 Jan;172(1):32–43. PMID:26538004
**4523.** McKee PH, Fletcher CD. Dermatofibrosarcoma protuberans presenting in infancy and childhood. J Cutan Pathol. 1991 Aug;18(4):241–6. PMID:1939782
**4524.** McKenney JK, Heerema-McKenney A, Rouse RV. Extragonadal germ cell tumors: a review with emphasis on pathologic features, clinical prognostic variables, and differential diagnostic considerations. Adv Anat Pathol. 2007 Mar;14(2):69–92. PMID:17471115
**4525.** McKenney JK, Przybycin CG, Trpkov K, et al. Eosinophilic solid and cystic renal cell carcinomas have metastatic potential. Histopathology. 2018 May;72(6):1066–7. PMID:29265482
**4526.** McKenney JK, Soslow RA, Longacre TA. Ovarian mature teratomas with mucinous epithelial neoplasms: morphologic heterogeneity and association with pseudomyxoma peritonei. Am J Surg Pathol. 2008 May;32(5):645–55. PMID:18344868
**4527.** McKinney M, Moffitt AB, Gaulard P, et al. The genetic basis of hepatosplenic T-cell lymphoma. Cancer Discov. 2017 Apr;7(4):369–79. PMID:28122867
**4528.** McLaughlin CC, Baptiste MS, Schymura MJ, et al. Maternal and infant birth characteristics and hepatoblastoma. Am J Epidemiol. 2006 May 1;163(9):818–28. PMID:16510543
**4529.** McLean CK, Squires JH, Reyes-Múgica M, et al. Hepatic vascular tumors in the neonate: angiosarcoma. J Pediatr. 2018 Feb;193:245–248.e1. PMID:29198544
**4530.** McLeod DS, Watters KF, Carpenter AD, et al. Thyrotropin and thyroid cancer diagnosis: a systematic review and dose-response meta-analysis. J Clin Endocrinol Metab. 2012 Aug;97(8):2682–92. PMID:22622023
**4531.** McLeod RA, Beabout JW. The roentgenographic features of chondroblastoma. Am J Roentgenol Radium Ther Nucl Med. 1973 Jun;118(2):464–71. PMID:4712761
**4532.** McMahon RT, Font RL, McLean IW. Phakomatous choristoma of eyelid: electron microscopical confirmation of lenticular derivation. Arch Ophthalmol. 1976 Oct;94(10):1778–81. PMID:973823
**4533.** McManamy CS, Lamont JM, Taylor RE, et al. Morphophenotypic variation predicts clinical behavior in childhood non-desmoplastic medulloblastomas. J Neuropathol Exp Neurol. 2003 Jun;62(6):627–32. PMID:12834107
**4534.** McManamy CS, Pears J, Weston CL, et al. Nodule formation and desmoplasia in medulloblastomas-defining the nodular/desmoplastic variant and its biological behavior. Brain Pathol. 2007 Apr;17(2):151–64. PMID:17388946
**4535.** McMaster ML, Goldstein AM, Parry DM. Clinical features distinguish childhood chordoma associated with tuberous sclerosis complex (TSC) from chordoma in the general paediatric population. J Med Genet. 2011 Jul;48(7):444–9. PMID:21266383
**4536.** McMenamin ME, Fletcher CD. Expanding the spectrum of malignant change in schwannomas: epithelioid malignant change, epithelioid malignant peripheral nerve sheath tumor, and epithelioid angiosarcoma: a study of 17 cases. Am J Surg Pathol. 2001 Jan;25(1):13–25. PMID:11145248
**4537.** McMenamin ME, Fletcher CD. Malignant myopericytoma: expanding the spectrum of tumours with myopericytic differentiation. Histopathology. 2002 Nov;41(5):450–60. PMID:12405913

4538. McNamara C, Davies J, Dyer M, et al. Guidelines on the investigation and management of follicular lymphoma. Br J Haematol. 2012 Feb;156(4):446–67. PMID:22211428
4539. McNulty SN, Evenson MJ, Corliss MM, et al. Diagnostic utility of next-generation sequencing for disorders of somatic mosaicism: a five-year cumulative cohort. Am J Hum Genet. 2019 Oct 3;105(4):734–46. PMID:31585106
4540. McQuillan SK, Grover SR, Pyman J, et al. Literature review of benign müllerian papilloma contrasted with vaginal rhabdomyosarcoma. J Pediatr Adolesc Gynecol. 2016 Aug;29(4):333–7. PMID:26948653
4541. McReynolds LJ, Savage SA. Pediatric leukemia susceptibility disorders: manifestations and management. Hematology Am Soc Hematol Educ Program. 2017 Dec 8;2017(1):242–50. PMID:29222262
4542. McThenia SS, Rawwas J, Oliveira JL, et al. Hepatosplenic γδ T-cell lymphoma of two adolescents: case report and retrospective literature review in children, adolescents, and young adults. Pediatr Transplant. 2018 Aug;22(5):e13213. PMID:29921021
4543. McWhinney SR, Pasini B, Stratakis CA, et al. Familial gastrointestinal stromal tumors and germ-line mutations. N Engl J Med. 2007 Sep 6;357(10):1054–6. PMID:17804857
4544. McWhorter HE, Woolner LB. Pigmented nevi, juvenile melanomas and malignant melanomas in children. Cancer. 1954 May;7(3):564–85. PMID:13160941
4545. McWilliams GD, SantaCruz K, Hart B, et al. Occurrence of DNET and other brain tumors in Noonan syndrome warrants caution with growth hormone therapy. Am J Med Genet A. 2016 Jan;170A(1):195–201. PMID:26377682
4546. Meadows AT, Friedman DL, Neglia JP, et al. Second neoplasms in survivors of childhood cancer: findings from the Childhood Cancer Survivor Study cohort. J Clin Oncol. 2009 May 10;27(14):2356–62. PMID:19255307
4547. Meadows AT, Strong LC, Li FP, et al. Bone sarcoma as a second malignant neoplasm in children: influence of radiation and genetic predisposition for the Late Effects Study Group. Cancer. 1980 Dec 15;46(12):2603–6. PMID:7448699
4548. Meany H, Dombi E, Reynolds J, et al. 18-fluorodeoxyglucose-positron emission tomography (FDG-PET) evaluation of nodular lesions in patients with Neurofibromatosis type 1 and plexiform neurofibromas (PN) or malignant peripheral nerve sheath tumors (MPNST). Pediatr Blood Cancer. 2013 Jan;60(1):59–64. PMID:22645095
4549. Meazza C, Bisogno G, Gronchi A, et al. Aggressive fibromatosis in children and adolescents: the Italian experience. Cancer. 2010 Jan 1;116(1):233–40. PMID:19950127
4550. Medeiros F, Erickson-Johnson MR, Keeney GL, et al. Frequency and characterization of HMGA2 and HMGA1 rearrangements in mesenchymal tumors of the lower genital tract. Genes Chromosomes Cancer. 2007 Nov;46(11):981–90. PMID:17654722
4551. Medeiros LJ, Palmedo G, Krigman HR, et al. Oncocytoid renal cell carcinoma after neuroblastoma: a report of four cases of a distinct clinicopathologic entity. Am J Surg Pathol. 1999 Jul;23(7):772–80. PMID:10403299
4552. Medhkour A, Traul D, Husain M. Neonatal subependymal giant cell astrocytoma. Pediatr Neurosurg. 2002 May;36(5):271–4. PMID:12053047
4553. Medvedev AE, Trufanova LV, Golubenko AV, et al. [The role of inner membrane in the realization of cAMP-dependent activation of mitochondrial enzymes]. Biokhimiia. 1990 Feb;55(2):225–31. Russian. PMID:2160290
4554. Meech SJ, McGavran L, Odom LF, et al. Unusual childhood extramedullary hematologic malignancy with natural killer cell properties that contains tropomyosin 4–anaplastic lymphoma kinase gene fusion. Blood. 2001 Aug 15;98(4):1209–16. PMID:11493472
4555. Mehollin-Ray AR, Kozinetz CA, Schlesinger AE, et al. Radiographic abnormalities in Rothmund-Thomson syndrome and genotype-phenotype correlation with RECQL4 mutation status. AJR Am J Roentgenol. 2008 Aug;191(2):W62-6. PMID:18647888
4556. Mehra R, Vats P, Cao X, et al. Somatic bi-allelic loss of TSC genes in eosinophilic solid and cystic renal cell carcinoma. Eur Urol. 2018 Oct;74(4):483–6. PMID:29941307
4557. Mei K, Liu A, Allan RW, et al. Diagnostic utility of SALL4 in primary germ cell tumors of the central nervous system: a study of 77 cases. Mod Pathol. 2009 Dec;22(12):1628–36. PMID:19820689
4558. Mei L, Smith SC, Faber AC, et al. Gastrointestinal stromal tumors: the GIST of precision medicine. Trends Cancer. 2018 Jan;4(1):74–91. PMID:29413424
4559. Meij BP, Lopes MB, Ellegala DB, et al. The long-term significance of microscopic dural invasion in 354 patients with pituitary adenomas treated with transsphenoidal surgery. J Neurosurg. 2002 Feb;96(2):195–208. PMID:11838791
4560. Meis JM, Dorfman HD, Nathanson SD, et al. Primary malignant giant cell tumor of bone: "dedifferentiated" giant cell tumor. Mod Pathol. 1989 Sep;2(5):541–6. PMID:2554283
4561. Meis JM, Enzinger FM, Martz KL, et al. Malignant peripheral nerve sheath tumors (malignant schwannomas) in children. Am J Surg Pathol. 1992 Jul;16(7):694–707. PMID:1530109
4562. Meis JM, Raymond AK, Evans HL, et al. "Dedifferentiated" chordoma. A clinicopathologic and immunohistochemical study of three cases. Am J Surg Pathol. 1987 Jul;11(7):516–25. PMID:2440324
4563. Meis-Kindblom JM, Bergh P, Gunterberg B, et al. Extraskeletal myxoid chondrosarcoma: a reappraisal of its morphologic spectrum and prognostic factors based on 117 cases. Am J Surg Pathol. 1999 Jun;23(6):636–50. PMID:10366145
4564. Meis-Kindblom JM, Kindblom LG, Enzinger FM. Sclerosing epithelioid fibrosarcoma. A variant of fibrosarcoma simulating carcinoma. Am J Surg Pathol. 1995 Sep;19(9):979–93. PMID:7661286
4565. Mejía Granados DM, de Baptista MB, Bonadia LC, et al. Clinical and molecular investigation of familial multiple lipomatosis: variants in the HMGA2 gene. Clin Cosmet Investig Dermatol. 2020 Jan 7;13:1–10. PMID:32021365
4566. Mejia-Guerrero S, Quejada M, Gokgoz N, et al. Characterization of the 12q15 MDM2 and 12q13-14 CDK4 amplicons and clinical correlations in osteosarcoma. Genes Chromosomes Cancer. 2010 Jun;49(6):518–25. PMID:20196171
4567. Mejía-Velázquez CP, Durán-Padilla MA, Gómez-Apo E, et al. Tumors of the salivary gland in Mexicans. A retrospective study of 360 cases. Med Oral Patol Oral Cir Bucal. 2012 Mar 1;17(2):e183–9. PMID:22143697
4568. Melani C, Jaffe ES, Wilson WH. Pathobiology and treatment of lymphomatoid granulomatosis, a rare EBV-driven disorder. Blood. 2020 Apr 16;135(16):1344–52. PMID:32107539
4569. Meletani T, Cantini L, Lanese A, et al. Are liver nested stromal epithelial tumors always low aggressive? World J Gastroenterol. 2017 Dec 14;23(46):8248–55. PMID:29290661
4570. Melkonian SC, Daniel CR, Ye Y, et al. Gene-environment interaction of genome-wide association study-identified susceptibility loci and meat-cooking mutagens in the etiology of renal cell carcinoma. Cancer. 2016 Jan 1;122(1):108–15. PMID:26551148
4571. Mellgren K, Attarbaschi A, Abla O, et al. Non-anaplastic peripheral T cell lymphoma in children and adolescents-an international review of 143 cases. Ann Hematol. 2016 Aug;95(8):1295–305. PMID:27270301
4572. Melloul S, Hélias-Rodzewicz Z, Cohen-Aubart F, et al. Highly sensitive methods are required to detect mutations in histiocytoses. Haematologica. 2019 Mar;104(3):e97–9. PMID:30262559
4573. Melnik BC, Vakilzadeh F, Aslanidis C, et al. Unilateral segmental acneiform naevus: a model disorder towards understanding fibroblast growth factor receptor 2 function in acne? Br J Dermatol. 2008 Jun;158(6):1397–9. PMID:18410418
4574. Melo JV. The diversity of BCR-ABL fusion proteins and their relationship to leukemia phenotype. Blood. 1996 Oct 1;88(7):2375–84. PMID:8839828
4575. Meloni-Ehrig AM, Riggott L, Christacos NC, et al. A case of lipoblastoma with seven copies of chromosome 8. Cancer Genet Cytogenet. 2009 Apr 1;190(1):49–51. PMID:19264235
4576. Mena H, Rushing EJ, Ribas JL, et al. Tumors of pineal parenchymal cells: a correlation of histological features, including nucleolar organizer regions, with survival in 35 cases. Hum Pathol. 1995 Jan;26(1):20–30. PMID:7821912
4577. Mendoza F, Kunitake H, Laks H, et al. Post-transplant lymphoproliferative disorder following pediatric heart transplantation. Pediatr Transplant. 2006 Feb;10(1):60–6. PMID:16499589
4578. Mendoza PR, Grossniklaus HE. The biology of retinoblastoma. Prog Mol Biol Transl Sci. 2015;134:503–16. PMID:26310174
4579. Mendoza PR, Specht CS, Hubbard GB, et al. Histopathologic grading of anaplasia in retinoblastoma. Am J Ophthalmol. 2015 Apr;159(4):764–76. PMID:25528954
4580. Meneses MF, Unni KK, Swee RG. Bizarre parosteal osteochondromatous proliferation of bone (Nora's lesion). Am J Surg Pathol. 1993 Jul;17(7):691–7. PMID:8317609
4581. Meng FJ, Zhou Y, Skakkebaek NE, et al. Detection and enrichment of carcinoma-in-situ cells in semen by an immunomagnetic method using monoclonal antibody M2A. Int J Androl. 1996 Dec;19(6):365–70. PMID:9051423
4582. Méni C, Bruneau J, Georgin-Lavialle S, et al. Paediatric mastocytosis: a systematic review of 1747 cases. Br J Dermatol. 2015 Mar;172(3):642–51. PMID:25662299
4583. Meni C, Georgin-Lavialle S, Le Saché de Peufeilhoux L, et al. Paediatric mastocytosis: long-term follow-up of 53 patients with whole sequencing of KIT. A prospective study. Br J Dermatol. 2018 Oct;179(4):925–32. PMID:29787623
4584. Menke JR, Raleigh DR, Gown AM, et al. Somatostatin receptor 2a is a more sensitive diagnostic marker of meningioma than epithelial membrane antigen. Acta Neuropathol. 2015 Sep;130(3):441–3. PMID:26195322
4585. Menter T, Gasser A, Juskevicius D, et al. Diagnostic utility of the germinal center-associated markers GCET1, HGAL, and LMO2 in hematolymphoid neoplasms. Appl Immunohistochem Mol Morphol. 2015 Aug;23(7):491–8. PMID:25203428
4586. Menter T, Juskevicius D, Alikian M, et al. Mutational landscape of B-cell post-transplant lymphoproliferative disorders. Br J Haematol. 2017 Jul;178(1):48–56. PMID:28419429
4587. Mentzel T, Beham A, Calonje E, et al. Epithelioid hemangioendothelioma of skin and soft tissues: clinicopathologic and immunohistochemical study of 30 cases. Am J Surg Pathol. 1997 Apr;21(4):363–74. PMID:9130982
4588. Mentzel T, Calonje E, Fletcher CD. Lipoblastoma and lipoblastomatosis: a clinicopathological study of 14 cases. Histopathology. 1993 Dec;23(6):527–33. PMID:8314236
4589. Mentzel T, Calonje E, Nascimento AG, et al. Infantile hemangiopericytoma versus infantile myofibromatosis. Study of a series suggesting a continuous spectrum of infantile myofibroblastic lesions. Am J Surg Pathol. 1994 Sep;18(9):922–30. PMID:8067513
4590. Mentzel T, Dei Tos AP, Sapi Z, et al. Myopericytoma of skin and soft tissues: clinicopathologic and immunohistochemical study of 54 cases. Am J Surg Pathol. 2006 Jan;30(1):104–13. PMID:16330949
4591. Mentzel T, Dry S, Katenkamp D, et al. Low-grade myofibroblastic sarcoma: analysis of 18 cases in the spectrum of myofibroblastic tumors. Am J Surg Pathol. 1998 Oct;22(10):1228–38. PMID:9777985
4592. Mentzel T, Katenkamp D. Intraneural angiosarcoma and angiosarcoma arising in benign and malignant peripheral nerve sheath tumours: clinicopathological and immunohistochemical analysis of four cases. Histopathology. 1999 Aug;35(2):114–20. PMID:10460655
4593. Mentzel T, Schildhaus HU, Palmedo G, et al. Postradiation cutaneous angiosarcoma after treatment of breast carcinoma is characterized by MYC amplification in contrast to atypical vascular lesions after radiotherapy and control cases: clinicopathological, immunohistochemical and molecular analysis of 66 cases. Mod Pathol. 2012 Jan;25(1):75–85. PMID:21909081
4594. Menze BH, Hamprecht FA. Multimodal medical image analysis: from visualization to disease modeling. Z Med Phys. 2011;21(1):1. PMID:21288704
4595. Meral Günes A, Millot F, Kalwak K, et al. Features and outcome of chronic myeloid leukemia at very young age: data from the International Pediatric Chronic Myeloid Leukemia Registry. Pediatr Blood Cancer. 2021 Jan;68(1):e28706. PMID:33034135
4596. Merard R, Ganesan R, Hirschowitz L. Growing teratoma syndrome: a report of 2 cases and review of the literature. Int J Gynecol Pathol. 2015 Sep;34(5):465–72. PMID:26262454
4597. Merchant TE, Bendel AE, Sabin ND, et al. Conformal radiation therapy for pediatric ependymoma, chemotherapy for incompletely resected ependymoma, and observation for completely resected, supratentorial ependymoma. J Clin Oncol. 2019 Apr 20;37(12):974–83. PMID:30811284
4598. Merchant TE, Li C, Xiong X, et al. Conformal radiotherapy after surgery for paediatric ependymoma: a prospective study. Lancet Oncol. 2009 Mar;10(3):258–66. PMID:19274783
4599. Merchant TE, Pollack IF, Loeffler JS. Brain tumors across the age spectrum: biology, therapy, and late effects. Semin Radiat Oncol. 2010 Jan;20(1):58–66. PMID:19959032
4600. Meredith DM, Fletcher CDM, Jo VY. Chondromyxoid fibroma arising in craniofacial sites: a clinicopathologic analysis of 25 cases. Am J Surg Pathol. 2018 Mar;42(3):392–400. PMID:29324473
4601. Mérel P, Hoang-Xuan K, Sanson M, et al. Screening for germ-line mutations in the NF2 gene. Genes Chromosomes Cancer. 1995 Feb;12(2):117–27. PMID:7535084
4602. Merfeld EC, Dahiya S, Perkins SM. Patterns of care and treatment outcomes of patients with astroblastoma: a National Cancer Database analysis. CNS Oncol. 2018 Apr;7(2):CNS13. PMID:29708401

**4603.** Meriden Z, Shi C, Edil BH, et al. Hyaline globules in neuroendocrine and solid-pseudopapillary neoplasms of the pancreas: a clue to the diagnosis. Am J Surg Pathol. 2011 Jul;35(7):981–8. PMID:21677537
**4604.** Merino DM, Shlien A, Villani A, et al. Molecular characterization of choroid plexus tumors reveals novel clinically relevant subgroups. Clin Cancer Res. 2015 Jan 1;21(1):184–92. PMID:25336695
**4605.** Merrow AC, Gupta A, Patel MN, et al. 2014 revised classification of vascular lesions from the International Society for the Study of Vascular Anomalies: radiologic-pathologic update. Radiographics. 2016 Sep-Oct;36(5):1494–516. PMID:27517361
**4606.** Mertens F, Fletcher CD, Antonescu CR, et al. Clinicopathologic and molecular genetic characterization of low-grade fibromyxoid sarcoma, and cloning of a novel FUS/CREB3L1 fusion gene. Lab Invest. 2005 Mar;85(3):408–15. PMID:15640831
**4607.** Mertens F, Möller E, Mandahl N, et al. The t(X;6) in subungual exostosis results in transcriptional deregulation of the gene for insulin receptor substrate 4. Int J Cancer. 2011 Jan 15;128(2):487–91. PMID:20340132
**4608.** Mertens F, Rydholm A, Brosjö O, et al. Hibernomas are characterized by rearrangements of chromosome bands 11q13-21. Int J Cancer. 1994 Aug 15;58(4):503–5. PMID:8056446
**4609.** Meru N, Davison S, Whitehead L, et al. Epstein-Barr virus infection in paediatric liver transplant recipients: detection of the virus in post-transplant tonsillectomy specimens. Mol Pathol. 2001 Aug;54(4):264–9. PMID:11477143
**4610.** Mervak TR, Unni KK, Pritchard DJ, et al. Telangiectatic osteosarcoma. Clin Orthop Relat Res. 1991 Sep; (270):135–9. PMID:1884532
**4611.** Meserve EE, Nucci MR. Peutz-Jeghers syndrome: pathobiology, pathologic manifestations, and suggestions for recommending genetic testing in pathology reports. Surg Pathol Clin. 2016 Jun;9(2):243–68. PMID:27241107
**4612.** Meshram GG, Kaur N, Hura KS. Pediatric pleomorphic adenoma of the parotid: case report, review of literature and novel therapeutic targets. Children (Basel). 2018 Sep 18;5(9):E127. PMID:30231590
**4613.** Messiaen L, Yao S, Brems H, et al. Clinical and mutational spectrum of neurofibromatosis type 1-like syndrome. JAMA. 2009 Nov 18;302(19):2111–8. PMID:19920235
**4614.** Messiaen LM, Callens T, Mortier G, et al. Exhaustive mutation analysis of the NF1 gene allows identification of 95% of mutations and reveals a high frequency of unusual splicing defects. Hum Mutat. 2000;15(6):541–55. PMID:10862084
**4615.** Messinger YH, Stewart DR, Priest JR, et al. Pleuropulmonary blastoma: a report on 350 central pathology-confirmed pleuropulmonary blastoma cases by the International Pleuropulmonary Blastoma Registry. Cancer. 2015 Jan 15;121(2):276–85. PMID:25209242
**4616.** Messing-Jünger AM, Floeth FW, Pauleit D, et al. Multimodal target point assessment for stereotactic biopsy in children with diffuse bithalamic astrocytomas. Childs Nerv Syst. 2002 Aug;18(8):445–9. PMID:12192504
**4617.** Mestach L, Polubothu S, Calder A, et al. Keratinocytic epidermal nevi associated with localized fibro-osseous lesions without hypophosphatemia. Pediatr Dermatol. 2020 Sep;37(5):890–5. PMID:32662096
**4618.** Mete O, Alshaikh OM, Cintosun A, et al. Synchronous multiple pituitary neuroendocrine tumors of different cell lineages. Endocr Pathol. 2018 Dec;29(4):332–8. PMID:30215160
**4619.** Mete O, Asa SL. Clinicopathological correlations in pituitary adenomas. Brain Pathol. 2012 Jul;22(4):443–53. PMID:22697380
**4620.** Mete O, Asa SL. Precursor lesions of endocrine system neoplasms. Pathology. 2013 Apr;45(3):316–30. PMID:23478233
**4621.** Mete O, Asa SL, Giordano TJ, et al. Immunohistochemical biomarkers of adrenal cortical neoplasms. Endocr Pathol. 2018 Jun;29(2):137–49. PMID:29542002
**4622.** Mete O, Cintosun A, Pressman I, et al. Epidemiology and biomarker profile of pituitary adenohypophysial tumors. Mod Pathol. 2018 Jun;31(6):900–9. PMID:29434339
**4623.** Mete O, Essa A, Bramdev A, et al. MEN2 syndrome-related medullary thyroid carcinoma with focal tyrosine hydroxylase expression: Does it represent a hybrid cellular phenotype or functional state of tumor cells? Endocr Pathol. 2017 Dec;28(4):362–6. PMID:28493102
**4624.** Mete O, Gomez-Hernandez K, Kucharczyk W, et al. Silent subtype 3 pituitary adenomas are not always silent and represent poorly differentiated monomorphous plurihormonal Pit-1 lineage adenomas. Mod Pathol. 2016 Feb;29(2):131–42. PMID:26743473
**4625.** Mete O, Kefeli M, Çalışkan S, et al. GATA3 immunoreactivity expands the transcription factor profile of pituitary neuroendocrine tumors. Mod Pathol. 2019 Apr;32(4):484–9. PMID:30390035
**4626.** Mete O, Lopes MB, Asa SL. Spindle cell oncocytomas and granular cell tumors of the pituitary are variants of pituicytoma. Am J Surg Pathol. 2013 Nov;37(11):1694–9. PMID:23887161
**4627.** Mete O, Tischler AS, de Krijger R, et al. Protocol for the examination of specimens from patients with pheochromocytomas and extra-adrenal paragangliomas. Arch Pathol Lab Med. 2014 Feb;138(2):182–8. PMID:24476517
**4628.** Metrock LK, Summers RJ, Park S, et al. Utility of peripheral blood immunophenotyping by flow cytometry in the diagnosis of pediatric acute leukemia. Pediatr Blood Cancer. 2017 Oct;64(10). PMID:28333411
**4629.** Metzger ML, Howard SC, Hudson MM, et al. Natural history of thyroid nodules in survivors of pediatric Hodgkin lymphoma. Pediatr Blood Cancer. 2006 Mar;46(3):314–9. PMID:16086425
**4630.** Metzger ML, Mauz-Körholz C. Epidemiology, outcome, targeted agents and immunotherapy in adolescent and young adult non-Hodgkin and Hodgkin lymphoma. Br J Haematol. 2019 Jun;185(6):1142–57. PMID:30729493
**4631.** Mewar P, González-Torres KE, Jacks TM, et al. Sinonasal myxoma: a distinct lesion of infants. Head Neck Pathol. 2020 Mar;14(1):212–9. PMID:30484069
**4632.** Meyer C, Burmeister T, Gröger D, et al. The MLL recombinome of acute leukemias in 2017. Leukemia. 2018 Feb;32(2):273–84. PMID:28701730
**4633.** Meyers PA, Gorlick R. Osteosarcoma. Pediatr Clin North Am. 1997 Aug;44(4):973–89. PMID:9286295
**4634.** Meyers SP, Khademian ZP, Biegel JA, et al. Primary intracranial atypical teratoid/rhabdoid tumors of infancy and childhood: MRI features and patient outcomes. AJNR Am J Neuroradiol. 2006 May;27(5):962–71. PMID:16687525
**4635.** Meyers SP, Khademian ZP, Chuang SH, et al. Choroid plexus carcinomas in children: MRI features and patient outcomes. Neuroradiology. 2004 Sep;46(9):770–80. PMID:15309348
**4636.** Meyran D, Petit A, Guilhot J, et al. Lymphoblastic predominance of blastic phase in children with chronic myeloid leukaemia treated with imatinib: a report from the I-CML-Ped Study. Eur J Cancer. 2020 Sep;137:224–34. PMID:32799036
**4637.** Meyronet D, Esteban-Mader M, Bonnet C, et al. Characteristics of H3 K27M-mutant gliomas in adults. Neuro Oncol. 2017 Aug 1;19(8):1127–34. PMID:28201752
**4638.** Mezmezian MB, Fernandez Ugazio G, Paparella ML. Histopathological features of malignant craniopharyngioma: case report and literature review. Clin Neuropathol. 2020 Jan/Feb;39(1):25–31. PMID:31661068
**4639.** Mhatre R, Sugur HS, Nandeesh BN, et al. MN1 rearrangement in astroblastoma: study of eight cases and review of literature. Brain Tumor Pathol. 2019 Jul;36(3):112–20. PMID:31111274
**4640.** Mialou V, Philip T, Kalifa C, et al. Metastatic osteosarcoma at diagnosis: prognostic factors and long-term outcome–the French pediatric experience. Cancer. 2005 Sep 1;104(5):1100–9. PMID:16015627
**4641.** Michael H, Lucia J, Foster RS, et al. The pathology of late recurrence of testicular germ cell tumors. Am J Surg Pathol. 2000 Feb;24(2):257–73. PMID:10680894
**4642.** Michal M, Berry RS, Rubin BP, et al. EWSR1-SMAD3-rearranged fibroblastic tumor: an emerging entity in an increasingly more complex group of fibroblastic/myofibroblastic neoplasms. Am J Surg Pathol. 2018 Oct;42(10):1325–33. PMID:29957732
**4643.** Michal M, Fanburg-Smith JC, Lasota J, et al. Minute synovial sarcomas of the hands and feet: a clinicopathologic study of 21 tumors less than 1 cm. Am J Surg Pathol. 2006 Jun;30(6):721–6. PMID:16723849
**4644.** Michal M, Kacerovska D, Mukensnabl P, et al. Ovarian fibromas with heavy deposition of hyaline globules: a diagnostic pitfall. Int J Gynecol Pathol. 2009 Jul;28(4):356–61. PMID:19483628
**4645.** Michal M, Kazakov DV, Belousova I, et al. A benign neoplasm with histopathological features of both schwannoma and retiform perineurioma (benign schwannoma-perineurioma): a report of six cases of a distinctive soft tissue tumor with a predilection for the fingers. Virchows Arch. 2004 Oct;445(4):347–53. PMID:15322875
**4646.** Michal M, Miettinen M. Myoepitheliomas of the skin and soft tissues. Report of 12 cases. Virchows Arch. 1999 May;434(5):393–400. PMID:10389622
**4647.** Michal M, Ptáková N, Martínek P, et al. S100 and CD34 positive spindle cell tumor with prominent perivascular hyalinization and a novel NCOA4-RET fusion. Genes Chromosomes Cancer. 2019 Sep;58(9):680–5. PMID:30938880
**4648.** Michalkiewicz E, Sandrini R, Figueiredo B, et al. Clinical and outcome characteristics of children with adrenocortical tumors: a report from the International Pediatric Adrenocortical Tumor Registry. J Clin Oncol. 2004 Mar 1;22(5):838–45. PMID:14990639
**4649.** Michel BC, D'Avino AR, Cassel SH, et al. A non-canonical SWI/SNF complex is a synthetic lethal target in cancers driven by BAF complex perturbation. Nat Cell Biol. 2018 Dec;20(12):1410–20. PMID:30397315
**4650.** Michonneau D, Petrella T, Ortonne N, et al. Subcutaneous panniculitis-like T-cell lymphoma: immunosuppressive drugs induce better response than polychemotherapy. Acta Derm Venereol. 2017 Mar 10;97(3):358–64. PMID:27722764
**4651.** Micko AS, Wöhrer A, Wolfsberger S, et al. Invasion of the cavernous sinus space in pituitary adenomas: endoscopic verification and its correlation with an MRI-based classification. J Neurosurg. 2015 Apr;122(4):803–11. PMID:25658782
**4652.** Middleton SB, Frayling IM, Phillips RK. Desmoids in familial adenomatous polyposis are monoclonal proliferations. Br J Cancer. 2000 Feb;82(4):827–32. PMID:10732754
**4653.** Miele E, De Vito R, Ciolfi A, et al. DNA methylation profiling for diagnosing undifferentiated sarcoma with capicua transcriptional receptor (CIC) alterations. Int J Mol Sci. 2020 Mar 6;21(5):E1818. PMID:32155762
**4654.** Miettinen M, Chatten J, Paetau A, et al. Monoclonal antibody NB84 in the differential diagnosis of neuroblastoma and other small round cell tumors. Am J Surg Pathol. 1998 Mar;22(3):327–32. PMID:9500774
**4655.** Miettinen M, Dow N, Lasota J, et al. A distinctive novel epitheliomesenchymal biphasic tumor of the stomach in young adults ("gastroblastoma"): a series of 3 cases. Am J Surg Pathol. 2009 Sep;33(9):1370–7. PMID:19718790
**4656.** Miettinen M, Fanburg-Smith JC, Virolainen M, et al. Epithelioid sarcoma: an immunohistochemical analysis of 112 classical and variant cases and a discussion of the differential diagnosis. Hum Pathol. 1999 Aug;30(8):934–42. PMID:10452506
**4657.** Miettinen M, Fetsch JF. Collagenous fibroma (desmoplastic fibroblastoma): a clinicopathologic analysis of 63 cases of a distinctive soft tissue lesion with stellate-shaped fibroblasts. Hum Pathol. 1998 Jul;29(7):676–82. PMID:9670823
**4658.** Miettinen M, Finnell V, Fetsch JF. Ossifying fibromyxoid tumor of soft parts–a clinicopathologic and immunohistochemical study of 104 cases with long-term follow-up and a critical review of the literature. Am J Surg Pathol. 2008 Jul;32(7):996–1005. PMID:18469710
**4659.** Miettinen M, Kahlos T. Undifferentiated (embryonal) sarcoma of the liver. Epithelial features as shown by immunohistochemical analysis and electron microscopic examination. Cancer. 1989 Nov 15;64(10):2096–103. PMID:2680050
**4660.** Miettinen M, Killian JK, Wang ZF, et al. Immunohistochemical loss of succinate dehydrogenase subunit A (SDHA) in gastrointestinal stromal tumors (GISTs) signals SDHA germline mutation. Am J Surg Pathol. 2013 Feb;37(2):234–40. PMID:23282968
**4661.** Miettinen M, Lasota J, Sobin LH. Gastrointestinal stromal tumors of the stomach in children and young adults: a clinicopathologic, immunohistochemical, and molecular genetic study of 44 cases with long-term follow-up and review of the literature. Am J Surg Pathol. 2005 Oct;29(10):1373–81. PMID:16160481
**4662.** Miettinen M, Lehto VP, Virtanen I. Malignant fibrous histiocytoma within a recurrent chordoma. A light microscopic, electron microscopic, and immunohistochemical study. Am J Clin Pathol. 1984 Dec;82(6):738–43. PMID:6095644
**4663.** Miettinen M, Lindenmayer AE, Chaubal A. Endothelial cell markers CD31, CD34, and BNH9 antibody to H- and Y-antigens–evaluation of their specificity and sensitivity in the diagnosis of vascular tumors and comparison with von Willebrand factor. Mod Pathol. 1994 Jan;7(1):82–90. PMID:7512718
**4664.** Miettinen M, McCue PA, Sarlomo-Rikala M, et al. GATA3: a multispecific but potentially useful marker in surgical pathology: a systematic analysis of 2500 epithelial and nonepithelial tumors. Am J Surg Pathol. 2014 Jan;38(1):13–22. PMID:24145643
**4665.** Miettinen M, McCue PA, Sarlomo-Rikala M, et al. Sox10–a marker for not only schwannian and melanocytic neoplasms but also myoepithelial cell tumors of soft tissue: a systematic analysis of 5134 tumors. Am J Surg Pathol. 2015 Jun;39(6):826–35. PMID:25724000
**4666.** Miettinen M, Paal E, Lasota J, et al. Gastrointestinal glomus tumors: a clinicopathologic,

immunohistochemical, and molecular genetic study of 32 cases. Am J Surg Pathol. 2002 Mar;26(3):301–11. PMID:11859201

4667. Miettinen M, Wang Z, Lasota J, et al. Nuclear brachyury expression is consistent in chordoma, common in germ cell tumors and small cell carcinomas, and rare in other carcinomas and sarcomas: an immunohistochemical study of 5229 cases. Am J Surg Pathol. 2015 Oct;39(10):1305–12. PMID:26099010

4668. Miettinen M, Wang Z, Sarlomo-Rikala M, et al. ERG expression in epithelioid sarcoma: a diagnostic pitfall. Am J Surg Pathol. 2013 Oct;37(10):1580–5. PMID:23774169

4669. Miettinen M, Wang ZF. Prox1 transcription factor as a marker for vascular tumors-evaluation of 314 vascular endothelial and 1086 nonvascular tumors. Am J Surg Pathol. 2012 Mar;36(3):351–9. PMID:22067331

4670. Miettinen M, Wang ZF, Paetau A, et al. ERG transcription factor as an immunohistochemical marker for vascular endothelial tumors and prostatic carcinoma. Am J Surg Pathol. 2011 Mar;35(3):432–41. PMID:21317715

4671. Miettinen M, Wang ZF, Sarlomo-Rikala M, et al. Succinate dehydrogenase-deficient GISTs: a clinicopathologic, immunohistochemical, and molecular genetic study of 66 gastric GISTs with predilection to young age. Am J Surg Pathol. 2011 Nov;35(11):1712–21. PMID:21997692

4672. Miettinen MM, Antonescu CR, Fletcher CDM, et al. Histopathologic evaluation of atypical neurofibromatous tumors and their transformation into malignant peripheral nerve sheath tumor in patients with neurofibromatosis 1-a consensus overview. Hum Pathol. 2017 Sep;67:1–10. PMID:28551330

4673. Migliavacca M, Assanelli A, Ponzoni M, et al. First occurrence of plasmablastic lymphoma in adenosine deaminase-deficient severe combined immunodeficiency disease patient and review of the literature. Front Immunol. 2018 Feb 2;9:113. PMID:29456531

4674. Mihaylova VT, Bindra RS, Yuan J, et al. Decreased expression of the DNA mismatch repair gene Mlh1 under hypoxic stress in mammalian cells. Mol Cell Biol. 2003 May;23(9):3265–73. PMID:12697826

4675. Miliaras D, Conroy J, Pervana S, et al. Karyotypic changes detected by comparative genomic hybridization in a stillborn infant with chorioangioma and liver hemangioma. Birth Defects Res A Clin Mol Teratol. 2007 Mar;79(3):236–41. PMID:17203486

4676. Miliauskas JR, Hunt JL. Primary unilateral multifocal pleomorphic adenoma of the parotid gland: molecular assessment and literature review. Head Neck Pathol. 2008 Dec;2(4):339–42. PMID:20614306

4677. Milković Periša M, Džombeta T, Stepan Giljević J, et al. Malignant peripheral nerve sheath tumor of the inguinum and angiosarcoma of the scalp in a child with neurofibromatosis type 1. Case Rep Pathol. 2017;2017:7542825. PMID:29138703

4678. Miller DD, Gupta A. Histopathology of vascular anomalies: update based on the revised 2014 ISSVA classification. Semin Cutan Med Surg. 2016 Sep;35(3):137–46. PMID:27607322

4679. Miller DR. A tribute to Sidney Farber– the father of modern chemotherapy. Br J Haematol. 2006 Jul;134(1):20–6. PMID:16803563

4680. Miller S, Rogers HA, Lyon P, et al. Genome-wide molecular characterization of central nervous system primitive neuroectodermal tumor and pineoblastoma. Neuro Oncol. 2011 Aug;13(8):866–79. PMID:21798848

4681. Miller S, Ward JH, Rogers HA, et al. Loss of INI1 protein expression defines a subgroup of aggressive central nervous system primitive neuroectodermal tumors. Brain Pathol. 2013 Jan;23(1):19–27. PMID:22672440

4682. Miller-Breslow A, Dorfman HD. Dupuytren's (subungual) exostosis. Am J Surg Pathol. 1988 May;12(5):368–78. PMID:3284396

4683. Millot F, Baruchel A, Guilhot J, et al. Imatinib is effective in children with previously untreated chronic myelogenous leukemia in early chronic phase: results of the French national phase IV trial. J Clin Oncol. 2011 Jul 10;29(20):2827–32. PMID:21670449

4684. Millot F, Facon T, Kerckaert JP, et al. Unusual recurrence of chronic myelogenous leukemia following bone marrow transplantation. Bone Marrow Transplant. 1991 May;7(5):393–5. PMID:2070150

4685. Millot F, Guilhot J, Baruchel A, et al. Impact of early molecular response in children with chronic myeloid leukemia treated in the French Glivec phase 4 study. Blood. 2014 Oct 9;124(15):2408–10. PMID:25170123

4686. Millot F, Guilhot J, Suttorp M, et al. Prognostic discrimination based on the EUTOS long-term survival score within the International Registry for Chronic Myeloid Leukemia in children and adolescents. Haematologica. 2017 Oct;102(10):1704–8. PMID:28838993

4687. Millot F, Maledon N, Guilhot J, et al. Favourable outcome of de novo advanced phases of childhood chronic myeloid leukaemia. Eur J Cancer. 2019 Jul;115:17–23. PMID:31082688

4688. Millot F, Traore P, Guilhot J, et al. Clinical and biological features at diagnosis in 40 children with chronic myeloid leukemia. Pediatrics. 2005 Jul;116(1):140–3. PMID:15995044

4689. Mills AE. Rhabdomyomatous mesenchymal hamartoma of skin. Am J Dermatopathol. 1989 Feb;11(1):58–63. PMID:2916743

4690. Mills SE, Cooper PH, Fechner RE. Lobular capillary hemangioma: the underlying lesion of pyogenic granuloma. A study of 73 cases from the oral and nasal mucous membranes. Am J Surg Pathol. 1980 Oct;4(5):470–9. PMID:7435775

4691. Milman T, Zhang Q, Ang S, et al. Conjunctival nevi and melanoma: multiparametric immunohistochemical analysis, including p16, SOX10, HMB45, and Ki-67. Hum Pathol. 2020 Sep;103:107–19. PMID:32707054

4692. Milne P, Bigley V, Bacon CM, et al. Hematopoietic origin of Langerhans cell histiocytosis and Erdheim-Chester disease in adults. Blood. 2017 Jul 13;130(2):167–75. PMID:28512190

4693. Min HS, Lee JY, Kim SK, et al. Genetic grouping of medulloblastomas by representative markers in pathologic diagnosis. Transl Oncol. 2013 Jun 1;6(3):265–72. PMID:23730405

4694. Min KW, Scheithauer BW. Pineal germinomas and testicular seminoma: a comparative ultrastructural study with special references to early carcinomatous transformation. Ultrastruct Pathol. 1990 Nov-Dec;14(6):483–96. PMID:2281547

4695. Min KW, Scheithauer BW, Bauserman SC. Pineal parenchymal tumors: an ultrastructural study with prognostic implications. Ultrastruct Pathol. 1994 Jan-Apr;18(1-2):69–85. PMID:8191649

4696. Minard-Colin V, Brugières L, Reiter A, et al. Non-Hodgkin lymphoma in children and adolescents: progress through effective collaboration, current knowledge, and challenges ahead. J Clin Oncol. 2015 Sep 20;33(27):2963–74. PMID:26304908

4697. Minehan KJ, Shaw EG, Scheithauer BW, et al. Spinal cord astrocytoma: pathological and treatment considerations. J Neurosurg. 1995 Oct;83(4):590–5. PMID:7674006

4698. Miquel J, Fraitag S, Hamel-Teillac D, et al. Lymphomatoid papulosis in children: a series of 25 cases. Br J Dermatol. 2014 Nov;171(5):1138–46. PMID:24749749

4699. Mir A, Agim NG, Kane AA, et al. Giant congenital melanocytic nevus treated with trametinib. Pediatrics. 2019 Mar;143(3):e20182469. PMID:30792255

4700. Mirabello L, Pfeiffer R, Murphy G, et al. Height at diagnosis and birth-weight as risk factors for osteosarcoma. Cancer Causes Control. 2011 Jun;22(6):899–908. PMID:21465145

4701. Mirabello L, Troisi RJ, Savage SA. Osteosarcoma incidence and survival rates from 1973 to 2004: data from the Surveillance, Epidemiology, and End Results Program. Cancer. 2009 Apr 1;115(7):1531–43. PMID:19197972

4702. Mirabello L, Yeager M, Mai PL, et al. Germline TP53 variants and susceptibility to osteosarcoma. J Natl Cancer Inst. 2015 Apr 20;107(7):djv101. PMID:25896519

4703. Miranda RN, Cousar JB, Hammer RD, et al. Somatic mutation analysis of IgH variable regions reveals that tumor cells of most parafollicular (monocytoid) B-cell lymphoma, splenic marginal zone B-cell lymphoma, and some hairy cell leukemia are composed of memory B lymphocytes. Hum Pathol. 1999 Mar;30(3):306–12. PMID:10088550

4704. Mirapoğlu SL, Aydogdu I, Gucin Z, et al. Traumatic rupture of solid pseudopapillary tumors of the pancreas in children: a case report. Mol Clin Oncol. 2016 Nov;5(5):587–9. PMID:27900090

4705. Mirkovic J, Calicchio M, Fletcher CD, et al. Diffuse and strong cyclin D1 immunoreactivity in clear cell sarcoma of the kidney. Histopathology. 2015 Sep;67(3):306–12. PMID:25556515

4706. Mirow C, Pietsch T, Berkefeld S, et al. Children <1 year show an inferior outcome when treated according to the traditional LGG treatment strategy: a report from the German multicenter trial HIT-LGG 1996 for children with low grade glioma (LGG). Pediatr Blood Cancer. 2014 Mar;61(3):457–63. PMID:24039013

4707. Mirra JM, Fain JS, Ward WG, et al. Extraskeletal telangiectatic osteosarcoma. Cancer. 1993 May 15;71(10):3014–9. PMID:8490830

4708. Mirra JM, Kessler S, Bhuta S, et al. The fibroma-like variant of epithelioid sarcoma. A fibrohistiocytic/myoid cell lesion often confused with benign and malignant spindle cell tumors. Cancer. 1992 Mar 15;69(6):1382–95. PMID:1371711

4709. Mirshahi UL, Kim J, Best AF, et al. A Genome-first approach to characterize DICER1 pathogenic variant prevalence, penetrance, and phenotype. JAMA Netw Open. 2021 Feb 1;4(2):e210112. PMID:33630087

4710. Mirza FN, Tuggle CT, Zogg CK, et al. Epidemiology of malignant cutaneous granular cell tumors: a US population-based cohort analysis using the Surveillance, Epidemiology, and End Results (SEER) database. J Am Acad Dermatol. 2018 Mar;78(3):490–7.e1. PMID:28989104

4711. Mishra A, Mehrotra PK, Agarwal G, et al. Pediatric and adolescent pheochromocytoma: clinical presentation and outcome of surgery. Indian Pediatr. 2014 Apr;51(4):299–302. PMID:24825268

4712. Misra A, Bakhshi S, Kumar R, et al. Pediatric plasmablastic lymphoma: diagnostic and therapeutic dilemma. Indian J Pathol Microbiol. 2017 Apr-Jun;60(2):303–4. PMID:28631667

4713. Mistry M, Zhukova N, Merico D, et al. BRAF mutation and CDKN2A deletion define a clinically distinct subgroup of childhood secondary high-grade glioma. J Clin Oncol. 2015 Mar 20;33(9):1015–22. PMID:25667294

4714. Mitchell A, Scheithauer BW, Doyon J, et al. Malignant perineurioma (malignant peripheral nerve sheath tumor with perineural differentiation). Clin Neuropathol. 2012 Nov-Dec;31(6):424–9. PMID:22762889

4715. Mitchell RT, Camacho-Moll M, Macdonald J, et al. Intratubular germ cell neoplasia of the human testis: heterogeneous protein expression and relation to invasive potential. Mod Pathol. 2014 Sep;27(9):1255–66. PMID:24457464

4716. Mito JK, Jo VY, Chiosea SI, et al. HMGA2 is a specific immunohistochemical marker for pleomorphic adenoma and carcinoma ex-pleomorphic adenoma. Histopathology. 2017 Oct;71(4):511–21. PMID:28463429

4717. Mitra A, MacIntyre DA, Ntritsos G, et al. The vaginal microbiota associates with the regression of untreated cervical intraepithelial neoplasia 2 lesions. Nat Commun. 2020 Apr 24;11(1):1999. PMID:32332850

4718. Mitry E, Ciccolallo L, Coleman MP, et al. Incidence of and survival from Wilms' tumour in adults in Europe: data from the EUROCARE study. Eur J Cancer. 2006 Sep;42(14):2363–8. PMID:16891111

4719. Mitsutake N, Knauf JA, Mitsutake S, et al. Conditional BRAFV600E expression induces DNA synthesis, apoptosis, dedifferentiation, and chromosomal instability in thyroid PCCL3 cells. Cancer Res. 2005 Mar 15;65(6):2465–73. PMID:15781663

4720. Mittal A, Vinay K, De D, et al. Tuberous sclerosis complex and diffuse lipomatosis: case report of a rare association. Indian Dermatol Online J. 2018 Jan-Feb;9(1):37–9. PMID:29441296

4721. Mittal P, Roberts CWM. The SWI/SNF complex in cancer - biology, biomarkers and therapy. Nat Rev Clin Oncol. 2020 Jul;17(7):435–48. PMID:32303701

4722. Mitter D, Ullmann R, Muradyan A, et al. Genotype-phenotype correlations in patients with retinoblastoma and interstitial 13q deletions. Eur J Hum Genet. 2011 Sep;19(9):947–58. PMID:21505449

4723. Miura T, Yamamoto T. Perforating pilomatricoma with anetodermic epidermis in an adolescent with lymphoma. Pediatr Dermatol. 2013 Jul-Aug;30(4):e68–9. PMID:22937738

4724. Miyahara H, Toyoshima Y, Natsumeda M, et al. Anaplastic astrocytoma with angiocentric ependymal differentiation. Neuropathology. 2011 Jun;31(3):292–8. PMID:21062363

4725. Miyake T, Yamamoto T, Hirai Y, et al. Survival rates and prognostic factors of Epstein-Barr virus-associated hydroa vacciniforme and hypersensitivity to mosquito bites. Br J Dermatol. 2015 Jan;172(1):56–63. PMID:25234411

4726. Miyake Y, Adachi JI, Suzuki T, et al. Craniospinal germinomas in patient with down syndrome successfully treated with standard-dose chemotherapy and craniospinal irradiation: case report and literature review. World Neurosurg. 2017 Dec;108:995.e9–15. PMID:28919233

4726A. Miyaki M, Iijima T, Ishii R, et al. Molecular evidence for multicentric development of thyroid carcinomas in patients with familial adenomatous polyposis. Am J Pathol. 2000 Dec;157(6):1825–7. PMID:11106555

4727. Miyano G, Hayashi T, Arakawa A, et al. Giant omental lipoblastoma and CD56 expression. Afr J Paediatr Surg. 2013 Jan-Apr;10(1):32–4. PMID:23519855

4728. Miyata H, Ryufuku M, Kubota Y, et al. Adult-onset angiocentric glioma of epithelioid cell-predominant type of the mesial temporal lobe suggestive of a rare but distinct clinicopathological subset within a spectrum of angiocentric cortical ependymal tumors.

Neuropathology. 2012 Oct;32(5):479–91. PMID:22151480

4729. Miyauchi J, Ito Y, Kawano T, et al. Unusual diffuse liver fibrosis accompanying transient myeloproliferative disorder in Down's syndrome: a report of four autopsy cases and proposal of a hypothesis. Blood. 1992 Sep 15;80(6):1521–7. PMID:1387814

4730. Mizoguchi Y, Fujita N, Taki T, et al. Juvenile myelomonocytic leukemia with t(7;11)(p15;p15) and NUP98-HOXA11 fusion. Am J Hematol. 2009 May;84(5):295–7. PMID:19338047

4731. Mizuguchi M, Ikeda K, Takashima S. Simultaneous loss of hamartin and tuberin from the cerebrum, kidney and heart with tuberous sclerosis. Acta Neuropathol. 2000 May;99(5):503–10. PMID:10805093

4732. Mizuguchi M, Kato M, Yamanouchi H, et al. Loss of tuberin from cerebral tissues with tuberous sclerosis and astrocytoma. Ann Neurol. 1996 Dec;40(6):941–4. PMID:9007104

4733. Mizuguchi M, Takashima S. Neuropathology of tuberous sclerosis. Brain Dev. 2001 Nov;23(7):508–15. PMID:11701246

4734. Mo D, Zhao Y, Balajee AS. Human RecQL4 helicase plays multifaceted roles in the genomic stability of normal and cancer cells. Cancer Lett. 2018 Jan 28;413:1–10. PMID:29080750

4735. Mobarki M, Dumollard JM, Dal Col P, et al. Granular cell tumor a study of 42 cases and systemic review of the literature. Pathol Res Pract. 2020 Apr;216(4):152865. PMID:32089415

4736. Möbius S, Schenk T, Himsel D, et al. Results of the European survey on the assessment of deep molecular response in chronic phase CML patients during tyrosine kinase inhibitor therapy (EUREKA registry). J Cancer Res Clin Oncol. 2019 Jun;145(6):1645–50. PMID:30941573

4737. Mobley BC, McKenney JK, Bangs CD, et al. Loss of SMARCB1/INI1 expression in poorly differentiated chordomas. Acta Neuropathol. 2010 Dec;120(6):745–53. PMID:21057957

4738. Modena P, Lualdi E, Facchinetti F, et al. SMARCB1/INI1 tumor suppressor gene is frequently inactivated in epithelioid sarcomas. Cancer Res. 2005 May 15;65(10):4012–9. PMID:15899790

4739. Moes-Sosnowska J, Szafron L, Nowakowska D, et al. Germline SMARCA4 mutations in patients with ovarian small cell carcinoma of hypercalcemic type. Orphanet J Rare Dis. 2015 Mar 15;10:32. PMID:25886974

4740. Mogul DB, Ling SC, Murray KF, et al. Characteristics of hepatitis B virus-associated hepatocellular carcinoma in children: a multi-center study. J Pediatr Gastroenterol Nutr. 2018 Oct;67(4):437–40. PMID:30063586

4741. Mohanty SK, Dey P, Ghoshal S, et al. Cytologic features of metastatic nasopharyngeal carcinoma. Diagn Cytopathol. 2002 Dec;27(6):340–2. PMID:12451563

4742. Mohindra S, Sakr H, Sturgis C, et al. LEF-1 is a sensitive marker of cribriform morular variant of papillary thyroid carcinoma. Head Neck Pathol. 2018 Dec;12(4):455–62. PMID:29243023

4743. Mohseni M, Uludag H, Brandwein JM. Advances in biology of acute lymphoblastic leukemia (ALL) and therapeutic implications. Am J Blood Res. 2018 Dec 10;8(4):29–56. PMID:30697448

4744. Mohseny AB, Szuhai K, Romeo S, et al. Osteosarcoma originates from mesenchymal stem cells in consequence of aneuploidization and genomic loss of Cdkn2. J Pathol. 2009 Nov;219(3):294–305. PMID:19718709

4745. Molitch ME. Diagnosis and treatment of pituitary adenomas: a review. JAMA. 2017 Feb 7;317(5):516–24. PMID:28170483

4746. Mollaoglu N, Tokman B, Kahraman S, et al. An unusual presentation of ossifying fibromyxoid tumor of the mandible: a case report. J Clin Pediatr Dent. 2006 Winter;31(2):136–8. PMID:17315811

4747. Möller E, Hornick JL, Magnusson L, et al. FUS-CREB3L2/L1-positive sarcomas show a specific gene expression profile with upregulation of CD24 and FOXL1. Clin Cancer Res. 2011 May 1;17(9):2646–56. PMID:21536545

4748. Möller I, Murali R, Müller H, et al. Activating cysteinyl leukotriene receptor 2 (CYSLTR2) mutations in blue nevi. Mod Pathol. 2017 Mar;30(3):350–6. PMID:27934878

4749. Möller P, Lämmler B, Herrmann B, et al. The primary mediastinal clear cell lymphoma of B-cell type has variable defects in MHC antigen expression. Immunology. 1986 Nov;59(3):411–7. PMID:3491784

4750. Möller P, Moldenhauer G, Momburg F, et al. Mediastinal lymphoma of clear cell type is a tumor corresponding to terminal steps of B cell differentiation. Blood. 1987 Apr;69(4):1087–95. PMID:3103712

4751. Møller P, Seppälä T, Bernstein I, et al. Cancer incidence and survival in Lynch syndrome patients receiving colonoscopic and gynaecological surveillance: first report from the Prospective Lynch Syndrome Database. Gut. 2017 Mar;66(3):464–72. PMID:26657901

4752. Møller P, Seppälä T, Bernstein I, et al. Incidence of and survival after subsequent cancers in carriers of pathogenic MMR variants with previous cancer: a report from the Prospective Lynch Syndrome Database. Gut. 2017 Sep;66(9):1657–64. PMID:27261338

4753. Møller P, Seppälä TT, Bernstein I, et al. Cancer risk and survival in path_MMR carriers by gene and gender up to 75 years of age: a report from the Prospective Lynch Syndrome Database. Gut. 2018 Jul;67(7):1306–16. PMID:28754778

4754. Molmenti EP, Nagata DE, Roden JS, et al. Post-transplant lymphoproliferative syndrome in the pediatric liver transplant population. Am J Transplant. 2001 Nov;1(4):356–9. PMID:12099380

4755. Molyneux E, Davidson A, Orem J, et al. The management of children with Kaposi sarcoma in resource limited settings. Pediatr Blood Cancer. 2013 Apr;60(4):538–42. PMID:23255282

4756. Momose S, Tamaru J, Kishi H, et al. Hyperactivated STAT3 in ALK-positive diffuse large B-cell lymphoma with clathrin-ALK fusion. Hum Pathol. 2009 Jan;40(1):75–82. PMID:18755494

4757. Momota H, Ichimiya S, Ikeda T, et al. Immunohistochemical analysis of the p53 family members in human craniopharyngiomas. Brain Tumor Pathol. 2003;20(2):73–7. PMID:14756444

4758. Monaco S, Tsao L, Murty VV, et al. Pediatric ALK+ anaplastic large cell lymphoma with t(3;8)(q26.2;q24) translocation and c-myc rearrangement terminating in a leukemic phase. Am J Hematol. 2007 Jan;82(1):59–64. PMID:16955462

4759. Monaco SE, Pantanowitz L, Khalbuss WE, et al. Cytomorphological and molecular genetic findings in pediatric thyroid fine-needle aspiration. Cancer Cytopathol. 2012 Oct 25;120(5):342–50. PMID:22605559

4760. Monaghan H, Salter DM, Al-Nafussi A. Giant cell tumour of tendon sheath (localised nodular tenosynovitis): clinicopathological features of 71 cases. J Clin Pathol. 2001 May;54(5):404–7. PMID:11328844

4761. Monclair T, Brodeur GM, Ambros PF, et al. The International Neuroblastoma Risk Group (INRG) staging system: an INRG Task Force report. J Clin Oncol. 2009 Jan 10;27(2):298–303. PMID:19047290

4762. Monda L, Wick MR. S-100 protein immunostaining in the differential diagnosis of chondroblastoma. Hum Pathol. 1985 Mar;16(3):287–93. PMID:2579018

4763. Mondal A, Das M, Chatterjee U, et al. Retiform hemangioendothelioma: an uncommon vascular neoplasm. Indian J Pathol Microbiol. 2020 Jan-Mar;63(1):122–4. PMID:32031140

4764. Mondal G, Lee JC, Ravindranathan A, et al. Pediatric bithalamic gliomas have a distinct epigenetic signature and frequent EGFR exon 20 insertions resulting in potential sensitivity to targeted kinase inhibition. Acta Neuropathol. 2020 Jun;139(6):1071–88. PMID:32303840

4765. Monfared A, Gorti G, Kim D. Microsurgical anatomy of the laryngeal nerves as related to thyroid surgery. Laryngoscope. 2002 Feb;112(2):386–92. PMID:11889402

4766. Monté AMC, D'Arco F, De Cocker LJL. Multinodular and vacuolating neuronal tumor in an adolescent with Klinefelter syndrome. Neuroradiology. 2017 Dec;59(12):1187–8. PMID:29038865

4767. Montella F, Giana M, Vigone A, et al. Angiomyofibroblastoma of the vulva: report of a case. Eur J Gynaecol Oncol. 2004;25(2):253–4. PMID:15032297

4768. Montes-Mojarro IA, Kim WY, Fend F, et al. Epstein - Barr virus positive T and NK-cell lymphoproliferations: morphological features and differential diagnosis. Semin Diagn Pathol. 2020 Jan;37(1):32–46. PMID:31889602

4769. Montes-Moreno S, Gonzalez-Medina AR, Rodriguez-Pinilla SM, et al. Aggressive large B-cell lymphoma with plasma cell differentiation: immunohistochemical characterization of plasmablastic lymphoma and diffuse large B-cell lymphoma with partial plasmablastic phenotype. Haematologica. 2010 Aug;95(8):1342–9. PMID:20418245

4770. Montes-Moreno S, Martinez-Magunacelaya N, Zecchini-Barrese T, et al. Plasmablastic lymphoma phenotype is determined by genetic alterations in MYC and PRDM1. Mod Pathol. 2017 Jan;30(1):85–94. PMID:27687004

4771. Montgomery BK, Alimchandani M, Mehta GU, et al. Tumors displaying hybrid schwannoma and neurofibroma features in patients with neurofibromatosis type 2. Clin Neuropathol. 2016 Mar-Apr;35(2):78–83. PMID:26709712

4772. Montgomery E, Goldblum JR, Fisher C. Myofibrosarcoma: a clinicopathologic study. Am J Surg Pathol. 2001 Feb;25(2):219–28. PMID:11176071

4773. Montgomery E, Lee JH, Abraham SC, et al. Superficial fibromatoses are genetically distinct from deep fibromatoses. Mod Pathol. 2001 Jul;14(7):695–701. PMID:11455002

4774. Montgomery EA, Meis JM. Nodular fasciitis. Its morphologic spectrum and immunohistochemical profile. Am J Surg Pathol. 1991 Oct;15(10):942–8. PMID:1928550

4775. Mooney EE, Nogales FF, Tavassoli FA. Hepatocytic differentiation in retiform Sertoli-Leydig cell tumors: distinguishing a heterologous element from Leydig cells. Hum Pathol. 1999 Jun;30(6):611–7. PMID:10374766

4776. Moore BD 3rd, Slopis JM, Jackson EF, et al. Brain volume in children with neurofibromatosis type 1: relation to neuropsychological status. Neurology. 2000 Feb 22;54(4):914–20. PMID:10690986

4777. Moore PS, Chang Y. Detection of herpesvirus-like DNA sequences in Kaposi's sarcoma in patients with and those without HIV infection. N Engl J Med. 1995 May 4;332(18):1181–5. PMID:7700310

4778. Moosavi C, Jha P, Fanburg-Smith JC. An update on plexiform fibrohistiocytic tumor and addition of 66 new cases from the Armed Forces Institute of Pathology, in honor of Franz M. Enzinger, MD. Ann Diagn Pathol. 2007 Oct;11(5):313–9. PMID:17870015

4779. Moosavi CA, Al-Nahar LA, Murphey MD, et al. Fibroosseous [corrected] pseudotumor of the digit: a clinicopathologic study of 43 new cases. Ann Diagn Pathol. 2008 Feb;12(1):21–8. PMID:18164411

4780. Moppett J, Oakhill A, Duncan AW. Second malignancies in children: the usual suspects? Eur J Radiol. 2001 Feb;37(2):95–108. PMID:11223476

4781. Moraes P, Pereira C, Almeida O, et al. Paediatric intraoral mucoepidermoid carcinoma mimicking a bone lesion. Int J Paediatr Dent. 2007 Mar;17(2):151–4. PMID:17263868

4782. Morak M, Koehler U, Schackert HK, et al. Biallelic MLH1 SNP cDNA expression or constitutional promoter methylation can hide genomic rearrangements causing Lynch syndrome. J Med Genet. 2011 Aug;48(8):513–9. PMID:21712435

4783. Morak M, Massdorf T, Sykora H, et al. First evidence for digenic inheritance in hereditary colorectal cancer by mutations in the base excision repair genes. Eur J Cancer. 2011 May;47(7):1046–55. PMID:21195604

4784. Moran CA, Suster S. Primary germ cell tumors of the mediastinum: I. Analysis of 322 cases with special emphasis on teratomatous lesions and a proposal for histopathologic classification and clinical staging. Cancer. 1997 Aug 15;80(4):681–90. PMID:9264351

4785. Moravová I, Hyánková E. [Experience with Vietnamese mothers and their children in an infant care facility]. Cesk Pediatr. 1990 Jun;45(6):366–8. Czech. PMID:2289259

4786. Moreau A, Galmiche L, Minard-Colin V, et al. Melanotic neuroectodermal tumor of infancy (MNTI) of the head and neck: a French multicenter study. J Craniomaxillofac Surg. 2018 Feb;46(2):201–6. PMID:29275074

4787. Moreira AL, Waisman J, Cangiarella JF. Aspiration cytology of the oncocytic variant of papillary adenocarcinoma of the thyroid gland. Acta Cytol. 2004 Mar-Apr;48(2):137–41. PMID:15085743

4788. Morerio C, Acquila M, Rosanda C, et al. HCMOGT-1 is a novel fusion partner to PDGFRB in juvenile myelomonocytic leukemia with t(5;17)(q33;p11.2). Cancer Res. 2004 Apr 15;64(8):2649–51. PMID:15087372

4789. Morerio C, Nozza P, Tassano E, et al. Differential diagnosis of lipoma-like lipoblastoma. Pediatr Blood Cancer. 2009 Jan;52(1):132–4. PMID:18798558

4790. Morerio C, Rapella A, Rosanda C, et al. PLAG1-HAS2 fusion in lipoblastoma with masked 8q intrachromosomal rearrangement. Cancer Genet Cytogenet. 2005 Jan 15;156(2):183–4. PMID:15642402

4791. Morgado JM, Perbellini O, Johnson RC, et al. CD30 expression by bone marrow mast cells from different diagnostic variants of systemic mastocytosis. Histopathology. 2013 Dec;63(6):780–7. PMID:24111625

4792. Mori N, Yamashita Y, Tsuzuki T, et al. Lymphomatous features of aggressive NK cell leukaemia/lymphoma with massive necrosis, haemophagocytosis and EB virus infection. Histopathology. 2000 Oct;37(4):363–71. PMID:11012744

4793. Moritake H, Ikeda T, Manabe A, et al. Cytomegalovirus infection mimicking juvenile myelomonocytic leukemia showing hypersensitivity to granulocyte-macrophage colony stimulating factor. Pediatr Blood Cancer. 2009 Dec 15;53(7):1324–6. PMID:19731324

4794. Moriwaki K, Manabe A, Taketani T, et al. Cytogenetics and clinical features of pediatric myelodysplastic syndrome in Japan. Int J Hematol. 2014 Nov;100(5):478–84. PMID:25261124

**4795.** Moriyama T, Metzger ML, Wu G, et al. Germline genetic variation in ETV6 and risk of childhood acute lymphoblastic leukaemia: a systematic genetic study. Lancet Oncol. 2015 Dec;16(16):1659–66. PMID:26522332

**4796.** Morohoshi T, Sagawa F, Mitsuya T. Pancreatoblastoma with marked elevation of serum alpha-fetoprotein. An autopsy case report with immunocytochemical study. Virchows Arch A Pathol Anat Histopathol. 1990;416(3):265–70. PMID:1689089

**4797.** Morowitz M, Huff D, von Allmen D. Epithelial ovarian tumors in children: a retrospective analysis. J Pediatr Surg. 2003 Mar;38(3):331–5. PMID:12632344

**4798.** Morris SM, Acosta MT, Garg S, et al. Disease burden and symptom structure of autism in neurofibromatosis type 1: a study of the International NF1-ASD Consortium Team (INFACT). JAMA Psychiatry. 2016 Dec 1;73(12):1276–84. PMID:27760236

**4799.** Morris SW, Kirstein MN, Valentine MB, et al. Fusion of a kinase gene, ALK, to a nucleolar protein gene, NPM, in non-Hodgkin's lymphoma. Science. 1994 Mar 4;263(5151):1281–4. PMID:8122112

**4800.** Morscio J, Dierickx D, Nijs J, et al. Clinicopathologic comparison of plasmablastic lymphoma in HIV-positive, immunocompetent, and posttransplant patients: single-center series of 25 cases and meta-analysis of 277 reported cases. Am J Surg Pathol. 2014 Jul;38(7):875–86. PMID:24832164

**4801.** Morse E, Fujiwara RJT, Husain Z, et al. Pediatric salivary cancer: epidemiology, treatment trends, and association of treatment modality with survival. Otolaryngol Head Neck Surg. 2018 Sep;159(3):553–63. PMID:29688836

**4802.** Moscicki AB, Shiboski S, Broering J, et al. The natural history of human papillomavirus infection as measured by repeated DNA testing in adolescent and young women. J Pediatr. 1998 Feb;132(2):277–84. PMID:9506641

**4803.** Moses MA, Green BC, Cugno S, et al. The management of midline frontonasal dermoids: a review of 55 cases at a tertiary referral center and a protocol for treatment. Plast Reconstr Surg. 2015 Jan;135(1):187–96. PMID:25285685

**4804.** Mosharafa AA, Foster RS, Leibovich BC, et al. Histology in mixed germ cell tumors. Is there a favorite pairing? J Urol. 2004 Apr;171(4):1471–3. PMID:15017200

**4805.** Mosquera JM, Dal Cin P, Mertz KD, et al. Validation of a TFE3 break-apart FISH assay for Xp11.2 translocation renal cell carcinomas. Diagn Mol Pathol. 2011 Sep;20(3):129–37. PMID:21817901

**4806.** Mosquera JM, Sboner A, Zhang L, et al. Novel MIR143-NOTCH fusions in benign and malignant glomus tumors. Genes Chromosomes Cancer. 2013 Nov;52(11):1075–87. PMID:23999936

**4807.** Mosquera JM, Sboner A, Zhang L, et al. Recurrent NCOA2 gene rearrangements in congenital/infantile spindle cell rhabdomyosarcoma. Genes Chromosomes Cancer. 2013 Jun;52(6):538–50. PMID:23463663

**4808.** Mossé YP. Anaplastic lymphoma kinase as a cancer target in pediatric malignancies. Clin Cancer Res. 2016 Feb 1;22(3):546–52. PMID:26503946

**4809.** Mosse YP, Laudenslager M, Khazi D, et al. Germline PHOX2B mutation in hereditary neuroblastoma. Am J Hum Genet. 2004 Oct;75(4):727–30. PMID:15338462

**4810.** Mossé YP, Laudenslager M, Longo L, et al. Identification of ALK as a major familial

neuroblastoma predisposition gene. Nature. 2008 Oct 16;455(7215):930–5. PMID:18724359

**4811.** Mossé YP, Voss SD, Lim MS, et al. Targeting ALK with crizotinib in pediatric anaplastic large cell lymphoma and inflammatory myofibroblastic tumor: a Children's Oncology Group Study. J Clin Oncol. 2017 Oct 1;35(28):3215–21. PMID:28787259

**4812.** Mostert M, Rosenberg C, Stoop H, et al. Comparative genomic and in situ hybridization of germ cell tumors of the infantile testis. Lab Invest. 2000 Jul;80(7):1055–64. PMID:10908150

**4813.** Mostofi FK. Proceedings: Testicular tumors. Epidemiologic, etiologic, and pathologic features. Cancer. 1973 Nov;32(5):1186–201. PMID:4148412

**4814.** Mostofi FK, Sesterhenn IA. Pathology of germ cell tumors of testes. Prog Clin Biol Res. 1985;203:1–34. PMID:3008176

**4815.** Mostofi FK, Sesterhenn IA, Davis CJ Jr. Developments in histopathology of testicular germ cell tumors. Semin Urol. 1988 Aug;6(3):171–88. PMID:2854295

**4816.** Mostofi FK, Sesterhenn IA, Davis CJ Jr. Immunopathology of germ cell tumors of the testis. Semin Diagn Pathol. 1987 Nov;4(4):320–41. PMID:2451261

**4817.** Mostoufi-Moab S, Labourier E, Sullivan L, et al. Molecular testing for oncogenic gene alterations in pediatric thyroid lesions. Thyroid. 2018 Jan;28(1):60–7. PMID:29108474

**4818.** Mota A, Argenziano G, Zalaudek I, et al. Clinical, dermoscopic and histopathologic findings of retiform hemangioendothelioma. Dermatol Pract Concept. 2013 Oct 31;3(4):11–4. PMID:24282657

**4819.** Mottok A, Hung SS, Chavez EA, et al. Integrative genomic analysis identifies key pathogenic mechanisms in primary mediastinal large B-cell lymphoma. Blood. 2019 Sep 5;134(10):802–13. PMID:31292115

**4820.** Mottok A, Renné C, Willenbrock K, et al. Somatic hypermutation of SOCS1 in lymphocyte-predominant Hodgkin lymphoma is accompanied by high JAK2 expression and activation of STAT6. Blood. 2007 Nov 1;110(9):3387–90. PMID:17652621

**4821.** Mottok A, Woolcock B, Chan FC, et al. Genomic alterations in CIITA are frequent in primary mediastinal large B cell lymphoma and are associated with diminished MHC class II expression. Cell Rep. 2015 Nov 17;13(7):1418–31. PMID:26549456

**4822.** Mottok A, Wright G, Rosenwald A, et al. Molecular classification of primary mediastinal large B-cell lymphoma using routinely available tissue specimens. Blood. 2018 Nov 29;132(22):2401–5. PMID:30257882

**4823.** Moul JW, McCarthy WF, Fernandez EB, et al. Percentage of embryonal carcinoma and of vascular invasion predicts pathological stage in clinical stage I nonseminomatous testicular cancer. Cancer Res. 1994 Jan 15;54(2):362–4. PMID:8275469

**4824.** Movahedi M, Bishop DT, Macrae F, et al. Obesity, aspirin, and risk of colorectal cancer in carriers of hereditary colorectal cancer: a prospective investigation in the CAPP2 study. J Clin Oncol. 2015 Nov 1;33(31):3591–7. PMID:26282643

**4825.** Movahedi-Lankarani S, Kurman RJ. Calretinin, a more sensitive but less specific marker than alpha-inhibin for ovarian sex cord-stromal neoplasms: an immunohistochemical study of 215 cases. Am J Surg Pathol. 2002 Nov;26(11):1477–83. PMID:12409724

**4826.** Mroczek EC, Weisenburger DD, Grierson HL, et al. Fatal infectious mononucleosis and virus-associated hemophagocytic syndrome. Arch Pathol Lab Med. 1987 Jun;111(6):530–5. PMID:3579509

**4827.** Msaouel P, Hong AL, Mullen EA, et al. Updated recommendations on the diagnosis, management, and clinical trial eligibility criteria for patients with renal medullary carcinoma. Clin Genitourin Cancer. 2019 Feb;17(1):1–6. PMID:30287223

**4828.** Msaouel P, Tannir NM, Walker CL. A model linking sickle Cell hemoglobinopathies and SMARCB1 loss in renal medullary carcinoma. Clin Cancer Res. 2018 May 1;24(9):2044–9. PMID:29440190

**4829.** Mucitelli DR, Charles EZ, Kraus FT. Chorioangiomas of intermediate size and intrauterine growth retardation. Pathol Res Pract. 1990 Aug;186(4):455–8. PMID:2247373

**4830.** Mudhar HS, Smith K, Talley P, et al. Fluorescence in situ hybridisation (FISH) in histologically challenging conjunctival melanocytic lesions. Br J Ophthalmol. 2013 Jan;97(1):40–6. PMID:23137666

**4831.** Mudry P, Slaby O, Neradil J, et al. Case report: rapid and durable response to PDGFR targeted therapy in a child with refractory multiple infantile myofibromatosis and a heterozygous germline mutation of the PDGFRB gene. BMC Cancer. 2017 Feb 10;17(1):119. PMID:28183292

**4832.** Muir TE, Cheville JC, Lager DJ. Metanephric adenoma, nephrogenic rests, and Wilms' tumor: a histologic and immunophenotypic comparison. Am J Surg Pathol. 2001 Oct;25(10):1290–6. PMID:11688464

**4833.** Mukai K, Seljeskog EL, Dehner LP. Pituitary adenomas in patients under 20 years old. A clinicopathological study of 12 cases. J Neurooncol. 1986;4(1):79–89. PMID:3018185

**4834.** Mukai M, Torikata C, Iri H, et al. Immunohistochemical identification of aggregated actin filaments in formalin-fixed, paraffin-embedded sections. I. A study of infantile digital fibromatosis by a new pretreatment. Am J Surg Pathol. 1992 Feb;16(2):110–5. PMID:1310240

**4835.** Mukai M, Torikata C, Iri H, et al. Infantile digital fibromatosis. An electron microscopic and immunohistochemical study. Acta Pathol Jpn. 1986 Nov;36(11):1605–15. PMID:3811906

**4836.** Mukherjee D, Chaichana KL, Gokaslan ZL, et al. Survival of patients with malignant primary osseous spinal neoplasms: results from the Surveillance, Epidemiology, and End Results (SEER) database from 1973 to 2003. J Neurosurg Spine. 2011 Feb;14(2):143–50. PMID:21184634

**4837.** Mukherjee S, Bandyopadhyay G, Saha S, et al. Cytodiagnosis of glomus tumor. J Cytol. 2010 Jul;27(3):104–5. PMID:21187877

**4838.** Mukherjee S, Bhadada SK, Arya AK, et al. Primary hyperparathyroidism in the young: comparison with adult primary hyperparathyroidism. Endocr Pract. 2018 Dec;24(12):1051–6. PMID:30289299

**4839.** Mukhopadhyay S, Valente AL, de la Roza G. Cystic nephroma: a histologic and immunohistochemical study of 10 cases. Arch Pathol Lab Med. 2004 Dec;128(12):1404–11. PMID:15578885

**4840.** Mukunyadzi P, Bardales RH, Palmer HE, et al. Tissue effects of salivary gland fine-needle aspiration. Does this procedure preclude accurate histologic diagnosis? Am J Clin Pathol. 2000 Nov;114(5):741–5. PMID:11068548

**4841.** Müller HL. Consequences of craniopharyngioma surgery in children. J Clin Endocrinol Metab. 2011 Jul;96(7):1981–91. PMID:21508127

**4842.** Müller HL, Bueb K, Bartels U, et al. Obesity after childhood craniopharyngioma–German multicenter study on pre-operative risk factors and quality of life. Klin Padiatr. 2001 Jul-Aug;213(4):244–9. PMID:11528558

**4843.** Müller HL, Emser A, Faldum A, et al. Longitudinal study on growth and body mass

index before and after diagnosis of childhood craniopharyngioma. J Clin Endocrinol Metab. 2004 Jul;89(7):3298–305. PMID:15240606

**4844.** Müller HL, Gebhardt U, Teske C, et al. Post-operative hypothalamic lesions and obesity in childhood craniopharyngioma: results of the multinational prospective trial Kraniopharyngeom 2000 after 3-year follow-up. Eur J Endocrinol. 2011 Jul;165(1):17–24. PMID:21490122

**4845.** Müller HL, Merchant TE, Warmuth-Metz M, et al. Craniopharyngioma. Nat Rev Dis Primers. 2019 Nov 7;5(1):75. PMID:31699993

**4846.** Müller S. Frictional keratosis, contact keratosis and smokeless tobacco keratosis: features of reactive white lesions of the oral mucosa. Head Neck Pathol. 2019 Mar;13(1):16–24. PMID:30671762

**4847.** Müller-Höcker J, Zietz CH, Sendelhofert A. Deregulated expression of cell cycle-associated proteins in solid pseudopapillary tumor of the pancreas. Mod Pathol. 2001 Feb;14(2):47–53. PMID:11235905

**4848.** Müller-Scholden J, Lehrnbecher T, Müller HL, et al. Radical surgery in a neonate with craniopharyngioma. report of a case. Pediatr Neurosurg. 2000 Nov;33(5):265–9. PMID:11155065

**4849.** Mullighan CG. The genomic landscape of acute lymphoblastic leukemia in children and young adults. Hematology Am Soc Hematol Educ Program. 2014 Dec 5;2014(1):174–80. PMID:25696852

**4850.** Mullighan CG, Miller CB, Radtke I, et al. BCR-ABL1 lymphoblastic leukaemia is characterized by the deletion of Ikaros. Nature. 2008 May 1;453(7191):110–4. PMID:18408710

**4851.** Mullighan CG, Su X, Zhang J, et al. Deletion of IKZF1 and prognosis in acute lymphoblastic leukemia. N Engl J Med. 2009 Jan 29;360(5):470–80. PMID:19129520

**4852.** Mulrooney DA, Carpenter B, Georgieff M, et al. Hepatic mesenchymal hamartoma in a neonate: a case report and review of the literature. J Pediatr Hematol Oncol. 2001 Jun-Jul;23(5):316–7. PMID:11464991

**4853.** Munden A, Butschek R, Tom WL, et al. Prospective study of infantile haemangiomas: incidence, clinical characteristics and association with placental anomalies. Br J Dermatol. 2014 Apr;170(4):907–13. PMID:24641194

**4854.** Mundo L, Ambrosio MR, Raimondi F, et al. Molecular switch from MYC to MYCN expression in MYC protein negative Burkitt lymphoma cases. Blood Cancer J. 2019 Nov 20;9(12):91. PMID:31748534

**4855.** Mungo DV, Zhang X, O'Keefe RJ, et al. COX-1 and COX-2 expression in osteoid osteomas. J Orthop Res. 2002 Jan;20(1):159–62. PMID:11853083

**4856.** Munier FL, Beck-Popovic M, Chantada GL, et al. Conservative management of retinoblastoma: challenging orthodoxy without compromising the state of metastatic grace. "Alive, with good vision and no comorbidity". Prog Retin Eye Res. 2019 Nov;73:100764. PMID:31173880

**4857.** Munier FL, Gaillard MC, Balmer A, et al. Intravitreal chemotherapy for vitreous disease in retinoblastoma revisited: from prohibition to conditional indications. Br J Ophthalmol. 2012 Aug;96(8):1078–83. PMID:22694968

**4858.** Mur TA, Pellegrini WR, Tracy LF, et al. Laryngeal granular cell tumors in children: a literature review. Int J Pediatr Otorhinolaryngol. 2020 Nov;138:110193. PMID:32705988

**4859.** Murakami N, Okuno Y, Yoshida K, et al. Integrated molecular profiling of juvenile myelomonocytic leukemia. Blood. 2018 Apr 5;131(14):1576–86. PMID:29437595

**4860.** Murali R, McCarthy SW, Scolyer RA. Blue nevi and related lesions: a review highlighting atypical and newly described variants, distinguishing features and diagnostic pitfalls.

Adv Anat Pathol. 2009 Nov;16(6):365–82. PMID:19851128

4861. Murali R, Wiesner T, Scolyer RA. Tumours associated with BAP1 mutations. Pathology. 2013 Feb;45(2):116–26. PMID:23277170

4862. Murawski M, Weeda VB, Maibach R, et al. Hepatocellular carcinoma in children: Does modified platinum- and doxorubicin-based chemotherapy increase tumor resectability and change outcome? Lessons learned from the SIOPEL 2 and 3 studies. J Clin Oncol. 2016 Apr 1;34(10):1050–6. PMID:26811523

4863. Mürbeth S, Rousarova M, Scherb H, et al. Thyroid cancer has increased in the adult populations of countries moderately affected by Chernobyl fallout. Med Sci Monit. 2004 Jul;10(7):CR300–6. PMID:15295858

4864. Murdock T, Orr B, Allen S, et al. Central nervous system-type neuroepithelial tumors and tumor-like proliferations developing in the gynecologic tract and pelvis: clinicopathologic analysis of 23 cases. Am J Surg Pathol. 2018 Nov;42(11):1429–44. PMID:30074494

4865. Murphey MD, Jelinek JS, Temple HT, et al. Imaging of periosteal osteosarcoma: radiologic-pathologic comparison. Radiology. 2004 Oct;233(1):129–38. PMID:15333772

4866. Murphey MD, Rhee JH, Lewis RB, et al. Pigmented villonodular synovitis: radiologic-pathologic correlation. Radiographics. 2008 Sep-Oct;28(5):1493–518. PMID:18794322

4867. Murphey MD, Vidal JA, Fanburg-Smith JC, et al. Imaging of synovial chondromatosis with radiologic-pathologic correlation. Radiographics. 2007 Sep-Oct;27(5):1465–88. PMID:17848703

4868. Murphey MD, wan Jaovisidha S, Temple HT, et al. Telangiectatic osteosarcoma: radiologic-pathologic comparison. Radiology. 2003 Nov;229(2):545–53. PMID:14512511

4869. Murphy SB. Classification, staging and end results of treatment of childhood non-Hodgkin's lymphomas: dissimilarities from lymphomas in adults. Semin Oncol. 1980 Sep;7(3):332–9. PMID:7414342

4870. Murray JC, Donahue DJ, Malik SI, et al. Temporal lobe pleomorphic xanthoastrocytoma and acquired BRAF mutation in an adolescent with the constitutional 22q11.2 deletion syndrome. J Neurooncol. 2011 May;102(3):509–14. PMID:20730472

4871. Murray MJ, Bartels U, Nishikawa R, et al. Consensus on the management of intracranial germ-cell tumours. Lancet Oncol. 2015 Sep;16(9):e470–7. PMID:26370356

4872. Murray MJ, Coleman N. Testicular cancer: a new generation of biomarkers for malignant germ cell tumours. Nat Rev Urol. 2012 May 1;9(6):298–300. PMID:22549310

4873. Murray N, Hanna B, Graf N, et al. The spectrum of infantile myofibromatosis includes both non-penetrance and adult recurrence. Eur J Med Genet. 2017 Jul;60(7):353–8. PMID:28286173

4874. Murshed K, Farghaly H. Multifocal epithelioid hemangioma of the penis in a 4-year-old child: a case report. Am J Dermatopathol. 2020 May;42(5):372–4. PMID:31693501

4875. Murthy A, Gonzalez-Agosti C, Cordero E, et al. NHE-RF, a regulatory cofactor for Na(+)-H+ exchange, is a common interactor for merlin and ERM (MERM) proteins. J Biol Chem. 1998 Jan 16;273(3):1273–6. PMID:9430655

4876. Murthy DP, SenGupta SK, Mola G, et al. Sclerosing stromal tumour of the ovary. P N G Med J. 1996 Mar;39(1):48–55. PMID:9522851

4877. Musani V, Sabol M, Car D, et al. PTCH1 gene polymorphisms in ovarian tumors: potential protective role of c.3944T allele. Gene. 2013 Mar 15;517(1):55–9. PMID:23313819

4878. Muscarella LA, Bisceglia M, Galliani CA, et al. Extraneuraxial hemangioblastoma: a clinicopathologic study of 10 cases with molecular analysis of the VHL gene. Pathol Res Pract. 2018 Aug;214(8):1156–65. PMID:29941223

4879. Mussa A, Duffy KA, Carli D, et al. Defining an optimal time window to screen for hepatoblastoma in children with Beckwith-Wiedemann syndrome. Pediatr Blood Cancer. 2019 Jan;66(1):e27492. PMID:30270492

4880. Mussa A, Molinatto C, Cerrato F, et al. Assisted reproductive techniques and risk of Beckwith-Wiedemann syndrome. Pediatrics. 2017 Jul;140(1):e20164311. PMID:28634246

4881. Mussa A, Russo S, De Crescenzo A, et al. Prevalence of Beckwith-Wiedemann syndrome in North West of Italy. Am J Med Genet A. 2013 Oct;161A(10):2481–6. PMID:23918458

4882. Mussavi M, Asadollahi K, Janbaz F, et al. The evaluation of red reflex sensitivity and specificity test among neonates in different conditions. Iran J Pediatr. 2014 Dec;24(6):697–702. PMID:26019774

4883. Musselman JR, Georgieff MK, Ross JA, et al. Maternal pregnancy events and exposures and risk of hepatoblastoma: a Children's Oncology Group (COG) study. Cancer Epidemiol. 2013 Jun;37(3):318–20. PMID:23312454

4884. Mussolin L, Damm-Welk C, Pillon M, et al. Use of minimal disseminated disease and immunity to NPM-ALK antigen to stratify ALK-positive ALCL patients with different prognosis. Leukemia. 2013 Feb;27(2):416–22. PMID:22907048

4885. Myers KA, Mandelstam SA, Ramantani G, et al. The epileptology of Koolen-de Vries syndrome: electro-clinico-radiologic findings in 31 patients. Epilepsia. 2017 Jun;58(6):1085–94. PMID:28440867

4886. Myers KC, Furutani E, Weller E, et al. Clinical features and outcomes of patients with Shwachman-Diamond syndrome and myelodysplastic syndrome or acute myeloid leukaemia: a multicentre, retrospective, cohort study. Lancet Haematol. 2020 Mar;7(3):e238–46. PMID:31879230

4887. Myhre-Jensen O. A consecutive 7-year series of 1331 benign soft tissue tumours. Clinicopathologic data. Comparison with sarcomas. Acta Orthop Scand. 1981 Jun;52(3):287–93. PMID:7282321

4888. Mylona S, Patsoura S, Galani P, et al. Osteoid osteomas in common and in technically challenging locations treated with computed tomography-guided percutaneous radiofrequency ablation. Skeletal Radiol. 2010 May;39(5):443–9. PMID:20066410

4889. Mylonas KS, Doulamis IP, Tsilimigras DI, et al. Solid pseudopapillary and malignant pancreatic tumors in childhood: a systematic review and evidence quality assessment. Pediatr Blood Cancer. 2018 Oct;65(10):e27114. PMID:29697193

4890. Mylonas KS, Kao CS, Levy D, et al. Clinicopathologic features and chromosome 12p status of pediatric sacrococcygeal teratomas: a multi-institutional analysis. Pediatr Dev Pathol. 2019 May-Jun;22(3):214–20. PMID:30176765

4891. Mynarek M, von Hoff K, Pietsch T, et al. Nonmetastatic medulloblastoma of early childhood: results from the prospective clinical trial HIT-2000 and an extended validation cohort. J Clin Oncol. 2020 Jun 20;38(18):2028–40. PMID:32330099

4892. Myssiorek D, Ruah CB, Hybels RL. Recurrent pleomorphic adenomas of the parotid gland. Head Neck. 1990 Jul-Aug;12(4):332–6. PMID:2361864

4893. Nabai H, Mehregan AH. Nevus comedonicus. A review of the literature and report of twelve cases. Acta Derm Venereol. 1973;53(1):71–4. PMID:4120812

4894. Nabavizadeh SA, Assadsangabi R, Hajmomenian M, et al. High accuracy of arterial spin labeling perfusion imaging in differentiation of pilomyxoid from pilocytic astrocytoma. Neuroradiology. 2015 May;57(5):527–33. PMID:25666232

4895. Nabbout R, Santos M, Rolland Y, et al. Early diagnosis of subependymal giant cell astrocytoma in children with tuberous sclerosis. J Neurol Neurosurg Psychiatry. 1999 Mar;66(3):370–5. PMID:10084537

4896. Nachman JB, Heerema NA, Sather H, et al. Outcome of treatment in children with hypodiploid acute lymphoblastic leukemia. Blood. 2007 Aug 15;110(4):1112–5. PMID:17473063

4897. Nador RG, Chadburn A, Gundappa G, et al. Human immunodeficiency virus (HIV)-associated polymorphic lymphoproliferative disorders. Am J Surg Pathol. 2003 Mar;27(3):293–302. PMID:12604885

4898. Nagai K, Nakano N, Iwai T, et al. Pediatric subcutaneous panniculitis-like T-cell lymphoma with favorable result by immunosuppressive therapy: a report of two cases. Pediatr Hematol Oncol. 2014 Sep;31(6):528–33. PMID:24684413

4899. Nagaishi M, Yokoo H, Nobusawa S, et al. Localized overexpression of alpha-internexin within nodules in multinodular and vacuolating neuronal tumors. Neuropathology. 2015 Dec;35(6):561–8. PMID:26073706

4900. Nagalakshmi VK, Ren Q, Pugh MM, et al. Dicer regulates the development of nephrogenic and ureteric compartments in the mammalian kidney. Kidney Int. 2011 Feb;79(3):317–30. PMID:20944551

4901. Nagano Y, Uchida K, Inoue M, et al. Mesenteric lipoblastoma presenting as a small intestinal volvulus in an infant: a case report and literature review. Asian J Surg. 2017 Jan;40(1):70–3. PMID:28034384

4902. Nagaraja S, Vitanza NA, Woo PJ, et al. Transcriptional dependencies in diffuse intrinsic pontine glioma. Cancer Cell. 2017 May 8;31(5):635–652.e6. PMID:28434841

4903. Nagorney DM, Adson MA, Weiland LH, et al. Fibrolamellar hepatoma. Am J Surg. 1985 Jan;149(1):113–9. PMID:2981486

4904. Naidu A, Chung B, Simon M, et al. Bilateral sclerosing stromal ovarian tumor in an adolescent. Case Rep Radiol. 2015;2015:271394. PMID:26064755

4905. Nair C, Chopra H, Shinde S, et al. Immunophenotype and ultrastructural studies in blast crisis of chronic myeloid leukemia. Leuk Lymphoma. 1995 Oct;19(3-4):309–13. PMID:8535224

4906. Naitoh Y, Sasajima T, Kinouchi H, et al. Medulloblastoma with extensive nodularity: single photon emission CT study with iodine-123 metaiodobenzylguanidine. AJNR Am J Neuroradiol. 2002 Oct;23(9):1564–7. PMID:12372749

4907. Nakagawara A, Li Y, Izumi H, et al. Neuroblastoma. Jpn J Clin Oncol. 2018 Mar 1;48(3):214–41. PMID:29378002

4908. Nakajima H, Sim FH, Bond JR, et al. Small cell osteosarcoma of bone. Review of 72 cases. Cancer. 1997 Jun 1;79(11):2095–106. PMID:9179055

4909. Nakajima N, Nobusawa S, Nakata S, et al. BRAF V600E, TERT promoter mutations and CDKN2A/B homozygous deletions are frequent in epithelioid glioblastomas: a histological and molecular analysis focusing on intratumoral heterogeneity. Brain Pathol. 2018 Sep;28(5):663–73. PMID:29105198

4910. Nakama S, Higashi T, Kimura A, et al. Double myxopapillary ependymoma of the cauda equina. J Orthop Sci. 2005 Sep;10(5):543–5. PMID:16193371

4911. Nakamura M, Chiba K, Matsumoto M, et al. Pleomorphic xanthoastrocytoma of the spinal cord. Case report. J Neurosurg Spine. 2006 Jul;5(1):72–5. PMID:16850961

4912. Nakamura M, Saeki N, Iwadate Y, et al. Neuroradiological characteristics of pineocytoma and pineoblastoma. Neuroradiology. 2000 Jul;42(7):509–14. PMID:10952183

4913. Nakamura M, Tokura Y. Superficial angiomyxoma on the scrotum of a child. Pediatr Dermatol. 2011 Mar-Apr;28(2):200–1. PMID:21504453

4914. Nakano Y, Hasegawa D, Stewart DR, et al. Presacral malignant teratoid neoplasm in association with pathogenic DICER1 variation. Mod Pathol. 2019 Dec;32(12):1744–50. PMID:31296931

4915. Nakashima Y, Miyagi-Shiohira C, Kobayashi N, et al. Adhesion characteristics of porcine pancreatic islets and exocrine tissue to coating materials. Islets. 2018 May 4;10(3):e1460294. PMID:29757700

4916. Nakashima Y, Tagawa H, Suzuki R, et al. Genome-wide array-based comparative genomic hybridization of natural killer cell lymphoma/leukemia: different genomic alteration patterns of aggressive NK-cell leukemia and extranodal Nk/T-cell lymphoma, nasal type. Genes Chromosomes Cancer. 2005 Nov;44(3):247–55. PMID:16049916

4917. Nakashima Y, Unni KK, Shives TC, et al. Mesenchymal chondrosarcoma of bone and soft tissue. A review of 111 cases. Cancer. 1986 Jun 15;57(12):2444–53. PMID:3697943

4918. Nakata K, Colombet M, Stiller CA, et al. Incidence of childhood renal tumours: an international population-based study. Int J Cancer. 2020 Dec 15;147(12):3313–27. PMID:32902866

4919. Nakata K, Ito Y, Magadi W, et al. Childhood cancer incidence and survival in Japan and England: a population-based study (1993-2010). Cancer Sci. 2018 Feb;109(2):422–34. PMID:29178401

4920. Nakaya M, Yoshihara S, Yoshitomi A, et al. Endoscopic endonasal excision of nasal chondromesenchymal hamartoma with intracranial extension. Eur Ann Otorhinolaryngol Head Neck Dis. 2017 Dec;134(6):423–5. PMID:28385583

4921. Nakaya T, Morita K, Kurata A, et al. Multifocal kaposiform hemangioendothelioma in multiple visceral organs: an autopsy of 9-day-old female baby. Hum Pathol. 2014 Aug;45(8):1773–7. PMID:24931465

4921A. Nakazawa T, Celestino R, Machado JC, et al. Cribriform-morular variant of papillary thyroid carcinoma displaying poorly differentiated features. Int J Surg Pathol. 2013 Aug;21(4):379–89. PMID:23349472

4922. Nakken S, Hovig E, Møller P, editors. Prospective Lynch Syndrome Database [Internet]. Edinburgh (UK): European Hereditary Tumour Group & Middlesex (UK): International Society for Gastrointestinal Hereditary Tumours; 2019. Available from https://www.lscarisk.org.

4923. Nalesnik MA, Jaffe R, Starzl TE, et al. The pathology of posttransplant lymphoproliferative disorders occurring in the setting of cyclosporine A-prednisone immunosuppression. Am J Pathol. 1988 Oct;133(1):173–92. PMID:2845789

4924. Nambirajan A, Sharma MC, Rajeshwari M, et al. A comparative immunohistochemical study of epithelial membrane antigen and NHERF1/EBP50 in the diagnosis of ependymomas. Appl Immunohistochem Mol Morphol. 2018 Jan;26(1):71–8. PMID:27753657

4925. Nambirajan A, Singh V, Irugu DVK, et al. Spindle epithelial tumour with thymus-like elements presenting with lymph node metastasis: an illustrative case report with review of literature. Cytopathology. 2019 Nov;30(6):657–61. PMID:31209931

4926. Nambirajan A, Suri V, Kedia S, et al. Paediatric diffuse leptomeningeal tumor with

glial and neuronal differentiation harbouring chromosome 1p/19q co-deletion and H3.3 K27M mutation: unusual molecular profile and its therapeutic implications. Brain Tumor Pathol. 2018 Jul;35(3):186–91. PMID:30030640
**4927.** Nambu M, Shimizu K, Ito S, et al. A case of juvenile myelomonocytic leukemia with ocular infiltration. Ann Hematol. 1999 Dec;78(12):568–70. PMID:10647883
**4928.** Nam-Cha SH, Montes-Moreno S, Salcedo MT, et al. Lymphocyte-rich classical Hodgkin's lymphoma: distinctive tumor and microenvironment markers. Mod Pathol. 2009 Aug;22(8):1006–15. PMID:19465900
**4929.** Nam-Cha SH, Roncador G, Sanchez-Verde L, et al. PD-1, a follicular T-cell marker useful for recognizing nodular lymphocyte-predominant Hodgkin lymphoma. Am J Surg Pathol. 2008 Aug;32(8):1252–7. PMID:18594468
**4930.** Naranjo A, Irwin MS, Hogarty MD, et al. Statistical framework in support of a revised Children's Oncology Group neuroblastoma risk classification system. JCO Clin Cancer Inform. 2018 Dec;2:1–15. PMID:30652588
**4931.** Narayan V, Savardekar AR, Mahadevan A, et al. Unusual occurrence of multifocal desmoplastic infantile astrocytoma: a case report and review of the literature. Pediatr Neurosurg. 2017;52(3):173–80. PMID:28222441
**4932.** Naresh KN, Ibrahim HA, Lazzi S, et al. Diagnosis of Burkitt lymphoma using an algorithmic approach–applicable in both resource-poor and resource-rich countries. Br J Haematol. 2011 Sep;154(6):770–6. PMID:21718280
**4933.** Narkewicz MR, Green M, Dunn S, et al. Decreasing incidence of symptomatic Epstein-Barr virus disease and posttransplant lymphoproliferative disorder in pediatric liver transplant recipients: report of the studies of pediatric liver transplantation experience. Liver Transpl. 2013 Jul;19(7):730–40. PMID:23696264
**4934.** Narla S, Govindraj J, Chandrasekar K, et al. Craniopharyngioma with malignant transformation: review of literature. Neurol India. 2017 Mar-Apr;65(2):418–20. PMID:28290422
**4935.** Narumi S, Amano N, Ishii T, et al. SAMD9 mutations cause a novel multisystem disorder, MIRAGE syndrome, and are associated with loss of chromosome 7. Nat Genet. 2016 Jul;48(7):792–7. PMID:27182967
**4936.** Nascimento AF, Fletcher CD. The controversial nosology of benign nerve sheath tumors: neurofilament protein staining demonstrates intratumoral axons in many sporadic schwannomas. Am J Surg Pathol. 2007 Sep;31(9):1363–70. PMID:17721192
**4937.** Nasit J, Vaghsiya V, Hiryur S, et al. Intraoperative squash cytologic features of subependymal giant cell astrocytoma. J Lab Physicians. 2016 Jan-Jun;8(1):58–61. PMID:27013816
**4938.** Nason GJ, Baker JF, O'Toole P, et al. Fibroma of the peroneus longus tendon sheath in a child: a case report. J Orthop Surg (Hong Kong). 2013 Dec;21(3):387–90. PMID:24366807
**4939.** Nassif S, Kaufman S, Vahdat S, et al. Clinicopathologic features of post-transplant lymphoproliferative disorders arising after pediatric small bowel transplant. Pediatr Transplant. 2013 Dec;17(8):765–73. PMID:24118781
**4940.** Nasu M, Emi M, Pastorino S, et al. High incidence of somatic BAP1 alterations in sporadic malignant mesothelioma. J Thorac Oncol. 2015 Apr;10(4):565–76. PMID:25658628
**4941.** Nathan N, Keppler-Noreuil KM, Biesecker LG, et al. Mosaic disorders of the PI3K/PTEN/AKT/TSC/mTORC1 signaling pathway. Dermatol Clin. 2017 Jan;35(1):51–60. PMID:27890237
**4942.** Nathanson S, Debray D, Delarue A, et al. Long-term survival after post-transplant lymphoproliferative disease in children. Pediatr Nephrol. 2002 Aug;17(8):668–72. PMID:12185479
**4943.** Nathany S, Chatterjee G, Ghai S, et al. Mutational landscape of Juvenile Myelomonocytic Leukemia (JMML)-A real-world context. Int J Lab Hematol. 2021 Dec;43(6):1531–8. PMID:34387930
**4944.** National Institute for Health and Care Excellence (NICE). Molecular testing strategies for Lynch syndrome in people with colorectal cancer: diagnostics guidance (DG27). London (UK): NICE; 2017 Feb. Available from: https://www.nice.org.uk/guidance/dg27.
**4945.** National Institutes of Health Consensus Development Conference. Neurofibromatosis. Conference statement. Arch Neurol. 1988 May;45(5):575–8. PMID:3128965
**4946.** Natkunam Y, Goodlad JR, Chadburn A, et al. EBV-positive B-cell proliferations of varied malignant potential: 2015 SH/EAHP workshop report-Part 1. Am J Clin Pathol. 2017 Feb 1;147(2):129–52. PMID:28395107
**4947.** Naudin ten Cate L, Vermeij-Keers C, Smit DA, et al. Intracranial teratoma with multiple fetuses: pre- and post-natal appearance. Hum Pathol. 1995 Jul;26(7):804–7. PMID:7628856
**4948.** Nault JC, Paradis V, Cherqui D, et al. Molecular classification of hepatocellular adenoma in clinical practice. J Hepatol. 2017 Nov;67(5):1074–83. PMID:28733222
**4949.** Navale P, Rooper LM, Bishop JA, et al. Mucoepidermoid carcinoma of the oropharynx: a tumor type with a propensity for regional metastasis unrelated to histologic grade. Hum Pathol. 2019 Nov;93:1–5. PMID:31442522
**4950.** Navalkele P, O'Dorisio MS, O'Dorisio TM, et al. Incidence, survival, and prevalence of neuroendocrine tumors versus neuroblastoma in children and young adults: nine standard SEER registries, 1975-2006. Pediatr Blood Cancer. 2011 Jan;56(1):50–7. PMID:21108439
**4951.** Naylor RM, Wohl A, Raghunathan A, et al. Novel suprasellar location of desmoplastic infantile astrocytoma and ganglioglioma: a single institution's experience. J Neurosurg Pediatr. 2018 Oct;22(4):397–403. PMID:29979130
**4952.** Nazira B, Gupta H, Chaturvedi AK, et al. Melanotic neuroectodermal tumor of infancy: discussion of a case and a review of the imaging findings. Cancer Imaging. 2009 Dec 24;9:121–5. PMID:20080455
**4953.** Neal MT, Ellis TL, Stanton CA. Pleomorphic xanthoastrocytoma in two siblings with neurofibromatosis type 1 (NF-1). Clin Neuropathol. 2012 Jan-Feb;31(1):54–6. PMID:22192706
**4954.** Neel HB 3rd, Whicker JH, Devine KD, et al. Juvenile angiofibroma. Review of 120 cases. Am J Surg. 1973 Oct;126(4):547–56. PMID:4355257
**4955.** Nelson AC, Pillay N, Henderson S, et al. An integrated functional genomics approach identifies the regulatory network directed by brachyury (T) in chordoma. J Pathol. 2012 Nov;228(3):274–85. PMID:22847733
**4956.** Nelson AJ, Zakaria R, Jenkinson MD, et al. Extent of resection predicts risk of progression in adult pilocytic astrocytoma. Br J Neurosurg. 2019 Jun;33(3):343–7. PMID:30653383
**4957.** Nelson BP, Nalesnik MA, Bahler DW, et al. Epstein-Barr virus-negative post-transplant lymphoproliferative disorders: a distinct entity? Am J Surg Pathol. 2000 Mar;24(3):375–85. PMID:10716151
**4958.** Nelson BP, Wolniak KL, Evens A, et al. Early posttransplant lymphoproliferative disease: clinicopathologic features and correlation with mTOR signaling pathway activation. Am J Clin Pathol. 2012 Oct;138(4):568–78. PMID:23010712
**4959.** Nelson JF, Felicio LS. Hormonal influences on reproductive aging in mice. Ann N Y Acad Sci. 1990;592:8–12. PMID:2197955
**4960.** Nelson S, Näthke IS. Interactions and functions of the adenomatous polyposis coli (APC) protein at a glance. J Cell Sci. 2013 Feb 15;126(Pt 4):873–7. PMID:23589686
**4961.** Nemcikova M, Vejvalkova S, Fencl F, et al. A novel heterozygous RIT1 mutation in a patient with Noonan syndrome, leukopenia, and transient myeloproliferation-a review of the literature. Eur J Pediatr. 2016 Apr;175(4):587–92. PMID:26518681
**4962.** Neou M, Villa C, Armignacco R, et al. Pangenomic classification of pituitary neuroendocrine tumors. Cancer Cell. 2020 Jan 13;37(1):123–134.e5. PMID:31883967
**4963.** Neri M, Di Donato S, Maglietta R, et al. Sudden death as presenting symptom caused by cardiac primary multicentric left ventricle rhabdomyoma, in an 11-month-old baby. An immunohistochemical study. Diagn Pathol. 2012 Dec 3;7:169. PMID:23206573
**4964.** Neskey DM, Klein JD, Hicks S, et al. Prognostic factors associated with decreased survival in patients with acinic cell carcinoma. JAMA Otolaryngol Head Neck Surg. 2013 Nov;139(11):1195–202. PMID:24076756
**4965.** Netherlands LOVD development team. InSiGHT DNA Variant Database [Internet]. Leiden (Netherlands): Leiden University Medical Center; 2018. Available from: https://www.insight-database.org.
**4966.** Nettersheim D, Biermann K, Gillis AJ, et al. NANOG promoter methylation and expression correlation during normal and malignant human germ cell development. Epigenetics. 2011 Jan;6(1):114–22. PMID:20930529
**4967.** Nettersheim D, Heimsoeth A, Jostes S, et al. SOX2 is essential for in vivo reprogramming of seminoma-like TCam-2 cells to an embryonal carcinoma-like fate. Oncotarget. 2016 Jul 26;7(30):47095–110. PMID:27283990
**4968.** Nettersheim D, Jostes S, Sharma R, et al. BMP inhibition in seminomas initiates acquisition of pluripotency via NODAL signaling resulting in reprogramming to an embryonal carcinoma. PLoS Genet. 2015 Jul 30;11(7):e1005415. PMID:26226633
**4969.** Nettersheim D, Westernströer B, Haas N, et al. Establishment of a versatile seminoma model indicates cellular plasticity of germ cell tumor cells. Genes Chromosomes Cancer. 2012 Jul;51(7):717–26. PMID:22489004
**4970.** Netto GJ, Nakai Y, Nakayama M, et al. Global DNA hypomethylation in intratubular germ cell neoplasia and seminoma, but not in nonseminomatous male germ cell tumors. Mod Pathol. 2008 Nov;21(11):1337–44. PMID:18622385
**4971.** Neubauer P, Weber AK, Miller NH, et al. Pigmented villonodular synovitis in children: a report of six cases and review of the literature. Iowa Orthop J. 2007;27:90–4. PMID:17907437
**4972.** Neubecker RD, Breen SL. Gynandroblastoma. A report of five cases, with a discussion of the histogenesis and classification of ovarian tumors. Am J Clin Pathol. 1962 Jul;38:60–9. PMID:14479145
**4973.** Neuhaus K, Landolt M, Vojvodic M, et al. Surgical treatment of children and youth with congenital melanocytic nevi: self- and proxy-reported opinions. Pediatr Surg Int. 2020 Apr;36(4):501–12. PMID:32125501
**4974.** Neuhold JC, Friesenhahn J, Gerdes N, et al. Case reports of fatal or metastasizing melanoma in children and adolescents: a systematic analysis of the literature. Pediatr Dermatol. 2015 Jan-Feb;32(1):13–22. PMID:25487565
**4975.** Neumann HP, Bausch B, McWhinney SR, et al. Germ-line mutations in nonsyndromic pheochromocytoma. N Engl J Med. 2002 May 9;346(19):1459–66. PMID:12000816
**4976.** Neumann JE, Spohn M, Obrecht D, et al. Molecular characterization of histopathological ependymoma variants. Acta Neuropathol. 2020 Feb;139(2):305–18. PMID:31679042
**4977.** Neuville A, Ranchère-Vince D, Dei Tos AP, et al. Impact of molecular analysis on the final sarcoma diagnosis: a study on 763 cases collected during a European epidemiological study. Am J Surg Pathol. 2013 Aug;37(8):1259–68. PMID:23774173
**4978.** Nevares RL, Mulliken JB, Robb RM. Ocular dermoids. Plast Reconstr Surg. 1988 Dec;82(6):959–64. PMID:3200959
**4979.** Neven B, Magerus-Chatinet A, Florkin B, et al. A survey of 90 patients with autoimmune lymphoproliferative syndrome related to TNFRSF6 mutation. Blood. 2011 Nov 3;118(18):4798–807. PMID:21885602
**4980.** Neven Q, Boulanger C, Bruwier A, et al. Clinical Spectrum of Ras-Associated Autoimmune Leukoproliferative Disorder (RALD). J Clin Immunol. 2021 Jan;41(1):51–8. PMID:33011939
**4981.** Neves RI, Stevenson J, Hancey MJ, et al. Endovascular papillary angioendothelioma (Dabska tumor): underrecognized malignant tumor in childhood. J Pediatr Surg. 2011 Jan;46(1):e25–8. PMID:21238627
**4982.** Neville H, Corpron C, Blakely ML, et al. Pediatric neurofibrosarcoma. J Pediatr Surg. 2003 Mar;38(3):343–6. PMID:12632346
**4983.** Newby R, Rowe D, Paterson L, et al. Cryptic EWSR1-FLI1 fusions in Ewing sarcoma: potential pitfalls in the diagnostic use of fluorescence in situ hybridization probes. Cancer Genet Cytogenet. 2010 Jul 1;200(1):60–4. PMID:20513536
**4984.** Newman DM, Walter JB. Multiple dermatofibromas in patients with systemic lupus erythematosus on immunosuppressive therapy. N Engl J Med. 1973 Oct 18;289(16):842–3. PMID:4763427
**4985.** Newman S, Fan L, Pribnow A, et al. Clinical genome sequencing uncovers potentially targetable truncations and fusions of MAP3K8 in spitzoid and other melanomas. Nat Med. 2019 Apr;25(4):597–602. PMID:30833747
**4986.** Newsome JR, Venkatramani R, Heczey A, et al. Cholangiocarcinoma among children and adolescents: a review of the literature and Surveillance, Epidemiology, and End Results Program database analysis. J Pediatr Gastroenterol Nutr. 2018 Jan;66(1):e12–8. PMID:28937543
**4987.** Newton JG, Horan JT, Newman S, et al. CD36-positive B-lymphoblasts predict poor outcome in children with B-lymphoblastic leukemia. Pediatr Dev Pathol. 2017 Jun;20(3):224–31. PMID:28521628
**4988.** Newton-Bishop JA, Chang YM, Iles MM, et al. Melanocytic nevi, nevus genes, and melanoma risk in a large case-control study in the United Kingdom. Cancer Epidemiol Biomarkers Prev. 2010 Aug;19(8):2043–54. PMID:20647408
**4989.** Ng A, Levy ML, Malicki DM, et al. Unusual high-grade and low-grade glioma in an infant with PPP1CB-ALK gene fusion. BMJ Case Rep. 2019 Feb 1;12(2):e228248. PMID:30709888
**4990.** Ng HK. Cytologic diagnosis of intracranial germinomas in smear preparations. Acta Cytol. 1995 Jul-Aug;39(4):693–7. PMID:7543235
**4991.** Ng TL, O'Sullivan MJ, Pallen CJ, et al. Ewing sarcoma with novel translocation t(2;16) producing an in-frame fusion of FUS and FEV. J Mol Diagn. 2007 Sep;9(4):459–63. PMID:17620387
**4992.** Ng WK, Ip P, Choy C, et al. Cytologic and immunocytochemical findings of anaplastic large

cell lymphoma: analysis of ten fine-needle aspiration specimens over a 9-year period. Cancer. 2003 Feb 25;99(1):33–43. PMID:12589644
**4993.** Ngan HL, Wang L, Lo KW, et al. Genomic landscapes of EBV-associated nasopharyngeal carcinoma vs. HPV-associated head and neck cancer. Cancers (Basel). 2018 Jun 21;10(7):E210. PMID:29933636
**4994.** Ngeow J, Mester J, Rybicki LA, et al. Incidence and clinical characteristics of thyroid cancer in prospective series of individuals with Cowden and Cowden-like syndrome characterized by germline PTEN, SDH, or KLLN alterations. J Clin Endocrinol Metab. 2011 Dec;96(12):E2063–71. PMID:21956414
**4995.** Toledo RA, Burnichon N, Cascon A, et al. Consensus statement on next-generation-sequencing-based diagnostic testing of hereditary phaeochromocytomas and paragangliomas. Nat Rev Endocrinol. 2017 Apr;13(4):233–47. PMID:27857127
**4996.** Nguyen D, Turner JT, Olsen C, et al. Cutaneous manifestations of proteus syndrome: correlations with general clinical severity. Arch Dermatol. 2004 Aug;140(8):947–53. PMID:15313810
**4997.** Nguyen HS, Doan N, Gelsomino M, et al. Dysembryoplastic neuroectodermal tumor: an analysis from the Surveillance, Epidemiology, and End Results Program, 2004-2013. World Neurosurg. 2017 Jul;103:380–5. PMID:28438654
**4998.** Nguyen HS, Doan NB, Gelsomino M, et al. Subependymal giant cell astrocytoma: a Surveillance, Epidemiology, and End Results Program-based analysis from 2004 to 2013. World Neurosurg. 2018 Oct;118:e263–8. PMID:29966782
**4999.** Nguyen NQ, Johns AL, Gill AJ, et al. Clinical and immunohistochemical features of 34 solid pseudopapillary tumors of the pancreas. J Gastroenterol Hepatol. 2011 Feb;26(2):267–74. PMID:21261715
**5000.** Ni HC, Chen SY, Chen L, et al. Angiocentric glioma: a report of nine new cases, including four with atypical histological features. Neuropathol Appl Neurobiol. 2015 Apr;41(3):333–46. PMID:24861831
**5001.** Ni YH, Chang MH, Wang KJ, et al. Clinical relevance of hepatitis B virus genotype in children with chronic infection and hepatocellular carcinoma. Gastroenterology. 2004 Dec;127(6):1733–8. PMID:15578511
**5002.** Niamba P, Léauté-Labrèze C, Boralevi F, et al. Further documentation of spontaneous regression of infantile digital fibromatosis. Pediatr Dermatol. 2007 May-Jun;24(3):280–4. PMID:17542881
**5003.** Nichols CR, Heerema NA, Palmer C, et al. Klinefelter's syndrome associated with mediastinal germ cell neoplasms. J Clin Oncol. 1987 Aug;5(8):1290–4. PMID:3040921
**5004.** Nichols JC, Amato JE, Chung SM. Characteristics of Lisch nodules in patients with neurofibromatosis type 1. J Pediatr Ophthalmol Strabismus. 2003 Sep-Oct;40(5):293–6. PMID:14560838
**5005.** Nicol K, Savell V, Moore J, et al. Distinguishing undifferentiated embryonal sarcoma of the liver from biliary tract rhabdomyosarcoma: a Children's Oncology Group study. Pediatr Dev Pathol. 2007 Mar-Apr;10(2):89–97. PMID:17378682
**5006.** Nicol KK, Geisinger KR. The cytomorphology of pleuropulmonary blastoma. Arch Pathol Lab Med. 2000 Mar;124(3):416–8. PMID:10705397
**5007.** Nicolae A, Ganapathi KA, Pham TH, et al. EBV-negative aggressive NK-cell leukemia/lymphoma: clinical, pathologic, and genetic features. Am J Surg Pathol. 2017 Jan;41(1):67–74. PMID:27631517
**5008.** Nicolae A, Pittaluga S, Abdullah S, et al. EBV-positive large B-cell lymphomas in young patients: a nodal lymphoma with evidence for a tolerogenic immune environment. Blood. 2015 Aug 13;126(7):863–72. PMID:25999451
**5009.** Nicolae A, Pittaluga S, Venkataraman G, et al. Peripheral T-cell lymphomas of follicular T-helper cell derivation with Hodgkin/Reed-Sternberg cells of B-cell lineage: both EBV-positive and EBV-negative variants exist. Am J Surg Pathol. 2013 Jun;37(6):816–26. PMID:23598959
**5010.** Nicolae A, Xi L, Pittaluga S, et al. Frequent STAT5B mutations in γδ hepatosplenic T-cell lymphomas. Leukemia. 2014 Nov;28(11):2244–8. PMID:24947020
**5011.** Nicolin G, Parkin P, Mabbott D, et al. Natural history and outcome of optic pathway gliomas in children. Pediatr Blood Cancer. 2009 Dec 15;53(7):1231–7. PMID:19621457
**5012.** Niehans GA, Manivel JC, Copland GT, et al. Immunohistochemistry of germ cell and trophoblastic neoplasms. Cancer. 1988 Sep 15;62(6):1113–23. PMID:2457424
**5013.** Nield LE, Mendelson M, Ahmad N, et al. Clinical review of obstructive primary cardiac tumors in childhood. Congenit Heart Dis. 2014 May-Jun;9(3):244–51. PMID:23962026
**5014.** Nielsen EH, Feldt-Rasmussen U, Poulsgaard L, et al. Incidence of craniopharyngioma in Denmark (n = 189) and estimated world incidence of craniopharyngioma in children and adults. J Neurooncol. 2011 Sep;104(3):755–63. PMID:21336771
**5015.** Nielsen GP, Fletcher CD, Smith MA, et al. Soft tissue aneurysmal bone cyst: a clinicopathologic study of five cases. Am J Surg Pathol. 2002 Jan;26(1):64–9. PMID:11756770
**5016.** Nielsen GP, Oliva E, Young RH, et al. Alveolar soft-part sarcoma of the female genital tract: a report of nine cases and review of the literature. Int J Gynecol Pathol. 1995 Oct;14(4):283–92. PMID:8598329
**5017.** Nielsen GP, Srivastava A, Kattapuram S, et al. Epithelioid hemangioma of bone revisited: a study of 50 cases. Am J Surg Pathol. 2009 Feb;33(2):270–7. PMID:18852673
**5018.** Nielsen GP, Young RH, Prat J, et al. Primary angiosarcoma of the ovary: a report of seven cases and review of the literature. Int J Gynecol Pathol. 1997 Oct;16(4):378–82. PMID:9421078
**5019.** Niemas-Teshiba R, Matsuno R, Wang LL, et al. MYC-family protein overexpression and prominent nucleolar formation represent prognostic indicators and potential therapeutic targets for aggressive high-MKI neuroblastomas: a report from the children's oncology group. Oncotarget. 2017 Dec 15;9(5):6416–32. PMID:29464082
**5020.** Niemeyer CM. RAS diseases in children. Haematologica. 2014 Nov;99(11):1653–62. PMID:25420281
**5021.** Niemeyer CM, Arico M, Basso G, et al. Chronic myelomonocytic leukemia in childhood: a retrospective analysis of 110 cases. Blood. 1997 May 15;89(10):3534–43. PMID:9160658
**5022.** Niemeyer CM, Baumann I. Classification of childhood aplastic anemia and myelodysplastic syndrome. Hematology Am Soc Hematol Educ Program. 2011;2011:84–9. PMID:22160017
**5023.** Niemeyer CM, Flotho C. Juvenile myelomonocytic leukemia: Who's the driver at the wheel? Blood. 2019 Mar 7;133(10):1060–70. PMID:30670449
**5024.** Niemeyer CM, Kang MW, Shin DH, et al. Germline CBL mutations cause developmental abnormalities and predispose to juvenile myelomonocytic leukemia. Nat Genet. 2010 Sep;42(9):794–800. PMID:20694012
**5024A.** Nieminen TT, Walker CJ, Olkinuora A, et al. Thyroid carcinomas that occur in familial adenomatous polyposis patients recurrently harbor somatic variants in APC, BRAF, and KTM2D. Thyroid. 2020 Mar;30(3):380–8. PMID:32024448
**5025.** Niewisch MR, Savage SA. An update on the biology and management of dyskeratosis congenita and related telomere biology disorders. Expert Rev Hematol. 2019 Dec;12(12):1037–52. PMID:31478401
**5026.** Nigam M, Aschebrook-Kilfoy B, Shikanov S, et al. Increasing incidence of testicular cancer in the United States and Europe between 1992 and 2009. World J Urol. 2015 May;33(5):623–31. PMID:25030752
**5027.** Nigawara K, Suzuki T, Tazawa H, et al. A case of recurrent malignant pheochromocytoma complicated by watery diarrhea, hypokalemia, achlorhydria syndrome. J Clin Endocrinol Metab. 1987 Nov;65(5):1053–6. PMID:3667875
**5028.** Niida Y, Stemmer-Rachamimov AO, Logrip M, et al. Survey of somatic mutations in tuberous sclerosis complex (TSC) hamartomas suggests different genetic mechanisms for pathogenesis of TSC lesions. Am J Hum Genet. 2001 Sep;69(3):493–503. PMID:11468687
**5029.** Nijsten T, Curiel-Lewandrowski C, Kadin ME. Lymphomatoid papulosis in children: a retrospective cohort study of 35 cases. Arch Dermatol. 2004 Mar;140(3):306–12. PMID:15023774
**5030.** Nikbakht H, Panditharatna E, Mikael LG, et al. Spatial and temporal homogeneity of driver mutations in diffuse intrinsic pontine glioma. Nat Commun. 2016 Apr 6;7:11185. PMID:27048880
**5031.** Nikiforov Y, Gnepp DR. Pediatric thyroid cancer after the Chernobyl disaster. Pathomorphologic study of 84 cases (1991-1992) from the Republic of Belarus. Cancer. 1994 Jul 15;74(2):748–66. PMID:8033057
**5032.** Nikiforov YE. Molecular diagnostics of thyroid tumors. Arch Pathol Lab Med. 2011 May;135(5):569–77. PMID:21526955
**5033.** Nikiforov YE, Erickson LA, Nikiforova MN, et al. Solid variant of papillary thyroid carcinoma: incidence, clinical-pathologic characteristics, molecular analysis, and biologic behavior. Am J Surg Pathol. 2001 Dec;25(12):1478–84. PMID:11717536
**5034.** Nikiforova MN, Nikiforov YE. Molecular diagnostics and predictors in thyroid cancer. Thyroid. 2009 Dec;19(12):1351–61. PMID:19895341
**5035.** Niktoreh N, Walter C, Zimmermann M, et al. Mutated WT1, FLT3-ITD, and NUP98-NSD1 fusion in various combinations define a poor prognostic group in pediatric acute myeloid leukemia. J Oncol. 2019 Jul 30;2019:1609128. PMID:31467532
**5036.** Nikumbh DB, Desai SR, Madan PS, et al. Bilateral giant juvenile fibroadenomas of breasts:a case report. Patholog Res Int. 2011;2011:482046. PMID:21660274
**5037.** Nilbert M, Planck M, Fernebro E, et al. Microsatellite instability is rare in rectal carcinomas and signifies hereditary cancer. Eur J Cancer. 1999 Jun;35(6):942–5. PMID:10533476
**5038.** Nilbert M, Rambech E. Beta-catenin activation through mutation is rare in rectal cancer. Cancer Genet Cytogenet. 2001 Jul 1;128(1):43–5. PMID:11454429
**5039.** Nilesh K, Mukherji S. Congenital muscular torticollis. Ann Maxillofac Surg. 2013 Jul;3(2):198–200. PMID:24205484
**5040.** Nilsson M, Domanski HA, Mertens F, et al. Molecular cytogenetic characterization of recurrent translocation breakpoints in bizarre parosteal osteochondromatous proliferation (Nora's lesion). Hum Pathol. 2004 Sep;35(9):1063–9. PMID:15343507
**5041.** Nishiguchi T, Mochizuki K, Ohsawa M, et al. Differentiating benign notochordal cell tumors from chordomas: radiographic features on MRI, CT, and tomography. AJR Am J Roentgenol. 2011 Mar;196(3):644–50. PMID:21343509
**5042.** Nishikawa H, Wu W, Koike A, et al. BRCA1-associated protein 1 interferes with BRCA1/BARD1 RING heterodimer activity. Cancer Res. 2009 Jan 1;69(1):111–9. PMID:19117993
**5043.** Nishio J, Iwasaki H, Nagatomo M, et al. Fibroma of tendon sheath with 11q rearrangements. Anticancer Res. 2014 Sep;34(9):5159–62. PMID:25202108
**5044.** Nishio J, Iwasaki H, Nishijima T, et al. Collagenous fibroma (desmoplastic fibroblastoma) of the finger in a child. Pathol Int. 2002 Apr;52(4):322–5. PMID:12031090
**5045.** Nishio J, Iwasaki H, Sakashita N, et al. Undifferentiated (embryonal) sarcoma of the liver in middle-aged adults: smooth muscle differentiation determined by immunohistochemistry and electron microscopy. Hum Pathol. 2003 Mar;34(3):246–52. PMID:12673559
**5046.** Nishio N, Takahashi Y, Tanaka M, et al. Aberrant phosphorylation of STAT5 by granulocyte-macrophage colony-stimulating factor in infant cytomegalovirus infection mimicking juvenile myelomonocytic leukemia. Leuk Res. 2011 Sep;35(9):1261–4. PMID:21571368
**5047.** Nishioka H, Inoshita N, Mete O, et al. The complementary role of transcription factors in the accurate diagnosis of clinically nonfunctioning pituitary adenomas. Endocr Pathol. 2015 Dec;26(4):349–55. PMID:26481628
**5048.** Nistal M, Codesal J, Paniagua R. Carcinoma in situ of the testis in infertile men. A histological, immunocytochemical, and cytophotometric study of DNA content. J Pathol. 1989 Nov;159(3):205–10. PMID:2593044
**5049.** Nistal M, Gonzalez-Peramato P, Regadera J, et al. Primary testicular lesions are associated with testicular germ cell tumors of adult men. Am J Surg Pathol. 2006 Oct;30(10):1260–8. PMID:17001157
**5050.** Nistal M, Paniagua R, González-Peramato P, et al. Perspectives in pediatric pathology, Chapter 25. Testicular and paratesticular tumors in the pediatric age group. Pediatr Dev Pathol. 2016 Nov/Dec;19(6):471–92. PMID:27626837
**5051.** Nistal M, Paniagua R, González-Peramato P, et al. Perspectives in pediatric pathology, Chapter 5. Gonadal dysgenesis. Pediatr Dev Pathol. 2015 Jul-Aug;18(4):259–78. PMID:25105336
**5052.** Nistal M, Rodríguez JI, García-Fernández E, et al. Fetal gonadoblastoid testicular dysplasia: a focal failure of testicular development. Pediatr Dev Pathol. 2007 Jul-Aug;10(4):274–81. PMID:17638428
**5053.** Nitta M, Hoshi A, Higure T, et al. A case of mixed germ cell tumor in the intramedullary spinal-cord. Tokai J Exp Clin Med. 2016 Sep 20;41(3):147–51. PMID:27628608
**5054.** Nitta Y, Miyachi M, Tomida A, et al. Identification of a novel BOC-PLAG1 fusion gene in a case of lipoblastoma. Biochem Biophys Res Commun. 2019 Apr 23;512(1):49–52. PMID:30857637
**5055.** Niu X, Wang T, Yang Y, et al. Prognostic factors for the survival outcome of bilateral thalamic glioma: an integrated survival analysis. World Neurosurg. 2018 Feb;110:e222–30. PMID:29102752
**5056.** Njauw CN, Kim I, Piris A, et al. Germline BAP1 inactivation is preferentially associated with metastatic ocular melanoma and cutaneous-ocular melanoma families. PLoS One. 2012;7(4):e35295. PMID:22545102
**5057.** Njei B, Konjeti VR, Ditah I. Prognosis of patients with fibrolamellar hepatocellular

carcinoma versus conventional hepatocellular carcinoma: a systematic review and meta-analysis. Gastrointest Cancer Res. 2014 Mar;7(2):49–54. PMID:24799971

**5058.** Njere I, Smith LL, Thurairasa D, et al. Systematic review and meta-analysis of appendiceal carcinoid tumors in children. Pediatr Blood Cancer. 2018 Aug;65(8):e27069. PMID:29745005

**5059.** Nobusawa S, Hirato J, Sugai T, et al. Atypical teratoid/rhabdoid tumor (AT/RT) arising from ependymoma: a type of AT/RT secondarily developing from other primary central nervous system tumors. J Neuropathol Exp Neurol. 2016 Feb;75(2):167–74. PMID:26769252

**5060.** Nobusawa S, Nakata S, Yoshida Y, et al. Secondary INI1-deficient rhabdoid tumors of the central nervous system: analysis of four cases and literature review. Virchows Arch. 2020 May;476(5):763–72. PMID:31707588

**5061.** Noda H, Okumura Y, Nakayama T, et al. Clinicopathological significance of MAML2 gene split in mucoepidermoid carcinoma. Cancer Sci. 2013 Jan;104(1):85–92. PMID:23035786

**5062.** Noetzli L, Lo RW, Lee-Sherick AB, et al. Germline mutations in ETV6 are associated with thrombocytopenia, red cell macrocytosis and predisposition to lymphoblastic leukemia. Nat Genet. 2015 May;47(5):535–8. PMID:25807284

**5063.** Nofal A, Sanad M, Assaf M, et al. Juvenile hyaline fibromatosis and infantile systemic hyalinosis: a unifying term and a proposed grading system. J Am Acad Dermatol. 2009 Oct;61(4):695–700. PMID:19344977

**5064.** Nogales FF, Aguilar D. Florid vascular proliferation in grade 0 glial implants from ovarian immature teratoma. Int J Gynecol Pathol. 2002 Jul;21(3):305–7. PMID:12068181

**5065.** Nogales FF, Dulcey I, Preda O. Germ cell tumors of the ovary: an update. Arch Pathol Lab Med. 2014 Mar;138(3):351–62. PMID:24576031

**5066.** Nogales FF Jr, Favara BE, Major FJ, et al. Immature teratoma of the ovary with a neural component ("solid" teratoma). A clinicopathologic study of 20 cases. Hum Pathol. 1976 Nov;7(6):625–42. PMID:992645

**5067.** Nogales FF, Goyenaga P, Preda O, et al. An analysis of five clear cell papillary cystadenomas of mesosalpinx and broad ligament: four associated with von Hippel-Lindau disease and one aggressive sporadic type. Histopathology. 2012 Apr;60(5):748–57. PMID:22296276

**5068.** Nogales FF Jr, Silverberg SG. Epidermoid cysts of the ovary: a report of five cases with histogenetic considerations and ultrastructural findings. Am J Obstet Gynecol. 1976 Mar 1;124(5):523–8. PMID:943942

**5069.** Nojima T, Unni KK, McLeod RA, et al. Periosteal chondroma and periosteal chondrosarcoma. Am J Surg Pathol. 1985 Sep;9(9):666–77. PMID:4051099

**5070.** Nolan A, Buza N, Margeta M, et al. Ovarian teratomas in women with anti-N-methyl-D-aspartate receptor encephalitis: topography and composition of immune cell and neuroglial populations is compatible with an autoimmune mechanism of disease. Am J Surg Pathol. 2019 Jul;43(7):949–64. PMID:31021857

**5071.** Nolan MA, Sakuta R, Chuang N, et al. Dysembryoplastic neuroepithelial tumors in childhood: long-term outcome and prognostic features. Neurology. 2004 Jun 22;62(12):2270–6. PMID:15210893

**5072.** Nölting S, Grossman AB. Signaling pathways in pheochromocytomas and paragangliomas: prospects for future therapies. Endocr Pathol. 2012 Mar;23(1):21–33. PMID:22391976

**5073.** Nonaka D. Differential expression of SOX2 and SOX17 in testicular germ cell tumors.

Am J Clin Pathol. 2009 May;131(5):731–6. PMID:19369635

**5074.** Nonaka D, Chiriboga L, Rubin BP. Sox10: a pan-schwannian and melanocytic marker. Am J Surg Pathol. 2008 Sep;32(9):1291–8. PMID:18636017

**5075.** Nonaka D, Tang Y, Chiriboga L, et al. Diagnostic utility of thyroid transcription factors Pax8 and TTF-2 (FoxE1) in thyroid epithelial neoplasms. Mod Pathol. 2008 Feb;21(2):192–200. PMID:18084247

**5076.** Noone AM, Cronin KA, Altekruse SF, et al. Cancer incidence and survival trends by subtype using data from the Surveillance Epidemiology and End Results Program, 1992-2013. Cancer Epidemiol Biomarkers Prev. 2017 Apr;26(4):632–41. PMID:27956436

**5077.** Noort S, Zimmermann M, Reinhardt D, et al. Prognostic impact of t(16;21)(p11;q22) and t(16;21)(q24;q22) in pediatric AML: a retrospective study by the I-BFM Study Group. Blood. 2018 Oct 11;132(15):1584–92. PMID:30150206

**5078.** Nord KH, Lilljebjörn H, Vezzi F, et al. GRM1 is upregulated through gene fusion and promoter swapping in chondromyxoid fibroma. Nat Genet. 2014 May;46(5):474–7. PMID:24658000

**5079.** Nord KM, Kandel J, Lefkowitch JH, et al. Multiple cutaneous infantile hemangiomas associated with hepatic angiosarcoma: case report and review of the literature. Pediatrics. 2006 Sep;118(3):e907–13. PMID:16880251

**5080.** Norman A, Abdelwahab IF, Buyon J, et al. Osteoid osteoma of the hip stimulating an early onset of osteoarthritis. Radiology. 1986 Feb;158(2):417–20. PMID:3941866

**5081.** Norman MG, Harrison KJ, Poskitt KJ, et al. Duplication of 9P and hyperplasia of the choroid plexus: a pathologic, radiologic, and molecular cytogenetics study. Pediatr Pathol Lab Med. 1995 Jan-Feb;15(1):109–20. PMID:8736601

**5082.** Norris HJ, Zirkin HJ, Benson WL. Immature (malignant) teratoma of the ovary: a clinical and pathologic study of 58 cases. Cancer. 1976 May;37(5):2359–72. PMID:1260722

**5083.** North PE. Classification and pathology of congenital and perinatal vascular anomalies of the head and neck. Otolaryngol Clin North Am. 2018 Feb;51(1):1–39. PMID:29217054

**5084.** North PE, Waner M, James CA, et al. Congenital nonprogressive hemangioma: a distinct clinicopathologic entity unlike infantile hemangioma. Arch Dermatol. 2001 Dec;137(12):1607–20. PMID:11735711

**5085.** North PE, Waner M, Mizeracki A, et al. GLUT1: a newly discovered immunohistochemical marker for juvenile hemangiomas. Hum Pathol. 2000 Jan;31(1):11–22. PMID:10665907

**5086.** Northcott PA, Buchhalter I, Morrissy AS, et al. The whole-genome landscape of medulloblastoma subtypes. Nature. 2017 Jul 19;547(7663):311–7. PMID:28726821

**5087.** Northcott PA, Jones DT, Kool M, et al. Medulloblastomics: the end of the beginning. Nat Rev Cancer. 2012 Dec;12(12):818–34. PMID:23175120

**5088.** Northcott PA, Lee C, Zichner T, et al. Enhancer hijacking activates GFI1 family oncogenes in medulloblastoma. Nature. 2014 Jul 24;511(7510):428–34. PMID:25043047

**5089.** Northcott PA, Nakahara Y, Wu X, et al. Multiple recurrent genetic events converge on control of histone lysine methylation in medulloblastoma. Nat Genet. 2009 Apr;41(4):465–72. PMID:19270706

**5090.** Northcott PA, Robinson GW, Kratz CP, et al. Medulloblastoma. Nat Rev Dis Primers. 2019 Feb 14;5(1):11. PMID:30765705

**5091.** Northcott PA, Shih DJ, Peacock J, et al. Subgroup-specific structural variation across

1,000 medulloblastoma genomes. Nature. 2012 Aug 2;488(7409):49–56. PMID:22832581

**5092.** Northrup H, Koenig MK, Pearson DA, et al. Tuberous sclerosis complex. In: Adam MP, Ardinger HH, Pagon RA, et al., editors. GeneReviews. Seattle (WA): University of Washington, Seattle; 1999 Jul 13. PMID:20301399

**5093.** Northrup H, Krueger DA, International Tuberous Sclerosis Complex Consensus Group. Tuberous sclerosis complex diagnostic criteria update: recommendations of the 2012 Iinternational Tuberous Sclerosis Complex Consensus Conference. Pediatr Neurol. 2013 Oct;49(4):243–54. PMID:24053982

**5093A.** Nosé V. Familial follicular cell tumors: classification and morphological characteristics. Endocr Pathol. 2010 Dec;21(4):219–26. PMID:20878367

**5094.** Nosé V. Familial thyroid cancer: a review. Mod Pathol. 2011 Apr;24 Suppl 2:S19–33. PMID:21455198

**5095.** Nosé V. Genodermatosis affecting the skin and mucosa of the head and neck: clinicopathologic, genetic, and molecular aspect–PTEN-hamartoma tumor syndrome/Cowden syndrome. Head Neck Pathol. 2016 Jun;10(2):131–8. PMID:26975628

**5095A.** Nosé V. Thyroid cancer of follicular cell origin in inherited tumor syndromes. Adv Anat Pathol. 2010 Nov;17(6):428–36. PMID:20966648

**5096.** Notohara K, Hamazaki S, Tsukayama C, et al. Solid-pseudopapillary tumor of the pancreas: immunohistochemical localization of neuroendocrine markers and CD10. Am J Surg Pathol. 2000 Oct;24(10):1361–71. PMID:11023097

**5097.** Nowak J, Jünger ST, Huflage H, et al. MRI phenotype of RELA-fused pediatric supratentorial ependymoma. Clin Neuroradiol. 2019 Dec;29(4):595–604. PMID:30027327

**5098.** Nowak J, Nemes K, Hohm A, et al. Magnetic resonance imaging surrogates of molecular subgroups in atypical teratoid/rhabdoid tumor. Neuro Oncol. 2018 Nov 12;20(12):1672–9. PMID:30010851

**5099.** Nowak J, Seidel C, Berg F, et al. MRI characteristics of ependymoblastoma: results from 22 centrally reviewed cases. AJNR Am J Neuroradiol. 2014 Oct;35(10):1996–2001. PMID:24948504

**5100.** Nseyo UO, Englander LS, Wajsman Z, et al. Histological patterns of treatment failures in testicular neoplasms. J Urol. 1985 Feb;133(2):219–20. PMID:2982043

**5101.** Nugent KP, Spigelman AD, Phillips RK. Life expectancy after colectomy and ileorectal anastomosis for familial adenomatous polyposis. Dis Colon Rectum. 1993 Nov;36(11):1059–62. PMID:8223060

**5102.** Numoto RT. Pineal parenchymal tumors: cell differentiation and prognosis. J Cancer Res Clin Oncol. 1994;120(11):683–90. PMID:7525594

**5103.** Nunes RH, Hsu CC, da Rocha AJ, et al. Multinodular and vacuolating neuronal tumor of the cerebrum: a new "leave me alone" lesion with a characteristic imaging pattern. AJNR Am J Neuroradiol. 2017 Oct;38(10):1899–904. PMID:28705817

**5104.** Nuovo MA, Norman A, Chumas J, et al. Myositis ossificans with atypical clinical, radiographic, or pathologic findings: a review of 23 cases. Skeletal Radiol. 1992;21(2):87–101. PMID:1566115

**5105.** Nusse R, Clevers H. Wnt/β-catenin signaling, disease, and emerging therapeutic modalities. Cell. 2017 Jun 1;169(6):985–99. PMID:28575679

**5106.** Nyström-Lahti M, Kristo P, Nicolaides NC, et al. Founding mutations and Alu-mediated recombination in hereditary colon

cancer. Nat Med. 1995 Nov;1(11):1203–6. PMID:7584997

**5107.** Oakley RH, Carty H, Cudmore RE. Multiple benign mesenchymomata of the chest wall. Pediatr Radiol. 1985;15(1):58–60. PMID:3969297

**5108.** Obari A, Sano T, Ohyama K, et al. Clinicopathological features of growth hormone-producing pituitary adenomas: difference among various types defined by cytokeratin distribution pattern including a transitional form. Endocr Pathol. 2008 Summer;19(2):82–91. PMID:18629656

**5109.** Oberlin O, Rey A, Lyden E, et al. Prognostic factors in metastatic rhabdomyosarcomas: results of a pooled analysis from United States and European cooperative groups. J Clin Oncol. 2008 May 10;26(14):2384–9. PMID:18467730

**5110.** Oberlin O, Rey A, Sanchez de Toledo J, et al. Randomized comparison of intensified six-drug versus standard three-drug chemotherapy for high-risk nonmetastatic rhabdomyosarcoma and other chemotherapy-sensitive childhood soft tissue sarcomas: long-term results from the International Society of Pediatric Oncology MMT95 study. J Clin Oncol. 2012 Jul 10;30(20):2457–65. PMID:22665534

**5111.** Obiorah IE, Brenholz P, Özdemirli M. Primary clear cell sarcoma of the dermis mimicking malignant melanoma. Balkan Med J. 2018 Mar 15;35(2):203–7. PMID:29072181

**5112.** O'Brien KP, Seroussi E, Dal Cin P, et al. Various regions within the alpha-helical domain of the COL1A1 gene are fused to the second exon of the PDGFB gene in dermatofibrosarcomas and giant-cell fibroblastomas. Genes Chromosomes Cancer. 1998 Oct;23(2):187–93. PMID:9739023

**5113.** Ocheni S, Kroeger N, Zabelina T, et al. EBV reactivation and post transplant lymphoproliferative disorders following allogeneic SCT. Bone Marrow Transplant. 2008 Aug;42(3):181–6. PMID:18516079

**5114.** O'Connell JX, Fanburg JC, Rosenberg AE. Giant cell tumor of tendon sheath and pigmented villonodular synovitis: immunophenotype suggests a synovial cell origin. Hum Pathol. 1995 Jul;26(7):771–5. PMID:7628850

**5115.** O'Connell JX, Kattapuram SV, Mankin HJ, et al. Epithelioid hemangioma of bone. A tumor often mistaken for low-grade angiosarcoma or malignant hemangioendothelioma. Am J Surg Pathol. 1993 Jun;17(6):610–7. PMID:8333560

**5116.** O'Connor DM, Norris HJ. The influence of grade on the outcome of stage I ovarian immature (malignant) teratomas and the reproducibility of grading. Int J Gynecol Pathol. 1994 Oct;13(4):283–9. PMID:7814189

**5117.** O'Connor N, Patel M, Umar T, et al. Head and neck pilomatricoma: an analysis of 201 cases. Br J Oral Maxillofac Surg. 2011 Jul;49(5):354–8. PMID:20594627

**5118.** Ocwieja KE, Vargas SO, Elisofon SA, et al. Pediatric post-transplant hepatic Kaposi sarcoma due to donor-derived human herpesvirus 8. Pediatr Transplant. 2019 May;23(3):e13384. PMID:30843320

**5119.** Oda Y, Tsuneyoshi M. Extrarenal rhabdoid tumors of soft tissue: clinicopathological and molecular genetic review and distinction from other soft-tissue sarcomas with rhabdoid features. Pathol Int. 2006 Jun;56(6):287–95. PMID:16704491

**5120.** Odell EW, Lombardi T, Barrett AW, et al. Hybrid central giant cell granuloma and central odontogenic fibroma-like lesions of the jaws. Histopathology. 1997 Feb;30(2):165–71. PMID:9067742

**5121.** Odell JM, Benjamin DR. Mesenchymal hamartoma of chest wall in infancy:

natural history of two cases. Pediatr Pathol. 1986;5(2):135–46. PMID:3763502
**5122.** O'Donnell PH, Jensen A, Posadas EM, et al. Renal medullary-like carcinoma in an adult without sickle cell hemoglobinopathy. Nat Rev Urol. 2010 Feb;7(2):110–4. PMID:20145663
**5122A.** Oetjen KA, Levoska MA, Tamura D, et al. Predisposition to hematologic malignancies in patients with xeroderma pigmentosum. Haematologica. 2020 Apr;105(4):e144–6. PMID:31439674
**5123.** Offergeld C, Brase C, Yaremchuk S, et al. Head and neck paragangliomas: clinical and molecular genetic classification. Clinics (Sao Paulo). 2012;67 Suppl 1:19–28. PMID:22584701
**5124.** O'Flynn O'Brien KL, Cortes-Santiago N, Patil NM, et al. A rare case of vulvar superficial angiomyxoma in a pediatric patient. J Pediatr Adolesc Gynecol. 2020 Dec;33(6):727–9. PMID:32739529
**5125.** Ogawa Y, Kishino M, Atsumi Y, et al. Plasmacytoid cells in salivary-gland pleomorphic adenomas: evidence of luminal cell differentiation. Virchows Arch. 2003 Nov;443(5):625–34. PMID:14614625
**5126.** Ogilvy KM, Jakubowski J, Shortland JR. Letter: Spinal subarachnoid spread of pituitary adenoma. J Neurol Neurosurg Psychiatry. 1974 Oct;37(10):1186. PMID:4443813
**5127.** Ogino H, Shibamoto Y, Takanaka T, et al. CNS germinoma with elevated serum human chorionic gonadotropin level: clinical characteristics and treatment outcome. Int J Radiat Oncol Biol Phys. 2005 Jul 1;62(3):803–8. PMID:15936563
**5128.** Ogino S, Redline RW. Villous capillary lesions of the placenta: distinctions between chorangioma, chorangiomatosis, and chorangiosis. Hum Pathol. 2000 Aug;31(8):945–54. PMID:10987255
**5129.** Ognjanovic S, Linabery AM, Charbonneau B, et al. Trends in childhood rhabdomyosarcoma incidence and survival in the United States, 1975-2005. Cancer. 2009 Sep 15;115(18):4218–26. PMID:19536876
**5130.** Ognjanovic S, Olivier M, Bergemann TL, et al. Sarcomas in TP53 germline mutation carriers: a review of the IARC TP53 database. Cancer. 2012 Mar 1;118(5):1387–96. PMID:21837677
**5131.** Ogose A, Hotta T, Emura I, et al. Recurrent malignant variant of phosphaturic mesenchymal tumor with oncogenic osteomalacia. Skeletal Radiol. 2001 Feb;30(2):99–103. PMID:11310207
**5132.** Ogose A, Unni KK, Swee RG, et al. Chondrosarcoma of small bones of the hands and feet. Cancer. 1997 Jul 1;80(1):50–9. PMID:9210708
**5133.** Ogose A, Yazawa Y, Ueda T, et al. Alveolar soft part sarcoma in Japan: multi-institutional study of 57 patients from the Japanese Musculoskeletal Oncology Group. Oncology. 2003;65(1):7–13. PMID:12837977
**5134.** Ogura K, Hosoda F, Nakamura H, et al. Highly recurrent H3F3A mutations with additional epigenetic regulator alterations in giant cell tumor of bone. Genes Chromosomes Cancer. 2017 Oct;56(10):711–8. PMID:28545165
**5135.** Ogwang MD, Bhatia K, Biggar RJ, et al. Incidence and geographic distribution of endemic Burkitt lymphoma in northern Uganda revisited. Int J Cancer. 2008 Dec 1;123(11):2658–63. PMID:18767045
**5153A.** Oh EJ, Lee S, Bae JS, et al. TERT promoter mutation in an aggressive cribriform morular variant of papillary thyroid carcinoma. Endocr Pathol. 2017 Mar;28(1):49–53. PMID:27688081
**5136.** Oh JE, Ohta T, Satomi K, et al. Alterations in the NF2/LATS1/LATS2/YAP pathway in schwannomas. J Neuropathol Exp Neurol. 2015 Oct;74(10):952–9. PMID:26360373
**5136A.** Oh MC, Tarapore PE, Kim JM, et al. Spinal ependymomas: benefits of extent of resection for different histological grades. J Clin Neurosci. 2013 Oct;20(10):1390–7. PMID:23768966
**5137.** Ohar JA, Cheung M, Talarchek J, et al. Germline BAP1 mutational landscape of asbestos-exposed malignant mesothelioma patients with family history of cancer. Cancer Res. 2016 Jan 15;76(2):206–15. PMID:26719535
**5138.** O'Hara BJ, Ehya H, Shields JA, et al. Fine needle aspiration biopsy in pediatric ophthalmic tumors and pseudotumors. Acta Cytol. 1993 Mar-Apr;37(2):125–30. PMID:8465629
**5139.** Ohashi R. Solid variant of papillary thyroid carcinoma: an under-recognized entity. Endocr J. 2020 Mar 28;67(3):241–8. PMID:31983699
**5140.** Ohashi R, Kawahara K, Namimatsu S, et al. Clinicopathological significance of a solid component in papillary thyroid carcinoma. Histopathology. 2017 Apr;70(5):775–81. PMID:27882585
**5141.** Ohashi R, Kawahara K, Namimatsu S, et al. Expression of MRP1 and ABCG2 is associated with adverse clinical outcomes of papillary thyroid carcinoma with a solid component. Hum Pathol. 2017 Sep;67:11–7. PMID:28411177
**5141A.** Ohki K, Kiyokawa N, Watanabe S, et al. Characteristics of genetic alterations of peripheral T-cell lymphoma in childhood including identification of novel fusion genes: the Japan Children's Cancer Group (JCCG). Br J Haematol. 2021 Aug;194(4):718–29. PMID:34258755
**5142.** Ohlinger R, Schwesinger G, Schimming A, et al. Juvenile papillomatosis (JP) of the female breast (Swiss Cheese Disease) – role of breast ultrasonography. Ultraschall Med. 2005 Feb;26(1):42–5. PMID:15700227
**5143.** Ohno Y, Amakawa R, Fukuhara S, et al. Acute transformation of chronic large granular lymphocyte leukemia associated with additional chromosome abnormality. Cancer. 1989 Jul 1;64(1):63–7. PMID:2731121
**5144.** Ohshima K, Kimura H, Yoshino T, et al. Proposed categorization of pathological states of EBV-associated T/natural killer-cell lymphoproliferative disorder (LPD) in children and young adults: overlap with chronic active EBV infection and infantile fulminant EBV T-LPD. Pathol Int. 2008 Apr;58(4):209–17. PMID:18324913
**5145.** Ohsugi H, Takizawa N, Kinoshita H, et al. Pheochromocytoma arising from an ectopic adrenal tissue in multiple endocrine neoplasia type 2A. Endocrinol Diabetes Metab Case Rep. 2019 Oct 12;2019:EDM190073. PMID:31610522
**5146.** Ohtomo R, Mori T, Shibata S, et al. SOX10 is a novel marker of acinus and intercalated duct differentiation in salivary gland tumors: a clue to the histogenesis for tumor diagnosis. Mod Pathol. 2013 Aug;26(8):1041–50. PMID:23558573
**5147.** Ojha SS, Naik LP, Fernandes GC, et al. Key cytological findings in FNA from infantile digital fibromatosis. Acta Cytol. 2011;55(5):481–4. PMID:21986179
**5148.** Okada E, Tamura A, Ishikawa O, et al. Tufted angioma (angioblastoma): case report and review of 41 cases in the Japanese literature. Clin Exp Dermatol. 2000 Nov;25(8):627–30. PMID:11167978
**5149.** Okada K, Frassica FJ, Sim FH, et al. Parosteal osteosarcoma. A clinicopathological study. J Bone Joint Surg Am. 1994 Mar;76(3):366–78. PMID:8126042
**5150.** Okada K, Hasegawa T, Yokoyama R, et al. Osteosarcoma with cytokeratin expression: a clinicopathological study of six cases with an emphasis on differential diagnosis from metastatic cancer. J Clin Pathol. 2003 Oct;56(10):742–6. PMID:14514776
**5151.** Okada K, Unni KK, Swee RG, et al. High grade surface osteosarcoma: a clinicopathologic study of 46 cases. Cancer. 1999 Mar 1;85(5):1044–54. PMID:10091787
**5152.** Okada Y, Nishikawa R, Matsutani M, et al. Hypomethylated X chromosome gain and rare isochromosome 12p in diverse intracranial germ cell tumors. J Neuropathol Exp Neurol. 2002 Jun;61(6):531–8. PMID:12071636
**5153.** Okamatsu C, London WB, Naranjo A, et al. Clinicopathological characteristics of ganglioneuroma and ganglioneuroblastoma: a report from the CCG and COG. Pediatr Blood Cancer. 2009 Oct;53(4):563–9. PMID:19530234
**5154.** Okamoto S, Machinami R, Tanizawa T, et al. Dedifferentiated liposarcoma with rhabdomyoblastic differentiation in an 8-year-old girl. Pathol Res Pract. 2010 Mar 15;206(3):191–6. PMID:19515501
**5155.** Okubo Y, Yoshioka E, Suzuki M, et al. Diagnosis, pathological findings, and clinical management of gangliocytic paraganglioma: a systematic review. Front Oncol. 2018 Jul 27;8:291. PMID:30101131
**5156.** Okudolo JO, Bagg A, Meghpara BB, et al. Conjunctival pediatric-type follicular lymphoma. Ophthalmic Plast Reconstr Surg. 2020 Mar/Apr;36(2):e46–9. PMID:31868792
**5157.** Olayiwola O, Hook K, Miller D, et al. Cutaneous granular cell tumors in children: case series and review of the literature. Pediatr Dermatol. 2017 Jul;34(4):e187–90. PMID:28543852
**5158.** Olesen IA, Hoei-Hansen CE, Skakkebaek NE, et al. Testicular carcinoma in situ in subfertile Danish men. Int J Androl. 2007 Aug;30(4):406–11. PMID:17705813
**5159.** Olgac S, Hutchinson B, Tickoo SK, et al. Alpha-methylacyl-CoA racemase as a marker in the differential diagnosis of metanephric adenoma. Mod Pathol. 2006 Feb;19(2):218–24. PMID:16424894
**5160.** Oliva E, Garcia-Miralles N, Vu Q, et al. CD10 expression in pure stromal and sex cord-stromal tumors of the ovary: an immunohistochemical analysis of 101 cases. Int J Gynecol Pathol. 2007 Oct;26(4):359–67. PMID:17885484
**5161.** Oliveira AM, Chou MM. USP6-induced neoplasms: the biologic spectrum of aneurysmal bone cyst and nodular fasciitis. Hum Pathol. 2014 Jan;45(1):1–11. PMID:23769422
**5162.** Oliveira AM, Hsi BL, Weremowicz S, et al. USP6 (Tre2) fusion oncogenes in aneurysmal bone cyst. Cancer Res. 2004 Mar 15;64(6):1920–3. PMID:15026324
**5163.** Oliveira AM, Perez-Atayde AR, Dal Cin P, et al. Aneurysmal bone cyst variant translocations upregulate USP6 transcription by promoter swapping with the ZNF9, COL1A1, TRAP150, and OMD genes. Oncogene. 2005 May 12;24(21):3419–26. PMID:15735689
**5164.** Oliver RT, Mead GM, Rustin GJ, et al. Randomized trial of carboplatin versus radiotherapy for stage I seminoma: mature results on relapse and contralateral testis cancer rates in MRC TE19/EORTC 30982 study (ISRCTN27163214). J Clin Oncol. 2011 Mar 10;29(8):957–62. PMID:21282539
**5165.** Olivier M, Goldgar DE, Sodha N, et al. Li-Fraumeni and related syndromes: correlation between tumor type, family structure, and TP53 genotype. Cancer Res. 2003 Oct 15;63(20):6643–50. PMID:14583457
**5166.** Olivier M, Hollstein M, Hainaut P. TP53 mutations in human cancers: origins, consequences, and clinical use. Cold Spring Harb Perspect Biol. 2010 Jan;2(1):a001008. PMID:20182602
**5167.** Olk-Batz C, Poetsch AR, Nöllke P, et al. Aberrant DNA methylation characterizes juvenile myelomonocytic leukemia with poor outcome. Blood. 2011 May 5;117(18):4871–80. PMID:21406719
**5168.** Olofson A, Marotti J, Tafe LJ, et al. Intranodal meningothelial proliferation in a patient with Cowden syndrome: a case report. Hum Pathol. 2017 Aug;66:183–7. PMID:28315423
**5169.** Olsen E, Vonderheid E, Pimpinelli N, et al. Revisions to the staging and classification of mycosis fungoides and Sezary syndrome: a proposal of the International Society for Cutaneous Lymphomas (ISCL) and the cutaneous lymphoma task force of the European Organization of Research and Treatment of Cancer (EORTC). Blood. 2007 Sep 15;110(6):1713–22. PMID:17540844
**5170.** Olsen SH, Thomas DG, Lucas DR. Cluster analysis of immunohistochemical profiles in synovial sarcoma, malignant peripheral nerve sheath tumor, and Ewing sarcoma. Mod Pathol. 2006 May;19(5):659–68. PMID:16528378
**5171.** Olsen TG, Helwig EB. Angiolymphoid hyperplasia with eosinophilia. A clinicopathologic study of 116 patients. J Am Acad Dermatol. 1985 May;12(5 Pt 1):781–96. PMID:4008683
**5172.** Olsen TK, Panagopoulos I, Meling TR, et al. Fusion genes with ALK as recurrent partner in ependymoma-like gliomas: a new brain tumor entity? Neuro Oncol. 2015 Oct;17(10):1365–73. PMID:25795305
**5173.** Olsson DS, Andersson E, Bryngelsson IL, et al. Excess mortality and morbidity in patients with craniopharyngioma, especially in patients with childhood onset: a population-based study in Sweden. J Clin Endocrinol Metab. 2015 Feb;100(2):467–74. PMID:25375987
**5174.** Olszewski AJ, Shrestha R, Cook NM. Race-specific features and outcomes of nodular lymphocyte-predominant Hodgkin lymphoma: analysis of the National Cancer Data Base. Cancer. 2015 Oct 1;121(19):3472–80. PMID:26149294
**5175.** O'Malley DP, Fedoriw Y, Weiss LM. Distinguishing classical Hodgkin lymphoma, gray zone lymphoma, and large B-cell lymphoma: a proposed scoring system. Appl Immunohistochem Mol Morphol. 2016 Sep;24(8):535–40. PMID:26447896
**5176.** O'Malley S, Weitman D, Olding M, et al. Multiple neoplasms following craniospinal irradiation for medulloblastoma in a patient with nevoid basal cell carcinoma syndrome. Case report. J Neurosurg. 1997 Feb;86(2):286–8. PMID:9010431
**5177.** Omar L, Gleason MK, Pfeifer CM, et al. Management of palpable pediatric breast masses with ultrasound characteristics of fibroadenoma: a more conservative approach. AJR Am J Roentgenol. 2019 Feb;212(2):450–5. PMID:30476459
**5178.** O'Marcaigh AS, Ledger GA, Roche PC, et al. Aromatase expression in human germinomas with possible biological effects. J Clin Endocrinol Metab. 1995 Dec;80(12):3763–6. PMID:8530631
**5179.** Omata M, Cheng AL, Kokudo N, et al. Asia-Pacific clinical practice guidelines on the management of hepatocellular carcinoma: a 2017 update. Hepatol Int. 2017 Jul;11(4):317–70. PMID:28620797
**5180.** O'Meara E, Stack D, Lee CH, et al. Characterization of the chromosomal translocation t(10;17)(q22;p13) in clear cell sarcoma of kidney. J Pathol. 2012 May;227(1):72–80. PMID:22294382
**5181.** Omenn GS. Ectopic hormone syndromes associated with tumors in childhood. Pediatrics. 1971 Mar;47(3):613–22. PMID:4323281
**5182.** Omland T, Akre H, Lie KA, et al. Risk factors for aggressive recurrent

respiratory papillomatosis in adults and juveniles. PLoS One. 2014 Nov 24;9(11):e113584. PMID:25419846
5183. Onadim Z, Hogg A, Baird PN, et al. Oncogenic point mutations in exon 20 of the RB1 gene in families showing incomplete penetrance and mild expression of the retinoblastoma phenotype. Proc Natl Acad Sci U S A. 1992 Jul 1;89(13):6177–81. PMID:1352883
5184. Onciu M, Behm FG, Downing JR, et al. ALK-positive plasmablastic B-cell lymphoma with expression of the NPM-ALK fusion transcript: report of 2 cases. Blood. 2003 Oct 1;102(7):2642–4. PMID:12816858
5185. Onder S, Hurdogan O, Bayram A, et al. The role of FOXL2, SOX9, and β-catenin expression and DICER1 mutation in differentiating sex cord tumor with annular tubules from other sex cord tumors of the ovary. Virchows Arch. 2021 Aug;479(2):317–24. PMID:33566167
5186. O'Neill AF, Hanto DW, Katzenstein HM. Cause and effect: the etiology of pediatric hepatocellular carcinoma and the role for liver transplantation. Pediatr Transplant. 2016 Nov;20(7):878–9. PMID:27726261
5187. Onerci M, Oğretmenoğlu O, Yücel T. Juvenile nasopharyngeal angiofibroma: a revised staging system. Rhinology. 2006 Mar;44(1):39–45. PMID:16550949
5188. Ong KW, Teo M, Lee V, et al. Expression of EBV latent antigens, mammalian target of rapamycin, and tumor suppression genes in EBV-positive smooth muscle tumors: clinical and therapeutic implications. Clin Cancer Res. 2009 Sep 1;15(17):5350–8. PMID:19706821
5189. Onishi S, Yamasaki F, Nakano Y, et al. RELA fusion-positive anaplastic ependymoma: molecular characterization and advanced MR imaging. Brain Tumor Pathol. 2018 Jan;35(1):41–5. PMID:29063976
5190. Online Mendelian Inheritance in Man. OMIM [Internet]. Baltimore (MD): Johns Hopkins University; 2016. MIM Number: 175100. Available from: https://omim.org/entry/175100.
5191. Onoda T, Kanno M, Sato H, et al. Identification of novel ALK rearrangement A2M-ALK in a neonate with fetal lung interstitial tumor. Genes Chromosomes Cancer. 2014 Oct;53(10):865–74. PMID:24965693
5192. Ooms AHAG, Vujanić GM, D'Hooghe E, et al. Renal tumors of childhood-A histopathologic pattern-based diagnostic approach. Cancers (Basel). 2020 Mar 19;12(3):E729. PMID:32204536
5193. Oosterhuis JW, Castedo SM, de Jong B, et al. Ploidy of primary germ cell tumors of the testis. Pathogenetic and clinical relevance. Lab Invest. 1989 Jan;60(1):14–21. PMID:2536126
5194. Oosterhuis JW, Kersemaekers AM, Jacobsen GK, et al. Morphology of testicular parenchyma adjacent to germ cell tumours. An interim report. APMIS. 2003 Jan;111(1):32–40. PMID:12752231
5195. Oosterhuis JW, Looijenga LH. Testicular germ-cell tumours in a broader perspective. Nat Rev Cancer. 2005 Mar;5(3):210–22. PMID:15738984
5196. Oosterhuis JW, Looijenga LH. The biology of human germ cell tumours: retrospective speculations and new prospectives. Eur Urol. 1993;23(1):245–50. PMID:8386656
5197. Oosterhuis JW, Looijenga LH, van Echten J, et al. Chromosomal constitution and developmental potential of human germ cell tumors and teratomas. Cancer Genet Cytogenet. 1997 May;95(1):96–102. PMID:9140458
5198. Oosterhuis JW, Looijenga LHJ. Human germ cell tumours from a developmental perspective. Nat Rev Cancer. 2019 Sep;19(9):522–37. PMID:31413324
5199. Oosterhuis JW, Looijenga LHJ. Germ cell tumors from a developmental perspective: cells of origin, pathogenesis, and molecular biology (emerging patterns). In: Nogales FF, Jimenez RE, editors. Pathology and biology of human germ cell tumors. Berlin (Germany): Springer; 2017. pp. 23–129.
5200. Oosterhuis JW, Stoop H, Dohle G, et al. A pathologist's view on the testis biopsy. Int J Androl. 2011 Aug;34(4 Pt 2):e14–9. PMID:21790650
5201. Oosterhuis JW, Stoop H, Honecker F, et al. Why human extragonadal germ cell tumours occur in the midline of the body: old concepts, new perspectives. Int J Androl. 2007 Aug;30(4):256–63. PMID:17705807
5202. Oosterhuis JW, Stoop JA, Rijlaarsdam MA, et al. Pediatric germ cell tumors presenting beyond childhood? Andrology. 2015 Jan;3(1):70–7. PMID:25427839
5203. Oparka R, Cassidy A, Reilly S, et al. The C134W (402 C>G) FOXL2 mutation is absent in ovarian gynandroblastoma: insights into the genesis of an unusual tumour. Histopathology. 2012 Apr;60(5):838–42. PMID:22296244
5204. Opelz G, Daniel V, Naujokat C, et al. Epidemiology of pretransplant EBV and CMV serostatus in relation to posttransplant non-Hodgkin lymphoma. Transplantation. 2009 Oct 27;88(8):962–7. PMID:19855238
5205. Opelz G, Döhler B. Lymphomas after solid organ transplantation: a collaborative transplant study report. Am J Transplant. 2004 Feb;4(2):222–30. PMID:14974943
5206. Opie J, Antel K, Koller A, et al. In the South African setting, HIV-associated Burkitt lymphoma is associated with frequent leukaemic presentation, complex cytogenetic karyotypes, and adverse clinical outcomes. Ann Hematol. 2020 Mar;99(3):571–8. PMID:31955214
5207. Opotowsky AR, Moko LE, Ginns J, et al. Pheochromocytoma and paraganglioma in cyanotic congenital heart disease. J Clin Endocrinol Metab. 2015 Apr;100(4):1325–34. PMID:25581599
5208. Opris I, Ducrotoy V, Bossut J, et al. Oligodendroglioma arising in an ovarian mature cystic teratoma. Int J Gynecol Pathol. 2009 Jul;28(4):367–71. PMID:19483626
5209. Orbach D, André N, Brecht IB, et al. Mesothelioma in children and adolescents: the European Cooperative Study Group for Pediatric Rare Tumors (EXPeRT) contribution. Eur J Cancer. 2020 Nov;140:63–70. PMID:33049597
5210. Orbach D, Brennan B, De Paoli A, et al. Conservative strategy in infantile fibrosarcoma is possible: the European Paediatric Soft Tissue Sarcoma Study Group experience. Eur J Cancer. 2016 Apr;57:1–9. PMID:26849118
5211. Orbach D, Mosseri V, Pissaloux D, et al. Genomic complexity in pediatric synovial sarcomas (Synobio study): the European pediatric soft tissue sarcoma group (EpSSG) experience. Cancer Med. 2018 Apr;7(4):1384–93. PMID:29533008
5212. Orbach D, Rey A, Cecchetto G, et al. Infantile fibrosarcoma: management based on the European experience. J Clin Oncol. 2010 Jan 10;28(2):318–23. PMID:19917847
5213. Ord RA, Carlson ER. Pediatric salivary gland malignancies. Oral Maxillofac Surg Clin North Am. 2016 Feb;28(1):83–9. PMID:26614703
5214. Ordóñez NG. Desmoplastic small round cell tumor: I: a histopathologic study of 39 cases with emphasis on unusual histological patterns. Am J Surg Pathol. 1998 Nov;22(11):1303–13. PMID:9808123
5215. Ordóñez NG. Value of GATA3 immunostaining in the diagnosis of parathyroid tumors. Appl Immunohistochem Mol Morphol. 2014 Nov-Dec;22(10):756–61. PMID:25046229
5216. Ordóñez-Rubiano EG, Forbes JA, Morgenstern PF, et al. Preserve or sacrifice the stalk? Endocrinological outcomes, extent of resection, and recurrence rates following endoscopic endonasal resection of craniopharyngiomas. J Neurosurg. 2018 Nov 1:1–9. PMID:30497145
5217. Ordulu Z, Young RH. Sertoli-Leydig cell tumors of the ovary with follicular differentiation often resembling juvenile granulosa cell tumor: a report of 38 cases including comments on sex cord-stromal tumors of mixed forms (so-called gynandroblastoma). Am J Surg Pathol. 2021 Jan;45(1):59–67. PMID:32815828
5218. Orem J, Maganda A, Mbidde EK, et al. Clinical characteristics and outcome of children with Burkitt lymphoma in Uganda according to HIV infection. Pediatr Blood Cancer. 2009 Apr;52(4):455–8. PMID:18802952
5219. Orlando CA, Bowman RL, Loose JH. Multicentric papillary-cystic neoplasm of the pancreas. Arch Pathol Lab Med. 1991 Sep;115(9):958–60. PMID:1718242
5220. Ormaechea N, Hernández-Martín A, Happle R, et al. Nevus of striated muscle: a new clinicopathologic entity. Pediatr Dermatol. 2014 Mar-Apr;31(2):254–6. PMID:24606209
5221. Orr BA, Clay MR, Pinto EM, et al. An update on the central nervous system manifestations of Li-Fraumeni syndrome. Acta Neuropathol. 2020 Apr;139(4):669–87. PMID:31468188
5222. Ortega-Monzó C, Molina-Gallardo I, Monteagudo-Castro C, et al. Precalcaneal congenital fibrolipomatous hamartoma: a report of four cases. Pediatr Dermatol. 2000 Nov-Dec;17(6):429–31. PMID:11123771
5223. Ortiz-Hidalgo C, de León-Bojorge B, Fernandez-Sobrino G, et al. Sialoblastoma: report of a congenital case with dysembryogenic alterations of the adjacent parotid gland. Histopathology. 2001 Jan;38(1):79–80. PMID:11210851
5224. Ortonne N, Wolkenstein P, Blakeley JO, et al. Cutaneous neurofibromas: current clinical and pathologic issues. Neurology. 2018 Jul 10;91(2 Suppl 1):S5–13. PMID:29987130
5225. Osborn AG, Blaser SI, Salzman KL, et al., editors. Diagnostic imaging: brain. 1st ed. Altona (MB): Amirsys; 2004.
5226. Oschlies I, Burkhardt B, Chassagne-Clement C, et al. Diagnosis and immunophenotype of 188 pediatric lymphoblastic lymphomas treated within a randomized prospective trial: experiences and preliminary recommendations from the European childhood lymphoma pathology panel. Am J Surg Pathol. 2011 Jun;35(6):836–44. PMID:21451365
5227. Oschlies I, Burkhardt B, Salaverria I, et al. Clinical, pathological and genetic features of primary mediastinal large B-cell lymphomas and mediastinal gray zone lymphomas in children. Haematologica. 2011 Feb;96(2):262–8. PMID:20971819
5228. Oschlies I, Klapper W, Zimmermann M, et al. Diffuse large B-cell lymphoma in pediatric patients belongs predominantly to the germinal-center type B-cell lymphomas: a clinicopathologic analysis of cases included in the German BFM (Berlin-Frankfurt-Munster) Multicenter Trial. Blood. 2006 May 15;107(10):4047–52. PMID:16424389
5229. Oschlies I, Lisfeld J, Lamant L, et al. ALK-positive anaplastic large cell lymphoma limited to the skin: clinical, histopathological and molecular analysis of 6 pediatric cases. A report from the ALCL99 study. Haematologica. 2013 Jan;98(1):50–6. PMID:22773605
5230. Oschlies I, Salaverria I, Mahn F, et al. Pediatric follicular lymphoma–a clinico-pathological study of a population-based series of patients treated within the Non-Hodgkin's Lymphoma–Berlin-Frankfurt-Munster (NHL-BFM) multicenter trials. Haematologica. 2010 Feb;95(2):253–9. PMID:19679882
5231. Oschlies I, Simonitsch-Klupp I, Maldyk J, et al. Subcutaneous panniculitis-like T-cell lymphoma in children: a detailed clinicopathological description of 11 multifocal cases with a high frequency of haemophagocytic syndrome. Br J Dermatol. 2015 Mar;172(3):793–7. PMID:25456748
5232. O'Shea R, Clarke R, Berkley E, et al. Next generation sequencing is informing phenotype: a TP53 example. Fam Cancer. 2018 Jan;17(1):123–8. PMID:28509937
5233. Oshimi K. Progress in understanding and managing natural killer-cell malignancies. Br J Haematol. 2007 Nov;139(4):532–44. PMID:17916099
5234. Osinga TE, Korpershoek E, de Krijger RR, et al. Catecholamine-synthesizing enzymes are expressed in parasympathetic head and neck paraganglioma tissue. Neuroendocrinology. 2015;101(4):289–95. PMID:25677368
5235. Osio A, Fraitag S, Hadj-Rabia S, et al. Clinical spectrum of tufted angiomas in childhood: a report of 13 cases and a review of the literature. Arch Dermatol. 2010 Jul;146(7):758–63. PMID:20644037
5236. Ostendorf AP, Gutmann DH, Weisenberg JL. Epilepsy in individuals with neurofibromatosis type 1. Epilepsia. 2013 Oct;54(10):1810–4. PMID:24032542
5237. Ostergaard P, Simpson MA, Connell FC, et al. Mutations in GATA2 cause primary lymphedema associated with a predisposition to acute myeloid leukemia (Emberger syndrome). Nat Genet. 2011 Sep 4;43(10):929–31. PMID:21892158
5238. Ostertun B, Wolf HK, Campos MG, et al. Dysembryoplastic neuroepithelial tumors: MR and CT evaluation. AJNR Am J Neuroradiol. 1996 Mar;17(3):419–30. PMID:8881234
5239. Ostrom QT, Chen Y, M de Blank P, et al. The descriptive epidemiology of atypical teratoid/rhabdoid tumors in the United States, 2001-2010. Neuro Oncol. 2014 Oct;16(10):1392–9. PMID:24847086
5240. Ostrom QT, Cioffi G, Gittleman H, et al. CBTRUS statistical report: primary brain and other central nervous system tumors diagnosed in the United States in 2012-2016. Neuro Oncol. 2019 Nov 1;21 Suppl 5:v1–100. PMID:31675094
5241. Ostrom QT, Gittleman H, Liao P, et al. CBTRUS statistical report: primary brain and central nervous system tumors diagnosed in the United States in 2007-2011. Neuro Oncol. 2014 Oct;16 Suppl 4:iv1–63. PMID:25304271
5242. Ostrom QT, Gittleman H, Truitt G, et al. CBTRUS statistical report: primary brain and other central nervous system tumors diagnosed in the United States in 2011-2015. Neuro Oncol. 2018 Oct 1;20 Suppl_4:iv1–86. PMID:30445539
5243. Ostrowski ML, McEnery KW. Cartilaginous lesions of the skeleton. Am J Clin Pathol. 2002 Jun;117 Suppl:S3–25. PMID:14569799
5244. Ostrzega N. Fine-needle aspiration cytology of juvenile papillomatosis of breast: a case report. Diagn Cytopathol. 1993 Aug;9(4):457–60. PMID:8261855
5245. Ostwal V, Rekhi B, Noronha V, et al. Primitive neuroectodermal tumor of ovary in a young lady, confirmed with molecular and cytogenetic results–a rare case report with a diagnostic and therapeutic challenge. Pathol Oncol Res. 2012 Oct;18(4):1101–6. PMID:22311546
5246. O'Sullivan MJ, Swanson PE, Knoll J, et al. Undifferentiated embryonal sarcoma with unusual features arising within mesenchymal hamartoma of the liver: report of a case and review of the literature. Pediatr Dev Pathol. 2001 Sep-Oct;4(5):482–9. PMID:11779051

**5247.** Osumi T, Tanaka F, Mori T, et al. Primary mediastinal large B-cell lymphoma in Japanese children and adolescents. Int J Hematol. 2017 Apr;105(4):440–4. PMID:27858330
**5248.** O'Suoji C, Welch JJ, Perkins SL, et al. Rare pediatric non-Hodgkin lymphomas: a report from Children's Oncology Group Study ANHL 04B1. Pediatr Blood Cancer. 2016 May;63(5):794–800. PMID:26728447
**5249.** Ota S, Hishinuma M, Yamauchi N, et al. Oncofetal protein glypican-3 in testicular germ-cell tumor. Virchows Arch. 2006 Sep;449(3):308–14. PMID:16896894
**5250.** Otero JJ, Rowitch D, Vandenberg S. OLIG2 is differentially expressed in pediatric astrocytic and in ependymal neoplasms. J Neurooncol. 2011 Sep;104(2):423–38. PMID:21193945
**5251.** Ottaviani G, Jaffe N. The epidemiology of osteosarcoma. Cancer Treat Res. 2009;152:3–13. PMID:20213383
**5252.** Ottesen AM, Skakkebaek NE, Lundsteen C, et al. High-resolution comparative genomic hybridization detects extra chromosome arm 12p material in most cases of carcinoma in situ adjacent to overt germ cell tumors, but not before the invasive tumor development. Genes Chromosomes Cancer. 2003 Oct;38(2):117–25. PMID:12939739
**5253.** Oudijk L, den Bakker MA, Hop WC, et al. Solitary, multifocal and generalized myofibromas: clinicopathological and immunohistochemical features of 114 cases. Histopathology. 2012 May;60 6B:E1–11. PMID:22486319
**5254.** Oudijk L, Gaal J, Korpershoek E, et al. SDHA mutations in adult and pediatric wild-type gastrointestinal stromal tumors. Mod Pathol. 2013 Mar;26(3):456–63. PMID:23174939
**5255.** Oudot C, Orbach D, Minard-Colin V, et al. Desmoid fibromatosis in pediatric patients: management based on a retrospective analysis of 59 patients and a review of the literature. Sarcoma. 2012;2012:475202. PMID:22924016
**5256.** Outani H, Imura Y, Tanaka T, et al. Clinical outcomes of patients with epithelioid sarcomas: impact and management of nodal metastasis. Int J Clin Oncol. 2018 Feb;23(1):181–8. PMID:28799063
**5257.** Owosho AA, Aguilar CE, Seethala RR. Comparison of p63 and p40 (ΔNp63) as basal, squamoid, and myoepithelial markers in salivary gland tumors. Appl Immunohistochem Mol Morphol. 2016 Aug;24(7):501–8. PMID:26230372
**5258.** Owosho AA, Zhang L, Rosenblum MK, et al. High sensitivity of FISH analysis in detecting homozygous SMARCB1 deletions in poorly differentiated chordoma: a clinicopathologic and molecular study of nine cases. Genes Chromosomes Cancer. 2018 Feb;57(2):89–95. PMID:29119645
**5259.** Oya S, Saito A, Okano A, et al. The pathogenesis of intracranial growing teratoma syndrome: proliferation of tumor cells or formation of multiple expanding cysts? Two case reports and review of the literature. Childs Nerv Syst. 2014 Aug;30(8):1455–61. PMID:24633581
**5260.** Ozaki Y, Suzuki-Inoue K, Inoue O. Novel interactions in platelet biology: CLEC-2/podoplanin and laminin/GPVI. J Thromb Haemost. 2009 Jul;7 Suppl 1:191–4. PMID:19630798
**5261.** Ozawa MG, Bhaduri A, Chisholm KM, et al. A study of the mutational landscape of pediatric-type follicular lymphoma and pediatric nodal marginal zone lymphoma. Mod Pathol. 2016 Oct;29(10):1212–20. PMID:27338637
**5262.** Ozawa T, Arora S, Szulzewsky F, et al. A de novo mouse model of C11orf95-RELA fusion-driven ependymoma identifies driver functions in addition to NF-κB. Cell Rep. 2018 Jun 26;23(13):3787–97. PMID:29949764
**5263.** Ozcan A, Shen SS, Hamilton C, et al. PAX 8 expression in non-neoplastic tissues, primary tumors, and metastatic tumors: a comprehensive immunohistochemical study. Mod Pathol. 2011 Jun;24(6):751–64. PMID:21317881
**5264.** Ozcanli H, Ozenci AM, Gurer EI, et al. Juxta-articular myxoma of the wrist: a case report. J Hand Surg Am. 2005 Jan;30(1):165–7. PMID:15680575
**5265.** Ozdemir I, Simsek E, Silan F, et al. Congenital sialoblastoma (embryoma) associated with premature centromere division and high level of alpha-fetoprotein. Prenat Diagn. 2005 Aug;25(8):687–9. PMID:16049999
**5266.** Ozek MM, Sav A, Pamir MN, et al. Pleomorphic xanthoastrocytoma associated with von Recklinghausen neurofibromatosis. Childs Nerv Syst. 1993 Feb;9(1):39–42. PMID:8481944
**5267.** Ozkoc G, Gonlusen G, Ozalay M, et al. Giant chondroblastoma of the scapula with pulmonary metastases. Skeletal Radiol. 2006 Jan;35(1):42–8. PMID:16007463
**5268.** Ozolek JA, Carrau R, Barnes EL, et al. Nasal chondromesenchymal hamartoma in older children and adults: series and immunohistochemical analysis. Arch Pathol Lab Med. 2005 Nov;129(11):1444–50. PMID:16253025
**5269.** Ozturk M. Genetic aspects of hepatocellular carcinogenesis. Semin Liver Dis. 1999;19(3):235–42. PMID:10518303
**5270.** Özyörük D, Kocayozgat A, Yaman-Bajin İ, et al. A synchronous occurrence of bifocal intracranial germinoma and bilateral testicular epidermoid cyst in an adolescent patient with Klinefelter's syndrome. Turk J Pediatr. 2019;61(3):456–9. PMID:31916730
**5271.** Özyurt J, Müller HL, Thiel CM. A systematic review of cognitive performance in patients with childhood craniopharyngioma. J Neurooncol. 2015 Oct;125(1):9–21. PMID:26369768
**5272.** Paaso A, Jaakola A, Syrjänen S, et al. From HPV infection to lesion progression: the role of HLA alleles and host immunity. Acta Cytol. 2019;63(2):148–58. PMID:30783048
**5273.** Paavonen J, Heinonen PK, Aine R, et al. Prevalence of nonspecific vaginitis and other cervicovaginal infections during the third trimester of pregnancy. Sex Transm Dis. 1986 Jan-Mar;13(1):5–8. PMID:3082020
**5274.** Pacifici M. The pathogenic roles of heparan sulfate deficiency in hereditary multiple exostoses. Matrix Biol. 2018 Oct;71-72:28–39. PMID:29277722
**5275.** Packer RJ, Iavarone A, Jones DTW, et al. Implications of new understandings of gliomas in children and adults with NF1: report of a consensus conference. Neuro Oncol. 2020 Jun 9;22(6):773–84. PMID:32055852
**5276.** Padalino MA, Vida VL, Bhattarai A, et al. Giant intramural left ventricular rhabdomyoma in a newborn. Circulation. 2011 Nov 15;124(20):2275–7. PMID:22083149
**5277.** Padalino MA, Vida VL, Boccuzzo G, et al. Surgery for primary cardiac tumors in children: early and late results in a multicenter European Congenital Heart Surgeons Association study. Circulation. 2012 Jul 3;126(1):22–30. PMID:22626745
**5278.** Paganini I, Chang VY, Capone GL, et al. Expanding the mutational spectrum of LZTR1 in schwannomatosis. Eur J Hum Genet. 2015 Jul;23(7):963–8. PMID:25335493
**5279.** Pagès M, Beccaria K, Boddaert N, et al. Co-occurrence of histone H3 K27M and BRAF V600E mutations in paediatric midline grade I ganglioglioma. Brain Pathol. 2018 Jan;28(1):103–11. PMID:27984673
**5280.** Pagès M, Pajtler KW, Puget S, et al. Diagnostics of pediatric supratentorial RELA ependymomas: integration of information from histopathology, genetics, DNA methylation and imaging. Brain Pathol. 2019 May;29(3):325–35. PMID:30325077
**5281.** Pagliai KA, Cohen BA. Pyogenic granuloma in children. Pediatr Dermatol. 2004 Jan-Feb;21(1):10–3. PMID:14871318
**5282.** Paietta E, Roberts KG, Wang V, et al. Molecular classification improves risk assessment in adult BCR-ABL1-negative B-ALL. Blood. 2021 Sep 16;138(11):948–58. PMID:33895809
**5283.** Pajtler KW, Wei Y, Okonechnikov K, et al. YAP1 subgroup supratentorial ependymoma requires TEAD and nuclear factor I-mediated transcriptional programmes for tumorigenesis. Nat Commun. 2019 Sep 2;10(1):3914. PMID:31477715
**5284.** Pajtler KW, Wen J, Sill M, et al. Molecular heterogeneity and CXorf67 alterations in posterior fossa group A (PFA) ependymomas. Acta Neuropathol. 2018 Aug;136(2):211–26. PMID:29909548
**5285.** Pajtler KW, Witt H, Sill M, et al. Molecular classification of ependymal tumors across all CNS compartments, histopathological grades, and age groups. Cancer Cell. 2015 May 11;27(5):728–43. PMID:25965575
**5286.** Pakbaz S, Asa SL, Mete O. Alpha-inhibin expression in paragangliomas and pheochromocytomas shows strong correlation in VHL- and SDHx-driven pseudohypoxic pathway disease. Mod Pathol. 2020 Mar 5;33(Suppl 2):591. Abstract no. 596. doi:10.1038/s41379-020-0469-4.
**5287.** Pakos EE, Nearchou AD, Grimer RJ, et al. Prognostic factors and outcomes for osteosarcoma: an international collaboration. Eur J Cancer. 2009 Sep;45(13):2367–75. PMID:19349163
**5288.** Pal P, Fernandes H, Ellison DW. Woman aged 24 years with fourth ventricular mass. Brain Pathol. 2005 Oct;15(4):367–8, 373. PMID:16389948
**5289.** Pal SK, Bergerot P, Dizman N, et al. Responses to alectinib in ALK-rearranged papillary renal cell carcinoma. Eur Urol. 2018 Jul;74(1):124–8. PMID:29685646
**5290.** Palacios G, Shaw TI, Li Y, et al. Novel ALK fusion in anaplastic large cell lymphoma involving EEF1G, a subunit of the eukaryotic elongation factor-1 complex. Leukemia. 2017 Mar;31(3):743–7. PMID:27840423
**5291.** Palaniappan K, Borkar VV, Safwan M, et al. Pediatric hepatocellular carcinoma in a developing country: Is the etiology changing? Pediatr Transplant. 2016 Nov;20(7):898–903. PMID:27392999
**5292.** Paller AS, Syder AJ, Chan YM, et al. Genetic and clinical mosaicism in a type of epidermal nevus. N Engl J Med. 1994 Nov 24;331(21):1408–15. PMID:7526210
**5292A.** Palmerini E, Gambarotti M, Italiano A, et al. A global collaboRAtive study of CIC-rearranged, BCOR::CCNB3-rearranged and other ultra-rare unclassified undifferentiated small round cell sarcomas (GRACefUl). Eur J Cancer. 2023 Apr;183:11–23. PMID:36791667
**5293.** Palsgrove DN, Brosnan-Cashman JA, Giannini C, et al. Subependymal giant cell astrocytoma-like astrocytoma: a neoplasm with a distinct phenotype and frequent neurofibromatosis type-1-association. Mod Pathol. 2018 Dec;31(12):1787–800. PMID:29973652
**5294.** Palsgrove DN, Li Y, Pratilas CA, et al. Eosinophilic solid and cystic (ESC) renal cell carcinomas harbor TSC mutations: molecular analysis supports an expanding clinicopathologic spectrum. Am J Surg Pathol. 2018 Sep;42(9):1166–81. PMID:29975249
**5295.** Paludo J, Fritchie K, Haddox CL, et al. Extraskeletal osteosarcoma: outcomes and the role of chemotherapy. Am J Clin Oncol. 2018 Sep;41(9):832–7. PMID:28622153
**5296.** Pamporaki C, Hamplova B, Peitzsch M, et al. Characteristics of pediatric vs adult pheochromocytomas and paragangliomas. J Clin Endocrinol Metab. 2017 Apr 1;102(4):1122–32. PMID:28324046
**5297.** Pan CC, Chung MY, Ng KF, et al. Constant allelic alteration on chromosome 16p (TSC2 gene) in perivascular epithelioid cell tumour (PEComa): genetic evidence for the relationship of PEComa with angiomyolipoma. J Pathol. 2008 Feb;214(3):387–93. PMID:18085521
**5298.** Pan J, Qi S, Liu Y, et al. Growth patterns of craniopharyngiomas: clinical analysis of 226 patients. J Neurosurg Pediatr. 2016 Apr;17(4):418–33. PMID:26636252
**5299.** Pan Z, Hu S, Li M, et al. ALK-positive large B-cell lymphoma: a clinicopathologic study of 26 cases with review of additional 108 cases in the literature. Am J Surg Pathol. 2017 Jan;41(1):25–38. PMID:27740969
**5300.** Pan Z, Xie Q, Repertinger S, et al. Plasmablastic transformation of low-grade CD5+ B-cell lymphoproliferative disorder with MYC gene rearrangements. Hum Pathol. 2013 Oct;44(10):2139–48. PMID:23791008
**5301.** Panagopoulos I, Gorunova L, Bjerkehagen B, et al. LAMTOR1-PRKCD and NUMA1-SFMBT1 fusion genes identified by RNA sequencing in aneurysmal benign fibrous histiocytoma with t(3;11)(p21;q13). Cancer Genet. 2015 Nov;208(11):545–51. PMID:26432191
**5302.** Panagopoulos I, Gorunova L, Zeller B, et al. Cryptic FUS-ERG fusion identified by RNA-sequencing in childhood acute myeloid leukemia. Oncol Rep. 2013 Dec;30(6):2587–92. PMID:24068373
**5303.** Panagopoulos I, Lobmaier I, Gorunova L, et al. Fusion of the genes WWTR1 and FOSB in pseudomyogenic hemangioendothelioma. Cancer Genomics Proteomics. 2019 Jul-Aug;16(4):293–8. PMID:31243110
**5304.** Panagopoulos I, Mertens F, Dêbiec-Rychter M, et al. Molecular genetic characterization of the EWS/ATF1 fusion gene in clear cell sarcoma of tendons and aponeuroses. Int J Cancer. 2002 Jun 1;99(4):560–7. PMID:11992546
**5305.** Panagopoulos I, Storlazzi CT, Fletcher CD, et al. The chimeric FUS/CREB3l2 gene is specific for low-grade fibromyxoid sarcoma. Genes Chromosomes Cancer. 2004 Jul;40(3):218–28. PMID:15139001
**5306.** Pande M, Lynch PM, Hopper JL, et al. Smoking and colorectal cancer in Lynch syndrome: results from the Colon Cancer Family Registry and the University of Texas M.D. Anderson Cancer Center. Clin Cancer Res. 2010 Feb 15;16(4):1331–9. PMID:20145170
**5307.** Pandey N, Singh PK, Mahapatra AK, et al. Pediatric bilateral large concurrent thalamic glioblastoma: an unusual case report. J Pediatr Neurosci. 2014 Jan;9(1):76–8. PMID:24891914
**5308.** Panea RI, Love CL, Shingleton JR, et al. The whole-genome landscape of Burkitt lymphoma subtypes. Blood. 2019 Nov 7;134(19):1598–607. PMID:31558468
**5309.** Pang C, Lim CS, Brookes J, et al. Emerging importance of molecular pathogenesis of vascular malformations in clinical practice and classifications. Vasc Med. 2020 Aug;25(4):364–77. PMID:32568624
**5310.** Pang Y, Gupta G, Yang C, et al. A novel splicing site IRP1 somatic mutation in a patient with pheochromocytoma and JAK2V617F positive polycythemia vera: a case report. BMC Cancer. 2018 Mar 13;18(1):286. PMID:29534684
**5311.** Panoutsakopoulos G, Pandis N, Kyriazoglou I, et al. Recurrent t(16;17)(q22;p13) in aneurysmal bone cysts. Genes Chromosomes Cancer. 1999 Nov;26(3):265–6. PMID:10502326

**5312.** Pansuriya TC, van Eijk R, d'Adamo P, et al. Somatic mosaic IDH1 and IDH2 mutations are associated with enchondroma and spindle cell hemangioma in Ollier disease and Maffucci syndrome. Nat Genet. 2011 Nov 6;43(12):1256–61. PMID:22057234
**5313.** Pantziarka P. Li Fraumeni syndrome, cancer and senescence: a new hypothesis. Cancer Cell Int. 2013 Apr 15;13(1):35. PMID:23587008
**5314.** Panwalkar P, Clark J, Ramaswamy V, et al. Immunohistochemical analysis of H3K27me3 demonstrates global reduction in group-A childhood posterior fossa ependymoma and is a powerful predictor of outcome. Acta Neuropathol. 2017 Nov;134(5):705–14. PMID:28733933
**5315.** Panwalkar P, Pratt D, Chung C, et al. SWI/SNF complex heterogeneity is related to polyphenotypic differentiation, prognosis, and immune response in rhabdoid tumors. Neuro Oncol. 2020 Jun 9;22(6):785–96. PMID:31912158
**5316.** Paoluzzi L, Maki RG. Diagnosis, prognosis, and treatment of alveolar soft-part sarcoma: a review. JAMA Oncol. 2019 Feb 1;5(2):254–60. PMID:30347044
**5317.** Papalas JA, Van Mater D, Wang E. Pyogenic variant of primary cutaneous anaplastic large-cell lymphoma: a lymphoproliferative disorder with a predilection for the immunocompromized and the young. Am J Dermatopathol. 2010 Dec;32(8):821–7. PMID:20881832
**5318.** Papathomas TG, de Krijger RR, Tischler AS. Paragangliomas: update on differential diagnostic considerations, composite tumors, and recent genetic developments. Semin Diagn Pathol. 2013 Aug;30(3):207–23. PMID:24144290
**5319.** Papathomas TG, Gaal J, Corssmit EP, et al. Non-pheochromocytoma (PCC)/paraganglioma (PGL) tumors in patients with succinate dehydrogenase-related PCC-PGL syndromes: a clinicopathological and molecular analysis. Eur J Endocrinol. 2013 Nov 22;170(1):1–12. PMID:24096523
**5320.** Papathomas TG, Oudijk L, Persu A, et al. SDHB/SDHA immunohistochemistry in pheochromocytomas and paragangliomas: a multicenter interobserver variation analysis using virtual microscopy: a Multinational Study of the European Network for the Study of Adrenal Tumors (ENS@T). Mod Pathol. 2015 Jun;28(6):807–21. PMID:25720320
**5321.** Papiani G, Einhorn LH. Salvage chemotherapy with high-dose carboplatin plus etoposide and autologous peripheral blood stem cell transplant in male pure choriocarcinoma: a retrospective analysis of 13 cases. Bone Marrow Transplant. 2007 Aug;40(3):235–7. PMID:17563738
**5322.** Papke DJ Jr, Al-Ibraheemi A, Fletcher CDM. Plexiform myofibroblastoma: clinicopathologic analysis of 36 cases of a distinctive benign tumor of soft tissue affecting mainly children and young adults. Am J Surg Pathol. 2020 Nov;44(11):1469–78. PMID:32618598
**5323.** Papp G, Krausz T, Stricker TP, et al. SMARCB1 expression in epithelioid sarcoma is regulated by miR-206, miR-381, and miR-671-5p on Both mRNA and protein levels. Genes Chromosomes Cancer. 2014 Feb;53(2):168–76. PMID:24327545
**5324.** Pappo AS, Devidas M, Jenkins J, et al. Phase II trial of neoadjuvant vincristine, ifosfamide, and doxorubicin with granulocyte colony-stimulating factor support in children and adolescents with advanced-stage nonrhabdomyosarcomatous soft tissue sarcomas: a Pediatric Oncology Group Study. J Clin Oncol. 2005 Jun 20;23(18):4031–8. PMID:15767644
**5325.** Pappo AS, Parham DM, Cain A, et al. Alveolar soft part sarcoma in children and adolescents: clinical features and outcome of 11 patients. Med Pediatr Oncol. 1996 Feb;26(2):81–4. PMID:8531857
**5326.** Papworth KE, Arroyo VM, Styring E, et al. Soft-tissue sarcoma in adolescents and young adults compared with older adults: a report among 5000 patients from the Scandinavian Sarcoma Group Central Register. Cancer. 2019 Oct 15;125(20):3595–602. PMID:31287163
**5327.** Paradela S, Fonseca E, Pita-Fernández S, et al. Prognostic factors for melanoma in children and adolescents: a clinicopathologic, single-center study of 137 patients. Cancer. 2010 Sep 15;116(18):4334–44. PMID:20549825
**5328.** Paradela S, Fonseca E, Prieto VG. Melanoma in children. Arch Pathol Lab Med. 2011 Mar;135(3):307–16. PMID:21366453
**5329.** Paradis J, Koltai PJ. Pediatric teratoma and dermoid cysts. Otolaryngol Clin North Am. 2015 Feb;48(1):121–36. PMID:25439551
**5330.** Parashar P, Baron E, Papadimitriou JC, et al. Basal cell adenocarcinoma of the oral minor salivary glands: review of the literature and presentation of two cases. Oral Surg Oral Med Oral Pathol Oral Radiol Endod. 2007 Jan;103(1):77–84. PMID:17178498
**5331.** Pardhe N, Singh N, Bharadwaj G, et al. Spindle cell lipoma. BMJ Case Rep. 2013 Aug 13;2013:bcr2013010438. PMID:23946512
**5332.** Pardo LM, Voigt AP, Alonzo TA, et al. Deciphering the significance of CD56 expression in pediatric acute myeloid leukemia: a report from the Children's Oncology Group. Cytometry B Clin Cytom. 2020 Jan;98(1):52–6. PMID:31294507
**5333.** Pareja F, Brandes AH, Basili T, et al. Loss-of-function mutations in ATP6AP1 and ATP6AP2 in granular cell tumors. Nat Commun. 2018 Aug 30;9(1):3533. PMID:30166553
**5334.** Pareja F, Da Cruz Paula A, Murray MP, et al. Recurrent MED12 exon 2 mutations in benign breast fibroepithelial lesions in adolescents and young adults. J Clin Pathol. 2019 Mar;72(3):258–62. PMID:30467240
**5335.** Paret C, Theruvath J, Russo A, et al. Activation of the basal cell carcinoma pathway in a patient with CNS HGNET-BCOR diagnosis: consequences for personalized targeted therapy. Oncotarget. 2016 Dec 13;7(50):83378–91. PMID:27825128
**5336.** Parfitt JR, McLean CA, Joseph MG, et al. Granular cell tumours of the gastrointestinal tract: expression of nestin and clinicopathological evaluation of 11 patients. Histopathology. 2006 Mar;48(4):424–30. PMID:16487364
**5337.** Parfitt T. Chernobyl's legacy. 20 years after the power station exploded, new cases of thyroid cancer are still rising, say experts. Lancet. 2004 May 8;363(9420):1534. PMID:15139340
**5338.** Parham DM, Alaggio R, Coffin CM. Myogenic tumors in children and adolescents. Pediatr Dev Pathol. 2012;15(1 Suppl):211–38. PMID:22420729
**5339.** Parham DM, Webber BL, Jenkins JJ 3rd, et al. Nonrhabdomyosarcomatous soft tissue sarcomas of childhood: formulation of a simplified system for grading. Mod Pathol. 1995 Sep;8(7):705–10. PMID:8539226
**5340.** Parilla M, Alikhan M, Al-Kawaaz M, et al. Genetic underpinnings of renal cell carcinoma with leiomyomatous stroma. Am J Surg Pathol. 2019 Aug;43(8):1135–44. PMID:30986793
**5341.** Parilla M, Kadri S, Patil SA, et al. Are sporadic eosinophilic solid and cystic renal cell carcinomas characterized by somatic tuberous sclerosis gene mutations? Am J Surg Pathol. 2018 Jul;42(7):911–7. PMID:29668487
**5342.** Parisi M, Grenda E, Hatziagorou E, et al. Chest wall lipoblastoma in a 3 year-old boy. Respir Med Case Rep. 2019 Jan 19;26:200–2. PMID:30723667
**5343.** Park CH, Kim KI, Lim YT, et al. Ruptured giant intrathoracic lipoblastoma in a 4-month-old infant: CT and MR findings. Pediatr Radiol. 2000 Jan;30(1):38–40. PMID:10663508
**5344.** Park CK, Kim HS. Clinicopathological characteristics of ovarian sclerosing stromal tumor with an emphasis on TFE3 overexpression. Anticancer Res. 2017 Oct;37(10):5441–7. PMID:28982854
**5344A.** Park J, Kim JW, Park H, et al. Multifocality in a patient with cribriform-morular variant of papillary thyroid carcinoma is an important clue for the diagnosis of familial adenomatous polyposis. Thyroid. 2019 Nov;29(11):1606–14. PMID:31469036
**5345.** Park JE. Long-term natural history of a neuromuscular choristoma of the sciatic nerve: a case report and literature review. Clin Imaging. 2019 May-Jun;55:18–22. PMID:30708195
**5346.** Park JR, Bagatell R, London WB, et al. Children's Oncology Group's 2013 blueprint for research: neuroblastoma. Pediatr Blood Cancer. 2013 Jun;60(6):985–93. PMID:23255319
**5347.** Park JY, Cohen C, Lopez D, et al. EGFR exon 20 insertion/duplication mutations characterize fibrous hamartoma of infancy. Am J Surg Pathol. 2016 Dec;40(12):1713–8. PMID:27631514
**5348.** Park JY, Kim E, Kim DW, et al. Cribriform neuroepithelial tumor in the third ventricle: a case report and literature review. Neuropathology. 2012 Oct;32(5):570–6. PMID:22239490
**5349.** Park M, Kim M, Hwang D, et al. Characterization of gene expression and activated signaling pathways in solid-pseudopapillary neoplasm of pancreas. Mod Pathol. 2014 Apr;27(4):580–93. PMID:24072181
**5350.** Park MS, Ravi V, Araujo DM. Inhibiting the VEGF-VEGFR pathway in angiosarcoma, epithelioid hemangioendothelioma, and hemangiopericytoma/solitary fibrous tumor. Curr Opin Oncol. 2010 Jul;22(4):351–5. PMID:20485168
**5351.** Park S, Ko YH. Epstein-Barr virus-associated T/natural killer-cell lymphoproliferative disorders. J Dermatol. 2014 Jan;41(1):29–39. PMID:24438142
**5352.** Park SM, Kim YN, Woo YJ, et al. A sclerosing stromal tumor of the ovary with masculinization in a premenarchal girl. Korean J Pediatr. 2011 May;54(5):224–7. PMID:21829415
**5353.** Park SY, Jin SP, Yeom B, et al. Multiple fibromas of tendon sheath: unusual presentation. Ann Dermatol. 2011 Sep;23 Suppl 1:S45–7. PMID:22028571
**5354.** Park WS, Dong SM, Kim SY, et al. Somatic mutations in the kinase domain of the Met/hepatocyte growth factor receptor gene in childhood hepatocellular carcinomas. Cancer Res. 1999 Jan 15;59(2):307–10. PMID:9927037
**5355.** Park YK, Unni KK, Kim YW, et al. Primary alveolar soft part sarcoma of bone. Histopathology. 1999 Nov;35(5):411–7. PMID:10583555
**5356.** Parker K, Venkataraman G. Challenges in the diagnosis of gray zone lymphomas. Surg Pathol Clin. 2019 Sep;12(3):709–18. PMID:31352983
**5357.** Parker M, Mohankumar KM, Punchihewa C, et al. C11orf95-RELA fusions drive oncogenic NF-κB signalling in ependymoma. Nature. 2014 Feb 27;506(7489):451–5. PMID:24553141
**5358.** Parkin JL, Arthur DC, Abramson CS, et al. Acute leukemia associated with the t(4;11) chromosome rearrangement: ultrastructural and immunologic characteristics. Blood. 1982 Dec;60(6):1321–31. PMID:6958337
**5359.** Parma J, Duprez L, Van Sande J, et al. Diversity and prevalence of somatic mutations in the thyrotropin receptor and Gs alpha genes as a cause of toxic thyroid adenomas. J Clin Endocrinol Metab. 1997 Aug;82(8):2695–701. PMID:9253356
**5360.** Parmar HA, Hawkins C, Ozelame R, et al. Fluid-attenuated inversion recovery ring sign as a marker of dysembryoplastic neuroepithelial tumors. J Comput Assist Tomogr. 2007 May-Jun;31(3):348–53. PMID:17538277
**5361.** Parmar V, Peters RT, Cheesman E, et al. Congenital infantile fibrosarcoma of the colon: a case series and literature review. Pediatr Surg Int. 2014 Oct;30(10):1079–85. PMID:25150723
**5362.** Parrington JM, West LF, Povey S. The origin of ovarian teratomas. J Med Genet. 1984 Feb;21(1):4–12. PMID:6363699
**5363.** Parrish A, Fenchel M, Storch GA, et al. Epstein-Barr viral loads do not predict post-transplant lymphoproliferative disorder in pediatric lung transplant recipients: a multicenter prospective cohort study. Pediatr Transplant. 2017 Sep;21(6):10.1111/petr.13011. PMID:28639398
**5364.** Parry DM, Eldridge R, Kaiser-Kupfer MI, et al. Neurofibromatosis 2 (NF2): clinical characteristics of 63 affected individuals and clinical evidence for heterogeneity. Am J Med Genet. 1994 Oct 1;52(4):450–61. PMID:7747758
**5365.** Parsons DW, Roy A, Yang Y, et al. Diagnostic yield of clinical tumor and germline whole-exome sequencing for children with solid tumors. JAMA Oncol. 2016 May 1;2(5):616–24. PMID:26822237
**5366.** Partap S, Curran EK, Propp JM, et al. Medulloblastoma incidence has not changed over time: a CBTRUS study. J Pediatr Hematol Oncol. 2009 Dec;31(12):970–1. PMID:19887963
**5367.** Parwani AV, Husain AN, Epstein JI, et al. Low-grade myxoid renal epithelial neoplasms with distal nephron differentiation. Hum Pathol. 2001 May;32(5):506–12. PMID:11381369
**5368.** Pascual JM, Prieto R, Castro-Dufourny I, et al. Craniopharyngiomas primarily involving the hypothalamus: a model of neurosurgical lesions to elucidate the neurobiological basis of psychiatric disorders. World Neurosurg. 2018 Dec;120:e1245–78. PMID:30240857
**5368A.** Pashankar F, Hanley K, Lockley M, et al. Addressing the diagnostic and therapeutic dilemmas of ovarian immature teratoma: report from a clinicopathologic consensus conference. Eur J Cancer. 2022 Sep;173:59–70. PMID:35863107
**5369.** Pasini B, McWhinney SR, Bei T, et al. Clinical and molecular genetics of patients with the Carney-Stratakis syndrome and germline mutations of the genes coding for the succinate dehydrogenase subunits SDHB, SDHC, and SDHD. Eur J Hum Genet. 2008 Jan;16(1):79–88. PMID:17667967
**5370.** Pasmant E, Parfait B, Luscan A, et al. Neurofibromatosis type 1 molecular diagnosis: What can NGS do for you when you have a large gene with loss of function mutations? Eur J Hum Genet. 2015 May;23(5):596–601. PMID:25074460
**5371.** Pasquier B, Péoc'H M, Fabre-Bocquentin B, et al. Surgical pathology of drug-resistant partial epilepsy. A 10-year-experience with a series of 327 consecutive resections. Epileptic Disord. 2002 Jun;4(2):99–119. PMID:12105073
**5372.** Passet M, Boissel N, Sigaux F, et al. PAX5 P80R mutation identifies a novel subtype of B-cell precursor acute lymphoblastic leukemia with favorable outcome. Blood. 2019 Jan 17;133(3):280–4. PMID:30510083
**5373.** Passmore SJ, Berry PJ, Oakhill A. Recurrent pancreatoblastoma with inappropriate adrenocorticotrophic hormone secretion. Arch Dis Child. 1988 Dec;63(12):1494–6. PMID:2852926

5374. Passmore SJ, Chessells JM, Kempski H, et al. Paediatric myelodysplastic syndromes and juvenile myelomonocytic leukaemia in the UK: a population-based study of incidence and survival. Br J Haematol. 2003 Jun;121(5):758–67. PMID:12780790
5375. Passmore SJ, Hann IM, Stiller CA, et al. Pediatric myelodysplasia: a study of 68 children and a new prognostic scoring system. Blood. 1995 Apr 1;85(7):1742–50. PMID:7703482
5376. Passos J, Quidet M, Brahimi A, et al. Familial adenomatous polyposis associated craniopharyngioma secondary to both germline and somatic mutations in the APC gene. Acta Neuropathol. 2020 Dec;140(6):967–9. PMID:33025138
5377. Pastor V, Hirabayashi S, Karow A, et al. Mutational landscape in children with myelodysplastic syndromes is distinct from adults: specific somatic drivers and novel germline variants. Leukemia. 2017 Mar;31(3):759–62. PMID:27876779
5378. Pastor VB, Sahoo SS, Boklan J, et al. Constitutional SAMD9L mutations cause familial myelodysplastic syndrome and transient monosomy 7. Haematologica. 2018 Mar;103(3):427–37. PMID:29217778
5379. Pastore G, Znaor A, Spreafico F, et al. Malignant renal tumours incidence and survival in European children (1978-1997): report from the Automated Childhood Cancer Information System project. Eur J Cancer. 2006 Sep;42(13):2103–14. PMID:16919774
5380. Pastorino S, Yoshikawa Y, Pass HI, et al. A subset of mesotheliomas with improved survival occurring in carriers of BAP1 and other germline mutations. J Clin Oncol. 2018 Oct 30;(Oct):JCO2018790352. PMID:30376426
5381. Patay Z, DeSain LA, Hwang SN, et al. MR imaging characteristics of wingless-type-subgroup pediatric medulloblastoma. AJNR Am J Neuroradiol. 2015 Dec;36(12):2386–93. PMID:26338912
5382. Patel A, Jhiang S, Dogra S, et al. Differentiated thyroid carcinoma that express sodium-iodide symporter have a lower risk of recurrence for children and adolescents. Pediatr Res. 2002 Nov;52(5):737–44. PMID:12409522
5383. Patel NR, Chrisinger JSA, Demicco EG, et al. USP6 activation in nodular fasciitis by promoter-swapping gene fusions. Mod Pathol. 2017 Nov;30(11):1577–88. PMID:28752842
5384. Patel PA, Anand AS, Parikh SK, et al. Primary central nervous system Burkitt lymphoma in HIV positive pediatric patient: a rare case report. J Pediatr Neurosci. 2019 Apr-Jun;14(2):86–9. PMID:31516626
5384A. Patel SS. Pediatric myelodysplastic syndromes. Clin Lab Med. 2021 Sep;41(3):517–28. PMID:34304779
5385. Pather S, MacKinnon D, Padayachee RS. Plasmablastic lymphoma in pediatric patients: clinicopathologic study of three cases. Ann Diagn Pathol. 2013 Feb;17(1):80–4. PMID:23036261
5386. Patil RB, Shanmukhaiah C, Jijina F, et al. Wiskott-Aldrich syndrome presenting with JMML-like blood picture and normal sized platelets. Case Rep Hematol. 2016;2016:8230786. PMID:27340577
5387. Patil S, Perry A, Maccollin M, et al. Immunohistochemical analysis supports a role for INI1/SMARCB1 in hereditary forms of schwannomas, but not in solitary, sporadic schwannomas. Brain Pathol. 2008 Oct;18(4):517–9. PMID:18422762
5388. Patrice SJ, Wiss K, Mulliken JB. Pyogenic granuloma (lobular capillary hemangioma): a clinicopathologic study of 178 cases. Pediatr Dermatol. 1991 Dec;8(4):267–76. PMID:1792196
5389. Patrick K, Wade R, Goulden N, et al. Outcome for children and young people with Early T-cell precursor acute lymphoblastic leukaemia treated on a contemporary protocol, UKALL 2003. Br J Haematol. 2014 Aug;166(3):421–4. PMID:24708207
5390. Patrizi A, Medri M, Raone B, et al. Clinical characteristics of Becker's nevus in children: report of 118 cases from Italy. Pediatr Dermatol. 2012 Sep-Oct;29(5):571–4. PMID:22471889
5391. Patronas NJ, Courcoutsakis N, Bromley CM, et al. Intramedullary and spinal canal tumors in patients with neurofibromatosis 2: MR imaging findings and correlation with genotype. Radiology. 2001 Feb;218(2):434–42. PMID:11161159
5392. Patterson AT, Kumar MG, Bayliss SJ, et al. Eccrine angiomatous hamartoma: a clinicopathologic review of 18 cases. Am J Dermatopathol. 2016 Jun;38(6):413–7. PMID:26760684
5393. Pattwell SS, Konnick EQ, Liu YJ, et al. Neurotrophic receptor tyrosine kinase 2 (NTRK2) alterations in low-grade gliomas: report of a novel gene fusion partner in a pilocytic astrocytoma and review of the literature. Case Rep Pathol. 2020 Jan 30;2020:5903863. PMID:32082673
5394. Paul P, Deka H, Malakar AK, et al. Nasopharyngeal carcinoma: understanding its molecular biology at a fine scale. Eur J Cancer Prev. 2018 Jan;27(1):33–41. PMID:27748661
5395. Paulli M, Sträter J, Gianelli U, et al. Mediastinal B-cell lymphoma: a study of its histomorphologic spectrum based on 109 cases. Hum Pathol. 1999 Feb;30(2):178–87. PMID:10029446
5396. Paulson VA, Rudzinski ER, Hawkins DS. Thyroid cancer in the pediatric population. Genes (Basel). 2019 Sep 18;10(9):E723. PMID:31540418
5397. Paulson VA, Stojanov IA, Wasman JK, et al. Recurrent and novel USP6 fusions in cranial fasciitis identified by targeted RNA sequencing. Mod Pathol. 2020 May;33(5):775–80. PMID:31827231
5398. Paulsson K, Forestier E, Lilljebjörn H, et al. Genetic landscape of high hyperdiploid childhood acute lymphoblastic leukemia. Proc Natl Acad Sci U S A. 2010 Dec 14;107(50):21719–24. PMID:21098271
5399. Paulsson K, Lilljebjörn H, Biloglav A, et al. The genomic landscape of high hyperdiploid childhood acute lymphoblastic leukemia. Nat Genet. 2015 Jun;47(6):672–6. PMID:25961940
5400. Paulus W, Honegger J, Keyvani K, et al. Xanthogranuloma of the sellar region: a clinicopathological entity different from adamantinomatous craniopharyngioma. Acta Neuropathol. 1999 Apr;97(4):377–82. PMID:10208277
5401. Paulus W, Jänisch W. Clinicopathologic correlations in epithelial choroid plexus neoplasms: a study of 52 cases. Acta Neuropathol. 1990;80(6):635–41. PMID:1703384
5402. Paulus W, Lisle DK, Tonn JC, et al. Molecular genetic alterations in pleomorphic xanthoastrocytoma. Acta Neuropathol. 1996;91(3):293–7. PMID:8834542
5403. Paulus W, Schlote W, Perentes E, et al. Desmoplastic supratentorial neuroepithelial tumours of infancy. Histopathology. 1992 Jul;21(1):43–9. PMID:1634201
5404. Paulus W, Stöckel C, Krauss J, et al. Odontogenic classification of craniopharyngiomas: a clinicopathological study of 54 cases. Histopathology. 1997 Feb;30(2):172–6. PMID:9067743
5405. Pauniaho SL, Heikinheimo O, Vettenranta K, et al. High prevalence of sacrococcygeal teratoma in Finland - a nationwide population-based study. Acta Paediatr. 2013 Jun;102(6):e251–6. PMID:23432104
5406. Pavlick D, Schrock AB, Malicki D, et al. Identification of NTRK fusions in pediatric mesenchymal tumors. Pediatr Blood Cancer. 2017 Aug;64(8). PMID:28097808
5407. Pavlova O, Fraitag S, Hohl D. 5-hydroxymethylcytosine expression in proliferative nodules arising within congenital nevi allows differentiation from malignant melanoma. J Invest Dermatol. 2016 Dec;136(12):2453–61. PMID:27456754
5408. Pavlus JD, Carter BW, Tolley MD, et al. Imaging of thoracic neurogenic tumors. AJR Am J Roentgenol. 2016 Sep;207(3):552–61. PMID:27340927
5409. Pawel BR. SMARCB1-deficient tumors of childhood: a practical guide. Pediatr Dev Pathol. 2018 Jan-Feb;21(1):6–28. PMID:29280680
5410. Peacock JD, Dykema KJ, Toriello HV, et al. Oculoectodermal syndrome is a mosaic RASopathy associated with KRAS alterations. Am J Med Genet A. 2015 Jul;167(7):1429–35. PMID:25808193
5411. Peard L, Cost NG, Saltzman AF. Pediatric pheochromocytoma: current status of diagnostic imaging and treatment procedures. Curr Opin Urol. 2019 Sep;29(5):493–9. PMID:31246590
5412. Pechalova PF, Bakardjiev AG, Beltcheva AB. Jaw cysts at children and adolescence: a single-center retrospective study of 152 cases in southern Bulgaria. Med Oral Patol Oral Cir Bucal. 2011 Sep 1;16(6):e767–71. PMID:21217618
5413. Pederiva F, Zanazzo GA, Gregori M, et al. Suprascapular lipoblastoma extending in to the thorax. APSP J Case Rep. 2013 May 27;4(2):20. PMID:24040598
5414. Pedersen M, Küsters-Vandevelde HVN, Viros A, et al. Primary melanoma of the CNS in children is driven by congenital expression of oncogenic NRAS in melanocytes. Cancer Discov. 2013 Apr;3(4):458–69. PMID:23303902
5415. Pedeutour F, Simon MP, Minoletti F, et al. Ring 22 chromosomes in dermatofibrosarcoma protuberans are low-level amplifiers of chromosome 17 and 22 sequences. Cancer Res. 1995 Jun 1;55(11):2400–3. PMID:7757993
5416. Pedeutour F, Simon MP, Minoletti F, et al. Translocation, t(17;22)(q22;q13), in dermatofibrosarcoma protuberans: a new tumor-associated chromosome rearrangement. Cytogenet Cell Genet. 1996;72(2-3):171–4. PMID:8978765
5417. Pei J, Cooper H, Flieder DB, et al. NEAT1-TFE3 and KAT6A-TFE3 renal cell carcinomas, new members of MiT family translocation renal cell carcinoma. Mod Pathol. 2019 May;32(5):710–6. PMID:30622287
5418. Pei J, Zhao X, Patchefsky AS, et al. Clinical application of RNA sequencing in sarcoma diagnosis: an institutional experience. Medicine (Baltimore). 2019 Jun;98(25):e16031. PMID:31232935
5419. Pei Y, Moore CE, Wang J, et al. An animal model of MYC-driven medulloblastoma. Cancer Cell. 2012 Feb 14;21(2):155–67. PMID:22340590
5420. Peifer M, Polakis P. Wnt signaling in oncogenesis and embryogenesis–a look outside the nucleus. Science. 2000 Mar 3;287(5458):1606–9. PMID:10733430
5421. Pekarski KL, Prayson RA. Suprasellar spindle cell lipoma. Ann Diagn Pathol. 2009 Jun;13(3):173–5. PMID:19433296
5422. Pekmezci M, Louie J, Gupta N, et al. Clinicopathological characteristics of adamantinomatous and papillary craniopharyngiomas: University of California, San Francisco experience 1985-2005. Neurosurgery. 2010 Nov;67(5):1341–9. PMID:20871436
5423. Pekmezci M, Reuss DE, Hirbe AC, et al. Morphologic and immunohistochemical features of malignant peripheral nerve sheath tumors and cellular schwannomas. Mod Pathol. 2015 Feb;28(2):187–200. PMID:25189642
5424. Pekmezci M, Stevers M, Phillips JJ, et al. Multinodular and vacuolating neuronal tumor of the cerebrum is a clonal neoplasm defined by genetic alterations that activate the MAP kinase signaling pathway. Acta Neuropathol. 2018 Mar;135(3):485–8. PMID:29428973
5425. Pekmezci M, Villanueva-Meyer JE, Goode B, et al. The genetic landscape of ganglioglioma. Acta Neuropathol Commun. 2018 Jun 7;6(1):47. PMID:29880043
5426. Pekova B, Sykorova V, Dvorakova S, et al. RET, NTRK, ALK, BRAF, and MET fusions in a large cohort of pediatric papillary thyroid carcinomas. Thyroid. 2020 Dec;30(12):1771–80. PMID:32495721
5427. Pelicci PG, Knowles DM 2nd, Magrath I, et al. Chromosomal breakpoints and structural alterations of the c-myc locus differ in endemic and sporadic forms of Burkitt lymphoma. Proc Natl Acad Sci U S A. 1986 May;83(9):2984–8. PMID:3458257
5428. Pelizzo G, Conoscenti G, Kalache KD, et al. Antenatal manifestation of congenital pancreatoblastoma in a fetus with Beckwith-Wiedemann syndrome. Prenat Diagn. 2003 Apr;23(4):292–4. PMID:12673632
5429. Pellegrini AE, Drake RD, Qualman SJ. Spindle cell hemangioendothelioma: a neoplasm associated with Maffucci's syndrome. J Cutan Pathol. 1995 Apr;22(2):173–6. PMID:7560353
5430. Pellegrino B, Terrier-Lacombe MJ, Oberlin O, et al. Lymphocyte-predominant Hodgkin's lymphoma in children: therapeutic abstention after initial lymph node resection–a study of the French Society of Pediatric Oncology. J Clin Oncol. 2003 Aug 1;21(15):2948–52. PMID:12885814
5431. Pelmus M, Guillou L, Hostein I, et al. Monophasic fibrous and poorly differentiated synovial sarcoma: immunohistochemical reassessment of 60 t(X;18)(SYT-SSX)-positive cases. Am J Surg Pathol. 2002 Nov;26(11):1434–40. PMID:12409719
5432. Pemberton LS, Dougal M, Magee B, et al. Experience of external beam radiotherapy given adjuvantly or at relapse following surgery for craniopharyngioma. Radiother Oncol. 2005 Oct;77(1):99–104. PMID:16216361
5433. Pemov A, Hansen NF, Sindiri S, et al. Low mutation burden and frequent loss of CDKN2A/B and SMARCA2, but not PRC2, define premalignant neurofibromatosis type 1-associated atypical neurofibromas. Neuro Oncol. 2019 Aug 5;21(8):981–92. PMID:30722027
5434. Pemov A, Li H, Patidar R, et al. The primacy of NF1 loss as the driver of tumorigenesis in neurofibromatosis type 1-associated plexiform neurofibromas. Oncogene. 2017 Jun 1;36(22):3168–77. PMID:28068329
5435. Peñarrocha M, Bonet J, Minguez JM, et al. Nerve sheath myxoma (neurothekeoma) in the tongue of a newborn. Oral Surg Oral Med Oral Pathol Oral Radiol Endod. 2000 Jul;90(1):74–7. PMID:10884639
5436. Pencalet P, Maixner W, Sainte-Rose C, et al. Benign cerebellar astrocytomas in children. J Neurosurg. 1999 Feb;90(2):265–73. PMID:9950497
5437. Pendleton C, Spinner RJ, Dyck PJB, et al. Association of intraneural perineurioma with neurofibromatosis type 2. Acta Neurochir (Wien). 2020 Aug;162(8):1891–7. PMID:32529330
5438. Peng R, Chen H, Yang X, et al. A novel sclerosing atypical lipomatous tumor/well-differentiated liposarcoma in a 7-year-old girl: report of a case with molecular confirmation. Hum Pathol. 2018 Jan;71:41–6. PMID:28705709

5439. Penkert J, Schmidt G, Hofmann W, et al. Breast cancer patients suggestive of Li-Fraumeni syndrome: mutational spectrum, candidate genes, and unexplained heredity. Breast Cancer Res. 2018 Aug 7;20(1):87. PMID:30086788
5440. Penko K, Livezey J, Fenton C, et al. BRAF mutations are uncommon in papillary thyroid cancer of young patients. Thyroid. 2005 Apr;15(4):320–5. PMID:15876153
5441. Pennacchia I, Kutzner H, Kazakov DV, et al. Fibroblastic connective tissue nevus: clinicopathological and immunohistochemical study of 14 cases. J Cutan Pathol. 2017 Oct;44(10):827–34. PMID:28632950
5442. Pennacchioli E, Fiore M, Collini P, et al. Alveolar soft part sarcoma: clinical presentation, treatment, and outcome in a series of 33 patients at a single institution. Ann Surg Oncol. 2010 Dec;17(12):3229–33. PMID:20593242
5443. Penta L, Cofini M, Lanciotti L, et al. Hashimoto's disease and thyroid cancer in children: Are they associated? Front Endocrinol (Lausanne). 2018 Oct 9;9:565. PMID:30356680
5444. Per H, Kontaş O, Kumandaş S, et al. A report of a desmoplastic non-infantile ganglioglioma in a 6-year-old boy with review of the literature. Neurosurg Rev. 2009 Jul;32(3):369–74. PMID:19280238
5445. Peraza A, Gómez R, Beltran J, et al. Mucoepidermoid carcinoma. An update and review of the literature. J Stomatol Oral Maxillofac Surg. 2020 Dec;121(6):713–20. PMID:32565266
5446. Pereira AM, Schmid EM, Schutte PJ, et al. High prevalence of long-term cardiovascular, neurological and psychosocial morbidity after treatment for craniopharyngioma. Clin Endocrinol (Oxf). 2005 Feb;62(2):197–204. PMID:15670196
5447. Pereira BD, Raimundo L, Mete O, et al. Monomorphous plurihormonal pituitary adenoma of Pit-1 lineage in a giant adolescent with central hyperthyroidism. Endocr Pathol. 2016 Mar;27(1):25–33. PMID:26330191
5448. Perez EA, Gutierrez JC, Koniaris LG, et al. Malignant pancreatic tumors: incidence and outcome in 58 pediatric patients. J Pediatr Surg. 2009 Jan;44(1):197–203. PMID:19159743
5449. Pérez-Gómez RM, Soria-Céspedes D, de León-Bojorge B, et al. Diffuse membranous immunoreactivity of CD56 and paranuclear dot-like staining pattern of cytokeratins AE1/3, CAM5.2, and OSCAR in undifferentiated (embryonal) sarcoma of the liver. Appl Immunohistochem Mol Morphol. 2010 Mar;18(2):195–8. PMID:19809302
5450. Pérez-Guillermo M, Masgrau NA, García-Solano J, et al. Cytologic aspect of fibrolamellar hepatocellular carcinoma in fine-needle aspirates. Diagn Cytopathol. 1999 Sep;21(3):180–7. PMID:10450103
5451. Perez-Rivas LG, Theodoropoulou M, Ferraù F, et al. The gene of the ubiquitin-specific protease 8 is frequently mutated in adenomas causing Cushing's disease. J Clin Endocrinol Metab. 2015 Jul;100(7):E997–1004. PMID:25942478
5452. Pérez-Rivas LG, Theodoropoulou M, Puar TH, et al. Somatic USP8 mutations are frequent events in corticotroph tumor progression causing Nelson's tumor. Eur J Endocrinol. 2018 Jan;178(1):57–63. PMID:28982703
5453. Perilongo G, Carollo C, Salviati L, et al. Diencephalic syndrome and disseminated juvenile pilocytic astrocytomas of the hypothalamic-optic chiasm region. Cancer. 1997 Jul 1;80(1):142–6. PMID:9210720
5454. Perka C, Labs K, Zippel H, et al. Localized pigmented villonodular synovitis of the knee joint: neoplasm or reactive granuloma? A review of 18 cases. Rheumatology (Oxford). 2000 Feb;39(2):172–8. PMID:10725067
5455. Perkins SL, Gross TG. Pediatric indolent lymphoma–Would less be better? Pediatr Blood Cancer. 2011 Aug;57(2):189–90. PMID:21495166
5456. Perkins SM, Mitra N, Fei W, et al. Patterns of care and outcomes of patients with pleomorphic xanthoastrocytoma: a SEER analysis. J Neurooncol. 2012 Oct;110(1):99–104. PMID:22843450
5457. Perlman EJ. Pediatric renal tumors: practical updates for the pathologist. Pediatr Dev Pathol. 2005 May-Jun;8(3):320–38. PMID:16010493
5458. Perlman EJ, Dickman PS, Askin FB, et al. Ewing's sarcoma–routine diagnostic utilization of MIC2 analysis: a Pediatric Oncology Group/Children's Cancer Group intergroup study. Hum Pathol. 1994 Mar;25(3):304–7. PMID:8150461
5459. Perlman EJ, Faria P, Soares A, et al. Hyperplastic perilobar nephroblastomatosis: long-term survival of 52 patients. Pediatr Blood Cancer. 2006 Feb;46(2):203–21. PMID:15816029
5460. Pernas FG, Younis RT, Lehman DA, et al. Management of pediatric airway granular cell tumor: role of laryngotracheal reconstruction. Int J Pediatr Otorhinolaryngol. 2006 Jun;70(6):957–63. PMID:16466812
5461. Pernicone PJ, Scheithauer BW, Sebo TJ, et al. Pituitary carcinoma: a clinicopathologic study of 15 cases. Cancer. 1997 Feb 15;79(4):804–12. PMID:9024719
5462. Pérot G, Chibon F, Montero A, et al. Constant p53 pathway inactivation in a large series of soft tissue sarcomas with complex genetics. Am J Pathol. 2010 Oct;177(4):2080–90. PMID:20884963
5463. Perreault S, Larouche V, Tabori U, et al. A phase 2 study of trametinib for patients with pediatric glioma or plexiform neurofibroma with refractory tumor and activation of the MAPK/ERK pathway: TRAM-01. BMC Cancer. 2019 Dec 27;19(1):1250. PMID:31881853
5464. Perreault S, Ramaswamy V, Achrol AS, et al. MRI surrogates for molecular subgroups of medulloblastoma. AJNR Am J Neuroradiol. 2014 Jul;35(7):1263–9. PMID:24831600
5465. Perret R, Escuriol J, Velasco V, et al. NFATc2-rearranged sarcomas: clinicopathologic, molecular, and cytogenetic study of 7 cases with evidence of AGGRECAN as a novel diagnostic marker. Mod Pathol. 2020 Oct;33(10):1930–44. PMID:32327700
5466. Perrone F, Bertolotti A, Montemurro G, et al. Frequent mutation and nuclear localization of β-catenin in sertoli cell tumors of the testis. Am J Surg Pathol. 2014 Jan;38(1):66–71. PMID:24061522
5467. Perrone S, D'Elia GM, Annechini G, et al. Infectious aetiology of marginal zone lymphoma and role of anti-infective therapy. Mediterr J Hematol Infect Dis. 2016 Jan 1;8(1):e2016006. PMID:26740867
5468. Perrotti D, Silvestri G, Stramucci L, et al. Cellular and molecular networks in chronic myeloid leukemia: the leukemic stem, progenitor and stromal cell interplay. Curr Drug Targets. 2017;18(4):377–88. PMID:27307150
5469. Perry A, Giannini C, Raghavan R, et al. Aggressive phenotypic and genotypic features in pediatric and NF2-associated meningiomas: a clinicopathologic study of 53 cases. J Neuropathol Exp Neurol. 2001 Oct;60(10):994–1003. PMID:11589430
5470. Perry A, Giannini C, Scheithauer BW, et al. Composite pleomorphic xanthoastrocytoma and ganglioglioma: report of four cases and review of the literature. Am J Surg Pathol. 1997 Jul;21(7):763–71. PMID:9236832
5471. Perry A, Kurtkaya-Yapicier O, Scheithauer BW, et al. Insights into meningioangiomatosis with and without meningioma: a clinicopathologic and genetic series of 24 cases with review of the literature. Brain Pathol. 2005 Jan;15(1):55–65. PMID:15779237
5472. Perry HD, Font RL. Iris nodules in von Recklinghausen's neurofibromatosis. Electron microscopic confirmation of their melanocytic origin. Arch Ophthalmol. 1982 Oct;100(10):1635–40. PMID:6814406
5473. Perry JA, Kiezun A, Tonzi P, et al. Complementary genomic approaches highlight the PI3K/mTOR pathway as a common vulnerability in osteosarcoma. Proc Natl Acad Sci U S A. 2014 Dec 23;111(51):E5564–73. PMID:25512523
5474. Persson F, Andrén Y, Winnes M, et al. High-resolution genomic profiling of adenomas and carcinomas of the salivary glands reveals amplification, rearrangement, and fusion of HMGA2. Genes Chromosomes Cancer. 2009 Jan;48(1):69–82. PMID:18828159
5475. Peruzzi L, Iuvone L, Ruggiero A, et al. Neuropsychological deterioration predicts tumor progression in a young boy with bithalamic glioma. Appl Neuropsychol Child. 2016;5(1):76–81. PMID:25650783
5476. Perwein T, Lackner H, Ebetsberger-Dachs G, et al. Management of children and adolescents with gray zone lymphoma: a case series. Pediatr Blood Cancer. 2020 May;67(5):e28206. PMID:32037692
5477. Pesatori AC, Baccarelli A, Consonni D, et al. Aryl hydrocarbon receptor-interacting protein and pituitary adenomas: a population-based study on subjects exposed to dioxin after the Seveso, Italy, accident. Eur J Endocrinol. 2008 Dec;159(6):699–703. PMID:18787049
5478. Pesce A, Palmieri M, Armocida D, et al. Spinal myxopapillary ependymoma: the Sapienza university experience and comprehensive literature review concerning the clinical course of 1602 patients. World Neurosurg. 2019 Sep;129:245–53. PMID:31152881
5479. Peshtani A, Kaliki S, Eagle RC, et al. Medulloepithelioma: a triad of clinical features. Oman J Ophthalmol. 2014 May;7(2):93–5. PMID:25136238
5480. Pession A, Masetti R, Rizzari C, et al. Results of the AIEOP AML 2002/01 multicenter prospective trial for the treatment of children with acute myeloid leukemia. Blood. 2013 Jul 11;122(2):170–8. PMID:23673857
5481. Peter S, Matevž S, Borut P. Spinal dumbbell lipoblastoma: a case-based update. Childs Nerv Syst. 2016 Nov;32(11):2069–73. PMID:27444294
5482. Peters TL, Kumar V, Polikepahad S, et al. BCOR-CCNB3 fusions are frequent in undifferentiated sarcomas of male children. Mod Pathol. 2015 Apr;28(4):575–86. PMID:25360585
5483. Peterson WF. Malignant degeneration of benign cystic teratomas of the overy; a collective review of the literature. Obstet Gynecol Surv. 1957 Dec;12(6):793–830. PMID:13493921
5484. Peterson WF. Solid, histologically benign teratomas of the ovary; a report of four cases and review of the literature. Am J Obstet Gynecol. 1956 Nov;72(5):1094–102. PMID:13362421
5485. Peterson WF, Prevost EC, Edmunds FT, et al. Benign cystic teratomas of the ovary; a clinico-statistical study of 1,007 cases with a review of the literature. Am J Obstet Gynecol. 1955 Aug;70(2):368–82. PMID:13238472
5486. Petit A, Trinquand A, Chevret S, et al. Oncogenetic mutations combined with MRD improve outcome prediction in pediatric T-cell acute lymphoblastic leukemia. Blood. 2018 Jan 18;131(3):289–300. PMID:29051182
5487. Petr EJ, Else T. Adrenocortical carcinoma (ACC): When and why should we consider germline testing? Presse Med. 2018 Jul-Aug;47(7-8 Pt 2):e119–25. PMID:30104051
5488. Petr EJ, Else T. Pheochromocytoma and paraganglioma in neurofibromatosis type 1: frequent surgeries and cardiovascular crises indicate the need for screening. Clin Diabetes Endocrinol. 2018 Jun 22;4:15. PMID:29977594
5489. Petrella G, Tamburrini G, Lauriola L, et al. Spinal epidural angiolipoma complicated by an intratumoral abscess. Case report. J Neurosurg. 2005 Aug;103(2 Suppl):166–9. PMID:16370284
5490. Petrossians P, Daly AF, Natchev E, et al. Acromegaly at diagnosis in 3173 patients from the Liège Acromegaly Survey (LAS) database. Endocr Relat Cancer. 2017 Oct;24(10):505–18. PMID:28733467
5491. Petruzzellis G, Valentini D, Del Bufalo F, et al. Vemurafenib treatment of pleomorphic xanthoastrocytoma in a child with down syndrome. Front Oncol. 2019 Apr 12;9:277. PMID:31032231
5492. Pettinato G, Di Vizio D, Manivel JC, et al. Solid-pseudopapillary tumor of the pancreas: a neoplasm with distinct and highly characteristic cytological features. Diagn Cytopathol. 2002 Dec;27(6):325–34. PMID:12451561
5493. Pettinato G, Manivel JC, d'Amore ES, et al. Melanotic neuroectodermal tumor of infancy. A reexamination of a histogenetic problem based on immunohistochemical, flow cytometric, and ultrastructural study of 10 cases. Am J Surg Pathol. 1991 Mar;15(3):233–45. PMID:1847607
5494. Pettinato G, Manivel JC, De Rosa N, et al. Inflammatory myofibroblastic tumor (plasma cell granuloma). Clinicopathologic study of 20 cases with immunohistochemical and ultrastructural observations. Am J Clin Pathol. 1990 Nov;94(5):538–46. PMID:2239820
5495. Pettinato G, Manivel JC, Ravetto C, et al. Papillary cystic tumor of the pancreas. A clinicopathologic study of 20 cases with cytologic, immunohistochemical, ultrastructural, and flow cytometric observations, and a review of the literature. Am J Clin Pathol. 1992 Nov;98(5):478–88. PMID:1283055
5496. Peuchmaur M, d'Amore ES, Joshi VV, et al. Revision of the International Neuroblastoma Pathology Classification: confirmation of favorable and unfavorable prognostic subsets in ganglioneuroblastoma, nodular. Cancer. 2003 Nov 15;98(10):2274–81. PMID:14601099
5497. Peyre M, Bah A, Kalamarides M. Multifocal choroid plexus papillomas: case report. Acta Neurochir (Wien). 2012 Feb;154(2):295–9. PMID:21953479
5498. Pfaff E, Aichmüller C, Sill M, et al. Molecular subgrouping of primary pineal parenchymal tumors reveals distinct subtypes correlated with clinical parameters and genetic alterations. Acta Neuropathol. 2020 Feb;139(2):243–57. PMID:31768671
5499. Pfeifer FM, Bridge JA, Neff JR, et al. Cytogenetic findings in aneurysmal bone cysts. Genes Chromosomes Cancer. 1991 Nov;3(6):416–9. PMID:1777412
5500. Pfirrmann M, Lauseker M, Hoffmann VS, et al. Prognostic scores for patients with chronic myeloid leukemia under particular consideration of competing causes of death. Ann Hematol. 2015 Apr;94 Suppl 2:S209–18. PMID:25814087
5501. Pfister S, Janzarik WG, Remke M, et al. BRAF gene duplication constitutes a mechanism of MAPK pathway activation in low-grade astrocytomas. J Clin Invest. 2008 May;118(5):1739–49. PMID:18398503
5502. Pfister SM, Reyes-Múgica M, Chan JKC, et al. A summary of the inaugural WHO classification of pediatric tumors: transitioning from the

optical into the molecular era. Cancer Discov. 2022 Feb;12(2):331–55. PMID:34921008

**5503.** Pflueger D, Sboner A, Storz M, et al. Identification of molecular tumor markers in renal cell carcinomas with TFE3 protein expression by RNA sequencing. Neoplasia. 2013 Nov;15(11):1231–40. PMID:24339735

**5504.** Pham NS, Poirier B, Fuller SC, et al. Pediatric lipoblastoma in the head and neck: a systematic review of 48 reported cases. Int J Pediatr Otorhinolaryngol. 2010 Jul;74(7):723–8. PMID:20472310

**5505.** Pham TH, Moir C, Thompson GB, et al. Pheochromocytoma and paraganglioma in children: a review of medical and surgical management at a tertiary care center. Pediatrics. 2006 Sep;118(3):1109–17. PMID:16951005

**5506.** Phi JH, Koh EJ, Kim SK, et al. Desmoplastic infantile astrocytoma: recurrence with malignant transformation into glioblastoma: a case report. Childs Nerv Syst. 2011 Dec;27(12):2177–81. PMID:21947035

**5507.** Phi JH, Park AK, Lee S, et al. Genomic analysis reveals secondary glioblastoma after radiotherapy in a subset of recurrent medulloblastomas. Acta Neuropathol. 2018 Jun;135(6):939–53. PMID:29644394

**5508.** Phi JH, Park SH, Chae JH, et al. Congenital subependymal giant cell astrocytoma: clinical considerations and expression of radial glial cell markers in giant cells. Childs Nerv Syst. 2008 Dec;24(12):1499–503. PMID:18629509

**5509.** Philippe-Chomette P, Kabbara N, Andre N, et al. Desmoplastic small round cell tumors with EWS-WT1 fusion transcript in children and young adults. Pediatr Blood Cancer. 2012 Jun;58(6):891–7. PMID:22162435

**5510.** Phillips CL, Miles L, Jones BV, et al. Medulloblastoma with melanotic differentiation: case report and review of the literature. J Neurooncol. 2011 Jul;103(3):759–64. PMID:20953660

**5511.** Phillips JJ, Gong H, Chen K, et al. The genetic landscape of anaplastic pleomorphic xanthoastrocytoma. Brain Pathol. 2019 Jan;29(1):85–96. PMID:30051528

**5512.** Phillips PP, Olsen KD. Recurrent pleomorphic adenoma of the parotid gland: report of 126 cases and a review of the literature. Ann Otol Rhinol Laryngol. 1995 Feb;104(2):100–4. PMID:7857010

**5513.** Phoenix TN, Patmore DM, Boop S, et al. Medulloblastoma genotype dictates blood brain barrier phenotype. Cancer Cell. 2016 Apr 11;29(4):508–22. PMID:27050100

**5514.** Picado O, Ferrantella A, Zabalo C, et al. Treatment patterns and outcomes for pancreatic tumors in children: an analysis of the National Cancer Database. Pediatr Surg Int. 2020 Mar;36(3):357–63. PMID:31989243

**5515.** Picard C, Orbach D, Carton M, et al. Revisiting the role of the pathological grading in pediatric adrenal cortical tumors: results from a national cohort study with pathological review. Mod Pathol. 2019 Apr;32(4):546–59. PMID:30401946

**5516.** Picard C, Silvy M, Gerard C, et al. Gs alpha overexpression and loss of Gs alpha imprinting in human somatotroph adenomas: association with tumor size and response to pharmacologic treatment. Int J Cancer. 2007 Sep 15;121(6):1245–52. PMID:17514647

**5517.** Picard D, Miller S, Hawkins CE, et al. Markers of survival and metastatic potential in childhood CNS primitive neuro-ectodermal brain tumours: an integrative genomic analysis. Lancet Oncol. 2012 Aug;13(8):838–48. PMID:22691720

**5518.** Picarsic J, Jaffe R. Nosology and pathology of Langerhans cell histiocytosis. Hematol Oncol Clin North Am. 2015 Oct;29(5):799–823. PMID:26461144

**5519.** Picarsic J, Pysher T, Zhou H, et al. BRAF V600E mutation in Juvenile Xanthogranuloma family neoplasms of the central nervous system (CNS-JXG): a revised diagnostic algorithm to include pediatric Erdheim-Chester disease. Acta Neuropathol Commun. 2019 Nov 4;7(1):168. PMID:31685033

**5520.** Piccaluga PP, De Falco G, Kustagi M, et al. Gene expression analysis uncovers similarity and differences among Burkitt lymphoma subtypes. Blood. 2011 Mar 31;117(13):3596–608. PMID:21245480

**5521.** Picci P, Manfrini M, Fabbri N, et al., editors. Atlas of musculoskeletal tumors and tumorlike lesions. The Rizzoli Case Archive. Cham (Switzerland): Springer International Publishing; 2014.

**5522.** Pickles JC, Fairchild AR, Stone TJ, et al. DNA methylation-based profiling for paediatric CNS tumour diagnosis and treatment: a population-based study. Lancet Child Adolesc Health. 2020 Feb;4(2):121–30. PMID:31786093

**5523.** Pickles JC, Mankad K, Aizpurua M, et al. A case series of diffuse glioneuronal tumours with oligodendroglioma-like features and nuclear clusters (DGONC). Neuropathol Appl Neurobiol. 2021 Apr;47(3):464–7. PMID:33325069

**5524.** Pienkowska M, Choufani S, Turinsky AL, et al. DNA methylation signature is prognostic of choroid plexus tumor aggressiveness. Clin Epigenetics. 2019 Aug 13;11(1):117. PMID:31409384

**5525.** Pierard GE, Lapiere CM. Nevi of connective tissue. A reappraisal of their classification. Am J Dermatopathol. 1985 Aug;7(4):325–33. PMID:3842789

**5526.** Pierre C, Agopiantz M, Brunaud L, et al. COPPS, a composite score integrating pathological features, PS100 and SDHB losses, predicts the risk of metastasis and progression-free survival in pheochromocytomas/paragangliomas. Virchows Arch. 2019 Jun;474(6):721–34. PMID:30868297

**5527.** Pierron G, Tirode F, Lucchesi C, et al. A new subtype of bone sarcoma defined by BCOR-CCNB3 gene fusion. Nat Genet. 2012 Mar 4;44(4):461–6. PMID:22387997

**5528.** Pieterse AS, Smith M, Smith LA, et al. Embryonal (undifferentiated) sarcoma of the liver. Fine-needle aspiration cytology and ultrastructural findings. Arch Pathol Lab Med. 1985 Jul;109(7):677–80. PMID:2990375

**5529.** Pietsch T, Haberler C. Update on the integrated histopathological and genetic classification of medulloblastoma - a practical diagnostic guideline. Clin Neuropathol. 2016 Nov/Dec;35(6):344–52. PMID:27781424

**5530.** Pietsch T, Schmidt R, Remke M, et al. Prognostic significance of clinical, histopathological, and molecular characteristics of medulloblastomas in the prospective HIT2000 multicenter clinical trial cohort. Acta Neuropathol. 2014 Jul;128(1):137–49. PMID:24791927

**5531.** Pietsch T, Waha A, Koch A, et al. Medulloblastomas of the desmoplastic variant carry mutations of the human homologue of Drosophila patched. Cancer Res. 1997 Jun 1;57(11):2085–8. PMID:9187099

**5532.** Pietsch T, Wohlers I, Goschzik T, et al. Supratentorial ependymomas of childhood carry C11orf95-RELA fusions leading to pathological activation of the NF-κB signaling pathway. Acta Neuropathol. 2014 Apr;127(4):609–11. PMID:24562983

**5533.** Pignolo RJ, Baujat G, Brown MA, et al. Natural history of fibrodysplasia ossificans progressiva: cross-sectional analysis of annotated baseline phenotypes. Orphanet J Rare Dis. 2019 May 3;14(1):98. PMID:31053156

**5534.** Pike AM, Oberman HA. Juvenile (cellular) adenofibromas. A clinicopathologic study.

Am J Surg Pathol. 1985 Oct;9(10):730–6. PMID:2998214

**5535.** Pilania K, Jankharia B, Memon FW. Fibroma of the patellar tendon sheath-a rare case in a young boy. Skeletal Radiol. 2019 Sep;48(9):1457–61. PMID:30783711

**5536.** Pilarski R, Burt R, Kohlman W, et al. Cowden syndrome and the PTEN hamartoma tumor syndrome: systematic review and revised diagnostic criteria. J Natl Cancer Inst. 2013 Nov 6;105(21):1607–16. PMID:24136893

**5537.** Pilarski R, Cebulla CM, Massengill JB, et al. Expanding the clinical phenotype of hereditary BAP1 cancer predisposition syndrome, reporting three new cases. Genes Chromosomes Cancer. 2014 Feb;53(2):177–82. PMID:24243779

**5538.** Pileri SA, Gaidano G, Zinzani PL, et al. Primary mediastinal B-cell lymphoma: high frequency of BCL-6 mutations and consistent expression of the transcription factors OCT-2, BOB.1, and PU.1 in the absence of immunoglobulins. Am J Pathol. 2003 Jan;162(1):243–53. PMID:12507907

**5539.** Pileri SA, Pulford K, Mori S, et al. Frequent expression of the NPM-ALK chimeric fusion protein in anaplastic large-cell lymphoma, lympho-histiocytic type. Am J Pathol. 1997 Apr;150(4):1207–11. PMID:9094977

**5540.** Pilichowska M, Pittaluga S, Ferry JA, et al. Clinicopathologic consensus study of gray zone lymphoma with features intermediate between DLBCL and classical HL. Blood Adv. 2017 Dec 11;1(26):2600–9. PMID:29296913

**5541.** Pillai S, Gopalan V, Smith RA, et al. Updates on the genetics and the clinical impacts on phaeochromocytoma and paraganglioma in the new era. Crit Rev Oncol Hematol. 2016 Apr;100:190–208. PMID:26839173

**5542.** Pillay K, Hendricks M, Davidson A. HHV-8 large T-cell lymphoma: an unusual malignancy amidst more common B-cell lymphomas in HIV-positive children treated at a single institution. J Pediatr Hematol Oncol. 2013 Aug;35(6):e246–8. PMID:23588335

**5543.** Pillay N, Plagnol V, Tarpey PS, et al. A common single-nucleotide variant in T is strongly associated with chordoma. Nat Genet. 2012 Nov;44(11):1185–7. PMID:23064415

**5544.** Pillon M, Di Tullio MT, Garaventa A, et al. Long-term results of the first Italian Association of Pediatric Hematology and Oncology protocol for the treatment of pediatric B-cell non-Hodgkin lymphoma (AIEOP LNH92). Cancer. 2004 Jul 15;101(2):385–94. PMID:15241838

**5545.** Pimenta FJ, Gontijo Silveira LF, Tavares GC, et al. HRPT2 gene alterations in ossifying fibroma of the jaws. Oral Oncol. 2006 Aug;42(7):735–9. PMID:16458039

**5546.** Pinato DJ, Ramachandran R, Toussi ST, et al. Immunohistochemical markers of the hypoxic response can identify malignancy in phaeochromocytomas and paragangliomas and optimize the detection of tumours with VHL germline mutations. Br J Cancer. 2013 Feb 5;108(2):429–37. PMID:23257898

**5547.** Pincus LB, LeBoit PE, McCalmont TH, et al. Subcutaneous panniculitis-like T-cell lymphoma with overlapping clinicopathologic features of lupus erythematosus: coexistence of 2 entities? Am J Dermatopathol. 2009 Aug;31(6):520–6. PMID:19590424

**5548.** Piñeros M, Mery L, Soerjomataram I, et al. Scaling up the surveillance of childhood cancer: a global roadmap. J Natl Cancer Inst. 2021 Jan 4;113(1):9–15. PMID:32433739

**5549.** Pinkel D. Differentiating juvenile myelomonocytic leukemia from infectious disease. Blood. 1998 Jan 1;91(1):365–7. PMID:9414312

**5550.** Pinna AD, Iwatsuki S, Lee RG, et al. Treatment of fibrolamellar hepatoma with subtotal hepatectomy or transplantation. Hepatology.

1997 Oct;26(4):877–83. PMID:9328308

**5551.** Pinna R, Cocco F, Campus G, et al. Genetic and developmental disorders of the oral mucosa: epidemiology; molecular mechanisms; diagnostic criteria; management. Periodontol 2000. 2019 Jun;80(1):12–27. PMID:31090139

**5552.** Pinna V, Lanari V, Daniele P, et al. p.Arg1809Cys substitution in neurofibromin is associated with a distinctive NF1 phenotype without neurofibromas. Eur J Hum Genet. 2015 Aug;23(8):1068–71. PMID:25370043

**5553.** Pinto A, Hutchison RE, Grant LH, et al. Follicular lymphomas in pediatric patients. Mod Pathol. 1990 May;3(3):308–13. PMID:2194214

**5554.** Pinto A, Signoretti S, Hirsch MS, et al. Immunohistochemical staining for BRAF V600E supports the diagnosis of metanephric adenoma. Histopathology. 2015 May;66(6):901–4. PMID:25130952

**5555.** Pinto EM, Chen X, Easton J, et al. Genomic landscape of paediatric adrenocortical tumours. Nat Commun. 2015 Mar 6;6:6302. PMID:25743702

**5556.** Pinto EM, Zambetti GP. What 20 years of research has taught us about the TP53 p.R337H mutation. Cancer. 2020 Nov 1;126(21):4678–86. PMID:32875577

**5557.** Pinto Gama HP, da Rocha AJ, Braga FT, et al. Comparative analysis of MR sequences to detect structural brain lesions in tuberous sclerosis. Pediatr Radiol. 2006 Feb;36(2):119–25. PMID:16283285

**5558.** Pinto RG, Couto F, Mandreker S. Infarction after fine needle aspiration. A report of four cases. Acta Cytol. 1996 Jul-Aug;40(4):739–41. PMID:8693896

**5559.** Piombo V, Jochmann K, Hoffmann D, et al. Signaling systems affecting the severity of multiple osteochondromas. Bone. 2018 Jun;111:71–81. PMID:29545125

**5560.** Piotrowski A, Xie J, Liu YF, et al. Germline loss-of-function mutations in LZTR1 predispose to an inherited disorder of multiple schwannomas. Nat Genet. 2014 Feb;46(2):182–7. PMID:24362817

**5561.** Piotrowski Z, Canter DJ, Kutikov A, et al. Metanephric adenofibroma: robotic partial nephrectomy of a large Wilms' tumor variant. Can J Urol. 2010 Aug;17(4):5309–12. PMID:20735912

**5562.** Pippucci T, Savoia A, Perrotta S, et al. Mutations in the 5' UTR of ANKRD26, the ankirin repeat domain 26 gene, cause an autosomal-dominant form of inherited thrombocytopenia, THC2. Am J Hum Genet. 2011 Jan 7;88(1):115–20. PMID:21211618

**5563.** Piquer Gibert M, Alsina L, Giner Muñoz MT, et al. Non-Hodgkin lymphoma in pediatric patients with common variable immunodeficiency. Eur J Pediatr. 2015 Aug;174(8):1069–76. PMID:25749928

**5564.** Piquero-Casals J, Okubo AY, Nico MM. Rothmund-Thomson syndrome in three siblings and development of cutaneous squamous cell carcinoma. Pediatr Dermatol. 2002 Jul-Aug;19(4):312–6. PMID:12220274

**5565.** Pirini MG, Mascalchi M, Salvi F, et al. Primary diffuse meningeal melanomatosis: radiologic-pathologic correlation. AJNR Am J Neuroradiol. 2003 Jan;24(1):115–8. PMID:12533338

**5566.** Piris MA, Medeiros LJ, Chang KC. Hodgkin lymphoma: a review of pathological features and recent advances in pathogenesis. Pathology. 2020 Jan;52(1):154–65. PMID:31699300

**5567.** Pitjadi TM, Grayson W. Epstein-Barr virus-associated smooth muscle tumour: a case series with a significant proportion of tumours showing proclivity for cutaneous soft tissues. Dermatopathology (Basel). 2019 Jun 26;6(2):133–46. PMID:31700854

**5568.** Pitjadi TM, Wadee R, Grayson W. Rhabdomyosarcoma arising in a giant congenital melanocytic naevus: case report and literature review. Dermatopathology (Basel). 2019 Jun 26;6(2):91–8. PMID:31700849
**5569.** Pitman MB, Faquin WC. The fine-needle aspiration biopsy cytology of pancreatoblastoma. Diagn Cytopathol. 2004 Dec;31(6):402–6. PMID:15540188
**5570.** Piunti A, Smith ER, Morgan MAJ, et al. CATACOMB: an endogenous inducible gene that antagonizes H3K27 methylation activity of Polycomb repressive complex 2 via an H3K27M-like mechanism. Sci Adv. 2019 Jul 3;5(7):eaax2887. PMID:31281901
**5571.** Pivonello R, Matrone C, Filippella M, et al. Dopamine receptor expression and function in clinically nonfunctioning pituitary tumors: comparison with the effectiveness of cabergoline treatment. J Clin Endocrinol Metab. 2004 Apr;89(4):1674–83. PMID:15070930
**5572.** Pizzi M, Tazzoli S, Carraro E, et al. Histology of pediatric classic Hodgkin lymphoma: from diagnosis to prognostic stratification. Pediatr Blood Cancer. 2020 May;67(5):e28230. PMID:32134194
**5573.** Planas-Ciudad S, Roé Crespo E, Sánchez-Carpintero I, et al. Infantile hemangiomas with minimal or arrested growth associated with soft tissue hypertrophy: a case series of 10 patients. J Eur Acad Dermatol Venereol. 2017 Nov;31(11):1924–9. PMID:28681397
**5574.** Plank TL, Logginidou H, Klein-Szanto A, et al. The expression of hamartin, the product of the TSC1 gene, in normal human tissues and in TSC1- and TSC2-linked angiomyolipomas. Mod Pathol. 1999 May;12(5):539–45. PMID:10349994
**5575.** Plank TL, Yeung RS, Henske EP. Hamartin, the product of the tuberous sclerosis 1 (TSC1) gene, interacts with tuberin and appears to be localized to cytoplasmic vesicles. Cancer Res. 1998 Nov 1;58(21):4766–70. PMID:9809973
**5576.** Plant AS, Busuttil RW, Rana A, et al. A single-institution retrospective cases series of childhood undifferentiated embryonal liver sarcoma (UELS): success of combined therapy and the use of orthotopic liver transplant. J Pediatr Hematol Oncol. 2013 Aug;35(6):451–5. PMID:23138115
**5577.** Płaszczyca A, Nilsson J, Magnusson L, et al. Fusions involving protein kinase C and membrane-associated proteins in benign fibrous histiocytoma. Int J Biochem Cell Biol. 2014 Aug;53:475–81. PMID:24721208
**5578.** Plaza JA, De Stefano D, Suster S, et al. Intradermal spitz nevi: a rare subtype of spitz nevi analyzed in a clinicopathologic study of 74 cases. Am J Dermatopathol. 2014 Apr;36(4):283–94. PMID:24736667
**5579.** Plaza JA, Sangueza M. Hydroa vacciniforme-like lymphoma with primarily periorbital swelling: 7 cases of an atypical clinical manifestation of this rare cutaneous T-cell lymphoma. Am J Dermatopathol. 2015 Jan;37(1):20–5. PMID:25162933
**5580.** Plevová P, Geržová H. Genetic causes of rare pediatric ovarian tumors. Klin Onkol. 2019 Summer;32 Supplementum2:79–91. PMID:31409083
**5581.** Plon SE, Lupo PJ. Genetic predisposition to childhood cancer in the genomic era. Annu Rev Genomics Hum Genet. 2019 Aug 31;20:241–63. PMID:31082280
**5582.** Plon SE, Pirics ML, Nuchtern J, et al. Multiple tumors in a child with germ-line mutations in TP53 and PTEN. N Engl J Med. 2008 Jul 31;359(5):537–9. PMID:18669439
**5583.** Plotkin SR, Blakeley JO, Evans DG, et al. Update from the 2011 International Schwannomatosis Workshop: from genetics to diagnostic criteria. Am J Med Genet A. 2013 Mar;161A(3):405–16. PMID:23401320
**5583A.** Plotkin SR, O'Donnell CC, Curry WT, et al. Spinal ependymomas in neurofibromatosis type 2: a retrospective analysis of 55 patients. J Neurosurg Spine. 2011 Apr;14(4):543–7. PMID:21294614
**5584.** Pogoriler J, O'Neill AF, Voss SD, et al. Hepatocellular carcinoma in Fanconi-Bickel syndrome. Pediatr Dev Pathol. 2018 Jan-Feb;21(1):84–90. PMID:28382841
**5585.** Poh B, Koso H, Momota H, et al. Foxr2 promotes formation of CNS-embryonal tumors in a Trp53-deficient background. Neuro Oncol. 2019 Aug 5;21(8):993–1004. PMID:30976792
**5586.** Pokorny KS, Hyman BM, Jakobiec FA, et al. Epibulbar choristomas containing lacrimal tissue. Clinical distinction from dermoids and histologic evidence of an origin from the palpebral lobe. Ophthalmology. 1987 Oct;94(10):1249–57. PMID:3684203
**5587.** Polchi A, Magini A, Meo DD, et al. mTOR signaling and neural stem cells: the tuberous sclerosis complex model. Int J Mol Sci. 2018 May 16;19(5):E1474. PMID:29772672
**5588.** Policarpio-Nicolas ML, Abbott TE, Dalkin AC, et al. Phosphaturic mesenchymal tumor diagnosed by fine-needle aspiration and core biopsy: a case report and review of literature. Diagn Cytopathol. 2008 Feb;36(2):115–9. PMID:18181193
**5589.** Pollack IF, Hurtt M, Pang D, et al. Dissemination of low grade intracranial astrocytomas in children. Cancer. 1994 Jun 1;73(11):2869–78. PMID:8194029
**5590.** Pollock BH, Jenson HB, Leach CT, et al. Risk factors for pediatric human immunodeficiency virus-related malignancy. JAMA. 2003 May 14;289(18):2393–9. PMID:12746363
**5591.** Pollock PM, Harper UL, Hansen KS, et al. High frequency of BRAF mutations in nevi. Nat Genet. 2003 Jan;33(1):19–20. PMID:12447372
**5592.** Polprasert C, Takeuchi Y, Kakiuchi N, et al. Frequent germline mutations of HAVCR2 in sporadic subcutaneous panniculitis-like T-cell lymphoma. Blood Adv. 2019 Feb 26;3(4):588–95. PMID:30792187
**5593.** Polsani A, Braithwaite KA, Alazraki AL, et al. NUT midline carcinoma: an imaging case series and review of literature. Pediatr Radiol. 2012 Feb;42(2):205–10. PMID:22033856
**5594.** Polubothu S, McGuire N, Al-Olabi L, et al. Does the gene matter? Genotype-phenotype and genotype-outcome associations in congenital melanocytic naevi. Br J Dermatol. 2020 Feb;182(2):434–43. PMID:31111470
**5595.** Pommert L, Bradley W. Pediatric gynecologic cancers. Curr Oncol Rep. 2017 Jul;19(7):44. PMID:28501984
**5596.** Pomposiello IM. [Juvenile elastoma. (Elastic nevus, connective nevus)]. Arch Argent Dermatol. 1963 Sep;13:329–30. Spanish. PMID:14155044
**5597.** Pontes FSC, de Souza LL, Uchôa DCC, et al. Melanotic neuroectodermal tumor of infancy of the jaw bones: update on the factors influencing survival and recurrence. Head Neck. 2018 Dec;40(12):2749–56. PMID:30390348
**5598.** Poon DS, Reich E, Smith VM, et al. Ruthenium-106 plaque brachytherapy in the primary management of ocular medulloepithelioma. Ophthalmology. 2015 Sep;122(9):1949–51. PMID:25863421
**5599.** Popova T, Hebert L, Jacquemin V, et al. Germline BAP1 mutations predispose to renal cell carcinomas. Am J Hum Genet. 2013 Jun 6;92(6):974–80. PMID:23684012
**5600.** Poretti A, Meoded A, Huisman TA. Neuroimaging of pediatric posterior fossa tumors including review of the literature. J Magn Reson Imaging. 2012 Jan;35(1):32–47. PMID:21989968
**5601.** Portera CA Jr, Ho V, Patel SR, et al. Alveolar soft part sarcoma: clinical course and patterns of metastasis in 70 patients treated at a single institution. Cancer. 2001 Feb 1;91(3):585–91. PMID:11169942
**5602.** Posnick JC, Bortoluzzi P, Armstrong DC, et al. Intracranial nasal dermoid sinus cysts: computed tomographic scan findings and surgical results. Plast Reconstr Surg. 1994 Apr;93(4):745–54. PMID:8134433
**5603.** Posso-De Los Rios CJ, Lara-Corrales I, Ho N. Dermatofibrosarcoma protuberans in pediatric patients: a report of 17 cases. J Cutan Med Surg. 2014 May-Jun;18(3):180–5. PMID:24800706
**5604.** Pothoulakis C. Pathogenesis of Clostridium difficile-associated diarrhoea. Eur J Gastroenterol Hepatol. 1996 Nov;8(11):1041–7. PMID:8944363
**5605.** Potorac I, Petrossians P, Daly AF, et al. T2-weighted MRI signal predicts hormone and tumor responses to somatostatin analogs in acromegaly. Endocr Relat Cancer. 2016 Nov;23(11):871–81. PMID:27649724
**5606.** Potter BK, Freedman BA, Lehman RA Jr, et al. Solitary epiphyseal enchondromas. J Bone Joint Surg Am. 2005 Jul;87(7):1551–60. PMID:15995123
**5607.** Poulogiannis G, Frayling IM, Arends MJ. DNA mismatch repair deficiency in sporadic colorectal cancer and Lynch syndrome. Histopathology. 2010 Jan;56(2):167–79. PMID:20102395
**5608.** Poulos C, Cheng L, Zhang S, et al. Analysis of ovarian teratomas for isochromosome 12p: evidence supporting a dual histogenetic pathway for teratomatous elements. Mod Pathol. 2006 Jun;19(6):766–71. PMID:16547466
**5609.** Powell SZ, Yachnis AT, Rorke LB, et al. Divergent differentiation in pleomorphic xanthoastrocytoma. Evidence for a neuronal element and possible relationship to ganglion cell tumors. Am J Surg Pathol. 1996 Jan;20(1):80–5. PMID:8540612
**5610.** Powers J, Pinto EM, Barnoud T, et al. A rare TP53 mutation predominant in Ashkenazi Jews confers risk of multiple cancers. Cancer Res. 2020 Sep 1;80(17):3732–44. PMID:32675277
**5611.** Pow-Sang J, Sánchez J, Benavente V, et al. Testicular yolk sac carcinoma in infants: natural history in 56 consecutive patients. Prog Clin Biol Res. 1985;203:623–37. PMID:3832112
**5612.** Poynter JN, Hooten AJ, Frazier AL, et al. Associations between variants in KITLG, SPRY4, BAK1, and DMRT1 and pediatric germ cell tumors. Genes Chromosomes Cancer. 2012 Mar;51(3):266–71. PMID:22072546
**5613.** Pozza C, Sesti F, Di Dato C, et al. A novel MAX gene mutation variant in a patient with multiple and "composite" neuroendocrine-neuroblastic tumors. Front Endocrinol (Lausanne). 2020 May 19;11:234. PMID:32508744
**5614.** Prabowo AS, Iyer AM, Veersema TJ, et al. BRAF V600E mutation is associated with mTOR signaling activation in glioneuronal tumors. Brain Pathol. 2014 Jan;24(1):52–66. PMID:23941441
**5615.** Prabowo AS, van Thuijl HF, Scheinin I, et al. Landscape of chromosomal copy number aberrations in gangliogliomas and dysembryoplastic neuroepithelial tumours. Neuropathol Appl Neurobiol. 2015 Oct;41(6):743–55. PMID:25764012
**5616.** Prada CE, Jousma E, Rizvi TA, et al. Neurofibroma-associated macrophages play roles in tumor growth and response to pharmacological inhibition. Acta Neuropathol. 2013 Jan;125(1):159–68. PMID:23099891
**5617.** Pradhan A, Grimer RJ, Abudu A, et al. Epithelioid sarcomas: How important is loco-regional control? Eur J Surg Oncol. 2017 Sep;43(9):1746–52. PMID:28756018
**5618.** Pradhan D, Schoedel K, McGough RL, et al. Pseudomyogenic hemangioendothelioma of skin, bone and soft tissue-a clinicopathological, immunohistochemical, and fluorescence in situ hybridization study. Hum Pathol. 2018 Jan;71:126–34. PMID:29104110
**5619.** Prakash S, Fountaine T, Raffeld M, et al. IgD positive L&H cells identify a unique subset of nodular lymphocyte predominant Hodgkin lymphoma. Am J Surg Pathol. 2006 May;30(5):585–92. PMID:16699312
**5620.** Prakash V, Batanian JR, Guzman MA, et al. Malignant transformation of a desmoplastic infantile ganglioglioma in an infant carrier of a nonsynonymous TP53 mutation. Pediatr Neurol. 2014 Jul;51(1):138–43. PMID:24768217
**5621.** Prasad AR, Savera AT, Gown AM, et al. The myoepithelial immunophenotype in 135 benign and malignant salivary gland tumors other than pleomorphic adenoma. Arch Pathol Lab Med. 1999 Sep;123(9):801–6. PMID:10458827
**5622.** Prasad ML, Pellegata NS, Huang Y, et al. Galectin-3, fibronectin-1, CITED-1, HBME1 and cytokeratin-19 immunohistochemistry is useful for the differential diagnosis of thyroid tumors. Mod Pathol. 2005 Jan;18(1):48–57. PMID:15272279
**5623.** Prasannan L, Warren L, Herzog CE, et al. Sinonasal myxoma: a pediatric case. J Pediatr Hematol Oncol. 2005 Feb;27(2):90–2. PMID:15701983
**5624.** Prat J, Scully RE. Cellular fibromas and fibrosarcomas of the ovary: a comparative clinicopathologic analysis of seventeen cases. Cancer. 1981 Jun 1;47(11):2663–70. PMID:7260859
**5625.** Prat J, Woodruff JM, Marcove RC. Epithelioid sarcoma: an analysis of 22 cases indicating the prognostic significance of vascular invasion and regional lymph node metastasis. Cancer. 1978 Apr;41(4):1472–87. PMID:639005
**5626.** Prat J, Young RH, Scully RE. Ovarian Sertoli-Leydig cell tumors with heterologous elements. II. Cartilage and skeletal muscle: a clinicopathologic analysis of twelve cases. Cancer. 1982 Dec 1;50(11):2465–75. PMID:7139538
**5627.** Prathap K, Looi LM, Prasad U. Localized amyloidosis in nasopharyngeal carcinoma. Histopathology. 1984 Jan;8(1):27–34. PMID:6706312
**5628.** Pratt CB, Pappo AS, Gieser P, et al. Role of adjuvant chemotherapy in the treatment of surgically resected pediatric nonrhabdomyosarcomatous soft tissue sarcomas: a Pediatric Oncology Group Study. J Clin Oncol. 1999 Apr;17(4):1219. PMID:10561182
**5629.** Pratt D, Natarajan SK, Banda A, et al. Circumscribed/non-diffuse histology confers a better prognosis in H3K27M-mutant gliomas. Acta Neuropathol. 2018 Feb;135(2):299–301. PMID:29302777
**5630.** Prayson RA. Myxopapillary ependymomas: a clinicopathologic study of 14 cases including MIB-1 and p53 immunoreactivity. Mod Pathol. 1997 Apr;10(4):304–10. PMID:9110291
**5631.** Prayson RA. Pleomorphic xanthoastrocytoma arising in neurofibromatosis Type 1. Clin Neuropathol. 2012 May-Jun;31(3):152–4. PMID:22551920
**5632.** Prayson RA, Khajavi K, Comair YG. Cortical architectural abnormalities and MIB1 immunoreactivity in gangliogliomas: a study of 60 patients with intracranial tumors. J Neuropathol Exp Neurol. 1995 Jul;54(4):513–20. PMID:7541447
**5633.** Preciado MV, Fallo A, Chabay P, et al. Epstein Barr virus-associated lymphoma

in HIV-infected children. Pathol Res Pract. 2002;198(5):327–32. PMID:12092768
5634. Premalata CS, Kumar RV, Saleem KM, et al. Fetal rhabdomyoma of the lower extremity. Pediatr Blood Cancer. 2009 Jul;52(7):881–3. PMID:19165887
5635. Prendergast N, Goldstein JD, Beier AD. Choroid plexus adenoma in a child: expanding the clinical and pathological spectrum. J Neurosurg Pediatr. 2018 Apr;21(4):428–33. PMID:29393815
5636. Presneau N, Baumhoer D, Behjati S, et al. Diagnostic value of H3F3A mutations in giant cell tumour of bone compared to osteoclast-rich mimics. J Pathol Clin Res. 2015 Mar 16;1(2):113–23. PMID:27499898
5637. Presneau N, Shalaby A, Ye H, et al. Role of the transcription factor T (brachyury) in the pathogenesis of sporadic chordoma: a genetic and functional-based study. J Pathol. 2011 Feb;223(3):327–35. PMID:21171078
5638. Preston DL, Ron E, Yonehara S, et al. Tumors of the nervous system and pituitary gland associated with atomic bomb radiation exposure. J Natl Cancer Inst. 2002 Oct 16;94(20):1555–63. PMID:12381708
5639. Pretell-Mazzini J, Murphy RF, Kushare I, et al. Unicameral bone cysts: general characteristics and management controversies. J Am Acad Orthop Surg. 2014 May;22(5):295–303. PMID:24788445
5640. Preuss M, Christiansen H, Merkenschlager A, et al. Disseminated oligodendroglial-like leptomeningeal tumors: preliminary diagnostic and therapeutic results for a novel tumor entity [corrected]. J Neurooncol. 2015 Aug;124(1):65–74. PMID:25672644
5641. Preusser M, Budka H, Rössler K, et al. OLIG2 is a useful immunohistochemical marker in differential diagnosis of clear cell primary CNS neoplasms. Histopathology. 2007 Feb;50(3):365–70. PMID:17257132
5642. Price HN, Schaffer JV. Congenital melanocytic nevi-when to worry and how to treat: facts and controversies. Clin Dermatol. 2010 May-Jun;28(3):293–302. PMID:20541682
5643. Price S, Shaw PA, Seitz A, et al. Natural history of autoimmune lymphoproliferative syndrome associated with FAS gene mutations. Blood. 2014 Mar 27;123(13):1989–99. PMID:24398331
5644. Price VE, Fletcher JA, Zielenska M, et al. Imatinib mesylate: an attractive alternative in young children with large, surgically challenging dermatofibrosarcoma protuberans. Pediatr Blood Cancer. 2005 May;44(5):511–5. PMID:15503291
5645. Priest JR, McDermott MB, Bhatia S, et al. Pleuropulmonary blastoma: a clinicopathologic study of 50 cases. Cancer. 1997 Jul 1;80(1):147–61. PMID:9210721
5646. Priest JR, Watterson J, Strong L, et al. Pleuropulmonary blastoma: a marker for familial disease. J Pediatr. 1996 Feb;128(2):220–4. PMID:8636815
5647. Priest JR, Williams GM, Manera R, et al. Ciliary body medulloepithelioma: four cases associated with pleuropulmonary blastoma–a report from the International Pleuropulmonary Blastoma Registry. Br J Ophthalmol. 2011 Jul;95(7):1001–5. PMID:21156700
5648. Priest JR, Williams GM, Mize WA, et al. Nasal chondromesenchymal hamartoma in children with pleuropulmonary blastoma–a report from the International Pleuropulmonary Blastoma Registry registry. Int J Pediatr Otorhinolaryngol. 2010 Nov;74(11):1240–4. PMID:20822816
5649. Priesterbach-Ackley LP, Boldt HB, Petersen JK, et al. Brain tumour diagnostics using a DNA methylation-based classifier as a diagnostic support tool. Neuropathol Appl Neurobiol. 2020 Aug;46(5):478–92. PMID:32072658
5650. Prieto R, Pascual JM, Barrios L. Optic chiasm distortions in craniopharyngiomas: a sign of hypothalamic involvement. Acta Neurochir (Wien). 2017 Aug;159(8):1533–5. PMID:28660394
5651. Prieto-Granada C, Zhang L, Chen HW, et al. A genetic dichotomy between pure sclerosing epithelioid fibrosarcoma (SEF) and hybrid SEF/low-grade fibromyxoid sarcoma: a pathologic and molecular study of 18 cases. Genes Chromosomes Cancer. 2015 Jan;54(1):28–38. PMID:25231134
5652. Prieto-Torres L, Rodriguez-Pinilla SM, Onaindia A, et al. CD30-positive primary cutaneous lymphoproliferative disorders: molecular alterations and targeted therapies. Haematologica. 2019 Feb;104(2):226–35. PMID:30630983
5653. Prindaville B, Lawrence H, Singh V, et al. Immunohistochemical staining of pediatric solitary angiokeratomas. Pediatr Dermatol. 2017 Mar;34(2):211–3. PMID:28297141
5654. Pritchard-Jones K, Fleming S. Cell types expressing the Wilms' tumour gene (WT1) in Wilms' tumours: implications for tumour histogenesis. Oncogene. 1991 Dec;6(12):2211–20. PMID:1722569
5655. Pritchard-Jones K, Fleming S, Davidson D, et al. The candidate Wilms' tumour gene is involved in genitourinary development. Nature. 1990 Jul 12;346(6280):194–7. PMID:2164159
5656. Prokurat A, Kluge P, Kościesza A, et al. Transitional liver cell tumors (TLCT) in older children and adolescents: a novel group of aggressive hepatic tumors expressing beta-catenin. Med Pediatr Oncol. 2002 Nov;39(5):510–8. PMID:12228909
5657. Prunotto G, Offor UT, Samarasinghe S, et al. HSCT provides effective treatment for lymphoproliferative disorders in children with primary immunodeficiency. J Allergy Clin Immunol. 2020 Aug;146(2):447–50. PMID:32371070
5658. Pryor SG, Lewis JE, Weaver AL, et al. Pediatric dermoid cysts of the head and neck. Otolaryngol Head Neck Surg. 2005 Jun;132(6):938–42. PMID:15944568
5659. Przygodzki RM, Finkelstein SD, Keohavong P, et al. Sporadic and Thorotrast-induced angiosarcomas of the liver manifest frequent and multiple point mutations in K-ras-2. Lab Invest. 1997 Jan;76(1):153–9. PMID:9010458
5660. Przygodzki RM, Hubbs AE, Zhao FQ, et al. Primary mediastinal seminomas: evidence of single and multiple KIT mutations. Lab Invest. 2002 Oct;82(10):1369–75. PMID:12379771
5661. Pugh TJ, Yu W, Yang J, et al. Exome sequencing of pleuropulmonary blastoma reveals frequent biallelic loss of TP53 and two hits in DICER1 resulting in retention of 5p-derived miRNA hairpin loop sequences. Oncogene. 2014 Nov 6;33(45):5295–302. PMID:24909177
5662. Pulford K, Lamant L, Morris SW, et al. Detection of anaplastic lymphoma kinase (ALK) and nucleolar protein nucleophosmin (NPM)-ALK proteins in normal and neoplastic cells with the monoclonal antibody ALK1. Blood. 1997 Feb 15;89(4):1394–404. PMID:9028963
5663. Pulitzer DR, Martin PC, Reed RJ. Fibroma of tendon sheath. A clinicopathologic study of 32 cases. Am J Surg Pathol. 1989 Jun;13(6):472–9. PMID:2729499
5664. Puliyel MM, Mascarenhas L, Zhou S, et al. Nuclear protein in testis midline carcinoma misdiagnosed as adamantinoma. J Clin Oncol. 2014 May 20;32(15):e57–60. PMID:24470009
5665. Puls F, Agaimy A, Flucke U, et al. Recurrent fusions between YAP1 and KMT2A in morphologically distinct neoplasms within the spectrum of low-grade fibromyxoid sarcoma and sclerosing epithelioid fibrosarcoma. Am J Surg Pathol. 2020 May;44(5):594–606. PMID:31913156
5666. Puls F, Hofvander J, Magnusson L, et al. FN1-EGF gene fusions are recurrent in calcifying aponeurotic fibroma. J Pathol. 2016 Mar;238(4):502–7. PMID:26691015
5667. Puls F, Niblett A, Marland G, et al. BCOR-CCNB3 (Ewing-like) sarcoma: a clinicopathologic analysis of 10 cases, in comparison with conventional Ewing sarcoma. Am J Surg Pathol. 2014 Oct;38(10):1307–18. PMID:24805859
5668. Punnett A, Tsang RW, Hodgson DC. Hodgkin lymphoma across the age spectrum: epidemiology, therapy, and late effects. Semin Radiat Oncol. 2010 Jan;20(1):30–44. PMID:19959029
5669. Pupulim LF, Vullierme MP, Paradis V, et al. Congenital portosystemic shunts associated with liver tumours. Clin Radiol. 2013 Jul;68(7):e362–9. PMID:23537576
5670. Puri A. Chondrosarcomas in children and adolescents. EFORT Open Rev. 2020 Feb 26;5(2):90–5. PMID:32175095
5671. Purnell CA, Skladman R, Alden TD, et al. Nasal dermoid cysts with intracranial extension: avoiding coronal incision through midline exposure and nasal bone osteotomy. J Neurosurg Pediatr. 2019 Dec 6:1–7. PMID:31812133
5672. Pushker N, Shrey D, Bajaj MS, et al. Malignant non-teratoid medulloepithelioma of the optic nerve with intraocular extension. Clin Exp Ophthalmol. 2010 Oct;38(7):731–3. PMID:20497433
5673. Pusztaszeri MP, Bongiovanni M, Faquin WC. Update on the cytologic and molecular features of medullary thyroid carcinoma. Adv Anat Pathol. 2014 Jan;21(1):26–35. PMID:24316908
5674. Putra J, Al-Ibraheemi A. Adipocytic tumors in Children: a contemporary review. Semin Diagn Pathol. 2019 Mar;36(2):95–104. PMID:30850231
5675. Pytel P, Taxy JB, Krausz T. Divergent differentiation in malignant soft tissue neoplasms: the paradigm of liposarcoma and malignant peripheral nerve sheath tumor. Int J Surg Pathol. 2005 Jan;13(1):19–28. PMID:15735851
5676. Qaddoumi I, Orisme W, Wen J, et al. Genetic alterations in uncommon low-grade neuroepithelial tumors: BRAF, FGFR1, and MYB mutations occur at high frequency and align with morphology. Acta Neuropathol. 2016 Jun;131(6):833–45. PMID:26810070
5677. Qi ST, Zhang H, Song Y, et al. Tumor cells forming sinusoids connected to vasculature are involved in hemorrhage of pineal choriocarcinoma. J Neurooncol. 2014 Aug;119(1):159–67. PMID:24847965
5678. Qiagen Bioinformatics. The Human Gene Mutation Database (HGMD) [Internet]. Hilden (Germany): Qiagen Bioinformatics; 2017. Available from: https://portal.biobase-international.com/.
5679. Qian M, Zhao X, Devidas M, et al. Genome-wide association study of susceptibility loci for T-cell acute lymphoblastic leukemia in children. J Natl Cancer Inst. 2019 Dec 1;111(12):1350–7. PMID:30938820
5680. Qian Q, You Y, Yang J, et al. Management and prognosis of patients with ovarian sex cord tumor with annular tubules: a retrospective study. BMC Cancer. 2015 Apr 12;15:270. PMID:25886261
5681. Qian X, Hornick JL, Cibas ES, et al. Angiomatoid fibrous histiocytoma a series of five cytologic cases with literature review and emphasis on diagnostic pitfalls. Diagn Cytopathol. 2012 Aug;40 Suppl 2:E86–93. PMID:22045622
5682. Qian ZJ, Jin MC, Meister KD, et al. Pediatric thyroid cancer incidence and mortality trends in the United States, 1973-2013. JAMA Otolaryngol Head Neck Surg. 2019 Jul 1;145(7):617–23. PMID:31120475
5683. Qin J, Wang Z, Hoogeveen-Westerveld M, et al. Structural basis of the interaction between tuberous sclerosis complex 1 (TSC1) and Tre2-Bub2-Cdc16 domain family member 7 (TBC1D7). J Biol Chem. 2016 Apr 15;291(16):8591–601. PMID:26893383
5684. Qin V, Verdijk RM, Paridaens D. Epibulbar osseous choristoma: a photo essay case report. Int Ophthalmol. 2019 May;39(5):1137–9. PMID:29589231
5685. Qing X, Qing A, Ji P, et al. Mixed phenotype (T/B/myeloid) extramedullary blast crisis as an initial presentation of chronic myelogenous leukemia. Exp Mol Pathol. 2018 Apr;104(2):130–3. PMID:29501750
5686. Qiu X, Montgomery E, Sun B. Inflammatory myofibroblastic tumor and low-grade myofibroblastic sarcoma: a comparative study of clinicopathologic features and further observations on the immunohistochemical profile of myofibroblasts. Hum Pathol. 2008 Jun;39(6):846–56. PMID:18400254
5687. Qualman S, Lynch J, Bridge J, et al. Prevalence and clinical impact of anaplasia in childhood rhabdomyosarcoma : a report from the Soft Tissue Sarcoma Committee of the Children's Oncology Group. Cancer. 2008 Dec 1;113(11):3242–7. PMID:18985676
5688. Quan VL, Panah E, Zhang B, et al. The role of gene fusions in melanocytic neoplasms. J Cutan Pathol. 2019 Nov;46(11):878–87. PMID:31152596
5689. Quan VL, Zhang B, Mohan LS, et al. Activating structural alterations in MAPK genes are distinct genetic drivers in a unique subgroup of Spitzoid neoplasms. Am J Surg Pathol. 2019 Apr;43(4):538–48. PMID:30640733
5690. Quan VL, Zhang B, Zhang Y, et al. Integrating next-generation sequencing with morphology improves prognostic and biologic classification of Spitz neoplasms. J Invest Dermatol. 2020 Aug;140(8):1599–608. PMID:32004563
5691. Quarello P, Bianchi M, Gambella A, et al. Pulmonary nodular lymphoid hyperplasia in pediatric patients with Hodgkin lymphoma. Pediatr Hematol Oncol. 2020 Aug;37(5):424–30. PMID:32131663
5692. Quarmyne MO, Gupta A, Adams DM. Lymphangiosarcoma of the thorax and thoracic vertebrae in a 16-year-old girl. J Clin Oncol. 2012 Oct 10;30(29):e294–8. PMID:22915659
5693. Qublan HS, Fayyad LM, Al-Ghoweri AS. Angiomyofibroblastoma of the vulva occurring in a teenaged girl. J Obstet Gynaecol. 2002 Sep;22(5):562–3. PMID:12521438
5694. Que SK, Weston G, Suchecki J, et al. Pigmentary disorders of the eyes and skin. Clin Dermatol. 2015 Mar-Apr;33(2):147–58. PMID:25704935
5695. Queisser A, Boon LM, Vikkula M. Etiology and genetics of congenital vascular lesions. Otolaryngol Clin North Am. 2018 Feb;51(1):41–53. PMID:29217067
5696. Quesada AE, Montalban-Bravo G, Luthra R, et al. Clinico-pathologic characteristics and outcomes of the World Health Organization (WHO) provisional entity de novo acute myeloid leukemia with mutated RUNX1. Mod Pathol. 2020 Sep;33(9):1678–89. PMID:32238878
5697. Quintanilla-Dieck L, Penn EB Jr. Congenital neck masses. Clin Perinatol. 2018 Dec;45(4):769–85. PMID:30396417
5698. Quintanilla-Martinez L, Fend F. Deciphering hydroa vacciniforme. Blood. 2019 Jun 27;133(26):2735–7. PMID:31248873
5699. Quintanilla-Martinez L, Kumar S, Fend F, et al. Fulminant EBV(+) T-cell lymphoproliferative disorder following acute/chronic EBV infection: a distinct clinicopathologic

syndrome. Blood. 2000 Jul 15;96(2):443–51. PMID:10887104
**5700.** Quintanilla-Martinez L, Ridaura C, Nagl F, et al. Hydroa vacciniforme-like lymphoma: a chronic EBV+ lymphoproliferative disorder with risk to develop a systemic lymphoma. Blood. 2013 Oct 31;122(18):3101–10. PMID:23982171
**5701.** Quintanilla-Martinez L, Sander B, Chan JK, et al. Indolent lymphomas in the pediatric population: follicular lymphoma, IRF4/MUM1+ lymphoma, nodal marginal zone lymphoma and chronic lymphocytic leukemia. Virchows Arch. 2016 Feb;468(2):141–57. PMID:26416032
**5702.** Quintini C, Kato T, Gaynor JJ, et al. Analysis of risk factors for the development of posttransplant lymphoprolipherative disorder among 119 children who received primary intestinal transplants at a single center. Transplant Proc. 2006 Jul-Aug;38(6):1755–8. PMID:16908272
**5703.** Qunaj L, Castillo JJ, Olszewski AJ. Survival of patients with CD20-negative variants of large B-cell lymphoma: an analysis of the National Cancer Data Base. Leuk Lymphoma. 2018 Jun;59(6):1375–83. PMID:29019447
**5704.** Qureshi SS, Bhagat M, Kurkure PA, et al. Ectopic Cushing syndrome secondary to recurrent pancreatoblastoma in a child: lessons learnt. J Cancer Res Ther. 2015 Oct-Dec;11(4):1027. PMID:26881602
**5705.** Raab SS, Silverman JF, McLeod DL, et al. Fine needle aspiration biopsy of fibromatoses. Acta Cytol. 1993 May-Jun;37(3):323–8. PMID:8498134
**5706.** Raabe EH, Laudenslager M, Winter C, et al. Prevalence and functional consequence of PHOX2B mutations in neuroblastoma. Oncogene. 2008 Jan 17;27(4):469–76. PMID:17637745
**5707.** Raafat F, Egan M. Benign cystic mesothelioma of the peritoneum: immunohistochemical and ultrastructural features in a child. Pediatr Pathol. 1988;8(3):321–9. PMID:3174512
**5708.** Rabban JT, Zaloudek CJ. A practical approach to immunohistochemical diagnosis of ovarian germ cell tumours and sex cord-stromal tumours. Histopathology. 2013 Jan;62(1):71–88. PMID:23240671
**5709.** Rabbie R, Rashid M, Arance AM, et al. Genomic analysis and clinical management of adolescent cutaneous melanoma. Pigment Cell Melanoma Res. 2017 May;30(3):307–16. PMID:28097802
**5710.** Racher H, Soliman S, Argiropoulos B, et al. Molecular analysis distinguishes metastatic disease from second cancers in patients with retinoblastoma. Cancer Genet. 2016 Jul-Aug;209(7-8):359–63. PMID:27318443
**5711.** Rachidi S, Sood AJ, Patel KG, et al. Melanotic neuroectodermal tumor of infancy: a systematic review. J Oral Maxillofac Surg. 2015 Oct;73(10):1946–56. PMID:25936939
**5712.** Raddaoui E, Donner LR, Panagopoulos I. Fusion of the FUS and ATF1 genes in a large, deep-seated angiomatoid fibrous histiocytoma. Diagn Mol Pathol. 2002 Sep;11(3):157–62. PMID:12218455
**5713.** Radich JP, Deininger M, Abboud CN, et al. Chronic myeloid leukemia, version 1.2019, NCCN clinical practice guidelines in oncology. J Natl Compr Canc Netw. 2018 Sep;16(9):1108–35. PMID:30181422
**5714.** Radivoyevitch T, Jankovic GM, Tiu RV, et al. Sex differences in the incidence of chronic myeloid leukemia. Radiat Environ Biophys. 2014 Mar;53(1):55–63. PMID:24337217
**5715.** Radkowski D, McGill T, Healy GB, et al. Angiofibroma. Changes in staging and treatment. Arch Otolaryngol Head Neck Surg. 1996 Feb;122(2):122–9. PMID:8630204
**5716.** Radu OM, Nikiforova MN, Farkas LM, et al. Challenging cases encountered in colorectal cancer screening for Lynch syndrome reveal novel findings: nucleolar MSH6 staining and impact of prior chemoradiation therapy. Hum Pathol. 2011 Sep;42(9):1247–58. PMID:21334712
**5717.** Raffaele A, Goruppi I, Mosconi M, et al. Juxta-articular myxoma of the hip: a rare pediatric tumor. J Am Acad Orthop Surg Glob Res Rev. 2019 Nov 12;3(11):e070. PMID:31875202
**5718.** Raffeld M, Abdullaev Z, Pack SD, et al. High level MYCN amplification and distinct methylation signature define an aggressive subtype of spinal cord ependymoma. Acta Neuropathol Commun. 2020 Jul 8;8(1):101. PMID:32641156
**5719.** Rafique MZ, Ahmad MN, Yaqoob N, et al. Diffuse bilateral thalamic astrocytoma. J Coll Physicians Surg Pak. 2007 Mar;17(3):170–2. PMID:17374306
**5720.** Ragazzini R, Pérez-Palacios R, Baymaz IH, et al. EZHIP constrains Polycomb Repressive Complex 2 activity in germ cells. Nat Commun. 2019 Aug 26;10(1):3858. PMID:31451685
**5721.** Ragel BT, Couldwell WT. Pituitary carcinoma: a review of the literature. Neurosurg Focus. 2004 Apr 15;16(4):E7. PMID:15191336
**5722.** Ragge NK, Acheson J, Murphree AL. Iris mammillations: significance and associations. Eye (Lond). 1996;10(Pt 1):86–91. PMID:8763309
**5723.** Raggi F, Russo D, Urbani C, et al. Divergent effects of dioxin- or non-dioxin-like polychlorinated biphenyls on the apoptosis of primary cell culture from the mouse pituitary gland. PLoS One. 2016 Jan 11;11(1):e0146729. PMID:26752525
**5724.** Raggio M, Kaplan AL, Harberg JF. Recurrent ovarian fibromas with basal cell nevus syndrome (Gorlin syndrome). Obstet Gynecol. 1983 Mar;61(3 Suppl):95S–6S. PMID:6823402
**5725.** Raghavan R, Dickey WT Jr, Margraf LR, et al. Proliferative activity in craniopharyngiomas: clinicopathological correlations in adults and children. Surg Neurol. 2000 Sep;54(3):241–7. PMID:11118571
**5726.** Raghunathan A, Olar A, Vogel H, et al. Isocitrate dehydrogenase 1 R132H mutation is not detected in angiocentric glioma. Ann Diagn Pathol. 2012 Aug;16(4):255–9. PMID:22445362
**5727.** Rahbar R, Grimmer JF, Vargas SO, et al. Mucoepidermoid carcinoma of the parotid gland in children: a 10-year experience. Arch Otolaryngol Head Neck Surg. 2006 Apr;132(4):375–80. PMID:16618905
**5728.** Rahbar R, Shah P, Mulliken JB, et al. The presentation and management of nasal dermoid: a 30-year experience. Arch Otolaryngol Head Neck Surg. 2003 Apr;129(4):464–71. PMID:12707196
**5729.** Rahemtullah A, Reichard KK, Preffer FI, et al. A double-positive CD4+CD8+ T-cell population is commonly found in nodular lymphocyte predominant Hodgkin lymphoma. Am J Clin Pathol. 2006 Nov;126(5):805–14. PMID:17050078
**5730.** Rai K, Pilarski R, Cebulla CM, et al. Comprehensive review of BAP1 tumor predisposition syndrome with report of two new cases. Clin Genet. 2016 Mar;89(3):285–94. PMID:26096145
**5731.** Raisanen J, Biegel JA, Hatanpaa KJ, et al. Chromosome 22q deletions in atypical teratoid/rhabdoid tumors in adults. Brain Pathol. 2005 Jan;15(1):23–8. PMID:15779233
**5732.** Raissaki MT, Segkos N, Prokopakis EP, et al. Congenital granular cell tumor (epulis): postnatal imaging appearances. J Comput Assist Tomogr. 2005 Jul-Aug;29(4):520–3. PMID:16012311
**5733.** Rajan PB, Cranor ML, Rosen PP. Cystosarcoma phyllodes in adolescent girls and young women: a study of 45 patients. Am J Surg Pathol. 1998 Jan;22(1):64–9. PMID:9422317
**5734.** Rajaram V, Knezevich S, Bove KE, et al. DNA sequence of the translocation breakpoints in undifferentiated embryonal sarcoma arising in mesenchymal hamartoma of the liver harboring the t(11;19)(q11;q13.4) translocation. Genes Chromosomes Cancer. 2007 May;46(5):508–13. PMID:17311249
**5735.** Rajpert-De Meyts E, Bartkova J, Samson M, et al. The emerging phenotype of the testicular carcinoma in situ germ cell. APMIS. 2003 Jan;111(1):267–78. PMID:12752272
**5736.** Rajpert-De Meyts E, Hanstein R, Jørgensen N, et al. Developmental expression of POU5F1 (OCT-3/4) in normal and dysgenetic human gonads. Hum Reprod. 2004 Jun;19(6):1338–44. PMID:15105401
**5737.** Rajpert-De Meyts E, McGlynn KA, Okamoto K, et al. Testicular germ cell tumours. Lancet. 2016 Apr 23;387(10029):1762–74. PMID:26651223
**5738.** Rajpert-De Meyts E. Developmental model for the pathogenesis of testicular carcinoma in situ: genetic and environmental aspects. Hum Reprod Update. 2006 May-Jun;12(3):303–23. PMID:16540528
**5739.** Rajpert-De Meyts E, Kvist M, Skakkebaek NE. Heterogeneity of expression of immunohistochemical tumour markers in testicular carcinoma in situ: pathogenetic relevance. Virchows Arch. 1996 Jun;428(3):133–9. PMID:8688967
**5740.** Rajpert-De Meyts E, Skakkebaek NE. Expression of the c-kit protein product in carcinoma-in-situ and invasive testicular germ cell tumours. Int J Androl. 1994 Apr;17(2):85–92. PMID:7517917
**5741.** Rajpert-De Meyts E, Skotheim RI. Complex polygenic nature of testicular germ cell cancer suggests multifactorial aetiology. Eur Urol. 2018 Jun;73(6):832–3. PMID:29530636
**5742.** Rajput DK, Mehrotra A, Srivastav AK, et al. Bilateral thalamic glioma in a 6-year-old child. J Pediatr Neurosci. 2010 Jan;5(1):45–8. PMID:21042509
**5743.** Raju GP, Urion DK, Sahin M. Neonatal subependymal giant cell astrocytoma: new case and review of literature. Pediatr Neurol. 2007 Feb;36(2):128–31. PMID:17275668
**5744.** Rakheja D, Lian F, Tomlinson GE, et al. Renal metanephric adenoma with previously unreported cytogenetic abnormalities: case report and review of the literature. Pediatr Dev Pathol. 2005 Mar-Apr;8(2):218–23. PMID:15747102
**5745.** Rakheja D, Margraf LR, Tomlinson GE, et al. Hepatic mesenchymal hamartoma with translocation involving chromosome band 19q13.4: a recurrent abnormality. Cancer Genet Cytogenet. 2004 Aug;153(1):60–3. PMID:15325096
**5746.** Ralte AM, Rao S, Sharma MC, et al. Myxopapillary ependymoma of the temporal lobe–report of a rare case of temporal lobe epilepsy. Clin Neuropathol. 2004 Mar-Apr;23(2):53–8. PMID:15074578
**5747.** Ramachandra S, Hollowood K, Bisceglia M, et al. Inflammatory pseudotumour of soft tissues: a clinicopathological and immunohistochemical analysis of 18 cases. Histopathology. 1995 Oct;27(4):313–23. PMID:8847061
**5748.** Ramamoorthy SK, Noutsos T, Wei D, et al. Recurrent and refractory hemophagocytic lymphohistiocytosis in an elderly. Role of immune aberration due to myeloid gene mutation. Blood. 2020 Nov 5;136(Suppl 1):24–6. doi:10.1182/blood-2020-133776.
**5749.** Ramani P, Cowell JK. The expression pattern of Wilms' tumour gene (WT1) product in normal tissues and paediatric renal tumours. J Pathol. 1996 Jun;179(2):162–8. PMID:8758208
**5750.** Ramanujam TM, Ramesh JC, Goh DW, et al. Malignant transformation of mesenchymal hamartoma of the liver: case report and review of the literature. J Pediatr Surg. 1999 Nov;34(11):1684–6. PMID:10591570
**5751.** Ramaswamy PV, Storm CA, Filiano JJ, et al. Multiple granular cell tumors in a child with Noonan syndrome. Pediatr Dermatol. 2010 Mar-Apr;27(2):209–11. PMID:20537083
**5752.** Ramaswamy V, Delaney H, Haque S, et al. Spectrum of central nervous system abnormalities in neurocutaneous melanocytosis. Dev Med Child Neurol. 2012 Jun;54(6):563–8. PMID:22469364
**5753.** Ramaswamy V, Hielscher T, Mack SC, et al. Therapeutic impact of cytoreductive surgery and irradiation of posterior fossa ependymoma in the molecular era: a retrospective multicohort analysis. J Clin Oncol. 2016 Jul 20;34(21):2468–77. PMID:27269943
**5754.** Ramaswamy V, Nör C, Taylor MD. p53 and Meduloblastoma. Cold Spring Harb Perspect Med. 2015 Dec 18;6(2):a026278. PMID:26684332
**5755.** Ramaswamy V, Remke M, Bouffet E, et al. Recurrence patterns across medulloblastoma subgroups: an integrated clinical and molecular analysis. Lancet Oncol. 2013 Nov;14(12):1200–7. PMID:24140199
**5756.** Ramaswamy V, Remke M, Bouffet E, et al. Risk stratification of childhood medulloblastoma in the molecular era: the current consensus. Acta Neuropathol. 2016 Jun;131(6):821–31. PMID:27040285
**5757.** Rambaldi A, Terao M, Bettoni S, et al. Differences in the expression of alkaline phosphatase mRNA in chronic myelogenous leukemia and paroxysmal nocturnal hemoglobinuria polymorphonuclear leukocytes. Blood. 1989 Apr;73(5):1113–5. PMID:2930836
**5758.** Ramdial PK, Sing Y, Deonarain J, et al. Extra-uterine myoid tumours in patients with acquired immunodeficiency syndrome: a clinicopathological reappraisal. Histopathology. 2011 Dec;59(6):1122–34. PMID:22175892
**5759.** Ramis-Zaldivar JE, Gonzalez-Farré B, Balagué O, et al. Distinct molecular profile of IRF4-rearranged large B-cell lymphoma. Blood. 2020 Jan 23;135(4):274–86. PMID:31738823
**5760.** Ramkissoon LA, Horowitz PM, Craig JM, et al. Genomic analysis of diffuse pediatric low-grade gliomas identifies recurrent oncogenic truncating rearrangements in the transcription factor MYBL1. Proc Natl Acad Sci U S A. 2013 May 14;110(20):8188–93. PMID:23633565
**5761.** Ramkumar HL, Brooks BP, Cao X, et al. Ophthalmic manifestations and histopathology of xeroderma pigmentosum: two clinicopathological cases and a review of the literature. Surv Ophthalmol. 2011 Jul-Aug;56(4):348–61. PMID:21684361
**5762.** Ramos E, Hernández F, Andres A, et al. Post-transplant lymphoproliferative disorders and other malignancies after pediatric intestinal transplantation: incidence, clinical features and outcome. Pediatr Transplant. 2013 Aug;17(5):472–8. PMID:23730927
**5763.** Ramos P, Karnezis AN, Craig DW, et al. Small cell carcinoma of the ovary, hypercalcemic type, displays frequent inactivating germline and somatic mutations in SMARCA4. Nat Genet. 2014 May;46(5):427–9. PMID:24658001
**5764.** Ramos P, Karnezis AN, Hendricks WP, et al. Loss of the tumor suppressor SMARCA4 in small cell carcinoma of the ovary, hypercalcemic type (SCCOHT). Rare Dis. 2014 Nov 3;2(1):e967148. PMID:26942101
**5765.** Ramphul K, Kota V, Mejias SG. Child syndrome. 2022 Jun 27. In: StatPearls. Treasure Island (FL): StatPearls Publishing; 2022 Jan–. PMID:29939590

5766. Rampp RD, Mancilla EE, Adzick NS, et al. Single gland, ectopic location: adenomas are common causes of primary hyperparathyroidism in children and adolescents. World J Surg. 2020 May;44(5):1518–25. PMID:31900569
5767. Randall BJ, Ritchie C, Hutchison RS. Paget's disease and invasive undifferentiated carcinoma occurring in a mature cystic teratoma of the ovary. Histopathology. 1991 May;18(5):469–70. PMID:1653182
5768. Raney RB, Meza J, Anderson JR, et al. Treatment of children and adolescents with localized parameningeal sarcoma: experience of the Intergroup Rhabdomyosarcoma Study Group protocols IRS-II through -IV, 1978-1997. Med Pediatr Oncol. 2002 Jan;38(1):22–32. PMID:11835233
5769. Ranga SM, Kuchangi NC, Shankar VS, et al. Retiform hemangioendothelioma: an uncommon pediatric vascular neoplasm. Indian J Dermatol. 2014 Nov;59(6):633. PMID:25484427
5770. Ranganathan S, Ningappa M, Ashokkumar C, et al. Loss of EGFR-ASAP1 signaling in metastatic and unresectable hepatoblastoma. Sci Rep. 2016 Dec 2;6:38347. PMID:27910913
5771. Rangel-Pozzo A, Sisdelli L, Cordioli MIV, et al. Genetic landscape of papillary thyroid carcinoma and nuclear architecture: an overview comparing pediatric and adult populations. Cancers (Basel). 2020 Oct 27;12(11):E3146. PMID:33120984
5772. Ranjan P, Naresh KN. CD30 expression in L&H cells of Hodgkin's disease, nodular lymphocyte predominant type. Histopathology. 2003 Apr;42(4):406–7. PMID:12653955
5773. Rao P, Tannir NM, Tamboli P. Expression of OCT3/4 in renal medullary carcinoma represents a potential diagnostic pitfall. Am J Surg Pathol. 2012 Apr;36(4):583–8. PMID:22301499
5774. Rao Q, Liu B, Cheng L, et al. Renal cell carcinomas with t(6;11)(p21;q12): a clinicopathologic study emphasizing unusual morphology, novel alpha-TFEB gene fusion point, immunobiomarkers, and ultrastructural features, as well as detection of the gene fusion by fluorescence in situ hybridization. Am J Surg Pathol. 2012 Sep;36(9):1327–38. PMID:22895266
5775. Rao Q, Shen Q, Xia QY, et al. PSF/SFPQ is a very common gene fusion partner in TFE3 rearrangement-associated perivascular epithelioid cell tumors (PEComas) and melanotic Xp11 translocation renal cancers: clinicopathologic, immunohistochemical, and molecular characteristics suggesting classification as a distinct entity. Am J Surg Pathol. 2015 Sep;39(9):1181–96. PMID:26274027
5776. Rao S, Yao Y, Soares de Brito J, et al. Dissecting ELANE neutropenia pathogenicity by human HSC gene editing. Cell Stem Cell. 2021 May 6;28(5):833–845.e5. PMID:33513358
5777. Rao SN, Bernet V. Indeterminate thyroid nodules in the era of molecular genomics. Mol Genet Genomic Med. 2020 Sep;8(9):e1288. PMID:32436637
5778. Rapisarda AMC, Cianci A, Caruso S, et al. Benign multicystic mesothelioma and peritoneal inclusion cysts: Are they the same clinical and histopathological entities? A systematic review to find an evidence-based management. Arch Gynecol Obstet. 2018 Jun;297(6):1353–75. PMID:29511797
5779. Rapkiewicz A, Wen H, Sen F, et al. Cytomorphologic examination of anaplastic large cell lymphoma by fine-needle aspiration cytology. Cancer. 2007 Dec 25;111(6):499–507. PMID:17941004
5780. Rapley EA, Turnbull C, Al Olama AA, et al. A genome-wide association study of testicular germ cell tumor. Nat Genet. 2009 Jul;41(7):807–10. PMID:19483681
5781. Rasche M, Zimmermann M, Borschel L, et al. Successes and challenges in the treatment of pediatric acute myeloid leukemia: a retrospective analysis of the AML-BFM trials from 1987 to 2012. Leukemia. 2018 Oct;32(10):2167–77. PMID:29550834
5782. Rashad MN, Fathalla MF, Kerr MG. Sex chromatin and chromosome analysis in ovarian teratomas. Am J Obstet Gynecol. 1966 Oct 15;96(4):461–5. PMID:5921072
5783. Rashid T, Bagatell R, Pawel B, et al. More than meets the eye? A cautionary tale of malignant ectomesenchymoma treated as low-risk orbital rhabdomyosarcoma. J Pediatr Hematol Oncol. 2021 Aug 1;43(6):e854–8. PMID:32769567
5784. Rasmussen SA, Yang Q, Friedman JM. Mortality in neurofibromatosis 1: an analysis using U.S. death certificates. Am J Hum Genet. 2001 May;68(5):1110–8. PMID:11283797
5785. Rassael H, Thompson LD, Heffess CS. A rationale for conservative management of microscopic papillary carcinoma of the thyroid gland: a clinicopathologic correlation of 90 cases. Eur Arch Otorhinolaryngol. 1998;255(9):462–7. PMID:9833215
5786. Rasul FT, Jaunmuktane Z, Khan AA, et al. Plurihormonal pituitary adenoma with concomitant adrenocorticotropic hormone (ACTH) and growth hormone (GH) secretion: a report of two cases and review of the literature. Acta Neurochir (Wien). 2014 Jan;156(1):141–6. PMID:24081787
5787. Rault-Petit B, Do Cao C, Guyétant S, et al. Current management and predictive factors of lymph node metastasis of appendix neuroendocrine tumors: a national study from the French Group of Endocrine Tumors (GTE). Ann Surg. 2019 Jul;270(1):165–71. PMID:29557879
5788. Rausch T, Jones DT, Zapatka M, et al. Genome sequencing of pediatric medulloblastoma links catastrophic DNA rearrangements with TP53 mutations. Cell. 2012 Jan 20;148(1-2):59–71. PMID:22265402
5789. Ravanpay AC, Barkley A, White-Dzuro GA, et al. Giant pediatric rhabdoid meningioma associated with a germline BAP1 pathogenic variation: a rare clinical case. World Neurosurg. 2018 Nov;119:402–15. PMID:29981911
5790. Ravell JC, Matsuda-Lennikov M, Chauvin SD, et al. Defective glycosylation and multisystem abnormalities characterize the primary immunodeficiency XMEN disease. J Clin Invest. 2020 Jan 2;130(1):507–22. PMID:31714901
5791. Raverot G, Burman P, McCormack A, et al. European Society of Endocrinology Clinical Practice Guidelines for the management of aggressive pituitary tumours and carcinomas. Eur J Endocrinol. 2018 Jan;178(1):G1–24. PMID:29046323
5792. Raverot G, Castinetti F, Jouanneau E, et al. Pituitary carcinomas and aggressive pituitary tumours: merits and pitfalls of temozolomide treatment. Clin Endocrinol (Oxf). 2012 Jun;76(6):769–75. PMID:22404748
5793. Raverot G, Wierinckx A, Jouanneau E, et al. Clinical, hormonal and molecular characterization of pituitary ACTH adenomas without (silent corticotroph adenomas) and with Cushing's disease. Eur J Endocrinol. 2010 Jul;163(1):35–43. PMID:20385723
5794. Ray S, Jones R, Pritchard-Jones K, et al. Pediatric and young adult renal cell carcinoma. Pediatr Blood Cancer. 2020 Nov;67(11):e28675. PMID:32869954
5795. Ray WZ, Blackburn SL, Casavilca-Zambrano S, et al. Clinicopathologic features of recurrent dysembryoplastic neuroepithelial tumor and rare malignant transformation: a report of 5 cases and review of the literature. J Neurooncol. 2009 Sep;94(2):283–92. PMID:19267228
5796. Raymond AA, Halpin SF, Alsanjari N, et al. Dysembryoplastic neuroepithelial tumor. Features in 16 patients. Brain. 1994 Jun;117(Pt 3):461–75. PMID:8032857
5797. Raza A, Cao H, Conrad R, et al. Nuclear protein in testis midline carcinoma with unusual elevation of α-fetoprotein and synaptophysin positivity: a case report and review of the literature. Expert Rev Anticancer Ther. 2015;15(10):1199–213. PMID:26402248
5798. Raza A, Kailash K, Malviya A. Rare cause of hip pain in a young girl. BMJ Case Rep. 2014 May 9;2014:bcr2014203802. PMID:24813200
5799. Razmpoosh M, Sansregret A, Oligny LL, et al. Assessment of correlation between p16INK4a staining, specific subtype of human papillomavirus, and progression of LSIL/CIN1 lesions: first comparative study. Am J Clin Pathol. 2014 Jul;142(1):104–10. PMID:24926093
5800. Reck-Burneo CA, Villanueva J, Velcek FT. Vaginal müllerian papilloma: an unusual cause of vaginal bleeding in a toddler. J Pediatr Adolesc Gynecol. 2009 Oct;22(5):e124–6. PMID:19616458
5801. Recondo G Jr, Busaidy N, Erasmus J, et al. Spindle epithelial tumor with thymus-like differentiation: a case report and comprehensive review of the literature and treatment options. Head Neck. 2015 May;37(5):746–54. PMID:24677409
5802. Redaelli A, Laskin BL, Stephens JM, et al. A systematic literature review of the clinical and epidemiological burden of acute lymphoblastic leukaemia (ALL). Eur J Cancer Care (Engl). 2005 Mar;14(1):53–62. PMID:15698386
5803. Reddy AT, Strother DR, Judkins AR, et al. Efficacy of high-dose chemotherapy and three-dimensional conformal radiation for atypical teratoid/rhabdoid tumor: a report from the Children's Oncology Group trial ACNS0333. J Clin Oncol. 2020 Apr 10;38(11):1175–85. PMID:32105509
5804. Reddy HS, Keene CD, Chang SH, et al. Immunohistochemical profiling including beta-catenin in conjunctival melanocytic lesions. Exp Mol Pathol. 2017 Apr;102(2):198–202. PMID:28161440
5805. Reddy N, Malipatil B, Kumar S. A rare case of familial multiple subcutaneous lipomatosis with novel PALB2 mutation and increased predilection to cancers. Hematol Oncol Stem Cell Ther. 2016 Dec;9(4):154–6. PMID:26845227
5806. Redmond LS, Ogwang MD, Kerchan P, et al. Endemic Burkitt lymphoma: a complication of asymptomatic malaria in sub-Saharan Africa based on published literature and primary data from Uganda, Tanzania, and Kenya. Malar J. 2020 Jul 28;19(1):239. PMID:32718346
5807. Rednam SP, Erez A, Druker H, et al. Von Hippel-Lindau and hereditary pheochromocytoma/paraganglioma syndromes: clinical features, genetics, and surveillance recommendations in childhood. Clin Cancer Res. 2017 Jun 15;23(12):e68–75. PMID:28620007
5808. Reed RC, Beischel L, Schoof J, et al. Androgenetic/biparental mosaicism in an infant with hepatic mesenchymal hamartoma and placental mesenchymal dysplasia. Pediatr Dev Pathol. 2008 Sep-Oct;11(5):377–83. PMID:18260692
5809. Reed RJ, Fine RM, Meltzer HD. Palisaded, encapsulated neuromas of the skin. Arch Dermatol. 1972 Dec;106(6):865–70. PMID:4639250
5810. Reed RJ, Ichinose H, Clark WH Jr, et al. Common and uncommon melanocytic nevi and borderline melanomas. Semin Oncol. 1975 Jun;2(2):119–47. PMID:1234372
5811. Reese TS. The molecular basis of axonal transport in the squid giant axon. Res Publ Assoc Res Nerv Ment Dis. 1987;65:89–102. PMID:2455314
5812. Reeves WC, Ruparelia SS, Swanson KI, et al. National registry for juvenile-onset recurrent respiratory papillomatosis. Arch Otolaryngol Head Neck Surg. 2003 Sep;129(9):976–82. PMID:12975271
5813. Regairaz M, Munier F, Sartelet H, et al. Mutation-independent activation of the anaplastic lymphoma kinase in neuroblastoma. Am J Pathol. 2016 Feb;186(2):435–45. PMID:26687816
5814. Regalbuto C, Malandrino P, Tumminia A, et al. A diffuse sclerosing variant of papillary thyroid carcinoma: clinical and pathologic features and outcomes of 34 consecutive cases. Thyroid. 2011 Apr;21(4):383–9. PMID:21309722
5815. Reichard KK, McKenna RW, Kroft SH. ALK-positive diffuse large B-cell lymphoma: report of four cases and review of the literature. Mod Pathol. 2007 Mar;20(3):310–9. PMID:17277765
5816. Reichart PA, Philipsen HP, Sonner S. Ameloblastoma: biological profile of 3677 cases. Eur J Cancer B Oral Oncol. 1995 Mar;31B(2):86–99. PMID:7633291
5817. Reid AG, De Melo VA, Elderfield K, et al. Phenotype of blasts in chronic myeloid leukemia in blastic phase-Analysis of bone marrow trephine biopsies and correlation with cytogenetics. Leuk Res. 2009 Mar;33(3):418–25. PMID:18760473
5818. Reid R, de Silva MV, Paterson L, et al. Low-grade fibromyxoid sarcoma and hyalinizing spindle cell tumor with giant rosettes share a common t(7;16)(q34;p11) translocation. Am J Surg Pathol. 2003 Sep;27(9):1229–36. PMID:12960807
5819. Reifenberger G, Kaulich K, Wiestler OD, et al. Expression of the CD34 antigen in pleomorphic xanthoastrocytomas. Acta Neuropathol. 2003 Apr;105(4):358–64. PMID:12624789
5820. Reijnders CM, Waaijer CJ, Hamilton A, et al. No haploinsufficiency but loss of heterozygosity for EXT in multiple osteochondromas. Am J Pathol. 2010 Oct;177(4):1946–57. PMID:20813973
5821. Reilly KM, Kim A, Blakely J, et al. Neurofibromatosis type 1-associated MPNST state of the science: outlining a research agenda for the future. J Natl Cancer Inst. 2017 Aug 1;109(8):djx124. PMID:29117388
5822. Reiman A, Srinivasan V, Barone G, et al. Lymphoid tumours and breast cancer in ataxia telangiectasia; substantial protective effect of residual ATM kinase activity against childhood tumours. Br J Cancer. 2011 Aug 9;105(4):586–91. PMID:21792198
5823. Reimann JD, Fletcher CD. Myxoid dermatofibrosarcoma protuberans: a rare variant analyzed in a series of 23 cases. Am J Surg Pathol. 2007 Sep;31(9):1371–7. PMID:17721193
5824. Reincke M, Sbiera S, Hayakawa A, et al. Mutations in the deubiquitinase gene USP8 cause Cushing's disease. Nat Genet. 2015 Jan;47(1):31–8. PMID:25485838
5825. Reinhardt A, Stichel D, Schrimpf D, et al. Anaplastic astrocytoma with piloid features, a novel molecular class of IDH wildtype glioma with recurrent MAPK pathway, CDKN2A/B and ATRX alterations. Acta Neuropathol. 2018 Aug;136(2):273–91. PMID:29564591
5826. Reinhardt A, Stichel D, Schrimpf D, et al. Tumors diagnosed as cerebellar glioblastoma comprise distinct molecular entities. Acta Neuropathol Commun. 2019 Oct 28;7(1):163. PMID:31661039
5827. Reis F, Faria AV, Zanardi VA, et al. Neuroimaging in pineal tumors. J Neuroimaging. 2006 Jan;16(1):52–8. PMID:16483277

5828. Reiseter T, Nordshus T, Borthne A, et al. Lipoblastoma: MRI appearances of a rare paediatric soft tissue tumour. Pediatr Radiol. 1999 Jul;29(7):542–5. PMID:10398794
5829. Reitamo JJ, Häyry P, Nykyri E, et al. The desmoid tumor. I. Incidence, sex-, age- and anatomical distribution in the Finnish population. Am J Clin Pathol. 1982 Jun;77(6):665–73. PMID:7091046
5830. Rejnmark L, Vestergaard P, Mosekilde L. Nephrolithiasis and renal calcifications in primary hyperparathyroidism. J Clin Endocrinol Metab. 2011 Aug;96(8):2377–85. PMID:21646371
5831. Rekhi B, Adamane S, Ghodke K, et al. Angiomatoid fibrous histiocytoma: clinicopathological spectrum of five cases, including EWSR1-CREB1 positive result in a single case. Indian J Pathol Microbiol. 2016 Apr-Jun;59(2):148–52. PMID:27166030
5832. Rekhi B, Deshmukh M, Jambhekar NA. Low-grade fibromyxoid sarcoma: a clinicopathologic study of 18 cases, including histopathologic relationship with sclerosing epithelioid fibrosarcoma in a subset of cases. Ann Diagn Pathol. 2011 Oct;15(5):303–11. PMID:21550274
5833. Rekhi B, Shetty O, Vora T, et al. Clinicopathologic, immunohistochemical, molecular cytogenetic profile with treatment and outcomes of 34 cases of Ewing sarcoma with epithelial differentiation, including 6 cases with "Adamantinoma-like" features, diagnosed at a single institution, India. Ann Diagn Pathol. 2020 Dec;49:151625. PMID:32932018
5834. Remacha L, Comino-Méndez I, Richter S, et al. Targeted exome sequencing of Krebs cycle genes reveals candidate cancer-predisposing mutations in pheochromocytomas and paragangliomas. Clin Cancer Res. 2017 Oct 15;23(20):6315–24. PMID:28720665
5835. Remacha L, Currás-Freixes M, Torres-Ruiz R, et al. Gain-of-function mutations in DNMT3A in patients with paraganglioma. Genet Med. 2018 Dec;20(12):1644–51. PMID:29740169
5836. Remacha L, Pirman D, Mahoney CE, et al. Recurrent Germline DLST Mutations in Individuals with Multiple Pheochromocytomas and Paragangliomas. Am J Hum Genet. 2019 Apr 4;104(4):651–64. PMID:30929736
5837. Reman O, Reznik Y, Casadevall N, et al. Polycythemia and steroid overproduction in a gonadotropin-secreting seminoma of the testis. Cancer. 1991 Nov 15;68(10):2224–9. PMID:1913460
5838. Remke M, Hielscher T, Northcott PA, et al. Adult medulloblastoma comprises three major molecular variants. J Clin Oncol. 2011 Jul 1;29(19):2717–23. PMID:21632505
5839. Remke M, Ramaswamy V, Peacock J, et al. TERT promoter mutations are highly recurrent in SHH subgroup medulloblastoma. Acta Neuropathol. 2013 Dec;126(6):917–29. PMID:24174164
5840. Remstein ED, Arndt CA, Nascimento AG. Plexiform fibrohistiocytic tumor: clinicopathologic analysis of 22 cases. Am J Surg Pathol. 1999 Jun;23(6):662–70. PMID:10366148
5841. Ren Q, Chen H, Wang Y, et al. Melanotic neuroectodermal tumor of infancy arising in the skull and brain: a systematic review. World Neurosurg. 2019 Oct;130:170–8. PMID:31295620
5842. Renaux-Petel M, Charbonnier F, Théry JC, et al. Contribution of de novo and mosaic TP53 mutations to Li-Fraumeni syndrome. J Med Genet. 2018 Mar;55(3):173–80. PMID:29070607
5843. Renehan A, Gleave EN, Hancock BD, et al. Long-term follow-up of over 1000 patients with salivary gland tumours treated in a single centre. Br J Surg. 1996 Dec;83(12):1750–4. PMID:9038559
5844. Renehan A, Gleave EN, McGurk M. An analysis of the treatment of 114 patients with recurrent pleomorphic adenomas of the parotid gland. Am J Surg. 1996 Dec;172(6):710–4. PMID:8988685
5845. Renshaw AA, Freyer DR, Hammers YA. Metastatic metanephric adenoma in a child. Am J Surg Pathol. 2000 Apr;24(4):570–4. PMID:10757405
5846. Repo P, Järvinen RS, Jäntti JE, et al. Population-based analysis of BAP1 germline variations in patients with uveal melanoma. Hum Mol Genet. 2019 Jul 15;28(14):2415–26. PMID:31058963
5847. Requena C, Requena L, Kutzner H, et al. Spitz nevus: a clinicopathological study of 349 cases. Am J Dermatopathol. 2009 Apr;31(2):107–16. PMID:19318795
5848. Requena C, Requena L, Sánchez-Yus E, et al. Hypopigmented Reed nevus. J Cutan Pathol. 2008 Oct;35 Suppl 1:87–9. PMID:18547345
5849. Requena L, Sanchez Yus E. Pigmented spindle cell naevus. Br J Dermatol. 1990 Dec;123(6):757–63. PMID:2265091
5850. Rescorla FJ, Breitfeld PP. Pediatric germ cell tumors. Curr Probl Cancer. 1999 Nov-Dec;23(6):257–303. PMID:10614561
5851. Rescorla FJ, Sawin RS, Coran AG, et al. Long-term outcome for infants and children with sacrococcygeal teratoma: a report from the Childrens Cancer Group. J Pediatr Surg. 1998 Feb;33(2):171–6. PMID:9498381
5852. Reuschenbach M, Kloor M, Morak M, et al. Serum antibodies against frameshift peptides in microsatellite unstable colorectal cancer patients with Lynch syndrome. Fam Cancer. 2010 Jun;9(2):173–9. PMID:19957108
5853. Revencu N, Boon LM, Mendola A, et al. RASA1 mutations and associated phenotypes in 68 families with capillary malformation-arteriovenous malformation. Hum Mutat. 2013 Dec;34(12):1632–41. PMID:24038909
5854. Revencu N, Fastre E, Ravoet M, et al. RASA1 mosaic mutations in patients with capillary malformation-arteriovenous malformation. J Med Genet. 2020 Jan;57(1):48–52. PMID:31300548
5855. Reye RD. Recurring digital fibrous tumors of childhood. Arch Pathol. 1965 Sep;80:228–31. PMID:14322942
5856. Reyes A, Moran CA, Suster S, et al. Neuroendocrine carcinomas (carcinoid tumor) of the testis. A clinicopathologic and immunohistochemical study of ten cases. Am J Clin Pathol. 2003 Aug;120(2):182–7. PMID:12931547
5857. Reyes-Múgica M, Arnsmeier SL, Backeljauw PF, et al. Phosphaturic mesenchymal tumor-induced rickets. Pediatr Dev Pathol. 2000 Jan-Feb;3(1):61–9. PMID:10594133
5858. Reyes-Mugica M, Chou P, Byrd S, et al. Nevomelanocytic proliferations in the central nervous system of children. Cancer. 1993 Oct 1;72(7):2277–85. PMID:8374887
5859. Reyes-Mugica M, Gonzalez-Crussi F, Bauer BS, et al. Bulky naevocytoma of the perineum: a singular variant of congenital giant pigmented naevus. Virchows Arch A Pathol Anat Histopathol. 1992;420(1):87–93. PMID:1539454
5860. Rezk SA, Weiss LM. EBV-associated lymphoproliferative disorders: update in classification. Surg Pathol Clin. 2019 Sep;12(3):745–70. PMID:31352986
5861. Rhiew RB, Manjila S, Lozen A, et al. Leptomeningeal dissemination of a pediatric neoplasm with 1p19q deletion showing mixed immunohistochemical features of an oligodendroglioma and neurocytoma. Acta Neurochir (Wien). 2010 Aug;152(8):1425–9. PMID:20446099
5862. Riad H, Mansour K, Sada HA, et al. Fatal metastatic cutaneous squamous cell carcinoma evolving from a localized verrucous epidermal nevus. Case Rep Dermatol. 2013 Oct 5;5(3):272–82. PMID:24403890
5863. Rialon KL, Murillo R, Fevurly RD, et al. Impact of screening for hepatic hemangiomas in patients with multiple cutaneous infantile hemangiomas. Pediatr Dermatol. 2015 Nov-Dec;32(6):808–12. PMID:26223454
5864. Rialon KL, Murillo R, Fevurly RD, et al. Risk factors for mortality in patients with multifocal and diffuse hepatic hemangiomas. J Pediatr Surg. 2015 May;50(5):837–41. PMID:25783331
5865. Riaz IB, Faridi W, Patnaik MM, et al. A systematic review on predisposition to lymphoid (B and T cell) neoplasias in patients with primary immunodeficiencies and immune dysregulatory disorders (inborn errors of immunity). Front Immunol. 2019 Apr 16;10:777. PMID:31057537
5866. Ribé A, McNutt NS. S100A6 protein expression is different in Spitz nevi and melanomas. Mod Pathol. 2003 May;16(5):505–11. PMID:12748257
5867. Ribeiro KdeC, Kowalski LP, Saba LM, et al. Epithelial salivary glands neoplasms in children and adolescents: a forty-four-year experience. Med Pediatr Oncol. 2002 Dec;39(6):594–600. PMID:12376983
5868. Ribeiro RC, Figueiredo B. Childhood adrenocortical tumours. Eur J Cancer. 2004 May;40(8):1117–26. PMID:15110875
5869. Ribeiro S, Napoli I, White IJ, et al. Injury signals cooperate with Nf1 loss to relieve the tumor-suppressive environment of adult peripheral nerve. Cell Rep. 2013 Oct 17;5(1):126–36. PMID:24075988
5870. Ribi S, Baumhoer D, Lee K, et al. TP53 intron 1 hotspot rearrangements are specific to sporadic osteosarcoma and can cause Li-Fraumeni syndrome. Oncotarget. 2015 Apr 10;6(10):7727–40. PMID:25762628
5871. Ricci F, Paradisi A, Annessi G, et al. Eruptive disseminated Spitz nevi. Eur J Dermatol. 2017 Feb 1;27(1):59–62. PMID:27758761
5872. Rice BH. Periapical radiopacities. J Md State Dent Assoc. 1978 Apr;21(1):21–5. PMID:285210
5873. Richards MK, Dahl JP, Gow K, et al. Factors associated with mortality in pediatric vs adult nasopharyngeal carcinoma. JAMA Otolaryngol Head Neck Surg. 2016 Mar;142(3):217–22. PMID:26769566
5874. Richards MK, Goldin AB, Beierle EA, et al. Breast malignancies in children: presentation, management, and survival. Ann Surg Oncol. 2017 Jun;24(6):1482–91. PMID:28058544
5875. Richards S, Aziz N, Bale S, et al. Standards and guidelines for the interpretation of sequence variants: a joint consensus recommendation of the American College of Medical Genetics and Genomics and the Association for Molecular Pathology. Genet Med. 2015 May;17(5):405–24. PMID:25741868
5876. Richardson MS, Muller S. Malignant odontogenic tumors: an update on selected tumors. Head Neck Pathol. 2014 Dec;8(4):411–20. PMID:25409848
5877. Richardson SK, Tannous ZS, Mihm MC Jr. Congenital and infantile melanoma: review of the literature and report of an uncommon variant, pigment-synthesizing melanoma. J Am Acad Dermatol. 2002 Jul;47(1):77–90. PMID:12077586
5878. Richardson TE, Butt YM, Torrealba JR, et al. Meningothelial-like nodules of the lung show SSTR2a Immunohistochemical Staining. Arch Pathol Lab Med. 2018 Jul;142(7):781–2. PMID:29939782
5879. Richardson TE, Tang K, Vasudevaraja V, et al. GOPC-ROS1 fusion due to microdeletion at 6q22 is an oncogenic driver in a subset of pediatric gliomas and glioneuronal tumors. J Neuropathol Exp Neurol. 2019 Dec 1;78(12):1089–99. PMID:31626289
5880. Richter J, John K, Staiger AM, et al. Epstein-Barr virus status of sporadic Burkitt lymphoma is associated with patient age and mutational features. Br J Haematol. 2022 Feb;196(3):681–9. PMID:34617271
5881. Richter J, Schlesner M, Hoffmann S, et al. Recurrent mutation of the ID3 gene in Burkitt lymphoma identified by integrated genome, exome and transcriptome sequencing. Nat Genet. 2012 Dec;44(12):1316–20. PMID:23143595
5882. Rickart AJ, Drummond-Hay V, Suchak A, et al. Melanotic neuroectodermal tumour of infancy: refining the surgical approach. Int J Oral Maxillofac Surg. 2019 Oct;48(10):1307–12. PMID:30871849
5883. Rickert CH, Paulus W. Tumors of the choroid plexus. Microsc Res Tech. 2001 Jan 1;52(1):104–11. PMID:11135453
5884. Rickert CH, Simon R, Bergmann M, et al. Comparative genomic hybridization in pineal parenchymal tumors. Genes Chromosomes Cancer. 2001 Jan;30(1):99–104. PMID:11107183
5885. Rickert CH, Wiestler OD, Paulus W. Chromosomal imbalances in choroid plexus tumors. Am J Pathol. 2002 Mar;160(3):1105–13. PMID:11891207
5886. Ricklefs FL, Fita KD, Rotermund R, et al. Genome-wide DNA methylation profiles distinguish silent from non-silent ACTH adenomas. Acta Neuropathol. 2020 Jul;140(1):95–7. PMID:32185515
5887. Riddler SA, Breinig MC, McKnight JL. Increased levels of circulating Epstein-Barr virus (EBV)-infected lymphocytes and decreased EBV nuclear antigen antibody responses are associated with the development of posttransplant lymphoproliferative disease in solid-organ transplant recipients. Blood. 1994 Aug 1;84(3):972–84. PMID:8043879
5888. Ridenour RV 3rd, Ahrens WA, Folpe AL, et al. Clinical and histopathologic features of chordomas in children and young adults. Pediatr Dev Pathol. 2010 Jan-Feb;13(1):9–17. PMID:19348512
5889. Rigaud C, Auperin A, Jourdain A, et al. Outcome of relapse in children and adolescents with B-cell non-Hodgkin lymphoma and mature acute leukemia: a report from the French LMB study. Pediatr Blood Cancer. 2019 Sep;66(9):e27873. PMID:31207026
5890. Righi A, Gambarotti M, Longo S, et al. Small cell osteosarcoma: clinicopathologic, immunohistochemical, and molecular analysis of 36 cases. Am J Surg Pathol. 2015 May;39(5):691–9. PMID:25723116
5891. Righi A, Sbaraglia M, Gambarotti M, et al. Primary vascular tumors of bone: a monoinstitutional morphologic and molecular analysis of 427 cases with emphasis on epithelioid variants. Am J Surg Pathol. 2020 Sep;44(9):1192–203. PMID:32271190
5892. Rijlaarsdam MA, Looijenga LH. An oncofetal and developmental perspective on testicular germ cell cancer. Semin Cancer Biol. 2014 Dec;29:59–74. PMID:25066859
5893. Rijlaarsdam MA, Tax DM, Gillis AJ, et al. Genome wide DNA methylation profiles provide clues to the origin and pathogenesis of germ cell tumors. PLoS One. 2015 Apr 10;10(4):e0122146. PMID:25859847
5894. Rijlaarsdam MA, van Herk HA, Gillis AJ, et al. Specific detection of OCT3/4 isoform A/B/B1 expression in solid (germ cell) tumours and cell lines: confirmation of OCT3/4 specificity for germ cell tumours. Br J Cancer. 2011 Sep 6;105(6):854–63. PMID:21847120
5895. Rimareix F, Bardot J, Andrac L, et al. Infantile digital fibroma–report on eleven cases.

Eur J Pediatr Surg. 1997 Dec;7(6):345–8. PMID:9493986
**5896.** Riminucci M, Collins MT, Fedarko NS, et al. FGF-23 in fibrous dysplasia of bone and its relationship to renal phosphate wasting. J Clin Invest. 2003 Sep;112(5):683–92. PMID:12952917
**5897.** Rindi G, Klimstra DS, Abedi-Ardekani B, et al. A common classification framework for neuroendocrine neoplasms: an International Agency for Research on Cancer (IARC) and World Health Organization (WHO) expert consensus proposal. Mod Pathol. 2018 Dec;31(12):1770–86. PMID:30140036
**5898.** Rio Frio T, Bahubeshi A, Kanellopoulou C, et al. DICER1 mutations in familial multinodular goiter with and without ovarian Sertoli-Leydig cell tumors. JAMA. 2011 Jan 5;305(1):68–77. PMID:21205968
**5899.** Riopel MA, Spellerberg A, Griffin CA, et al. Genetic analysis of ovarian germ cell tumors by comparative genomic hybridization. Cancer Res. 1998 Jul 15;58(14):3105–10. PMID:9679978
**5900.** Rioux JP, Myers RA. Hyperbaric oxygen for methylene chloride poisoning: report on two cases. Ann Emerg Med. 1989 Jun;18(6):691–5. PMID:2729697
**5901.** Ripperger T, Bielack SS, Borkhardt A, et al. Childhood cancer predisposition syndromes-A concise review and recommendations by the Cancer Predisposition Working Group of the Society for Pediatric Oncology and Hematology. Am J Med Genet A. 2017 Apr;173(4):1017–37. PMID:28168833
**5902.** Ritter MR, Dorrell MI, Edmonds J, et al. Insulin-like growth factor 2 and potential regulators of hemangioma growth and involution identified by large-scale expression analysis. Proc Natl Acad Sci U S A. 2002 May 28;99(11):7455–60. PMID:12032304
**5903.** Riva G, Cima L, Villanova M, et al. Low-grade neuroepithelial tumor: unusual presentation in an adult without history of seizures. Neuropathology. 2018 Oct;38(5):557–60. PMID:30051533
**5904.** Rivera B, Gayden T, Carrot-Zhang J, et al. Germline and somatic FGFR1 abnormalities in dysembryoplastic neuroepithelial tumors. Acta Neuropathol. 2016 Jun;131(6):847–63. PMID:26920151
**5905.** Rix M, Hertel NT, Nielsen FC, et al. Cushing's disease in childhood as the first manifestation of multiple endocrine neoplasia syndrome type 1. Eur J Endocrinol. 2004 Dec;151(6):709–15. PMID:15588237
**5906.** Rizzo KA, Streubel B, Pittaluga S, et al. Marginal zone lymphomas in children and the young adult population; characterization of genetic aberrations by FISH and RT-PCR. Mod Pathol. 2010 Jun;23(6):866–73. PMID:20305621
**5907.** Ro JY, Dexeus FH, el-Naggar A, et al. Testicular germ cell tumors. Clinically relevant pathologic findings. Pathol Annu. 1991;26(Pt 2):59–87. PMID:1650448
**5908.** Roach ES, Sparagana SP. Diagnostic criteria for tuberous sclerosis complex. In: Kwiatkowski DJ, Whittemore VH, Thiele EA, editors. Tuberous sclerosis complex: genes, clinical features, and therapeutics. Weinheim (Germany): Wiley-Blackwell; 2010. pp. 21–5.
**5909.** Roake CM, Artandi SE. DNA repair: telomere-lengthening mechanism revealed. Nature. 2016 Nov 3;539(7627):35–6. PMID:27760112
**5910.** Robbiani DF, Deroubaix S, Feldhahn N, et al. Plasmodium infection promotes genomic instability and AID-dependent B cell lymphoma. Cell. 2015 Aug 13;162(4):727–37. PMID:26276629
**5911.** Robbins P, Papadimitriou J. Glandular peripheral nerve sheath tumours. Pathol Res Pract. 1994 Apr;190(4):412–5. PMID:8078812
**5912.** Robboy SJ, Norris HJ, Scully RE. Insular carcinoid primary in the ovary. A clinicopathologic analysis of 48 cases. Cancer. 1975 Aug;36(2):404–18. PMID:1157010
**5913.** Robboy SJ, Scully RE. Ovarian teratoma with glial implants on the peritoneum. An analysis of 12 cases. Hum Pathol. 1970 Dec;1(4):643–53. PMID:5521737
**5914.** Robboy SJ, Scully RE. Strumal carcinoid of the ovary: an analysis of 50 cases of a distinctive tumor composed of thyroid tissue and carcinoid. Cancer. 1980 Nov 1;46(9):2019–34. PMID:7427909
**5915.** Robboy SJ, Scully RE, Norris HJ. Primary trabecular carcinoid of the ovary. Obstet Gynecol. 1977 Feb;49(2):202–7. PMID:834404
**5916.** Robboy SJ, Shaco-Levy R, Peng RY, et al. Malignant struma ovarii: an analysis of 88 cases, including 27 with extraovarian spread. Int J Gynecol Pathol. 2009 Sep;28(5):405–22. PMID:19696610
**5917.** Roberts CW, Biegel JA. The role of SMARCB1/INI1 in development of rhabdoid tumor. Cancer Biol Ther. 2009 Mar;8(5):412–6. PMID:19305156
**5918.** Roberts I, Alford K, Hall G, et al. GATA1-mutant clones are frequent and often unsuspected in babies with Down syndrome: identification of a population at risk of leukemia. Blood. 2013 Dec 5;122(24):3908–17. PMID:24021668
**5919.** Roberts I, Fordham NJ, Rao A, et al. Neonatal leukaemia. Br J Haematol. 2018 Jul;182(2):170–84. PMID:29806701
**5920.** Roberts KG, Li Y, Payne-Turner D, et al. Targetable kinase-activating lesions in Ph-like acute lymphoblastic leukemia. N Engl J Med. 2014 Sep 11;371(11):1005–15. PMID:25207766
**5921.** Roberts RO, Lynch CF, Jones MP, et al. Medulloblastoma: a population-based study of 532 cases. J Neuropathol Exp Neurol. 1991 Mar;50(2):134–44. PMID:2010773
**5922.** Robinson G, Parker M, Kranenburg TA, et al. Novel mutations target distinct subgroups of medulloblastoma. Nature. 2012 Aug 2;488(7409):43–8. PMID:22722829
**5923.** Robinson GW, Gajjar A. Genomics paves the way for better infant medulloblastoma therapy. J Clin Oncol. 2020 Jun 20;38(18):2010–3. PMID:32352857
**5924.** Robinson GW, Rudneva VA, Buchhalter I, et al. Risk-adapted therapy for young children with medulloblastoma (SJYC07): therapeutic and molecular outcomes from a multicentre, phase 2 trial. Lancet Oncol. 2018 Jun;19(6):768–84. PMID:29778738
**5925.** Robinson MR, Salit RB, Bryant-Greenwood PK, et al. Burkitt's/Burkitt's-like lymphoma presenting as bacterial sinusitis in two HIV-infected children. AIDS Patient Care STDS. 2001 Sep;15(9):453–8. PMID:11587630
**5926.** Rock MG, Sim FH, Unni KK, et al. Secondary malignant giant-cell tumor of bone. Clinicopathological assessment of nineteen patients. J Bone Joint Surg Am. 1986 Sep;68(7):1073–9. PMID:3745247
**5927.** Roden RBS, Stern PL. Opportunities and challenges for human papillomavirus vaccination in cancer. Nat Rev Cancer. 2018 Apr;18(4):240–54. PMID:29497146
**5928.** Rodgers B, Zeim S, Crawford B, et al. Splenic papillary angioendothelioma in a 6-year-old girl. J Pediatr Hematol Oncol. 2007 Dec;29(12):808–10. PMID:18090926
**5929.** Rodig SJ, Vergilio JA, Shahsafaei A, et al. Characteristic expression patterns of TCL1, CD38, and CD44 identify aggressive lymphomas harboring a MYC translocation. Am J Surg Pathol. 2008 Jan;32(1):113–22. PMID:18162778
**5930.** Rodrigues-Fernandes CI, Pérez-de-Oliveira ME, Aristizabal Arboleda LP, et al. Clinicopathological analysis of oral Burkitt's lymphoma in pediatric patients: a systematic review. Int J Pediatr Otorhinolaryngol. 2020 Jul;134:110033. PMID:32302884
**5931.** Rodriguez DP, Orscheln ES, Koch BL. Masses of the nose, nasal cavity, and nasopharynx in children. Radiographics. 2017 Oct;37(6):1704–30. PMID:29019747
**5932.** Rodriguez E, Sreekantaiah C, Gerald W, et al. A recurring translocation, t(11;22)(p13;q11.2), characterizes intra-abdominal desmoplastic small round-cell tumors. Cancer Genet Cytogenet. 1993 Aug;69(1):17–21. PMID:8374894
**5933.** Rodriguez FJ, Brosnan-Cashman JA, Allen SJ, et al. Alternative lengthening of telomeres, ATRX loss and H3-K27M mutations in histologically defined pilocytic astrocytoma with anaplasia. Brain Pathol. 2019 Jan;29(1):126–40. PMID:30192422
**5934.** Rodriguez FJ, Graham MK, Brosnan-Cashman JA, et al. Telomere alterations in neurofibromatosis type 1-associated solid tumors. Acta Neuropathol Commun. 2019 Aug 28;7(1):139. PMID:31462295
**5935.** Rodriguez FJ, Ligon AH, Horkayne-Szakaly I, et al. BRAF duplications and MAPK pathway activation are frequent in gliomas of the optic nerve proper. J Neuropathol Exp Neurol. 2012 Sep;71(9):789–94. PMID:22892521
**5936.** Rodriguez FJ, Perry A, Gutmann DH, et al. Gliomas in neurofibromatosis type 1: a clinicopathologic study of 100 patients. J Neuropathol Exp Neurol. 2008 Mar;67(3):240–9. PMID:18344915
**5937.** Rodriguez FJ, Perry A, Rosenblum MK, et al. Disseminated oligodendroglial-like leptomeningeal tumor of childhood: a distinctive clinicopathologic entity. Acta Neuropathol. 2012 Nov;124(5):627–41. PMID:22941225
**5938.** Rodriguez FJ, Scheithauer BW, Burger PC, et al. Anaplasia in pilocytic astrocytoma predicts aggressive behavior. Am J Surg Pathol. 2010 Feb;34(2):147–60. PMID:20061938
**5939.** Rodriguez FJ, Scheithauer BW, Tsunoda S, et al. The spectrum of malignancy in craniopharyngioma. Am J Surg Pathol. 2007 Jul;31(7):1020–8. PMID:17592268
**5940.** Rodriguez FJ, Schniederjan MJ, Nicolaides T, et al. High rate of concurrent BRAF-KIAA1549 gene fusion and 1p deletion in disseminated oligodendroglioma-like leptomeningeal neoplasms (DOLN). Acta Neuropathol. 2015 Apr;129(4):609–10. PMID:25720745
**5941.** Rodriguez FJ, Tihan T, Lin D, et al. Clinicopathologic features of pediatric oligodendrogliomas: a series of 50 patients. Am J Surg Pathol. 2014 Aug;38(8):1058–70. PMID:24805856
**5942.** Rodriguez FJ, Vizcaino MA, Blakeley J, et al. Frequent alternative lengthening of telomeres and ATRX loss in adult NF1-associated diffuse and high-grade astrocytomas. Acta Neuropathol. 2016 Nov;132(5):761–3. PMID:27650176
**5943.** Rodriguez HA, Berthrong M. Multiple primary intracranial tumors in von Recklinghausen's neurofibromatosis. Arch Neurol. 1966 May;14(5):467–75. PMID:4957904
**5944.** Rodriguez LA, Edwards MS, Levin VA. Management of hypothalamic gliomas in children: an analysis of 33 cases. Neurosurgery. 1990 Feb;26(2):242–6. PMID:2308672
**5945.** Rodriguez PN, Hafez GR, Messing EM. Nonseminomatous germ cell tumor of the testicle: Does extensive staging of the primary tumor predict the likelihood of metastatic disease? J Urol. 1986 Sep;136(3):604–8. PMID:3016346
**5946.** Rodriguez-Galindo C, Figueiredo BC, Zambetti GP, et al. Biology, clinical characteristics, and management of adrenocortical tumors in children. Pediatr Blood Cancer. 2005 Sep;45(3):265–73. PMID:15747338
**5947.** Rodriguez-Galindo C, Wilson MW, Haik BG, et al. Treatment of metastatic retinoblastoma. Ophthalmology. 2003 Jun;110(6):1237–40. PMID:12799253
**5948.** Rodríguez-Jurado R, Palacios C, Durán-McKinster C, et al. Medallion-like dermal dendrocyte hamartoma: a new clinically and histopathologically distinct lesion. J Am Acad Dermatol. 2004 Sep;51(3):359–63. PMID:15337977
**5949.** Rodríguez-Pinilla SM, Barrionuevo C, García J, et al. Epstein-Barr virus-positive systemic NK/T-cell lymphomas in children: report of six cases. Histopathology. 2011 Dec;59(6):1183–93. PMID:22175898
**5950.** Roebuck DJ, Aronson D, Clapuyt P, et al. 2005 PRETEXT: a revised staging system for primary malignant liver tumours of childhood developed by the SIOPEL group. Pediatr Radiol. 2007 Feb;37(2):123–32. PMID:17186233
**5951.** Roemer MGM, Redd RA, Cader FZ, et al. Major histocompatibility complex class II and programmed death ligand 1 expression predict outcome after programmed death 1 blockade in classic Hodgkin lymphoma. J Clin Oncol. 2018 Apr 1;36(10):942–50. PMID:29394125
**5952.** Rogers PC, Olson TA, Cullen JW, et al. Treatment of children and adolescents with stage II testicular and stages I and II ovarian malignant germ cell tumors: a Pediatric Intergroup Study–Pediatric Oncology Group 9048 and Children's Cancer Group 8891. J Clin Oncol. 2004 Sep 1;22(17):3563–9. PMID:15337806
**5953.** Rogers S, Jones DTW, Ireland A, et al. Unusual paediatric spinal myxopapillary ependymomas: unique molecular entities or pathological variations on a theme? J Clin Neurosci. 2018 Apr;50:144–8. PMID:29402569
**5954.** Röhrich M, Koelsche C, Schrimpf D, et al. Methylation-based classification of benign and malignant peripheral nerve sheath tumors. Acta Neuropathol. 2016 Jun;131(6):877–87. PMID:26857854
**5955.** Roithmann S, Toledano M, Tourani JM, et al. HIV-associated non-Hodgkin's lymphomas: clinical characteristics and outcome. The experience of the French Registry of HIV-associated tumors. Ann Oncol. 1991 Apr;2(4):289–95. PMID:1868025
**5956.** Roizen J, Levine MA. A meta-analysis comparing the biochemistry of primary hyperparathyroidism in youths to the biochemistry of primary hyperparathyroidism in adults. J Clin Endocrinol Metab. 2014 Dec;99(12):4555–64. PMID:25181388
**5957.** Rojas Y, Slater BJ, Braverman RM, et al. Extrarenal Wilms tumor: a case report and review of the literature. J Pediatr Surg. 2013 Jun;48(6):E33–5. PMID:23845655
**5958.** Rojnueangnit K, Xie J, Gomes A, et al. High incidence of Noonan syndrome features including short stature and pulmonic stenosis in patients carrying NF1 missense mutations affecting p.Arg1809: genotype-phenotype correlation. Hum Mutat. 2015 Nov;36(11):1052–63. PMID:26178382
**5959.** Roma AA, Goyal A, Yang B. Differential expression patterns of GATA3 in uterine mesonephric and nonmesonephric lesions. Int J Gynecol Pathol. 2015 Sep;34(5):480–6. PMID:25851711
**5960.** Romanet P, Guerin C, Pedini P, et al. Pathological and genetic characterization of bilateral adrenomedullary hyperplasia in a patient with germline MAX mutation. Endocr Pathol. 2017 Dec;28(4):302–7. PMID:27838885

5961. Romano F, Stroppa P, Bravi M, et al. Favorable outcome of primary liver transplantation in children with cirrhosis and hepatocellular carcinoma. Pediatr Transplant. 2011 Sep;15(6):573–9. PMID:21797955
5962. Romberg N, Le Coz C, Glauzy S, et al. Patients with common variable immunodeficiency with autoimmune cytopenias exhibit hyperplastic yet inefficient germinal center responses. J Allergy Clin Immunol. 2019 Jan;143(1):258–65. PMID:29935219
5963. Romeo S, Bovée JV, Grogan SP, et al. Chondromyxoid fibroma resembles in vitro chondrogenesis, but differs in expression of signalling molecules. J Pathol. 2005 Jun;206(2):135–42. PMID:15880456
5964. Romeo S, Hogendoorn PC, Dei Tos AP. Benign cartilaginous tumors of bone: from morphology to somatic and germ-line genetics. Adv Anat Pathol. 2009 Sep;16(5):307–15. PMID:19700940
5965. Ron E, Lubin JH, Shore RE, et al. Thyroid cancer after exposure to external radiation: a pooled analysis of seven studies. Radiat Res. 1995 Mar;141(3):259–77. PMID:7871153
5966. Ron E, Modan B, Boice JD Jr, et al. Tumors of the brain and nervous system after radiotherapy in childhood. N Engl J Med. 1988 Oct 20;319(16):1033–9. PMID:3173432
5967. Ronceray L, Abla O, Barzilai-Birenboim S, et al. Children and adolescents with marginal zone lymphoma have an excellent prognosis with limited chemotherapy or a watch-and-wait strategy after complete resection. Pediatr Blood Cancer. 2018 Apr;65(4). PMID:29286565
5968. Ronchi A, Di Martino M, Caputo A, et al. Fine-needle aspiration cytology is an effective diagnostic tool in paediatric patients with mucoepidermoid carcinoma as secondary neoplasm. Acta Cytol. 2020;64(6):520–31. PMID:32526741
5969. Ronellenfitsch MW, Harter PN, Kirchner M, et al. Targetable ERBB2 mutations identified in neurofibroma/schwannoma hybrid nerve sheath tumors. J Clin Invest. 2020 May 1;130(5):2488–95. PMID:32017710
5970. Ronnett BM, Seidman JD. Mucinous tumors arising in ovarian mature cystic teratomas: relationship to the clinical syndrome of pseudomyxoma peritonei. Am J Surg Pathol. 2003 May;27(5):650–7. PMID:12717249
5971. Rooper LM, Jo VY, Antonescu CR, et al. Adamantinoma-like Ewing sarcoma of the salivary glands: a newly recognized mimicker of basaloid salivary carcinomas. Am J Surg Pathol. 2019 Feb;43(2):187–94. PMID:30285997
5972. Rorke LB, Packer RJ, Biegel JA. Central nervous system atypical teratoid/rhabdoid tumors of infancy and childhood: definition of an entity. J Neurosurg. 1996 Jul;85(1):56–65. PMID:8683283
5973. Rørth M, Rajpert-De Meyts E, Andersson L, et al. Carcinoma in situ in the testis. Scand J Urol Nephrol Suppl. 2000; (205):166–86. PMID:11144894
5974. Rosario M, Kim HS, Yun JY, et al. Surveillance for lung metastasis from giant cell tumor of bone. J Surg Oncol. 2017 Dec;116(7):907–13. PMID:28650536
5975. Rosario PW, Mourão GF. Noninvasive follicular thyroid neoplasm with papillary-like nuclear features (NIFTP) in children and adolescents. Endocrine. 2018 Sep;61(3):542–4. PMID:29974337
5976. Roschewski M, Dunleavy K, Abramson JS, et al. Multicenter study of risk-adapted therapy with dose-adjusted EPOCH-R in adults with untreated Burkitt lymphoma. J Clin Oncol. 2020 Aug 1;38(22):2519–29. PMID:32453640
5977. Rosemberg S, Fujiwara D. Epidemiology of pediatric tumors of the nervous system according to the WHO 2000 classification: a report of 1,195 cases from a single institution. Childs Nerv Syst. 2005 Nov;21(11):940–4. PMID:16044344
5978. Rosen G, Caparros B, Huvos AG, et al. Preoperative chemotherapy for osteogenic sarcoma: selection of postoperative adjuvant chemotherapy based on the response of the primary tumor to preoperative chemotherapy. Cancer. 1982 Mar 15;49(6):1221–30. PMID:6174200
5979. Rosen PP, Cantrell B, Mullen DL, et al. Juvenile papillomatosis (Swiss cheese disease) of the breast. Am J Surg Pathol. 1980 Feb;4(1):3–12. PMID:7361994
5980. Rosen PP, Holmes G, Lesser ML, et al. Juvenile papillomatosis and breast carcinoma. Cancer. 1985 Mar 15;55(6):1345–52. PMID:3971303
5981. Rosen PP, Kimmel M. Juvenile papillomatosis of the breast. A follow-up study of 41 patients having biopsies before 1979. Am J Clin Pathol. 1990 May;93(5):599–603. PMID:2158224
5982. Rosen PP, Lyngholm B, Kinne DW, et al. Juvenile papillomatosis of the breast and family history of breast carcinoma. Cancer. 1982 Jun 15;49(12):2591–5. PMID:7074576
5983. Rosenbaum E, Jadeja B, Xu B, et al. Prognostic stratification of clinical and molecular epithelioid hemangioendothelioma subsets. Mod Pathol. 2020 Apr;33(4):591–602. PMID:31537895
5984. Rosenberg C, Van Gurp RJ, Geelen E, et al. Overrepresentation of the short arm of chromosome 12 is related to invasive growth of human testicular seminomas and nonseminomas. Oncogene. 2000 Nov 30;19(51):5858–62. PMID:11127816
5985. Rosenberg HS, Stenback WA, Spjut HJ. The fibromatoses of infancy and childhood. Perspect Pediatr Pathol. 1978;4:269–348. PMID:215963
5986. Rosenberg T, Philipsen BB, Mehlum CS, et al. Therapeutic use of the human papillomavirus vaccine on recurrent respiratory papillomatosis: a systematic review and meta-analysis. J Infect Dis. 2019 Mar 15;219(7):1016–25. PMID:30358875
5987. Rosenthal AK, Klausmeier M, Cronin ME, et al. Hepatic angiosarcoma occurring after cyclophosphamide therapy: case report and review of the literature. Am J Clin Oncol. 2000 Dec;23(6):581–3. PMID:11202801
5988. Rosenthal MS, Angelos P, Cooper DS, et al. Clinical and professional ethics guidelines for the practice of thyroidology. Thyroid. 2013 Oct;23(10):1203–10. PMID:23750916
5989. Rosenthal MS, Diekema DS. Pediatric ethics guidelines for hereditary medullary thyroid cancer. Int J Pediatr Endocrinol. 2011;2011:847603. PMID:21436957
5990. Rosenwald A, Wright G, Leroy K, et al. Molecular diagnosis of primary mediastinal B cell lymphoma identifies a clinically favorable subgroup of diffuse large B cell lymphoma related to Hodgkin lymphoma. J Exp Med. 2003 Sep 15;198(6):851–62. PMID:12975453
5991. Rosenzweig M, Ali SM, Wong V, et al. A case of advanced infantile myofibromatosis harboring a novel MYH10-RET fusion. Pediatr Blood Cancer. 2017 Jul;64(7). PMID:28028925
5992. Roser M, Ritchie H, Dadonaite B. Our World In Data [Internet]. 2013. Child and infant mortality; updated 2019 Nov. Available from: https://ourworldindata.org/child-mortality.
5993. Rosh JR, Gross T, Mamula P, et al. Hepatosplenic T-cell lymphoma in adolescents and young adults with Crohn's disease: a cautionary tale? Inflamm Bowel Dis. 2007 Aug;13(8):1024–30. PMID:17480018
5994. Rosolen A, Perkins SL, Pinkerton CR, et al. Revised international pediatric non-Hodgkin lymphoma staging system. J Clin Oncol. 2015 Jun 20;33(18):2112–8. PMID:25940716
5995. Rosolen A, Pillon M, Garaventa A, et al. Anaplastic large cell lymphoma treated with a leukemia-like therapy: report of the Italian Association of Pediatric Hematology and Oncology (AIEOP) LNH-92 protocol. Cancer. 2005 Nov 15;104(10):2133–40. PMID:16211546
5996. Ross DS, Giri DD, Akram MM, et al. Fibroepithelial lesions in the breast of adolescent females: a clinicopathological study of 54 cases. Breast J. 2017 Mar;23(2):182–92. PMID:28299887
5997. Ross HM, Daniel HD, Vivekanandan P, et al. Fibrolamellar carcinomas are positive for CD68. Mod Pathol. 2011 Mar;24(3):390–5. PMID:21113139
5998. Ross JH, Rybicki L, Kay R. Clinical behavior and a contemporary management algorithm for prepubertal testis tumors: a summary of the Prepubertal Testis Tumor Registry. J Urol. 2002 Oct;168(4 Pt 2):1675–8. PMID:12352332
5999. Rossi ED, Bizzarro T, Martini M, et al. Morphological features that can predict BRAFV600E -mutated carcinoma in paediatric thyroid cytology. Cytopathology. 2017 Feb;28(1):55–64. PMID:27256275
6000. Rossi ED, Martini M, Capodimonti S, et al. Analysis of immunocytochemical and molecular BRAF expression in thyroid carcinomas: a cytohistologic institutional experience. Cancer Cytopathol. 2014 Jul;122(7):527–35. PMID:24639117
6001. Rossi ED, Martini M, Cenci T, et al. The role of thyroid FNA cytology in pediatric malignant lesions: an overview of the literature. Cancer Cytopathol. 2017 Aug;125(8):594–603. PMID:28581673
6002. Rossi ED, Mehrotra S, Kilic AI, et al. Noninvasive follicular thyroid neoplasm with papillary-like nuclear features in the pediatric age group. Cancer Cytopathol. 2018 Jan;126(1):27–35. PMID:29024469
6003. Rossi ED, Raffaelli M, Mule' A, et al. Simultaneous immunohistochemical expression of HBME-1 and galectin-3 differentiates papillary carcinomas from hyperfunctioning lesions of the thyroid. Histopathology. 2006 Jun;48(7):795–800. PMID:16722927
6004. Rossi ED, Revelli L, Martini M, et al. Cribriform-morular variant of papillary thyroid carcinoma in an 8-year-old girl: a case report with immunohistochemical and molecular testing. Int J Surg Pathol. 2012 Dec;20(6):629–32. PMID:22494995
6005. Rossi ED, Straccia P, Martini M, et al. The role of thyroid fine-needle aspiration cytology in the pediatric population: an institutional experience. Cancer Cytopathol. 2014 May;122(5):359–67. PMID:24474727
6006. Rossi S, Rodriguez FJ, Mota RA, et al. Primary leptomeningeal oligodendroglioma with documented progression to anaplasia and t(1;19)(q10;p10) in a child. Acta Neuropathol. 2009 Oct;118(4):575–7. PMID:19562354
6007. Rossi S, Szuhai K, Ijszenga M, et al. EWSR1-CREB1 and EWSR1-ATF1 fusion genes in angiomatoid fibrous histiocytoma. Clin Cancer Res. 2007 Dec 15;13(24):7322–8. PMID:18094413
6008. Rotenberg BW, Daniel SJ, Nish IA, et al. Myxomatous lesions of the maxilla in children: a case series and review of management. Int J Pediatr Otorhinolaryngol. 2004 Oct;68(10):1251–6. PMID:15364495
6009. Roth A, Micheau C. Embryoma (or embryonal tumor) of the parotid gland: report of two cases. Pediatr Pathol. 1986;5(1):9–15. PMID:3725707
6010. Roth J, Roach ES, Bartels U, et al. Subependymal giant cell astrocytoma: diagnosis, screening, and treatment. Recommendations from the International Tuberous Sclerosis Complex Consensus Conference 2012. Pediatr Neurol. 2013 Dec;49(6):439–44. PMID:24138953
6011. Roth LM, Cheng L. Gonadoblastoma: origin and outcome. Hum Pathol. 2020 Jun;100:47–53. PMID:31805291
6012. Roth LM, Czernobilsky B, Akgul M, et al. Gonadoblastoma in individuals with a normal karyotype and no evidence of a disorder of sex development. Pathology. 2020 Aug;52(5):605–7. PMID:32616344
6013. Roth LM, Eglen DE. Gonadoblastoma. Immunohistochemical and ultrastructural observations. Int J Gynecol Pathol. 1989;8(1):72–81. PMID:2707955
6014. Roth LM, Karseladze AI. Highly differentiated follicular carcinoma arising from struma ovarii: a report of 3 cases, a review of the literature, and a reassessment of so-called peritoneal strumosis. Int J Gynecol Pathol. 2008 Apr;27(2):213–22. PMID:18317221
6015. Roth LM, Miller AW 3rd, Talerman A. Typical thyroid-type carcinoma arising in struma ovarii: a report of 4 cases and review of the literature. Int J Gynecol Pathol. 2008 Oct;27(4):496–506. PMID:18753973
6016. Roth LM, Talerman A. Recent advances in the pathology and classification of ovarian germ cell tumors. Int J Gynecol Pathol. 2006 Oct;25(4):305–20. PMID:16990705
6017. Rothenberg AB, Berdon WE, D'Angio GJ, et al. The association between neuroblastoma and opsoclonus-myoclonus syndrome: a historical review. Pediatr Radiol. 2009 Jul;39(7):723–6. PMID:19430769
6018. Rothman IL. Michelin tire baby syndrome: a review of the literature and a proposal for diagnostic criteria with adoption of the name circumferential skin folds syndrome. Pediatr Dermatol. 2014 Nov-Dec;31(6):659–63. PMID:25424205
6019. Röttgers S, Gombert M, Teigler-Schlegel A, et al. ALK fusion genes in children with atypical myeloproliferative leukemia. Leukemia. 2010 Jun;24(6):1197–200. PMID:20428197
6020. Rotunno M, McMaster ML, Boland J, et al. Whole exome sequencing in families at high risk for Hodgkin lymphoma: identification of a predisposing mutation in the KDR gene. Haematologica. 2016 Jul;101(7):853–60. PMID:27365461
6021. Rougemont AL, Sartelet H, Oligny LL, et al. Accessory liver lobe with mesothelial inclusion cysts in an omphalocele: a new malformative association. Pediatr Dev Pathol. 2007 May-Jun;10(3):224–8. PMID:17535091
6022. Rouleau GA, Merel P, Lutchman M, et al. Alteration in a new gene encoding a putative membrane-organizing protein causes neuro-fibromatosis type 2. Nature. 1993 Jun 10;363(6429):515–21. PMID:8379998
6023. Roussel-Gervais A, Couture C, Langlais D, et al. The cables1 gene in glucocorticoid regulation of pituitary corticotrope growth and cushing disease. J Clin Endocrinol Metab. 2016 Feb;101(2):513–22. PMID:26695862
6024. Routman DM, Raghunathan A, Giannini C, et al. Anaplastic ependymoma and posterior fossa grouping in a patient With H3K27ME3 loss of expression but chromosomal imbalance. Adv Radiat Oncol. 2019 Mar 14;4(3):466–72. PMID:31360801
6025. Roux A, Pallud J, Saffroy R, et al. High-grade gliomas in adolescents and young adults highlight histomolecular differences from their adult and pediatric counterparts. Neuro Oncol. 2020 Aug 17;22(8):1190–202. PMID:32025728
6026. Rove KO, Maroni PD, Cost CR, et al. Pathologic risk factors in pediatric and adolescent patients with clinical stage I testicular stromal tumors. J Pediatr Hematol Oncol. 2015 Nov;37(8):e441–6. PMID:26479987

6027. Rowe DT, Qu L, Reyes J, et al. Use of quantitative competitive PCR to measure Epstein-Barr virus genome load in the peripheral blood of pediatric transplant patients with lymphoproliferative disorders. J Clin Microbiol. 1997 Jun;35(6):1612–5. PMID:9163497
6028. Roy A, Kumar V, Zorman B, et al. Recurrent internal tandem duplications of BCOR in clear cell sarcoma of the kidney. Nat Commun. 2015 Nov 17;6:8891. PMID:26573325
6029. Rozas-Muñoz E, Frieden IJ, Roé E, et al. Vascular stains: proposal for a clinical classification to improve diagnosis and management. Pediatr Dermatol. 2016 Nov;33(6):570–84. PMID:27456075
6030. Rozmaryn LM, Sadler AH, Dorfman HD. Intraosseous glomus tumor in the ulna. A case report. Clin Orthop Relat Res. 1987 Jul;(220):126–9. PMID:3036410
6031. Ruan Y, Shen X, Shi R, et al. Hydroa vacciniforme-like lymphoproliferative disorder treated with intravenous immunoglobulin: long-term remission without haematopoietic stem cell transplantation or chemotherapy. Acta Derm Venereol. 2020 Jun 18;100(13):adv00192. PMID:32516422
6032. Rubin T, Schwartz A, Fornari E, et al. Novel pathologic finding of digital soft tissue chondroma in a child: a case report and review of literature. Int J Surg Pathol. 2015 Oct;23(7):589–92. PMID:26113665
6033. Rubinstein JC, Visa A, Zhang L, et al. Primary low-grade fibromyxoid sarcoma of the kidney in a child with the alternative EWSR1-CREB3L1 gene fusion. Pediatr Dev Pathol. 2014 Jul-Aug;17(4):321–6. PMID:24896634
6034. Rubinstein LJ. The malformative central nervous system lesions in the central and peripheral forms of neurofibromatosis. A neuropathological study of 22 cases. Ann N Y Acad Sci. 1986;486:14–29. PMID:3105387
6035. Rubio GA, Alvarado A, Gerth DJ, et al. Incidence and outcomes of dermatofibrosarcoma protuberans in the US pediatric population. J Craniofac Surg. 2017 Jan;28(1):182–4. PMID:27922973
6036. Rubnitz JE. How I treat pediatric acute myeloid leukemia. Blood. 2012 Jun 21;119(25):5980–8. PMID:22566607
6037. Rubnitz JE, Gibson B, Smith FO. Acute myeloid leukemia. Hematol Oncol Clin North Am. 2010 Feb;24(1):35–63. PMID:20113895
6038. Rubnitz JE, Inaba H, Dahl G, et al. Minimal residual disease-directed therapy for childhood acute myeloid leukaemia: results of the AML02 multicentre trial. Lancet Oncol. 2010 Jun;11(6):543–52. PMID:20451454
6039. Rubnitz JE, Lacayo NJ, Inaba H, et al. Clofarabine can replace anthracyclines and etoposide in remission induction therapy for childhood acute myeloid leukemia: the AML08 multicenter, randomized phase III trial. J Clin Oncol. 2019 Aug 10;37(23):2072–81. PMID:31246522
6040. Rud CN, Daugaard G, Rajpert-De Meyts E, et al. Sperm concentration, testicular volume and age predict risk of carcinoma in situ in contralateral testis of men with testicular germ cell cancer. J Urol. 2013 Dec;190(6):2074–80. PMID:23770148
6041. Rudà R, Gilbert M, Soffietti R. Ependymomas of the adult: molecular biology and treatment. Curr Opin Neurol. 2008 Dec;21(6):754–61. PMID:18989122
6042. Rudà R, Reifenberger G, Frappaz D, et al. EANO guidelines for the diagnosis and treatment of ependymal tumors. Neuro Oncol. 2018 Mar 27;20(4):445–56. PMID:29194500
6043. Rudzinski ER, Anderson JR, Chi YY, et al. Histology, fusion status, and outcome in metastatic rhabdomyosarcoma: a report from the Children's Oncology Group. Pediatr Blood Cancer. 2017 Dec;64(12):10.1002/pbc.26645. PMID:28521080
6044. Rudzinski ER, Anderson JR, Lyden ER, et al. Myogenin, AP2β, NOS-1, and HMGA2 are surrogate markers of fusion status in rhabdomyosarcoma: a report from the soft tissue sarcoma committee of the children's oncology group. Am J Surg Pathol. 2014 May;38(5):654–9. PMID:24618610
6045. Rudzinski ER, Kelsey A, Vokuhl C, et al. Pathology of childhood rhabdomyosarcoma: a consensus opinion document from the Children's Oncology Group, European Paediatric Soft Tissue Sarcoma Study Group, and the Cooperative Weichteilsarkom Studiengruppe. Pediatr Blood Cancer. 2021 Mar;68(3):e28798. PMID:33306276
6046. Rudzinski ER, Lockwood CM, Stohr BA, et al. Pan-Trk immunohistochemistry identifies NTRK rearrangements in pediatric mesenchymal tumors. Am J Surg Pathol. 2018 Jul;42(7):927–35. PMID:29683818
6047. Rudzinski ER, Teot LA, Anderson JR, et al. Dense pattern of embryonal rhabdomyosarcoma, a lesion easily confused with alveolar rhabdomyosarcoma: a report from the Soft Tissue Sarcoma Committee of the Children's Oncology Group. Am J Clin Pathol. 2013 Jul;140(1):82–90. PMID:23765537
6048. Rueckert J, Devitt K, Kalof A, et al. "Lipoblastoma" has a nice ring to it. J Assoc Genet Technol. 2018;44(2):45–8. PMID:29897891
6049. Rueda-Pedraza ME, Heifetz SA, Sesterhenn IA, et al. Primary intracranial germ cell tumors in the first two decades of life. A clinical, light-microscopic, and immunohistochemical analysis of 54 cases. Perspect Pediatr Pathol. 1987;10:160–207. PMID:3588245
6050. Ruiz-Maldonado R, Parrilla FM, Orozco-Covarrubias ML, et al. Edematous, scarring vasculitic panniculitis: a new multisystemic disease with malignant potential. J Am Acad Dermatol. 1995 Jan;32(1):37–44. PMID:7822515
6051. Ruland V, Hartung S, Kordes U, et al. Choroid plexus carcinomas are characterized by complex chromosomal alterations related to patient age and prognosis. Genes Chromosomes Cancer. 2014 May;53(5):373–80. PMID:24478045
6052. Ruo L, Coit DG, Brennan MF, et al. Long-term follow-up of patients with familial adenomatous polyposis undergoing pancreaticoduodenal surgery. J Gastrointest Surg. 2002 Sep-Oct;6(5):671–5. PMID:12399055
6053. Rusch A, Ziltener G, Nackaerts K, et al. Prevalence of BRCA-1 associated protein 1 germline mutation in sporadic malignant pleural mesothelioma cases. Lung Cancer. 2015 Jan;87(1):77–9. PMID:25468148
6054. Ruschel HC, Beilke LP, Beilke RP, et al. Congential epulis of newborn: report of a spontaneous regression case. J Clin Pediatr Dent. 2008 Winter;33(2):167–9. PMID:19358386
6055. Rush S, Foreman N, Liu A. Brainstem ganglioglioma successfully treated with vemurafenib. J Clin Oncol. 2013 Apr 1;31(10):e159–60. PMID:23358987
6056. Rushing EJ, Thompson LD, Mena H. Malignant transformation of a dysembryoplastic neuroepithelial tumor after radiation and chemotherapy. Ann Diagn Pathol. 2003 Aug;7(4):240–4. PMID:12913847
6057. Rushlow D, Piovesan B, Zhang K, et al. Detection of mosaic RB1 mutations in families with retinoblastoma. Hum Mutat. 2009 May;30(5):842–51. PMID:19280657
6058. Rushlow DE, Mol BM, Kennett JY, et al. Characterisation of retinoblastomas without RB1 mutations: genomic, gene expression, and clinical studies. Lancet Oncol. 2013 Apr;14(4):327–34. PMID:23498719
6059. Ruskova A, Thula R, Chan G. Aggressive Natural Killer-Cell Leukemia: report of five cases and review of the literature. Leuk Lymphoma. 2004 Dec;45(12):2427–38. PMID:15621755
6060. Russano de Paiva Silva G, Tournier E, Sarian LO, et al. Prevalence of CD30 immunostaining in neoplastic mast cells: a retrospective immunohistochemical study. Medicine (Baltimore). 2018 May;97(21):e10642. PMID:29794740
6061. Russell DS, Rubinstein LJ. Pathology of tumours of the nervous system. 5th ed. London (UK): Edward Arnold; 1989.
6062. Russell-Goldman E, Hornick JL, Qian X, et al. NKX2.2 immunohistochemistry in the distinction of Ewing sarcoma from cytomorphologic mimics: diagnostic utility and pitfalls. Cancer Cytopathol. 2018 Nov;126(11):942–9. PMID:30376220
6063. Russo C, Nastro A, Cicala D, et al. Neuroimaging in tuberous sclerosis complex. Childs Nerv Syst. 2020 Oct;36(10):2497–509. PMID:32519125
6064. Russo C, Pellarin M, Tingby O, et al. Comparative genomic hybridization in patients with supratentorial and infratentorial primitive neuroectodermal tumors. Cancer. 1999 Jul 15;86(2):331–9. PMID:10421270
6065. Russo M, Malandrino P, Moleti M, et al. Differentiated thyroid cancer in children: heterogeneity of predictive risk factors. Pediatr Blood Cancer. 2018 Sep;65(9):e27226. PMID:29768715
6066. Rustin GJ, Vogelzang NJ, Sleijfer DT, et al. Consensus statement on circulating tumour markers and staging patients with germ cell tumours. Prog Clin Biol Res. 1990;357:277–84. PMID:2170994
6067. Rutenberg MS, Rotondo RL, Rao D, et al. Clinical outcomes following proton therapy for adult craniopharyngioma: a single-institution cohort study. J Neurooncol. 2020 Apr;147(2):387–95. PMID:32086697
6068. Ruteshouser EC, Huff V. Familial Wilms tumor. Am J Med Genet C Semin Med Genet. 2004 Aug 15;129C(1):29–34. PMID:15264270
6069. Rutkowski S, Bode U, Deinlein F, et al. Treatment of early childhood medulloblastoma by postoperative chemotherapy alone. N Engl J Med. 2005 Mar 10;352(10):978–86. PMID:15758008
6070. Rutkowski S, von Hoff K, Emser A, et al. Survival and prognostic factors of early childhood medulloblastoma: an international meta-analysis. J Clin Oncol. 2010 Nov 20;28(33):4961–8. PMID:20940197
6071. Rutnin S, Porntharukcharoen S, Boonsakan P. Clinicopathologic, immunophenotypic, and molecular analysis of subcutaneous panniculitis-like T-cell lymphoma: a retrospective study in a tertiary care center. J Cutan Pathol. 2019 Jan;46(1):44–51. PMID:30350476
6072. Rutter J, Winge DR, Schiffman JD. Succinate dehydrogenase - Assembly, regulation and role in human disease. Mitochondrion. 2010 Jun;10(4):393–401. PMID:20226277
6073. Ruzevick J, Koh EK, Gonzalez-Cuyar LF, et al. Clival paragangliomas: a report of two cases involving the midline skull base and review of the literature. J Neurooncol. 2017 May;132(3):473–8. PMID:28299533
6074. Ryall S, Guzman M, Elbabaa SK, et al. H3 K27M mutations are extremely rare in posterior fossa group A ependymoma. Childs Nerv Syst. 2017 Jul;33(7):1047–51. PMID:28623522
6075. Ryall S, Krishnatry R, Arnoldo A, et al. Targeted detection of genetic alterations reveal the prognostic impact of H3K27M and MAPK pathway aberrations in paediatric thalamic glioma. Acta Neuropathol Commun. 2016 Aug 31;4(1):93. PMID:27577993
6076. Ryall S, Tabori U, Hawkins C. Pediatric low-grade glioma in the era of molecular diagnostics. Acta Neuropathol Commun. 2020 Mar 12;8(1):30. PMID:32164789
6077. Ryall S, Zapotocky M, Fukuoka K, et al. Integrated molecular and clinical analysis of 1,000 pediatric low-grade gliomas. Cancer Cell. 2020 Apr 13;37(4):569–583.e5. PMID:32289278
6078. Ryan JT, El-Naggar AK, Huh W, et al. Primacy of surgery in the management of mucoepidermoid carcinoma in children. Head Neck. 2011 Dec;33(12):1769–73. PMID:21284057
6079. Ryan RJ, Akin C, Castells M, et al. Mast cell sarcoma: a rare and potentially under-recognized diagnostic entity with specific therapeutic implications. Mod Pathol. 2013 Apr;26(4):533–43. PMID:23196796
6080. Rybak LD, Abramovici L, Kenan S, et al. Cortico-medullary continuity in bizarre parosteal osteochondromatous proliferation mimicking osteochondroma on imaging. Skeletal Radiol. 2007 Sep;36(9):829–34. PMID:17437102
6081. Rybak LD, Rosenthal DI, Wittig JC. Chondroblastoma: radiofrequency ablation–alternative to surgical resection in selected cases. Radiology. 2009 May;251(2):599–604. PMID:19304917
6082. Ryder J, Wang X, Bao L, et al. Aggressive natural killer cell leukemia: report of a Chinese series and review of the literature. Int J Hematol. 2007 Jan;85(1):18–25. PMID:17261497
6083. Ryman W, Bale P. Recurring digital fibromas of infancy. Australas J Dermatol. 1985 Dec;26(3):113–7. PMID:3835952
6084. Rymkiewicz G, Grygalewicz B, Chechlinska M, et al. A comprehensive flow-cytometry-based immunophenotypic characterization of Burkitt-like lymphoma with 11q aberration. Mod Pathol. 2018 May;31(5):732–43. PMID:29327714
6086. Saab ST, Hornick JL, Fletcher CD, et al. IgG4 plasma cells in inflammatory myofibroblastic tumor: inflammatory marker or pathogenic link? Mod Pathol. 2011 Apr;24(4):606–12. PMID:21297584
6087. Saab ST, McClain CM, Coffin CM. Fibrous hamartoma of infancy: a clinicopathologic analysis of 60 cases. Am J Surg Pathol. 2014 Mar;38(3):394–401. PMID:24525510
6088. Saad AA, Beshlawi I, Zachariah M, et al. KMT2A-MLLT3 AML masquerading as JMML may disguise fatal leukemia. Oman Med J. 2019 Nov;34(6):553–5. PMID:31745420
6089. Saad AG, Kumar S, Ron E, et al. Proliferative activity of human thyroid cells in various age groups and its correlation with the risk of thyroid cancer after radiation exposure. J Clin Endocrinol Metab. 2006 Jul;91(7):2672–7. PMID:16670159
6090. Saadat E, Vargas SO, Anderson M, et al. Pediatric intra-articular localized tenosynovial giant cell tumor presenting as an acutely irritable hip: a case report. JBJS Case Connect. 2016 Jul-Sep;6(3):e60. PMID:29252637
6091. Saade RE, Bell D, Garcia J, et al. Role of CRTC1/MAML2 translocation in the prognosis and clinical outcomes of mucoepidermoid carcinoma. JAMA Otolaryngol Head Neck Surg. 2016 Mar;142(3):234–40. PMID:26796488
6092. Saarinen S, Kaasinen E, Karjalainen-Lindsberg ML, et al. Primary mediastinal large B-cell lymphoma segregating in a family: exome sequencing identifies MLL as a candidate predisposition gene. Blood. 2013 Apr 25;121(17):3428–30. PMID:23457195
6093. Saarinen S, Pukkala E, Vahteristo P, et al. High familial risk in nodular lymphocyte-predominant Hodgkin lymphoma. J Clin Oncol. 2013 Mar 1;31(7):938–43. PMID:23284040
6094. Saarinen S, Vahteristo P, Launonen V, et al. Analysis of KLHDC8B in familial nodular

lymphocyte predominant Hodgkin lymphoma. Br J Haematol. 2011 Aug;154(3):413–5. PMID:21517803
**6095.** Saavedra HI, Knauf JA, Shirokawa JM, et al. The RAS oncogene induces genomic instability in thyroid PCCL3 cells via the MAPK pathway. Oncogene. 2000 Aug 10;19(34):3948–54. PMID:10951588
**6096.** Sabbaghian N, Hamel N, Srivastava A, et al. Germline DICER1 mutation and associated loss of heterozygosity in a pineoblastoma. J Med Genet. 2012 Jul;49(7):417–9. PMID:22717647
**6097.** Sachdeva MU, Vankalakunti M, Rangan A, et al. The role of immunohistochemistry in medullomyoblastoma–a case series highlighting divergent differentiation. Diagn Pathol. 2008 Apr 25;3:18. PMID:18439235
**6098.** Sack MJ, Astengo-Osuna C, Lin BT, et al. HBME-1 immunostaining in thyroid fine-needle aspirations: a useful marker in the diagnosis of carcinoma. Mod Pathol. 1997 Jul;10(7):668–74. PMID:9237176
**6099.** Sadashivam S, Menon G, Abraham M, et al. Adult craniopharyngioma: the role of extent of resection in tumor recurrence and long-term functional outcome. Clin Neurol Neurosurg. 2020 May;192:105711. PMID:32036264
**6100.** Saeger W, Ebrahimi A, Beschorner R, et al. Teratoma of the sellar region: a case report. Endocr Pathol. 2017 Dec;28(4):315–9. PMID:28102527
**6101.** Saeger W, Lüdecke DK, Buchfelder M, et al. Pathohistological classification of pituitary tumors: 10 years of experience with the German Pituitary Tumor Registry. Eur J Endocrinol. 2007 Feb;156(2):203–16. PMID:17287410
**6102.** Safadi A, Fliss DM, Issakov J, et al. Infantile sinonasal myxoma: a unique variant of maxillofacial myxoma. J Oral Maxillofac Surg. 2011 Feb;69(2):553–8. PMID:21168253
**6103.** Sagebiel RW, Chinn EK, Egbert BM. Pigmented spindle cell nevus. Clinical and histologic review of 90 cases. Am J Surg Pathol. 1984 Sep;8(9):645–53. PMID:6476194
**6104.** Saglam M, Kurt H, Meral C. An unusual location for intracranial lipoma: lateral pontomesencephalic lipoma in an infant. Pediatr Neurol. 2015 Nov;53(5):464–5. PMID:26255751
**6105.** Saglietti C, Schneider V, Bongiovanni M, et al. Acinar cell carcinoma of the pancreas with thyroid-like follicular features: first description of a new diagnostic challenging subtype. Virchows Arch. 2019 Dec;475(6):789–94. PMID:31338587
**6106.** Saha K, Sarkar S, Jash D, et al. Aggressive angiomyxoma of greater omentum with pleural effusion in a young male. J Cancer Res Ther. 2014 Apr-Jun;10(2):371–3. PMID:25022396
**6107.** Sahai S, Rajan S, Singh N, et al. Congenital infiltrating lipomatosis of the face with exophytic temporomandibular joint ankylosis: a case report and review of the literature. Dentomaxillofac Radiol. 2013;42(3):16128745. PMID:22241871
**6108.** Sahakitrungruang T, Srichomthong C, Pornkunwilai S, et al. Germline and somatic DICER1 mutations in a pituitary blastoma causing infantile-onset Cushing's disease. J Clin Endocrinol Metab. 2014 Aug;99(8):E1487–92. PMID:24823459
**6109.** Sahin G, Palanduz A, Aydogan G, et al. Classic Kaposi sarcoma in 3 unrelated Turkish children born to consanguineous kindreds. Pediatrics. 2010 Mar;125(3):e704–8. PMID:20156905
**6110.** Sahm F, Jakobiec FA, Meyer J, et al. Somatic mutations of DICER1 and KMT2D are frequent in intraocular medulloepitheliomas. Genes Chromosomes Cancer. 2016 May;55(5):418–27. PMID:26841698
**6111.** Sahoo S, Hoda SA, Rosai J, et al. Cytokeratin 19 immunoreactivity in the diagnosis of papillary thyroid carcinoma: a note of caution. Am J Clin Pathol. 2001 Nov;116(5):696–702. PMID:11710686
**6112.** Sahoo SS, Kozyra EJ, Wlodarski MW. Germline predisposition in myeloid neoplasms: unique genetic and clinical features of GATA2 deficiency and SAMD9/SAMD9L syndromes. Best Pract Res Clin Haematol. 2020 Sep;33(3):101197. PMID:33038986
**6113.** Sailhan F, Chotel F, Parot R, et al. Chondroblastoma of bone in a pediatric population. J Bone Joint Surg Am. 2009 Sep;91(9):2159–68. PMID:19723993
**6114.** Sainz J, Figueroa K, Baser ME, et al. High frequency of nonsense mutations in the NF2 gene caused by C to T transitions in five CGA codons. Hum Mol Genet. 1995 Jan;4(1):137–9. PMID:7711726
**6115.** Saito K, Kobayashi E, Yoshida A, et al. Angiomatoid fibrous histiocytoma: a series of seven cases including genetically confirmed aggressive cases and a literature review. BMC Musculoskelet Disord. 2017 Jan 23;18(1):31. PMID:28114920
**6116.** Saito Y, Hinoi T, Ueno H, et al. Risk factors for the development of desmoid tumor after colectomy in patients with familial adenomatous polyposis: multicenter retrospective cohort study in Japan. Ann Surg Oncol. 2016 Aug;23 Suppl 4:559–65. PMID:27387679
**6117.** Sakaguchi H, Okuno Y, Muramatsu H, et al. Exome sequencing identifies secondary mutations of SETBP1 and JAK3 in juvenile myelomonocytic leukemia. Nat Genet. 2013 Aug;45(8):937–41. PMID:23832011
**6118.** Sakamoto A, Imamura S, Matsumoto Y, et al. Bizarre parosteal osteochondromatous proliferation with an inversion of chromosome 7. Skeletal Radiol. 2011 Nov;40(11):1487–90. PMID:21509435
**6119.** Sakamoto A, Tanaka K, Yoshida T, et al. Nonossifying fibroma accompanied by pathological fracture in a 12-year-old runner. J Orthop Sports Phys Ther. 2008 Jul;38(7):434–8. PMID:18591758
**6120.** Sakamoto K, Nakasone H, Togashi Y, et al. ALK-positive large B-cell lymphoma: identification of EML4-ALK and a review of the literature focusing on the ALK immunohistochemical staining pattern. Int J Hematol. 2016 Apr;103(4):399–408. PMID:26781614
**6121.** Sakharpe A, Lahat G, Gulamhusein T, et al. Epithelioid sarcoma and unclassified sarcoma with epithelioid features: clinicopathological variables, molecular markers, and a new experimental model. Oncologist. 2011;16(4):512–22. PMID:21357725
**6122.** Sakuntabhai A, Dhitavat J, Burge S, et al. Mosaicism for ATP2A2 mutations causes segmental Darier's disease. J Invest Dermatol. 2000 Dec;115(6):1144–7. PMID:11121153
**6123.** Sakuta R, Otsubo H, Nolan MA, et al. Recurrent intractable seizures in children with cortical dysplasia adjacent to dysembryoplastic neuroepithelial tumor. J Child Neurol. 2005 Apr;20(4):377–84. PMID:15921242
**6124.** Salama ME, Rajan Mariappan M, Inamdar K, et al. The value of CD23 expression as an additional marker in distinguishing mediastinal (thymic) large B-cell lymphoma from Hodgkin lymphoma. Int J Surg Pathol. 2010 Apr;18(2):121–8. PMID:19223373
**6125.** Salama Y, Albanyan S, Szybowska M, et al. Comprehensive characterization of a Canadian cohort of von Hippel-Lindau disease patients. Clin Genet. 2019 Nov;96(5):461–7. PMID:31368132
**6126.** Salas S, Dufresne A, Bui B, et al. Prognostic factors influencing progression-free survival determined from a series of sporadic desmoid tumors: a wait-and-see policy according to tumor presentation. J Clin Oncol. 2011 Sep 10;29(26):3553–8. PMID:21844500
**6127.** Salaverria I, Martin-Guerrero I, Burkhardt B, et al. High resolution copy number analysis of IRF4 translocation-positive diffuse large B-cell and follicular lymphomas. Genes Chromosomes Cancer. 2013 Feb;52(2):150–5. PMID:23073988
**6128.** Salaverria I, Martin-Guerrero I, Wagener R, et al. A recurrent 11q aberration pattern characterizes a subset of MYC-negative high-grade B-cell lymphomas resembling Burkitt lymphoma. Blood. 2014 Feb 20;123(8):1187–98. PMID:24398325
**6129.** Salaverria I, Philipp C, Oschlies I, et al. Translocations activating IRF4 identify a subtype of germinal center-derived B-cell lymphoma affecting predominantly children and young adults. Blood. 2011 Jul 7;118(1):139–47. PMID:21487109
**6130.** Saletta F, Dalla Pozza L, Byrne JA. Genetic causes of cancer predisposition in children and adolescents. Transl Pediatr. 2015 Apr;4(2):67–75. PMID:26835363
**6131.** Saleva-Stateva M, Hess M, Technau-Hafsi K, et al. Molecular characterization and natural history of linear porokeratosis: a case series. J Am Acad Dermatol. 2021 Dec;85(6):1603–6. PMID:33279647
**6131A.** Salgado CM, Alaggio R, Ciolfi A, et al. Pediatric BCOR-altered tumors from soft tissue/kidney display specific DNA methylation profiles. Mod Pathol. 2023 Feb;36(2):100039. PMID:36853789
**6132.** Salgado CM, Basu D, Nikiforova M, et al. Amplification of mutated NRAS leading to congenital melanoma in neurocutaneous melanocytosis. Melanoma Res. 2015 Oct;25(5):453–60. PMID:26266759
**6133.** Salgado CM, Basu D, Nikiforova M, et al. BRAF mutations are also associated with neurocutaneous melanocytosis and large/giant congenital melanocytic nevi. Pediatr Dev Pathol. 2015 Jan-Feb;18(1):1–9. PMID:25490715
**6134.** Salgado CM, Silver RB, Bauer BS, et al. Skin of patients with large/giant congenital melanocytic nevi shows increased mast cells. Pediatr Dev Pathol. 2014 May-Jun;17(3):198–203. PMID:24679055
**6135.** Salgado CM, Zin A, Garrido M, et al. Pediatric soft tissue tumors with BCOR ITD express EGFR but not OLIG2. Pediatr Dev Pathol. 2020 Nov-Dec;23(6):424–30. PMID:32790583
**6136.** Salhany KE, Macon WR, Choi JK, et al. Subcutaneous panniculitis-like T-cell lymphoma: clinicopathologic, immunophenotypic, and genotypic analysis of alpha/beta and gamma/delta subtypes. Am J Surg Pathol. 1998 Jul;22(7):881–93. PMID:9669350
**6137.** Salib C, Edelman M, Lilly J, et al. USP6 gene rearrangement by FISH analysis in cranial fasciitis: a report of three cases. Head Neck Pathol. 2020 Mar;14(1):257–61. PMID:30758758
**6138.** Salinas-Souza C, De Andrea C, Bihl M, et al. GNAS mutations are not detected in parosteal and low-grade central osteosarcomas. Mod Pathol. 2015 Oct;28(10):1336–42. PMID:26248895
**6138A.** Salmeron-Villalobos J, Egan C, Borgmann V, et al. A unifying hypothesis for PNMZL and PTFL: morphological variants with a common molecular profile. Blood Adv. 2022 Aug 23;6(16):4661–74. PMID:35609565
**6139.** Salomao DR, Nascimento AG. Plexiform fibrohistiocytic tumor with systemic metastases: a case report. Am J Surg Pathol. 1997 Apr;21(4):469–76. PMID:9130995
**6140.** Salzburg J, Burkhardt B, Zimmermann M, et al. Prevalence, clinical pattern, and outcome of CNS involvement in childhood and adolescent non-Hodgkin's lymphoma differ by non-Hodgkin's lymphoma subtype: a Berlin-Frankfurt-Munster Group Report. J Clin Oncol. 2007 Sep 1;25(25):3915–22. PMID:17761975
**6141.** Salzer-Kuntschik M, Delling G, Beron G, et al. Morphological grades of regression in osteosarcoma after polychemotherapy - study COSS 80. J Cancer Res Clin Oncol. 1983;106 Suppl:21–4. PMID:6577010
**6142.** Samad A, Shah AA, Stelow EB, et al. Cercariform cells: another cytologic feature distinguishing solid pseudopapillary neoplasms from pancreatic endocrine neoplasms and acinar cell carcinomas in endoscopic ultrasound-guided fine-needle aspirates. Cancer Cytopathol. 2013 Jun;121(6):298–310. PMID:23765692
**6143.** Sampaio MS, Cho YW, Shah T, et al. Impact of Epstein-Barr virus donor and recipient serostatus on the incidence of post-transplant lymphoproliferative disorder in kidney transplant recipients. Nephrol Dial Transplant. 2012 Jul;27(7):2971–9. PMID:22273720
**6144.** Sampson JR, Scahill SJ, Stephenson JB, et al. Genetic aspects of tuberous sclerosis in the west of Scotland. J Med Genet. 1989 Jan;26(1):28–31. PMID:2918523
**6145.** Samuels SL, Surrey LF, Hawkes CP, et al. Characteristics of follicular variant papillary thyroid carcinoma in a Pediatric Cohort. J Clin Endocrinol Metab. 2018 Apr 1;103(4):1639–48. PMID:29438531
**6146.** Sanada Y, Mizuta K, Niki T, et al. Hepatocellular nodules resulting from congenital extrahepatic portosystemic shunts can differentiate into potentially malignant hepatocellular adenomas. J Hepatobiliary Pancreat Sci. 2015 Oct;22(10):746–56. PMID:26138244
**6147.** Sancak O, Nellist M, Goedbloed M, et al. Mutational analysis of the TSC1 and TSC2 genes in a diagnostic setting: genotype–phenotype correlations and comparison of diagnostic DNA techniques in tuberous sclerosis complex. Eur J Hum Genet. 2005 Jun;13(6):731–41. PMID:15798777
**6148.** Sanchez R, Ladino-Torres MF, Bernat JA, et al. Breast fibroadenomas in the pediatric population: common and uncommon sonographic findings. Pediatr Radiol. 2010 Oct;40(10):1681–9. PMID:20449731
**6149.** Sánchez-Romero C, Carlos R, Díaz Molina JP, et al. Nasopharyngeal angiofibroma: a clinical, histopathological and immunohistochemical study of 42 cases with emphasis on stromal features. Head Neck Pathol. 2018 Mar;12(1):52–61. PMID:28508272
**6150.** Sandahl JD, Kjeldsen E, Abrahamsson J, et al. The applicability of the WHO classification in paediatric AML. A NOPHO-AML study. Br J Haematol. 2015 Jun;169(6):859–67. PMID:25819835
**6151.** Sandberg AA, Bridge JA. Updates on the cytogenetics and molecular genetics of bone and soft tissue tumors. Dermatofibrosarcoma protuberans and giant cell fibroblastoma. Cancer Genet Cytogenet. 2003 Jan 1;140(1):1–12. PMID:12550751
**6152.** Sander CA, Medeiros LJ, Weiss LM, et al. Lymphoproliferative lesions in patients with common variable immunodeficiency syndrome. Am J Surg Pathol. 1992 Dec;16(12):1170–82. PMID:1334378
**6153.** Sander S, Calado DP, Srinivasan L, et al. Synergy between PI3K signaling and MYC in Burkitt lymphomagenesis. Cancer Cell. 2012 Aug 14;22(2):167–79. PMID:22897848
**6154.** Sanderson EA, Killoran CE, Pedvis-Leftick A, et al. Localized Darier's disease in a Blaschkoid distribution: two cases of phenotypic mosaicism and a review of mosaic Darier's disease. J Dermatol. 2007 Nov;34(11):761–4. PMID:17973816

6155. Sandrini R, Ribeiro RC, DeLacerda L. Childhood adrenocortical tumors. J Clin Endocrinol Metab. 1997 Jul;82(7):2027–31. PMID:9215267
6156. Sandvik U, Svensdotter E, Gustavsson B. Spinal cavernous extradural angiolipoma manifesting as a spontaneous spinal epidural hematoma in a child. Childs Nerv Syst. 2015 Aug;31(8):1223–6. PMID:26065860
6157. Sanerkin NG, Mott MG, Roylance J. An unusual intraosseous lesion with fibroblastic, osteoclastic, osteoblastic, aneurysmal and fibromyxoid elements. "Solid" variant of aneurysmal bone cyst. Cancer. 1983 Jun 15;51(12):2278–86. PMID:6850506
6158. Sanford LJ, Gordon S, Travers JB. Familial granular cell tumors: a case report and review of the literature. Pediatr Dermatol. 2013 May-Jun;30(3):e8–11. PMID:22994929
6159. Sangueza M, Plaza JA. Hydroa vacciniforme-like cutaneous T-cell lymphoma: clinicopathologic and immunohistochemical study of 12 cases. J Am Acad Dermatol. 2013 Jul;69(1):112–9. PMID:23541598
6160. Sanjay BK, Sim FH, Unni KK, et al. Giant-cell tumours of the spine. J Bone Joint Surg Br. 1993 Jan;75(1):148–54. PMID:8421014
6161. Sanjuan-Pla A, Bueno C, Prieto C, et al. Revisiting the biology of infant t(4;11)/MLL-AF4+ B-cell acute lymphoblastic leukemia. Blood. 2015 Dec 17;126(25):2676–85. PMID:26463423
6162. Sankar B, Ng BY, Hopgood P, et al. Subungual exostosis following toe nail removal–case report. Int J Clin Pract Suppl. 2005 Apr;(147):132–3. PMID:15875652
6163. Sankar S, Lessnick SL. Promiscuous partnerships in Ewing's sarcoma. Cancer Genet. 2011 Jul;204(7):351–65. PMID:21872822
6164. Sano H, Gonzalez-Gomez I, Wu SQ, et al. A case of composite neuroblastoma composed of histologically and biologically distinct clones. Pediatr Dev Pathol. 2007 May-Jun;10(3):229–32. PMID:17535087
6165. Sano H, Kobayashi R, Suzuki D, et al. Wiskott-Aldrich syndrome with unusual clinical features similar to juvenile myelomonocytic leukemia. Int J Hematol. 2012 Aug;96(2):279–83. PMID:22736231
6166. Sano T, Kovacs K, Asa SL, et al. Immunoreactive luteinizing hormone in functioning corticotroph adenomas of the pituitary. Immunohistochemical and tissue culture studies of two cases. Virchows Arch A Pathol Anat Histopathol. 1990;417(4):361–7. PMID:2173251
6167. Sano T, Ohshima T, Yamada S. Expression of glycoprotein hormones and intracytoplasmic distribution of cytokeratin in growth hormone-producing pituitary adenomas. Pathol Res Pract. 1991 Jun;187(5):530–3. PMID:1717959
6168. Santagata S, Ligon KL, Hornick JL. Embryonic stem cell transcription factor signatures in the diagnosis of primary and metastatic germ cell tumors. Am J Surg Pathol. 2007 Jun;31(6):836–45. PMID:17527070
6169. Santiago T, Clay MR, Allen SJ, et al. Recurrent BCOR internal tandem duplication and BCOR or BCL6 expression distinguish primitive myxoid mesenchymal tumor of infancy from congenital infantile fibrosarcoma. Mod Pathol. 2017 Jun;30(6):884–91. PMID:28256570
6170. Santiago T, Clay MR, Allen SJ, et al. Recurrent BCOR internal tandem duplication and BCOR or BCL6 expression distinguish primitive myxoid mesenchymal tumor of infancy from congenital infantile fibrosarcoma. Mod Pathol. 2018 Feb;31(2):374. PMID:29430000
6171. Santora DC, Biglan AW, Johnson BL. Episcleral osteocartilaginous choristoma. Am J Ophthalmol. 1995 May;119(5):654–5. PMID:7733194
6172. Santos GC, Carvalho KC, Falzoni R, et al. Glial fibrillary acidic protein in tumor types with cartilaginous differentiation. Mod Pathol. 2009 Oct;22(10):1321–7. PMID:19668151
6173. Sanusi T, Li Y, Sun L, et al. Eccrine angiomatous hamartoma: a clinicopathological study of 26 cases. Dermatology. 2015;231(1):63–9. PMID:25895513
6174. Sanz-Trelles A, Rodrigo-Fernandez I, Ayala-Carbonero A, et al. Retiform hemangioendothelioma. A new case in a child with diffuse endovascular papillary endothelial proliferation. J Cutan Pathol. 1997 Aug;24(7):440–4. PMID:9274963
6175. Sápi Z, Papp G, Szendrői M, et al. Epigenetic regulation of SMARCB1 By miR-206, -381 and -671-5p is evident in a variety of SMARCB1 immunonegative soft tissue sarcomas, while miR-765 appears specific for epithelioid sarcoma. A miRNA study of 223 soft tissue sarcomas. Genes Chromosomes Cancer. 2016 Oct;55(10):786–802. PMID:27223121
6176. Sara AS, Evans HL, Benjamin RS. Malignant melanoma of soft parts (clear cell sarcoma). A study of 17 cases, with emphasis on prognostic factors. Cancer. 1990 Jan 15;65(2):367–74. PMID:2295060
6177. Sarasin A, Quentin S, Droin N, et al. Familial predisposition to TP53/complex karyotype MDS and leukemia in DNA repair-deficient xeroderma pigmentosum. Blood. 2019 Jun 20;133(25):2718–24. PMID:30914417
6178. Sargar K, Kao SC, Spunt SL, et al. MRI and CT of low-grade fibromyxoid sarcoma in children: a report from Children's Oncology Group Study ARST0332. AJR Am J Roentgenol. 2015 Aug;205(2):414–20. PMID:26204295
6179. Sarin KY, Sun BK, Bangs CD, et al. Activating HRAS mutation in agminated Spitz nevi arising in a nevus spilus. JAMA Dermatol. 2013 Sep;149(9):1077–81. PMID:23884457
6180. Sarkozy C, Chong L, Takata K, et al. Gene expression profiling of gray zone lymphoma. Blood Adv. 2020 Jun 9;4(11):2523–35. PMID:32516416
6181. Sarkozy C, Copie-Bergman C, Damotte D, et al. Gray-zone lymphoma between cHL and large B-cell lymphoma: a histopathologic series from the LYSA. Am J Surg Pathol. 2019 Mar;43(3):341–51. PMID:30540571
6182. Sarkozy C, Hung SS, Chavez EA, et al. Mutational landscape of gray zone lymphoma. Blood. 2021 Apr 1;137(13):1765–76. PMID:32961552
6183. Sarkozy C, Molina T, Ghesquières H, et al. Mediastinal gray zone lymphoma: clinico-pathological characteristics and outcomes of 99 patients from the Lymphoma Study Association. Haematologica. 2017 Jan;102(1):150–9. PMID:27758822
6184. Sarungbam J, Agaram N, Hwang S, et al. Symplastic/pseudoanaplastic giant cell tumor of the bone. Skeletal Radiol. 2016 Jul;45(7):929–35. PMID:27020452
6185. Sasaki H, Manabe A, Kojima S, et al. Myelodysplastic syndrome in childhood: a retrospective study of 189 patients in Japan. Leukemia. 2001 Nov;15(11):1713–20. PMID:11681412
6186. Sastre X, Chantada GL, Doz F, et al. Proceedings of the consensus meetings from the International Retinoblastoma Staging Working Group on the pathology guidelines for the examination of enucleated eyes and evaluation of prognostic risk factors in retinoblastoma. Arch Pathol Lab Med. 2009 Aug;133(8):1199–202. PMID:19653709
6187. Sathe PA, Ghodke RK, Kandalkar BM. Fetus in fetu: an institutional experience. Pediatr Dev Pathol. 2014 Jul-Aug;17(4):243–9. PMID:24689738
6188. Sato K, Oka H, Utsuki S, et al. Ciliated craniopharyngioma may arise from Rathke cleft cyst. Clin Neuropathol. 2006 Jan-Feb;25(1):25–8. PMID:16465771
6189. Sato M, Tanaka N, Sato T, et al. Oral and maxillofacial tumours in children: a review. Br J Oral Maxillofac Surg. 1997 Apr;35(2):92–5. PMID:9146865
6190. Satou A, Asano N, Kato S, et al. Prognostic impact of MUM1/IRF4 expression in Burkitt Lymphoma (BL): a reappraisal of 88 BL patients in Japan. Am J Surg Pathol. 2017 Mar;41(3):389–95. PMID:28079574
6191. Sau P, Graham JH, Helwig EB. Pigmented spindle cell nevus: a clinicopathologic analysis of ninety-five cases. J Am Acad Dermatol. 1993 Apr;28(4):565–71. PMID:8463457
6192. Saunders J, Ingley K, Wang XQ, et al. Loss of BRG1 (SMARCA4) immunoexpression in a pediatric non-central nervous system tumor cohort. Pediatr Dev Pathol. 2020 Mar-Apr;23(2):132–8. PMID:31403913
6193. Saunders T, Margo CE. Intraocular medulloepithelioma. Arch Pathol Lab Med. 2012 Feb;136(2):212–6. PMID:22288972
6194. Saussine A, Marrou K, Delanoé P, et al. Connective tissue nevi: an entity revisited. J Am Acad Dermatol. 2012 Aug;67(2):233–9. PMID:22014540
6195. Sausville JE, Hernandez DJ, Argani P, et al. Pediatric renal cell carcinoma. J Pediatr Urol. 2009 Aug;5(4):308–14. PMID:19443274
6196. Savage DG, Szydlo RM, Goldman JM. Clinical features at diagnosis in 430 patients with chronic myeloid leukaemia seen at a referral centre over a 16-year period. Br J Haematol. 1997 Jan;96(1):111–6. PMID:9012696
6197. Savage KJ, Monti S, Kutok JL, et al. The molecular signature of mediastinal large B-cell lymphoma differs from that of other diffuse large B-cell lymphomas and shares features with classical Hodgkin lymphoma. Blood. 2003 Dec 1;102(12):3871–9. PMID:12933571
6198. Savage MO, Lowe DG. Gonadal neoplasia and abnormal sexual differentiation. Clin Endocrinol (Oxf). 1990 Apr;32(4):519–33. PMID:2189603
6199. Savage SA, Mirabello L. Using epidemiology and genomics to understand osteosarcoma etiology. Sarcoma. 2011;2011:548151. PMID:21437228
6200. Savera AT, Gown AM, Zarbo RJ. Immunolocalization of three novel smooth muscle-specific proteins in salivary gland pleomorphic adenoma: assessment of the morphogenetic role of myoepithelium. Mod Pathol. 1997 Nov;10(11):1093–100. PMID:9388059
6201. Savitchi E, Rao S. Squamous cell carcinoma and pleomorphic sarcoma (MFH) arising in a mature cystic teratoma of the ovary. Int J Gynecol Pathol. 2012 Sep;31(5):443–6. PMID:22833084
6202. Savoie A, Perpête C, Carpentier L, et al. Direct correlation between the load of Epstein-Barr virus-infected lymphocytes in the peripheral blood of pediatric transplant patients and risk of lymphoproliferative disease. Blood. 1994 May 1;83(9):2715–22. PMID:8167350
6203. Sawamura Y, Ikeda J, Shirato H, et al. Germ cell tumours of the central nervous system: treatment consideration based on 111 cases and their long-term clinical outcomes. Eur J Cancer. 1998 Jan;34(1):104–10. PMID:9624246
6204. Sawh RN, Malpica A, Deavers MT, et al. Benign cystic mesothelioma of the peritoneum: a clinicopathologic study of 17 cases and immunohistochemical analysis of estrogen and progesterone receptor status. Hum Pathol. 2003 Apr;34(4):369–74. PMID:12733118
6205. Sawyer JR, Tryka AF, Lewis JM. A novel reciprocal chromosome translocation t(11;22)(p13;q12) in an intraabdominal desmoplastic small round-cell tumor. Am J Surg Pathol. 1992 Apr;16(4):411–6. PMID:1314522
6206. Sayegh ET, Aranda D, Kim JM, et al. Prognosis by tumor location in adults with intracranial ependymomas. J Clin Neurosci. 2014 Dec;21(12):2096–101. PMID:25037313
6207. Sayles LC, Breese MR, Koehne AL, et al. Genome-informed targeted therapy for osteosarcoma. Cancer Discov. 2019 Jan;9(1):46–63. PMID:30266815
6208. Sbiera S, Perez-Rivas LG, Taranets L, et al. Driver mutations in USP8 wild-type Cushing's disease. Neuro Oncol. 2019 Oct 9;21(10):1273–83. PMID:31222332
6209. Schaefer IM, Dong F, Garcia EP, et al. Recurrent SMARCB1 inactivation in epithelioid malignant peripheral nerve sheath tumors. Am J Surg Pathol. 2019 Jun;43(6):835–43. PMID:30864974
6210. Schaefer IM, Fletcher CD. Malignant peripheral nerve sheath tumor (MPNST) arising in diffuse-type neurofibroma: clinicopathologic characterization in a series of 9 cases. Am J Surg Pathol. 2015 Sep;39(9):1234–41. PMID:25929351
6211. Schaefer IM, Fletcher CD. Myxoid variant of so-called angiomatoid "malignant fibrous histiocytoma": clinicopathologic characterization in a series of 21 cases. Am J Surg Pathol. 2014 Jun;38(6):816–23. PMID:24503754
6212. Schaefer IM, Ströbel P, Thiha A, et al. Soft tissue perineurioma and other unusual tumors in a patient with neurofibromatosis type 1. Int J Clin Exp Pathol. 2013 Nov 15;6(12):3003–8. PMID:24294391
6213. Schäfer M, Kadmon M, Schmidt W, et al. Neonatal gardner fibroma leads to detection of familial adenomatous polyposis: two case reports. European J Pediatr Surg Rep. 2016 Dec;4(1):17–21. PMID:28018803
6214. Schaffer JV. Update on melanocytic nevi in children. Clin Dermatol. 2015 May-Jun;33(3):368–86. PMID:25889140
6215. Schaison F, Anract P, Coste F, et al. [Chondrosarcoma secondary to multiple cartilage diseases. Study of 29 clinical cases and review of the literature]. Rev Chir Orthop Repar Appar Mot. 1999 Dec;85(8):834–45. French. PMID:10637885
6216. Schajowicz F, Gallardo H. Epiphysial chondroblastoma of bone. A clinico-pathological study of sixty-nine cases. J Bone Joint Surg Br. 1970 May;52(2):205–26. PMID:5445403
6217. Schecter AK, Lester B, Pan TD, et al. Linear nevus comedonicus with epidermolytic hyperkeratosis. J Cutan Pathol. 2004 Aug;31(7):502–5. PMID:15239681
6218. Scheer M, Vokuhl C, Veit-Friedrich I, et al. Low-grade fibromyxoid sarcoma: a report of the Cooperative Weichteilsarkom Studiengruppe (CWS). Pediatr Blood Cancer. 2020 Feb;67(2):e28009. PMID:31736251
6219. Scheers I, Bachy V, Stephenne X, et al. Risk of hepatocellular carcinoma in liver mitochondrial respiratory chain disorders. J Pediatr. 2005 Mar;146(3):414–7. PMID:15756232
6220. Scheil S, Brüderlein S, Eicker M, et al. Low frequency of chromosomal imbalances in anaplastic ependymomas as detected by comparative genomic hybridization. Brain Pathol. 2001 Apr;11(2):133–43. PMID:11303789
6221. Scheimann AO, Strautnieks SS, Knisely AS, et al. Mutations in bile salt export pump (ABCB11) in two children with progressive familial intrahepatic cholestasis and cholangiocarcinoma. J Pediatr. 2007 May;150(5):556–9. PMID:17452236
6222. Scheipl S, Barnard M, Cottone L, et al. EGFR inhibitors identified as a potential treatment for chordoma in a focused compound

screen. J Pathol. 2016 Jul;239(3):320–34. PMID:27102572
6223. Scheithauer BW. Pathobiology of the pineal gland with emphasis on parenchymal tumors. Brain Tumor Pathol. 1999;16(1):1–9. PMID:10532417
6224. Scheithauer BW, Amrami KK, Folpe AL, et al. Synovial sarcoma of nerve. Hum Pathol. 2011 Apr;42(4):568–77. PMID:21295819
6225. Scheithauer BW, Horvath E, Abel TW, et al. Pituitary blastoma: a unique embryonal tumor. Pituitary. 2012 Sep;15(3):365–73. PMID:21805093
6226. Scheithauer BW, Kovacs K, Horvath E, et al. Pituitary blastoma. Acta Neuropathol. 2008 Dec;116(6):657–66. PMID:18551299
6227. Schelfhout LJ, Van Muijen GN, Fleuren GJ. Expression of keratin 19 distinguishes papillary thyroid carcinoma from follicular carcinomas and follicular thyroid adenoma. Am J Clin Pathol. 1989 Nov;92(5):654–8. PMID:2479256
6228. Schenker K, Blumer S, Jaramillo D, et al. Epithelioid hemangioma of bone: radiologic and magnetic resonance imaging characteristics with histopathological correlation. Pediatr Radiol. 2017 Nov;47(12):1631–7. PMID:28721475
6229. Scheri KC, Leonetti E, Laino L, et al. c-MET receptor as potential biomarker and target molecule for malignant testicular germ cell tumors. Oncotarget. 2018 Aug 7;9(61):31842–60. PMID:30159127
6230. Scheurlen WG, Schwabe GC, Joos S, et al. Molecular analysis of childhood primitive neuroectodermal tumors defines markers associated with poor outcome. J Clin Oncol. 1998 Jul;16(7):2478–85. PMID:9667267
6231. Schick B, Rippel C, Brunner C, et al. Numerical sex chromosome aberrations in juvenile angiofibromas: genetic evidence for an androgen-dependent tumor? Oncol Rep. 2003 Sep-Oct;10(5):1251–5. PMID:12883689
6232. Schiffman JD, Geller JI, Mundt E, et al. Update on pediatric cancer predisposition syndromes. Pediatr Blood Cancer. 2013 Aug;60(8):1247–52. PMID:23625733
6233. Schild SE, Scheithauer BW, Schomberg PJ, et al. Pineal parenchymal tumors. Clinical, pathologic, and therapeutic aspects. Cancer. 1993 Aug 1;72(3):870–80. PMID:8334641
6234. Schiller PI, Itin PH. Angiokeratomas: an update. Dermatology. 1996;193(4):275–82. PMID:8993949
6235. Schindeler A, Little DG. Recent insights into bone development, homeostasis, and repair in type 1 neurofibromatosis (NF1). Bone. 2008 Apr;42(4):616–22. PMID:18248783
6236. Schindler G, Capper D, Meyer J, et al. Analysis of BRAF V600E mutation in 1,320 nervous system tumors reveals high mutation frequencies in pleomorphic xanthoastrocytoma, ganglioglioma and extra-cerebellar pilocytic astrocytoma. Acta Neuropathol. 2011 Mar;121(3):397–405. PMID:21274720
6237. Schittenhelm J, Roser F, Tatagiba M, et al. Diagnostic value of EAAT-1 and Kir7.1 for distinguishing endolymphatic sac tumors from choroid plexus tumors. Am J Clin Pathol. 2012 Jul;138(1):85–9. PMID:22706862
6238. Schlaffer SM, Buchfelder M, Stoehr R, et al. Rathke's cleft cyst as origin of a pediatric papillary craniopharyngioma. Front Genet. 2018 Feb 22;9:49. PMID:29520296
6239. Schlegelberger B, Heller PG. RUNX1 deficiency (familial platelet disorder with predisposition to myeloid leukemia, FPDMM). Semin Hematol. 2017 Apr;54(2):75–80. PMID:28637620
6240. Schleiermacher G, Delattre O, Peter M, et al. Clinical relevance of loss heterozygosity of the short arm of chromosome 1 in neuroblastoma: a single-institution study. Int J Cancer. 1996 Apr 22;69(2):73–8. PMID:8608986
6241. Schleiermacher G, Mosseri V, London WB, et al. Segmental chromosomal alterations have prognostic impact in neuroblastoma: a report from the INRG project. Br J Cancer. 2012 Oct 9;107(8):1418–22. PMID:22976801
6242. Schlitter AM, Konukiewitz B, Kleeff J, et al. [Recurrent duodenal ulcer bleeding as the first manifestation of a solid pseudopapillary neoplasm of the pancreas with hepatic metastases]. Dtsch Med Wochenschr. 2013 May;138(20):1050–3. German. PMID:23670260
6243. Schmale GA, Conrad EU 3rd, Raskind WH. The natural history of hereditary multiple exostoses. J Bone Joint Surg Am. 1994 Jul;76(7):986–92. PMID:8027127
6244. Schmalisch K, Beschorner R, Psaras T, et al. Postoperative intracranial seeding of craniopharyngiomas–report of three cases and review of the literature. Acta Neurochir (Wien). 2010 Feb;152(2):313–9. PMID:19859655
6245. Schmelz M, Montes-Moreno S, Piris M, et al. Lack and/or aberrant localization of major histocompatibility class II (MHCII) protein in plasmablastic lymphoma. Haematologica. 2012 Oct;97(10):1614–6. PMID:22689685
6246. Schmidbauer M, Budka H, Pilz P. Neuroepithelial and ectomesenchymal differentiation in a primitive pineal tumor ("pineal anlage tumor"). Clin Neuropathol. 1989 Jan-Feb;8(1):7–10. PMID:2650944
6247. Schmidt J, Derr V, Heinrich MC, et al. BRAF in papillary thyroid carcinoma of ovary (struma ovarii). Am J Surg Pathol. 2007 Sep;31(9):1337–43. PMID:17721188
6248. Schmidt J, Gong S, Marafioti T, et al. Genome-wide analysis of pediatric-type follicular lymphoma reveals low genetic complexity and recurrent alterations of TNFRSF14 gene. Blood. 2016 Aug 25;128(8):1101–11. PMID:27257180
6249. Schmidt J, Ramis-Zaldivar JE, Nadeu F, et al. Mutations of MAP2K1 are frequent in pediatric-type follicular lymphoma and result in ERK pathway activation. Blood. 2017 Jul 20;130(3):323–7. PMID:28533310
6250. Schmidt ML, Salwen HR, Chagnovich D, et al. Evidence for molecular heterogeneity in human ganglioneuroblastoma. Pediatr Pathol. 1993 Nov-Dec;13(6):787–96. PMID:8108298
6251. Schmitz R, Wright GW, Huang DW, et al. Genetics and pathogenesis of diffuse large B-cell lymphoma. N Engl J Med. 2018 Apr 12;378(15):1396–407. PMID:29641966
6252. Schmitz R, Young RM, Ceribelli M, et al. Burkitt lymphoma pathogenesis and therapeutic targets from structural and functional genomics. Nature. 2012 Oct 4;490(7418):116–20. PMID:22885699
6253. Schneider AB, Ron E, Lubin J, et al. Dose-response relationships for radiation-induced thyroid cancer and thyroid nodules: evidence for the prolonged effects of radiation on the thyroid. J Clin Endocrinol Metab. 1993 Aug;77(2):362–9. PMID:8345040
6254. Schneider BF, Glass WF 2nd, Brooks CH, et al. Membranous glomerulonephritis associated with testicular seminoma. J Intern Med. 1995 Jun;237(6):599–602. PMID:7782733
6255. Schneider DT, Calaminus G, Koch S, et al. Epidemiologic analysis of 1,442 children and adolescents registered in the German germ cell tumor protocols. Pediatr Blood Cancer. 2004 Feb;42(2):169–75. PMID:14752882
6256. Schneider DT, Jänig U, Calaminus G, et al. Ovarian sex cord-stromal tumors–a clinicopathological study of 72 cases from the Kiel Pediatric Tumor Registry. Virchows Arch. 2003 Oct;443(4):549–60. PMID:12910419
6257. Schneider DT, Orbach D, Cecchetto G, et al. Ovarian Sertoli Leydig cell tumours in children and adolescents: an analysis of the European Cooperative Study Group on Pediatric Rare Tumors (EXPeRT). Eur J Cancer. 2015 Mar;51(4):543–50. PMID:25514863
6258. Schneider DT, Schuster AE, Fritsch MK, et al. Multipoint imprinting analysis indicates a common precursor cell for gonadal and nongonadal pediatric germ cell tumors. Cancer Res. 2001 Oct 1;61(19):7268–76. PMID:11585765
6259. Schneider DT, Zahn S, Sievers S, et al. Molecular genetic analysis of central nervous system germ cell tumors with comparative genomic hybridization. Mod Pathol. 2006 Jun;19(6):864–73. PMID:16607373
6260. Schneider H, Vesell M. Dysgerminoma and pregnancy. Am J Obstet Gynecol. 1947 Apr;53(4):688–91. PMID:20291244
6261. Schneppenheim R, Frühwald MC, Gesk S, et al. Germline nonsense mutation and somatic inactivation of SMARCA4/BRG1 in a family with rhabdoid tumor predisposition syndrome. Am J Hum Genet. 2010 Feb 12;86(2):279–84. PMID:20137775
6262. Schniederjan MJ, Alghamdi S, Castellano-Sanchez A, et al. Diffuse leptomeningeal neuroepithelial tumor: 9 pediatric cases with chromosome 1p/19q deletion status and IDH1 (R132H) immunohistochemistry. Am J Surg Pathol. 2013 May;37(5):763–71. PMID:23588371
6263. Schöffski P, Wozniak A, Kasper B, et al. Activity and safety of crizotinib in patients with alveolar soft part sarcoma with rearrangement of TFE3: European Organization for Research and Treatment of Cancer (EORTC) phase II trial 90101 'CREATE'. Ann Oncol. 2018 Mar 1;29(3):758–65. PMID:29216400
6264. Schofield D, West DC, Anthony DC, et al. Correlation of loss of heterozygosity at chromosome 9q with histological subtype in medulloblastomas. Am J Pathol. 1995 Feb;146(2):472–80. PMID:7856756
6265. Scholfield DW, Sadozai Z, Ghali C, et al. Does osteofibrous dysplasia progress to adamantinoma and how should they be treated? Bone Joint J. 2017 Mar;99-B(3):409–16. PMID:28249983
6266. Scholtysik R, Kreuz M, Klapper W, et al. Detection of genomic aberrations in molecularly defined Burkitt's lymphoma by array-based, high resolution, single nucleotide polymorphism analysis. Haematologica. 2010 Dec;95(12):2047–55. PMID:20823134
6267. Schon K, Tischkowitz M. Clinical implications of germline mutations in breast cancer: TP53. Breast Cancer Res Treat. 2018 Jan;167(2):417–23. PMID:29039119
6268. Schönung M, Meyer J, Nöllke P, et al. International consensus definition of DNA methylation subgroups in juvenile myelomonocytic leukemia. Clin Cancer Res. 2021 Jan 1;27(1):158–68. PMID:33139265
6269. Schooler GR, Squires JH, Alazraki A, et al. Pediatric hepatoblastoma, hepatocellular carcinoma, and other hepatic neoplasms: consensus imaging recommendations from American College of Radiology Pediatric Liver Reporting and Data System (LI-RADS) Working Group. Radiology. 2020 Sep;296(3):493–7. PMID:32602829
6270. Schoolmeester JK, Xing D, Keeney GL, et al. Genital rhabdomyoma of the lower female genital tract: a study of 12 cases with molecular cytogenetic findings. Int J Gynecol Pathol. 2018 Jul;37(4):349–55. PMID:28700439
6271. Schrader KA, Nelson TN, De Luca A, et al. Multiple granular cell tumors are an associated feature of LEOPARD syndrome caused by mutation in PTPN11. Clin Genet. 2009 Feb;75(2):185–9. PMID:19054014
6272. Schramm J, Luyken C, Urbach H, et al. Evidence for a clinically distinct new subtype of grade II astrocytomas in patients with long-term epilepsy. Neurosurgery. 2004 Aug;55(2):340–7. PMID:15271240
6273. Schrappe M, Valsecchi MG, Bartram CR, et al. Late MRD response determines relapse risk overall and in subsets of childhood T-cell ALL: results of the AIEOP-BFM-ALL 2000 study. Blood. 2011 Aug 25;118(8):2077–84. PMID:21719599
6274. Schraw JM, Desrosiers TA, Nembhard WN, et al. Cancer diagnostic profile in children with structural birth defects: an assessment in 15,000 childhood cancer cases. Cancer. 2020 Aug 1;126(15):3483–92. PMID:32469081
6275. Schropp KP, Lobe TE, Rao B, et al. Sacrococcygeal teratoma: the experience of four decades. J Pediatr Surg. 1992 Aug;27(8):1075–8. PMID:1403540
6276. Schubbert S, Zenker M, Rowe SL, et al. Germline KRAS mutations cause Noonan syndrome. Nat Genet. 2006 Mar;38(3):331–6. PMID:16474405
6277. Schubert S, Abdul-Khaliq H, Lehmkuhl HB, et al. Diagnosis and treatment of post-transplantation lymphoproliferative disorder in pediatric heart transplant patients. Pediatr Transplant. 2009 Feb;13(1):54–62. PMID:18518912
6278. Schuettpelz LG, McDonald S, Whitesell K, et al. Pilocytic astrocytoma in a child with Noonan syndrome. Pediatr Blood Cancer. 2009 Dec;53(6):1147–9. PMID:19621452
6279. Schuhmacher B, Bein J, Rausch T, et al. JUNB, DUSP2, SGK1, SOCS1 and CREBBP are frequently mutated in T-cell/histiocyte-rich large B-cell lymphoma. Haematologica. 2019 Feb;104(2):330–7. PMID:30213827
6280. Schüller U, Heine VM, Mao J, et al. Acquisition of granule neuron precursor identity is a critical determinant of progenitor cell competence to form Shh-induced medulloblastoma. Cancer Cell. 2008 Aug 12;14(2):123–34. PMID:18691547
6281. Schulte JH, Schulte S, Heukamp LC, et al. Targeted therapy for neuroblastoma: ALK inhibitors. Klin Padiatr. 2013 Nov;225(6):303–8. PMID:24166094
6282. Schulte SL, Waha A, Steiger B, et al. CNS germinomas are characterized by global demethylation, chromosomal instability and mutational activation of the Kit-, Ras/Raf/Erk- and Akt-pathways. Oncotarget. 2016 Aug 23;7(34):55026–42. PMID:27391150
6283. Schultz KA, Pacheco MC, Yang J, et al. Ovarian sex cord-stromal tumors, pleuropulmonary blastoma and DICER1 mutations: a report from the International Pleuropulmonary Blastoma Registry. Gynecol Oncol. 2011 Aug;122(2):246–50. PMID:21501861
6284. Schultz KA, Yang J, Doros L, et al. DICER1-pleuropulmonary blastoma familial tumor predisposition syndrome: a unique constellation of neoplastic conditions. Pathol Case Rev. 2014 Mar;19(2):90–100. PMID:25356068
6285. Schultz KAP, Harris AK, Finch M, et al. DICER1-related Sertoli-Leydig cell tumor and gynandroblastoma: clinical and genetic findings from the International Ovarian and Testicular Stromal Tumor Registry. Gynecol Oncol. 2017 Dec;147(3):521–7. PMID:29037807
6286. Schultz KAP, Rednam SP, Kamihara J, et al. PTEN, DICER1, FH, and their associated tumor susceptibility syndromes: clinical features, genetics, and surveillance recommendations in childhood. Clin Cancer Res. 2017 Jun 15;23(12):e76–82. PMID:28620008
6287. Schultz KAP, Williams GM, Kamihara J, et al. DICER1 and associated conditions: identification of at-risk individuals and recommended surveillance strategies. Clin Cancer Res. 2018 May 15;24(10):2251–61. PMID:29343557
6288. Schutgens EM, Picci P, Baumhoer D, et al. Surgical outcome and oncological survival

of osteofibrous dysplasia-like and classic adamantinomas: an international multicenter study of 318 cases. J Bone Joint Surg Am. 2020 Oct 7;102(19):1703–13. PMID:33027124
**6289.** Schütte P, Möricke A, Zimmermann M, et al. Preexisting conditions in pediatric ALL patients: spectrum, frequency and clinical impact. Eur J Med Genet. 2016 Mar;59(3):143–51. PMID:26732628
**6290.** Schwab C, Gabrysch A, Olbrich P, et al. Phenotype, penetrance, and treatment of 133 cytotoxic T-lymphocyte antigen 4-insufficient subjects. J Allergy Clin Immunol. 2018 Dec;142(6):1932–46. PMID:29729943
**6291.** Schwab JH, Antonescu CR, Athanasian EA, et al. A comparison of intramedullary and juxtacortical low-grade osteogenic sarcoma. Clin Orthop Relat Res. 2008 Jun;466(6):1318–22. PMID:18425560
**6292.** Schwalbe EC, Hicks D, Rafiee G, et al. Minimal methylation classifier (MIMIC): a novel method for derivation and rapid diagnostic detection of disease-associated DNA methylation signatures. Sci Rep. 2017 Oct 18;7(1):13421. PMID:29044166
**6293.** Schwalbe EC, Lindsey JC, Nakjang S, et al. Novel molecular subgroups for clinical classification and outcome prediction in childhood medulloblastoma: a cohort study. Lancet Oncol. 2017 Jul;18(7):958–71. PMID:28545823
**6294.** Schwalbe EC, Williamson D, Lindsey JC, et al. DNA methylation profiling of medulloblastoma allows robust subclassification and improved outcome prediction using formalin-fixed biopsies. Acta Neuropathol. 2013 Mar;125(3):359–71. PMID:23291781
**6295.** Schwartz HS, Walker R. Recognizable magnetic resonance imaging characteristics of intramuscular myxoma. Orthopedics. 1997 May;20(5):431–5. PMID:9172250
**6296.** Schwartz HS, Zimmerman NB, Simon MA, et al. The malignant potential of enchondromatosis. J Bone Joint Surg Am. 1987 Feb;69(2):269–74. PMID:3805090
**6297.** Schwartz JR, Ma J, Lamprecht T, et al. The genomic landscape of pediatric myelodysplastic syndromes. Nat Commun. 2017 Nov 16;8(1):1557. PMID:29146900
**6298.** Schwartz RA, Torre DP. The Muir-Torre syndrome: a 25-year retrospect. J Am Acad Dermatol. 1995 Jul;33(1):90–104. PMID:7601953
**6299.** Schwartzentruber J, Korshunov A, Liu XY, et al. Driver mutations in histone H3.3 and chromatin remodelling genes in paediatric glioblastoma. Nature. 2012 Jan 29;482(7384):226–31. PMID:22286061
**6300.** Schwarz S, Zenk J, Müller M, et al. The many faces of acinic cell carcinomas of the salivary glands: a study of 40 cases relating histological and immunohistological subtypes to clinical parameters and prognosis. Histopathology. 2012 Sep;61(3):395–408. PMID:22551398
**6301.** Schwarz Y, Pitaro J, Waissbluth S, et al. Review of pediatric head and neck pilomatrixoma. Int J Pediatr Otorhinolaryngol. 2016 Jun;85:148–53. PMID:27240514
**6302.** Schwock J, Geddie WR. Diagnosis of B-cell non-hodgkin lymphomas with small-/intermediate-sized cells in cytopathology. Patholog Res Int. 2012;2012:164934. PMID:22693682
**6303.** Sciot R, Dorfman H, Brys P, et al. Cytogenetic-morphologic correlations in aneurysmal bone cyst, giant cell tumor of bone and combined lesions. A report from the CHAMP study group. Mod Pathol. 2000 Nov;13(11):1206–10. PMID:11106078
**6304.** Scognamiglio T, Hyjek E, Kao J, et al. Diagnostic usefulness of HBME1, galectin-3, CK19, and CITED1 and evaluation of their expression in encapsulated lesions with questionable features of papillary thyroid carcinoma. Am J Clin Pathol. 2006 Nov;126(5):700–8. PMID:17050067
**6305.** Scollon S, Anglin AK, Thomas M, et al. A comprehensive review of pediatric tumors and associated cancer predisposition syndromes. J Genet Couns. 2017 Jun;26(3):387–434. PMID:28357779
**6306.** Scott A, Upadhyay V. Carcinoid tumours of the appendix in children in Auckland, New Zealand: 1965-2008. N Z Med J. 2011 Mar 25;124(1331):56–60. PMID:21725413
**6307.** Scott JX, Krishnan S, Bourne AJ, et al. Treatment of metastatic sialoblastoma with chemotherapy and surgery. Pediatr Blood Cancer. 2008 Jan;50(1):134–7. PMID:16514617
**6308.** Scott RH, Stiller CA, Walker L, et al. Syndromes and constitutional chromosomal abnormalities associated with Wilms tumour. J Med Genet. 2006 Sep;43(9):705–15. PMID:16690728
**6309.** Scully RE. Gonadoblastoma. A review of 74 cases. Cancer. 1970 Jun;25(6):1340–56. PMID:4193741
**6310.** Scully RE. Gonadoblastoma; a gonadal tumor related to the dysgerminoma (seminoma) and capable of sex-hormone production. Cancer. 1953 May;6(3):455–63. PMID:13042769
**6311.** Scully RE. Sex cord tumor with annular tubules a distinctive ovarian tumor of the Peutz-Jeghers syndrome. Cancer. 1970 May;25(5):1107–21. PMID:5429475
**6312.** Scully RE. The prolonged gestation, birth, and early life of the sex cord tumor with annular tubules and how it joined a syndrome. Int J Surg Pathol. 2000 Jul;8(3):233–8. PMID:11493995
**6313.** Scully RE, Young RH, Clement PB. Tumors of the ovary, maldeveloped gonads, fallopian tube and broad ligament. Washington, DC: Armed Forces Institute of Pathology; 1998. (AFIP atlas of tumor pathology, series 3; fascicle 23).
**6314.** Sebire NJ, Ramsay AD, Malone M, et al. Extensive posttreatment ganglioneuromatous differentiation of rhabdomyosarcoma: malignant ectomesenchymoma in an infant. Pediatr Dev Pathol. 2003 Jan-Feb;6(1):94–6. PMID:12469232
**6315.** Sebro R, DeLaney T, Hornicek F, et al. Differences in sex distribution, anatomic location and MR imaging appearance of pediatric compared to adult chordomas. BMC Med Imaging. 2016 Sep 8;16(1):53. PMID:27609115
**6316.** Seefelder C, Sparks JW, Chirnomas D, et al. Perioperative management of a child with severe hypertension from a catecholamine secreting neuroblastoma. Paediatr Anaesth. 2005 Jul;15(7):606–10. PMID:15960647
**6317.** Seeger RC, Brodeur GM, Sather H, et al. Association of multiple copies of the N-myc oncogene with rapid progression of neuroblastomas. N Engl J Med. 1985 Oct 31;313(18):1111–6. PMID:4047115
**6318.** Seegmiller AC, Kroft SH, Karandikar NJ, et al. Characterization of immunophenotypic aberrancies in 200 cases of B acute lymphoblastic leukemia. Am J Clin Pathol. 2009 Dec;132(6):940–9. PMID:19926587
**6319.** Seemayer TA, Gross TG, Egeler RM, et al. X-linked lymphoproliferative disease: twenty-five years after the discovery. Pediatr Res. 1995 Oct;38(4):471–8. PMID:8559596
**6320.** Seethala RR, Chiosea SI. MAML2 Status in mucoepidermoid carcinoma can no longer be considered a prognostic marker. Am J Surg Pathol. 2016 Aug;40(8):1151–3. PMID:27299797
**6321.** Seethala RR, Dacic S, Cieply K, et al. A reappraisal of the MECT1/MAML2 translocation in salivary mucoepidermoid carcinomas. Am J Surg Pathol. 2010 Aug;34(8):1106–21. PMID:20588178
**6321A.** Seguí N, Mina LB, Lázaro C, et al. Germline mutations in FAN1 cause hereditary colorectal cancer by impairing DNA repair. Gastroenterology. 2015 Sep;149(3):563–6. PMID:26052075
**6322.** Séguier-Lipszyc E, Baazov A, Fichman S, et al. Current management of lipoblastoma. Eur J Pediatr. 2018 Feb;177(2):237–41. PMID:29243188
**6323.** Seidemann K, Tiemann M, Henze G, et al. Therapy for non-Hodgkin lymphoma in children with primary immunodeficiency: analysis of 19 patients from the BFM trials. Med Pediatr Oncol. 1999 Dec;33(6):536–44. PMID:10573576
**6324.** Seidemann K, Tiemann M, Schrappe M, et al. Short-pulse B-non-Hodgkin lymphoma-type chemotherapy is efficacious treatment for pediatric anaplastic large cell lymphoma: a report of the Berlin-Frankfurt-Münster Group Trial NHL-BFM 90. Blood. 2001 Jun 15;97(12):3699–706. PMID:11389005
**6325.** Seifert G, Donath K. Classification of the pathohistology of diseases of the salivary glands - review of 2,600 cases in the Salivary Gland Register. Beitr Pathol. 1976 Oct;159(1):1–32. PMID:999595
**6326.** Seifert G, Langrock I, Donath K. [A pathological classification of pleomorphic adenoma of the salivary glands (author's transl)]. HNO. 1976 Dec;24(12):415–26. German. PMID:1002574
**6327.** Seijas R, Ares O, Sierra J, et al. Oncogenic osteomalacia: two case reports with surprisingly different outcomes. Arch Orthop Trauma Surg. 2009 Apr;129(4):533–9. PMID:19125258
**6328.** Seket B, Saurin JC, Scoazec JY, et al. [Pancreatic acinar cell carcinoma in a patient with familial adenomatous polyposis]. Gastroenterol Clin Biol. 2003 Aug-Sep;27(8-9):818–20. French. PMID:14586255
**6329.** Seki M, Yoshida K, Shiraishi Y, et al. Biallelic DICER1 mutations in sporadic pleuropulmonary blastoma. Cancer Res. 2014 May 15;74(10):2742–9. PMID:24675358
**6330.** Sekimizu M, Yoshida A, Mitani S, et al. Frequent mutations of genes encoding vacuolar H+ -ATPase components in granular cell tumors. Genes Chromosomes Cancer. 2019 Jun;58(6):373–80. PMID:30597645
**6331.** Sekine S, Ogawa R, Saito S, et al. Cytoplasmic MSH2 immunoreactivity in a patient with Lynch syndrome with an EPCAM-MSH2 fusion. Histopathology. 2017 Mar;70(4):664–9. PMID:27896849
**6332.** Sekine S, Shibata T, Kokubu A, et al. Craniopharyngiomas of adamantinomatous type harbor beta-catenin gene mutations. Am J Pathol. 2002 Dec;161(6):1997–2001. PMID:12466115
**6333.** Šekoranja D, Boštjančič E, Salapura V, et al. Primary aneurysmal bone cyst with a novel SPARC-USP6 translocation identified by next-generation sequencing. Cancer Genet. 2018 Dec;228-229:12–6. PMID:30553465
**6334.** Šekoranja D, Vergot K, Hawlina G, et al. Combined deep penetrating nevi of the conjunctiva are relatively common lesions characterised by BRAFV600E mutation and activation of the beta catenin pathway: a clinicopathological analysis of 34 lesions. Br J Ophthalmol. 2020 Jul;104(7):1016–21. PMID:31558492
**6335.** Šekoranja D, Zupan A, Mavčič B, et al. Novel ASAP1-USP6, FAT1-USP6, SAR1A-USP6, and TNC-USP6 fusions in primary aneurysmal bone cyst. Genes Chromosomes Cancer. 2020 Jun;59(6):357–65. PMID:32011035
**6336.** Selby DM, Stocker JT, Ishak KG. Angiosarcoma of the liver in childhood: a clinicopathologic and follow-up study of 10 cases. Pediatr Pathol. 1992 Jul-Aug;12(4):485–98. PMID:1409148
**6337.** Selenica P, Raj N, Kumar R, et al. Solid pseudopapillary neoplasms of the pancreas are dependent on the Wnt pathway. Mol Oncol. 2019 Aug;13(8):1684–92. PMID:30972907
**6338.** Selle B, Furtwängler R, Graf N, et al. Population-based study of renal cell carcinoma in children in Germany, 1980-2005: more frequently localized tumors and underlying disorders compared with adult counterparts. Cancer. 2006 Dec 15;107(12):2906–14. PMID:17109448
**6339.** Semmelink HJ, Pruszczynski M, Wiersma-van Tilburg A, et al. Cytokeratin expression in chondroblastomas. Histopathology. 1990 Mar;16(3):257–63. PMID:1692005
**6340.** Sencan A, Mir E, Sencan AB, et al. Intrascrotal paratesticular rhabdomyoma: a case report. Acta Paediatr. 2000 Aug;89(8):1020–2. PMID:10976850
**6341.** Senoo H, Iida S, Kishino M, et al. Solitary congenital granular cell lesion of the tongue. Oral Surg Oral Med Oral Pathol Oral Radiol Endod. 2007 Jul;104(1):e45–8. PMID:17577543
**6342.** Seppälä T, Pylvänäinen K, Evans DG, et al. Colorectal cancer incidence in path_MLH1 carriers subjected to different follow-up protocols: a Prospective Lynch Syndrome Database report. Hered Cancer Clin Pract. 2017 Oct 10;15:18. PMID:29046738
**6343.** Septer S, Slowik V, Morgan R, et al. Thyroid cancer complicating familial adenomatous polyposis: mutation spectrum of at-risk individuals. Hered Cancer Clin Pract. 2013 Oct 5;11(1):13. PMID:24093640
**6344.** Seregard S. Phakomatous choristoma may be located in the eyelid or orbit or both. Acta Ophthalmol Scand. 1999 Jun;77(3):343–6. PMID:10406159
**6345.** Serrano-Villar S, Vásquez-Domínguez E, Pérez-Molina JA, et al. HIV, HPV, and microbiota: partners in crime? AIDS. 2017 Feb 20;31(4):591–4. PMID:27922858
**6346.** Sethi S, Tageja N, Singh J, et al. Hyperammonemic encephalopathy: a rare presentation of fibrolamellar hepatocellular carcinoma. Am J Med Sci. 2009 Dec;338(6):522–4. PMID:20010160
**6347.** Sethia R, Rawlins KW, Aljasser A, et al. Pediatric nasopharyngeal fibrolipoma: a case report and review of the literature. Int J Pediatr Otorhinolaryngol. 2019 Oct;125:103–6. PMID:31276891
**6348.** Settas N, Faucz FR, Stratakis CA. Succinate dehydrogenase (SDH) deficiency, Carney triad and the epigenome. Mol Cell Endocrinol. 2018 Jul 5;469:107–11. PMID:28739378
**6349.** Setty BA, Jinesh GG, Arnold M, et al. The genomic landscape of undifferentiated embryonal sarcoma of the liver is typified by C19MC structural rearrangement and overexpression combined with TP53 mutation or loss. PLoS Genet. 2020 Apr 20;16(4):e1008642. PMID:32310940
**6350.** Sévenet N, Sheridan E, Amram D, et al. Constitutional mutations of the hSNF5/INI1 gene predispose to a variety of cancers. Am J Hum Genet. 1999 Nov;65(5):1342–8. PMID:10521299
**6351.** Sevinir B, Ozkan TB. Infantile hepatic hemangioendothelioma: clinical presentation and treatment. Turk J Gastroenterol. 2007 Sep;18(3):182–7. PMID:17891692
**6352.** Sferopoulos NK, Kotakidou R, Petropoulos AS. Myositis ossificans in children: a review. Eur J Orthop Surg Traumatol. 2017 May;27(4):491–502. PMID:28275867
**6353.** Sforza-Huffman C. Cytology of fibrous hamartoma of infancy: a helpful approach for an uncommon soft tissue lesion. Acta Cytol. 2008 Mar-Apr;52(2):123. PMID:18499982
**6354.** Shabani M, Nichols KE, Rezaei N. Primary immunodeficiencies associated with

EBV-Induced lymphoproliferative disorders. Crit Rev Oncol Hematol. 2016 Dec;108:109–27. PMID:27931829
6355. Shaco-Levy R, Peng RY, Snyder MJ, et al. Malignant struma ovarii: a blinded study of 86 cases assessing which histologic features correlate with aggressive clinical behavior. Arch Pathol Lab Med. 2012 Feb;136(2):172–8. PMID:22288964
6356. Shafizadeh N, Ferrell LD, Kakar S. Utility and limitations of glypican-3 expression for the diagnosis of hepatocellular carcinoma at both ends of the differentiation spectrum. Mod Pathol. 2008 Aug;21(8):1011–8. PMID:18536657
6357. Shah AH, Khatib Z, Niazi T. Extracranial extra-CNS spread of embryonal tumor with multilayered rosettes (ETMR): case series and systematic review. Childs Nerv Syst. 2018 Apr;34(4):649–54. PMID:29177676
6358. Shah AY, Karam JA, Malouf GG, et al. Management and outcomes of patients with renal medullary carcinoma: a multicentre collaborative study. BJU Int. 2017 Dec;120(6):782–92. PMID:27860149
6359. Shah KK, McHugh JB, Folpe AL, et al. Dermatofibrosarcoma protuberans of distal extremities and acral sites: a clinicopathologic analysis of 27 cases. Am J Surg Pathol. 2018 Mar;42(3):413–9. PMID:29240584
6360. Shah R, Xia C, Krailo M, et al. Is carboplatin-based chemotherapy as effective as cisplatin-based chemotherapy in the treatment of advanced-stage dysgerminoma in children, adolescents and young adults? Gynecol Oncol. 2018 Aug;150(2):253–60. PMID:29884437
6361. Shah S, Schrader KA, Waanders E, et al. A recurrent germline PAX5 mutation confers susceptibility to pre-B cell acute lymphoblastic leukemia. Nat Genet. 2013 Oct;45(10):1226–31. PMID:24013638
6362. Shah SP, Köbel M, Senz J, et al. Mutation of FOXL2 in granulosa-cell tumors of the ovary. N Engl J Med. 2009 Jun 25;360(26):2719–29. PMID:19516027
6363. Shah SS, Chandan VS, Wilbur DC, et al. Glial fibrillary acidic protein and CD57 immunolocalization in cell block preparations is a useful adjunct in the diagnosis of pleomorphic adenoma. Arch Pathol Lab Med. 2007 Sep;131(9):1373–7. PMID:17824792
6364. Shah U, Giubellino A, Pacak K. Pheochromocytoma: implications in tumorigenesis and the actual management. Minerva Endocrinol. 2012 Jun;37(2):141–56. PMID:22691888
6365. Shaher RM, Mintzer J, Farina M, et al. Clinical presentation of rhabdomyoma of the heart in infancy and childhood. Am J Cardiol. 1972 Jul 11;30(1):95–103. PMID:4260837
6366. Shahid M, Dhillon VS, Khalil HS, et al. A SRY-HMG box frame shift mutation inherited from a mosaic father with a mild form of testicular dysgenesis syndrome in Turner syndrome patient. BMC Med Genet. 2010 Sep 19;11:131. PMID:20849656
6367. Shain AH, Yeh I, Kovalyshyn I, et al. The genetic evolution of melanoma from precursor lesions. N Engl J Med. 2015 Nov 12;373(20):1926–36. PMID:26559571
6368. Shakur SF, McGirt MJ, Johnson MW, et al. Angiocentric glioma: a case series. J Neurosurg Pediatr. 2009 Mar;3(3):197–202. PMID:19338465
6369. Shalaby A, Presneau N, Ye H, et al. The role of epidermal growth factor receptor in chordoma pathogenesis: a potential therapeutic target. J Pathol. 2011 Feb;223(3):336–46. PMID:21171079
6370. Shallop B, Abraham JA. Synovial chondromatosis of pes anserine bursa secondary to osteochondroma. Orthopedics. 2014 Aug;37(8):e735–8. PMID:25102510
6371. Sham JS, Poon YF, Wei WI, et al. Nasopharyngeal carcinoma in young patients. Cancer. 1990 Jun 1;65(11):2606–10. PMID:2337878
6372. Shankar AG, Kirkwood AA, Depani S, et al. Relapsed or poorly responsive nodular lymphocyte predominant Hodgkin lymphoma in children and adolescents - a report from the United Kingdom's Children's Cancer and Leukaemia Study Group. Br J Haematol. 2016 May;173(3):421–31. PMID:26996288
6373. Shankar AG, Kirkwood AA, Hall GW, et al. Childhood and adolescent nodular lymphocyte predominant Hodgkin lymphoma - a review of clinical outcome based on the histological variants. Br J Haematol. 2015 Oct;171(2):254–62. PMID:26115355
6374. Shankar GM, Abedalthagafi M, Vaubel RA, et al. Germline and somatic BAP1 mutations in high-grade rhabdoid meningiomas. Neuro Oncol. 2017 Apr 1;19(4):535–45. PMID:28170043
6375. Shankar GM, Santagata S. BAP1 mutations in high-grade meningioma: implications for patient care. Neuro Oncol. 2017 Oct 19;19(11):1447–56. PMID:28482042
6376. Shanley S, Ratcliffe J, Hockey A, et al. Nevoid basal cell carcinoma syndrome: review of 118 affected individuals. Am J Med Genet. 1994 Apr 15;50(3):282–90. PMID:8042673
6377. Shanmuganathan N, Branford S. The hidden pathogenesis of CML: Is BCR-ABL1 the first event? Curr Hematol Malig Rep. 2019 Dec;14(6):501–6. PMID:31696382
6378. Shanmugaratnam K, Chan SH, de-Thé G, et al. Histopathology of nasopharyngeal carcinoma: correlations with epidemiology, survival rates and other biological characteristics. Cancer. 1979 Sep;44(3):1029–44. PMID:225002
6379. Shapiro RS, Stool SE, Snow JB Jr, et al. Parapharyngeal rhabdomyoma. Arch Otolaryngol. 1975 May;101(5):323–6. PMID:1131092
6380. Sharaf AF, Hamouda ES, Teo JG. Bilateral thalamic and right fronto-temporo-parietal gliomas in a 4 years old child diagnosed by magnetic resonance imaging. J Radiol Case Rep. 2016 Jan 31;10(1):1–13. PMID:27200150
6381. Sharara NA, Alexander RA, Luthert PJ, et al. Differential immunoreactivity of melanocytic lesions of the conjunctiva. Histopathology. 2001 Oct;39(4):426–31. PMID:11683945
6382. Sharif K, Ramani P, Lochbühler H, et al. Recurrent mesenchymal hamartoma associated with 19q translocation. A call for more radical surgical resection. Eur J Pediatr Surg. 2006 Feb;16(1):64–7. PMID:16544232
6383. Sharif S, Ferner R, Birch JM, et al. Second primary tumors in neurofibromatosis 1 patients treated for optic glioma: substantial risks after radiotherapy. J Clin Oncol. 2006 Jun 1;24(16):2570–5. PMID:16735710
6384. Sharma H, Jane MJ, Reid R. Pigmented villonodular synovitis of the foot and ankle: forty years of experience from the Scottish bone tumor registry. J Foot Ankle Surg. 2006 Sep-Oct;45(5):329–36. PMID:16949531
6385. Sharma H, Rana B, Mahendra A, et al. Outcome of 17 pigmented villonodular synovitis (PVNS) of the knee at 6 years mean follow-up. Knee. 2007 Oct;14(5):390–4. PMID:17600720
6386. Sharma M, Ralte A, Arora R, et al. Subependymal giant cell astrocytoma: a clinicopathological study of 23 cases with special emphasis on proliferative markers and expression of p53 and retinoblastoma gene proteins. Pathology. 2004 Apr;36(2):139–44. PMID:15203749
6387. Sharma MC, Ralte AM, Gaekwad S, et al. Subependymal giant cell astrocytoma–a clinicopathological study of 23 cases with special emphasis on histogenesis. Pathol Oncol Res. 2004;10(4):219–24. PMID:15619643
6388. Sharma MK, Mansur DB, Reifenberger G, et al. Distinct genetic signatures among pilocytic astrocytomas relate to their brain region origin. Cancer Res. 2007 Feb 1;67(3):890–900. PMID:17283119
6389. Sharma MK, Zehnbauer BA, Watson MA, et al. RAS pathway activation and an oncogenic RAS mutation in sporadic pilocytic astrocytoma. Neurology. 2005 Oct 25;65(8):1335–6. PMID:16247081
6390. Sharma P, Shakya U, Sayami G, et al. Lipoblastoma: an unusual tumour of the left ventricle. Eur J Cardiothorac Surg. 2016 May;49(5):e147–8. PMID:26819289
6391. Sharma P, Shields CL, Turaka K, et al. Ciliary body medulloepithelioma with neoplastic cyclitic membrane imaging with fluorescein angiography and ultrasound biomicroscopy. Graefes Arch Clin Exp Ophthalmol. 2011 Aug;249(8):1259–61. PMID:21505878
6392. Sharma S, Mishra K, Khanna G. Fibromatosis colli in infants. A cytologic study of eight cases. Acta Cytol. 2003 May-Jun;47(3):359–62. PMID:12789914
6393. Sharma T, Schwalbe EC, Williamson D, et al. Second-generation molecular subgrouping of medulloblastoma: an international meta-analysis of Group 3 and Group 4 subtypes. Acta Neuropathol. 2019 Aug;138(2):309–26. PMID:31076851
6394. Shaw RK, Issekutz AC, Fraser R, et al. Bilateral adrenal EBV-associated smooth muscle tumors in a child with a natural killer cell deficiency. Blood. 2012 Apr 26;119(17):4009–12. PMID:22427204
6395. Shehata BM, Gupta NA, Katzenstein HM, et al. Undifferentiated embryonal sarcoma of the liver is associated with mesenchymal hamartoma and multiple chromosomal abnormalities: a review of eleven cases. Pediatr Dev Pathol. 2011 Mar-Apr;14(2):111–6. PMID:20925497
6396. Shehata BM, Steelman CK, Abramowsky CR, et al. NUT midline carcinoma in a newborn with multiorgan disseminated tumor and a 2-year-old with a pancreatic/hepatic primary. Pediatr Dev Pathol. 2010 Nov-Dec;13(6):481–5. PMID:20017639
6397. Shelekhova KV, Kazakov DV, Hes O, et al. Phosphaturic mesenchymal tumor (mixed connective tissue variant): a case report with spectral analysis. Virchows Arch. 2006 Feb;448(2):232–5. PMID:16447065
6398. Shen C, Gao Y, Xu T, et al. Carcinoma of the nasopharynx in young patients: a single institution experience. Clin Oncol (R Coll Radiol). 2009 Oct;21(8):617–22. PMID:19660923
6399. Shen H, Shih J, Hollern DP, et al. Integrated molecular characterization of testicular germ cell tumors. Cell Rep. 2018 Jun 12;23(11):3392–406. PMID:29898407
6400. Shen LY, Amin SM, Chamlin SL, et al. Varied presentations of pediatric lipoblastoma: case series and review of the literature. Pediatr Dermatol. 2017 Mar;34(2):180–6. PMID:28111780
6401. Shen T, Zhuang Z, Gersell DJ, et al. Allelic deletion of VHL gene detected in papillary tumors of the broad ligament, epididymis, and retroperitoneum in von Hippel-Lindau disease patients. Int J Surg Pathol. 2000 Jul;8(3):207–12. PMID:11493991
6402. Shepherd CW, Gomez MR, Lie JT, et al. Causes of death in patients with tuberous sclerosis. Mayo Clin Proc. 1991 Aug;66(8):792–6. PMID:1861550
6403. Shepherd CW, Houser OW, Gomez MR. MR findings in tuberous sclerosis complex and correlation with seizure development and mental impairment. AJNR Am J Neuroradiol. 1995 Jan;16(1):149–55. PMID:7900584
6404. Shern JF, Chen L, Chmielecki J, et al. Comprehensive genomic analysis of rhabdomyosarcoma reveals a landscape of alterations affecting a common genetic axis in fusion-positive and fusion-negative tumors. Cancer Discov. 2014 Feb;4(2):216–31. PMID:24436047
6405. Shern JF, Selfe J, Izquierdo E, et al. Genomic classification and clinical outcome in rhabdomyosarcoma: a report from an international consortium. J Clin Oncol. 2021 Sep 10;39(26):2859–71. PMID:34166060
6406. Shern JF, Yohe ME, Khan J. Pediatric rhabdomyosarcoma. Crit Rev Oncog. 2015;20(3-4):227–43. PMID:26349418
6407. Shet NS, Cole BL, Iyer RS. Imaging of pediatric pancreatic neoplasms with radiologic-histopathologic correlation. AJR Am J Roentgenol. 2014 Jun;202(6):1337–48. PMID:24848833
6408. Shet T, Borges A, Nair C, et al. Two unusual lesions in the nasal cavity of infants–a nasal chondromesenchymal hamartoma and an aneurysmal bone cyst like lesion. More closely related than we think? Int J Pediatr Otorhinolaryngol. 2004 Mar;68(3):359–64. PMID:15129948
6409. Shet T, Ramadwar M, Sharma S, et al. An eyelid sialoblastoma-like tumor with a sarcomatoid myoepithelial component. Pediatr Dev Pathol. 2007 Jul-Aug;10(4):309–14. PMID:17638426
6410. Shi M, Roemer MG, Chapuy B, et al. Expression of programmed cell death 1 ligand 2 (PD-L2) is a distinguishing feature of primary mediastinal (thymic) large B-cell lymphoma and associated with PDCD1LG2 copy gain. Am J Surg Pathol. 2014 Dec;38(12):1715–23. PMID:25025450
6411. Shi Y, Rojas Y, Zhang W, et al. Characteristics and outcomes in children with undifferentiated embryonal sarcoma of the liver: a report from the National Cancer Database. Pediatr Blood Cancer. 2017 Apr;64(4):e26272. PMID:27781381
6412. Shia J, Holck S, Depetris G, et al. Lynch syndrome-associated neoplasms: a discussion on histopathology and immunohistochemistry. Fam Cancer. 2013 Jun;12(2):241–60. PMID:23435936
6413. Shia J, Zhang L, Shike M, et al. Secondary mutation in a coding mononucleotide tract in MSH6 causes loss of immunoexpression of MSH6 in colorectal carcinomas with MLH1/PMS2 deficiency. Mod Pathol. 2013 Jan;26(1):131–8. PMID:22918162
6414. Shiba N, Yoshida K, Hara Y, et al. Transcriptome analysis offers a comprehensive illustration of the genetic background of pediatric acute myeloid leukemia. Blood Adv. 2019 Oct 22;3(20):3157–69. PMID:31648321
6415. Shibamoto Y, Takahashi M, Sasai K. Prognosis of intracranial germinoma with syncytiotrophoblastic giant cells treated by radiation therapy. Int J Radiat Oncol Biol Phys. 1997 Feb 1;37(3):505–10. PMID:9112445
6416. Shibata Y, Yamazaki M, Takei M, et al. Early-onset, severe, and recurrent primary hyperparathyroidism associated with a novel CDC73 mutation. Endocr J. 2015;62(7):627–32. PMID:25959515
6417. Shibayama T, Okamoto T, Nakashima Y, et al. Screening of BCOR-CCNB3 sarcoma using immunohistochemistry for CCNB3: a clinicopathological report of three pediatric cases. Pathol Int. 2015 Aug;65(8):410–4. PMID:26037154
6418. Shibuya R, Matsuyama A, Shiba E, et al. CAMTA1 is a useful immunohistochemical marker for diagnosing epithelioid haemangioendothelioma. Histopathology. 2015 Dec;67(6):827–35. PMID:25879300
6419. Shields CL, Demirci H, Karatza E, et al. Clinical survey of 1643 melanocytic

and nonmelanocytic conjunctival tumors. Ophthalmology. 2004 Sep;111(9):1747–54. PMID:15350332
6420. Shields CL, Douglass AM, Beggache M, et al. Intravitreous chemotherapy for active vitreous seeding from retinoblastoma: outcomes after 192 consecutive injections. The 2015 Howard Naquin Lecture. Retina. 2016 Jun;36(6):1184–90. PMID:26630319
6421. Shields CL, Fasiuddin AF, Mashayekhi A, et al. Conjunctival nevi: clinical features and natural course in 410 consecutive patients. Arch Ophthalmol. 2004 Feb;122(2):167–75. PMID:14769591
6422. Shields CL, Ghassemi F, Tuncer S, et al. Clinical spectrum of diffuse infiltrating retinoblastoma in 34 consecutive eyes. Ophthalmology. 2008 Dec;115(12):2253–8. PMID:18962920
6423. Shields CL, Mashayekhi A, Cater J, et al. Chemoreduction for retinoblastoma: analysis of tumor control and risks for recurrence in 457 tumors. Trans Am Ophthalmol Soc. 2004;102:35–44. PMID:15747743
6424. Shields CL, Qureshi A, Eagle RC Jr, et al. Epibulbar osseous choristoma in 8 patients. Cornea. 2012 Jul;31(7):756–60. PMID:22516954
6425. Shields JA, Eagle RC Jr, Ferguson K, et al. Tumors of the nonpigmented epithelium of the ciliary body: the Lorenz E. Zimmerman Tribute Lecture. Retina. 2015 May;35(5):957–65. PMID:25545484
6426. Shields JA, Eagle RC Jr, Shields CL, et al. Congenital neoplasms of the nonpigmented ciliary epithelium (medulloepithelioma). Ophthalmology. 1996 Dec;103(12):1998–2006. PMID:9003333
6427. Shields JA, Eagle RC Jr, Shields CL, et al. Pigmented medulloepithelioma of the ciliary body. Arch Ophthalmol. 2002 Feb;120(2):207–10. PMID:11831926
6428. Shields JA, Shields CL, Suvarnamani C, et al. Retinoblastoma manifesting as orbital cellulitis. Am J Ophthalmol. 1991 Oct 15;112(4):442–9. PMID:1928248
6429. Shih AR, Chebib I, Deshpande V, et al. Molecular characteristics of poorly differentiated chordoma. Genes Chromosomes Cancer. 2019 Nov;58(11):804–8. PMID:31135077
6430. Shih AR, Cote GM, Chebib I, et al. Clinicopathologic characteristics of poorly differentiated chordoma. Mod Pathol. 2018 Aug;31(8):1237–45. PMID:29483606
6431. Shih DJ, Northcott PA, Remke M, et al. Cytogenetic prognostication within medulloblastoma subgroups. J Clin Oncol. 2014 Mar 20;32(9):886–96. PMID:24493713
6432. Shimada H. In situ neuroblastoma: an important concept related to the natural history of neural crest tumors. Pediatr Dev Pathol. 2005 May-Jun;8(3):305–6. PMID:16010489
6433. Shimada H, Ambros IM, Dehner LP, et al. Terminology and morphologic criteria of neuroblastic tumors: recommendations by the International Neuroblastoma Pathology Committee. Cancer. 1999 Jul 15;86(2):349–63. PMID:10421272
6434. Shimada H, Ambros IM, Dehner LP, et al. The International Neuroblastoma Pathology Classification (the Shimada system). Cancer. 1999 Jul 15;86(2):364–72. PMID:10421273
6435. Shimada H, Aoyama C, Chiba T, et al. Prognostic subgroups for undifferentiated neuroblastoma: immunohistochemical study with anti-S-100 protein antibody. Hum Pathol. 1985 May;16(5):471–6. PMID:3886523
6436. Shimada H, Stram DO, Chatten J, et al. Identification of subsets of neuroblastomas by combined histopathologic and N-myc analysis. J Natl Cancer Inst. 1995 Oct 4;87(19):1470–6. PMID:7674334
6437. Shimada H, Umehara S, Monobe Y, et al. International neuroblastoma pathology classification for prognostic evaluation of patients with peripheral neuroblastic tumors: a report from the Children's Cancer Group. Cancer. 2001 Nov 1;92(9):2451–61. PMID:11745303
6438. Shimada T, Mizutani S, Muto T, et al. Cloning and characterization of FGF23 as a causative factor of tumor-induced osteomalacia. Proc Natl Acad Sci U S A. 2001 May 22;98(11):6500–5. PMID:11344269
6439. Shimada T, Urakawa I, Yamazaki Y, et al. FGF-23 transgenic mice demonstrate hypophosphatemic rickets with reduced expression of sodium phosphate cotransporter type IIa. Biochem Biophys Res Commun. 2004 Feb 6;314(2):409–14. PMID:14733920
6440. Shimizu S, Hashimoto H, Enjoji M. Nodular fasciitis: an analysis of 250 patients. Pathology. 1984 Apr;16(2):161–6. PMID:6462780
6441. Shin BK, Kim MK, Park SH, et al. Fine-needle aspiration cytology of pleuropulmonary blastoma: a case report with unusual features. Diagn Cytopathol. 2001 Dec;25(6):397–402. PMID:11747237
6442. Shin DH, Lee JH, Kang HJ, et al. Novel epitheliomesenchymal biphasic stomach tumour (gastroblastoma) in a 9-year-old: morphological, ultrastructural and immunohistochemical findings. J Clin Pathol. 2010 Mar;63(3):270–4. PMID:20203230
6443. Shin SA, Ahn B, Kim SK, et al. Brainstem astroblastoma with MN1 translocation. Neuropathology. 2018 Dec;38(6):631–7. PMID:30238518
6444. Shinar E, Gershon ZL, Leiserowitz R, et al. Coexistence of Gaucher disease and Philadelphia positive chronic granulocytic leukemia. Am J Hematol. 1982 Apr;12(2):199–202. PMID:6951408
6445. Shing DC, McMullan DJ, Roberts P, et al. FUS/ERG gene fusions in Ewing's tumors. Cancer Res. 2003 Aug 1;63(15):4568–76. PMID:12907633
6446. Shinkai T, Masumoto K, Ono K, et al. A case of unusual histology of infantile lipoblastoma confirmed by PLAG1 rearrangement. Surg Case Rep. 2015 Dec;1(1):42. PMID:26943407
6447. Shinoda J, Sakai N, Yano H, et al. Prognostic factors and therapeutic problems of primary intracranial choriocarcinoma/germ-cell tumors with high levels of HCG. J Neurooncol. 2004 Jan;66(1-2):225–40. PMID:15015791
6448. Shinohara M, Komatsu H, Kawamura T, et al. Familial testicular teratoma in 2 children: familial report and review of the literature. J Urol. 1980 Apr;123(4):552–5. PMID:7365898
6449. Shinohara M, Shitara T, Hatakeyama SI, et al. An infant with systemic hypertension, renal artery stenosis, and neuroblastoma. J Pediatr Surg. 2004 Jan;39(1):103–6. PMID:14694383
6450. Shirahata M, Ono T, Stichel D, et al. Novel, improved grading system(s) for IDH-mutant astrocytic gliomas. Acta Neuropathol. 2018 Jul;136(1):153–66. PMID:29687258
6451. Shiran SI, Ben-Sira L, Elhasid R, et al. Multiple brain developmental venous anomalies as a marker for constitutional mismatch repair deficiency syndrome. AJNR Am J Neuroradiol. 2018 Oct;39(10):1943–6. PMID:30166433
6452. Shirley MD, Tang H, Gallione CJ, et al. Sturge-Weber syndrome and port-wine stains caused by somatic mutation in GNAQ. N Engl J Med. 2013 May 23;368(21):1971–9. PMID:23656586
6453. Shitara S, Tokime T, Akiyama Y. Multinodular and vacuolating neuronal tumor: a case report and literature review. Surg Neurol Int. 2018 Mar 19;9:63. PMID:29629230
6454. Shkalim Zemer V, Toledano H, Kornreich L, et al. Sporadic desmoid tumors in the pediatric population: a single center experience and review of the literature. J Pediatr Surg. 2017 Oct;52(10):1637–41. PMID:28209418
6455. Shlien A, Campbell BB, de Borja R, et al. Combined hereditary and somatic mutations of replication error repair genes result in rapid onset of ultra-hypermutated cancers. Nat Genet. 2015 Mar;47(3):257–62. PMID:25642631
6456. Shmookler BM, Enzinger FM, Weiss SW. Giant cell fibroblastoma. A juvenile form of dermatofibrosarcoma protuberans. Cancer. 1989 Nov 15;64(10):2154–61. PMID:2804904
6457. Shore EM, Xu M, Feldman GJ, et al. A recurrent mutation in the BMP type I receptor ACVR1 causes inherited and sporadic fibrodysplasia ossificans progressiva. Nat Genet. 2006 May;38(5):525–7. PMID:16642017
6458. Shore RE, Hildreth N, Dvoretsky P, et al. Thyroid cancer among persons given X-ray treatment in infancy for an enlarged thymus gland. Am J Epidemiol. 1993 May 15;137(10):1068–80. PMID:8317436
6459. Short MP, Richardson EP Jr, Haines JL, et al. Clinical, neuropathological and genetic aspects of the tuberous sclerosis complex. Brain Pathol. 1995 Apr;5(2):173–9. PMID:7670658
6460. Shorter NA, Glick RD, Klimstra DS, et al. Malignant pancreatic tumors in childhood and adolescence: the Memorial Sloan-Kettering experience, 1967 to present. J Pediatr Surg. 2002 Jun;37(6):887–92. PMID:12037756
6461. Shuch B, Ricketts CJ, Metwalli AR, et al. The genetic basis of pheochromocytoma and paraganglioma: implications for management. Urology. 2014 Jun;83(6):1225–32. PMID:24642075
6462. Shukla S, Sehgal S, Prabhat P, et al. Congenital presentation of a solitary superficial angiomyxoma in the parotid region masquerading as parotid tumor. Turk Patoloji Derg. 2018;34(3):262–4. PMID:28272665
6463. Shulman SC, Katzenstein H, Bridge J, et al. Ewing sarcoma with 7;22 translocation: three new cases and clinicopathological characterization. Fetal Pediatr Pathol. 2012 Dec;31(6):341–8. PMID:22432475
6464. Shupnik MA, Pitt LK, Soh AY, et al. Selective expression of estrogen receptor alpha and beta isoforms in human pituitary tumors. J Clin Endocrinol Metab. 1998 Nov;83(11):3965–72. PMID:9814476
6465. Siannis F, Farewell VT, Head J. A multi-state model for joint modelling of terminal and non-terminal events with application to Whitehall II. Stat Med. 2007 Jan 30;26(2):426–42. PMID:16220522
6466. Sibley CD, Brown HA, Harrop AR, et al. Exophytic nodule on the scalp. Superficial angiomyxoma. JAMA Dermatol. 2013 Jun;149(6):751–6. PMID:23783153
6467. Siddiqui S, Naaz S, Ahmad M, et al. Encephalocraniocutaneous lipomatosis: a case report with review of literature. Neuroradiol J. 2017 Dec;30(6):578–82. PMID:28707961
6468. Side L, Taylor B, Cayouette M, et al. Homozygous inactivation of the NF1 gene in bone marrow cells from children with neurofibromatosis type 1 and malignant myeloid disorders. N Engl J Med. 1997 Jun 12;336(24):1713–20. PMID:9180088
6469. Sidwell RU, Rouse P, Owen RA, et al. Granular cell tumor of the scrotum in a child with Noonan syndrome. Pediatr Dermatol. 2008 May-Jun;25(3):341–3. PMID:18577039
6470. Sie AS, Mensenkamp AR, Adang EMM, et al. Fourfold increased detection of Lynch syndrome by raising age limit for tumour genetic testing from 50 to 70 years is cost-effective. Ann Oncol. 2014 Oct;25(10):2001–7. PMID:25081898
6471. Sieber OM, Segditsas S, Knudsen AL, et al. Disease severity and genetic pathways in attenuated familial adenomatous polyposis vary greatly but depend on the site of the germline mutation. Gut. 2006 Oct;55(10):1440–8. PMID:16461775
6472. Siegel HJ, Rock MG. Occult phosphaturic mesenchymal tumor detected by Tc-99m sestamibi scan. Clin Nucl Med. 2002 Aug;27(8):608–9. PMID:12170016
6473. Siegel RL, Miller KD, Jemal A. Cancer Statistics, 2017. CA Cancer J Clin. 2017 Jan;67(1):7–30. PMID:28055103
6474. Siegel RL, Miller KD, Jemal A. Cancer statistics, 2018. CA Cancer J Clin. 2018 Jan;68(1):7–30. PMID:29313949
6475. Siegfried A, Cances C, Denuelle M, et al. Noonan syndrome, PTPN11 mutations, and brain tumors. A clinical report and review of the literature. Am J Med Genet A. 2017 Apr;173(4):1061–5. PMID:28328117
6476. Siegfried A, Morin S, Munzer C, et al. A French retrospective study on clinical outcome in 102 choroid plexus tumors in children. J Neurooncol. 2017 Oct;135(1):151–60. PMID:28677107
6477. Siegfried A, Rousseau A, Maurage CA, et al. EWSR1-PATZ1 gene fusion may define a new glioneuronal tumor entity. Brain Pathol. 2019 Jan;29(1):53–62. PMID:29679497
6478. Sievers P, Schrimpf D, Stichel D, et al. Posterior fossa pilocytic astrocytomas with oligodendroglial features show frequent FGFR1 activation via fusion or mutation. Acta Neuropathol. 2020 Feb;139(2):403–6. PMID:31729570
6479. Sievers P, Sill M, Schrimpf D, et al. A subset of pediatric-type thalamic gliomas share a distinct DNA methylation profile, H3K27me3 loss and frequent alteration of EGFR. Neuro Oncol. 2021 Jan 30;23(1):34–43. PMID:33130881
6480. Sievers S, Alemazkour K, Zahn S, et al. IGF2/H19 imprinting analysis of human germ cell tumors (GCTs) using the methylation-sensitive single-nucleotide primer extension method reflects the origin of GCTs in different stages of primordial germ cell development. Genes Chromosomes Cancer. 2005 Nov;44(3):256–64. PMID:16001432
6481. Sievert AJ, Jackson EM, Gai X, et al. Duplication of 7q34 in pediatric low-grade astrocytomas detected by high-density single-nucleotide polymorphism-based genotype arrays results in a novel BRAF fusion gene. Brain Pathol. 2009 Jul;19(3):449–58. PMID:19016743
6482. Sigismondi C, Gadducci A, Lorusso D, et al. Ovarian Sertoli-Leydig cell tumors. a retrospective MITO study. Gynecol Oncol. 2012 Jun;125(3):673–6. PMID:22446621
6483. Siitonen HA, Sotkasiira J, Biervliet M, et al. The mutation spectrum in RECQL4 diseases. Eur J Hum Genet. 2009 Feb;17(2):151–8. PMID:18716613
6484. Silva VW, Askan G, Daniel TD, et al. Biliary carcinomas: pathology and the role of DNA mismatch repair deficiency. Chin Clin Oncol. 2016 Oct;5(5):62. PMID:27829276
6485. Silve C, Jüppner H. Ollier disease. Orphanet J Rare Dis. 2006 Sep 22;1:37. PMID:16995932
6486. Silveira AB, Kasper LH, Fan Y, et al. H3.3 K27M depletion increases differentiation and extends latency of diffuse intrinsic pontine glioma growth in vivo. Acta Neuropathol. 2019 Apr;137(4):637–55. PMID:30770999
6487. Silver RT. The blast phase of chronic myeloid leukaemia. Best Pract Res Clin Haematol. 2009 Sep;22(3):387–94. PMID:19959089
6488. Silverman JF, Holbrook CT, Pories WJ, et al. Fine needle aspiration cytology of pancreatoblastoma with immunocytochemical and ultrastructural studies. Acta Cytol. 1990 Sep-Oct;34(5):632–40. PMID:2220242

6489. Simanshu DK, Nissley DV, McCormick F. RAS proteins and their regulators in human disease. Cell. 2017 Jun 29;170(1):17–33. PMID:28666118
6490. Simon MP, Pedeutour F, Sirvent N, et al. Deregulation of the platelet-derived growth factor B-chain gene via fusion with collagen gene COL1A1 in dermatofibrosarcoma protuberans and giant-cell fibroblastoma. Nat Genet. 1997 Jan;15(1):95–8. PMID:8988177
6491. Simons A, Schepens M, Jeuken J, et al. Frequent loss of 9p21 (p16(INK4A)) and other genomic imbalances in human malignant fibrous histiocytoma. Cancer Genet Cytogenet. 2000 Apr 15;118(2):89–98. PMID:10748288
6492. Simpson PR, Rutledge JC, Schaefer SD, et al. Congenital hybrid basal cell adenoma–adenoid cystic carcinoma of the salivary gland. Pediatr Pathol. 1986;6(2-3):199–208. PMID:3029739
6493. Sinclair TJ, Thorson CM, Alvarez E, et al. Pleomorphic myxoid liposarcoma in an adolescent with Li-Fraumeni syndrome. Pediatr Surg Int. 2017 May;33(5):631–5. PMID:28160093
6494. Singh A, Joshi V, Jindal AK, et al. An updated review on activated PI3 kinase delta syndrome (APDS). Genes Dis. 2019 Oct 14;7(1):67–74. PMID:32181277
6495. Singh AD, Santos CM, Shields CL, et al. Observations on 17 patients with retinocytoma. Arch Ophthalmol. 2000 Feb;118(2):199–205. PMID:10676785
6496. Singhal S, Birch JM, Kerr B, et al. Neurofibromatosis type 1 and sporadic optic gliomas. Arch Dis Child. 2002 Jul;87(1):65–70. PMID:12089128
6497. Singhi AD, Lilo M, Hruban RH, et al. Overexpression of lymphoid enhancer-binding factor 1 (LEF1) in solid-pseudopapillary neoplasms of the pancreas. Mod Pathol. 2014 Oct;27(10):1355–63. PMID:24658583
6498. Singhi AD, McGrath K, Brand RE, et al. Preoperative next-generation sequencing of pancreatic cyst fluid is highly accurate in cyst classification and detection of advanced neoplasia. Gut. 2018 Dec;67(12):2131–41. PMID:28970292
6499. Sinicrope FA, Sargent DJ. Molecular pathways: microsatellite instability in colorectal cancer: prognostic, predictive, and therapeutic implications. Clin Cancer Res. 2012 Mar 15;18(6):1506–12. PMID:22302899
6500. Sinnott BP, Patel M. Giant cell lesion of the jaw as a presenting feature of Noonan syndrome. BMJ Case Rep. 2018 May 30;2018:bcr-2017-224115. PMID:29848529
6501. Sio TT, Vu CC, Sohawon S, et al. Extraskeletal osteosarcoma: an international rare cancer network study. Am J Clin Oncol. 2016 Feb;39(1):32–6. PMID:24401667
6502. Sirohi D, Smith SC, Epstein JI, et al. Pericytic tumors of the kidney-a clinicopathologic analysis of 17 cases. Hum Pathol. 2017 Jun;64:106–17. PMID:28438616
6503. Sirotkina M, Douroudis K, Westgren M, et al. Association of chorangiomas to hypoxia-related placental changes in singleton and multiple pregnancy placentas. Placenta. 2016 Mar;39:154–9. PMID:26992689
6504. Sirotkina M, Douroudis K, Westgren M, et al. Genetic analysis of copy number variation in large chorangiomas. Pediatr Dev Pathol. 2019 May-Jun;22(3):236–42. PMID:30428272
6505. Sirvent N, Coindre JM, Maire G, et al. Detection of MDM2-CDK4 amplification by fluorescence in situ hybridization in 200 paraffin-embedded tumor samples: utility in diagnosing adipocytic lesions and comparison with immunohistochemistry and real-time PCR. Am J Surg Pathol. 2007 Oct;31(10):1476–89. PMID:17895748
6506. Sirvent N, Maire G, Pedeutour F. Genetics of dermatofibrosarcoma protuberans family of tumors: from ring chromosomes to tyrosine kinase inhibitor treatment. Genes Chromosomes Cancer. 2003 May;37(1):1–19. PMID:12661001
6507. Siskin GP, Haller JO, Miller S, et al. AIDS-related lymphoma: radiologic features in pediatric patients. Radiology. 1995 Jul;196(1):63–6. PMID:7784591
6508. Sitthichaiyakul P, Somran J, Oilmungmool N, et al. Sialoblastoma of the cheek: a case report and review of the literature. Mol Clin Oncol. 2016 Jun;4(6):925–8. PMID:27284424
6509. Sitthinamsuwan P, Pattanaprichakul P, Treetipsatit J, et al. Subcutaneous panniculitis-like T-cell lymphoma versus lupus erythematosus panniculitis: distinction by means of the periadipocytic cell proliferation index. Am J Dermatopathol. 2018 Aug;40(8):567–74. PMID:29742552
6510. Skakkebaek NE. Possible carcinoma-in-situ of the testis. Lancet. 1972 Sep 9;2(7776):516–7. PMID:4115573
6511. Skakkebaek NE, Berthelsen JG, Giwercman A, et al. Carcinoma-in-situ of the testis: possible origin from gonocytes and precursor of all types of germ cell tumours except spermatocytoma. Int J Androl. 1987 Feb;10(1):19–28. PMID:3034791
6512. Skakkebaek NE, Holm M, Hoei-Hansen C, et al. Association between testicular dysgenesis syndrome (TDS) and testicular neoplasia: evidence from 20 adult patients with signs of maldevelopment of the testis. APMIS. 2003 Jan;111(1):1–9. PMID:12752226
6513. Skakkebaek NE, Rajpert-De Meyts E, Main KM. Testicular dysgenesis syndrome: an increasingly common developmental disorder with environmental aspects. Hum Reprod. 2001 May;16(5):972–8. PMID:11331648
6514. Skala SL, Wang X, Zhang Y, et al. Next-generation RNA sequencing-based biomarker characterization of chromophobe renal cell carcinoma and related oncocytic neoplasms. Eur Urol. 2020 Jul;78(1):63–74. PMID:32299640
6515. Skala SL, Xiao H, Udager AM, et al. Detection of 6 TFEB-amplified renal cell carcinomas and 25 renal cell carcinomas with MITF translocations: systematic morphologic analysis of 85 cases evaluated by clinical TFE3 and TFEB FISH assays. Mod Pathol. 2018 Jan;31(1):179–97. PMID:28840857
6516. Skalet AH, Gombos DS, Gallie BL, et al. Screening children at risk for retinoblastoma: consensus report from the American Association of Ophthalmic Oncologists and Pathologists. Ophthalmology. 2018 Mar;125(3):453–8. PMID:29056300
6516A. Skálová A, Agaimy A, Stanowska O, et al. Molecular profiling of salivary oncocytic mucoepidermoid carcinomas helps to resolve differential diagnostic dilemma with low-grade oncocytic lesions. Am J Surg Pathol. 2020 Dec;44(12):1612–22. PMID:33002921
6517. Skálová A, Weinreb I, Hyrcza M, et al. Clear cell myoepithelial carcinoma of salivary glands showing EWSR1 rearrangement: molecular analysis of 94 salivary gland carcinomas with prominent clear cell component. Am J Surg Pathol. 2015 Mar;39(3):338–48. PMID:25581728
6518. Skapek SX, Ferrari A, Gupta AA, et al. Rhabdomyosarcoma. Nat Rev Dis Primers. 2019 Jan 7;5(1):1. PMID:30617281
6519. Skaria PE, Ahmed AA, Yin H, et al. Expression of HBME-1 and CD56 in follicular variant of papillary carcinoma in children: an immunohistochemical study and their diagnostic utility. Pathol Res Pract. 2019 May;215(5):880–4. PMID:30711197
6520. Skidmore RA, Ivker RA, Resnick SD. Upper extremity atrophy associated with a giant congenital melanocytic nevus. Pediatr Dermatol. 1995 Sep;12(3):272–4. PMID:7501564
6521. Sklar C, Whitton J, Mertens A, et al. Abnormalities of the thyroid in survivors of Hodgkin's disease: data from the Childhood Cancer Survivor Study. J Clin Endocrinol Metab. 2000 Sep;85(9):3227–32. PMID:10999813
6522. Skullerud K, Stenwig AE, Brandtzaeg P, et al. Intracranial primary leiomyosarcoma arising in a teratoma of the pineal area. Clin Neuropathol. 1995 Jul-Aug;14(4):245–8. PMID:8521631
6523. Slack GW, Ferry JA, Hasserjian RP, et al. Lymphocyte depleted Hodgkin lymphoma: an evaluation with immunophenotyping and genetic analysis. Leuk Lymphoma. 2009 Jun;50(6):937–43. PMID:19455461
6524. Slade I, Bacchelli C, Davies H, et al. DICER1 syndrome: clarifying the diagnosis, clinical features and management implications of a pleiotropic tumour predisposition syndrome. J Med Genet. 2011 Apr;48(4):273–8. PMID:21266384
6525. Slegers RJ, Blumcke I. Low-grade developmental and epilepsy associated brain tumors: a critical update 2020. Acta Neuropathol Commun. 2020 Mar 9;8(1):27. PMID:32151273
6526. Sloan EA, Hilz S, Gupta R, et al. Gliomas arising in the setting of Li-Fraumeni syndrome stratify into two molecular subgroups with divergent clinicopathologic features. Acta Neuropathol. 2020 May;139(5):953–7. PMID:32157385
6527. Slowik V, Attard T, Dai H, et al. Desmoid tumors complicating familial adenomatous polyposis: a meta-analysis mutation spectrum of affected individuals. BMC Gastroenterol. 2015 Jul 16;15:84. PMID:26179480
6528. Słowikowska-Hilczer J, Romer TE, Kula K. Neoplastic potential of germ cells in relation to disturbances of gonadal organogenesis and changes in karyotype. J Androl. 2003 Mar-Apr;24(2):270–8. PMID:12634315
6529. Slupianek A, Nieborowska-Skorska M, Hoser G, et al. Role of phosphatidylinositol 3-kinase-Akt pathway in nucleophosmin/anaplastic lymphoma kinase-mediated lymphomagenesis. Cancer Res. 2001 Mar 1;61(5):2194–9. PMID:11280786
6530. Smeland S, Bielack SS, Whelan J, et al. Survival and prognosis with osteosarcoma: outcomes in more than 2000 patients in the EURAMOS-1 (European and American Osteosarcoma Study) cohort. Eur J Cancer. 2019 Mar;109:36–50. PMID:30685685
6531. Smets F, Sokal EM. Epstein-Barr virus-related lymphoproliferation in children after liver transplant: role of immunity, diagnosis, and management. Pediatr Transplant. 2002 Aug;6(4):280–7. PMID:12234267
6532. Smith AB, Rushing EJ, Smirniotopoulos JG. From the archives of the AFIP: lesions of the pineal region: radiologic-pathologic correlation. Radiographics. 2010 Nov;30(7):2001–20. PMID:21057132
6533. Smith AB, Rushing EJ, Smirniotopoulos JG. Pigmented lesions of the central nervous system: radiologic-pathologic correlation. Radiographics. 2009 Sep-Oct;29(5):1503–24. PMID:19755608
6534. Smith AN, Miller LA, Song N, et al. The duality of beta-catenin function: a requirement in lens morphogenesis and signaling suppression of lens fate in periocular ectoderm. Dev Biol. 2005 Sep 15;285(2):477–89. PMID:16102745
6535. Smith AR, Christiansen EC, Wagner JE, et al. Early hematopoietic stem cell transplant is associated with favorable outcomes in children with MDS. Pediatr Blood Cancer. 2013 Apr;60(4):705–10. PMID:23152304
6536. Smith DM, Mahmoud HH, Jenkins JJ 3rd, et al. Myofibrosarcoma of the head and neck in children. Pediatr Pathol Lab Med. 1995 May-Jun;15(3):403–18. PMID:8597827
6537. Smith EJ, Rezeanu L, Carron J. Case presentation of soft tissue parapharyngeal chondroma in a pediatric patient. Am J Otolaryngol. 2013 Nov-Dec;34(6):720–3. PMID:24035183
6538. Smith HO, Berwick M, Verschraegen CF, et al. Incidence and survival rates for female malignant germ cell tumors. Obstet Gynecol. 2006 May;107(5):1075–85. PMID:16648414
6539. Smith JD, Harvey RN, Darr OA, et al. Head and neck paragangliomas: a two-decade institutional experience and algorithm for management. Laryngoscope Investig Otolaryngol. 2017 Nov 11;2(6):380–9. PMID:29299512
6540. Smith JR, Marqusee E, Webb S, et al. Thyroid nodules and cancer in children with PTEN hamartoma tumor syndrome. J Clin Endocrinol Metab. 2011 Jan;96(1):34–7. PMID:20962022
6541. Smith KJ, Barrett TL, Skelton HG 3rd, et al. Spindle cell and epithelioid cell nevi with atypia and metastasis (malignant Spitz nevus). Am J Surg Pathol. 1989 Nov;13(11):931–9. PMID:2802011
6542. Smith LB, Valdes Y, Check WE, et al. Juvenile myelomonocytic leukemia presenting with facial nerve paresis: a unique presentation. J Pediatr Hematol Oncol. 2007 Nov;29(11):770–3. PMID:17984696
6543. Smith MC, Cohen DN, Greig B, et al. The ambiguous boundary between EBV-related hemophagocytic lymphohistiocytosis and systemic EBV-driven T cell lymphoproliferative disorder. Int J Clin Exp Pathol. 2014 Aug 15;7(9):5738–49. PMID:25337215
6544. Smith MH. NP shares experiences in ARNP Program. Nurse Pract. 1992 Aug;17(8):15. PMID:1501791
6545. Smith MJ, Beetz C, Williams SG, et al. Germline mutations in SUFU cause Gorlin syndrome-associated childhood medulloblastoma and redefine the risk associated with PTCH1 mutations. J Clin Oncol. 2014 Dec 20;32(36):4155–61. PMID:25403219
6546. Smith MJ, Higgs JE, Bowers NL, et al. Cranial meningiomas in 411 neurofibromatosis type 2 (NF2) patients with proven gene mutations: clear positional effect of mutations, but absence of female severity effect on age at onset. J Med Genet. 2011 Apr;48(4):261–5. PMID:21278391
6547. Smith MJ, Isidor B, Beetz C, et al. Mutations in LZTR1 add to the complex heterogeneity of schwannomatosis. Neurology. 2015 Jan 13;84(2):141–7. PMID:25480913
6548. Smith MJ, Wallace AJ, Bowers NL, et al. SMARCB1 mutations in schwannomatosis and genotype correlations with rhabdoid tumors. Cancer Genet. 2014 Sep;207(9):373–8. PMID:24933152
6549. Smith ML, Cavenagh JD, Lister TA, et al. Mutation of CEBPA in familial acute myeloid leukemia. N Engl J Med. 2004 Dec 2;351(23):2403–7. PMID:15575056
6550. Smith NE, Deyrup AT, Mariño-Enriquez A, et al. VCL-ALK renal cell carcinoma in children with sickle-cell trait: the eighth sickle-cell nephropathy? Am J Surg Pathol. 2014 Jun;38(6):858–63. PMID:24698962
6551. Smith NE, Illei PB, Allaf M, et al. t(6;11) renal cell carcinoma (RCC): expanded immunohistochemical profile emphasizing novel RCC markers and report of 10 new genetically confirmed cases. Am J Surg Pathol. 2014 May;38(5):604–14. PMID:24618616
6552. Smith SC, Buehler D, Choi EY, et al. CIC-DUX sarcomas demonstrate frequent MYC amplification and ETS-family transcription factor

expression. Mod Pathol. 2015 Jan;28(1):57–68. PMID:24947144
6553. Smith YR, Quint EH, Hinton EL. Recurrent benign müllerian papilloma of the cervix. J Pediatr Adolesc Gynecol. 1998 Feb;11(1):29–31. PMID:9526823
6554. Smoll NR, Drummond KJ. The incidence of medulloblastomas and primitive neurectodermal tumours in adults and children. J Clin Neurosci. 2012 Nov;19(11):1541–4. PMID:22981874
6555. Smolle E, Al-Qubati S, Stefanits H, et al. Medullomyoblastoma: a case report and literature review of a rare tumor entity. Anticancer Res. 2012 Nov;32(11):4939–44. PMID:23155263
6556. Smrkolj S, Sorc L, Sinkovec J, et al. Müllerian papilloma in a patient with Proteus syndrome: case report and review of the literature. Eur J Gynaecol Oncol. 2012;33(4):428–32. PMID:23091906
6557. Snir OL, DeJoseph M, Wong S, et al. Frequent homozygosity in both mature and immature ovarian teratomas: a shared genetic basis of tumorigenesis. Mod Pathol. 2017 Oct;30(10):1467–75. PMID:28664933
6558. Snowsill T, Coelho H, Huxley N, et al. Molecular testing for Lynch syndrome in people with colorectal cancer: systematic reviews and economic evaluation. Health Technol Assess. 2017 Sep;21(51):1–238. PMID:28895526
6559. Snowsill T, Huxley N, Hoyle M, et al. A systematic review and economic evaluation of diagnostic strategies for Lynch syndrome. Health Technol Assess. 2014 Sep;18(58):1–406. PMID:25244061
6560. Snuderl M, Kannan K, Pfaff E, et al. Recurrent homozygous deletion of DROSHA and microduplication of PDE4DIP in pineoblastoma. Nat Commun. 2018 Jul 20;9(1):2868. PMID:30030436
6561. Snyder RE. A radiolabelled pulse for the simultaneous study of anterograde and retrograde axonal transport. J Neurosci Methods. 1986 Aug;17(2-3):109–19. PMID:2429122
6562. Snyderman CH, Pant H, Carrau RL, et al. A new endoscopic staging system for angiofibromas. Arch Otolaryngol Head Neck Surg. 2010 Jun;136(6):588–94. PMID:20566910
6563. So JS, Epstein JI. GATA3 expression in paragangliomas: a pitfall potentially leading to misdiagnosis of urothelial carcinoma. Mod Pathol. 2013 Oct;26(10):1365–70. PMID:23599157
6564. Sobel RA. Vestibular (acoustic) schwannomas: histologic features in neurofibromatosis 2 and in unilateral cases. J Neuropathol Exp Neurol. 1993 Mar;52(2):106–13. PMID:8440992
6565. Soblet J, Kangas J, Nätynki M, et al. Blue rubber bleb nevus (BRBN) syndrome is caused by somatic TEK (TIE2) mutations. J Invest Dermatol. 2017 Jan;137(1):207–16. PMID:27519652
6566. Sobrinho-Simões M, Máximo V, Rocha AS, et al. Intragenic mutations in thyroid cancer. Endocrinol Metab Clin North Am. 2008 Jun;37(2):333–62, viii. PMID:18502330
6567. Söder S, Inwards C, Müller S, et al. Cell biology and matrix biochemistry of chondromyxoid fibroma. Am J Clin Pathol. 2001 Aug;116(2):271–7. PMID:11488075
6568. Sofela AA, Hettige S, Curran O, et al. Malignant transformation in craniopharyngiomas. Neurosurgery. 2014 Sep;75(3):306–14. PMID:24978859
6569. Sogani PC, Fair WR. Surveillance alone in the treatment of clinical stage I nonseminomatous germ cell tumor of the testis (NSGCT). Semin Urol. 1988 Feb;6(1):53–6. PMID:2838876
6570. Sohani AR, Jaffe ES, Harris NL, et al. Nodular lymphocyte-predominant hodgkin lymphoma with atypical T cells: a morphologic variant mimicking peripheral T-cell lymphoma. Am J Surg Pathol. 2011 Nov;35(11):1666–78. PMID:21997687
6571. Soler J, Bordes R, Ortūno F, et al. Aggressive natural killer cell leukaemia/lymphoma in two patients with lethal midline granuloma. Br J Haematol. 1994 Mar;86(3):659–62. PMID:8043452
6572. Soler JM, Pizà G, Aliaga F. Special characteristics of osteoid osteoma in the proximal phalanx. J Hand Surg Br. 1997 Dec;22(6):793–7. PMID:9457591
6573. Soliman SE, Racher H, Zhang C, et al. Genetics and molecular diagnostics in retinoblastoma–an update. Asia Pac J Ophthalmol (Phila). 2017 Mar-Apr;6(2):197–207. PMID:28399338
6574. Solomon DA, Wood MD, Tihan T, et al. Diffuse midline gliomas with histone H3-K27M mutation: a series of 47 cases assessing the spectrum of morphologic variation and associated genetic alterations. Brain Pathol. 2016 Sep;26(5):569–80. PMID:26517431
6575. Soluk Tekkesin M, Tuna EB, Olgac V, et al. Odontogenic lesions in a pediatric population: review of the literature and presentation of 745 cases. Int J Pediatr Otorhinolaryngol. 2016 Jul;86:196–9. PMID:27260607
6576. Som PM, Brandwein M, Silvers AR, et al. Sialoblastoma (embryoma): MR findings of a rare pediatric salivary gland tumor. AJNR Am J Neuroradiol. 1997 May;18(5):847–50. PMID:9159361
6577. Somerhausen NS, Fletcher CD. Diffuse-type giant cell tumor: clinicopathologic and immunohistochemical analysis of 50 cases with extraarticular disease. Am J Surg Pathol. 2000 Apr;24(4):479–92. PMID:10757395
6578. Son EJ, Nosé V. Familial follicular cell-derived thyroid carcinoma. Front Endocrinol (Lausanne). 2012 May 3;3:61. PMID:22654876
6579. Song JY, Egan C, Bouska AC, et al. Genomic characterization of diffuse large B-cell lymphoma transformation of nodular lymphocyte-predominant Hodgkin lymphoma. Leukemia. 2020 Aug;34(8):2238–42. PMID:32054999
6580. Song JY, Pittaluga S, Dunleavy K, et al. Lymphomatoid granulomatosis–a single institute experience: pathologic findings and clinical correlations. Am J Surg Pathol. 2015 Feb;39(2):141–56. PMID:25321327
6581. Song SY, Kim WS, Ko YH, et al. Aggressive natural killer cell leukemia: clinical features and treatment outcome. Haematologica. 2002 Dec;87(12):1343–5. PMID:12495907
6582. Song W, Suurmeijer AJH, Bollen SM, et al. Soft tissue aneurysmal bone cyst: six new cases with imaging details, molecular pathology, and review of the literature. Skeletal Radiol. 2019 Jul;48(7):1059–67. PMID:30603771
6583. Song WJ, Sullivan MG, Legare RD, et al. Haploinsufficiency of CBFA2 causes familial thrombocytopenia with propensity to develop acute myelogenous leukaemia. Nat Genet. 1999 Oct;23(2):166–75. PMID:10508512
6584. Songu M, Adibelli H, Diniz G. White sponge nevus: clinical suspicion and diagnosis. Pediatr Dermatol. 2012 Jul-Aug;29(4):495–7. PMID:22352924
6585. Sonigo G, Battistella M, Beylot-Barry M, et al. HAVCR2 mutations are associated with severe hemophagocytic syndrome in subcutaneous panniculitis-like T-cell lymphoma. Blood. 2020 Mar 26;135(13):1058–61. PMID:32005988
6586. Sonne SB, Almstrup K, Dalgaard M, et al. Analysis of gene expression profiles of microdissected cell populations indicates that testicular carcinoma in situ is an arrested gonocyte. Cancer Res. 2009 Jun 15;69(12):5241–50. PMID:19491264
6587. Sonne SB, Herlihy AS, Hoei-Hansen CE, et al. Identity of M2A (D2-40) antigen and gp36 (Aggrus, T1A-2, podoplanin) in human developing testis, testicular carcinoma in situ and germ-cell tumours. Virchows Arch. 2006 Aug;449(2):200–6. PMID:16736189
6588. Sonneland PR, Scheithauer BW, Onofrio BM. Myxopapillary ependymoma. A clinicopathologic and immunocytochemical study of 77 cases. Cancer. 1985 Aug 15;56(4):883–93. PMID:4016681
6589. Sonnex TS, Hawk JL. Hydroa vacciniforme: a review of ten cases. Br J Dermatol. 1988 Jan;118(1):101–8. PMID:3342168
6589A. Soravia C, Sugg SL, Berk T, et al. Familial adenomatous polyposis-associated thyroid cancer: a clinical, pathological, and molecular genetics study. Am J Pathol. 1999 Jan;154(1):127–35. PMID:9916927
6590. Sordillo PP, Epremian B, Koziner B, et al. Lymphomatoid granulomatosis: an analysis of clinical and immunologic characteristics. Cancer. 1982 May 15;49(10):2070–6. PMID:6978760
6591. Sorensen PH, Lessnick SL, Lopez-Terrada D, et al. A second Ewing's sarcoma translocation, t(21;22), fuses the EWS gene to another ETS-family transcription factor, ERG. Nat Genet. 1994 Feb;6(2):146–51. PMID:8162068
6592. Sorge C, Costa LJ, Taub JW, et al. Incidence and outcomes of rare paediatric non-hodgkin lymphomas. Br J Haematol. 2019 Mar;184(5):864–7. PMID:29611181
6593. Sorkin T, Strautnieks S, Foskett P, et al. Multiple β-catenin mutations in hepatocellular lesions arising in Abernethy malformation. Hum Pathol. 2016 Jul;53:153–8. PMID:27038679
6594. Sorrell AD, Alonzo TA, Hilden JM, et al. Favorable survival maintained in children who have myeloid leukemia associated with Down syndrome using reduced-dose chemotherapy on Children's Oncology Group trial A2971: a report from the Children's Oncology Group. Cancer. 2012 Oct 1;118(19):4806–14. PMID:22392565
6595. Sorrell AD, Espenschied CR, Culver JO, et al. Tumor protein p53 (TP53) testing and Li-Fraumeni syndrome : current status of clinical applications and future directions. Mol Diagn Ther. 2013 Feb;17(1):31–47. PMID:23355100
6596. Sorrentino S, Conte M, Nozza P, et al. Simultaneous occurrence of pancreatoblastoma and neuroblastoma in a newborn with beckwith-wiedemann syndrome. J Pediatr Hematol Oncol. 2010 Jul;32(5):e207–9. PMID:20495482
6597. Sorrentino S, Gigliotti AR, Sementa AR, et al. Neuroblastoma in the adult: the Italian experience with 21 patients. J Pediatr Hematol Oncol. 2014 Nov;36(8):e499–505. PMID:24633299
6598. Sotelo-Avila C, Gonzalez-Crussi F, Sadowinski S, et al. Clear cell sarcoma of the kidney: a clinicopathologic study of 21 patients with long-term follow-up evaluation. Hum Pathol. 1985 Dec;16(12):1219–30. PMID:4065884
6599. Sotlar K, Cerny-Reiterer S, Petat-Dutter K, et al. Aberrant expression of CD30 in neoplastic mast cells in high-grade mastocytosis. Mod Pathol. 2011 Apr;24(4):585–95. PMID:21186345
6600. Sotlar K, Escribano L, Landt O, et al. One-step detection of c-kit point mutations using peptide nucleic acid-mediated polymerase chain reaction clamping and hybridization probes. Am J Pathol. 2003 Mar;162(3):737–46. PMID:12598308
6601. Soufir N, Ribojad M, Magnaldo T, et al. Germline and somatic mutations of the INK4a-ARF gene in a xeroderma pigmentosum group C patient. J Invest Dermatol. 2002 Dec;119(6):1355–60. PMID:12485439
6602. Soukup J, Česák T, Hornychová H, et al. Stem cell transcription factor Sox2 is expressed in a subset of folliculo-stellate cells of growth hormone-producing pituitary neuroendocrine tumours and its expression shows no association with tumour size or IGF1 levels: a clinicopathological study of 109 cases. Endocr Pathol. 2020 Dec;31(4):337–47. PMID:32632839
6603. Soule EH, Pritchard DJ. Fibrosarcoma in infants and children: a review of 110 cases. Cancer. 1977 Oct;40(4):1711–21. PMID:561651
6604. Sowery RD, Jensen C, Morrison KB, et al. Comparative genomic hybridization detects multiple chromosomal amplifications and deletions in undifferentiated embryonal sarcoma of the liver. Cancer Genet Cytogenet. 2001 Apr 15;126(2):128–33. PMID:11376805
6605. Spada A, Arosio M, Bochicchio D, et al. Clinical, biochemical, and morphological correlates in patients bearing growth hormone-secreting pituitary tumors with or without constitutively active adenylyl cyclase. J Clin Endocrinol Metab. 1990 Dec;71(6):1421–6. PMID:1977758
6606. Spans L, Fletcher CD, Antonescu CR, et al. Recurrent MALAT1-GLI1 oncogenic fusion and GLI1 up-regulation define a subset of plexiform fibromyxoma. J Pathol. 2016 Jul;239(3):335–43. PMID:27101025
6607. Sparber-Sauer M, Koscielniak E, Vokuhl C, et al. Endothelial cell malignancies in infants, children and adolescents: treatment results of three Cooperative Weichteilsarkom Studiengruppe (CWS) trials and one registry. Pediatr Blood Cancer. 2020 Mar;67(3):e28095. PMID:31814291
6608. Spatz A, Calonje E, Handfield-Jones S, et al. Spitz tumors in children: a grading system for risk stratification. Arch Dermatol. 1999 Mar;135(3):282–5. PMID:10086449
6609. Spaun E, Rix P. Benign cystic monodermal teratoma of neurogenic type. Int J Gynecol Pathol. 1990;9(3):283–90. PMID:2373589
6610. Spear GS, Martin CG. Fetal gonadoblastoid testicular dysplasia. Hum Pathol. 1986 May;17(5):531–3. PMID:3699814
6611. Specht K, Sung YS, Zhang L, et al. Distinct transcriptional signature and immunoprofile of CIC-DUX4 fusion-positive round cell tumors compared to EWSR1-rearranged Ewing sarcomas: further evidence toward distinct pathologic entities. Genes Chromosomes Cancer. 2014 Jul;53(7):622–33. PMID:24723486
6612. Specht K, Zhang L, Sung YS, et al. Novel BCOR-MAML3 and ZC3H7B-BCOR gene fusions in undifferentiated small blue round cell sarcomas. Am J Surg Pathol. 2016 Apr;40(4):433–42. PMID:26752546
6613. Spector LG, Birch J. The epidemiology of hepatoblastoma. Pediatr Blood Cancer. 2012 Nov;59(5):776–9. PMID:22692949
6614. Spector LG, Feusner JH, Ross JA. Hepatoblastoma and low birth weight. Pediatr Blood Cancer. 2004 Nov;43(6):706. PMID:15390302
6615. Spector LG, Johnson KJ, Soler JT, et al. Perinatal risk factors for hepatoblastoma. Br J Cancer. 2008 May 6;98(9):1570–3. PMID:18392049
6616. Speer AL, Schofield DE, Wang KS, et al. Contemporary management of lipoblastoma. J Pediatr Surg. 2008 Jul;43(7):1295–300. PMID:18639685
6617. Speicher DJ, Johnson NW. Detection of human herpesvirus 8 by quantitative polymerase chain reaction: development and standardisation of methods. BMC Infect Dis. 2012 Sep 11;12:210. PMID:22963082
6618. Spence T, Perotti C, Sin-Chan P, et al. A novel C19MC amplified cell line links Lin28/let-7 to mTOR signaling in embryonal tumor with multilayered rosettes. Neuro Oncol. 2014 Jan;16(1):62–71. PMID:24311633

6619. Spence T, Sin-Chan P, Picard D, et al. CNS-PNETs with C19MC amplification and/or LIN28 expression comprise a distinct histogenetic diagnostic and therapeutic entity. Acta Neuropathol. 2014 Aug;128(2):291–303. PMID:24839957
6620. Sperfeld AD, Hein C, Schröder JM, et al. Occurrence and characterization of peripheral nerve involvement in neurofibromatosis type 2. Brain. 2002 May;125(Pt 5):996–1004. PMID:11960890
6622. Spiegel A, Paillard C, Ducassou S, et al. Paediatric anaplastic large cell lymphoma with leukaemic presentation in children: a report of nine French cases. Br J Haematol. 2014 May;165(4):545–51. PMID:24666317
6623. Spiers AS, Bain BJ, Turner JE. The peripheral blood in chronic granulocytic leukaemia. Study of 50 untreated Philadelphia-positive cases. Scand J Haematol. 1977 Jan;18(1):25–38. PMID:265093
6624. Spigelman AD, Williams CB, Talbot IC, et al. Upper gastrointestinal cancer in patients with familial adenomatous polyposis. Lancet. 1989 Sep 30;2(8666):783–5. PMID:2571019
6625. Spina V, Bruscaggin A, Cuccaro A, et al. Circulating tumor DNA reveals genetics, clonal evolution, and residual disease in classical Hodgkin lymphoma. Blood. 2018 May 31;131(22):2413–25. PMID:29449275
6626. Spina V, Rossi D. Molecular pathogenesis of splenic and nodal marginal zone lymphoma. Best Pract Res Clin Haematol. 2017 Mar-Jun;30(1-2):5–12. PMID:28288716
6627. Spinelli C, Rossi L, Barbetta A, et al. Incidental ganglioneuromas: a presentation of 14 surgical cases and literature review. J Endocrinol Invest. 2015 May;38(5):547–54. PMID:25501841
6628. Spingardi O, Zoccolan A, Venturino E. Infantile digital fibromatosis: our experience and long-term results. Chir Main. 2011 Feb;30(1):62–5. PMID:21276743
6629. Spiro RH. Salivary neoplasms: overview of a 35-year experience with 2,807 patients. Head Neck Surg. 1986 Jan-Feb;8(3):177–84. PMID:3744850
6630. Spouge AR, Thain LM. Osteoid osteoma: MR imaging revisited. Clin Imaging. 2000 Jan-Feb;24(1):19–27. PMID:11120413
6631. Spunt SL, Francotte N, De Salvo GL, et al. Clinical features and outcomes of young patients with epithelioid sarcoma: an analysis from the Children's Oncology Group and the European paediatric soft tissue Sarcoma Study Group prospective clinical trials. Eur J Cancer. 2019 May;112:98–106. PMID:30954717
6632. Spunt SL, Poquette CA, Hurt YS, et al. Prognostic factors for children and adolescents with surgically resected nonrhabdomyosarcoma soft tissue sarcoma: an analysis of 121 patients treated at St Jude Children's Research Hospital. J Clin Oncol. 1999 Dec;17(12):3697–705. PMID:10577841
6633. Spunt SL, Pratt CB, Rao BN, et al. Childhood carcinoid tumors: the St Jude Children's Research Hospital experience. J Pediatr Surg. 2000 Sep;35(9):1282–6. PMID:10999679
6634. Squillaro AI, Zhou S, Thomas SM, et al. A 10-month-old infant presenting with signs of precocious puberty secondary to a sclerosing stromal tumor of the ovary in the absence of hormonal elevation. Pediatr Dev Pathol. 2019 Jul-Aug;22(4):375–9. PMID:30577720
6635. Sreetharan V, Kangesu L, Sommerlad BC. Atypical congenital dermoids of the face: a 25-year experience. J Plast Reconstr Aesthet Surg. 2007;60(9):1025–9. PMID:17662465
6636. Srirangam Nadhamuni V, Korbonits M. Novel insights into pituitary tumorigenesis: genetic and epigenetic mechanisms. Endocr Rev. 2020 Dec 1;41(6):bnaa006. PMID:32201880
6637. Srivastava P, Ahluwalia C, Zaheer S, et al. Aggressive angiomyxoma of vulva in a 13-year-old female. J Cancer Res Ther. 2015 Oct-Dec;11(4):937–9. PMID:26881549
6638. Srivastava S, Zou ZQ, Pirollo K, et al. Germ-line transmission of a mutated p53 gene in a cancer-prone family with Li-Fraumeni syndrome. Nature. 1990 Dec 20-27;348(6303):747–9. PMID:2259385
6639. Srouji MN, Chatten J, Schulman WM, et al. Mesenchymal hamartoma of the liver in infants. Cancer. 1978 Nov;42(5):2483–9. PMID:363258
6640. St. Jude Children's Research Hospital [Internet]. Memphis (TN): St. Jude Children's Research Hospital; 2021. WHO Global Initiative for Childhood Cancer. Available from: https://www.stjude.org/global/collaborating-to-cure/global-initiative.html.
6641. Staals EL, Bacchini P, Bertoni F. High-grade surface osteosarcoma: a review of 25 cases from the Rizzoli Institute. Cancer. 2008 Apr 1;112(7):1592–9. PMID:18300258
6642. Stafford JM, Lee CH, Voigt P, et al. Multiple modes of PRC2 inhibition elicit global chromatin alterations in H3K27M pediatric glioma. Sci Adv. 2018 Oct 31;4(10):eaau5935. PMID:30402543
6643. Stagner AM, Jakobiec FA. Updates on the molecular pathology of selected ocular and ocular adnexal tumors: potential targets for future therapy. Semin Ophthalmol. 2016;31(1-2):188–96. PMID:26959146
6644. Stanelle EJ, Christison-Lagay ER, Healey JH, et al. Pediatric and adolescent synovial sarcoma: multivariate analysis of prognostic factors and survival outcomes. Ann Surg Oncol. 2013 Jan;20(1):73–9. PMID:22878620
6645. Stanescu Cosson R, Varlet P, Beuvon F, et al. Dysembryoplastic neuroepithelial tumors: CT, MR findings and imaging follow-up: a study of 53 cases. J Neuroradiol. 2001 Dec;28(4):230–40. PMID:11924137
6646. Stang A, Trabert B, Wentzensen N, et al. Gonadal and extragonadal germ cell tumours in the United States, 1973-2007. Int J Androl. 2012 Aug;35(4):616–25. PMID:22320869
6647. Stanley CC, Westmoreland KD, Heimlich BJ, et al. Outcomes for paediatric Burkitt lymphoma treated with anthracycline-based therapy in Malawi. Br J Haematol. 2016 Jun;173(5):705–12. PMID:26914979
6648. Star P, Goodwin A, Kapoor R, et al. Germline BAP1-positive patients: the dilemmas of cancer surveillance and a proposed interdisciplinary consensus monitoring strategy. Eur J Cancer. 2018 Mar;92:48–53. PMID:29413689
6649. Starenki D, Park JI. Pediatric medullary thyroid carcinoma. J Pediatr Oncol. 2015;3(2):29–37. PMID:27014708
6650. Starzyk J, Starzyk B, Bartnik-Mikuta A, et al. Gonadotropin releasing hormone-independent precocious puberty in a 5 year-old girl with suprasellar germ cell tumor secreting beta-hCG and alpha-fetoprotein. J Pediatr Endocrinol Metab. 2001 Jun;14(6):789–96. PMID:11453531
6651. Stavropoulos F, Katz J. Central giant cell granulomas: a systematic review of the radiographic characteristics with the addition of 20 new cases. Dentomaxillofac Radiol. 2002 Jul;31(4):213–7. PMID:12087437
6652. Stavrou T, Bromley CM, Nicholson HS, et al. Prognostic factors and secondary malignancies in childhood medulloblastoma. J Pediatr Hematol Oncol. 2001 Oct;23(7):431–6. PMID:11878577
6653. Stawarski A, Maleika P. Neuroendocrine tumors of the gastrointestinal tract and pancreas: Is it also a challenge for pediatricians? Adv Clin Exp Med. 2020 Feb;29(2):265–70. PMID:32091671
6654. Steele CD, Tarabichi M, Oukrif D, et al. Undifferentiated sarcomas develop through distinct evolutionary pathways. Cancer Cell. 2019 Mar 18;35(3):441–456.e8. PMID:30889380
6655. Steelman C, Katzenstein H, Parham D, et al. Unusual presentation of congenital infantile fibrosarcoma in seven infants with molecular-genetic analysis. Fetal Pediatr Pathol. 2011;30(5):329–37. PMID:21843073
6656. Stefanaki C, Chardalias L, Soura E, et al. Paediatric melanoma. J Eur Acad Dermatol Venereol. 2017 Oct;31(10):1604–15. PMID:28449284
6657. Stefanko NS, Davies OMT, Beato MJ, et al. Hamartomas and midline anomalies in association with infantile hemangiomas, PHACE, and LUMBAR syndromes. Pediatr Dermatol. 2020 Jan;37(1):78–85. PMID:31631401
6658. Steffen-Smith EA, Baker EH, Venzon D, et al. Measurements of the pons as a biomarker of progression for pediatric DIPG. J Neurooncol. 2014 Jan;116(1):127–33. PMID:24113877
6659. Steidl C, Connors JM, Gascoyne RD. Molecular pathogenesis of Hodgkin's lymphoma: increasing evidence of the importance of the microenvironment. J Clin Oncol. 2011 May 10;29(14):1812–26. PMID:21483001
6660. Steidl C, Gascoyne RD. The molecular pathogenesis of primary mediastinal large B-cell lymphoma. Blood. 2011 Sep 8;118(10):2659–69. PMID:21700770
6661. Steidl C, Lee T, Shah SP, et al. Tumor-associated macrophages and survival in classic Hodgkin's lymphoma. N Engl J Med. 2010 Mar 11;362(10):875–85. PMID:20220182
6662. Steidl C, Shah SP, Woolcock BW, et al. MHC class II transactivator CIITA is a recurrent gene fusion partner in lymphoid cancers. Nature. 2011 Mar 17;471(7338):377–81. PMID:21368758
6663. Stein H, Foss HD, Dürkop H, et al. CD30(+) anaplastic large cell lymphoma: a review of its histopathologic, genetic, and clinical features. Blood. 2000 Dec 1;96(12):3681–95. PMID:11090048
6664. Stein H, Mason DY, Gerdes J, et al. The expression of the Hodgkin's disease associated antigen Ki-1 in reactive and neoplastic lymphoid tissue: evidence that Reed-Sternberg cells and histiocytic malignancies are derived from activated lymphoid cells. Blood. 1985 Oct;66(4):848–58. PMID:3876124
6665. Steinbok P, Gopalakrishnan CV, Hengel AR, et al. Pediatric thalamic tumors in the MRI era: a Canadian perspective. Childs Nerv Syst. 2016 Feb;32(2):269–80. PMID:26597682
6666. Steinemann D, Arning L, Praulich I, et al. Mitotic recombination and compound-heterozygous mutations are predominant NF1-inactivating mechanisms in children with juvenile myelomonocytic leukemia and neurofibromatosis type 1. Haematologica. 2010 Feb;95(2):320–3. PMID:20015894
6667. Steiner MA, Giles HW. Mesenchymal hamartoma of the liver demonstrating peripheral calcification in a 12-year-old boy. Pediatr Radiol. 2008 Nov;38(11):1232–4. PMID:18648751
6668. Stein-Wexler R. Pediatric soft tissue sarcomas. Semin Ultrasound CT MR. 2011 Oct;32(5):470–88. PMID:21963167
6669. Steliarova-Foucher E, Colombet M, Ries LAG, et al. International incidence of childhood cancer, 2001-10: a population-based registry study. Lancet Oncol. 2017 Jun;18(6):719–31. PMID:28410997
6670. Steliarova-Foucher E, Stiller CA, Pukkala E, et al. Thyroid cancer incidence and survival among European children and adolescents (1978-1997): report from the Automated Childhood Cancer Information System project. Eur J Cancer. 2006 Sep;42(13):2150–69. PMID:16919778
6671. Stelow EB, Bellizzi AM, Taneja K, et al. NUT rearrangement in undifferentiated carcinomas of the upper aerodigestive tract. Am J Surg Pathol. 2008 Jun;32(6):828–34. PMID:18391746
6672. Stemmer-Rachamimov AO, Gonzalez-Agosti C, Xu L, et al. Expression of NF2-encoded merlin and related ERM family proteins in the human central nervous system. J Neuropathol Exp Neurol. 1997 Jun;56(6):735–42. PMID:9184664
6673. Stemmer-Rachamimov AO, Horgan MA, Taratuto AL, et al. Meningioangiomatosis is associated with neurofibromatosis 2 but not with somatic alterations of the NF2 gene. J Neuropathol Exp Neurol. 1997 May;56(5):485–9. PMID:9143261
6674. Stemmer-Rachamimov AO, Ino Y, Lim ZY, et al. Loss of the NF2 gene and merlin occur by the tumorlet stage of schwannoma development in neurofibromatosis 2. J Neuropathol Exp Neurol. 1998 Dec;57(12):1164–7. PMID:9862639
6675. Stemmer-Rachamimov AO, Xu L, Gonzalez-Agosti C, et al. Universal absence of merlin, but not other ERM family members, in schwannomas. Am J Pathol. 1997 Dec;151(6):1649–54. PMID:9403715
6676. Stenman A, Zedenius J, Juhlin CC. Over-diagnosis of potential malignant behavior in MEN 2A-associated pheochromocytomas using the PASS and GAPP algorithms. Langenbecks Arch Surg. 2018 Sep;403(6):785–90. PMID:29779047
6677. Stenman A, Zedenius J, Juhlin CC. The value of histological algorithms to predict the malignancy potential of pheochromocytomas and abdominal paragangliomas-a meta-analysis and systematic review of the literature. Cancers (Basel). 2019 Feb 15;11(2):E225. PMID:30769931
6678. Stenman G, Kindblom LG, Angervall L. Reciprocal translocation t(12;22)(q13;q13) in clear-cell sarcoma of tendons and aponeuroses. Genes Chromosomes Cancer. 1992 Mar;4(2):122–7. PMID:1373311
6679. Stennert E, Guntinas-Lichius O, Klussmann JP, et al. Histopathology of pleomorphic adenoma in the parotid gland: a prospective unselected series of 100 cases. Laryngoscope. 2001 Dec;111(12):2195–200. PMID:11802025
6680. Stennert E, Wittekindt C, Klussmann JP, et al. Recurrent pleomorphic adenoma of the parotid gland: a prospective histopathological and immunohistochemical study. Laryngoscope. 2004 Jan;114(1):158–63. PMID:14710014
6681. Stephenson CA, Kletzel M, Seibert JJ, et al. Pancreatoblastoma: MR appearance. J Comput Assist Tomogr. 1990 May-Jun;14(3):492–3. PMID:2159494
6682. Stergiopoulos P, Link B, Naumann GO, et al. Solid corneal dermoids and subconjunctival lipodermoids: impact of differentiated surgical therapy on the functional long-term outcome. Cornea. 2009 Jul;28(6):644–51. PMID:19512907
6683. Sterkenburg AS, Hoffmann A, Gebhardt U, et al. Survival, hypothalamic obesity, and neuropsychological/psychosocial status after childhood-onset craniopharyngioma: newly reported long-term outcomes. Neuro Oncol. 2015 Jul;17(7):1029–38. PMID:25838139
6684. Steven MJ, Howatson A, Hanretty K, et al. A mesothelial-lined cyst: an unusual presentation. J Pediatr Surg. 2009 May;44(5):e25–7. PMID:19433156
6685. Stevens MC, Rey A, Bouvet N, et al. Treatment of nonmetastatic rhabdomyosarcoma in childhood and adolescence: third study of the International Society of Paediatric Oncology–SIOP Malignant Mesenchymal Tumor 89.

J Clin Oncol. 2005 Apr 20;23(12):2618–28. PMID:15728225
6686. Stevens TM, Morlote D, Swensen J, et al. Spindle epithelial tumor with thymus-like differentiation (SETTLE): a next-generation sequencing study. Head Neck Pathol. 2019 Jun;13(2):162–8. PMID:29736783
6687. Stevens WR, Johnson CD, Stephens DH, et al. Fibrolamellar hepatocellular carcinoma: stage at presentation and results of aggressive surgical management. AJR Am J Roentgenol. 1995 May;164(5):1153–8. PMID:7717223
6688. Stewart CJ, Farquharson MA, Foulis AK. Characterization of the inflammatory infiltrate in ovarian dysgerminoma: an immunocytochemical study. Histopathology. 1992 Jun;20(6):491–7. PMID:1607150
6689. Stewart DR, Best AF, Williams GM, et al. Neoplasm risk among individuals with a pathogenic germline variant in DICER1. J Clin Oncol. 2019 Mar 10;37(8):668–76. PMID:30715996
6690. Stewart DR, Messinger Y, Williams GM, et al. Nasal chondromesenchymal hamartomas arise secondary to germline and somatic mutations of DICER1 in the pleuropulmonary blastoma tumor predisposition disorder. Hum Genet. 2014 Nov;133(11):1443–50. PMID:25118636
6691. Stewart DR, Pemov A, Van Loo P, et al. Mitotic recombination of chromosome arm 17q as a cause of loss of heterozygosity of NF1 in neurofibromatosis type 1-associated glomus tumors. Genes Chromosomes Cancer. 2012 May;51(5):429–37. PMID:22250039
6692. Stichel D, Ebrahimi A, Reuss D, et al. Distribution of EGFR amplification, combined chromosome 7 gain and chromosome 10 loss, and TERT promoter mutation in brain tumors and their potential for the reclassification of IDHwt astrocytoma to glioblastoma. Acta Neuropathol. 2018 Nov;136(5):793–803. PMID:30187121
6693. Stieglitz E, Liu YL, Emanuel PD, et al. Mutations in GATA2 are rare in juvenile myelomonocytic leukemia. Blood. 2014 Feb 27;123(9):1426–7. PMID:24578498
6694. Stieglitz E, Mazor T, Olshen AB, et al. Genome-wide DNA methylation is predictive of outcome in juvenile myelomonocytic leukemia. Nat Commun. 2017 Dec 19;8(1):2127. PMID:29259179
6695. Stieglitz E, Taylor-Weiner AN, Chang TY, et al. The genomic landscape of juvenile myelomonocytic leukemia. Nat Genet. 2015 Nov;47(11):1326–33. PMID:26457647
6696. Stieglitz E, Troup CB, Gelston LC, et al. Subclonal mutations in SETBP1 confer a poor prognosis in juvenile myelomonocytic leukemia. Blood. 2015 Jan 15;125(3):516–24. PMID:25395418
6697. Stiles CE, Korbonits M. Familial isolated pituitary adenoma. In: Feingold KR, Anawalt B, Boyce A, et al., editors. Endotext. South Dartmouth (MA): MDText.com, Inc.; 2000–. PMID:25905184
6698. Stinco G, Governatori G, Mattighello P, et al. Multiple cutaneous neoplasms in a patient with Rothmund-Thomson syndrome: case report and published work review. J Dermatol. 2008 Mar;35(3):154–61. PMID:18346259
6699. Stinner B, Rothmund M. Neuroendocrine tumours (carcinoids) of the appendix. Best Pract Res Clin Gastroenterol. 2005 Oct;19(5):729–38. PMID:16253897
6700. Stipa F, Yoon SS, Liau KH, et al. Outcome of patients with fibrolamellar hepatocellular carcinoma. Cancer. 2006 Mar 15;106(6):1331–8. PMID:16475212
6701. Stivaros SM, Stemmer-Rachamimov AO, Alston R, et al. Multiple synchronous sites of origin of vestibular schwannomas in neurofibromatosis Type 2. J Med Genet. 2015 Aug;52(8):557–62. PMID:26104281
6702. Stocker JT, Ishak KG. Mesenchymal hamartoma of the liver: report of 30 cases and review of the literature. Pediatr Pathol. 1983 Jul-Sep;1(3):245–67. PMID:6687279
6703. Stocker JT, Ishak KG. Undifferentiated (embryonal) sarcoma of the liver: report of 31 cases. Cancer. 1978 Jul;42(1):336–48. PMID:208754
6704. Stockman DL, Ali SM, He J, et al. Sclerosing epithelioid fibrosarcoma presenting as intraabdominal sarcomatosis with a novel EWSR1-CREB3L1 gene fusion. Hum Pathol. 2014 Oct;45(10):2173–8. PMID:25123073
6705. Stockman DL, Hornick JL, Deavers MT, et al. ERG and FLI1 protein expression in epithelioid sarcoma. Mod Pathol. 2014 Apr;27(4):496–501. PMID:24072183
6706. Stockman DL, Miettinen M, Suster S, et al. Malignant gastrointestinal neuroectodermal tumor: clinicopathologic, immunohistochemical, ultrastructural, and molecular analysis of 16 cases with a reappraisal of clear cell sarcoma-like tumors of the gastrointestinal tract. Am J Surg Pathol. 2012 Jun;36(6):857–68. PMID:22592145
6708. Stojanova A, Penn LZ. The role of INI1/hSNF5 in gene regulation and cancer. Biochem Cell Biol. 2009 Feb;87(1):163–77. PMID:19234532
6709. Stojsic Z, Jankovic R, Jovanovic B, et al. Benign cystic mesothelioma of the peritoneum in a male child. J Pediatr Surg. 2012 Oct;47(10):e45–9. PMID:23084231
6710. Stoll LM, Li QK. Cytology of fine-needle aspiration of inflammatory myofibroblastic tumor. Diagn Cytopathol. 2011 Sep;39(9):663–72. PMID:20730898
6711. Stömmer P, Kraus J, Stolte M, et al. Solid and cystic pancreatic tumors. Clinical, histochemical, and electron microscopic features in ten cases. Cancer. 1991 Mar 15;67(6):1635–41. PMID:1900454
6712. Stomp W, Reijnierse M, Kloppenburg M, et al. Prevalence of cartilaginous tumours as an incidental finding on MRI of the knee. Eur Radiol. 2015 Dec;25(12):3480–7. PMID:25994192
6713. Stone AM, Shenker IR, McCarthy K. Adolescent breast masses. Am J Surg. 1977 Aug;134(2):275–7. PMID:889047
6714. Stone DM, Hynes M, Armanini M, et al. The tumour-suppressor gene patched encodes a candidate receptor for Sonic hedgehog. Nature. 1996 Nov 14;384(6605):129–34. PMID:8906787
6715. Stone DM, Murone M, Luoh S, et al. Characterization of the human suppressor of fused, a negative regulator of the zinc-finger transcription factor Gli. J Cell Sci. 1999 Dec;112(Pt 23):4437–48. PMID:10564661
6716. Stone JJ, Prasad NK, Laumonerie P, et al. Recurrent desmoid-type fibromatosis associated with underlying neuromuscular choristoma. J Neurosurg. 2018 Aug 31;131(1):175–83. PMID:30168738
6717. Stone TJ, Keeley A, Virasami A, et al. Comprehensive molecular characterisation of epilepsy-associated glioneuronal tumours. Acta Neuropathol. 2018 Jan;135(1):115–29. PMID:29058119
6718. Stone TJ, Rowell R, Jayasekera BAP, et al. Review: Molecular characteristics of long-term epilepsy-associated tumours (LEATs) and mechanisms for tumour-related epilepsy (TRE). Neuropathol Appl Neurobiol. 2018 Feb;44(1):56–69. PMID:29315734
6719. Stoop H, Honecker F, van de Geijn GJ, et al. Stem cell factor as a novel diagnostic marker for early malignant germ cells. J Pathol. 2008 Sep;216(1):43–54. PMID:18566970
6720. Stoop H, Kirkels W, Dohle GR, et al. Diagnosis of testicular carcinoma in situ '(intratubular and microinvasive)' seminoma and embryonal carcinoma using direct enzymatic alkaline phosphatase reactivity on frozen histological sections. Histopathology. 2011 Feb;58(3):440–6. PMID:21323965
6721. Storlazzi CT, Mertens F, Mandahl N, et al. A novel fusion gene, SS18L1/SSX1, in synovial sarcoma. Genes Chromosomes Cancer. 2003 Jun;37(2):195–200. PMID:12696068
6722. Storlazzi CT, Wozniak A, Panagopoulos I, et al. Rearrangement of the COL12A1 and COL4A5 genes in subungual exostosis: molecular cytogenetic delineation of the tumor-specific translocation t(X;6)(q13-14;q22). Int J Cancer. 2006 Apr 15;118(8):1972–6. PMID:16284948
6723. Stow P, Key L, Chen X, et al. Clinical significance of low levels of minimal residual disease at the end of remission induction therapy in childhood acute lymphoblastic leukemia. Blood. 2010 Jun 10;115(23):4657–63. PMID:20304809
6724. Stowe IB, Mercado EL, Stowe TR, et al. A shared molecular mechanism underlies the human rasopathies Legius syndrome and Neurofibromatosis-1. Genes Dev. 2012 Jul 1;26(13):1421–6. PMID:22751498
6725. Strahm B, Locatelli F, Bader P, et al. Reduced intensity conditioning in unrelated donor transplantation for refractory cytopenia in childhood. Bone Marrow Transplant. 2007 Aug;40(4):329–33. PMID:17589538
6726. Strahm B, Nöllke P, Zecca M, et al. Hematopoietic stem cell transplantation for advanced myelodysplastic syndrome in children: results of the EWOG-MDS 98 study. Leukemia. 2011 Mar;25(3):455–62. PMID:21212791
6727. Stratakis CA, Carney JA. The triad of paragangliomas, gastric stromal tumours and pulmonary chondromas (Carney triad), and the dyad of paragangliomas and gastric stromal sarcomas (Carney-Stratakis syndrome): molecular genetics and clinical implications. J Intern Med. 2009 Jul;266(1):43–52. PMID:19522824
6728. Stratmann R, Krieg M, Haas R, et al. Putative control of angiogenesis in hemangioblastomas by the von Hippel-Lindau tumor suppressor gene. J Neuropathol Exp Neurol. 1997 Nov;56(11):1242–52. PMID:9370235
6729. Straus SE, Jaffe ES, Puck JM, et al. The development of lymphomas in families with autoimmune lymphoproliferative syndrome with germline Fas mutations and defective lymphocyte apoptosis. Blood. 2001 Jul 1;98(1):194–200. PMID:11418480
6730. Strauss A, Furlan I, Steinmann S, et al. Unmistakable morphology? Infantile malignant osteopetrosis resembling juvenile myelomonocytic leukemia in infants. J Pediatr. 2015 Aug;167(2):486–8. PMID:25982139
6731. Streblow RC, Dafferner AJ, Nelson M, et al. Imbalances of chromosomes 4, 9, and 12 are recurrent in the thecoma-fibroma group of ovarian stromal tumors. Cancer Genet Cytogenet. 2007 Oct 15;178(2):135–40. PMID:17954269
6732. Strickland KC, Howitt BE, Barletta JA, et al. Suggesting the cytologic diagnosis of noninvasive follicular thyroid neoplasm with papillary-like nuclear features (NIFTP): a retrospective analysis of atypical and suspicious nodules. Cancer Cytopathol. 2018 Feb;126(2):86–93. PMID:28914983
6733. Stringer MD, Alizai NK. Mesenchymal hamartoma of the liver: a systematic review. J Pediatr Surg. 2005 Nov;40(11):1681–90. PMID:16291152
6734. Strobbe L, Valke LL, Diets IJ, et al. A 20-year population-based study on the epidemiology, clinical features, treatment, and outcome of nodular lymphocyte predominant Hodgkin lymphoma. Ann Hematol. 2016 Feb;95(3):417–23. PMID:26732883
6735. Stroosma OB, Delaere KP. Carcinoid tumours of the testis. BJU Int. 2008 May;101(9):1101–5. PMID:18190641
6736. Strullu M, Caye A, Lachenaud J, et al. Juvenile myelomonocytic leukaemia and Noonan syndrome. J Med Genet. 2014 Oct;51(10):689–97. PMID:25097206
6737. Stuart LN, Hiatt KM, Zaki Z, et al. Plaque-like CD34-positive dermal fibroma/medallion-like dermal dendrocyte hamartoma: an unusual spindle cell neoplasm. J Cutan Pathol. 2014 Aug;41(8):625–9. PMID:25065391
6738. Stubbins RJ, Alami Laroussi N, Peters AC, et al. Epstein-Barr virus associated smooth muscle tumors in solid organ transplant recipients: incidence over 31 years at a single institution and review of the literature. Transpl Infect Dis. 2019 Feb;21(1):e13010. PMID:30298678
6739. Stuivenvolt M, Mandl E, Verheul J, et al. Atypical transformation in sacral drop metastasis from posterior fossa choroid plexus papilloma. BMJ Case Rep. 2012 Aug 24;2012:bcr0120125681. PMID:22922909
6740. Sturm D, Orr BA, Toprak UH, et al. New brain tumor entities emerge from molecular classification of CNS-PNETs. Cell. 2016 Feb 25;164(5):1060–72. PMID:26919435
6741. Sturm D, Witt H, Hovestadt V, et al. Hotspot mutations in H3F3A and IDH1 define distinct epigenetic and biological subgroups of glioblastoma. Cancer Cell. 2012 Oct 16;22(4):425–37. PMID:23079654
6742. Styczynski J, van der Velden W, Fox CP, et al. Management of Epstein-Barr virus infections and post-transplant lymphoproliferative disorders in patients after allogeneic hematopoietic stem cell transplantation: Sixth European Conference on Infections in Leukemia (ECIL-6) guidelines. Haematologica. 2016 Jul;101(7):803–11. PMID:27365460
6743. Su IJ, Chen RL, Lin DT, et al. Epstein-Barr virus (EBV) infects T lymphocytes in childhood EBV-associated hemophagocytic syndrome in Taiwan. Am J Pathol. 1994 Jun;144(6):1219–25. PMID:8203462
6744. Su L, Beals T, Bernacki EG, et al. Spindle epithelial tumor with thymus-like differentiation: a case report with cytologic, histologic, immunohistologic, and ultrastructural findings. Mod Pathol. 1997 May;10(5):510–4. PMID:9160319
6745. Su WP. Histopathologic varieties of epidermal nevus. A study of 160 cases. Am J Dermatopathol. 1982 Apr;4(2):161–70. PMID:7048967
6746. Suarez F, Lortholary O, Hermine O, et al. Infection-associated lymphomas derived from marginal zone B cells: a model of antigen-driven lymphoproliferation. Blood. 2006 Apr 15;107(8):3034–44. PMID:16397126
6747. Suarez F, Mahlaoui N, Canioni D, et al. Incidence, presentation, and prognosis of malignancies in ataxia-telangiectasia: a report from the French national registry of primary immune deficiencies. J Clin Oncol. 2015 Jan 10;33(2):202–8. PMID:25488969
6748. Subbiah V, Lamhamedi-Cherradi SE, Cuglievan B, et al. Multimodality treatment of desmoplastic small round cell tumor: chemotherapy and complete cytoreductive surgery improve patient survival. Clin Cancer Res. 2018 Oct 1;24(19):4865–73. PMID:29871905
6749. Subramaniam K, Yeung D, Grimpen F, et al. Hepatosplenic T-cell lymphoma, immunosuppressive agents and biologicals: What are the risks? Intern Med J. 2014 Mar;44(3):287–90. PMID:24621284
6750. Sudduth CL, McGuire AM, Smits PJ, et al. Arteriovenous malformation phenotype resembling congenital hemangioma contains KRAS mutations. Clin Genet. 2020 Dec;98(6):595–7. PMID:32799314

6751. Suen KC, Magee JF, Halparin LS, et al. Fine needle aspiration cytology of fibrolamellar hepatocellular carcinoma. Acta Cytol. 1985 Sep-Oct;29(5):867–72. PMID:2996274
6752. Suerink M, Ripperger T, Messiaen L, et al. Constitutional mismatch repair deficiency as a differential diagnosis of neurofibromatosis type 1: consensus guidelines for testing a child without malignancy. J Med Genet. 2019 Feb;56(2):53–62. PMID:30415209
6753. Sugai M, Kimura N, Umehara M, et al. A case of pancreatoblastoma prenatally diagnosed as intraperitoneal cyst. Pediatr Surg Int. 2006 Oct;22(10):845–7. PMID:16896817
6754. Suganuma R, Wang LL, Sano H, et al. Peripheral neuroblastic tumors with genotype-phenotype discordance: a report from the Children's Oncology Group and the International Neuroblastoma Pathology Committee. Pediatr Blood Cancer. 2013 Mar;60(3):363–70. PMID:22744966
6755. Sugawara E, Togashi Y, Kuroda N, et al. Identification of anaplastic lymphoma kinase fusions in renal cancer: large-scale immunohistochemical screening by the intercalated antibody-enhanced polymer method. Cancer. 2012 Sep 15;118(18):4427–36. PMID:22252991
6756. Sugino K, Nagahama M, Kitagawa W, et al. Papillary thyroid carcinoma in children and adolescents: long-term follow-up and clinical characteristics. World J Surg. 2015 Sep;39(9):2259–65. PMID:25802237
6757. Sugita S, Arai Y, Aoyama T, et al. NUT-M2A-CIC fusion small round cell sarcoma: a genetically distinct variant of CIC-rearranged sarcoma. Hum Pathol. 2017 Jul;65:225–30. PMID:28188754
6758. Sugita S, Arai Y, Tonooka A, et al. A novel CIC-FOXO4 gene fusion in undifferentiated small round cell sarcoma: a genetically distinct variant of Ewing-like sarcoma. Am J Surg Pathol. 2014 Nov;38(11):1571–6. PMID:25007147
6759. Suh JK, Gao YJ, Tang JY, et al. Clinical characteristics and treatment outcomes of pediatric patients with non-Hodgkin lymphoma in East Asia. Cancer Res Treat. 2020 Apr;52(2):359–68. PMID:31352772
6760. Suh KY, Frieden IJ. Infantile hemangiomas with minimal or arrested growth: a retrospective case series. Arch Dermatol. 2010 Sep;146(9):971–6. PMID:20855695
6761. Suijker J, Baelde HJ, Roelofs H, et al. The oncometabolite D-2-hydroxyglutarate induced by mutant IDH1 or -2 blocks osteoblast differentiation in vitro and in vivo. Oncotarget. 2015 Jun 20;6(17):14832–42. PMID:26046462
6762. Sukov WR, Cheville JC, Giannini C, et al. Isochromosome 12p and polysomy 12 in primary central nervous system germ cell tumors: frequency and association with clinicopathologic features. Hum Pathol. 2010 Feb;41(2):232–8. PMID:19801160
6763. Sukov WR, Franco MF, Erickson-Johnson M, et al. Frequency of USP6 rearrangements in myositis ossificans, brown tumor, and cherubism: molecular cytogenetic evidence that a subset of "myositis ossificans-like lesions" are the early phases in the formation of soft-tissue aneurysmal bone cyst. Skeletal Radiol. 2008 Apr;37(4):321–7. PMID:18265974
6764. Sukov WR, Hodge JC, Lohse CM, et al. ALK alterations in adult renal cell carcinoma: frequency, clinicopathologic features and outcome in a large series of consecutively treated patients. Mod Pathol. 2012 Nov;25(11):1516–25. PMID:22743654
6765. Sukov WR, Hodge JC, Lohse CM, et al. TFE3 rearrangements in adult renal cell carcinoma: clinical and pathologic features with outcome in a large series of consecutively treated patients. Am J Surg Pathol. 2012 May;36(5):663–70. PMID:22498819
6766. Sullivan KE, Mullen CA, Blaese RM, et al. A multiinstitutional survey of the Wiskott-Aldrich syndrome. J Pediatr. 1994 Dec;125(6 Pt 1):876–85. PMID:7996359
6767. Sullivan LM, Folpe AL, Pawel BR, et al. Epithelioid sarcoma is associated with a high percentage of SMARCB1 deletions. Mod Pathol. 2013 Mar;26(3):385–92. PMID:23060122
6768. Sultan I, Casanova M, Ferrari A, et al. Differential features of nasopharyngeal carcinoma in children and adults: a SEER study. Pediatr Blood Cancer. 2010 Aug;55(2):279–84. PMID:20582982
6769. Sultan I, Qaddoumi I, Rodriguez-Galindo C, et al. Age, stage, and radiotherapy, but not primary tumor site, affects the outcome of patients with malignant rhabdoid tumors. Pediatr Blood Cancer. 2010 Jan;54(1):35–40. PMID:19798737
6770. Sultan I, Rodriguez-Galindo C, Al-Sharabati S, et al. Salivary gland carcinomas in children and adolescents: a population-based study, with comparison to adult cases. Head Neck. 2011 Oct;33(10):1476–81. PMID:21928420
6771. Sultan I, Rodriguez-Galindo C, Saab R, et al. Comparing children and adults with synovial sarcoma in the Surveillance, Epidemiology, and End Results Program, 1983 to 2005: an analysis of 1268 patients. Cancer. 2009 Aug 1;115(15):3537–47. PMID:19514087
6772. Sumazin P, Chen Y, Treviño LR, et al. Genomic analysis of hepatoblastoma identifies distinct molecular and prognostic subgroups. Hepatology. 2017 Jan;65(1):104–21. PMID:27775819
6773. Sumegi J, Streblow R, Frayer RW, et al. Recurrent t(2;2) and t(2;8) translocations in rhabdomyosarcoma without the canonical PAX-FOXO1 fuse PAX3 to members of the nuclear receptor transcriptional coactivator family. Genes Chromosomes Cancer. 2010 Mar;49(3):224–36. PMID:19953635
6774. Sun C, Zhang W, Ma H, et al. Main traits of breast fibroadenoma among adolescent girls. Cancer Biother Radiopharm. 2020 May;35(4):271–6. PMID:32267738
6775. Sun R, Sun L, Li G, et al. Congenital infiltrating lipomatosis of the face: a subtype of hemifacial hyperplasia. Int J Pediatr Otorhinolaryngol. 2019 Oct;125:107–12. PMID:31280031
6776. Sun Y, Zhao M, Lao IW, et al. The clinicopathological spectrum of pseudomyogenic hemangioendothelioma: report of an additional series with review of the literature. Virchows Arch. 2020 Aug;477(2):231–40. PMID:31980959
6777. Suneja R, Grimer RJ, Belthur M, et al. Chondroblastoma of bone: long-term results and functional outcome after intralesional curettage. J Bone Joint Surg Br. 2005 Jul;87(7):974–8. PMID:15972914
6779. Sung MS, Lee GK, Kang HS, et al. Sacrococcygeal chordoma: MR imaging in 30 patients. Skeletal Radiol. 2005 Feb;34(2):87–94. PMID:15480648
6780. Sung MT, Maclennan GT, Lopez-Beltran A, et al. Primary mediastinal seminoma: a comprehensive assessment integrated with histology, immunohistochemistry, and fluorescence in situ hybridization for chromosome 12p abnormalities in 23 cases. Am J Surg Pathol. 2008 Jan;32(1):146–55. PMID:18162782
6781. Sunitsch S, Gilg MM, Kashofer K, et al. Detection of GNAS mutations in intramuscular / cellular myxomas as diagnostic tool in the classification of myxoid soft tissue tumors. Diagn Pathol. 2018 Aug 15;13(1):52. PMID:30111377
6782. Suresh S, Saifuddin A. Radiological appearances of appendicular osteosarcoma: a comprehensive pictorial review. Clin Radiol. 2007 Apr;62(4):314–23. PMID:17331824
6783. Surrey LF, Jain P, Zhang B, et al. Genomic analysis of dysembryoplastic neuroepithelial tumor spectrum reveals a diversity of molecular alterations dysregulating the MAPK and PI3K/mTOR pathways. J Neuropathol Exp Neurol. 2019 Dec 1;78(12):1100–11. PMID:31617914
6784. Surun A, Varlet P, Brugières L, et al. Medulloblastomas associated with an APC germline pathogenic variant share the good prognosis of CTNNB1-mutated medulloblastomas. Neuro Oncol. 2020 Jan 11;22(1):128–38. PMID:31504825
6785. Surveillance, Epidemiology, and End Results (SEER) Program [Internet]. Bethesda (MD): National Cancer Institute; 2017. International Classification of Childhood Cancer (ICCC) recode third edition ICD-O-3/IARC 2017. Available from: https://seer.cancer.gov/iccc/iccc-iarc-2017.html
6786. Surveillance, Epidemiology, and End Results (SEER) Program [Internet]. Bethesda (MD): National Cancer Institute; 2018. Cancer Stat Facts: leukemia - chronic myeloid leukemia (CML). Available from: https://seer.cancer.gov/statfacts/html/cmyl.html.
6787. Surveillance, Epidemiology, and End Results (SEER) Program [Internet]. Bethesda (MD): National Cancer Institute; 2020. SEER Cancer Statistics Review (CSR) 1975-2017. Available from: https://seer.cancer.gov/archive/csr/1975_2017/.
6788. Surveillance, Epidemiology, and End Results (SEER) Program [Internet]. Bethesda (MD): National Cancer Institute; 2020. SEER Explorer. Available from: https://seer.cancer.gov/explorer/.
6789. Susam-Sen H, Yalcin B, Kutluk T, et al. Lipoblastoma in children: review of 12 cases. Pediatr Int. 2017 May;59(5):545–50. PMID:28083971
6790. Sussman W, Stasney J. Congenital glycogenic tumor of the heart. Am Heart J. 1950 Aug;40(2):312–5. PMID:15432292
6791. Suster S. Hyalinizing spindle and epithelioid cell nevus. A study of five cases of a distinctive histologic variant of Spitz's nevus. Am J Dermatopathol. 1994 Dec;16(6):593–8. PMID:7532378
6792. Suttorp M, Eckardt L, Tauer JT, et al. Management of chronic myeloid leukemia in childhood. Curr Hematol Malig Rep. 2012 Jun;7(2):116–24. PMID:22395816
6793. Suttorp M, Metzler M, Millot F. Horn of plenty: value of the international registry for pediatric chronic myeloid leukemia. World J Clin Oncol. 2020 Jun 24;11(6):308–19. PMID:32874947
6794. Suttorp M, Schulze P, Glauche I, et al. Front-line imatinib treatment in children and adolescents with chronic myeloid leukemia: results from a phase III trial. Leukemia. 2018 Jul;32(7):1657–69. PMID:29925908
6795. Suurmeijer AJ, Dickson BC, Swanson D, et al. The histologic spectrum of soft tissue spindle cell tumors with NTRK3 gene rearrangements. Genes Chromosomes Cancer. 2019 Nov;58(11):739–46. PMID:31112350
6796. Suurmeijer AJH, Dickson BC, Swanson D, et al. A morphologic and molecular reappraisal of myoepithelial tumors of soft tissue, bone, and viscera with EWSR1 and FUS gene rearrangements. Genes Chromosomes Cancer. 2020 Jun;59(6):348–56. PMID:31994243
6797. Suurmeijer AJH, Dickson BC, Swanson D, et al. A novel group of spindle cell tumors defined by S100 and CD34 co-expression shows recurrent fusions involving RAF1, BRAF, and NTRK1/2 genes. Genes Chromosomes Cancer. 2018 Dec;57(12):611–21. PMID:30276917
6798. Suzuki H, Kumar SA, Shuai S, et al. Recurrent noncoding U1 snRNA mutations drive cryptic splicing in SHH medulloblastoma. Nature. 2019 Oct;574(7780):707–11. PMID:31664194
6799. Suzuki K, Ohshima K, Karube K, et al. Clinicopathological states of Epstein-Barr virus-associated T/NK-cell lymphoproliferative disorders (severe chronic active EBV infection) of children and young adults. Int J Oncol. 2004 May;24(5):1165–74. PMID:15067338
6800. Suzuki R, Kagami Y, Takeuchi K, et al. Prognostic significance of CD56 expression for ALK-positive and ALK-negative anaplastic large-cell lymphoma of T/null cell phenotype. Blood. 2000 Nov 1;96(9):2993–3000. PMID:11049976
6801. Suzuki R, Suzumiya J, Nakamura S, et al. Aggressive natural killer-cell leukemia revisited: large granular lymphocyte leukemia of cytotoxic NK cells. Leukemia. 2004 Apr;18(4):763–70. PMID:14961041
6802. Suzuki-Inoue K, Tsukiji N, Shirai T, et al. Platelet CLEC-2: roles beyond hemostasis. Semin Thromb Hemost. 2018 Mar;44(2):126–34. PMID:28992650
6803. Švajdler M, Michal M, Martínek P, et al. Fibro-osseous pseudotumor of digits and myositis ossificans show consistent COL1A1-USP6 rearrangement: a clinicopathological and genetic study of 27 cases. Hum Pathol. 2019 Jun;88:39–47. PMID:30946936
6804. Swaminathan R, Rama R, Shanta V. Childhood cancers in Chennai, India, 1990-2001: incidence and survival. Int J Cancer. 2008 Jun 1;122(11):2607–11. PMID:18324630
6805. Swamy R, Embleton N, Hale J. Sacrococcygeal teratoma over two decades: birth prevalence, prenatal diagnosis and clinical outcomes. Prenat Diagn. 2008 Nov;28(11):1048–51. PMID:18973151
6806. Swanson AA, Raghunathan A, Jenkins RB, et al. Spinal cord ependymomas with MYCN amplification show aggressive clinical behavior. J Neuropathol Exp Neurol. 2019 Sep 1;78(9):791–7. PMID:31373367
6807. Sweeney CJ, Hermans BP, Heilman DK, et al. Results and outcome of retroperitoneal lymph node dissection for clinical stage I embryonal carcinoma–predominant testis cancer. J Clin Oncol. 2000 Jan;18(2):358–62. PMID:10637250
6808. Sweeney RT, McClary AC, Myers BR, et al. Identification of recurrent SMO and BRAF mutations in ameloblastomas. Nat Genet. 2014 Jul;46(7):722–5. PMID:24859340
6809. Sweet-Cordero EA, Biegel JA. The genomic landscape of pediatric cancers: implications for diagnosis and treatment. Science. 2019 Mar 15;363(6432):1170–5. PMID:30872516
6810. Swensen JJ, Keyser J, Coffin CM, et al. Familial occurrence of schwannomas and malignant rhabdoid tumour associated with a duplication in SMARCB1. J Med Genet. 2009 Jan;46(1):68–72. PMID:19124645
6811. Swerdlow SH. Pediatric follicular lymphomas, marginal zone lymphomas, and marginal zone hyperplasia. Am J Clin Pathol. 2004 Dec;122 Suppl:S98–109. PMID:15690646
6812. Swerdlow SH, Campo E, Harris NL, et al., editors. WHO classification of tumours of haematopoietic and lymphoid tissues. Lyon (France): International Agency for Research on Cancer; 2017. (WHO classification of tumours series, 4th rev. ed.; vol. 2). https://publications.iarc.fr/556.
6813. Swerdlow SH, Campo E, Pileri SA, et al. The 2016 revision of the World Health Organization classification of lymphoid neoplasms. Blood. 2016 May 19;127(20):2375–90. PMID:26980727

6814. Syed JS, Nguyen KA, Wu CQ, et al. Distinguishing pediatric and adolescent renal cell carcinoma from other renal malignancies. Pediatr Blood Cancer. 2017 May;64(5). PMID:27805307
6815. Syngal S, Brand RE, Church JM, et al. ACG clinical guideline: genetic testing and management of hereditary gastrointestinal cancer syndromes. Am J Gastroenterol. 2015 Feb;110(2):223–62. PMID:25645574
6816. Syrjänen S. Current concepts on human papillomavirus infections in children. APMIS. 2010 Jun;118(6-7):494–509. PMID:20553530
6817. Szczepanowski M, Lange J, Kohler CW, et al. Cell-of-origin classification by gene expression and MYC-rearrangements in diffuse large B-cell lymphoma of children and adolescents. Br J Haematol. 2017 Oct;179(1):116–9. PMID:28643426
6818. Szeifert GT, Pásztor E. Could craniopharyngiomas produce pituitary hormones? Neurol Res. 1993 Feb;15(1):68–9. PMID:8098858
6819. Szuhai K, de Jong D, Leung WY, et al. Transactivating mutation of the MYOD1 gene is a frequent event in adult spindle cell rhabdomyosarcoma. J Pathol. 2014 Feb;232(3):300–7. PMID:24272621
6820. Szuhai K, Ijszenga M, de Jong D, et al. The NFATc2 gene is involved in a novel cloned translocation in a Ewing sarcoma variant that couples its function in immunology to oncology. Clin Cancer Res. 2009 Apr 1;15(7):2259–68. PMID:19318479
6821. Szuhai K, IJszenga M, Tanke HJ, et al. Detection and molecular cytogenetic characterization of a novel ring chromosome in a histological variant of Ewing sarcoma. Cancer Genet Cytogenet. 2007 Jan 1;172(1):12–22. PMID:17175374
6822. Szyfelbein WM, Young RH, Scully RE. Cystic struma ovarii: a frequently unrecognized tumor. A report of 20 cases. Am J Surg Pathol. 1994 Aug;18(8):785–8. PMID:8037292
6823. Szyfelbein WM, Young RH, Scully RE. Struma ovarii simulating ovarian tumors of other types. A report of 30 cases. Am J Surg Pathol. 1995 Jan;19(1):21–9. PMID:7802134
6824. Szymanska J, Mandahl N, Mertens F, et al. Ring chromosomes in parosteal osteosarcoma contain sequences from 12q13-15: a combined cytogenetic and comparative genomic hybridization study. Genes Chromosomes Cancer. 1996 May;16(1):31–4. PMID:9162194
6825. Tabareau-Delalande F, Collin C, Gomez-Brouchet A, et al. Chromosome 12 long arm rearrangement covering MDM2 and RASAL1 is associated with aggressive craniofacial juvenile ossifying fibroma and extracranial psammomatoid fibro-osseous lesions. Mod Pathol. 2015 Jan;28(1):48–56. PMID:24925056
6826. Tabori U, Baskin B, Shago M, et al. Universal poor survival in children with medulloblastoma harboring somatic TP53 mutations. J Clin Oncol. 2010 Mar 10;28(8):1345–50. PMID:20142599
6827. Tabori U, Shlien A, Baskin B, et al. TP53 alterations determine clinical subgroups and survival of patients with choroid plexus tumors. J Clin Oncol. 2010 Apr 20;28(12):1995–2001. PMID:20308654
6828. Tabouret E, Bequet C, Denicolaï E, et al. BRAF mutation and anaplasia may be predictive factors of progression-free survival in adult pleomorphic xanthoastrocytoma. Eur J Surg Oncol. 2015 Dec;41(12):1685–90. PMID:26454767
6829. Tachibana O, Yamashima T, Yamashita J, et al. Immunohistochemical expression of human chorionic gonadotropin and P-glycoprotein in human pituitary glands and craniopharyngiomas. J Neurosurg. 1994 Jan;80(1):79–84. PMID:7903692
6830. Tacke ZC, Eikelenboom MJ, Vermeulen RJ, et al. Childhood lymphomatoid granulomatosis: a report of 2 cases and review of the literature. J Pediatr Hematol Oncol. 2014 Oct;36(7):e416–22. PMID:24390446
6831. Taddesse-Heath L, Pittaluga S, Sorbara L, et al. Marginal zone B-cell lymphoma in children and young adults. Am J Surg Pathol. 2003 Apr;27(4):522–31. PMID:12657939
6832. Tadini G, Boldrini MP, Brena M, et al. Nevoid follicular mucinosis: a new type of hair follicle nevus. J Cutan Pathol. 2013 Sep;40(9):844–7. PMID:23621858
6833. Taggard DA, Menezes AH. Three choroid plexus papillomas in a patient with Aicardi syndrome. A case report. Pediatr Neurosurg. 2000 Oct;33(4):219–23. PMID:11124640
6834. Tai CC, Curtis JL, Szmuszkovicz JR, et al. Abdominal involvement in pediatric heart and lung transplant recipients with posttransplant lymphoproliferative disease increases the risk of mortality. J Pediatr Surg. 2008 Dec;43(12):2174–7. PMID:19040929
6835. Tajima S, Fukayama M. Fibroblast growth factor receptor 1 (FGFR1) expression in phosphaturic mesenchymal tumors. Int J Clin Exp Pathol. 2015 Aug 1;8(8):9422–7. PMID:26464698
6836. Tajima Y, Kohara N, Maeda J, et al. Peritoneal and nodal recurrence 7 years after the excision of a ruptured solid pseudopapillary neoplasm of the pancreas: report of a case. Surg Today. 2012 Aug;42(8):776–80. PMID:22706721
6836A. Tajima S, Namiki I, Koda K. A clear cell variant of mucoepidermoid carcinoma harboring CRTC1-MAML2 fusion gene found in buccal mucosa: report of a case showing a large clear cell component and lacking typical epidermoid cells and intermediate cells. Med Mol Morphol. 2017 Jun;50(2):117–21. PMID:26297211
6837. Takagi N, Hirokawa M, Nobuoka Y, et al. Diffuse sclerosing variant of papillary thyroid carcinoma: a study of fine needle aspiration cytology in 20 patients. Cytopathology. 2014 Jun;25(3):199–204. PMID:23781895
6838. Takahashi H, Hida T. Carney complex: report of a Japanese case associated with cutaneous superficial angiomyxomas, labial lentigines, and a pituitary adenoma. J Dermatol. 2002 Dec;29(12):790–6. PMID:12532046
6839. Takahashi K, Mulliken JB, Kozakewich HP, et al. Cellular markers that distinguish the phases of hemangioma during infancy and childhood. J Clin Invest. 1994 Jun;93(6):2357–64. PMID:7911127
6840. Takahashi M, Yamamoto J, Aoyama Y, et al. Efficacy of multi-staged surgery and adjuvant chemotherapy for successful treatment of atypical choroid plexus papilloma in an infant: case report. Neurol Med Chir (Tokyo). 2009 Oct;49(10):484–7. PMID:19855149
6841. Takami H, Fukuoka K, Fukushima S, et al. Integrated clinical, histopathological, and molecular data analysis of 190 central nervous system germ cell tumors from the iGCT Consortium. Neuro Oncol. 2019 Dec 17;21(12):1565–77. PMID:31420671
6842. Takami H, Fukushima S, Aoki K, et al. Intratumoural immune cell landscape in germinoma reveals multipotent lineages and exhibits prognostic significance. Neuropathol Appl Neurobiol. 2020 Feb;46(2):111–24. PMID:31179566
6843. Takami H, Perry A, Graffeo CS, et al. Comparison on epidemiology, tumor location, histology, and prognosis of intracranial germ cell tumors between Mayo Clinic and Japanese consortium cohorts. J Neurosurg. 2020 Jan 31:1–11. PMID:32005022
6844. Takeda A, Watanabe K, Hayashi S, et al. Gynandroblastoma with a juvenile granulosa cell component in an adolescent: case report and literature review. J Pediatr Adolesc Gynecol. 2017 Apr;30(2):251–5. PMID:27751908
6845. Takeda S, Miyoshi S, Ohta M, et al. Primary germ cell tumors in the mediastinum: a 50-year experience at a single Japanese institution. Cancer. 2003 Jan 15;97(2):367–76. PMID:12518361
6846. Takeda Y, Shimono M. Pleomorphic adenoma with nuclear palisading arrangement of modified myoepithelial cells: histopathologic and immunohistochemical study. Bull Tokyo Dent Coll. 1999 Feb;40(1):27–34. PMID:10522175
6847. Takei H, Dauser RC, Adesina AM. Cytomorphologic characteristics, differential diagnosis and utility during intraoperative consultation for medulloblastoma. Acta Cytol. 2007 Mar-Apr;51(2):183–92. PMID:17425200
6848. Takeshima H, Kawahara Y, Hirano H, et al. Postoperative regression of desmoplastic infantile gangliogliomas: report of two cases. Neurosurgery. 2003 Oct;53(4):979–83. PMID:14519230
6849. Takeuchi K, Soda M, Togashi Y, et al. Identification of a novel fusion, SQSTM1-ALK, in ALK-positive large B-cell lymphoma. Haematologica. 2011 Mar;96(3):464–7. PMID:21134980
6850. Takeuchi K, Soda M, Togashi Y, et al. Pulmonary inflammatory myofibroblastic tumor expressing a novel fusion, PPFIBP1-ALK: reappraisal of anti-ALK immunohistochemistry as a tool for novel ALK fusion identification. Clin Cancer Res. 2011 May 15;17(10):3341–8. PMID:21430068
6851. Talbert RJ, Laor T, Yin H. Proliferative myositis: expanding the differential diagnosis of a soft tissue mass in infancy. Skeletal Radiol. 2011 Dec;40(12):1623–7. PMID:21912882
6852. Talbot C, Khan T, Smith M. Infantile digital fibromatosis. J Pediatr Orthop B. 2007 Mar;16(2):110–2. PMID:17273037
6853. Talerman A. Carcinoid tumors of the ovary. J Cancer Res Clin Oncol. 1984;107(2):125–35. PMID:6715397
6854. Talerman A, Evans MI. Primary trabecular carcinoid tumor of the ovary. Cancer. 1982 Oct 1;50(7):1403–7. PMID:7104979
6855. Talmon GA, Cohen SM. Mesenchymal hamartoma of the liver with an interstitial deletion involving chromosome band 19q13.4: a theory as to pathogenesis? Arch Pathol Lab Med. 2006 Aug;130(8):1216–8. PMID:16879027
6856. Tamimi HK, Bolen JW. Enchondromatosis (Ollier's disease) and ovarian juvenile granulosa cell tumor. Cancer. 1984 Apr 1;53(7):1605–8. PMID:6365306
6857. Tampourlou M, Ntali G, Ahmed S, et al. Outcome of nonfunctioning pituitary adenomas that regrow after primary treatment: a study from two large UK centers. J Clin Endocrinol Metab. 2017 Jun 1;102(6):1889–97. PMID:28323946
6858. Tamura D, DiGiovanna JJ, Khan SG, et al. Living with xeroderma pigmentosum: comprehensive photoprotection for highly photosensitive patients. Photodermatol Photoimmunol Photomed. 2014 Apr-Jun;30(2-3):146–52. PMID:24417420
6859. Tamura D, Khan SG, DiGiovanna JJ. Molecular diagnosis of xeroderma pigmentosum variant in an isolated population: the interface between precision medicine and public health. Br J Dermatol. 2017 May;176(5):1125–6. PMID:28504392
6860. Tan A, Stewart CJ, Garrett KL, et al. Novel BRAF and KRAS mutations in papillary thyroid carcinoma arising in struma ovarii. Endocr Pathol. 2015 Dec;26(4):296–301. PMID:26362194
6861. Tan C, Scotting PJ. Stem cell research points the way to the cell of origin for intracranial germ cell tumours. J Pathol. 2013 Jan;229(1):4–11. PMID:22926997
6862. Tan CS, Loh HL, Foo MW, et al. Epstein-Barr virus-associated smooth muscle tumors after kidney transplantation: treatment and outcomes in a single center. Clin Transplant. 2013 Jul-Aug;27(4):E462–8. PMID:23682851
6863. Tan H, Mei L, Huang Y, et al. Three novel mutations of STK11 gene in Chinese patients with Peutz-Jeghers syndrome. BMC Med Genet. 2016 Nov 8;17(1):77. PMID:27821076
6864. Tan KL, Scott DW, Hong F, et al. Tumor-associated macrophages predict inferior outcomes in classic Hodgkin lymphoma: a correlative study from the E2496 Intergroup trial. Blood. 2012 Oct 18;120(16):3280–7. PMID:22948049
6865. Tan SY, Szymanski LJ, Galliani C, et al. Solitary fibrous tumors in pediatric patients: a rare and potentially overdiagnosed neoplasm, confirmed by STAT6 immunohistochemistry. Pediatr Dev Pathol. 2018 Jul-Aug;21(4):389–400. PMID:29228868
6866. Tan TSE, Patel L, Gopal-Kothandapani JS, et al. The neuroendocrine sequelae of paediatric craniopharyngioma: a 40-year meta-data analysis of 185 cases from three UK centres. Eur J Endocrinol. 2017 Mar;176(3):359–69. PMID:28073908
6867. Tanaka A, Hirokawa M, Higuchi M, et al. Diagnostic clues indicating tall cell variants of papillary thyroid carcinoma in fine needle aspiration. Diagn Cytopathol. 2019 May;47(5):452–7. PMID:30582297
6868. Tanaka M, Kato K, Gomi K, et al. NUT midline carcinoma: report of 2 cases suggestive of pulmonary origin. Am J Surg Pathol. 2012 Mar;36(3):381–8. PMID:22301500
6869. Tanaka M, Kohashi K, Kushitani K, et al. Inflammatory myofibroblastic tumors of the lung carrying a chimeric A2M-ALK gene: report of 2 infantile cases and review of the differential diagnosis of infantile pulmonary lesions. Hum Pathol. 2017 Aug;66:177–82. PMID:28705706
6870. Tanaka M, Suda T, Haze K, et al. Fas ligand in human serum. Nat Med. 1996 Mar;2(3):317–22. PMID:8612231
6871. Tanaka N, Ueno T, Takama Y, et al. Fibroadenoma in adolescent females after living donor liver transplantation. Pediatr Transplant. 2017 Sep;21(6). PMID:28556594
6872. Tanaka T, Fumino S, Shirai T, et al. Mesenchymal hamartoma of the chest wall in a 10-year-old girl mimicking malignancy: a case report. Skeletal Radiol. 2019 Apr;48(4):643–7. PMID:30374636
6873. Tanaka Y, Ijiri R, Yamanaka S, et al. Pancreatoblastoma: optically clear nuclei in squamoid corpuscles are rich in biotin. Mod Pathol. 1998 Oct;11(10):945–9. PMID:9796720
6874. Tanaka Y, Kato K, Notohara K, et al. Frequent beta-catenin mutation and cytoplasmic/nuclear accumulation in pancreatic solid-pseudopapillary neoplasm. Cancer Res. 2001 Dec 1;61(23):8401–4. PMID:11731417
6875. Tanaka Y, Kato K, Notohara K, et al. Significance of aberrant (cytoplasmic/nuclear) expression of beta-catenin in pancreatoblastoma. J Pathol. 2003 Feb;199(2):185–90. PMID:12533831
6876. Tanaka Y, Notohara K, Kato K, et al. Usefulness of beta-catenin immunostaining for the differential diagnosis of solid-pseudopapillary neoplasm of the pancreas. Am J Surg Pathol. 2002 Jun;26(6):818–20. PMID:12023593
6877. Tanaka Y, Sasaki Y, Nishihira H, et al. Ovarian juvenile granulosa cell tumor associated with Maffucci's syndrome. Am J Clin Pathol. 1992 Apr;97(4):523–7. PMID:1553918
6878. Tanas MR, Ma S, Jadaan FO, et al. Mechanism of action of a WWTR1(TAZ)-CAMTA1 fusion oncoprotein. Oncogene. 2016 Feb 18;35(7):929–38. PMID:25961935

**6879.** Tanas MR, Sboner A, Oliveira AM, et al. Identification of a disease-defining gene fusion in epithelioid hemangioendothelioma. Sci Transl Med. 2011 Aug 31;3(98):98ra82. PMID:21885404
**6880.** Tanase A, Schmitz N, Stein H, et al. Allogeneic and autologous stem cell transplantation for hepatosplenic T-cell lymphoma: a retrospective study of the EBMT Lymphoma Working Party. Leukemia. 2015 Mar;29(3):686–8. PMID:25234166
**6881.** Tang LH, Aydin H, Brennan MF, et al. Clinically aggressive solid pseudopapillary tumors of the pancreas: a report of two cases with components of undifferentiated carcinoma and a comparative clinicopathologic analysis of 34 conventional cases. Am J Surg Pathol. 2005 Apr;29(4):512–9. PMID:15767807
**6882.** Tang TT, Segura AD, Oechler HW, et al. Inflammatory myofibrohistiocytic proliferation simulating sarcoma in children. Cancer. 1990 Apr 1;65(7):1626–34. PMID:2311072
**6883.** Tang YT, Wang D, Luo H, et al. Aggressive NK-cell leukemia: clinical subtypes, molecular features, and treatment outcomes. Blood Cancer J. 2017 Dec 21;7(12):660. PMID:29263371
**6884.** Tangye SG, Al-Herz W, Bousfiha A, et al. Human inborn errors of immunity: 2019 update on the classification from the International Union of Immunological Societies Expert Committee. J Clin Immunol. 2020 Jan;40(1):24–64. PMID:31953710
**6885.** Tangye SG, Latour S. Primary immunodeficiencies reveal the molecular requirements for effective host defense against EBV infection. Blood. 2020 Feb 27;135(9):644–55. PMID:31942615
**6886.** Tanizaki Y, Jin L, Scheithauer BW, et al. P53 gene mutations in pituitary carcinomas. Endocr Pathol. 2007 Winter;18(4):217–22. PMID:18026859
**6887.** Tanizawa A. Optimal management for pediatric chronic myeloid leukemia. Pediatr Int. 2016 Mar;58(3):171–9. PMID:26646444
**6888.** Tannenbaum M, Colucci PG, Baad M, et al. Chondroid lipoma: multimodality imaging in a 9-year-old female. Skeletal Radiol. 2020 Jan;49(1):161–9. PMID:31230114
**6889.** Tantcheva-Poor I, Marathovouniotis N, Kutzner H, et al. Vascular congenital dermatofibrosarcoma protuberans: a new histological variant of dermatofibrosarcoma protuberans. Am J Dermatopathol. 2012 Jun;34(4):e46–9. PMID:22257899
**6890.** Tantcheva-Poor I, Reinhold K, Krieg T, et al. Trichilemmal cyst nevus: a new complex organoid epidermal nevus. J Am Acad Dermatol. 2007 Nov;57(5 Suppl):S72–7. PMID:17097381
**6891.** Tao J, Calvisi DF, Ranganathan S, et al. Activation of β-catenin and Yap1 in human hepatoblastoma and induction of hepatocarcinogenesis in mice. Gastroenterology. 2014 Sep;147(3):690–701. PMID:24837480
**6892.** Tao J, Valderrama E. Epstein-Barr virus-associated polymorphic B-cell lymphoproliferative disorders in the lungs of children with AIDS: a report of two cases. Am J Surg Pathol. 1999 May;23(5):560–6. PMID:10328088
**6893.** Tao R, Murad N, Xu Z, et al. MYC drives Group 3 medulloblastoma through transformation of Sox2+ astrocyte progenitor cells. Cancer Res. 2019 Apr 15;79(8):1967–80. PMID:30862721
**6894.** Tap WD, Gelderblom H, Palmerini E, et al. Pexidartinib versus placebo for advanced tenosynovial giant cell tumour (ENLIVEN): a randomised phase 3 trial. Lancet. 2019 Aug 10;394(10197):478–87. PMID:31229240
**6895.** Tapella L, Sesta A, Cassarino MF, et al. Benzene and 2-ethyl-phthalate induce proliferation in normal rat pituitary cells. Pituitary. 2017 Jun;20(3):311–8. PMID:27853917
**6896.** Taratuto AL, Monges J, Lylyk P, et al. Superficial cerebral astrocytoma attached to dura. Report of six cases in infants. Cancer. 1984 Dec 1;54(11):2505–12. PMID:6498740
**6897.** Tariq MU, Din NU, Bashir MR. Hairy polyp, a clinicopathologic study of four cases. Head Neck Pathol. 2013 Sep;7(3):232–5. PMID:23494895
**6898.** Tarlock K, Lamble AJ, Wang YC, et al. CEBPA-bZip mutations are associated with favorable prognosis in de novo AML: a report from the Children's Oncology Group. Blood. 2021 Sep 30;138(13):1137–47. PMID:33951732
**6899.** Tarpey PS, Behjati S, Young MD, et al. The driver landscape of sporadic chordoma. Nat Commun. 2017 Oct 12;8(1):890. PMID:29026114
**6900.** Tarrant WP, Czerniak BA, Guo CC. Relationship between primary and metastatic testicular germ cell tumors: a clinicopathologic analysis of 100 cases. Hum Pathol. 2013 Oct;44(10):2220–6. PMID:23856516
**6901.** Tarulli GA, Stanton PG, Loveland KL, et al. A survey of Sertoli cell differentiation in men after gonadotropin suppression and in testicular cancer. Spermatogenesis. 2013 Jan 1;3(1):e24014. PMID:23687617
**6902.** Taruscio D, Paradisi S, Zamboni G, et al. Pancreatic acinar carcinoma shows a distinct pattern of chromosomal imbalances by comparative genomic hybridization. Genes Chromosomes Cancer. 2000 Jul;28(3):294–9. PMID:10862035
**6903.** Taskinen M, Ranki A, Pukkala E, et al. Extended follow-up of the Finnish cartilage-hair hypoplasia cohort confirms high incidence of non-Hodgkin lymphoma and basal cell carcinoma. Am J Med Genet A. 2008 Sep 15;146A(18):2370–5. PMID:18698627
**6904.** Taskinen S, Fagerholm R, Aronniemi J, et al. Testicular tumors in children and adolescents. J Pediatr Urol. 2008 Apr;4(2):134–7. PMID:18631909
**6905.** Tate G, Suzuki T, Mitsuya T. Mutation of the PTEN gene in a human hepatic angiosarcoma. Cancer Genet Cytogenet. 2007 Oct 15;178(2):160–2. PMID:17954274
**6906.** Tate M, Sughrue ME, Rutkowski MJ, et al. The long-term postsurgical prognosis of patients with pineoblastoma. Cancer. 2012 Jan 1;118(1):173–9. PMID:21717450
**6907.** Tateishi U, Müller NL, Johkoh T, et al. Primary mediastinal lymphoma: characteristic features of the various histological subtypes on CT. J Comput Assist Tomogr. 2004 Nov-Dec;28(6):782–9. PMID:15538151
**6908.** Tatekawa Y, Muraji T, Nishijima E, et al. Composite pheochromocytoma associated with adrenal neuroblastoma in an infant: a case report. J Pediatr Surg. 2006 Feb;41(2):443–5. PMID:16481267
**6909.** Tateno T, Zhu X, Asa SL, et al. Chromatin remodeling and histone modifications in pituitary tumors. Mol Cell Endocrinol. 2010 Sep 15;326(1-2):66–70. PMID:20060434
**6910.** Tatevossian RG, Tang B, Dalton J, et al. MYB upregulation and genetic aberrations in a subset of pediatric low-grade gliomas. Acta Neuropathol. 2010 Dec;120(6):731–43. PMID:21046410
**6911.** Tateyama H, Tada T, Okabe M, et al. Different keratin profiles in craniopharyngioma subtypes and ameloblastomas. Pathol Res Pract. 2001;197(11):735–42. PMID:11770017
**6912.** Tatlidede S, Karsidag S, Ugurlu K, et al. Sialoblastoma: a congenital epithelial tumor of the salivary gland. J Pediatr Surg. 2006 Jul;41(7):1322–5. PMID:16818073
**6913.** Tatsi C, Bacopoulou F, Lyssikatos C, et al. Sporadic melanotic schwannoma with overlapping features of melanocytoma bearing a GNA11 mutation in an adolescent girl. Pediatr Blood Cancer. 2017 Jun;64(6):10.1002/pbc.26400. PMID:28012237
**6914.** Taub JW, Berman JN, Hitzler JK, et al. Improved outcomes for myeloid leukemia of Down syndrome: a report from the Children's Oncology Group AAML0431 trial. Blood. 2017 Jun 22;129(25):3304–13. PMID:28389462
**6915.** Taub JW, Ge Y. Down syndrome, drug metabolism and chromosome 21. Pediatr Blood Cancer. 2005 Jan;44(1):33–9. PMID:15390307
**6916.** Tauziède-Espariat A, Debily MA, Castel D, et al. An integrative radiological, histopathological and molecular analysis of pediatric pontine histone-wildtype glioma with MYCN amplification (HGG-MYCN). Acta Neuropathol Commun. 2019 Jun 10;7(1):87. PMID:31177990
**6917.** Tauziède-Espariat A, Debily MA, Castel D, et al. The pediatric supratentorial MYCN-amplified high-grade gliomas methylation class presents the same radiological, histopathological and molecular features as their pontine counterparts. Acta Neuropathol Commun. 2020 Jul 9;8(1):104. PMID:32646492
**6918.** Tauziède-Espariat A, Pagès M, Roux A, et al. Pediatric methylation class HGNET-MN1: unresolved issues with terminology and grading. Acta Neuropathol Commun. 2019 Nov 10;7(1):176. PMID:31707996
**6919.** Tawana K, Rio-Machin A, Preudhomme C, et al. Familial CEBPA-mutated acute myeloid leukemia. Semin Hematol. 2017 Apr;54(2):87–93. PMID:28637622
**6920.** Taweevisit M, Trinavarat P, Thorner PS. Aspiration cytology of mesenchymal hamartoma of the chest wall: a case report and literature review. Diagn Cytopathol. 2014 Oct;42(10):890–4. PMID:24574377
**6921.** Tay TK, Chang KT, Thike AA, et al. Paediatric fibroepithelial lesions revisited: pathological insights. J Clin Pathol. 2015 Aug;68(8):633–41. PMID:25998513
**6922.** Tay TKY, Guan P, Loke BN, et al. Molecular insights into paediatric breast fibroepithelial tumours. Histopathology. 2018 Nov;73(5):809–18. PMID:29969836
**6923.** Taylor GP. Congenital epithelial tumor of the parotid-sialoblastoma. Pediatr Pathol. 1988;8(4):447–52. PMID:3211816
**6924.** Taylor J, McCluggage WG. Ovarian sex cord-stromal tumors with melanin pigment: report of a previously undescribed phenomenon. Int J Gynecol Pathol. 2019 Jan;38(1):92–6. PMID:29140884
**6925.** Taylor JB, Solomon DH, Levine RE, et al. Exophthalmos in seminoma. Regression with steroids and orcheictomy. JAMA. 1978 Sep 1;240(9):860–2. PMID:671734
**6926.** Taylor KR, Mackay A, Truffaux N, et al. Recurrent activating ACVR1 mutations in diffuse intrinsic pontine glioma. Nat Genet. 2014 May;46(5):457–61. PMID:24705252
**6927.** Taylor MD, Gokgoz N, Andrulis IL, et al. Familial posterior fossa brain tumors of infancy secondary to germline mutation of the hSNF5 gene. Am J Hum Genet. 2000 Apr;66(4):1403–6. PMID:10739763
**6928.** Taylor MD, Jones DR. Genetic markers of mediastinal tumors. Thorac Surg Clin. 2009 Feb;19(1):17–27. PMID:19288817
**6929.** Taylor MD, Liu L, Raffel C, et al. Mutations in SUFU predispose to medulloblastoma. Nat Genet. 2002 Jul;31(3):306–10. PMID:12068298
**6930.** Taylor MD, Northcott PA, Korshunov A, et al. Molecular subgroups of medulloblastoma: the current consensus. Acta Neuropathol. 2012 Apr;123(4):465–72. PMID:22134537
**6931.** Taylor MD, Poppleton H, Fuller C, et al. Radial glia cells are candidate stem cells of ependymoma. Cancer Cell. 2005 Oct;8(4):323–35. PMID:16226707
**6932.** Taylor-Weiner A, Zack T, O'Donnell E, et al. Genomic evolution and chemoresistance in germ-cell tumours. Nature. 2016 Nov 30;540(7631):114–8. PMID:27905446
**6933.** Tcheng WY, Said J, Hall T, et al. Post-transplant multiple myeloma in a pediatric renal transplant patient. Pediatr Blood Cancer. 2006 Aug;47(2):218–23. PMID:16086426
**6934.** Tchoghandjian A, Fernandez C, Colin C, et al. Pilocytic astrocytoma of the optic pathway: a tumour deriving from radial glia cells with a specific gene signature. Brain. 2009 Jun;132(Pt 6):1523–35. PMID:19336457
**6935.** Techavichit P, Hicks MJ, López-Terrada DH, et al. Mucoepidermoid carcinoma in children: a single institutional experience. Pediatr Blood Cancer. 2016 Jan;63(1):27–31. PMID:26221861
**6936.** Techavichit P, Masand PM, Himes RW, et al. Undifferentiated embryonal sarcoma of the liver (UESL): a single-center experience and review of the literature. J Pediatr Hematol Oncol. 2016 May;38(4):261–8. PMID:26925712
**6937.** Tee AR, Fingar DC, Manning BD, et al. Tuberous sclerosis complex-1 and -2 gene products function together to inhibit mammalian target of rapamycin (mTOR)-mediated downstream signaling. Proc Natl Acad Sci U S A. 2002 Oct 15;99(21):13571–6. PMID:12271141
**6938.** Telfeian AE, Judkins A, Younkin D, et al. Subependymal giant cell astrocytoma with cranial and spinal metastases in a patient with tuberous sclerosis. Case report. J Neurosurg. 2004 May;100(5 Suppl Pediatrics):498–500. PMID:15287462
**6939.** Telugu RB, Prabhu AJ, Kalappurayil NB, et al. Clinicopathological study of 18 cases of inflammatory myofibroblastic tumors with reference to ALK-1 Expression: 5-year experience in a tertiary care center. J Pathol Transl Med. 2017 May;51(3):255–63. PMID:28415158
**6940.** Tembo R, Kaile T, Kafita D, et al. Detection of human herpes virus 8 in Kaposi's sarcoma tissues at the University Teaching Hospital, Lusaka, Zambia. Pan Afr Med J. 2017 Jun 22;27:137. PMID:28904666
**6941.** Temming P, Arendt M, Viehmann A, et al. How eye-preserving therapy affects long-term overall survival in heritable retinoblastoma survivors. J Clin Oncol. 2016 Sep 10;34(26):3183–8. PMID:27382102
**6942.** Tempark T, Shwayder T. Mucinous eccrine naevus: case report and review of the literature. Clin Exp Dermatol. 2013 Jan;38(1):1–4. PMID:23252751
**6943.** Ten Broek RW, Koelsche C, Eijkelenboom A, et al. Kaposiform hemangioendothelioma and tufted angioma - (epi)genetic analysis including genome-wide methylation profiling. Ann Diagn Pathol. 2020 Feb;44:151434. PMID:31887709
**6944.** ten Heuvel SE, Hoekstra HJ, Bastiaannet E, et al. The classic prognostic factors tumor stage, tumor size, and tumor grade are the strongest predictors of outcome in synovial sarcoma: no role for SSX fusion type or ezrin expression. Appl Immunohistochem Mol Morphol. 2009 May;17(3):189–95. PMID:18997619
**6945.** Teo JY, Cheong CS, Wong CY. Low local recurrence rates in young Asian patients with phyllodes tumours: less is more. ANZ J Surg. 2012 May;82(5):325–8. PMID:22507352
**6946.** Teo WY, Shen J, Su JM, et al. Implications of tumor location on subtypes of medulloblastoma. Pediatr Blood Cancer. 2013 Sep;60(9):1408–10. PMID:23512859
**6947.** Terashima K, Yu A, Chow WY, et al. Genome-wide analysis of DNA copy number alterations and loss of heterozygosity

in intracranial germ cell tumors. Pediatr Blood Cancer. 2014 Apr;61(4):593–600. PMID:24249158

**6948.** Terenziani M, D'Angelo P, Bisogno G, et al. Teratoma with a malignant somatic component in pediatric patients: the Associazione Italiana Ematologia Oncologia Pediatrica (AIEOP) experience. Pediatr Blood Cancer. 2010 Apr;54(4):532–7. PMID:20049928

**6949.** Terenziani M, Piva L, Spreafico F, et al. Clinical stage I nonseminomatous germ cell tumors of the testis in childhood and adolescence: an analysis of 31 cases. J Pediatr Hematol Oncol. 2002 Aug-Sep;24(6):454–8. PMID:12218592

**6950.** Terrier LM, Bauchet L, Rigau V, et al. Natural course and prognosis of anaplastic gangliogliomas: a multicenter retrospective study of 43 cases from the French Brain Tumor Database. Neuro Oncol. 2017 May 1;19(5):678–88. PMID:28453747

**6951.** Terrier-Lacombe MJ, Guillou L, Maire G, et al. Dermatofibrosarcoma protuberans, giant cell fibroblastoma, and hybrid lesions in children: clinicopathologic comparative analysis of 28 cases with molecular data–a study from the French Federation of Cancer Centers Sarcoma Group. Am J Surg Pathol. 2003 Jan;27(1):27–39. PMID:12502925

**6952.** Teruya-Feldstein J, Jaffe ES, Burd PR, et al. The role of Mig, the monokine induced by interferon-gamma, and IP-10, the interferon-gamma-inducible protein-10, in tissue necrosis and vascular damage associated with Epstein-Barr virus-positive lymphoproliferative disease. Blood. 1997 Nov 15;90(10):4099–105. PMID:9354680

**6953.** Teruya-Feldstein J, Temeck BK, Sloas MM, et al. Pulmonary malignant lymphoma of mucosa-associated lymphoid tissue (MALT) arising in a pediatric HIV-positive patient. Am J Surg Pathol. 1995 Mar;19(3):357–63. PMID:7872434

**6954.** Tesher MS, Esteban Y, Henderson TO, et al. Mucosal-associated lymphoid tissue (MALT) lymphoma in association with pediatric primary Sjogren syndrome: 2 cases and review. J Pediatr Hematol Oncol. 2019 Jul;41(5):413–6. PMID:30371536

**6955.** Tesileanu CMS, Dirven L, Wijnenga MMJ, et al. Survival of diffuse astrocytic glioma, IDH1/2 wildtype, with molecular features of glioblastoma, WHO grade IV: a confirmation of the cIMPACT-NOW criteria. Neuro Oncol. 2020 Apr 15;22(4):515–23. PMID:31637414

**6956.** Tessler FN, Middleton WD, Grant EG, et al. ACR Thyroid Imaging, Reporting and Data System (TI-RADS): white paper of the ACR TI-RADS Committee. J Am Coll Radiol. 2017 May;14(5):587–95. PMID:28372962

**6957.** Testa JR, Cheung M, Pei J, et al. Germline BAP1 mutations predispose to malignant mesothelioma. Nat Genet. 2011 Aug 28;43(10):1022–5. PMID:21874000

**6958.** Thaung C, Bonshek RE, Leatherbarrow B. Phakomatous choristoma of the eyelid: a case with associated eye abnormalities. Br J Ophthalmol. 2006 Feb;90(2):245–6. PMID:16424545

**6959.** Theilen TM, Soerensen J, Bochennek K, et al. Crizotinib in ALK+ inflammatory myofibroblastic tumors-current experience and future perspectives. Pediatr Blood Cancer. 2018 Apr;65(4). PMID:29286567

**6960.** Thériault BL, Dimaras H, Gallie BL, et al. The genomic landscape of retinoblastoma: a review. Clin Exp Ophthalmol. 2014 Jan-Feb;42(1):33–52. PMID:24433356

**6961.** Thiagalingam S, Johnson MM, Colby KA, et al. Juvenile conjunctival nevus: clinicopathologic analysis of 33 cases. Am J Surg Pathol. 2008 Mar;32(3):399–406. PMID:18300811

**6962.** Thiel EL, Trost BA, Tower RL. A composite pheochromocytoma/ganglioneuroblastoma of the adrenal gland. Pediatr Blood Cancer. 2010 Jul 1;54(7):1032–4. PMID:20162688

**6963.** Thiele EA. Managing and understanding epilepsy in tuberous sclerosis complex. Epilepsia. 2010 Feb;51 Suppl 1:90–1. PMID:20331728

**6964.** Thiessen B, Finlay J, Kulkarni R, et al. Astroblastoma: Does histology predict biologic behavior? J Neurooncol. 1998 Oct;40(1):59–65. PMID:9874187

**6965.** Thimsen V, John N, Buchfelder M, et al. Expression of SRY-related HMG box transcription factors (Sox) 2 and 9 in Craniopharyngioma subtypes and surrounding brain tissue. Sci Rep. 2017 Nov 20;7(1):15856. PMID:29158570

**6966.** Thiollier C, Lopez CK, Gerby B, et al. Characterization of novel genomic alterations and therapeutic approaches using acute megakaryoblastic leukemia xenograft models. J Exp Med. 2012 Oct 22;209(11):2017–31. PMID:23045605

**6967.** Thom M, Blümcke I, Aronica E. Long-term epilepsy-associated tumors. Brain Pathol. 2012 May;22(3):350–79. PMID:22497610

**6968.** Thom M, Gomez-Anson B, Revesz T, et al. Spontaneous intralesional haemorrhage in dysembryoplastic neuroepithelial tumours: a series of five cases. J Neurol Neurosurg Psychiatry. 1999 Jul;67(1):97–101. PMID:10369831

**6969.** Thom M, Liu J, Bongaarts A, et al. Multinodular and vacuolating neuronal tumors in epilepsy: dysplasia or neoplasia? Brain Pathol. 2018 Mar;28(2):155–71. PMID:28833756

**6970.** Thom M, Toma A, An S, et al. One hundred and one dysembryoplastic neuroepithelial tumors: an adult epilepsy series with immunohistochemical, molecular genetic, and clinical correlations and a review of the literature. J Neuropathol Exp Neurol. 2011 Oct;70(10):859–78. PMID:21937911

**6971.** Thoman PJ, Shaw SL, Collins JF. Isolation and characterization of fibronectin from baboon plasma. Connect Tissue Res. 1985;13(2):135–43. PMID:3157541

**6972.** Thomas C, Ruland V, Kordes U, et al. Pediatric atypical choroid plexus papilloma reconsidered: increased mitotic activity is prognostic only in older children. Acta Neuropathol. 2015 Jun;129(6):925–7. PMID:25935663

**6973.** Thomas C, Sill M, Ruland V, et al. Methylation profiling of choroid plexus tumors reveals 3 clinically distinct subgroups. Neuro Oncol. 2016 Jun;18(6):790–6. PMID:26826203

**6974.** Thomas C, Wefers A, Bens S, et al. Desmoplastic myxoid tumor, SMARCB1-mutant: clinical, histopathological and molecular characterization of a pineal region tumor encountered in adolescents and adults. Acta Neuropathol. 2020 Feb;139(2):277–86. PMID:31732806

**6975.** Thomas CM, Asa SL, Ezzat S, et al. Diagnosis and pathologic characteristics of medullary thyroid carcinoma-review of current guidelines. Curr Oncol. 2019 Oct;26(5):338–44. PMID:31708652

**6976.** Thomas PK, King RH, Chiang TR, et al. Neurofibromatous neuropathy. Muscle Nerve. 1990 Feb;13(2):93–101. PMID:2156160

**6977.** Thompson BA, Spurdle AB, Plazzer JP, et al. Application of a 5-tiered scheme for standardized classification of 2,360 unique mismatch repair gene variants in the InSiGHT locus-specific database. Nat Genet. 2014 Feb;46(2):107–15. PMID:24362816

**6978.** Thompson LD. Pheochromocytoma of the Adrenal gland Scaled Score (PASS) to separate benign from malignant neoplasms: a clinicopathologic and immunophenotypic study of 100 cases. Am J Surg Pathol. 2002 May;26(5):551–66. PMID:11979086

**6979.** Thompson LD, Aslam MN, Stall JN, et al. Clinicopathologic and immunophenotypic characterization of 25 cases of acinic cell carcinoma with high-grade transformation. Head Neck Pathol. 2016 Jun;10(2):152–60. PMID:26245749

**6980.** Thompson LD, Gyure KA. Extracranial sinonasal tract meningiomas: a clinicopathologic study of 30 cases with a review of the literature. Am J Surg Pathol. 2000 May;24(5):640–50. PMID:10800982

**6981.** Thompson LD, Nelson BL, Barnes EL. Ceruminous adenomas: a clinicopathologic study of 41 cases with a review of the literature. Am J Surg Pathol. 2004 Mar;28(3):308–18. PMID:15104293

**6982.** Thompson LD, Wieneke JA, Heffess CS. Diffuse sclerosing variant of papillary thyroid carcinoma: a clinicopathologic and immunophenotypic analysis of 22 cases. Endocr Pathol. 2005 Winter;16(4):331–48. PMID:16627920

**6983.** Thompson LDR, Gill AJ, Asa SL, et al. Data set for the reporting of pheochromocytoma and paraganglioma: explanations and recommendations of the guidelines from the International Collaboration on Cancer Reporting. Hum Pathol. 2021 Apr;110:83–97. PMID:32407815

**6984.** Thompson LDR, Herrera HB, Lau SK. Thyroglossal duct cyst carcinomas in pediatric patients: report of two cases with a comprehensive literature review. Head Neck Pathol. 2017 Dec;11(4):442–9. PMID:28293858

**6985.** Thorer H, Zimmermann M, Makarova O, et al. Primary central nervous system lymphoma in children and adolescents: low relapse rate after treatment according to Non-Hodgkin-Lymphoma Berlin-Frankfurt-Münster protocols for systemic lymphoma. Haematologica. 2014 Nov;99(11):e238–41. PMID:25107886

**6986.** Thosani S, Ayala-Ramirez M, Palmer L, et al. The characterization of pheochromocytoma and its impact on overall survival in multiple endocrine neoplasia type 2. J Clin Endocrinol Metab. 2013 Nov;98(11):E1813–9. PMID:24030942

**6987.** Thway K. Well-differentiated liposarcoma and dedifferentiated liposarcoma: an updated review. Semin Diagn Pathol. 2019 Mar;36(2):112–21. PMID:30852045

**6988.** Thway K, Fisher C. Angiomatoid fibrous histiocytoma: the current status of pathology and genetics. Arch Pathol Lab Med. 2015 May;139(5):674–82. PMID:25927151

**6989.** Thway K, Fisher C, Debiec-Rychter M, et al. Claudin-1 is expressed in perineurioma-like low-grade fibromyxoid sarcoma. Hum Pathol. 2009 Nov;40(11):1586–90. PMID:19540561

**6990.** Thway K, Fisher C, Sebire NJ. Pediatric fibroblastic and myofibroblastic lesions. Adv Anat Pathol. 2012 Jan;19(1):54–65. PMID:22156834

**6991.** Thway K, Jones RL, Noujaim J, et al. Epithelioid Sarcoma: diagnostic Features and Genetics. Adv Anat Pathol. 2016 Jan;23(1):41–9. PMID:26645461

**6992.** Tiacci E, Ladewig E, Schiavoni G, et al. Pervasive mutations of JAK-STAT pathway genes in classical Hodgkin lymphoma. Blood. 2018 May 31;131(22):2454–65. PMID:29650799

**6993.** Tian L, Cui CY, Lu SY, et al. Clinical presentation and CT/MRI findings of alveolar soft part sarcoma: a retrospective single-center analysis of 14 cases. Acta Radiol. 2016 Apr;57(4):475–80. PMID:26231949

**6994.** Tiemann K, Heitling U, Kosmahl M, et al. Solid pseudopapillary neoplasms of the pancreas show an interruption of the Wnt-signaling pathway and express gene products of 11q. Mod Pathol. 2007 Sep;20(9):955–60. PMID:17632456

**6995.** Tien RD, Barkovich AJ, Edwards MS. MR imaging of pineal tumors. AJR Am J Roentgenol. 1990 Jul;155(1):143–51. PMID:2162137

**6996.** Tihan T, Ersen A, Qaddoumi I, et al. Pathologic characteristics of pediatric intracranial pilocytic astrocytomas and their impact on outcome in 3 countries: a multi-institutional study. Am J Surg Pathol. 2012 Jan;36(1):43–55. PMID:21989351

**6997.** Tihan T, Fisher PG, Kepner JL, et al. Pediatric astrocytomas with monomorphous pilomyxoid features and a less favorable outcome. J Neuropathol Exp Neurol. 1999 Oct;58(10):1061–8. PMID:10515229

**6998.** Tilakaratne WM, Jayasooriya PR, Tennakoon TM, et al. Epithelial salivary tumors in Sri Lanka: a retrospective study of 713 cases. Oral Surg Oral Med Oral Pathol Oral Radiol Endod. 2009 Jul;108(1):90–8. PMID:19403317

**6999.** Tirabosco R, Mangham DC, Rosenberg AE, et al. Brachyury expression in extra-axial skeletal and soft tissue chordomas: a marker that distinguishes chordoma from mixed tumor/myoepithelioma/parachordoma in soft tissue. Am J Surg Pathol. 2008 Apr;32(4):572–80. PMID:18301055

**7000.** Tirode F, Surdez D, Ma X, et al. Genomic landscape of Ewing sarcoma defines an aggressive subtype with co-association of STAG2 and TP53 mutations. Cancer Discov. 2014 Nov;4(11):1342–53. PMID:25223734

**7001.** Tischkowitz M, Huang S, Banerjee S, et al. Small-cell carcinoma of the ovary, hypercalcemic type-genetics, new treatment targets, and current management guidelines. Clin Cancer Res. 2020 Aug 1;26(15):3908–17. PMID:32156746

**7002.** Tischler AS. Pheochromocytoma and extra-adrenal paraganglioma: updates. Arch Pathol Lab Med. 2008 Aug;132(8):1272–84. PMID:18684026

**7003.** Tischler AS, deKrijger RR. 15 years of paraganglioma: pathology of pheochromocytoma and paraganglioma. Endocr Relat Cancer. 2015 Aug;22(4):T123–33. PMID:26136457

**7004.** Titgemeyer C, Grois N, Minkov M, et al. Pattern and course of single-system disease in Langerhans cell histiocytosis data from the DAL-HX 83- and 90-study. Med Pediatr Oncol. 2001 Aug;37(2):108–14. PMID:11496348

**7005.** Titsinides S, Nikitakis NG, Tasoulas J, et al. Ossifying fibromyxoid tumor of the retromolar trigone: a case report and systematic review of the literature. Int J Surg Pathol. 2017 Sep;25(6):526–32. PMID:28436288

**7006.** Togo T, Araki E, Ota M, et al. Fibrous hamartoma of infancy in a patient with Williams syndrome. Br J Dermatol. 2007 May;156(5):1052–5. PMID:17326745

**7007.** Toki S, Wakai S, Sekimizu M, et al. PAX7 immunohistochemical evaluation of Ewing sarcoma and other small round cell tumours. Histopathology. 2018 Oct;73(4):645–52. PMID:29920735

**7008.** Tolbert VP, Coggins GE, Maris JM. Genetic susceptibility to neuroblastoma. Curr Opin Genet Dev. 2017 Feb;42:81–90. PMID:28458126

**7009.** Toledano H, Orenstein N, Sofrin E, et al. Paediatric systemic lupus erythematosus as a manifestation of constitutional mismatch repair deficiency. J Med Genet. 2020 Jul;57(7):505–8. PMID:31501241

**7010.** Tomić TT, Olausson J, Wilzén A, et al. A new GTF2I-BRAF fusion mediating MAPK pathway activation in pilocytic astrocytoma. PLoS One. 2017 Apr 27;12(4):e0175638. PMID:28448514

**7011.** Tomlinson GE, Breslow NE, Dome J, et al. Rhabdoid tumor of the kidney in the National Wilms' Tumor Study: age at diagnosis as a prognostic factor. J Clin Oncol. 2005 Oct 20;23(30):7641–5. PMID:16234525

**7012.** Tong Y, Merino D, Nimmervoll B, et al. Cross-Species Genomics Identifies TAF12, NFYC, and RAD54L as Choroid Plexus Carcinoma Oncogenes. Cancer Cell. 2015 May 11;27(5):712–27. PMID:25965574

**7013.** Tono C, Xu G, Toki T, et al. JAK2 Val617Phe activating tyrosine kinase mutation in juvenile myelomonocytic leukemia. Leukemia. 2005 Oct;19(10):1843–4. PMID:16079889

**7014.** Tonon G, Modi S, Wu L, et al. t(11;19)(q21;p13) translocation in mucoepidermoid carcinoma creates a novel fusion product that disrupts a Notch signaling pathway. Nat Genet. 2003 Feb;33(2):208–13. PMID:12539049

**7015.** Tonorezos ES, Friedman DN, Barnea D, et al. Recommendations for long-term follow-up of adults with heritable retinoblastoma. Ophthalmology. 2020 Nov;127(11):1549–57. PMID:32422154

**7016.** Topka S, Vijai J, Walsh MF, et al. Germline ETV6 mutations confer susceptibility to acute lymphoblastic leukemia and thrombocytopenia. PLoS Genet. 2015 Jun 23;11(6):e1005262. PMID:26102509

**7017.** Torabinia N, Khalesi S. Clinicopathological study of 229 cases of salivary gland tumors in Isfahan population. Dent Res J (Isfahan). 2014 Sep;11(5):559–63. PMID:25426146

**7018.** Torbenson M. Review of the clinicopathologic features of fibrolamellar carcinoma. Adv Anat Pathol. 2007 May;14(3):217–23. PMID:17452818

**7019.** Torbidoni AV, Laurent VE, Sampor C, et al. Association of cone-rod homeobox transcription factor messenger RNA with pediatric metastatic retinoblastoma. JAMA Ophthalmol. 2015 Jul;133(7):805–12. PMID:25928893

**7020.** Torchia D, Schachner LA, Izakovic J. Segmental acne versus mosaic conditions with acne lesions. Dermatology. 2012;224(1):10–4. PMID:22456681

**7021.** Torchia J, Golbourn B, Feng S, et al. Integrated (epi)-genomic analyses identify subgroup-specific therapeutic targets in CNS rhabdoid tumors. Cancer Cell. 2016 Dec 12;30(6):891–908. PMID:27960086

**7022.** Torchia J, Picard D, Lafay-Cousin L, et al. Molecular subgroups of atypical teratoid rhabdoid tumours in children: an integrated genomic and clinicopathological analysis. Lancet Oncol. 2015 May;16(5):569–82. PMID:25882982

**7023.** Tordjman KM, Greenman Y, Ram Z, et al. Plurihormonal pituitary tumor of Pit-1 and SF-1 lineages, with synchronous collision corticotroph tumor: a possible stem cell phenomenon. Endocr Pathol. 2019 Mar;30(1):74–80. PMID:30610567

**7024.** Tordjman M, Dubois M, de Malherbe M, et al. Clear cell sarcoma of the tongue on MRI and PET/CT. Clin Nucl Med. 2018 Apr;43(4):e118–21. PMID:29401145

**7025.** Torlakovic E, Tierens A, Dang HD, et al. The transcription factor PU.1, necessary for B-cell development is expressed in lymphocyte predominance, but not classical Hodgkin's disease. Am J Pathol. 2001 Nov;159(5):1807–14. PMID:11696441

**7026.** Tornóczky T, Kálmán E, Kajtár PG, et al. Large cell neuroblastoma: a distinct phenotype of neuroblastoma with aggressive clinical behavior. Cancer. 2004 Jan 15;100(2):390–7. PMID:14716776

**7027.** Tornóczky T, Semjén D, Shimada H, et al. Pathology of peripheral neuroblastic tumors: significance of prominent nucleoli in undifferentiated/poorly differentiated neuroblastoma. Pathol Oncol Res. 2007;13(4):269–75. PMID:18158560

**7028.** Torre M, Meredith DM, Dubuc A, et al. Recurrent EP300-BCOR fusions in pediatric gliomas with distinct clinicopathologic features. J Neuropathol Exp Neurol. 2019 Apr 1;78(4):305–14. PMID:30816933

**7029.** Torrelo A, Colmenero I, Kristal L, et al. Papular epidermal nevus with "skyline" basal cell layer (PENS). J Am Acad Dermatol. 2011 May;64(5):888–92. PMID:21315481

**7030.** Torrelo A, Hadj-Rabia S, Colmenero I, et al. Folliculocystic and collagen hamartoma of tuberous sclerosis complex. J Am Acad Dermatol. 2012 Apr;66(4):617–21. PMID:21839539

**7031.** Torresan F, Iacobone M. Clinical features, treatment, and surveillance of hyperparathyroidism-jaw tumor syndrome: an up-to-date and review of the literature. Int J Endocrinol. 2019 Dec 18;2019:1761030. PMID:31929790

**7032.** Torres-Mora J, Dry S, Li X, et al. Malignant melanotic schwannian tumor: a clinicopathologic, immunohistochemical, and gene expression profiling study of 40 cases, with a proposal for the reclassification of "melanotic schwannoma". Am J Surg Pathol. 2014 Jan;38(1):94–105. PMID:24145644

**7034.** Tort F, Pinyol M, Pulford K, et al. Molecular characterization of a new ALK translocation involving moesin (MSN-ALK) in anaplastic large cell lymphoma. Lab Invest. 2001 Mar;81(3):419–26. PMID:11310834

**7035.** Tortosa F, Webb SM. Atypical pituitary adenomas: 10 years of experience in a reference centre in Portugal. Neurologia. 2016 Mar;31(2):97–105. PMID:26300499

**7036.** Tostar U, Malm CJ, Meis-Kindblom JM, et al. Deregulation of the hedgehog signalling pathway: a possible role for the PTCH and SUFU genes in human rhabdomyoma and rhabdomyosarcoma development. J Pathol. 2006 Jan;208(1):17–25. PMID:16294371

**7037.** Totonchy MB, Tamura D, Pantell MS, et al. Auditory analysis of xeroderma pigmentosum 1971-2012: hearing function, sun sensitivity and DNA repair predict neurological degeneration. Brain. 2013 Jan;136(Pt 1):194–208. PMID:23365097

**7038.** Touat M, Gratieux J, Condette Auliac S, et al. Vemurafenib and cobimetinib overcome resistance to vemurafenib in BRAF-mutant ganglioglioma. Neurology. 2018 Sep 11;91(11):523–5. PMID:30120137

**7039.** Toumi O, Ammar H, Korbi I, et al. Gastroblastoma, a biphasic neoplasm of stomach: a case report. Int J Surg Case Rep. 2017;39:72–6. PMID:28822310

**7040.** Touquet R, Mackenzie IJ, Carruth JA. Management of the parotid pleomorphic adenoma, the problem of exposing tumour tissue at operation. The logical pursuit of treatment policies. Br J Oral Maxillofac Surg. 1990 Dec;28(6):404–8. PMID:2177656

**7041.** Touriol C, Greenland C, Lamant L, et al. Further demonstration of the diversity of chromosomal changes involving 2p23 in ALK-positive lymphoma: 2 cases expressing ALK kinase fused to CLTCL (clathrin chain polypeptide-like). Blood. 2000 May 15;95(10):3204–7. PMID:10807789

**7042.** Towbin AJ, Meyers RL, Woodley H, et al. 2017 PRETEXT: radiologic staging system for primary hepatic malignancies of childhood revised for the Paediatric Hepatic International Tumour Trial (PHITT). Pediatr Radiol. 2018 Apr;48(4):536–54. PMID:29427028

**7043.** Traisrisilp K, Srisupundit K, Suwansirikul S, et al. Intracranial fetus-in-fetu with numerous fully developed organs. J Clin Ultrasound. 2018 Sep;46(7):487–93. PMID:29193240

**7044.** Tran L, Fitzpatrick C, Cohn SL, et al. Composite tumor with pheochromocytoma and immature neuroblastoma: report of two cases with cytogenetic analysis and discussion of current terminology. Virchows Arch. 2017 Oct;471(4):553–7. PMID:28864906

**7045.** Tran TA, Fabre M, Pariente D, et al. Erdheim-Chester disease in childhood: a challenging diagnosis and treatment. J Pediatr Hematol Oncol. 2009 Oct;31(10):782–6. PMID:19755920

**7046.** Tranvinh E, Yeom KW, Iv M. Imaging neck masses in the neonate and young infant. Semin Ultrasound CT MR. 2015 Apr;36(2):120–37. PMID:26001942

**7047.** Trapido EJ, Brinton LA, Schairer C, et al. Estrogen replacement therapy and benign breast disease. J Natl Cancer Inst. 1984 Nov;73(5):1101–5. PMID:6092767

**7048.** Trassard M, Le Doussal V, Bui BN, et al. Angiosarcoma arising in a solitary schwannoma (neurilemoma) of the sciatic nerve. Am J Surg Pathol. 1996 Nov;20(11):1412–7. PMID:8898847

**7049.** Traum AZ, Rodig NM, Pilichowska ME, et al. Central nervous system lymphoproliferative disorder in pediatric kidney transplant recipients. Pediatr Transplant. 2006 Jun;10(4):505–12. PMID:16712612

**7050.** Traverse-Glehen A, Davi F, Ben Simon E, et al. Analysis of VH genes in marginal zone lymphoma reveals marked heterogeneity between splenic and nodal tumors and suggests the existence of clonal selection. Haematologica. 2005 Apr;90(4):470–8. PMID:15820942

**7051.** Traverse-Glehen A, Pittaluga S, Gaulard P, et al. Mediastinal gray zone lymphoma: the missing link between classic Hodgkin's lymphoma and mediastinal large B-cell lymphoma. Am J Surg Pathol. 2005 Nov;29(11):1411–21. PMID:16224207

**7052.** Travert M, Huang Y, de Leval L, et al. Molecular features of hepatosplenic T-cell lymphoma unravels potential novel therapeutic targets. Blood. 2012 Jun 14;119(24):5795–806. PMID:22510872

**7053.** Treffel M, Lardenois E, Larousserie F, et al. Denosumab-treated giant cell tumors of bone: a clinicopathologic analysis of 35 cases from the French Group of Bone Pathology. Am J Surg Pathol. 2020 Jan;44(1):1–10. PMID:31651524

**7054.** Treger TD, Chowdhury T, Pritchard-Jones K, et al. The genetic changes of Wilms tumour. Nat Rev Nephrol. 2019 Apr;15(4):240–51. PMID:30705419

**7055.** Trehan G, Bruge H, Vinchon M, et al. MR imaging in the diagnosis of desmoplastic infantile tumor: retrospective study of six cases. AJNR Am J Neuroradiol. 2004 Jun-Jul;25(6):1028–33. PMID:15205142

**7056.** Trenor CC 3rd, Chaudry G. Complex lymphatic anomalies. Semin Pediatr Surg. 2014 Aug;23(4):186–90. PMID:25241096

**7057.** Tretiakova MS. Eosinophilic solid and cystic renal cell carcinoma mimicking epithelioid angiomyolipoma: series of 4 primary tumors and 2 metastases. Hum Pathol. 2018 Oct;80:65–75. PMID:29885406

**7058.** Trevisson E, Cassina M, Opocher E, et al. Natural history of optic pathway gliomas in a cohort of unselected patients affected by Neurofibromatosis 1. J Neurooncol. 2017 Sep;134(2):279–87. PMID:28577031

**7059.** Triana P, Rodríguez-Laguna L, Giacaman A, et al. Congenital hepatic hemangiomas: clinical, histologic, and genetic correlation. J Pediatr Surg. 2020 Oct;55(10):2170–6. PMID:32115227

**7060.** Triantafyllou A, Thompson LD, Devaney KO, et al. Functional histology of salivary gland pleomorphic adenoma: an appraisal. Head Neck Pathol. 2015 Sep;9(3):387–404. PMID:25380577

**7061.** Triggiani V, Guastamacchia E, Renzulli G, et al. Papillary thyroid carcinoma in Peutz-Jeghers syndrome. Thyroid. 2011 Nov;21(11):1273–7. PMID:21877933

**7062.** Trimboli P, Guidobaldi L, Bongiovanni M, et al. Use of fine-needle aspirate calcitonin to detect medullary thyroid carcinoma: a systematic review. Diagn Cytopathol. 2016 Jan;44(1):45–51. PMID:26481456

**7063.** Trindade F, Tellechea O, Torrelo A, et al. Wilms tumor 1 expression in vascular neoplasms and vascular malformations. Am J Dermatopathol. 2011 Aug;33(6):569–72. PMID:21697701

**7064.** Trindade F, Torrelo A, Kutzner H, et al. An immunohistochemical study of angiokeratomas of children. Am J Dermatopathol. 2014 Oct;36(10):796–9. PMID:25243395

**7065.** Trisolini E, Wardighi DE, Giry M, et al. Actionable FGFR1 and BRAF mutations in adult circumscribed gliomas. J Neurooncol. 2019 Nov;145(2):241–5. PMID:31673897

**7066.** Tritou I, Vakaki M, Sfakiotaki R, et al. Pediatric thyroid ultrasound: a radiologist's checklist. Pediatr Radiol. 2020 Apr;50(4):563–74. PMID:32166365

**7067.** Trivellin G, Daly AF, Faucz FR, et al. Gigantism and acromegaly due to Xq26 microduplications and GPR101 mutation. N Engl J Med. 2014 Dec 18;371(25):2363–74. PMID:25470569

**7068.** Trobaugh-Lotrario A, Katzenstein HM, Ranganathan S, et al. Small cell undifferentiated histology does not adversely affect outcome in hepatoblastoma: a report from the Children's Oncology Group (COG) AHEP0731 Study Committee. J Clin Oncol. 2022 Feb 10;40(5):459–67. PMID:34874751

**7069.** Trobaugh-Lotrario AD, Finegold MJ, Feusner JH. Rhabdoid tumors of the liver: rare, aggressive, and poorly responsive to standard cytotoxic chemotherapy. Pediatr Blood Cancer. 2011 Sep;57(3):423–8. PMID:21744471

**7070.** Trobaugh-Lotrario AD, Tomlinson GE, Finegold MJ, et al. Small cell undifferentiated variant of hepatoblastoma: adverse clinical and molecular features similar to rhabdoid tumors. Pediatr Blood Cancer. 2009 Mar;52(3):328–34. PMID:18985717

**7071.** Trofatter JA, MacCollin MM, Rutter JL, et al. A novel moesin-, ezrin-, radixin-like gene is a candidate for the neurofibromatosis 2 tumor suppressor. Cell. 1993 Mar 12;72(5):791–800. PMID:8453669

**7072.** Tron V, Bellamy C, Wood W. Familial cutaneous heterotopic meningeal nodules. J Am Acad Dermatol. 1993 Jun;28(6):1015–7. PMID:8496446

**7073.** Trouillas J, Jaffrain-Rea ML, Vasiljevic A, et al. Are aggressive pituitary tumors and carcinomas two sides of the same coin? Pathologists reply to clinician's questions. Rev Endocr Metab Disord. 2020 Jun;21(2):243–51. PMID:32504268

**7074.** Trouillas J, Roy P, Sturm N, et al. A new prognostic clinicopathological classification of pituitary adenomas: a multicentric case-control study of 410 patients with 8 years post-operative follow-up. Acta Neuropathol. 2013 Jul;126(1):123–35. PMID:23400299

**7075.** Trouillas J, Vasiljevic A, Lapoirie M, et al. Pathological markers of somatotroph pituitary neuroendocrine tumors predicting the response to medical treatment. Minerva Endocrinol. 2019 Jun;44(2):129–36. PMID:30531694

**7076.** Troum S, Dalton ML, Donner RS, et al. Multifocal mesenchymal hamartoma of the chest wall in infancy. J Pediatr Surg. 1996 May;31(5):713–5. PMID:8861490

**7077.** Trpkov K, Hes O, Bonert M, et al. Eosinophilic, solid, and cystic renal cell carcinoma: clinicopathologic study of 16 unique, sporadic neoplasms occurring in women. Am J Surg Pathol. 2016 Jan;40(1):60–71. PMID:26414221

**7078.** Trubnik V, Conley R, Ritterband DC, et al. Progressive growth in epibulbar complex choristomas: report of 2 cases and review of literature. Cornea. 2011 Nov;30(11):1267–9. PMID:21885965

**7079.** Trülzsch B, Krohn K, Wonerow P, et al. Detection of thyroid-stimulating hormone receptor and Gsalpha mutations: in 75 toxic thyroid nodules by denaturing gradient gel electrophoresis. J Mol Med (Berl). 2001;78(12):684–91. PMID:11434721

**7080.** Truta B, Chen YY, Blanco AM, et al. Tumor histology helps to identify Lynch syndrome among colorectal cancer patients. Fam Cancer. 2008;7(3):267–74. PMID:18283560

**7081.** Tsagarakis NJ, Papadhimitriou SI, Pavlidis D, et al. Contribution of immunophenotype to the investigation and differential diagnosis of Burkitt lymphoma, double-hit high-grade B-cell lymphoma, and single-hit MYC-rearranged diffuse large B-cell lymphoma. Cytometry B Clin Cytom. 2020 Sep;98(5):412–20. PMID:32497402

**7082.** Tsai AS, Lee KY, Al Jajeh I, et al. Epibulbar osseous choristoma: a report of two cases. Orbit. 2008;27(3):231–3. PMID:18569837

**7083.** Tsai LL, Drubach L, Fahey F, et al. [18F]-Fluorodeoxyglucose positron emission tomography in children with neurofibromatosis type 1 and plexiform neurofibromas: correlation with malignant transformation. J Neurooncol. 2012 Jul;108(3):469–75. PMID:22407214

**7084.** Tsang CM, Lui VWY, Bruce JP, et al. Translational genomics of nasopharyngeal cancer. Semin Cancer Biol. 2020 Apr;61:84–100. PMID:31521748

**7085.** Tsang P, Cesarman E, Chadburn A, et al. Molecular characterization of primary mediastinal B cell lymphoma. Am J Pathol. 1996 Jun;148(6):2017–25. PMID:8669486

**7086.** Tsao L, Hsi ED. The clinicopathologic spectrum of posttransplantation lymphoproliferative disorders. Arch Pathol Lab Med. 2007 Aug;131(8):1209–18. PMID:17683183

**7087.** Tso MO. Clues to the cells of origin in retinoblastoma. Int Ophthalmol Clin. 1980 Summer;20(2):191–210. PMID:6995387

**7088.** Ts'o MO, Fine BS, Zimmerman LE. The Flexner-Wintersteiner rosettes in retinoblastoma. Arch Pathol. 1969 Dec;88(6):664–71. PMID:5357720

**7089.** Ts'o MO, Fine BS, Zimmerman LE. The nature of retinoblastoma. II. Photoreceptor differentiation: an electron microscopic study. Am J Ophthalmol. 1970 Mar;69(3):350–9. PMID:5418851

**7090.** Ts'o MO, Zimmerman LE, Fine BS. The nature of retinoblastoma. I. Photoreceptor differentiation: a clinical and histopathologic study. Am J Ophthalmol. 1970 Mar;69(3):339–49. PMID:4190798

**7091.** Tsubota A, Akiyama M, Sakai K, et al. Keratin 1 gene mutation detected in epidermal nevus with epidermolytic hyperkeratosis. J Invest Dermatol. 2007 Jun;127(6):1371–4. PMID:17255957

**7092.** Tsuchiya K, Reijo R, Page DC, et al. Gonadoblastoma: molecular definition of the susceptibility region on the Y chromosome. Am J Hum Genet. 1995 Dec;57(6):1400–7. PMID:8533770

**7093.** Tsuda M, Davis IJ, Argani P, et al. TFE3 fusions activate MET signaling by transcriptional up-regulation, defining another class of tumors as candidates for therapeutic MET inhibition. Cancer Res. 2007 Feb 1;67(3):919–29. PMID:17283122

**7094.** Tsuda Y, Zhang L, Meyers P, et al. The clinical heterogeneity of round cell sarcomas with EWSR1/FUS gene fusions: impact of gene fusion type on clinical features and outcome. Genes Chromosomes Cancer. 2020 Sep;59(9):525–34. PMID:32362012

**7095.** Tsugu H, Oshiro S, Ueno Y, et al. Primary yolk sac tumor within the lateral ventricle. Neurol Med Chir (Tokyo). 2009 Nov;49(11):528–31. PMID:19940403

**7095A.** Tsuji H, Yasuoka H, Nakamura Y, et al. Aggressive cribriform-morular variant of papillary thyroid carcinoma: report of an unusual case with pulmonary metastasis displaying poorly differentiated features. Pathol Int. 2018 Dec;68(12):700–5. PMID:30376202

**7096.** Tsuji K, Ishikawa Y, Imamura T. Technique for differentiating alveolar soft part sarcoma from other tumors in paraffin-embedded tissue: comparison of immunohistochemistry for TFE3 and CD147 and of reverse transcription polymerase chain reaction for ASP-SCR1-TFE3 fusion transcript. Hum Pathol. 2012 Mar;43(3):356–63. PMID:21835426

**7097.** Tsujimura T, Sakaguchi K, Aozasa K. Phosphaturic mesenchymal tumor, mixed connective tissue variant (oncogenic osteomalacia). Pathol Int. 1996 Mar;46(3):238–41. PMID:10846577

**7098.** Tsukada T, Yoshida H, Ishikawa M, et al. Malignant struma ovarii presenting with follicular carcinoma: a case report with molecular analysis. Gynecol Oncol Rep. 2019 Sep 9;30:100498. PMID:31538107

**7099.** Tsukamoto K, Murakami M, Seo Y, et al. Energetic recovery from hypothermic preservation in the rat liver. J Surg Res. 1990 Jan;48(1):46–50. PMID:2296180

**7100.** Tsuruta T, Ogawa A, Ishii K, et al. CA19-9: a possible serum marker for embryonal carcinoma. Urol Int. 1997;58(1):20–4. PMID:9058515

**7101.** Tsuyuguchi S, Sugiyama K, Kinoshita Y, et al. Primary and recurrent growing teratoma syndrome in central nervous system nongerminomatous germ cell tumors: case series and review of the literature. World Neurosurg. 2020 Feb;134:e360–71. PMID:31751614

**7102.** Tsuzuki T, Magi-Galluzzi C, Epstein JI. ALK-1 expression in inflammatory myofibroblastic tumor of the urinary bladder. Am J Surg Pathol. 2004 Dec;28(12):1609–14. PMID:15577680

**7103.** Tucker MA, D'Angio GJ, Boice JD Jr, et al. Bone sarcomas linked to radiotherapy and chemotherapy in children. N Engl J Med. 1987 Sep 3;317(10):588–93. PMID:3475572

**7104.** Tufton N, Shapiro L, Srirangalingam U, et al. Outcomes of annual surveillance imaging in an adult and paediatric cohort of succinate dehydrogenase B mutation carriers. Clin Endocrinol (Oxf). 2017 Feb;86(2):286–96. PMID:27678251

**7105.** Tumini S, Carinci S, Anzellotti MT, et al. Genital sanguineous discharge in prepuberty: a case of mullerian papilloma of vagina in a nine-year-old girl. J Pediatr Endocrinol Metab. 2010 Aug;23(8):831–2. PMID:21073126

**7106.** Tumwine LK, Orem J, Kerchan P, et al. EBV, HHV8 and HIV in B cell non Hodgkin lymphoma in Kampala, Uganda. Infect Agent Cancer. 2010 Jun 30;5:12. PMID:20591151

**7107.** Tunstall O, Bhatnagar N, James B, et al. Guidelines for the investigation and management of transient leukaemia of Down syndrome. Br J Haematol. 2018 Jul;182(2):200–11. PMID:29916557

**7108.** Turchini J, Cheung VKY, Tischler AS, et al. Pathology and genetics of phaeochromocytoma and paraganglioma. Histopathology. 2018 Jan;72(1):97–105. PMID:29239044

**7109.** Turchini J, Gill AJ. Hereditary parathyroid disease: sometimes pathologists do not know what they are missing. Endocr Pathol. 2020 Sep;31(3):218–30. PMID:32468209

**7110.** Turchini J, Gill AJ. Morphologic clues to succinate dehydrogenase (SDH) deficiency in pheochromocytomas and paragangliomas. Am J Surg Pathol. 2020 Mar;44(3):422–4. PMID:31789631

**7111.** Turchini J, Sioson L, Clarkson A, et al. Utility of GATA-3 expression in the analysis of pituitary neuroendocrine tumour (PitNET) transcription factors. Endocr Pathol. 2020 Jun;31(2):150–5. PMID:32193825

**7112.** Turcot J, Despres JP, St Pierre F. Malignant tumors of the central nervous system associated with familial polyposis of the colon: report of two cases. Dis Colon Rectum. 1959 Sep-Oct;2:465–8. PMID:13839882

**7113.** Turcotte RE, Kurt AM, Sim FH, et al. Chondroblastoma. Hum Pathol. 1993 Sep;24(9):944–9. PMID:8253461

**7114.** Turgut M. Spinal extradural angiolipoma, with a literature review. Childs Nerv Syst. 2004 Feb;20(2):73–4. PMID:14634778

**7115.** Turkoglu E, Kertmen H, Sanli AM, et al. Clinical outcome of adult choroid plexus tumors: retrospective analysis of a single institute. Acta Neurochir (Wien). 2014 Aug;156(8):1461–8. PMID:24866474

**7116.** Turner AL, D'Souza P, Belirgen M, et al. Atypical Presentation of multinodular and vacuolating neuronal tumor of the cerebrum in a boy. J Neurosci Rural Pract. 2020 Jan;11(1):214–5. PMID:32140033

**7117.** Turner Ii RM, Tomaszewski JJ, Fox JA, et al. Metanephric adenofibroma. Can J Urol. 2013 Apr;20(2):6737–8. PMID:23587517

**7118.** Turner SD, Alexander DR. Fusion tyrosine kinase mediated signalling pathways in the transformation of haematopoietic cells. Leukemia. 2006 Apr;20(4):572–82. PMID:16482213

**7119.** Tuttle RM, Ball DW, Byrd D, et al. Medullary carcinoma. J Natl Compr Canc Netw. 2010 May;8(5):512–30. PMID:20495082

**7120.** Twa DD, Chan FC, Ben-Neriah S, et al. Genomic rearrangements involving programmed death ligands are recurrent in primary mediastinal large B-cell lymphoma. Blood. 2014 Mar 27;123(13):2062–5. PMID:24497532

**7121.** Tyburczy ME, Dies KA, Glass J, et al. Mosaic and intronic mutations in TSC1/TSC2 explain the majority of TSC patients with no mutation identified by conventional testing. PLoS Genet. 2015 Nov 5;11(11):e1005637. PMID:26540169

**7122.** Tymen R, Forestier JF, Boutet B, et al. [Late Becker's nevus. One hundred cases (author's transl)]. Ann Dermatol Venereol. 1981;108(1):41–6. French. PMID:7235503

**7123.** Tzankov A, Bourgau C, Kaiser A, et al. Rare expression of T-cell markers in classical Hodgkin's lymphoma. Mod Pathol. 2005 Dec;18(12):1542–9. PMID:16056244

**7124.** Uccini S, Al-Jadiry MF, Scarpino S, et al. Epstein-Barr virus-positive diffuse large B-cell lymphoma in children: a disease reminiscent of Epstein-Barr virus-positive diffuse large B-cell lymphoma of the elderly. Hum Pathol. 2015 May;46(5):716–24. PMID:25704629

**7125.** Ud Din N, Ahmad Z, Zreik R, et al. Abdominopelvic and retroperitoneal low-grade fibromyxoid sarcoma: a clinicopathologic study of 13 cases. Am J Clin Pathol. 2018 Jan 29;149(2):128–34. PMID:29385413

**7126.** Udager AM, Chiosea SI. Salivary duct carcinoma: an update on morphologic mimics and diagnostic use of androgen receptor immunohistochemistry. Head Neck Pathol. 2017 Sep;11(3):288–94. PMID:28321773

**7127.** Udager AM, Magers MJ, Goerke DM, et al. The utility of SDHB and FH immunohistochemistry in patients evaluated for hereditary paraganglioma-pheochromocytoma syndromes. Hum Pathol. 2018 Jan;71:47–54. PMID:29079178

**7128.** Udager AM, Pan J, Magers MJ, et al. Molecular and immunohistochemical characterization reveals novel BRAF mutations in metanephric adenoma. Am J Surg Pathol. 2015 Apr;39(4):549–57. PMID:25602792

**7129.** Ueno-Yokohata H, Okita H, Nakasato K, et al. Consistent in-frame internal tandem duplications of BCOR characterize clear cell sarcoma of the kidney. Nat Genet. 2015 Aug;47(8):861–3. PMID:26098867

**7130.** Uffmann M, Rasche M, Zimmermann M, et al. Therapy reduction in patients with Down syndrome and myeloid leukemia: the international ML-DS 2006 trial. Blood. 2017 Jun 22;129(25):3314–21. PMID:28400376

**7131.** Uglietta JP, Boyko OB, Rippe DJ, et al. Intracerebral extension of nasal dermoid cyst: CT appearance. J Comput Assist Tomogr. 1989 Nov-Dec;13(6):1061–4. PMID:2584485

**7132.** UICC [Internet]. Geneva (Switzerland): Union for International Cancer Control; 2020. TNM Publications and Resources – Errata; updated 2020 Oct 6. Available from: https://www.uicc.org/resources/tnm/publications-resources.

**7133.** UICC [Internet]. Geneva (Switzerland): Union for International Cancer Control; 2020. TNM Publications and Resources – Errata; updated 2020 Oct 6. Available from: https://www.uicc.org/resources/tnm/publications-resources.

**7134.** Uitto J, Santa Cruz DJ, Eisen AZ. Connective tissue nevi of the skin. Clinical, genetic, and histopathologic classification of hamartomas of the collagen, elastin, and proteoglycan type. J Am Acad Dermatol. 1980 Nov;3(5):441–61. PMID:7217375

**7135.** Ulbright TM. Germ cell tumors of the gonads: a selective review emphasizing problems in differential diagnosis, newly appreciated, and controversial issues. Mod Pathol. 2005 Feb;18 Suppl 2:S61–79. PMID:15761467

**7136.** Ulbright TM, Alexander RW, Kraus FT. Intramural papilloma of the vagina: evidence of Müllerian histogenesis. Cancer. 1981 Nov 15;48(10):2260–6. PMID:6170416

**7137.** Ulbright TM, Hattab EM, Zhang S, et al. Primitive neuroectodermal tumors in patients with testicular germ cell tumors usually resemble pediatric-type central nervous system embryonal neoplasms and lack chromosome 22 rearrangements. Mod Pathol. 2010 Jul;23(7):972–80. PMID:20348883

**7138.** Ulbright TM, Tickoo SK, Berney DM, et al. Best practices recommendations in the application of immunohistochemistry in testicular tumors: report from the International Society of Urological Pathology consensus conference. Am J Surg Pathol. 2014 Aug;38(8):e50–9. PMID:24832161

**7139.** Ulbright TM, Young RH. Gonadoblastoma and selected other aspects of gonadal pathology in young patients with disorders of sex development. Semin Diagn Pathol. 2014 Sep;31(5):427–40. PMID:25129544

**7140.** Ulbright TM, Young RH. Seminoma with conspicuous signet ring cells: a rare, previously uncharacterized morphologic variant. Am J Surg Pathol. 2008 Aug;32(8):1175–81. PMID:18580681

**7141.** Ulbright TM, Young RH. Testicular and paratesticular tumors and tumor-like lesions in the first 2 decades. Semin Diagn Pathol. 2014 Sep;31(5):323–81. PMID:25440720

**7142.** Ulbright TM, Young RH, Scully RE. Trophoblastic tumors of the testis other than classic choriocarcinoma: "monophasic" choriocarcinoma and placental site trophoblastic tumor: a report of two cases. Am J Surg Pathol. 1997 Mar;21(3):282–8. PMID:9060597

**7143.** Unal S, Cetin M, Kutlay NY, et al. Hemophagocytosis associated with leukemia: a striking association with juvenile myelomonocytic leukemia. Ann Hematol. 2010 Apr;89(4):359–64. PMID:19798502

**7144.** Unger P, Hoffman K, Pertsemlidis D, et al. S100 protein-positive sustentacular cells in

malignant and locally aggressive adrenal pheochromocytomas. Arch Pathol Lab Med. 1991 May;115(5):484–7. PMID:1673596
7145. Unger S, Seidl M, Schmitt-Graeff A, et al. Ill-defined germinal centers and severely reduced plasma cells are histological hallmarks of lymphadenopathy in patients with common variable immunodeficiency. J Clin Immunol. 2014 Aug;34(6):615–26. PMID:24789743
7146. Ungewickell A, Bhaduri A, Rios E, et al. Genomic analysis of mycosis fungoides and Sézary syndrome identifies recurrent alterations in TNFR2. Nat Genet. 2015 Sep;47(9):1056–60. PMID:26258847
7147. Unni KK, Dahlin DC, Beabout JW. Periosteal osteogenic sarcoma. Cancer. 1976 May;37(5):2476–85. PMID:1063059
7148. Uno K, Takita J, Yokomori K, et al. Aberrations of the hSNF5/INI1 gene are restricted to malignant rhabdoid tumors or atypical teratoid/rhabdoid tumors in pediatric solid tumors. Genes Chromosomes Cancer. 2002 May;34(1):33–41. PMID:11921280
7149. Untanu RV, Back J, Appel B, et al. Variant histology, IgD and CD30 expression in low-risk pediatric nodular lymphocyte predominant Hodgkin lymphoma: a report from the Children's Oncology Group. Pediatr Blood Cancer. 2018 Jan;65(1):10.1002/pbc.26753. PMID:28802087
7150. Upadhyaya M, Huson SM, Davies M, et al. An absence of cutaneous neurofibromas associated with a 3-bp inframe deletion in exon 17 of the NF1 gene (c.2970-2972 delAAT): evidence of a clinically significant NF1 genotype-phenotype correlation. Am J Hum Genet. 2007 Jan;80(1):140–51. PMID:17160901
7151. Upadhyaya SA, Robinson GW, Onar-Thomas A, et al. Molecular grouping and outcomes of young children with newly diagnosed ependymoma treated on the multi-institutional SJYC07 trial. Neuro Oncol. 2019 Oct 9;21(10):1319–30. PMID:30976811
7152. Uramoto N, Furukawa M, Yoshizaki T. Malignant phosphaturic mesenchymal tumor, mixed connective tissue variant of the tongue. Auris Nasus Larynx. 2009 Feb;36(1):104–5. PMID:18329207
7153. Urayama KY, Jarrett RF, Hjalgrim H, et al. Genome-wide association study of classical Hodgkin lymphoma and Epstein-Barr virus status-defined subgroups. J Natl Cancer Inst. 2012 Feb 8;104(3):240–53. PMID:22286212
7153A. Urbina F, Sazunic I, Murray G. Infantile systemic hyalinosis or juvenile hyaline fibromatosis? Pediatr Dermatol. 2004 Mar-Apr;21(2):154–9. PMID:15078358
7154. Uro-Coste E, Masliah-Planchon J, Siegfried A, et al. ETMR-like infantile cerebellar embryonal tumors in the extended morphologic spectrum of DICER1-related tumors. Acta Neuropathol. 2019 Jan;137(1):175–7. PMID:30446821
7155. Urth A, Remacle JM, Levie P, et al. Nasal dermoid cyst: diagnosis and management of five cases. Acta Otorhinolaryngol Belg. 2002;56(3):325–9. PMID:12244897
7156. Ushijima M, Tsuneyoshi M, Enjoji M. Dupuytren type fibromatoses. A clinicopathologic study of 62 cases. Acta Pathol Jpn. 1984 Sep;34(5):991–1001. PMID:6507097
7157. Usyk M, Zolnik CP, Castle PE, et al. Cervicovaginal microbiome and natural history of HPV in a longitudinal study. PLoS Pathog. 2020 Mar 26;16(3):e1008376. PMID:32214382
7158. Utashima D, Matsumura N, Suzuki T, et al. Clinical results of surgical resection and histopathological evaluation of synovial chondromatosis in the shoulder: a retrospective study and literature review. Clin Orthop Surg. 2020 Mar;12(1):68–75. PMID:32117541
7159. Uusitalo E, Leppävirta J, Koffert A, et al. Incidence and mortality of neurofibromatosis: a total population study in Finland. J Invest Dermatol. 2015 Mar;135(3):904–6. PMID:25354145
7160. Vaccaro M, Romeo U, Romeo C, et al. Spitz nevus: a rare lesion of the oral cavity. Pediatr Dermatol. 2016 Mar-Apr;33(2):e154–5. PMID:27001333
7161. Vachette M, Moulin A, Zografos L, et al. Epibulbar osseous choristoma: a clinicopathological case series and review of the literature. Klin Monbl Augenheilkd. 2012 Apr;229(4):420–3. PMID:22496017
7162. Vagge A, Camicione P, Capris C, et al. Choroidal abnormalities in neurofibromatosis type 1 detected by near-infrared reflectance imaging in paediatric population. Acta Ophthalmol. 2015 Dec;93(8):e667–71. PMID:25990002
7163. Vaillant V, Reiter A, Zimmermann M, et al. Seroepidemiological analysis and literature review of the prevalence of Epstein-Barr virus and herpesvirus infections in pediatric cases with non-Hodgkin lymphoma in Central Europe. Pediatr Blood Cancer. 2019 Jul;66(7):e27752. PMID:30977593
7164. Vajdic CM, Mao L, van Leeuwen MT, et al. Are antibody deficiency disorders associated with a narrower range of cancers than other forms of immunodeficiency? Blood. 2010 Aug 26;116(8):1228–34. PMID:20466855
7165. Vakiani E, Basso K, Klein U, et al. Genetic and phenotypic analysis of B-cell post-transplant lymphoproliferative disorders provides insights into disease biology. Hematol Oncol. 2008 Dec;26(4):199–211. PMID:18457340
7166. Vakiani E, Nandula SV, Subramaniyam S, et al. Cytogenetic analysis of B-cell posttransplant lymphoproliferations validates the World Health Organization classification and suggests inclusion of florid follicular hyperplasia as a precursor lesion. Hum Pathol. 2007 Feb;38(2):315–25. PMID:17134734
7167. Valdebran M, Wine Lee L. Hemangioma-related syndromes. Curr Opin Pediatr. 2020 Aug;32(4):498–505. PMID:32692048
7168. Valdez JM, Nichols KE, Kesserwan C. Li-Fraumeni syndrome: a paradigm for the understanding of hereditary cancer predisposition. Br J Haematol. 2017 Feb;176(4):539–52. PMID:27984644
7169. Valdez R, McKeever P, Finn WG, et al. Composite germ cell tumor and B-cell non-Hodgkin's lymphoma arising in the sella turcica. Hum Pathol. 2002 Oct;33(10):1044–7. PMID:12395379
7170. Valdez TA, Desai U, Volk MS. Recurrent fetal rhabdomyoma of the head and neck. Int J Pediatr Otorhinolaryngol. 2006 Jun;70(6):1115–8. PMID:16406074
7171. Valdivielso-Ramos M, Burdaspal A, Conde E, et al. Balloon-cell variant of the Spitz nevus. J Eur Acad Dermatol Venereol. 2016 Sep;30(9):1621–2. PMID:26147249
7172. Valdivielso-Ramos M, Torrelo A, Campos M, et al. Pediatric dermatofibrosarcoma protuberans in Madrid, Spain: multi-institutional outcomes. Pediatr Dermatol. 2014 Nov-Dec;31(6):676–82. PMID:25424208
7173. Valencia Ocampo OJ, Julio L, Zapata V, et al. Mycosis fungoides in children and adolescents: a series of 23 cases. Actas Dermosifiliogr (Engl Ed). 2020 Mar;111(2):149–56. PMID:31277835
7174. Valent P, Horny HP, Arock M. The underestimated role of basophils in Ph+ chronic myeloid leukaemia. Eur J Clin Invest. 2018 Oct;48(10):e13000. PMID:30019447
7175. Valent P, Horny HP, Escribano L, et al. Diagnostic criteria and classification of mastocytosis: a consensus proposal. Leuk Res. 2001 Jul;25(7):603–25. PMID:11377686
7176. Valente PT, Hoober JK, Phillips SJ. Tyrosine-rich crystalloids in pleomorphic adenoma: SEM findings and partial biochemical characterization. Ultrastruct Pathol. 1988 Nov-Dec;12(6):613–20. PMID:2853475
7177. Valentijn LJ, Koster J, Zwijnenburg DA, et al. TERT rearrangements are frequent in neuroblastoma and identify aggressive tumors. Nat Genet. 2015 Dec;47(12):1411–4. PMID:26523776
7178. Valera A, Balagué O, Colomo L, et al. IG/MYC rearrangements are the main cytogenetic alteration in plasmablastic lymphomas. Am J Surg Pathol. 2010 Nov;34(11):1686–94. PMID:20962620
7179. Valera A, Colomo L, Martínez A, et al. ALK-positive large B-cell lymphomas express a terminal B-cell differentiation program and activated STAT3 but lack MYC rearrangements. Mod Pathol. 2013 Oct;26(10):1329–37. PMID:23599149
7180. Valera ET, McConechy MK, Gayden T, et al. Methylome analysis and whole-exome sequencing reveal that brain tumors associated with encephalocraniocutaneous lipomatosis are midline pilocytic astrocytomas. Acta Neuropathol. 2018 Oct;136(4):657–60. PMID:30143858
7181. Valera ET, Neder L, Queiroz RG, et al. Perinatal complex low- and high-grade glial tumor harboring a novel GIGYF2-ALK fusion. Pediatr Blood Cancer. 2020 Jan;67(1):e28015. PMID:31556208
7182. Valery PC, Laversanne M, Bray F. Bone cancer incidence by morphological subtype: a global assessment. Cancer Causes Control. 2015 Aug;26(8):1127–39. PMID:26054913
7183. Valeton JM, Van Norren D. Retinal site of transient tritanopia. Nature. 1979 Aug 9;280(5722):488–90. PMID:111147
7183A. Valle L. Recent discoveries in the genetics of familial colorectal cancer and polyposis. Clin Gastroenterol Hepatol. 2017 Jun;15(6):809–19. PMID:27712984
7184. Valle L, Hernández-Illán E, Bellido F, et al. New insights into POLE and POLD1 germline mutations in familial colorectal cancer and polyposis. Hum Mol Genet. 2014 Jul 1;23(13):3506–12. PMID:24501277
7185. Vallerie AM, Lerner JP, Wright JD, et al. Peritoneal inclusion cysts: a review. Obstet Gynecol Surv. 2009 May;64(5):321–34. PMID:19386139
7186. Valls J, Ottolenghi CE, Schajowicz F. Epiphyseal chondroblastoma of bone. J Bone Joint Surg Am. 1951 Oct;33-A(4):997–1009. PMID:14880556
7187. Valstar MH, de Ridder M, van den Broek EC, et al. Salivary gland pleomorphic adenoma in the Netherlands: a nationwide observational study of primary tumor incidence, malignant transformation, recurrence, and risk factors for recurrence. Oral Oncol. 2017 Mar;66:93–9. PMID:28249655
7188. van Casteren NJ, Boellaard WP, Dohle GR, et al. Heterogeneous distribution of ITGCNU in an adult testis: consequences for biopsy-based diagnosis. Int J Surg Pathol. 2008 Jan;16(1):21–4. PMID:18203779
7189. van Casteren NJ, de Jong J, Stoop H, et al. Evaluation of testicular biopsies for carcinoma in situ: immunohistochemistry is mandatory. Int J Androl. 2009 Dec;32(6):666–74. PMID:18798762
7190. van Casteren NJ, Stoop H, Dohle GR, et al. Noninvasive detection of testicular carcinoma in situ in semen using OCT3/4. Eur Urol. 2008 Jul;54(1):153–8. PMID:17996359
7191. Van Damme A, Seront E, Dekeuleneer V, et al. New and emerging targeted therapies for vascular malformations. Am J Clin Dermatol. 2020 Oct;21(5):657–68. PMID:32557381
7192. van de Nes J, Wrede K, Ringelstein A, et al. Diagnosing a primary leptomeningeal melanoma by gene mutation signature. J Invest Dermatol. 2016 Jul;136(7):1526–8. PMID:27060446
7193. van de Nes JA, Nelles J, Kreis S, et al. Comparing the prognostic value of BAP1 mutation pattern, chromosome 3 status, and BAP1 immunohistochemistry in uveal melanoma. Am J Surg Pathol. 2016 Jun;40(6):796–805. PMID:27015033
7194. van de Rijn M, Barr FG, Xiong QB, et al. Poorly differentiated synovial sarcoma: an analysis of clinical, pathologic, and molecular genetic features. Am J Surg Pathol. 1999 Jan;23(1):106–12. PMID:9888710
7195. van den Akker EL, de Krijger RR, de Herder WW, et al. Congenital hemihypertrophy and pheochromocytoma, not a coincidental combination? Eur J Pediatr. 2002 Mar;161(3):157–60. PMID:11998914
7196. van den Berg H, Kroon HM, Slaar A, et al. Incidence of biopsy-proven bone tumors in children: a report based on the Dutch pathology registration "PALGA". J Pediatr Orthop. 2008 Jan-Feb;28(1):29–35. PMID:18157043
7197. van den Heuvel-Eibrink MM, Grundy P, Graf N, et al. Characteristics and survival of 750 children diagnosed with a renal tumor in the first seven months of life: a collaborative study by the SIOP/GPOH/SFOP, NWTSG, and UKCCSG Wilms tumor study groups. Pediatr Blood Cancer. 2008 Jun;50(6):1130–4. PMID:18095319
7198. van den Heuvel-Eibrink MM, van Tinteren H, Rehorst H, et al. Malignant rhabdoid tumours of the kidney (MRTKs), registered on recent SIOP protocols from 1993 to 2005: a report of the SIOP renal tumour study group. Pediatr Blood Cancer. 2011 May;56(5):733–7. PMID:21370404
7199. van den Hoek J, de Krijger R, van de Ven K, et al. Cystic nephroma, cystic partially differentiated nephroblastoma and cystic Wilms' tumor in children: a spectrum with therapeutic dilemmas. Urol Int. 2009;82(1):65–70. PMID:19172100
7200. van der Graaf WTA, Orbach D, Judson IR, et al. Soft tissue sarcomas in adolescents and young adults: a comparison with their paediatric and adult counterparts. Lancet Oncol. 2017 Mar;18(3):e166–75. PMID:28271871
7201. van der Heijden L, Gibbons CL, Hassan AB, et al. A multidisciplinary approach to giant cell tumors of tendon sheath and synovium–a critical appraisal of literature and treatment proposal. J Surg Oncol. 2013 Mar;107(4):433–45. PMID:22806927
7202. van der Maten J, Blaauwgeers JL, Sutedja TG, et al. Granular cell tumors of the tracheobronchial tree. J Thorac Cardiovasc Surg. 2003 Sep;126(3):740–3. PMID:14502147
7203. van der Velden VH, Beverloo HB, Hoogeveen PG, et al. A novel BCR-ABL fusion transcript (e18a2) in a child with chronic myeloid leukemia. Leukemia. 2007 Apr;21(4):833–5. PMID:17268511
7204. van der Zwan YG, Biermann K, Wolffenbuttel KP, et al. Gonadal maldevelopment as risk factor for germ cell cancer: towards a clinical decision model. Eur Urol. 2015 Apr;67(4):692–701. PMID:25240975
7205. Van Dievel J, Sciot R, Delcroix M, et al. Single-center experience with intimal sarcoma, an ultra-orphan, commonly fatal mesenchymal malignancy. Oncol Res Treat. 2017;40(6):353–9. PMID:28501860
7206. Van Dorpe J, Sciot R, De Vos R, et al. Neuromuscular choristoma (hamartoma) with smooth and striated muscle component: case report with immunohistochemical and ultrastructural analysis. Am J Surg Pathol. 1997 Sep;21(9):1090–5. PMID:9298886
7207. van Echten J, Oosterhuis JW, Looijenga LH, et al. No recurrent structural abnormalities

apart from i(12p) in primary germ cell tumors of the adult testis. Genes Chromosomes Cancer. 1995 Oct;14(2):133–44. PMID:8527395

**7208.** van Engelen K, Villani A, Wasserman JD, et al. DICER1 syndrome: approach to testing and management at a large pediatric tertiary care center. Pediatr Blood Cancer. 2018 Jan;65(1). PMID:28960912

**7209.** van Engen-van Grunsven AC, Rabold K, Küsters-Vandevelde HV, et al. Copy number variations as potential diagnostic and prognostic markers for CNS melanocytic neoplasms in neurocutaneous melanosis. Acta Neuropathol. 2017 Feb;133(2):333–5. PMID:27988846

**7210.** van Esser JW, van der Holt B, Meijer E, et al. Epstein-Barr virus (EBV) reactivation is a frequent event after allogeneic stem cell transplantation (SCT) and quantitatively predicts EBV-lymphoproliferative disease following T-cell–depleted SCT. Blood. 2001 Aug 15;98(4):972–8. PMID:11493441

**7211.** van Gaal JC, Flucke UE, Roeffen MH, et al. Anaplastic lymphoma kinase aberrations in rhabdomyosarcoma: clinical and prognostic implications. J Clin Oncol. 2012 Jan 20;30(3):308–15. PMID:22184391

**7212.** Van Geertruyden J, Lorea P, Goldschmidt D, et al. Glomus tumours of the hand. A retrospective study of 51 cases. J Hand Surg Br. 1996 Apr;21(2):257–60. PMID:8732413

**7213.** van Iersel L, Brokke KE, Adan RAH, et al. Pathophysiology and individualized treatment of hypothalamic obesity following craniopharyngioma and other suprasellar tumors: a systematic review. Endocr Rev. 2019 Feb 1;40(1):193–235. PMID:30247642

**7214.** van IJzendoorn DG, de Jong D, Romagosa C, et al. Fusion events lead to truncation of FOS in epithelioid hemangioma of bone. Genes Chromosomes Cancer. 2015 Sep;54(9):565–74. PMID:26173738

**7215.** van IJzendoorn DGP, Forghany Z, Liebelt F, et al. Functional analyses of a human vascular tumor FOS variant identify a novel degradation mechanism and a link to tumorigenesis. J Biol Chem. 2017 Dec 29;292(52):21282–90. PMID:29150442

**7216.** van Lier MG, Leenen CH, Wagner A, et al. Yield of routine molecular analyses in colorectal cancer patients ≤70 years to detect underlying Lynch syndrome. J Pathol. 2012 Apr;226(5):764–74. PMID:22081473

**7217.** van Nederveen FH, Gaal J, Favier J, et al. An immunohistochemical procedure to detect patients with paraganglioma and phaeochromocytoma with germline SDHB, SDHC, or SDHD gene mutations: a retrospective and prospective analysis. Lancet Oncol. 2009 Aug;10(8):764–71. PMID:19576851

**7218.** Van Neer FJ, Toonstra J, Van Voorst Vader PC, et al. Lymphomatoid papulosis in children: a study of 10 children registered by the Dutch Cutaneous Lymphoma Working Group. Br J Dermatol. 2001 Feb;144(2):351–4. PMID:11251571

**7219.** van Nguyen JM, Bouchard-Fortier G, Ferguson SE, et al. How common is the growing teratoma syndrome in patients with ovarian immature teratoma? Int J Gynecol Cancer. 2016 Sep;26(7):1201–6. PMID:27258729

**7220.** Van Nieuwenhuysen E, Busschaert P, Neven P, et al. The genetic landscape of 87 ovarian germ cell tumors. Gynecol Oncol. 2018 Oct;151(1):61–8. PMID:30170975

**7221.** van Noesel MM, Orbach D, Brennan B, et al. Outcome and prognostic factors in pediatric malignant peripheral nerve sheath tumors: an analysis of the European Pediatric Soft Tissue Sarcoma Group (EpSSG) NRSTS-2005 prospective study. Pediatr Blood Cancer. 2019 Oct;66(10):e27833. PMID:31241238

**7222.** Van Raamsdonk CD, Bezrookove V, Green G, et al. Frequent somatic mutations of GNAQ in uveal melanoma and blue naevi. Nature. 2009 Jan 29;457(7229):599–602. PMID:19078957

**7223.** Van Raamsdonk CD, Griewank KG, Crosby MB, et al. Mutations in GNA11 in uveal melanoma. N Engl J Med. 2010 Dec 2;363(23):2191–9. PMID:21083380

**7224.** Van Roosbroeck K, Cools J, Dierickx D, et al. ALK-positive large B-cell lymphomas with cryptic SEC31A-ALK and NPM1-ALK fusions. Haematologica. 2010 Mar;95(3):509–13. PMID:20207848

**7225.** van Slegtenhorst M, de Hoogt R, Hermans C, et al. Identification of the tuberous sclerosis gene TSC1 on chromosome 9q34. Science. 1997 Aug 8;277(5327):805–8. PMID:9242607

**7226.** van Slegtenhorst M, Verhoef S, Tempelaars A, et al. Mutational spectrum of the TSC1 gene in a cohort of 225 tuberous sclerosis complex patients: no evidence for genotype-phenotype correlation. J Med Genet. 1999 Apr;36(4):285–9. PMID:10227394

**7227.** Van Vlierberghe P, Ambesi-Impiombato A, Perez-Garcia A, et al. ETV6 mutations in early immature human T cell leukemias. J Exp Med. 2011 Dec 19;208(13):2571–9. PMID:22162831

**7228.** van Vugt LJ, van der Vleuten CJM, Flucke U, et al. The utility of GLUT1 as a diagnostic marker in cutaneous vascular anomalies: a review of literature and recommendations for daily practice. Pathol Res Pract. 2017 Jun;213(6):591–7. PMID:28552538

**7229.** van den Berg H, van Rijn RR, Merks JH. Management of tumors of the chest wall in childhood: a review. J Pediatr Hematol Oncol. 2008 Mar;30(3):214–21. PMID:18376284

**7230.** VandenBerg SR. Desmoplastic infantile ganglioglioma and desmoplastic cerebral astrocytoma of infancy. Brain Pathol. 1993 Jul;3(3):275–81. PMID:8293187

**7231.** VandenBerg SR, May EE, Rubinstein LJ, et al. Desmoplastic supratentorial neuroepithelial tumors of infancy with divergent differentiation potential ("desmoplastic infantile gangliogliomas"). Report on 11 cases of a distinctive embryonal tumor with favorable prognosis. J Neurosurg. 1987 Jan;66(1):58–71. PMID:3097276

**7232.** VandenBoom T, Quan VL, Zhang B, et al. Genomic fusions in pigmented spindle cell nevus of reed. Am J Surg Pathol. 2018 Aug;42(8):1042–51. PMID:29794873

**7233.** Vander Poorten V, Triantafyllou A, Thompson LD, et al. Salivary acinic cell carcinoma: reappraisal and update. Eur Arch Otorhinolaryngol. 2016 Nov;273(11):3511–31. PMID:26685679

**7234.** Vanderveen KA, Thompson SM, Callstrom MR, et al. Biopsy of pheochromocytomas and paragangliomas: potential for disaster. Surgery. 2009 Dec;146(6):1158–66. PMID:19958944

**7235.** Vandeva S, Daly AF, Petrossians P, et al. Somatic and germline mutations in the pathogenesis of pituitary adenomas. Eur J Endocrinol. 2019 Dec;181(6):R235–54. PMID:31658440

**7236.** Van Effenterre R, Boch AL. Craniopharyngioma in adults and children: a study of 122 surgical cases. J Neurosurg. 2002 Jul;97(1):3–11. PMID:12134929

**7237.** Vanel D, Picci P, De Paolis M, et al. Radiological study of 12 high-grade surface osteosarcomas. Skeletal Radiol. 2001 Dec;30(12):667–71. PMID:11810163

**7238.** Vang R, Gown AM, Zhao C, et al. Ovarian mucinous tumors associated with mature cystic teratomas: morphologic and immunohistochemical analysis identifies a subset of

potential teratomatous origin that shares features of lower gastrointestinal tract mucinous tumors more commonly encountered as secondary tumors in the ovary. Am J Surg Pathol. 2007 Jun;31(6):854–69. PMID:17527072

**7239.** van Hemel BM, Suurmeijer AJ. Effective application of the methanol-based PreservCyt(™) fixative and the Cellient(™) automated cell block processor to diagnostic cytopathology, immunocytochemistry, and molecular biology. Diagn Cytopathol. 2013 Aug;41(8):734–41. PMID:23444168

**7240.** Vanhentenrijk V, Vanden Bempt I, Dierickx D, et al. Relationship between classic Hodgkin lymphoma and overlapping large cell lymphoma investigated by comparative expressed sequence hybridization expression profiling. J Pathol. 2006 Oct;210(2):155–62. PMID:16874743

**7241.** van IJzendoorn DGP, Bovée JVMG. Vascular tumors of bone: the evolvement of a classification based on molecular developments. Surg Pathol Clin. 2017 Sep;10(3):621–35. PMID:28797505

**7242.** Van Maldergem L, Piard J, Larizza L, et al. Baller-Gerold syndrome. In: Adam MP, Ardinger HH, Pagon RA, et al., editors. GeneReviews. Seattle (WA): University of Washington, Seattle; 2007 Aug 13. PMID:20301383

**7243.** Varano G, Raffel S, Sormani M, et al. The B-cell receptor controls fitness of MYC-driven lymphoma cells via GSK3β inhibition. Nature. 2017 Jun 8;546(7657):302–6. PMID:28562582

**7244.** Varela-Duran J, Enzinger FM. Calcifying synovial sarcoma. Cancer. 1982 Jul 15;50(2):345–52. PMID:6282441

**7245.** Vargas SO, French CA, Faul PN, et al. Upper respiratory tract carcinoma with chromosomal translocation 15;19: evidence for a distinct disease entity of young patients with a rapidly fatal course. Cancer. 2001 Sep 1;92(5):1195–203. PMID:11571733

**7246.** Vargas-Parra GM, González-Acosta M, Thompson BA, et al. Elucidating the molecular basis of MSH2-deficient tumors by combined germline and somatic analysis. Int J Cancer. 2017 Oct 1;141(7):1365–80. PMID:28577310

**7247.** Varlet P, Le Teuff G, Le Deley MC, et al. WHO grade has no prognostic value in the pediatric high-grade glioma included in the HERBY trial. Neuro Oncol. 2020 Jan 11;22(1):116–27. PMID:31419298

**7248.** Varley JM. Germline TP53 mutations and Li-Fraumeni syndrome. Hum Mutat. 2003 Mar;21(3):313–20. PMID:12619118

**7249.** Varoquaux A, Kebebew E, Sebag F, et al. Endocrine tumors associated with the vagus nerve. Endocr Relat Cancer. 2016 Sep;23(9):R371–9. PMID:27406876

**7250.** Vase MØ, Maksten EF, Bendix K, et al. Occurrence and prognostic relevance of CD30 expression in post-transplant lymphoproliferative disorders. Leuk Lymphoma. 2015 Jun;56(6):1677–85. PMID:25248878

**7251.** Vasen HF, Blanco I, Aktan-Collan K, et al. Revised guidelines for the clinical management of Lynch syndrome (HNPCC): recommendations by a group of European experts. Gut. 2013 Jun;62(6):812–23. PMID:23408351

**7252.** Vasen HF, Ghorbanoghli Z, Bourdeaut F, et al. Guidelines for surveillance of individuals with constitutional mismatch repair-deficiency proposed by the European Consortium "Care for CMMR-D" (C4CMMR-D). J Med Genet. 2014 May;51(5):283–93. PMID:24556086

**7253.** Vasen HF, Möslein G, Alonso A, et al. Guidelines for the clinical management of familial adenomatous polyposis (FAP). Gut. 2008 May;57(5):704–13. PMID:18194984

**7254.** Vasko V, Bauer AJ, Tuttle RM, et al. Papillary and follicular thyroid cancers in children. Endocr Dev. 2007;10:140–72. PMID:17684395

**7255.** Vassallo J, Lamant L, Brugieres L, et al. ALK-positive anaplastic large cell lymphoma mimicking nodular sclerosis Hodgkin's lymphoma: report of 10 cases. Am J Surg Pathol. 2006 Feb;30(2):223–9. PMID:16434897

**7256.** Vaubel R, Zschernack V, Tran QT, et al. Biology and grading of pleomorphic xanthoastrocytoma-What have we learned about it? Brain Pathol. 2021 Jan;31(1):20–32. PMID:32619305

**7257.** Vaubel RA, Caron AA, Yamada S, et al. Recurrent copy number alterations in low-grade and anaplastic pleomorphic xanthoastrocytoma with and without BRAF V600E mutation. Brain Pathol. 2018 Mar;28(2):172–82. PMID:28181325

**7258.** Vaubell JI, Sing Y, Ramburan A, et al. Pediatric plasmablastic lymphoma: a clinicopathologic study. Int J Surg Pathol. 2014 Oct;22(7):607–16. PMID:24771257

**7259.** Védrine PO, Coffinet L, Temam S, et al. Mucoepidermoid carcinoma of salivary glands in the pediatric age group: 18 clinical cases, including 11 second malignant neoplasms. Head Neck. 2006 Sep;28(9):827–33. PMID:16783829

**7260.** Vega F, Medeiros LJ, Bueso-Ramos CE, et al. Hematolymphoid neoplasms associated with rearrangements of PDGFRA, PDGFRB, and FGFR1. Am J Clin Pathol. 2015 Sep;144(3):377–92. PMID:26276769

**7261.** Vega F, Medeiros LJ, Gaulard P. Hepatosplenic and other gammadelta T-cell lymphomas. Am J Clin Pathol. 2007 Jun;127(6):869–80. PMID:17509984

**7262.** Vege KD, Giannini C, Scheithauer BW. The immunophenotype of ependymomas. Appl Immunohistochem Mol Morphol. 2000 Mar;8(1):25–31. PMID:10937045

**7263.** Veldman J, Visser L, Huberts-Kregel M, et al. Rosetting T cells in Hodgkin lymphoma are activated by immunological synapse components HLA class II and CD58. Blood. 2020 Nov 19;136(21):2437–41. PMID:32589698

**7264.** Velez MJ, Billings SD, Weaver JA. Fibroblastic connective tissue nevus. J Cutan Pathol. 2016 Jan;43(1):75–9. PMID:26268513

**7265.** Vellios F, Baez J, Shumacker HB. Lipoblastomatosis: a tumor of fetal fat different from hibernoma; report of a case, with observations on the embryogenesis of human adipose tissue. Am J Pathol. 1958 Nov-Dec;34(6):1149–59. PMID:13583102

**7266.** Vellone VG, Calamaro P, Vignale C, et al. Atypical cellular chorangioma: a potential diagnostic pitfall with worrisome aspects but a favorable prognosis. Int J Surg Pathol. 2015 Aug;23(5):364–8. PMID:25998317

**7267.** Veltman IM, Schepens MT, Looijenga LH, et al. Germ cell tumours in neonates and infants: a distinct subgroup? APMIS. 2003 Jan;111(1):152–60. PMID:12752256

**7268.** Velz J, Agaimy A, Frontzek K, et al. Molecular and clinicopathologic heterogeneity of intracranial tumors mimicking extraskeletal myxoid chondrosarcoma. J Neuropathol Exp Neurol. 2018 Aug 1;77(8):727–35. PMID:29924341

**7269.** Vencio EF, Reeve CM, Unni KK, et al. Mesenchymal chondrosarcoma of the jaw bones: clinicopathologic study of 19 cases. Cancer. 1998 Jun 15;82(12):2350–5. PMID:9635527

**7270.** Venencie PY, Boffa GA, Delmas PD, et al. Pachydermoperiostosis with gastric hypertrophy, anemia, and increased serum bone Gla-protein levels. Arch Dermatol. 1988 Dec;124(12):1831–4. PMID:3263841

**7271.** Venkataraman G, Raffeld M, Pittaluga S, et al. CD15-expressing nodular lymphocyte-predominant Hodgkin lymphoma. Histopathology. 2011 Apr;58(5):803–5. PMID:21457163

7272. Venneti S, Santi M, Felicella MM, et al. A sensitive and specific histopathologic prognostic marker for H3F3A K27M mutant pediatric glioblastomas. Acta Neuropathol. 2014 Nov;128(5):743–53. PMID:25200322
7273. Ventii KH, Devi NS, Friedrich KL, et al. BRCA1-associated protein-1 is a tumor suppressor that requires deubiquitinating activity and nuclear localization. Cancer Res. 2008 Sep 1;68(17):6953–62. PMID:18757409
7274. Vera-Bolanos E, Aldape K, Yuan Y, et al. Clinical course and progression-free survival of adult intracranial and spinal ependymoma patients. Neuro Oncol. 2015 Mar;17(3):440–7. PMID:25121770
7275. Verbeke SL, Bovée JV. Primary vascular tumors of bone: a spectrum of entities? Int J Clin Exp Pathol. 2011 Aug 15;4(6):541–51. PMID:21904630
7276. Verbeke SL, de Jong D, Bertoni F, et al. Array CGH analysis identifies two distinct subgroups of primary angiosarcoma of bone. Genes Chromosomes Cancer. 2015 Feb;54(2):72–81. PMID:25231439
7277. Verburg FA, Van Santen HM, Luster M. Pediatric papillary thyroid cancer: current management challenges. Onco Targets Ther. 2016 Dec 28;10:165–75. PMID:28096684
7278. Verdegaal SH, Bovée JV, Pansuriya TC, et al. Incidence, predictive factors, and prognosis of chondrosarcoma in patients with Ollier disease and Maffucci syndrome: an international multicenter study of 161 patients. Oncologist. 2011;16(12):1771–9. PMID:22147000
7279. Verdijk RM. On the classification and grading of medulloepithelioma of the eye. Ocul Oncol Pathol. 2016 Apr;2(3):190–3. PMID:27239464
7280. Vered M, Dobriyan A, Buchner A. Congenital granular cell epulis presents an immunohistochemical profile that distinguishes it from the granular cell tumor of the adult. Virchows Arch. 2009 Mar;454(3):303–10. PMID:19205730
7281. Vergamini LB, Frazier AL, Abrantes FL, et al. Increase in the incidence of differentiated thyroid carcinoma in children, adolescents, and young adults: a population-based study. J Pediatr. 2014 Jun;164(6):1481–5. PMID:24630354
7282. Vergel De Dios AM, Bond JR, Shives TC, et al. Aneurysmal bone cyst. A clinicopathologic study of 238 cases. Cancer. 1992 Jun 15;69(12):2921–31. PMID:1591685
7283. Vergier B, Laharanne E, Prochazkova-Carlotti M, et al. Proliferative nodules vs melanoma arising in giant congenital melanocytic nevi during childhood. JAMA Dermatol. 2016 Oct 1;152(10):1147–51. PMID:27486690
7284. Verma J, Teh BS, Paulino AC. Characteristics and outcome of radiation and chemotherapy-related mucoepidermoid carcinoma of the salivary glands. Pediatr Blood Cancer. 2011 Dec 15;57(7):1137–41. PMID:21280198
7285. Verma K, Kapila K. Role of fine needle aspiration cytology in diagnosis of pleomorphic adenomas. Cytopathology. 2002 Apr;13(2):121–7. PMID:11952751
7286. Veronese F, Miglino B, Boggio P, et al. Gorlin-Goltz syndrome: a case series from north Italy. Eur J Dermatol. 2018 Oct 1;28(5):687–8. PMID:30129523
7287. Verp MS, Simpson JL. Abnormal sexual differentiation and neoplasia. Cancer Genet Cytogenet. 1987 Apr;25(2):191–218. PMID:3548944
7288. Verrill C, Yilmaz A, Srigley JR, et al. Reporting and staging of testicular germ cell tumors: the International Society of Urological Pathology (ISUP) Testicular Cancer Consultation Conference Recommendations. Am J Surg Pathol. 2017 Jun;41(6):e22–32. PMID:28368923
7289. Verschoor AJ, Bovée JVMG, Mastboom MJL, et al. Incidence and demographics of giant cell tumor of bone in the Netherlands: first nationwide Pathology Registry Study. Acta Orthop. 2018 Oct;89(5):570–4. PMID:29987945
7290. Versteege I, Sévenet N, Lange J, et al. Truncating mutations of hSNF5/INI1 in aggressive paediatric cancer. Nature. 1998 Jul 9;394(6689):203–6. PMID:9671307
7291. Vervaet N, Van Ginderdeuren R, Van Den Oord JJ, et al. A rare conjunctival Spitz nevus: a case report and literature review. Bull Soc Belge Ophtalmol. 2007; (303):63–7. PMID:17894290
7292. Vestergaard P, Mollerup CL, Frøkjaer VG, et al. [Cohort study of fracture risk before and after surgery of primary hyperparathyroidism]. Ugeskr Laeger. 2001 Sep 3;163(36):4875–8. Danish. PMID:11571864
7293. Vettermann FJ, Felsberg J, Reifenberger G, et al. Characterization of diffuse gliomas with histone H3-G34 mutation by MRI and dynamic 18F-FET PET. Clin Nucl Med. 2018 Dec;43(12):895–8. PMID:30358620
7294. Viana A, Aguinaga F, Marinho F, et al. Basal cell carcinoma arising on a verrucous epidermal nevus: a case report. Case Rep Dermatol. 2015 Feb 20;7(1):20–4. PMID:25848348
7295. Vicus D, Beiner ME, Clarke B, et al. Ovarian immature teratoma: treatment and outcome in a single institutional cohort. Gynecol Oncol. 2011 Oct;123(1):50–3. PMID:21764111
7296. Vidyadhar M, Amanda C, Thuan Q, et al. Sialoblastoma. J Pediatr Surg. 2008 Oct;43(10):e11–3. PMID:18926196
7297. Vieira J, Pinto C, Afonso M, et al. Identification of previously unrecognized FAP in children with Gardner fibroma. Eur J Hum Genet. 2015 May;23(5):715–8. PMID:25074465
7298. Viguer JM, Vicandi B, Jiménez-Heffernan JA, et al. Fine needle aspiration cytology of pleomorphic adenoma. An analysis of 212 cases. Acta Cytol. 1997 May-Jun;41(3):786–94. PMID:9167703
7299. Vij M, Shanmugam NP, Reddy MS, et al. Hepatocarcinogenesis in multidrug-resistant P-glycoprotein 3 deficiency. Pediatr Transplant. 2017 May;21(3). PMID:28127842
7300. Vij M, Shanmugam NP, Reddy MS, et al. Paediatric hepatocellular carcinoma in tight junction protein 2 (TJP2) deficiency. Virchows Arch. 2017 Nov;471(5):679–83. PMID:28733884
7301. Vilarinho S, Erson-Omay EZ, Harmanci AS, et al. Paediatric hepatocellular carcinoma due to somatic CTNNB1 and NFE2L2 mutations in the setting of inherited bi-allelic ABCB11 mutations. J Hepatol. 2014 Nov;61(5):1178–83. PMID:25016225
7302. Villà S, Miller RC, Krengli M, et al. Primary pineal tumors: outcome and prognostic factors–a study from the Rare Cancer Network (RCN). Clin Transl Oncol. 2012 Nov;14(11):827–34. PMID:22914906
7302A. Villa C, Lagonigro MS, Magri F, et al. Hyperplasia-adenoma sequence in pituitary tumorigenesis related to aryl hydrocarbon receptor interacting protein gene mutation. Endocr Relat Cancer. 2011 Jun 8;18(3):347–56. PMID:21450940
7303. Villani A, Shore A, Wasserman JD, et al. Biochemical and imaging surveillance in germline TP53 mutation carriers with Li-Fraumeni syndrome: 11 year follow-up of a prospective observational study. Lancet Oncol. 2016 Sep;17(9):1295–305. PMID:27501770
7304. Villar-Taibo R, Peteiro-González D, Cabezas-Agrícola JM, et al. Aggressiveness of the tall cell variant of papillary thyroid carcinoma is independent of the tumor size and patient age. Oncol Lett. 2017 May;13(5):3501–7. PMID:28529577
7305. Vinayak R, Cruz RJ Jr, Ranganathan S, et al. Pediatric liver transplantation for hepatocellular cancer and rare liver malignancies: US multicenter and single-center experience (1981-2015). Liver Transpl. 2017 Dec;23(12):1577–88. PMID:28834194
7306. Vin-Christian K, McCalmont TH, Frieden IJ. Kaposiform hemangioendothelioma. An aggressive, locally invasive vascular tumor that can mimic hemangioma of infancy. Arch Dermatol. 1997 Dec;133(12):1573–8. PMID:9420544
7307. Vinci M, Burford A, Molinari V, et al. Functional diversity and cooperativity between subclonal populations of pediatric glioblastoma and diffuse intrinsic pontine glioma cells. Nat Med. 2018 Aug;24(8):1204–15. PMID:29967352
7308. Vinters HV, Park SH, Johnson MW, et al. Cortical dysplasia, genetic abnormalities and neurocutaneous syndromes. Dev Neurosci. 1999 Nov;21(3-5):248–59. PMID:10575248
7309. Viola F, Villani E, Natacci F, et al. Choroidal abnormalities detected by near-infrared reflectance imaging as a new diagnostic criterion for neurofibromatosis 1. Ophthalmology. 2012 Feb;119(2):369–75. PMID:21963267
7310. Virgone C, Andreetta M, Avanzini S, et al. Pheochromocytomas and paragangliomas in children: data from the Italian Cooperative Study (TREP). Pediatr Blood Cancer. 2020 Aug;67(8):e28332. PMID:32491270
7311. Virgone C, Cecchetto G, Dall'Igna P, et al. Mesenchymal hamartoma of the liver in older children: an adult variant or a different entity? Report of a case with review of the literature. Appl Immunohistochem Mol Morphol. 2015 Oct;23(9):667–73. PMID:22935827
7312. Viskochil D, Buchberg AM, Xu G, et al. Deletions and a translocation interrupt a cloned gene at the neurofibromatosis type 1 locus. Cell. 1990 Jul 13;62(1):187–92. PMID:1694727
7313. Visser J, Hukin J, Sargent M, et al. Late mortality in pediatric patients with craniopharyngioma. J Neurooncol. 2010 Oct;100(1):105–11. PMID:20204458
7314. Viswanathan K, McMillen B, Cheng E, et al. Juvenile papillomatosis (Swiss-cheese disease) of breast in an adult male with sequential diagnoses of ipsilateral intraductal, invasive, and widely metastatic carcinoma: a case report and review of the disease in males. Int J Surg Pathol. 2017 Sep;25(6):536–42. PMID:28420303
7315. Vitorovic D, Rosenblum J, Thomas C, et al. Primary CNS teratocarcinoma. Front Neurol. 2012 Feb 6;3:14. PMID:22363315
7316. Vivekanandan P, Daniel H, Yeh MM, et al. Mitochondrial mutations in hepatocellular carcinomas and fibrolamellar carcinomas. Mod Pathol. 2010 Jun;23(6):790–8. PMID:20228784
7317. Vivekanandan P, Micchelli ST, Torbenson M. Anterior gradient-2 is overexpressed by fibrolamellar carcinomas. Hum Pathol. 2009 Mar;40(3):293–9. PMID:18973922
7318. Vladoiu MC, El-Hamamy I, Donovan LK, et al. Childhood cerebellar tumours mirror conserved fetal transcriptional programs. Nature. 2019 Aug;572(7767):67–73. PMID:31043743
7319. Vo KT, Matthay KK, Neuhaus J, et al. Clinical, biologic, and prognostic differences on the basis of primary tumor site in neuroblastoma: a report from the international neuroblastoma risk group project. J Clin Oncol. 2014 Oct 1;32(28):3169–76. PMID:25154816
7320. Vogel WH. Li-Fraumeni syndrome. J Adv Pract Oncol. 2017 Nov-Dec;8(7):742–6. PMID:30333936
7321. Vogelstein B, Lane D, Levine AJ. Surfing the p53 network. Nature. 2000 Nov 16;408(6810):307–10. PMID:11099028
7322. Vogt PH, Besikoglu B, Bettendorf M, et al. Gonadoblastoma Y locus genes expressed in germ cells of individuals with dysgenetic gonads and a Y chromosome in their karyotypes include DDX3Y and TSPY. Hum Reprod. 2019 Apr 1;34(4):770–9. PMID:30753444
7323. Vokuhl C, Nourkami-Tutdibi N, Furtwängler R, et al. ETV6-NTRK3 in congenital mesoblastic nephroma: a report of the SIOP/GPOH nephroblastoma study. Pediatr Blood Cancer. 2018 Apr;65(4). PMID:29286563
7324. Vokuhl C, Oyen F, Häberle B, et al. Small cell undifferentiated (SCUD) hepatoblastomas: all malignant rhabdoid tumors? Genes Chromosomes Cancer. 2016 Dec;55(12):925–31. PMID:27356182
7325. Volante M, Collini P, Nikiforov YE, et al. Poorly differentiated thyroid carcinoma: the Turin proposal for the use of uniform diagnostic criteria and an algorithmic diagnostic approach. Am J Surg Pathol. 2007 Aug;31(8):1256–64. PMID:17667551
7326. Volante M, Daniele L, Asioli S, et al. Tumor staging but not grading is associated with adverse clinical outcome in neuroendocrine tumors of the appendix: a retrospective clinical pathologic analysis of 138 cases. Am J Surg Pathol. 2013 Apr;37(4):606–12. PMID:23426123
7327. Völkl TM, Langer T, Aigner T, et al. Klinefelter syndrome and mediastinal germ cell tumors. Am J Med Genet A. 2006 Mar 1;140(5):471–81. PMID:16470792
7328. Volsen SG, Barrass N, Scott MP, et al. Cellular and molecular effects of di-n-octyltin dichloride on the rat thymus. Int J Immunopharmacol. 1989;11(6):703–15. PMID:2681007
7329. Voltaggio L, Murray R, Lasota J, et al. Gastric schwannoma: a clinicopathologic study of 51 cases and critical review of the literature. Hum Pathol. 2012 May;43(5):650–9. PMID:22137423
7330. von der Maase H, Rørth M, Walbom-Jørgensen S, et al. Carcinoma in situ of contralateral testis in patients with testicular germ cell cancer: study of 27 cases in 500 patients. Br Med J (Clin Res Ed). 1986 Nov 29;293(6559):1398–401. PMID:3026550
7331. von Hochstetter AR, Sigg C, Saremaslani P, et al. The significance of giant cells in human testicular seminomas. A clinico-pathological study. Virchows Arch A Pathol Anat Histopathol. 1985;407(3):309–22. PMID:2412341
7332. von Hoff K, Hinkes B, Dannenmann-Stern E, et al. Frequency, risk-factors and survival of children with atypical teratoid rhabdoid tumors (AT/RT) of the CNS diagnosed between 1988 and 2004, and registered to the German HIT database. Pediatr Blood Cancer. 2011 Dec 1;57(6):978–85. PMID:21796761
7333. von Salomé J, Liu T, Keihäs M, et al. Haplotype analysis suggest that the MLH1 c.2059C > T mutation is a Swedish founder mutation. Fam Cancer. 2018 Oct;17(4):531–7. PMID:29288294
7334. von Hochstetter AR, Hedinger CE. The differential diagnosis of testicular germ cell tumors in theory and practice. A critical analysis of two major systems of classifiction and review of 389 cases. Virchows Arch A Pathol Anat Histol. 1982 Aug;396(3):247–77. PMID:6291228
7335. Vortmeyer AO, Devouassoux-Shisheboran M, Li G, et al. Microdissection-based analysis of mature ovarian teratoma. Am J Pathol. 1999 Apr;154(4):987–91. PMID:10233836
7336. Vortmeyer AO, Frank S, Jeong SY, et al. Developmental arrest of angioblastic lineage initiates tumorigenesis in von Hippel-Lindau disease. Cancer Res. 2003 Nov 1;63(21):7051–5. PMID:14612494
7337. Vortmeyer AO, Tran MG, Zeng W, et al. Evolution of VHL tumourigenesis in nerve root tissue. J Pathol. 2006 Nov;210(3):374–82. PMID:16981244
7338. Vortmeyer AO, Yuan Q, Lee YS, et al. Developmental effects of von Hippel-Lindau gene

deficiency. Ann Neurol. 2004 May;55(5):721–8. PMID:15122713
**7338A.** Vose J, Armitage J, Weisenburger D, et al. International peripheral T-cell and natural killer/T-cell lymphoma study: pathology findings and clinical outcomes. J Clin Oncol. 2008 Sep 1;26(25):4124–30. PMID:18626005
**7339.** Voss MH, Lunning MA, Maragulia JC, et al. Intensive induction chemotherapy followed by early high-dose therapy and hematopoietic stem cell transplantation results in improved outcome for patients with hepatosplenic T-cell lymphoma: a single institution experience. Clin Lymphoma Myeloma Leuk. 2013 Feb;13(1):8–14. PMID:23107915
**7340.** Voz ML, Agten NS, Van de Ven WJ, et al. PLAG1, the main translocation target in pleomorphic adenoma of the salivary glands, is a positive regulator of IGF-II. Cancer Res. 2000 Jan 1;60(1):106–13. PMID:10646861
**7341.** Voz ML, Aström AK, Kas K, et al. The recurrent translocation t(5;8)(p13;q12) in pleomorphic adenomas results in upregulation of PLAG1 gene expression under control of the LIFR promoter. Oncogene. 1998 Mar;16(11):1409–16. PMID:9525740
**7342.** Vujanić GM, Apps JR, Moroz V, et al. Nephrogenic rests in Wilms tumors treated with preoperative chemotherapy: the UK SIOP Wilms Tumor 2001 Trial experience. Pediatr Blood Cancer. 2017 Nov;64(11). PMID:28383760
**7343.** Vujanić GM, D'Hooghe E, Popov SD, et al. The effect of preoperative chemotherapy on histological subtyping and staging of Wilms tumors: the United Kingdom Children's Cancer Study Group (UKCCSG) Wilms tumor trial 3 (UKW3) experience. Pediatr Blood Cancer. 2019 Mar;66(3):e27549. PMID:30408319
**7344.** Vujanić GM, Gessler M, Ooms AHAG, et al. The UMBRELLA SIOP-RTSG 2016 Wilms tumour pathology and molecular biology protocol. Nat Rev Urol. 2018 Nov;15(11):693–701. PMID:30310143
**7345.** Vujanić GM, Harms D, Sandstedt B, et al. New definitions of focal and diffuse anaplasia in Wilms tumor: the International Society of Paediatric Oncology (SIOP) experience. Med Pediatr Oncol. 1999 May;32(5):317–23. PMID:10219330
**7346.** Vujanić GM, Kelsey A, Perlman EJ, et al. Anaplastic sarcoma of the kidney: a clinicopathologic study of 20 cases of a new entity with polyphenotypic features. Am J Surg Pathol. 2007 Oct;31(10):1459–68. PMID:17895746
**7347.** Vujanić GM, Sandstedt B, Harms D, et al. Revised International Society of Paediatric Oncology (SIOP) working classification of renal tumors of childhood. Med Pediatr Oncol. 2002 Feb;38(2):79–82. PMID:11813170
**7348.** Vujanić GM, Sandstedt B, Kelsey A, et al. Central pathology review in multicenter trials and studies: lessons from the nephroblastoma trials. Cancer. 2009 May 1;115(9):1977–83. PMID:19241454
**7349.** Vujanić GM, Schiavo Lena M, Sebire NJ. Botryoid Wilms tumor: a non-existent "entity" causing diagnostic and staging difficulties. Virchows Arch. 2019 Feb;474(2):227–34. PMID:30515564
**7350.** Vujovic S, Henderson S, Presneau N, et al. Brachyury, a crucial regulator of notochordal development, is a novel biomarker for chordomas. J Pathol. 2006 Jun;209(2):157–65. PMID:16538613
**7351.** Vuong HG, Odate T, Duong UNP, et al. Prognostic importance of solid variant papillary thyroid carcinoma: a systematic review and meta-analysis. Head Neck. 2018 Jul;40(7):1588–97. PMID:29509280
**7352.** Vyas M, Hechtman JF, Zhang Y, et al. DNAJB1-PRKACA fusions occur in oncocytic pancreatic and biliary neoplasms and are not specific for fibrolamellar hepatocellular carcinoma. Mod Pathol. 2020 Apr;33(4):648–56. PMID:31676785
**7353.** Wadt KA, Aoude LG, Johansson P, et al. A recurrent germline BAP1 mutation and extension of the BAP1 tumor predisposition spectrum to include basal cell carcinoma. Clin Genet. 2015 Sep;88(3):267–72. PMID:25225168
**7353A.** Wagenblast E, Araújo J, Gan OI, et al. Mapping the cellular origin and early evolution of leukemia in Down syndrome. Science. 2021 Jul 9;373(6551):eabf6202. PMID:34244384
**7354.** Wagener R, Bens S, Toprak UH, et al. Cryptic insertion of MYC exons 2 and 3 into the immunoglobulin heavy chain locus detected by whole genome sequencing in a case of "MYC-negative" Burkitt lymphoma. Haematologica. 2020 Apr;105(4):e202–5. PMID:31073073
**7355.** Wagener R, Seufert J, Raimondi F, et al. The mutational landscape of Burkitt-like lymphoma with 11q aberration is distinct from that of Burkitt lymphoma. Blood. 2019 Feb 28;133(9):962–6. PMID:30567752
**7356.** Wagner AJ, Remillard SP, Zhang YX, et al. Loss of expression of SDHA predicts SDHA mutations in gastrointestinal stromal tumors. Mod Pathol. 2013 Feb;26(2):289–94. PMID:22955521
**7357.** Wagner EF, Eferl R. Fos/AP-1 proteins in bone and the immune system. Immunol Rev. 2005 Dec;208:126–40. PMID:16313345
**7358.** Wagner J, Portwine C, Rabin K, et al. High frequency of germline p53 mutations in childhood adrenocortical cancer. J Natl Cancer Inst. 1994 Nov 16;86(22):1707–10. PMID:7966399
**7359.** Wagner VP, Carlos R, Romañach MJ, et al. Malignant transformation of craniomaxillofacial fibro-osseous lesions: a systematic review. J Oral Pathol Med. 2019 Jul;48(6):441–50. PMID:31062892
**7360.** Waguespack SG, Rich T, Grubbs E, et al. A current review of the etiology, diagnosis, and treatment of pediatric pheochromocytoma and paraganglioma. J Clin Endocrinol Metab. 2010 May;95(5):2023–37. PMID:20215394
**7361.** Waguespack SG, Rich TA, Perrier ND, et al. Management of medullary thyroid carcinoma and MEN2 syndromes in childhood. Nat Rev Endocrinol. 2011 Aug 23;7(10):596–607. PMID:21862994
**7362.** Wakely PE Jr, McDermott JE, Ali SZ. Cytopathology of alveolar soft part sarcoma: a report of 10 cases. Cancer. 2009 Dec 25;117(6):500–7. PMID:19787801
**7363.** Wakely PE Jr, Price WG, Frable WJ. Sternomastoid tumor of infancy (fibromatosis colli): diagnosis by aspiration cytology. Mod Pathol. 1989 Jul;2(4):378–81. PMID:2762289
**7364.** Walczak BE, Johnson CN, Howe BM. Myositis ossificans. J Am Acad Orthop Surg. 2015 Oct;23(10):612–22. PMID:26320160
**7365.** Waldman JS, Marcus AJ, Soter NA, et al. Cutaneous inflammation: effects of hydroxy acids and eicosanoid pathway inhibitors on vascular permeability. J Invest Dermatol. 1989 Jan;92(1):112–6. PMID:2491876
**7366.** Waldmann TA, Bradley JE. Polycythemia secondary to a pheochromocytoma with production of an erythropoiesis stimulating factor by the tumor. Proc Soc Exp Biol Med. 1961 Nov;108:425–7. PMID:14004535
**7367.** Waldron CA, el-Mofty SK, Gnepp DR. Tumors of the intraoral minor salivary glands: a demographic and histologic study of 426 cases. Oral Surg Oral Med Oral Pathol. 1988 Sep;66(3):323–33. PMID:2845326
**7368.** Wali GN, Halliday D, Dua J, et al. Cutaneous hyperpigmentation and familial gastrointestinal stromal tumour associated with KIT mutation. Clin Exp Dermatol. 2019 Jun;44(4):418–21. PMID:30280421
**7369.** Walker BA, Saltzman BS, Herlihy EP, et al. Phenotypic characterization of epibulbar dermoids. Int Ophthalmol. 2017 Jun;37(3):499–505. PMID:27405313
**7370.** Walker EA, Murphey MD, Fetsch JF. Imaging characteristics of tenosynovial and bursal chondromatosis. Skeletal Radiol. 2011 Mar;40(3):317–25. PMID:20711779
**7371.** Wallace AJ, Watson CJ, Oward E, et al. Mutation scanning of the NF2 gene: an improved service based on meta-PCR/sequencing, dosage analysis, and loss of heterozygosity analysis. Genet Test. 2004 Winter;8(4):368–80. PMID:15684865
**7372.** Wallace MR, Marchuk DA, Andersen LB, et al. Type 1 neurofibromatosis gene: identification of a large transcript disrupted in three NF1 patients. Science. 1990 Jul 13;249(4965):181–6. PMID:2134734
**7373.** Wallace PW, Conrad C, Brückmann S, et al. Metabolomics, machine learning and immunohistochemistry to predict succinate dehydrogenase mutational status in phaeochromocytomas and paragangliomas. J Pathol. 2020 Aug;251(4):378–87. PMID:32462735
**7374.** Walpole S, Pritchard AL, Cebulla CM, et al. Comprehensive study of the clinical phenotype of germline BAP1 variant-carrying families worldwide. J Natl Cancer Inst. 2018 Dec 1;110(12):1328–41. PMID:30517737
**7375.** Walsh TJ, Grady RW, Porter MP, et al. Incidence of testicular germ cell cancers in U.S. children: SEER Program experience 1973 to 2000. Urology. 2006 Aug;68(2):402–5. PMID:16904461
**7376.** Walter JW, North PE, Waner M, et al. Somatic mutation of vascular endothelial growth factor receptors in juvenile hemangioma. Genes Chromosomes Cancer. 2002 Mar;33(3):295–303. PMID:11807987
**7377.** Walterhouse DO, Pappo AS, Meza JL, et al. Shorter-duration therapy using vincristine, dactinomycin, and lower-dose cyclophosphamide with or without radiotherapy for patients with newly diagnosed low-risk rhabdomyosarcoma: a report from the Soft Tissue Sarcoma Committee of the Children's Oncology Group. J Clin Oncol. 2014 Nov 1;32(31):3547–52. PMID:25267746
**7378.** Walther C, Hofvander J, Nilsson J, et al. Gene fusion detection in formalin-fixed paraffin-embedded benign fibrous histiocytomas using fluorescence in situ hybridization and RNA sequencing. Lab Invest. 2015 Sep;95(9):1071–6. PMID:26121314
**7379.** Walther C, Tayebwa J, Lilljebjörn H, et al. A novel SERPINE1-FOSB fusion gene results in transcriptional up-regulation of FOSB in pseudomyogenic haemangioendothelioma. J Pathol. 2014 Apr;232(5):534–40. PMID:24374978
**7380.** Wan MJ, Ullrich NJ, Manley PE, et al. Long-term visual outcomes of optic pathway gliomas in pediatric patients without neurofibromatosis type 1. J Neurooncol. 2016 Aug;129(1):173–8. PMID:27311725
**7381.** Wan YCE, Liu J, Chan KM. Histone H3 mutations in cancer. Curr Pharmacol Rep. 2018;4(4):292–300. PMID:30101054
**7382.** Wanat KA, Reid E, Kamiyango W, et al. Tumoral bacillary angiomatosis in a child with human immunodeficiency virus. JAMA Dermatol. 2014 Sep;150(9):1015–6. PMID:25076357
**7383.** Wang AC, Jones DTW, Abecassis IJ, et al. Desmoplastic infantile ganglioglioma/astrocytoma (DIG/DIA) are distinct entities with frequent BRAFV600 mutations. Mol Cancer Res. 2018 Oct;16(10):1491–8. PMID:30006355
**7384.** Wang AH, Wang YY, Yao Y, et al. Summary of 615 patients of chronic myeloid leukemia in Shanghai from 2001 to 2006. J Exp Clin Cancer Res. 2010 Mar 3;29:20. PMID:20199658
**7385.** Wang C, Mao M, Li B, et al. Surgery alone is effective in the management of pediatric salivary gland acinic cell carcinoma. J Oral Maxillofac Surg. 2019 Aug;77(8):1713–23. PMID:30825434
**7386.** Wang CH, Hsu TR, Yang TY, et al. Primary yolk sac tumor of bilateral basal ganglia. J Chin Med Assoc. 2010 Aug;73(8):444–8. PMID:20728859
**7387.** Wang CP, Chang YH, Chang YT. Fetal rhabdomyoma of the right tonsil with polyp-like appearance. Case Rep Otolaryngol. 2015;2015:713278. PMID:26246927
**7388.** Wang F, He Y, Li C, et al. Malignant craniopharyngioma: a report of seven cases and review of the literature. World Neurosurg. 2020 Mar;135:e194–201. PMID:31785438
**7389.** Wang G, Tucker T, Ng TL, et al. Fine-needle aspiration of soft tissue myoepithelioma. Diagn Cytopathol. 2016 Feb;44(2):152–5. PMID:26644362
**7390.** Wang G, Wu C, Wang Y, et al. A girl with a giant fibrolipoma in her thoracic cavity: a rare case report. J Med Case Rep. 2019 May 7;13(1):140. PMID:31060610
**7391.** Wang G, Zhang X, Feng M, et al. Comparing survival outcomes of gross total resection and subtotal resection with radiotherapy for craniopharyngioma: a meta-analysis. J Surg Res. 2018 Jun;226:131–9. PMID:29661278
**7392.** Wang GN, Cui Y, Zhao WG, et al. Clinicopathological analysis of the hydroa vacciniforme-like lymphoproliferative disorder with natural killer cell phenotype compared with cutaneous natural killer T-cell lymphoma. Exp Ther Med. 2018 Dec;16(6):4772–8. PMID:30542432
**7393.** Wang GY, Thomas DG, Davis JL, et al. EWSR1-NFATC2 translocation-associated sarcoma clinicopathologic findings in a rare aggressive primary bone or soft tissue tumor. Am J Surg Pathol. 2019 Aug;43(8):1112–22. PMID:30994538
**7394.** Wang H, Correa H, Sanders M, et al. Noninvasive follicular thyroid neoplasm with papillary-like nuclear features in children: an institutional experience and literature review. Pediatr Dev Pathol. 2020 Mar-Apr;23(2):121–6. PMID:31483741
**7395.** Wang H, Jacobson A, Harmon DC, et al. Prognostic factors in alveolar soft part sarcoma: a SEER analysis. J Surg Oncol. 2016 Apr;113(5):581–6. PMID:26804150
**7396.** Wang H, Mehrad M, Ely KA, et al. Incidence and malignancy rates of indeterminate pediatric thyroid nodules. Cancer Cytopathol. 2019 Apr;127(4):231–9. PMID:30768868
**7397.** Wang H, Weiss VL, Hoffman RD, et al. Salivary gland NUT carcinoma with prolonged survival in children: case illustration and systematic review of literature. Head Neck Pathol. 2021 Mar;15(1):236–43. PMID:32077054
**7398.** Wang HH, Chen YL, Kao HL, et al. Extra-adrenal paraganglioma of the prostate. Can Urol Assoc J. 2013 May-Jun;7(5-6):E370–2. PMID:23766843
**7399.** Wang HW, Balakrishna JP, Pittaluga S, et al. Diagnosis of Hodgkin lymphoma in the modern era. Br J Haematol. 2019 Jan;184(1):45–59. PMID:30407610
**7400.** Wang J, Liu Z, Fang J, et al. Atypical teratoid/rhabdoid tumors with multilayered rosettes in the pineal region. Brain Tumor Pathol. 2016 Oct;33(4):261–6. PMID:27307151
**7401.** Wang J, Zhu XZ, Zhang RY. [Malignant granular cell tumor: a clinicopathologic analysis of 10 cases with review of literature]. Zhonghua Bing Li Xue Za Zhi. 2004 Dec;33(6):497–502. Chinese. PMID:15634442

7402. Wang JH, Dhillon AP, Sankey EA, et al. 'Neuroendocrine' differentiation in primary neoplasms of the liver. J Pathol. 1991 Jan;163(1):61–7. PMID:1848280
7403. Wang KH, Kupa J, Duffy KA, et al. Diagnosis and management of Beckwith-Wiedemann syndrome. Front Pediatr. 2020 Jan 21;7:562. PMID:32039119
7404. Wang KK, Glenn RL, Adams DM, et al. Surgical management of fibroadipose vascular anomaly of the lower extremities. J Pediatr Orthop. 2020 Mar;40(3):e227–36. PMID:31181028
7405. Wang L, Basturk O, Wang J, et al. A FISH assay efficiently screens for BRAF gene rearrangements in pancreatic acinar-type neoplasms. Mod Pathol. 2018 Jan;31(1):132–40. PMID:28884748
7406. Wang L, Liu L, Wang G, et al. Congenital disseminated tufted angioma. J Cutan Pathol. 2013 Apr;40(4):405–8. PMID:23373432
7407. Wang L, Motoi T, Khanin R, et al. Identification of a novel, recurrent HEY1-NCOA2 fusion in mesenchymal chondrosarcoma based on a genome-wide screen of exon-level expression data. Genes Chromosomes Cancer. 2012 Feb;51(2):127–39. PMID:22034177
7408. Wang L, Yamaguchi S, Burstein MD, et al. Novel somatic and germline mutations in intracranial germ cell tumours. Nature. 2014 Jul 10;511(7508):241–5. PMID:24896186
7409. Wang LL, Gannavarapu A, Kozinetz CA, et al. Association between osteosarcoma and deleterious mutations in the RECQL4 gene in Rothmund-Thomson syndrome. J Natl Cancer Inst. 2003 May 7;95(9):669–74. PMID:12734318
7410. Wang LL, Levy ML, Lewis RA, et al. Clinical manifestations in a cohort of 41 Rothmund-Thomson syndrome patients. Am J Med Genet. 2001 Jul 22;102(1):11–7. PMID:11471165
7411. Wang LL, Levy ML. Chapter 140: Rothmund–Thomson syndrome, Bloom syndrome, dyskeratosis congenita, Fanconi anaemia and poikiloderma with neutropenia. In: Hoeger P, Kinsler V, Yan A, et al., editors. Harper's textbook of pediatric dermatology. 4th ed. Hoboken (NJ): John Wiley & Sons; 2020. pp. 1786–801.
7412. Wang LL, Perlman EJ, Vujanic GM, et al. Desmoplastic small round cell tumor of the kidney in childhood. Am J Surg Pathol. 2007 Apr;31(4):576–84. PMID:17414105
7413. Wang LL, Plon SE. Rothmund-Thomson syndrome. In: Adam MP, Ardinger HH, Pagon RA, et al., editors. GeneReviews. Seattle (WA): University of Washington, Seattle; 1999 Oct 6. PMID:20301415
7414. Wang LL, Suganuma R, Ikegaki N, et al. Neuroblastoma of undifferentiated subtype, prognostic significance of prominent nucleolar formation, and MYC/MYCN protein expression: a report from the Children's Oncology Group. Cancer. 2013 Oct 15;119(20):3718–26. PMID:23901000
7415. Wang LL, Teshiba R, Ikegaki N, et al. Augmented expression of MYC and/or MYCN protein defines highly aggressive MYC-driven neuroblastoma: a Children's Oncology Group study. Br J Cancer. 2015 Jun 30;113(1):57–63. PMID:26035700
7416. Wang M, Tihan T, Rojiani AM, et al. Monomorphous angiocentric glioma: a distinctive epileptogenic neoplasm with features of infiltrating astrocytoma and ependymoma. J Neuropathol Exp Neurol. 2005 Oct;64(10):875–81. PMID:16215459
7417. Wang M, Zhang R, Liu X, et al. Supratentorial extraventricular ependymomas: a retrospective study focused on long-term outcomes and prognostic factors. Clin Neurol Neurosurg. 2018 Feb;165:1–6. PMID:29253745
7418. Wang Q, Ma S, Chen H, et al. Sialoblastoma in chin and management of treatment. Int J Pediatr Otorhinolaryngol. 2018 Jun;109:168–73. PMID:29728174
7419. Wang T, Li W, Wu X, et al. Nasal chondromesenchymal hamartoma in young children: CT and MRI findings and review of the literature. World J Surg Oncol. 2014 Aug 12;12:257. PMID:25117604
7420. Wang T, Li YQ, Liu H, et al. Bifocal juvenile papillomatosis as a marker of breast cancer: a case report and review of the literature. Oncol Lett. 2014 Dec;8(6):2587–90. PMID:25364432
7421. Wang WH, Grigoriou E, Dormans JP. Synovial chondromatosis of the spine in the skeletally immature: case report and updated review of the literature. J Pediatr Orthop B. 2015 May;24(3):255–61. PMID:25493704
7422. Wang WL, Evans HL, Meis JM, et al. FUS rearrangements are rare in 'pure' sclerosing epithelioid fibrosarcoma. Mod Pathol. 2012 Jun;25(6):846–53. PMID:22388756
7423. Wang WL, Patel NR, Caragea M, et al. Expression of ERG, an Ets family transcription factor, identifies ERG-rearranged Ewing sarcoma. Mod Pathol. 2012 Oct;25(10):1378–83. PMID:22766791
7424. Wang WP, Guo C, Berney DM, et al. Primary carcinoid tumors of the testis: a clinicopathologic study of 29 cases. Am J Surg Pathol. 2010 Apr;34(4):519–24. PMID:20351489
7425. Wang X, Chen Z, Qiu S, et al. Evaluating the effect of cryptorchidism on clinical stage of testicular seminoma. Cancer Manag Res. 2020 Jun 23;12:4883–8. PMID:32606976
7426. Wang X, Dubuc AM, Ramaswamy V, et al. Medulloblastoma subgroups remain stable across primary and metastatic compartments. Acta Neuropathol. 2015 Mar;129(3):449–57. PMID:25689980
7427. Wang X, Lee RS, Alver BH, et al. SMARCB1-mediated SWI/SNF complex function is essential for enhancer regulation. Nat Genet. 2017 Feb;49(2):289–95. PMID:27941797
7428. Wang Y, Chen J, Yang W, et al. The oncogenic roles of DICER1 RNase IIIb domain mutations in ovarian Sertoli-Leydig cell tumors. Neoplasia. 2015 Aug;17(8):650–60. PMID:26408257
7429. Wang Y, Chen SY, Karnezis AN, et al. The histone methyltransferase EZH2 is a therapeutic target in small cell carcinoma of the ovary, hypercalcaemic type. J Pathol. 2017 Jul;242(3):371–83. PMID:28444909
7430. Wang Y, Karnezis AN, Magrill J, et al. DICER1 hot-spot mutations in ovarian gynandroblastoma. Histopathology. 2018 Aug;73(2):306–13. PMID:29660837
7431. Wang Y, Wenzl K, Manske MK, et al. Amplification of 9p24.1 in diffuse large B-cell lymphoma identifies a unique subset of cases that resemble primary mediastinal large B-cell lymphoma. Blood Cancer J. 2019 Aug 30;9(9):73. PMID:31471540
7432. Wang YL, Zhu YX, Chen TZ, et al. Clinicopathologic study of 1176 salivary gland tumors in a Chinese population: experience of one cancer center 1997-2007. Acta Otolaryngol. 2012 Aug;132(8):879–86. PMID:22497626
7433. Wang Z, McGlynn KA, Rajpert-De Meyts E, et al. Meta-analysis of five genome-wide association studies identifies multiple new loci associated with testicular germ cell tumor. Nat Genet. 2017 Jul;49(7):1141–7. PMID:28604732
7434. Wang Z, Yuan Y, Zhuang H, et al. Hepatic haemangiomas: possible association with IL-17. J Clin Pathol. 2012 Feb;65(2):146–51. PMID:22031591
7435. Wang ZB, Wei LX. [Primary hepatic angiosarcoma: a clinical and pathological analysis]. Zhonghua Bing Li Xue Za Zhi. 2013 Jun;42(6):376–80. Chinese. PMID:24060070
7436. Wang ZB, Yuan J, Chen W, et al. Transcription factor ERG is a specific and sensitive diagnostic marker for hepatic angiosarcoma. World J Gastroenterol. 2014 Apr 7;20(13):3672–9. PMID:24707153
7437. Ward E, DeSantis C, Robbins A, et al. Childhood and adolescent cancer statistics, 2014. CA Cancer J Clin. 2014 Mar-Apr;64(2):83–103. PMID:24488779
7438. Ward SC, Huang J, Tickoo SK, et al. Fibrolamellar carcinoma of the liver exhibits immunohistochemical evidence of both hepatocyte and bile duct differentiation. Mod Pathol. 2010 Sep;23(9):1180–90. PMID:20495535
7439. Ward SC, Thung SN, Lim KH, et al. Hepatic progenitor cells in liver cancers from Asian children. Liver Int. 2010 Jan;30(1):102–11. PMID:19793197
7440. Ward ZJ, Yeh JM, Bhakta N, et al. Estimating the total incidence of global childhood cancer: a simulation-based analysis. Lancet Oncol. 2019 Apr;20(4):483–93. PMID:30824204
7441. Wardinsky TD, Pagon RA, Kropp RJ, et al. Nasal dermoid sinus cysts: association with intracranial extension and multiple malformations. Cleft Palate Craniofac J. 1991 Jan;28(1):87–95. PMID:2004099
7442. Warmke LM, Meis JM. Sclerosing epithelioid fibrosarcoma: a distinct sarcoma with aggressive features. Am J Surg Pathol. 2021 Mar 1;45(3):317–28. PMID:32769431
7443. Warmuth-Metz M, Gnekow AK, Müller H, et al. Differential diagnosis of suprasellar tumors in children. Klin Padiatr. 2004 Nov-Dec;216(6):323–30. PMID:15565547
7444. Warner J, Jones EW. Pyogenic granuloma recurring with multiple satellites. A report of 11 cases. Br J Dermatol. 1968 Apr;80(4):218–27. PMID:5647967
7445. Warner TF, Seo IS, Azen EA, et al. Immunocytochemistry of acinic cell carcinomas and mixed tumors of salivary glands. Cancer. 1985 Nov 1;56(9):2221–7. PMID:2413984
7446. Warnick RE, Raisanen J, Adornato BT, et al. Intracranial myxopapillary ependymoma: case report. J Neurooncol. 1993 Mar;15(3):251–6. PMID:8360710
7447. Warren AJ. Molecular basis of the human ribosomopathy Shwachman-Diamond syndrome. Adv Biol Regul. 2018 Jan;67:109–27. PMID:28942353
7448. Warren M, Matsuno R, Tran H, et al. Utility of Phox2b immunohistochemical stain in neural crest tumours and non-neural crest tumours in paediatric patients. Histopathology. 2018 Mar;72(4):685–96. PMID:28986989
7449. Warren M, Turpin BK, Mark M, et al. Undifferentiated myxoid lipoblastoma with PLAG1-HAS2 fusion in an infant; morphologically mimicking primitive myxoid mesenchymal tumor of infancy (PMMTI)–diagnostic importance of cytogenetic and molecular testing and literature review. Cancer Genet. 2016 Jan-Feb;209(1-2):21–9. PMID:26701195
7450. Warren M, Xu D, Li X. Gene fusions PAFAH1B1-USP6 and RUNX2-USP6 in aneurysmal bone cysts identified by next generation sequencing. Cancer Genet. 2017 Apr;212-213:13–8. PMID:28449806
7451. Warrick E, Garcia M, Chagnoleau C, et al. Preclinical corrective gene transfer in xeroderma pigmentosum human skin stem cells. Mol Ther. 2012 Apr;20(4):798–807. PMID:22068429
7452. Wartchow EP, Trost BA, Tucker JA, et al. Renal medullary carcinoma: ultrastructural studies may benefit diagnosis. Ultrastruct Pathol. 2008 Nov-Dec;32(6):252–6. PMID:19117267
7453. Warthin AS. Classics in oncology. Heredity with reference to carcinoma as shown by the study of the cases examined in the pathological laboratory of the University of Michigan, 1895-1913. By Aldred Scott Warthin. 1913. CA Cancer J Clin. 1985 Nov-Dec;35(6):348–59. PMID:3931868
7454. Wassef M, Blei F, Adams D, et al. Vascular anomalies classification: recommendations from the International Society for the Study of Vascular Anomalies. Pediatrics. 2015 Jul;136(1):e203–14. PMID:26055853
7455. Wästerlid T, Nordström L, Freiburghaus C, et al. Frequency and clinical implications of SOX11 expression in Burkitt lymphoma. Leuk Lymphoma. 2017 Jul;58(7):1760–3. PMID:27869516
7456. Waszak SM, Northcott PA, Buchhalter I, et al. Spectrum and prevalence of genetic predisposition in medulloblastoma: a retrospective genetic study and prospective validation in a clinical trial cohort. Lancet Oncol. 2018 Jun;19(6):785–98. PMID:29753700
7457. Waszak SM, Robinson GW, Gudenas BL, et al. Germline elongator mutations in sonic hedgehog medulloblastoma. Nature. 2020 Apr;580(7803):396–401. PMID:32296180
7458. Watanabe IC, Billis A, Guimarães MS, et al. Renal medullary carcinoma: report of seven cases from Brazil. Mod Pathol. 2007 Sep;20(9):914–20. PMID:17643096
7459. Watanabe K, Suzuki T. Epithelioid fibrosarcoma of the ovary. Virchows Arch. 2004 Oct;445(4):410–3. PMID:15322876
7460. Waters AM, Russell RT, Maizlin II, et al. Comparison of pediatric and adult solid pseudopapillary neoplasms of the pancreas. J Surg Res. 2019 Oct;242:312–7. PMID:31129239
7461. Watson GH. Cardiac rhabdomyomas in tuberous sclerosis. Ann N Y Acad Sci. 1991;615:50–7. PMID:2039167
7462. Watson S, Perrin V, Guillemot D, et al. Transcriptomic definition of molecular subgroups of small round cell sarcomas. J Pathol. 2018 May;245(1):29–40. PMID:29431183
7463. Wcislak SM, King WS, Waller BR 3rd, et al. Multifocal pheochromocytoma-paraganglioma in a 29-year-old woman with cyanotic congenital heart disease. Surgery. 2019 Jan;165(1):228–31. PMID:30340856
7464. Weaver KJ, Crawford LM, Bennett JA, et al. Brainstem angiocentric glioma: report of 2 cases. J Neurosurg Pediatr. 2017 Oct;20(4):347–51. PMID:28753090
7465. Webber SA, Naftel DC, Fricker FJ, et al. Lymphoproliferative disorders after paediatric heart transplantation: a multi-institutional study. Lancet. 2006 Jan 21;367(9506):233–9. PMID:16427492
7466. Weber A, Langhanki L, Schütz A, et al. Expression profiles of p53, p63, and p73 in benign salivary gland tumors. Virchows Arch. 2002 Nov;441(5):428–36. PMID:12447671
7467. Weber DC, Wang Y, Miller R, et al. Long-term outcome of patients with spinal myxopapillary ependymoma: treatment results from the MD Anderson Cancer Center and institutions from the Rare Cancer Network. Neuro Oncol. 2015 Apr;17(4):588–95. PMID:25301811
7468. Wechsler J, Greene M, McDevitt MA, et al. Acquired mutations in GATA1 in the megakaryoblastic leukemia of Down syndrome. Nat Genet. 2002 Sep;32(1):148–52. PMID:12172547
7469. Wechsler-Reya RJ, Scott MP. Control of neuronal precursor proliferation in the cerebellum by sonic hedgehog. Neuron. 1999 Jan;22(1):103–14. PMID:10027293
7470. Weeda VB, Murawski M, McCabe AJ, et al. Fibrolamellar variant of hepatocellular carcinoma does not have a better survival than conventional hepatocellular carcinoma–results

and treatment recommendations from the Childhood Liver Tumour Strategy Group (SIOPEL) experience. Eur J Cancer. 2013 Aug;49(12):2698–704. PMID:23683550
**7471.** Weedon D, Little JH. Spindle and epithelioid cell nevi in children and adults. A review of 211 cases of the Spitz nevus. Cancer. 1977 Jul;40(1):217–25. PMID:880553
**7472.** Weeks DA, Beckwith JB, Mierau GW, et al. Rhabdoid tumor of kidney. A report of 111 cases from the National Wilms' Tumor Study Pathology Center. Am J Surg Pathol. 1989 Jun;13(6):439–58. PMID:2543225
**7473.** Wefers AK, Stichel D, Schrimpf D, et al. Isomorphic diffuse glioma is a morphologically and molecularly distinct tumour entity with recurrent gene fusions of MYBL1 or MYB and a benign disease course. Acta Neuropathol. 2020 Jan;139(1):193–209. PMID:31563982
**7474.** Wefers AK, Warmuth-Metz M, Pöschl J, et al. Subgroup-specific localization of human medulloblastoma based on pre-operative MRI. Acta Neuropathol. 2014;127(6):931–3. PMID:24699697
**7475.** Wegert J, Vokuhl C, Collord G, et al. Recurrent intragenic rearrangements of EGFR and BRAF in soft tissue tumors of infants. Nat Commun. 2018 Jun 18;9(1):2378. PMID:29915264
**7476.** Wehner MS, Humphreys JL, Sharkey FE. Epididymal rhabdomyoma: report of a case, including histologic and immunohistochemical findings. Arch Pathol Lab Med. 2000 Oct;124(10):1518–9. PMID:11035587
**7477.** Wehrli BM, Weiss SW, Yandow S, et al. Gardner-associated fibromas (GAF) in young patients: a distinct fibrous lesion that identifies unsuspected Gardner syndrome and risk for fibromatosis. Am J Surg Pathol. 2001 May;25(5):645–51. PMID:11342777
**7478.** Wei J, Liao Z, Zhao G, et al. Clinicopathological features of pseudomyogenic hemangioendothelioma and precision therapy based on whole exome sequencing. Cancer Commun (Lond). 2020 Apr;40(4):197–201. PMID:32227592
**7479.** Wei S, Baloch ZW, LiVolsi VA. Pathology of Struma Ovarii: a Report of 96 Cases. Endocr Pathol. 2015 Dec;26(4):342–8. PMID:26374222
**7480.** Wei SJ, Nguyen TH, Yang IH, et al. MYC transcription activation mediated by OCT4 as a mechanism of resistance to 13-cisRA-mediated differentiation in neuroblastoma. Cell Death Dis. 2020 May 14;11(5):368. PMID:32409685
**7481.** Weidner N. Germ-cell tumors of the mediastinum. Semin Diagn Pathol. 1999 Feb;16(1):42–50. PMID:10355653
**7482.** Weidner N. Review and update: oncogenic osteomalacia-rickets. Ultrastruct Pathol. 1991 Jul-Oct;15(4-5):317–33. PMID:1755097
**7483.** Weidner N, Santa Cruz D. Phosphaturic mesenchymal tumors. A polymorphous group causing osteomalacia or rickets. Cancer. 1987 Apr 15;59(8):1442–54. PMID:3545439
**7484.** Weihrauch M, Bader M, Lehnert G, et al. Mutation analysis of K-ras-2 in liver angiosarcoma and adjacent nonneoplastic liver tissue from patients occupationally exposed to vinyl chloride. Environ Mol Mutagen. 2002;40(1):36–40. PMID:12211074
**7485.** Weil SC, Hrisinko MA. A hybrid eosinophilic-basophilic granulocyte in chronic granulocytic leukemia. Am J Clin Pathol. 1987 Jan;87(1):66–70. PMID:2432775
**7486.** Weiland LH. The histopathological spectrum of nasopharyngeal carcinoma. IARC Sci Publ (1971). 1978; (20):41–50. PMID:730199
**7487.** Weinberg AG, Finegold MJ. Primary hepatic tumors of childhood. Hum Pathol. 1983 Jun;14(6):512–37. PMID:6303939
**7488.** Weingart MF, Roth JJ, Hutt-Cabezas M, et al. Disrupting LIN28 in atypical teratoid rhabdoid tumors reveals the importance of the mitogen activated protein kinase pathway as a therapeutic target. Oncotarget. 2015 Feb 20;6(5):3165–77. PMID:25638158
**7489.** Weinstein JM, Drolet BA, Esterly NB, et al. Congenital dermatofibrosarcoma protuberans: variability in presentation. Arch Dermatol. 2003 Feb;139(2):207–11. PMID:12588227
**7490.** Weiss A, Khoury JD, Hoffer FA, et al. Telangiectatic osteosarcoma: the St. Jude Children's Research Hospital's experience. Cancer. 2007 Apr 15;109(8):1627–37. PMID:17351949
**7491.** Weiss SW, Enzinger FM. Epithelioid hemangioendothelioma: a vascular tumor often mistaken for a carcinoma. Cancer. 1982 Sep 1;50(5):970–81. PMID:7093931
**7492.** Weiss VL, Antonescu CR, Alaggio R, et al. Myxoinflammatory fibroblastic sarcoma in children and adolescents: clinicopathologic aspects of a rare neoplasm. Pediatr Dev Pathol. 2013 Nov-Dec;16(6):425–31. PMID:23919754
**7493.** Weitz NA, Lauren CT, Starc TJ, et al. Congenital cutaneous hemangioma causing cardiac failure: a case report and review of the literature. Pediatr Dermatol. 2013 Nov-Dec;30(6):e180–90. PMID:23025620
**7494.** Welch Dinauer CA, Tuttle RM, Robie DK, et al. Clinical features associated with metastasis and recurrence of differentiated thyroid cancer in children, adolescents and young adults. Clin Endocrinol (Oxf). 1998 Nov;49(5):619–28. PMID:10197078
**7495.** Weller M, van den Bent M, Tonn JC, et al. European Association for Neuro-Oncology (EANO) guideline on the diagnosis and treatment of adult astrocytic and oligodendroglial gliomas. Lancet Oncol. 2017 Jun;18(6):e315–29. PMID:28483413
**7496.** Wells SA Jr, Asa SL, Dralle H, et al. Revised American Thyroid Association guidelines for the management of medullary thyroid carcinoma. Thyroid. 2015 Jun;25(6):567–610. PMID:25810047
**7497.** Wemmert S, Willnecker V, Kulas P, et al. Identification of CTNNB1 mutations, CTNNB1 amplifications, and an Axin2 splice variant in juvenile angiofibromas. Tumour Biol. 2016 Apr;37(4):5539–49. PMID:26572152
**7498.** Wen J, Liu H, Xiao S, et al. Synovial chondromatosis of the hip joint in childhood: a case report and literature review. Medicine (Baltimore). 2018 Dec;97(51):e13199. PMID:30572428
**7499.** Wendling-Keim D, Vokuhl C, Walz C, et al. Activation of hedgehog signaling in aggressive hepatic hemangioma in newborns and infants. Anticancer Res. 2019 May;39(5):2351–60. PMID:31092427
**7500.** Wenger DE, Wold LE. Benign vascular lesions of bone: radiologic and pathologic features. Skeletal Radiol. 2000 Feb;29(2):63–74. PMID:10741493
**7501.** Wenig BM, Vinh TN, Smirniotopoulos JG, et al. Aggressive psammomatoid ossifying fibromas of the sinonasal region: a clinicopathologic study of a distinct group of fibro-osseous lesions. Cancer. 1995 Oct 1;76(7):1155–65. PMID:8630892
**7502.** Werbrouck C, Evangelista CCS, Lobón-Iglesias MJ, et al. TP53 pathway alterations drive radioresistance in diffuse intrinsic pontine gliomas (DIPG). Clin Cancer Res. 2019 Nov 15;25(22):6788–800. PMID:31481512
**7502A.** Weren RD, Ligtenberg MJ, Kets CM, et al. A germline homozygous mutation in the base-excision repair gene NTHL1 causes adenomatous polyposis and colorectal cancer. Nat Genet. 2015 Jun;47(6):668–71. PMID:25938944
**7503.** Wermann H, Stoop H, Gillis AJ, et al. Global DNA methylation in fetal human germ cells and germ cell tumours: association with differentiation and cisplatin resistance. J Pathol. 2010 Aug;221(4):433–42. PMID:20593487
**7504.** Werness BA, Guccion JG. Tumor of the broad ligament in von Hippel-Lindau disease of probable mullerian origin. Int J Gynecol Pathol. 1997 Jul;16(3):282–5. PMID:9421096
**7505.** Wesseler K, Kraft F, Eggermann T. Molecular and clinical opposite findings in 11p15.5 associated imprinting disorders: characterization of basic mechanisms to improve clinical management. Int J Mol Sci. 2019 Aug 28;20(17):E4219. PMID:31466347
**7506.** Wessendorf S, Barth TF, Viardot A, et al. Further delineation of chromosomal consensus regions in primary mediastinal B-cell lymphomas: an analysis of 37 tumor samples using high-resolution genomic profiling (array-CGH). Leukemia. 2007 Dec;21(12):2463–9. PMID:17728785
**7507.** West AN, Neale GA, Pounds S, et al. Gene expression profiling of childhood adrenocortical tumors. Cancer Res. 2007 Jan 15;67(2):600–8. PMID:17234769
**7508.** West JA, Viswanathan SR, Yabuuchi A, et al. A role for Lin28 in primordial germ-cell development and germ-cell malignancy. Nature. 2009 Aug 13;460(7257):909–13. PMID:19578360
**7509.** Westfal ML, Chang DC, Kelleher CM. A population-based analysis of pediatric breast cancer. J Pediatr Surg. 2019 Jan;54(1):140–4. PMID:30352693
**7510.** Westin M, Rekabdar E, Blomstrand L, et al. Mutations in the genes for keratin-4 and keratin-13 in Swedish patients with white sponge nevus. J Oral Pathol Med. 2018 Feb;47(2):152–7. PMID:29047160
**7511.** Wey EA, Britton AJ, Sferra JJ, et al. Gastroblastoma in a 28-year-old man with nodal metastasis: proof of the malignant potential. Arch Pathol Lab Med. 2012 Aug;136(8):961–4. PMID:22849746
**7512.** White B, Belzberg A, Ahlawat S, et al. Intraneural perineurioma in neurofibromatosis type 2 with molecular analysis. Clin Neuropathol. 2020 Jul/Aug;39(4):167–71. PMID:32271143
**7513.** White FV, Dehner LP, Belchis DA, et al. Congenital disseminated malignant rhabdoid tumor: a distinct clinicopathologic entity demonstrating abnormalities of chromosome 22q11. Am J Surg Pathol. 1999 Mar;23(3):249–56. PMID:10078913
**7514.** White G. Congenital rhabdomyomatous mesenchymal hamartoma. Am J Dermatopathol. 1990 Oct;12(5):539–40. PMID:2244670
**7515.** White J, Chan YF. Aggressive angiomyxoma of the vulva in an 11-year-old girl. Pediatr Pathol. 1994 Jan-Feb;14(1):27–37. PMID:8159617
**7516.** White W, Shiu MH, Rosenblum MK, et al. Cellular schwannoma. A clinicopathologic study of 57 patients and 58 tumors. Cancer. 1990 Sep 15;66(6):1266–75. PMID:2400975
**7517.** Whittle SB, Hicks MJ, Roy A, et al. Congenital spindle cell rhabdomyosarcoma. Pediatr Blood Cancer. 2019 Nov;66(11):e27935. PMID:31339226
**7518.** Whitworth J, Skytte AB, Sunde L, et al. Multilocus inherited neoplasia alleles syndrome: a case series and review. JAMA Oncol. 2016 Mar;2(3):373–9. PMID:26659639
**7519.** WHO Classification of Tumours Editorial Board. Breast tumours. Lyon (France): International Agency for Research on Cancer; 2019. (WHO classification of tumours series, 5th ed.; vol. 2). https://publications.iarc.fr/581.
**7520.** WHO Classification of Tumours Editorial Board. Central nervous system tumours. Lyon (France): International Agency for Research on Cancer; 2021. (WHO classification of tumours series, 5th ed.; vol. 6). https://publications.iarc.fr/601.
**7521.** WHO Classification of Tumours Editorial Board. Digestive system tumours. Lyon (France): International Agency for Research on Cancer; 2019. (WHO classification of tumours series, 5th ed.; vol. 1). https://publications.iarc.fr/579.
**7522.** WHO Classification of Tumours Editorial Board. Endocrine and neuroendocrine tumours. Lyon (France): International Agency for Research on Cancer; forthcoming. (WHO classification of tumours series, 5th ed.). https://publications.iarc.fr/.
**7522A.** WHO Classification of Tumours Editorial Board. Haematolymphoid tumours. Lyon (France): International Agency for Research on Cancer; forthcoming. (WHO classification of tumours series, 5th ed.). https://publications.iarc.fr/.
**7523.** WHO Classification of Tumours Editorial Board. Soft tissue and bone tumours. Lyon (France): International Agency for Research on Cancer; 2020. (WHO classification of tumours series, 5th ed.; vol. 3). https://publications.iarc.fr/588.
**7524.** WHO. Technical Report: WHO guidelines for the health sector response to child maltreatment. Geneva (Switzerland): WHO; 2019. Available from: https://www.who.int/violence_injury_prevention/publications/violence/Technical-Report-WHO-Guidelines-for-the-health-sector-response-to-child-maltreatment-2.pdf.
**7525.** Wiatrak BJ, Wiatrak DW, Broker TR, et al. Recurrent respiratory papillomatosis: a longitudinal study comparing severity associated with human papilloma viral types 6 and 11 and other risk factors in a large pediatric population. Laryngoscope. 2004 Nov;114(11 Pt 2 Suppl 104):1–23. PMID:15514560
**7526.** Wick A, Kessler T, Platten M, et al. Superiority of temozolomide over radiotherapy for elderly patients with RTK II methylation class, MGMT promoter methylated malignant astrocytoma. Neuro Oncol. 2020 Aug 17;22(8):1162–72. PMID:32064499
**7527.** Wick MR, Ritter JH, Dehner LP. Malignant rhabdoid tumors: a clinicopathologic review and conceptual discussion. Semin Diagn Pathol. 1995 Aug;12(3):233–48. PMID:8545590
**7528.** Wicking C, Gillies S, Smyth I, et al. De novo mutations of the Patched gene in nevoid basal cell carcinoma syndrome help to define the clinical phenotype. Am J Med Genet. 1997 Dec 19;73(3):304–7. PMID:9415689
**7529.** Wicking C, Shanley S, Smyth I, et al. Most germ-line mutations in the nevoid basal cell carcinoma syndrome lead to a premature termination of the PATCHED protein, and no genotype-phenotype correlations are evident. Am J Hum Genet. 1997 Jan;60(1):21–6. PMID:8981943
**7530.** Wicklund CL, Pauli RM, Johnston D, et al. Natural history study of hereditary multiple exostoses. Am J Med Genet. 1995 Jan 2;55(1):43–6. PMID:7702095
**7531.** Widemann BC, Italiano A. Biology and management of undifferentiated pleomorphic sarcoma, myxofibrosarcoma, and malignant peripheral nerve sheath tumors: state of the art and perspectives. J Clin Oncol. 2018 Jan 10;36(2):160–7. PMID:29220302
**7532.** Widhe B, Widhe T. Initial symptoms and clinical features in osteosarcoma and Ewing sarcoma. J Bone Joint Surg Am. 2000 May;82(5):667–74. PMID:10819277
**7533.** Wiechers T, Rabenhorst A, Schick T, et al. Large maculopapular cutaneous lesions are associated with favorable outcome in childhood-onset mastocytosis. J Allergy Clin Immunol. 2015 Dec;136(6):1581–1590.e3. PMID:26152315
**7534.** Wieland I, Tinschert S, Zenker M. High-level somatic mosaicism of AKT1 c.49G>A

mutation in skin scrapings from epidermal nevi enables non-invasive molecular diagnosis in patients with Proteus syndrome. Am J Med Genet A. 2013 Apr;161A(4):889–91. PMID:23436452
**7535.** Wieneke JA, Thompson LD, Heffess CS. Adrenal cortical neoplasms in the pediatric population: a clinicopathologic and immunophenotypic analysis of 83 patients. Am J Surg Pathol. 2003 Jul;27(7):867–81. PMID:12826878
**7536.** Wieser I, Wohlmuth C, Nunez CA, et al. Lymphomatoid papulosis in children and adolescents: a systematic review. Am J Clin Dermatol. 2016 Aug;17(4):319–27. PMID:27138554
**7537.** Wiesner T, Kutzner H, Cerroni L, et al. Genomic aberrations in spitzoid melanocytic tumours and their implications for diagnosis, prognosis and therapy. Pathology. 2016 Feb;48(2):113–31. PMID:27020384
**7538.** Wiesner T, Murali R, Fried I, et al. A distinct subset of atypical Spitz tumors is characterized by BRAF mutation and loss of BAP1 expression. Am J Surg Pathol. 2012 Jun;36(6):818–30. PMID:22367297
**7539.** Wiesner T, Obenauf AC, Murali R, et al. Germline mutations in BAP1 predispose to melanocytic tumors. Nat Genet. 2011 Aug 28;43(10):1018–21. PMID:21874003
**7540.** Wiestler OD, von Siebenthal K, Schmitt HP, et al. Distribution and immunoreactivity of cerebral micro-hamartomas in bilateral acoustic neurofibromatosis (neurofibromatosis 2). Acta Neuropathol. 1989;79(2):137–43. PMID:2596263
**7541.** Wilding A, Ingham SL, Lalloo F, et al. Life expectancy in hereditary cancer predisposing diseases: an observational study. J Med Genet. 2012 Apr;49(4):264–9. PMID:22362873
**7542.** Wilentz RE, Goggins M, Redston M, et al. Genetic, immunohistochemical, and clinical features of medullary carcinoma of the pancreas: a newly described and characterized entity. Am J Pathol. 2000 May;156(5):1641–51. PMID:10793075
**7543.** Wilkerson BW, Crim JR, Hung M, et al. Characterization of synovial sarcoma calcification. AJR Am J Roentgenol. 2012 Dec;199(6):W730-4. PMID:23169746
**7544.** Willemze R. Mycosis fungoides variants-clinicopathologic features, differential diagnosis, and treatment. Semin Cutan Med Surg. 2018 Mar;37(1):11–7. PMID:29719015
**7545.** Willemze R, Hodak E, Zinzani PL, et al. Primary cutaneous lymphomas: ESMO Clinical Practice Guidelines for diagnosis, treatment and follow-up. Ann Oncol. 2018 Oct 1;29 Suppl 4:iv30–40. PMID:29878045
**7546.** Willemze R, Jansen PM, Cerroni L, et al. Subcutaneous panniculitis-like T-cell lymphoma: definition, classification, and prognostic factors: an EORTC Cutaneous Lymphoma Group Study of 83 cases. Blood. 2008 Jan 15;111(2):838–45. PMID:17934071
**7547.** William J, Laskin W, Nayar R, et al. Diagnosis of phosphaturic mesenchymal tumor (mixed connective tissue type) by cytopathology. Diagn Cytopathol. 2012 Aug;40 Suppl 2:E109–13. PMID:22927293
**7548.** Williams DM, Hobson R, Imeson J, et al. Anaplastic large cell lymphoma in childhood: analysis of 72 patients treated on the United Kingdom Children's Cancer Study Group chemotherapy regimens. Br J Haematol. 2002 Jun;117(4):812–20. PMID:12060115
**7549.** Williams EA, Wakimoto H, Shankar GM, et al. Frequent inactivating mutations of the PBAF complex gene PBRM1 in meningioma with papillary features. Acta Neuropathol. 2020 Jul;140(1):89–93. PMID:32405805
**7550.** Williams ED, Abrosimov A, Bogdanova T, et al. Thyroid carcinoma after Chernobyl latent period, morphology and aggressiveness. Br J Cancer. 2004 Jun 1;90(11):2219–24. PMID:15150580
**7551.** Williams K, Chernetsova E, Michaud J, et al. Neurogenic ovarian cyst–a rare, monodermal teratoma. Pediatr Dev Pathol. 2015 Jul-Aug;18(4):341–2. PMID:26261871
**7552.** Williams L, Thompson LD, Seethala RR, et al. Salivary duct carcinoma: the predominance of apocrine morphology, prevalence of histologic variants, and androgen receptor expression. Am J Surg Pathol. 2015 May;39(5):705–13. PMID:25871467
**7553.** Williams LA, Pankratz N, Lane J, et al. Klinefelter syndrome in males with germ cell tumors: a report from the Children's Oncology Group. Cancer. 2018 Oct 1;124(19):3900–8. PMID:30291793
**7554.** Williams MD. Paragangliomas of the head and neck: an overview from diagnosis to genetics. Head Neck Pathol. 2017 Sep;11(3):278–87. PMID:28321772
**7555.** Williams MD, DeLellis RA, Erickson LA, et al. Pathology data set for reporting parathyroid carcinoma and atypical parathyroid neoplasm: recommendations from the International Collaboration on Cancer Reporting. Hum Pathol. 2021 Apr;110:73–82. PMID:32687943
**7556.** Williams MD, Tischler AS. Update from the 4th edition of the World Health Organization classification of head and neck tumours: paragangliomas. Head Neck Pathol. 2017 Mar;11(1):88–95. PMID:28247224
**7557.** Williamson SR, Grignon DJ, Cheng L, et al. Renal cell carcinoma with chromosome 6p amplification including the TFEB gene: a novel mechanism of tumor pathogenesis? Am J Surg Pathol. 2017 Mar;41(3):287–98. PMID:28009604
**7558.** Williamson TH, Garner A, Moore AT. Structure of Lisch nodules in neurofibromatosis type 1. Ophthalmic Paediatr Genet. 1991 Mar;12(1):11–7. PMID:1908964
**7559.** Willis RA. The borderland of embryology and pathology. Bull N Y Acad Med. 1950 Jul;26(7):440–60. PMID:15426876
**7560.** Willis RA. Chapter 11: The embryonic tumours and teratomas. In: The borderland of embryology and pathology. 2nd ed. London (UK): Butterworth & Co.; 1962. pp. 410–54.
**7561.** Wilson BG, Roberts CW. SWI/SNF nucleosome remodellers and cancer. Nat Rev Cancer. 2011 Jun 9;11(7):481–92. PMID:21654818
**7562.** Wilson BG, Wang X, Shen X, et al. Epigenetic antagonism between polycomb and SWI/SNF complexes during oncogenic transformation. Cancer Cell. 2010 Oct 19;18(4):316–28. PMID:20951942
**7563.** Wilson C, Bonnet C, Guy C, et al. Tsc1 haploinsufficiency without mammalian target of rapamycin activation is sufficient for renal cyst formation in Tsc1+/- mice. Cancer Res. 2006 Aug 15;66(16):7934–8. PMID:16912167
**7564.** Wilson DB, Michalski JM, Grossman WJ, et al. Isolated CNS relapse following stem cell transplantation for juvenile myelomonocytic leukemia. J Pediatr Hematol Oncol. 2003 Nov;25(11):910–3. PMID:14608204
**7565.** Wilson RD, Hedrick H, Flake AW, et al. Sacrococcygeal teratomas: prenatal surveillance, growth and pregnancy outcome. Fetal Diagn Ther. 2009;25(1):15–20. PMID:19122459
**7566.** Wilson TJ, Amrami KK, Howe BM, et al. Clinical and radiological follow-up of intraneural perineuriomas. Neurosurgery. 2019 Dec 1;85(6):786–92. PMID:30481319
**7567.** Wilson WH, Kingma DW, Raffeld M, et al. Association of lymphomatoid granulomatosis with Epstein-Barr viral infection of B lymphocytes and response to interferon-alpha 2b. Blood. 1996 Jun 1;87(11):4531–7. PMID:8639820
**7568.** Wimmer K, Kratz CP, Vasen HF, et al. Diagnostic criteria for constitutional mismatch repair deficiency syndrome: suggestions of the European consortium 'Care for CMMRD' (C4CMMRD). J Med Genet. 2014 Jun;51(6):355–65. PMID:24737826
**7569.** Win AK, Dowty JG, English DR, et al. Body mass index in early adulthood and colorectal cancer risk for carriers and non-carriers of germline mutations in DNA mismatch repair genes. Br J Cancer. 2011 Jun 28;105(1):162–9. PMID:21559014
**7570.** Windsor R, Stiller C, Webb D. Peripheral T-cell lymphoma in childhood: population-based experience in the United Kingdom over 20 years. Pediatr Blood Cancer. 2008 Apr;50(4):784–7. PMID:18022899
**7571.** Wingerchuk DM, Noseworthy JH, Kimmel DW. Paraneoplastic encephalomyelitis and seminoma: importance of testicular ultrasonography. Neurology. 1998 Nov;51(5):1504–7. PMID:9818899
**7572.** Wishnow KI, Johnson DE, Swanson DA, et al. Identifying patients with low-risk clinical stage I nonseminomatous testicular tumors who should be treated by surveillance. Urology. 1989 Dec;34(6):339–43. PMID:2480680
**7573.** Wisniewski M, Deppisch LM. Solid teratomas of the ovary. Cancer. 1973 Aug;32(2):440–6. PMID:4722922
**7574.** Witkowski L, Carrot-Zhang J, Albrecht S, et al. Germline and somatic SMARCA4 mutations characterize small cell carcinoma of the ovary, hypercalcemic type. Nat Genet. 2014 May;46(5):438–43. PMID:24658002
**7575.** Witkowski L, Goudie C, Ramos P, et al. The influence of clinical and genetic factors on patient outcome in small cell carcinoma of the ovary, hypercalcemic type. Gynecol Oncol. 2016 Jun;141(3):454–60. PMID:26975901
**7576.** Witkowski L, Lalonde E, Zhang J, et al. Familial rhabdoid tumour 'avant la lettre'–from pathology review to exome sequencing and back again. J Pathol. 2013 Sep;231(1):35–43. PMID:23775540
**7577.** Witkowski L, Mattina J, Schönberger S, et al. DICER1 hotspot mutations in non-epithelial gonadal tumours. Br J Cancer. 2013 Nov 12;109(10):2744–50. PMID:24136150
**7578.** Witkowski L, McCluggage WG, Foulkes WD. Recently characterized molecular events in uncommon gynaecological neoplasms and their clinical importance. Histopathology. 2016 Dec;69(6):903–13. PMID:27504996
**7579.** Witt H, Gramatzki D, Hentschel B, et al. DNA methylation-based classification of ependymomas in adulthood: implications for diagnosis and treatment. Neuro Oncol. 2018 Nov 12;20(12):1616–24. PMID:30053291
**7580.** Witt H, Mack SC, Ryzhova M, et al. Delineation of two clinically and molecularly distinct subgroups of posterior fossa ependymoma. Cancer Cell. 2011 Aug 16;20(2):143–57. PMID:21840481
**7581.** Witt RL. The significance of the margin in parotid surgery for pleomorphic adenoma. Laryngoscope. 2002 Dec;112(12):2141–54. PMID:12461331
**7582.** Witt RL, Eisele DW, Morton RP, et al. Etiology and management of recurrent parotid pleomorphic adenoma. Laryngoscope. 2015 Apr;125(4):888–93. PMID:25289881
**7583.** Witt TR, Shah JP, Sternberg SS. Juvenile nasopharyngeal angiofibroma. A 30 year clinical review. Am J Surg. 1983 Oct;146(4):521–5. PMID:6312826
**7584.** Wittekind C, Brierley JD, Lee A, et al., editors. TNM supplement: a commentary on uniform use. 5th ed. Oxford (UK): Wiley-Blackwell; 2019.
**7585.** Wittekindt C, Streubel K, Arnold G, et al. Recurrent pleomorphic adenoma of the parotid gland: analysis of 108 consecutive patients. Head Neck. 2007 Sep;29(9):822–8. PMID:17563905
**7586.** Wizigmann-Voos S, Breier G, Risau W, et al. Up-regulation of vascular endothelial growth factor and its receptors in von Hippel-Lindau disease-associated and sporadic hemangioblastomas. Cancer Res. 1995 Mar 15;55(6):1358–64. PMID:7533661
**7587.** Wlodarska I, Martin-Garcia N, Achten R, et al. Fluorescence in situ hybridization study of chromosome 7 aberrations in hepatosplenic T-cell lymphoma: isochromosome 7q as a common abnormality accumulating in forms with features of cytologic progression. Genes Chromosomes Cancer. 2002 Mar;33(3):243–51. PMID:11807981
**7588.** Wlodarska I, Nooyen P, Maes B, et al. Frequent occurrence of BCL6 rearrangements in nodular lymphocyte predominance Hodgkin lymphoma but not in classical Hodgkin lymphoma. Blood. 2003 Jan 15;101(2):706–10. PMID:12393409
**7589.** Wlodarski MW, Hirabayashi S, Pastor V, et al. Prevalence, clinical characteristics, and prognosis of GATA2-related myelodysplastic syndromes in children and adolescents. Blood. 2016 Mar 17;127(11):1387–97. PMID:26702063
**7590.** Wlodarski MW, Sahoo SS, Niemeyer CM. Monosomy 7 in pediatric myelodysplastic syndromes. Hematol Oncol Clin North Am. 2018 Aug;32(4):729–43. PMID:30047423
**7591.** Wnorowski M, Prosch H, Prayer D, et al. Pattern and course of neurodegeneration in Langerhans cell histiocytosis. J Pediatr. 2008 Jul;153(1):127–32. PMID:18571550
**7592.** Wobker SE, Matoso A, Pratilas CA, et al. Metanephric adenoma-epithelial wilms tumor overlap lesions: an analysis of BRAF status. Am J Surg Pathol. 2019 Sep;43(9):1157–69. PMID:31192863
**7593.** Woehrer A, Slavc I, Peyrl A, et al. Embryonal tumor with abundant neuropil and true rosettes (ETANTR) with loss of morphological but retained genetic key features during progression. Acta Neuropathol. 2011 Dec;122(6):787–90. PMID:22057788
**7594.** Woessmann W, Lisfeld J, Burkhardt B, et al. Therapy in primary mediastinal B-cell lymphoma. N Engl J Med. 2013 Jul 18;369(3):282. PMID:23863060
**7595.** Woessmann W, Quintanilla-Martinez L. Rare mature B-cell lymphomas in children and adolescents. Hematol Oncol. 2019 Jun;37 Suppl 1:53–61. PMID:31187530
**7596.** Woessmann W, Seidemann K, Mann G, et al. The impact of the methotrexate administration schedule and dose in the treatment of children and adolescents with B-cell neoplasms: a report of the BFM Group Study NHL-BFM95. Blood. 2005 Feb 1;105(3):948–58. PMID:15486066
**7597.** Woessmann W, Zimmermann M, Meinhardt A, et al. Progressive or relapsed Burkitt lymphoma or leukemia in children and adolescents after BFM-type first-line therapy. Blood. 2020 Apr 2;135(14):1124–32. PMID:31961927
**7598.** Wojcik JB, Bellizzi AM, Dal Cin P, et al. Primary sclerosing epithelioid fibrosarcoma of bone: analysis of a series. Am J Surg Pathol. 2014 Nov;38(11):1538–44. PMID:24921641
**7599.** Wold LE, Laws ER Jr. Cranial chordomas in children and young adults. J Neurosurg. 1983 Dec;59(6):1043–7. PMID:6631498
**7600.** Wolf HK, Müller MB, Spänle M, et al. Ganglioglioma: a detailed histopathological and immunohistochemical analysis of 61 cases. Acta Neuropathol. 1994;88(2):166–73. PMID:7985497
**7601.** Wolf RE, Enneking WF. The staging and surgery of musculoskeletal neoplasms. Orthop Clin North Am. 1996 Jul;27(3):473–81. PMID:8649730

7602. Wolff JE, Sajedi M, Brant R, et al. Choroid plexus tumours. Br J Cancer. 2002 Nov 4;87(10):1086–91. PMID:12402146
7603. Wolff K, Komar M, Petzelbauer P. Clinical and histopathological aspects of cutaneous mastocytosis. Leuk Res. 2001 Jul;25(7):519–28. PMID:11377676
7604. Wolfswinkel EM, Imahiyerobo TA, McComb JG, et al. Proteus syndrome with a cranial intraosseous lipoma. J Craniofac Surg. 2017 Nov;28(8):e771–3. PMID:28938315
7605. Wolska-Kuśnierz B, Gregorek H, Chrzanowska K, et al. Nijmegen breakage syndrome: clinical and immunological features, long-term outcome and treatment options - a retrospective analysis. J Clin Immunol. 2015 Aug;35(6):538–49. PMID:26271390
7606. Wolter NE, Adil E, Irace AL, et al. Malignant glomus tumors of the head and neck in children and adults: evaluation and management. Laryngoscope. 2017 Dec;127(12):2873–82. PMID:28294349
7607. Won JH, Lee JY, Hong HS, et al. Thyroid nodules and cancer in children and adolescents affected by Hashimoto's thyroiditis. Br J Radiol. 2018 Jul;91(1087):20180014. PMID:29595320
7608. Wong FL, Boice JD Jr, Abramson DH, et al. Cancer incidence after retinoblastoma. Radiation dose and sarcoma risk. JAMA. 1997 Oct 15;278(15):1262–7. PMID:9333268
7609. Wong GC, Li KK, Wang WW, et al. Clinical and mutational profiles of adult medulloblastoma groups. Acta Neuropathol Commun. 2020 Nov 10;8(1):191. PMID:33172502
7610. Wong JC, Bryant V, Lamprecht T, et al. Germline SAMD9 and SAMD9L mutations are associated with extensive genetic evolution and diverse hematologic outcomes. JCI Insight. 2018 Jul 26;3(14):121086. PMID:30046003
7611. Wong JR, Morton LM, Tucker MA, et al. Risk of subsequent malignant neoplasms in long-term hereditary retinoblastoma survivors after chemotherapy and radiotherapy. J Clin Oncol. 2014 Oct 10;32(29):3284–90. PMID:25185089
7612. Wong KK, Miller BS, Viglianti BL, et al. Molecular imaging in the management of adrenocortical cancer: a systematic review. Clin Nucl Med. 2016 Aug;41(8):e368–82. PMID:26825212
7613. Wong MK, Ng CCY, Kuick CH, et al. Clear cell sarcomas of the kidney are characterised by BCOR gene abnormalities, including exon 15 internal tandem duplications and BCOR-CCNB3 gene fusion. Histopathology. 2018 Jan;72(2):320–9. PMID:28833375
7614. Wong MY, Andrews KA, Challis BG, et al. Clinical practice guidance: surveillance for phaeochromocytoma and paraganglioma in paediatric succinate dehydrogenase gene mutation carriers. Clin Endocrinol (Oxf). 2019 Apr;90(4):499–505. PMID:30589099
7615. Wong NL, Di F. Pseudosarcomatous fasciitis and myositis: diagnosis by fine-needle aspiration cytology. Am J Clin Pathol. 2009 Dec;132(6):857–65. PMID:19926576
7616. Wong TT, Ho DM, Chang KP, et al. Primary pediatric brain tumors: statistics of Taipei VGH, Taiwan (1975-2004). Cancer. 2005 Nov 15;104(10):2156–67. PMID:16220552
7617. Wood MD, Tihan T, Perry A, et al. Multimodal molecular analysis of astroblastoma enables reclassification of most cases into more specific molecular entities. Brain Pathol. 2018 Mar;28(2):192–202. PMID:28960623
7618. Woodruff JM, Christensen WN. Glandular peripheral nerve sheath tumors. Cancer. 1993 Dec 15;72(12):3618–28. PMID:8252477
7619. Woodruff JM, Perino G. Non-germ-cell or teratomatous malignant tumors showing additional rhabdomyoblastic differentiation, with emphasis on the malignant triton tumor. Semin Diagn Pathol. 1994 Feb;11(1):69–81. PMID:8202648
7620. Woodruff JM, Scheithauer BW, Kurtkaya-Yapicier O, et al. Congenital and childhood plexiform (multinodular) cellular schwannoma: a troublesome mimic of malignant peripheral nerve sheath tumor. Am J Surg Pathol. 2003 Oct;27(10):1321–9. PMID:14508393
7621. Woodruff JM, Selig AM, Crowley K, et al. Schwannoma (neurilemoma) with malignant transformation. A rare, distinctive peripheral nerve tumor. Am J Surg Pathol. 1994 Sep;18(9):882–95. PMID:8067509
7622. Woods WG, Barnard DR, Alonzo TA, et al. Prospective study of 90 children requiring treatment for juvenile myelomonocytic leukemia or myelodysplastic syndrome: a report from the Children's Cancer Group. J Clin Oncol. 2002 Jan 15;20(2):434–40. PMID:11786571
7622A. Woolgar JA, Rippin JW, Browne RM. A comparative histological study of odontogenic keratocysts in basal cell naevus syndrome and control patients. J Oral Pathol. 1987 Feb;16(2):75–80. PMID:2441019
7622B. Woolgar JA, Rippin JW, Browne RM. A comparative study of the clinical and histological features of recurrent and non-recurrent odontogenic keratocysts. J Oral Pathol. 1987 Mar;16(3):124–8. PMID:2442330
7623. Worawongvasu R, Songkampol K. Fibro-osseous lesions of the jaws: an analysis of 122 cases in Thailand. J Oral Pathol Med. 2010 Oct;39(9):703–8. PMID:20819127
7624. Worch J, Cyrus J, Goldsby R, et al. Racial differences in the incidence of mesenchymal tumors associated with EWSR1 translocation. Cancer Epidemiol Biomarkers Prev. 2011 Mar;20(3):449–53. PMID:21212061
7625. Woyach JA, Shah MH. New therapeutic advances in the management of progressive thyroid cancer. Endocr Relat Cancer. 2009 Sep;16(3):715–31. PMID:19218279
7626. Wozniak LJ, Mauer TL, Venick RS, et al. Clinical characteristics and outcomes of PTLD following intestinal transplantation. Clin Transplant. 2018 Aug;32(8):e13313. PMID:29888807
7627. Wrede B, Hasselblatt M, Peters O, et al. Atypical choroid plexus papilloma: clinical experience in the CPT-SIOP-2000 study. J Neurooncol. 2009 Dec;95(3):383–92. PMID:19543851
7628. Wright DH. What is Burkitt's lymphoma and when is it endemic? Blood. 1999 Jan 15;93(2):758. PMID:10215347
7629. Wu CC, Shete S, Amos CI, et al. Joint effects of germ-line p53 mutation and sex on cancer risk in Li-Fraumeni syndrome. Cancer Res. 2006 Aug 15;66(16):8287–92. PMID:16912210
7630. Wu CT, Inwards CY, O'Laughlin S, et al. Chondromyxoid fibroma of bone: a clinicopathologic review of 278 cases. Hum Pathol. 1998 May;29(5):438–46. PMID:9596266
7631. Wu D, Sherwood A, Fromm JR, et al. High-throughput sequencing detects minimal residual disease in acute T lymphoblastic leukemia. Sci Transl Med. 2012 May 16;4(134):134ra63. PMID:22593176
7632. Wu G, Broniscer A, McEachron TA, et al. Somatic histone H3 alterations in pediatric diffuse intrinsic pontine gliomas and non-brainstem glioblastomas. Nat Genet. 2012 Jan 29;44(3):251–3. PMID:22286216
7633. Wu G, Diaz AK, Paugh BS, et al. The genomic landscape of diffuse intrinsic pontine glioma and pediatric non-brainstem high-grade glioma. Nat Genet. 2014 May;46(5):444–50. PMID:24705251
7634. Wu H, Bui MM, Zhou L, et al. Phosphaturic mesenchymal tumor with an admixture of epithelial and mesenchymal elements in the jaws: clinicopathological and immunohistochemical analysis of 22 cases with literature review. Mod Pathol. 2019 Feb;32(2):189–204. PMID:30206408
7635. Wu H, Wasik MA, Przybylski G, et al. Hepatosplenic gamma-delta T-cell lymphoma as a late-onset posttransplant lymphoproliferative disorder in renal transplant recipients. Am J Clin Pathol. 2000 Apr;113(4):487–96. PMID:10761449
7636. Wu J, Jiao Y, Dal Molin M, et al. Whole-exome sequencing of neoplastic cysts of the pancreas reveals recurrent mutations in components of ubiquitin-dependent pathways. Proc Natl Acad Sci U S A. 2011 Dec 27;108(52):21188–93. PMID:22158988
7637. Wu JT, Book L, Sudar K. Serum alpha fetoprotein (AFP) levels in normal infants. Pediatr Res. 1981 Jan;15(1):50–2. PMID:6163129
7638. Wu MK, Cotter MB, Pears J, et al. Tumor progression in DICER1-mutated cystic nephroma-witnessing the genesis of anaplastic sarcoma of the kidney. Hum Pathol. 2016 Jul;53:114–20. PMID:27036314
7639. Wu MK, Goudie C, Druker H, et al. Evolution of renal cysts to anaplastic sarcoma of kidney in a child with DICER1 syndrome. Pediatr Blood Cancer. 2016 Jul;63(7):1272–5. PMID:26928971
7640. Wu MK, Vujanic GM, Fahiminiya S, et al. Anaplastic sarcomas of the kidney are characterized by DICER1 mutations. Mod Pathol. 2018 Jan;31(1):169–78. PMID:28862265
7641. Wu S, Zou X, Sun Z, et al. Unilateral retinocytoma associated with a variant in the RB1 gene. Mol Genet Genomic Med. 2020 Apr;8(4):e1156. PMID:31997559
7642. Wu TT, Swerdlow SH, Locker J, et al. Recurrent Epstein-Barr virus-associated lesions in organ transplant recipients. Hum Pathol. 1996 Feb;27(2):157–64. PMID:8617457
7643. Wu XC, Chen VW, Steele B, et al. Cancer incidence in adolescents and young adults in the United States, 1992-1997. J Adolesc Health. 2003 Jun;32(6):405–15. PMID:12782451
7644. Wunder JS, Eppert K, Burrow SR, et al. Co-amplification and overexpression of CDK4, SAS and MDM2 occurs frequently in human parosteal osteosarcomas. Oncogene. 1999 Jan 21;18(3):783–8. PMID:9989829
7645. Wünsche L, Kiesel B, Fischer H. [Lysogeny and lysogenic conversion in methylotrophic bacteria. II. Lysogenic conversion in facultative methanol-assimilating Acetobacter strains]. Z Allg Mikrobiol. 1983;23(3):189–96. German. PMID:6880251
7646. Wysozan TR, Khelifa S, Turchan K, et al. The morphologic spectrum of germline-mutated BAP1-inactivated melanocytic tumors includes lesions with conventional nevic melanocytes: a case report and review of literature. J Cutan Pathol. 2019 Nov;46(11):852–7. PMID:31206729
7647. Xi S, Sai K, Hu W, et al. Clinical significance of the histological and molecular characteristics of ependymal tumors: a single institution case series from China. BMC Cancer. 2019 Jul 19;19(1):717. PMID:31324163
7648. Xia M, Singhi AD, Dudley B, et al. Small bowel adenocarcinoma frequently exhibits Lynch syndrome-associated mismatch repair protein deficiency but does not harbor sporadic MLH1 deficiency. Appl Immunohistochem Mol Morphol. 2017 Jul;25(6):399–406. PMID:27258561
7649. Xiao GH, Jin F, Yeung RS. Identification of tuberous sclerosis 2 messenger RNA splice variants that are conserved and differentially expressed in rat and human tissues. Cell Growth Differ. 1995 Sep;6(9):1185–91. PMID:8519695
7650. Xiao Y, Jiang Y, Xiong Y, et al. Pediatric malignant phyllodes tumors of the breast: characteristics and outcomes based on the Surveillance Epidemiology and End Results database. J Surg Res. 2020 May;249:205–15. PMID:31991330
7651. Xiao Y, van Halteren AGS, Lei X, et al. Bone marrow-derived myeloid progenitors as driver mutation carriers in high- and low-risk Langerhans cell histiocytosis. Blood. 2020 Nov 5;136(19):2188–99. PMID:32750121
7652. Xin W, Rubin MA, McKeever PE. Differential expression of cytokeratins 8 and 20 distinguishes craniopharyngioma from Rathke cleft cyst. Arch Pathol Lab Med. 2002 Oct;126(10):1174–8. PMID:12296753
7653. Xing D, Banet N, Sharma R, et al. Aberrant Pax-8 expression in well-differentiated papillary mesothelioma and malignant mesothelioma of the peritoneum: a clinicopathologic study. Hum Pathol. 2018 Feb;72:160–6. PMID:29241740
7654. Xing M. Molecular pathogenesis and mechanisms of thyroid cancer. Nat Rev Cancer. 2013 Mar;13(3):184–99. PMID:23429735
7655. Xing Y, Lerario AM, Rainey W, et al. Development of adrenal cortex zonation. Endocrinol Metab Clin North Am. 2015 Jun;44(2):243–74. PMID:26038200
7656. Xu B, Aneja A, Ghossein R, et al. Salivary gland epithelial neoplasms in pediatric population: a single-institute experience with a focus on the histologic spectrum and clinical outcome. Hum Pathol. 2017 Sep;67:37–44. PMID:28739497
7657. Xu B, Hirokawa M, Yoshimoto K, et al. Spindle epithelial tumor with thymus-like differentiation of the thyroid: a case report with pathological and molecular genetics study. Hum Pathol. 2003 Feb;34(2):190–3. PMID:12612889
7658. Xu HM, Gutmann DH. Merlin differentially associates with the microtubule and actin cytoskeleton. J Neurosci Res. 1998 Feb 1;51(3):403–15. PMID:9486775
7659. Xu L, Polski A, Prabakar RK, et al. Chromosome 6p amplification in aqueous humor cell-free DNA is a prognostic biomarker for retinoblastoma ocular survival. Mol Cancer Res. 2020 Aug;18(8):1166–75. PMID:32434859
7660. Xu P, Shen P, Jin Y, et al. Epithelioid inflammatory myofibroblastic sarcoma of stomach: diagnostic pitfalls and clinical characteristics. Int J Clin Exp Pathol. 2019 May 1;12(5):1738–44. PMID:31933992
7661. Xu Q, Pearce MS, Parker L. Incidence and survival for testicular germ cell tumor in young males: a report from the Northern Region Young Person's Malignant Disease Registry, United Kingdom. Urol Oncol. 2007 Jan-Feb;25(1):32–7. PMID:17208136
7662. Xu T, Wu Y, Wu RX, et al. Validation and comparison of three newly-released thyroid imaging reporting and data systems for cancer risk determination. Endocrine. 2019 May;64(2):299–307. PMID:30474824
7663. Xu XL, Fang Y, Lee TC, et al. Retinoblastoma has properties of a cone precursor tumor and depends upon cone-specific MDM2 signaling. Cell. 2009 Jun 12;137(6):1018–31. PMID:19524506
7664. Xu XL, Singh HP, Wang L, et al. Rb suppresses human cone-precursor-derived retinoblastoma tumours. Nature. 2014 Oct 16;514(7522):385–8. PMID:25252974
7665. Xu Z, Lian S. Epstein-Barr virus-associated hydroa vacciniforme-like cutaneous lymphoma in seven Chinese children. Pediatr Dermatol. 2010 Sep-Oct;27(5):463–9. PMID:20497358
7666. Yabe M, Medeiros LJ, Daneshbod Y, et al. Hepatosplenic T-cell lymphoma arising in patients with immunodysregulatory disorders: a study of 7 patients who did not receive tumor necrosis factor-α inhibitor therapy and literature

review. Ann Diagn Pathol. 2017 Feb;26:16–22. PMID:28038706
**7667.** Yagnik VD. Juvenile giant fibroadenoma. Clin Pract. 2011 Jul 1;1(3):e49. PMID:24765310
**7668.** Yakaboski E, Fuleihan RL, Sullivan KE, et al. Lymphoproliferative disease in CVID: a report of types and frequencies from a US patient registry. J Clin Immunol. 2020 Apr;40(3):524–30. PMID:32185577
**7669.** Yalamanchili V, Entezami P, Langenburg S, et al. Consider benign Müllerian papilloma: a rare cause of vaginal bleeding in children. Pediatr Surg Int. 2014 Dec;30(12):1285–7. PMID:25330952
**7670.** Yamada H, Haratake J, Narasaki T, et al. Embryonal craniopharyngioma. Case report of the morphogenesis of a craniopharyngioma. Cancer. 1995 Jun 15;75(12):2971–7. PMID:7773950
**7671.** Yamada S, Aiba T, Sano T, et al. Growth hormone-producing pituitary adenomas: correlations between clinical characteristics and morphology. Neurosurgery. 1993 Jul;33(1):20–7. PMID:7689191
**7672.** Yamada S, Fukuhara N, Horiguchi K, et al. Clinicopathological characteristics and therapeutic outcomes in thyrotropin-secreting pituitary adenomas: a single-center study of 90 cases. J Neurosurg. 2014 Dec;121(6):1462–73. PMID:25237847
**7673.** Yamada Y, Kinoshita I, Kenichi K, et al. Histopathological and genetic review of phosphaturic mesenchymal tumours, mixed connective tissue variant. Histopathology. 2018 Feb;72(3):460–71. PMID:28858396
**7674.** Yamada Y, Kuda M, Kohashi K, et al. Histological and immunohistochemical characteristics of undifferentiated small round cell sarcomas associated with CIC-DUX4 and BCOR-CCNB3 fusion genes. Virchows Arch. 2017 Apr;470(4):373–80. PMID:28197724
**7675.** Yamada Y, Ohmi K, Tsunematu R, et al. Gynandroblastoma of the ovary having a typical morphological appearance: a case study. Jpn J Clin Oncol. 1991 Feb;21(1):62–8. PMID:2067122
**7676.** Yamaguchi T, Dorfman HD. Radiographic and histologic patterns of calcification in chondromyxoid fibroma. Skeletal Radiol. 1998 Oct;27(10):559–64. PMID:9840392
**7677.** Yamaguchi T, Suzuki S, Ishiiwa H, et al. Intraosseous benign notochordal cell tumours: overlooked precursors of classic chordomas? Histopathology. 2004 Jun;44(6):597–602. PMID:15186275
**7678.** Yamaguchi U, Hasegawa T, Hirose T, et al. Sclerosing perineurioma: a clinicopathological study of five cases and diagnostic utility of immunohistochemical staining for GLUT1. Virchows Arch. 2003 Aug;443(2):159–63. PMID:12836021
**7679.** Yamamoto H, Iwasaki T, Yamada Y, et al. Diagnostic utility of histone H3.3 G34W, G34R, and G34V mutant-specific antibodies for giant cell tumors of bone. Hum Pathol. 2018 Mar;73:41–50. PMID:29241742
**7680.** Yamamoto H, Kohashi K, Oda Y, et al. Absence of human herpesvirus-8 and Epstein-Barr virus in inflammatory myofibroblastic tumor with anaplastic large cell lymphoma kinase fusion gene. Pathol Int. 2006 Oct;56(10):584–90. PMID:16984614
**7681.** Yamamoto H, Yoshida A, Taguchi K, et al. ALK, ROS1 and NTRK3 gene rearrangements in inflammatory myofibroblastic tumours. Histopathology. 2016 Jul;69(1):72–83. PMID:26647767
**7682.** Yamamoto K, Yamada K, Nakahara T, et al. Rapid regrowth of solitary subependymal giant cell astrocytoma–case report. Neurol Med Chir (Tokyo). 2002 May;42(5):224–7. PMID:12064158
**7683.** Yamane Y, Mena H, Nakazato Y. Immunohistochemical characterization of pineal parenchymal tumors using novel monoclonal antibodies to the pineal body. Neuropathology. 2002 Jun;22(2):66–76. PMID:12075938
**7684.** Yamanouchi H, Ho M, Jay V, et al. Giant cells in cortical tubers in tuberous sclerosis showing synaptophysin-immunoreactive halos. Brain Dev. 1997 Jan;19(1):21–4. PMID:9071486
**7685.** Yamaoka H, Ohtsu K, Sueda T, et al. Diagnostic and prognostic impact of beta-catenin alterations in pediatric liver tumors. Oncol Rep. 2006 Mar;15(3):551–6. PMID:16465411
**7686.** Yamasaki K, Nakano Y, Nobusawa S, et al. Spinal cord astroblastoma with an EWSR1-BEND2 fusion classified as a high-grade neuroepithelial tumour with MN1 alteration. Neuropathol Appl Neurobiol. 2020 Feb;46(2):190–3. PMID:31863478
**7687.** Yamasaki T, Sakai N, Shinmura K, et al. Anaplastic changes of diffuse leptomeningeal glioneuronal tumor with polar spongioblastoma pattern. Brain Tumor Pathol. 2018 Oct;35(4):209–16. PMID:30051174
**7688.** Yamashita S, Saenko V. Mechanisms of disease: molecular genetics of childhood thyroid cancers. Nat Clin Pract Endocrinol Metab. 2007 May;3(5):422–9. PMID:17452969
**7689.** Yamashita S, Vauthey JN, Kaseb AO, et al. Prognosis of fibrolamellar carcinoma compared to non-cirrhotic conventional hepatocellular carcinoma. J Gastrointest Surg. 2016 Oct;20(10):1725–31. PMID:27456016
**7689A.** Yamato G, Deguchi T, Terui K, et al. Predictive factors for the development of leukemia in patients with transient abnormal myelopoiesis and Down syndrome. Leukemia. 2021 May;35(5):1480–4. PMID:33654203
**7690.** Yamazaki F, Nakatani F, Asano N, et al. Novel NTRK3 fusions in fibrosarcomas of adults. Am J Surg Pathol. 2019 Apr;43(4):523–30. PMID:30520818
**7691.** Yamazaki F, Nakazawa A, Osumi T, et al. Two cases of neuroblastoma comprising two distinct clones. Pediatr Blood Cancer. 2014 Apr;61(4):760–2. PMID:24108545
**7692.** Yan AC, Chamlin SL, Liang MG, et al. Congenital infantile fibrosarcoma: a masquerader of ulcerated hemangioma. Pediatr Dermatol. 2006 Jul-Aug;23(4):330–4. PMID:16918626
**7693.** Yan Z, Xia L, Huang Y, et al. Nasopharyngeal carcinoma in children and adolescents in an endemic area: a report of 185 cases. Int J Pediatr Otorhinolaryngol. 2013 Sep;77(9):1454–60. PMID:23830224
**7694.** Yanai-Inbar I, Scully RE. Relation of ovarian dermoid cysts and immature teratomas: an analysis of 350 cases of immature teratoma and 10 cases of dermoid cyst with microscopic foci of immature tissue. Int J Gynecol Pathol. 1987;6(3):203–12. PMID:3429105
**7695.** Yancoskie AE, Reebye UN, Segal JD, et al. Congenital granular cell lesion of the tongue: a report of two cases and review of the literature. Oral Surg Oral Med Oral Pathol Oral Radiol. 2016 Jul;122(1):e14–8. PMID:26712684
**7696.** Yang A, Sisson R, Gupta A, et al. Germline APC mutations in hepatoblastoma. Pediatr Blood Cancer. 2018 Apr;65(4). PMID:29251405
**7697.** Yang C, Siebert JR, Burns R, et al. Heterogeneity of human bone marrow and blood natural killer cells defined by single-cell transcriptome. Nat Commun. 2019 Sep 2;10(1):3931. PMID:31477722
**7698.** Yang FC, Ingram DA, Chen S, et al. Nf1-dependent tumors require a microenvironment containing Nf1+/– and c-kit-dependent bone marrow. Cell. 2008 Oct 31;135(3):437–48. PMID:18984156
**7699.** Yang P, Cornejo KM, Sadow PM, et al. Renal cell carcinoma in tuberous sclerosis complex. Am J Surg Pathol. 2014 Jul;38(7):895–909. PMID:24832166
**7700.** Yang S, Zheng X, Lu C, et al. Molecular basis for oncohistone H3 recognition by SETD2 methyltransferase. Genes Dev. 2016 Jul 15;30(14):1611–6. PMID:27474439
**7701.** Yang W, Zhang P, Hama A, et al. Diagnosis of acquired bone marrow failure syndrome during childhood using the 2008 World Health Organization classification system. Int J Hematol. 2012 Jul;96(1):34–8. PMID:22562435
**7702.** Yang X, Wang X. Imaging findings of pancreatoblastoma in 4 children including a case of ectopic pancreatoblastoma. Pediatr Radiol. 2010 Oct;40(10):1609–14. PMID:20686762
**7703.** Yang XR, Ng D, Alcorta DA, et al. T (brachyury) gene duplication confers major susceptibility to familial chordoma. Nat Genet. 2009 Nov;41(11):1176–8. PMID:19801981
**7704.** Yang ZJ, Ellis T, Markant SL, et al. Medulloblastoma can be initiated by deletion of Patched in lineage-restricted progenitors or stem cells. Cancer Cell. 2008 Aug 12;14(2):135–45. PMID:18691548
**7705.** Yao DX, Soslow RA, Hedvat CV, et al. Melan-A (A103) and inhibin expression in ovarian neoplasms. Appl Immunohistochem Mol Morphol. 2003 Sep;11(3):244–9. PMID:12966351
**7706.** Yao K, Duan Z, Wang Y, et al. Detection of H3K27M mutation in cases of brain stem subependymoma. Hum Pathol. 2019 Feb;84:262–9. PMID:30389438
**7707.** Yasir S, Torbenson MS. Angiosarcoma of the liver: clinicopathologic features and morphologic patterns. Am J Surg Pathol. 2019 May;43(5):581–90. PMID:30986799
**7708.** Yasmeen S, Rajkumar A, Grossman H, et al. Terminal deoxynucleotidyl transferase (TdT)-negative lymphoblastic leukemia in pediatric patients: incidence and clinical significance. Pediatr Dev Pathol. 2017 Nov-Dec;20(6):463–8. PMID:29187045
**7709.** Yasunaga M, Saito T, Eto T, et al. Dedifferentiated chondrosarcoma arising in a mature cystic teratoma of the ovary: a case report and review of the literature. Int J Gynecol Pathol. 2011 Jul;30(4):391–4. PMID:21623194
**7710.** Yasunari T, Shiraki K, Hattori H, et al. Frequency of choroidal abnormalities in neurofibromatosis type 1. Lancet. 2000 Sep 16;356(9234):988–92. PMID:11041400
**7711.** Yau DTW, Chan JKC, Bao S, et al. Bone sarcoma with EWSR1-NFATC2 fusion: sarcoma with varied morphology and amplification of fusion gene distinct from Ewing sarcoma. Int J Surg Pathol. 2019 Aug;27(5):561–7. PMID:30714449
**7712.** Yazdan P, Cooper C, Sholl LM, et al. Comparative analysis of atypical spitz tumors with heterozygous versus homozygous 9p21 deletions for clinical outcomes, histomorphology, BRAF mutation, and p16 expression. Am J Surg Pathol. 2014 May;38(5):638–45. PMID:24451276
**7713.** Yazganoglu KD, Topkarci Z, Buyukbabani N, et al. Childhood mycosis fungoides: a report of 20 cases from Turkey. J Eur Acad Dermatol Venereol. 2013 Mar;27(3):295–300. PMID:22176010
**7714.** Yde CW, Sehested A, Mateu-Regué À, et al. A new NFIA:RAF1 fusion activating the MAPK pathway in pilocytic astrocytoma. Cancer Genet. 2016 Oct;209(10):440–4. PMID:27810072
**7715.** Yeh I, Botton T, Talevich E, et al. Activating MET kinase rearrangements in melanoma and Spitz tumours. Nat Commun. 2015 May 27;6:7174. PMID:26013381
**7716.** Yeh I, Tee MK, Botton T, et al. NTRK3 kinase fusions in Spitz tumours. J Pathol. 2016 Nov;240(3):282–90. PMID:27477320
**7717.** Yeh IT, Lenci RE, Qin Y, et al. A germline mutation of the KIF1B beta gene on 1p36 in a family with neural and nonneural tumors. Hum Genet. 2008 Oct;124(3):279–85. PMID:18726616
**7718.** Yen E, Deen M, Marshall I. Youngest reported patient presenting with an androgen producing sclerosing stromal ovarian tumor. J Pediatr Adolesc Gynecol. 2014 Oct;27(5):e121–4. PMID:24656709
**7719.** Yen JB, Kong MS, Lin JN. Hepatic mesenchymal hamartoma. J Paediatr Child Health. 2003 Nov;39(8):632–4. PMID:14629534
**7720.** Yesil S, Tanyildiz HG, Akyurek N, et al. A rare presentation of paraovarian sclerosing stromal tumor with high mitotic activity. J Pediatr Adolesc Gynecol. 2016 Feb;29(1):e13–5. PMID:26327562
**7721.** Yesim G, Gupse T, Zafer U, et al. Mesenchymal hamartoma of the liver in adulthood: immunohistochemical profiles, clinical and histopathological features in two patients. J Hepatobiliary Pancreat Surg. 2005;12(6):502–7. PMID:16365828
**7722.** Yi JW, Park YK, Choi YM, et al. Bulbous urethra involved in perineal extraskeletal myxoid chondrosarcoma in a child. Int J Urol. 2004 Jun;11(6):436–9. PMID:15157219
**7723.** Yibulayin F, Feng L, Wang M, et al. Head & neck acinar cell carcinoma: a population-based study using the SEER registry. BMC Cancer. 2020 Jul 8;20(1):631. PMID:32641007
**7724.** Yikilmaz A, Ngan BY, Navarro OM. Imaging of childhood angiomatoid fibrous histiocytoma with pathological correlation. Pediatr Radiol. 2015 Nov;45(12):1796–802. PMID:26162466
**7725.** Yıldızer EK, Gungor K, Kahraman SA. Cyst-like lesion in mandibular coronoid process: an unusual location. Oral Surg Oral Med Oral Pathol Oral Radiol. 2017 Apr;123(4):414–8. PMID:27496575
**7726.** Yilmaz E, Sal S, Lebe B. Differentiation of phyllodes tumors versus fibroadenomas. Acta Radiol. 2002 Jan;43(1):34–9. PMID:11972459
**7727.** Yilmaz R, Bayramoglu Z, Bicen F, et al. Sonographic and magnetic resonance imaging characteristics of juvenile papillomatosis: three cases with different manifestations. Ultrasound Q. 2017 Jun;33(2):174–8. PMID:28538449
**7728.** Yin WH, Guo N, Tian XY, et al. Pediatric anaplastic lymphoma kinase-positive large B-cell lymphoma: a case report and review of the literature. Pediatr Dev Pathol. 2012 Jul-Aug;15(4):318–23. PMID:22394191
**7729.** Yip FW, Reeve TS, Poole AG, et al. Thyroid nodules in childhood and adolescence. Aust N Z J Surg. 1994 Oct;64(10):676–8. PMID:7945063
**7730.** Yoder N, Marks A, Hui P, et al. Low-grade astrocytoma within a mature cystic teratoma in an adolescent patient. J Pediatr Adolesc Gynecol. 2018 Jun;31(3):325–7. PMID:29107097
**7730A.** Yokota T, Tachizawa T, Fukino K, et al. A family with spinal anaplastic ependymoma: evidence of loss of chromosome 22q in tumor. J Hum Genet. 2003;48(11):598–602. PMID:14566482
**7731.** Yokoyama M, Ozeki M, Nozawa A, et al. Low-dose sirolimus for a patient with blue rubber bleb nevus syndrome. Pediatr Int. 2020 Jan;62(1):112–3. PMID:31879989
**7732.** Yonemoto T, Hosono A, Iwata S, et al. The prognosis of osteosarcoma occurring as second malignancy of childhood cancers may be favorable: experience of two cancer centers in Japan. Int J Clin Oncol. 2015 Jun;20(3):613–6. PMID:25022788
**7733.** Yonese I, Sakashita C, Imadome KI, et al. Nationwide survey of systemic chronic active EBV infection in Japan in accordance with the

new WHO classification. Blood Adv. 2020 Jul 14;4(13):2918–26. PMID:32598475
**7734.** Yonkof JR, Gupta A, Rueda CM, et al. A novel pathogenic variant in CARMIL2 (RLTPR) causing CARMIL2 deficiency and EBV-associated smooth muscle tumors. Front Immunol. 2020 Jun 18;11:884. PMID:32625199
**7735.** Yoo SC, Chang KH, Lyu MO, et al. Clinical characteristics of struma ovarii. J Gynecol Oncol. 2008 Jun;19(2):135–8. PMID:19471561
**7736.** Yoon NR, Lee JW, Kim BG, et al. Gliomatosis peritonei is associated with frequent recurrence, but does not affect overall survival in patients with ovarian immature teratoma. Virchows Arch. 2012 Sep;461(3):299–304. PMID:22820986
**7737.** Yoshida A, Arai Y, Kobayashi E, et al. CIC break-apart fluorescence in-situ hybridization misses a subset of CIC-DUX4 sarcomas: a clinicopathological and molecular study. Histopathology. 2017 Sep;71(3):461–9. PMID:28493604
**7738.** Yoshida A, Asano N, Kawai A, et al. Differential SALL4 immunoexpression in malignant rhabdoid tumours and epithelioid sarcomas. Histopathology. 2015 Jan;66(2):252–61. PMID:24827994
**7739.** Yoshida A, Goto K, Kodaira M, et al. CIC-rearranged sarcomas: a study of 20 cases and comparisons with Ewing sarcomas. Am J Surg Pathol. 2016 Mar;40(3):313–23. PMID:26685084
**7740.** Yoshida A, Sekine S, Tsuta K, et al. NKX2.2 is a useful immunohistochemical marker for Ewing sarcoma. Am J Surg Pathol. 2012 Jul;36(7):993–9. PMID:22446943
**7741.** Yoshida A, Ushiku T, Motoi T, et al. Immunohistochemical analysis of MDM2 and CDK4 distinguishes low-grade osteosarcoma from benign mimics. Mod Pathol. 2010 Sep;23(9):1279–88. PMID:20601938
**7742.** Yoshida A, Ushiku T, Motoi T, et al. MDM2 and CDK4 immunohistochemical coexpression in high-grade osteosarcoma: correlation with a dedifferentiated subtype. Am J Surg Pathol. 2012 Mar;36(3):423–31. PMID:22301501
**7743.** Yoshida A, Wakai S, Ryo E, et al. Expanding the phenotypic spectrum of mesenchymal tumors harboring the EWSR1-CREM fusion. Am J Surg Pathol. 2019 Dec;43(12):1622–30. PMID:31305268
**7744.** Yoshida EJ, García J, Eisele DW, et al. Salivary gland malignancies in children. Int J Pediatr Otorhinolaryngol. 2014 Feb;78(2):174–8. PMID:24332197
**7745.** Yoshida H, Miyachi M, Ouchi K, et al. Identification of COL3A1 and RAB2A as novel translocation partner genes of PLAG1 in lipoblastoma. Genes Chromosomes Cancer. 2014 Jul;53(7):606–11. PMID:24700772
**7746.** Yoshida K, Toki T, Okuno Y, et al. The landscape of somatic mutations in Down syndrome-related myeloid disorders. Nat Genet. 2013 Nov;45(11):1293–9. PMID:24056718
**7747.** Yoshida KI, Machado I, Motoi T, et al. NKX3-1 is a useful immunohistochemical marker of EWSR1-NFATC2 sarcoma and mesenchymal chondrosarcoma. Am J Surg Pathol. 2020 Jun;44(6):719–28. PMID:31972596
**7748.** Yoshida M, Fushiki S, Takeuchi Y, et al. Diffuse bilateral thalamic astrocytomas as examined serially by MRI. Childs Nerv Syst. 1998 Aug;14(8):384–8. PMID:9753406
**7749.** Yoshida N, Takahashi Y, Yabe H, et al. Conditioning regimen for allogeneic bone marrow transplantation in children with acquired bone marrow failure: fludarabine/melphalan vs. fludarabine/cyclophosphamide. Bone Marrow Transplant. 2020 Jul;55(7):1272–81. PMID:32444864
**7750.** Yoshida Y, Nobusawa S, Nakata S, et al. CNS high-grade neuroepithelial tumor with BCOR internal tandem duplication: a comparison with its counterparts in the kidney and soft tissue. Brain Pathol. 2018 Sep;28(5):710–20. PMID:29226988
**7751.** Yoshimi A, Kamachi Y, Imai K, et al. Wiskott-Aldrich syndrome presenting with a clinical picture mimicking juvenile myelomonocytic leukaemia. Pediatr Blood Cancer. 2013 May;60(5):836–41. PMID:23023736
**7752.** Yoshimi A, Niemeyer C, Baumann I, et al. High incidence of Fanconi anaemia in patients with a morphological picture consistent with refractory cytopenia of childhood. Br J Haematol. 2013 Jan;160(1):109–11. PMID:23043447
**7753.** Yoshimi A, Strahm B, Baumann I, et al. Hematopoietic stem cell transplantation in children and young adults with secondary myelodysplastic syndrome and acute myelogenous leukemia after aplastic anemia. Biol Blood Marrow Transplant. 2014 Mar;20(3):425–9. PMID:24316460
**7754.** Yoshimi A, van den Heuvel-Eibrink MM, Baumann I, et al. Comparison of horse and rabbit antithymocyte globulin in immunosuppressive therapy for refractory cytopenia of childhood. Haematologica. 2014 Apr;99(4):656–63. PMID:24162791
**7755.** Yoshimoto M, Graham C, Chilton-MacNeill S, et al. Detailed cytogenetic and array analysis of pediatric primitive sarcomas reveals a recurrent CIC-DUX4 fusion gene event. Cancer Genet Cytogenet. 2009 Nov;195(1):1–11. PMID:19837261
**7756.** Yoshimoto T, Tanaka M, Homme M, et al. CIC-DUX4 induces small round cell sarcomas distinct from Ewing sarcoma. Cancer Res. 2017 Jun 1;77(11):2927–37. PMID:28404587
**7757.** Yoshizato T, Nannya Y, Atsuta Y, et al. Genetic abnormalities in myelodysplasia and secondary acute myeloid leukemia: impact on outcome of stem cell transplantation. Blood. 2017 Apr 27;129(17):2347–58. PMID:28223278
**7758.** You H, Kim YI, Im SY, et al. Immunohistochemical study of central neurocytoma, subependymoma, and subependymal giant cell astrocytoma. J Neurooncol. 2005 Aug;74(1):1–8. PMID:16078101
**7759.** Young CL, Sim FH, Unni KK, et al. Chondrosarcoma of bone in children. Cancer. 1990 Oct 1;66(7):1641–8. PMID:2208016
**7760.** Young EE, Brown CT, Merguerian PA, et al. Pediatric and adolescent renal cell carcinoma. Urol Oncol. 2016 Jan;34(1):42–9. PMID:26299882
**7761.** Young KZ, Fossum SL, Lowe L, et al. An adolescent with uveal melanoma and BAP1 tumor predisposition syndrome. JAAD Case Rep. 2020 Apr 25;6(6):563–6. PMID:32509949
**7762.** Young LS, Rickinson AB. Epstein-Barr virus: 40 years on. Nat Rev Cancer. 2004 Oct;4(10):757–68. PMID:15510157
**7763.** Young RH. New and unusual aspects of ovarian germ cell tumors. Am J Surg Pathol. 1993 Dec;17(12):1210–24. PMID:7694512
**7764.** Young RH. Ovarian tumors and tumor-like lesions in the first three decades. Semin Diagn Pathol. 2014 Sep;31(5):382–426. PMID:25440719
**7765.** Young RH, Dickersin GR, Scully RE. Juvenile granulosa cell tumor of the ovary. A clinicopathological analysis of 125 cases. Am J Surg Pathol. 1984 Aug;8(8):575–96. PMID:6465418
**7766.** Young RH, Kozakewich HP, Scully RE. Metastatic ovarian tumors in children: a report of 14 cases and review of the literature. Int J Gynecol Pathol. 1993 Jan;12(1):8–19. PMID:8418081
**7767.** Young RH, Oliva E, Scully RE. Small cell carcinoma of the ovary, hypercalcemic type. A clinicopathological analysis of 150 cases. Am J Surg Pathol. 1994 Nov;18(11):1102–16. PMID:7943531
**7768.** Young RH, Prat J, Scully RE. Epidermoid cyst of the ovary. A report of three cases with comments on histogenesis. Am J Clin Pathol. 1980 Feb;73(2):272–6. PMID:7355867
**7769.** Young RH, Prat J, Scully RE. Ovarian Sertoli-Leydig cell tumors with heterologous elements. I. Gastrointestinal epithelium and carcinoid: a clinicopathologic analysis of thirty-six cases. Cancer. 1982 Dec 1;50(11):2448–56. PMID:7139537
**7770.** Young RH, Scully RE. Ovarian Sertoli-Leydig cell tumors with a retiform pattern: a problem in histopathologic diagnosis. A report of 25 cases. Am J Surg Pathol. 1983 Dec;7(8):755–71. PMID:6660351
**7771.** Young RH, Scully RE. Ovarian Sertoli-Leydig cell tumors. A clinicopathological analysis of 207 cases. Am J Surg Pathol. 1985 Aug;9(8):543–69. PMID:3911780
**7772.** Young RH, Welch WR, Dickersin GR, et al. Ovarian sex cord tumor with annular tubules: review of 74 cases including 27 with Peutz-Jeghers syndrome and four with adenoma malignum of the cervix. Cancer. 1982 Oct 1;50(7):1384–402. PMID:7104978
**7773.** Young RJ, Brown NJ, Reed MW, et al. Angiosarcoma. Lancet Oncol. 2010 Oct;11(10):983–91. PMID:20537949
**7774.** Yousem SA, Weiss LM, Warnke RA. Primary mediastinal non-Hodgkin's lymphomas: a morphologic and immunologic study of 19 cases. Am J Clin Pathol. 1985 Jun;83(6):676–80. PMID:3923821
**7775.** Youssef N, Vabres P, Buisson T, et al. Two unusual tumors in a patient with xeroderma pigmentosum: atypical fibroxanthoma and basosquamous carcinoma. J Cutan Pathol. 1999 Oct;26(9):430–5. PMID:10563498
**7776.** Youssefian L, Vahidnezhad H, Touati A, et al. The genetic basis of hyaline fibromatosis syndrome in patients from a consanguineous background: a case series. BMC Med Genet. 2018 May 25;19(1):87. PMID:29801470
**7777.** Yu CL, Tucker MA, Abramson DH, et al. Cause-specific mortality in long-term survivors of retinoblastoma. J Natl Cancer Inst. 2009 Apr 15;101(8):581–91. PMID:19351917
**7778.** Yu L, Liu J, Lao IW, et al. Epithelioid inflammatory myofibroblastic sarcoma: a clinicopathological, immunohistochemical and molecular cytogenetic analysis of five additional cases and review of the literature. Diagn Pathol. 2016 Jul 27;11(1):67. PMID:27460384
**7779.** Yu Y, Flint AF, Mulliken JB, et al. Endothelial progenitor cells in infantile hemangioma. Blood. 2004 Feb 15;103(4):1373–5. PMID:14576053
**7780.** Yu Y, Wylie-Sears J, Boscolo E, et al. Genomic imprinting of IGF2 is maintained in infantile hemangioma despite its high level of expression. Mol Med. 2004 Jul-Dec;10(7-12):117–23. PMID:15706404
**7781.** Yu YR, Espinoza J, Mehta DK, et al. Perinatal diagnosis and management of oropharyngeal fetus in fetu: a case report. J Clin Ultrasound. 2018 May;46(4):286–91. PMID:28949025
**7782.** Yue Q, Yu Y, Shi Z, et al. Prediction of BRAF mutation status of craniopharyngioma using magnetic resonance imaging features. J Neurosurg. 2018 Jul;129(1):27–34. PMID:28984520
**7783.** Yun SJ, Hwang SY, Jin W, et al. Intramuscular diffuse-type tenosynovial giant cell tumor of the deltoid muscle in a child. Skeletal Radiol. 2014 Aug;43(8):1179–83. PMID:24676801
**7784.** Yurgelun MB, Kulke MH, Fuchs CS, et al. Cancer susceptibility gene mutations in individuals with colorectal cancer. J Clin Oncol. 2017 Apr 1;35(10):1086–95. PMID:28135145
**7785.** Yust Katz S, Cachia D, Kamiya-Matsuoka C, et al. Ependymomas arising outside of the central nervous system: a case series and literature review. J Clin Neurosci. 2018 Jan;47:202–7. PMID:29054328
**7786.** Yust-Katz S, Anderson MD, Liu D, et al. Clinical and prognostic features of adult patients with gangliogliomas. Neuro Oncol. 2014 Mar;16(3):409–13. PMID:24305706
**7787.** Zacharia BE, Bruce SS, Goldstein H, et al. Incidence, treatment and survival of patients with craniopharyngioma in the Surveillance, Epidemiology and End Results program. Neuro Oncol. 2012 Aug;14(8):1070–8. PMID:22735773
**7788.** Zackheim HS, McCalmont TH, Deanovic FW, et al. Mycosis fungoides with onset before 20 years of age. J Am Acad Dermatol. 1997 Apr;36(4):557–62. PMID:9092741
**7789.** Zada G, Woodmansee WW, Ramkissoon S, et al. Atypical pituitary adenomas: incidence, clinical characteristics, and implications. J Neurosurg. 2011 Feb;114(2):336–44. PMID:20868211
**7790.** Zafar M, Ezzat S, Ramyar L, et al. Cell-specific expression of estrogen receptor in the human pituitary and its adenomas. J Clin Endocrinol Metab. 1995 Dec;80(12):3621–7. PMID:8530610
**7791.** Zagzag D, Zhong H, Scalzitti JM, et al. Expression of hypoxia-inducible factor 1alpha in brain tumors: association with angiogenesis, invasion, and progression. Cancer. 2000 Jun 1;88(11):2606–18. PMID:10861440
**7792.** Zaidi HA, Cote DJ, Dunn IF, et al. Predictors of aggressive clinical phenotype among immunohistochemically confirmed atypical adenomas. J Clin Neurosci. 2016 Dec;34:246–51. PMID:27765563
**7793.** Zajac V, Kirchhoff T, Levy ER, et al. Characterisation of X;17(q12;p13) translocation breakpoints in a female patient with hypomelanosis of Ito and choroid plexus papilloma. Eur J Hum Genet. 1997 Mar-Apr;5(2):61–8. PMID:9195154
**7794.** Zakrzewska M, Wojcik I, Zakrzewski K, et al. Mutational analysis of hSNF5/INI1 and TP53 genes in choroid plexus carcinomas. Cancer Genet Cytogenet. 2005 Jan 15;156(2):179–82. PMID:15642401
**7795.** Zaky W, Dhall G, Khatua S, et al. Choroid plexus carcinoma in children: the Head Start experience. Pediatr Blood Cancer. 2015 May;62(5):784–9. PMID:25662896
**7796.** Zaky W, Patil SS, Park M, et al. Ganglioglioma in children and young adults: single institution experience and review of the literature. J Neurooncol. 2018 Sep;139(3):739–47. PMID:29882043
**7797.** Zaliova M, Kotrova M, Bresolin S, et al. ETV6/RUNX1-like acute lymphoblastic leukemia: a novel B-cell precursor leukemia subtype associated with the CD27/CD44 immunophenotype. Genes Chromosomes Cancer. 2017 Aug;56(8):608–16. PMID:28395118
**7798.** Zaloudek C, Norris HJ. Sertoli-Leydig tumors of the ovary. A clinicopathologic study of 64 intermediate and poorly differentiated neoplasms. Am J Surg Pathol. 1984 Jun;8(6):405–18. PMID:6731664
**7799.** Zamani M, Grønhøj C, Schmidt Jensen J, et al. Survival and characteristics of pediatric salivary gland cancer: a systematic review and meta-analysis. Pediatr Blood Cancer. 2019 Mar;66(3):e27543. PMID:30378272
**7800.** Zambrano E, Nosé V, Perez-Atayde AR, et al. Distinct chromosomal rearrangements in subungual (Dupuytren) exostosis and bizarre parosteal osteochondromatous proliferation (Nora lesion). Am J Surg Pathol. 2004 Aug;28(8):1033–9. PMID:15252309
**7801.** Zámecník M, Michal M, Simpson RH, et al. Ossifying fibromyxoid tumor of soft parts: a

report of 17 cases with emphasis on unusual histological features. Ann Diagn Pathol. 1997 Dec;1(2):73–81. PMID:9869828

**7802.** Zamir E, Mechoulam H, Micera A, et al. Inflamed juvenile conjunctival naevus: clinicopathological characterisation. Br J Ophthalmol. 2002 Jan;86(1):28–30. PMID:11801498

**7803.** Zanation AM, Mitchell CA, Rose AS. Endoscopic skull base techniques for juvenile nasopharyngeal angiofibroma. Otolaryngol Clin North Am. 2012 Jun;45(3):711–30, ix. PMID:22588045

**7804.** Zand DJ, Huff D, Everman D, et al. Autosomal dominant inheritance of infantile myofibromatosis. Am J Med Genet A. 2004 Apr 30;126A(3):261–6. PMID:15054839

**7805.** Zanello M, Pages M, Tauziède-Espariat A, et al. Clinical, imaging, histopathological and molecular characterization of anaplastic ganglioglioma. J Neuropathol Exp Neurol. 2016 Oct;75(10):971–80. PMID:27539475

**7806.** Zapata S, Kearns DB. Nasal dermoids. Curr Opin Otolaryngol Head Neck Surg. 2006 Dec;14(6):406–11. PMID:17099348

**7807.** Zapotocky M, Beera K, Adamski J, et al. Survival and functional outcomes of molecularly defined childhood posterior fossa ependymoma: cure at a cost. Cancer. 2019 Jun 1;125(11):1867–76. PMID:30768777

**7808.** Zapotocky M, Mata-Mbemba D, Sumerauer D, et al. Differential patterns of metastatic dissemination across medulloblastoma subgroups. J Neurosurg Pediatr. 2018 Feb;21(2):145–52. PMID:29219788

**7809.** Zarate JO, Sampaolesi R. Pleomorphic xanthoastrocytoma of the retina. Am J Surg Pathol. 1999 Jan;23(1):79–81. PMID:9888706

**7810.** Zarbo RJ, Prasad AR, Regezi JA, et al. Salivary gland basal cell and canalicular adenomas: immunohistochemical demonstration of myoepithelial cell participation and morphogenetic considerations. Arch Pathol Lab Med. 2000 Mar;124(3):401–5. PMID:10705394

**7811.** Zare SY, Leivo M, Fadare O. Recurrent pleomorphic myxoid liposarcoma in a patient with Li-Fraumeni syndrome. Int J Surg Pathol. 2020 Apr;28(2):225–8. PMID:31559875

**7812.** Zatelli MC, Piccin D, Tagliati F, et al. Dopamine receptor subtype 2 and somatostatin receptor subtype 5 expression influences somatostatin analogs effects on human somatotroph pituitary adenomas in vitro. J Mol Endocrinol. 2005 Oct;35(2):333–41. PMID:16216913

**7813.** Zauderer MG, Jayakumaran G, DuBoff M, et al. Prevalence and preliminary validation of screening criteria to identify carriers of germline BAP1 mutations. J Thorac Oncol. 2019 Nov;14(11):1989–94. PMID:31323388

**7814.** Zayour M, Bolognia JL, Lazova R. Multiple Spitz nevi: a clinicopathologic study of 9 patients. J Am Acad Dermatol. 2012 Sep;67(3):451–8.e1–2. PMID:22300833

**7815.** Zec N, De Girolami U, Schofield DE, et al. Giant cell ependymoma of the filum terminale. A report of two cases. Am J Surg Pathol. 1996 Sep;20(9):1091–101. PMID:8764746

**7816.** Zecca M, Bergamaschi G, Kratz C, et al. JAK2 V617F mutation is a rare event in juvenile myelomonocytic leukemia. Leukemia. 2007 Feb;21(2):367–9. PMID:17151700

**7817.** Zehetgruber H, Bittner B, Gruber D, et al. Prevalence of aneurysmal and solitary bone cysts in young patients. Clin Orthop Relat Res. 2005 Oct;439(439):136–43. PMID:16205152

**7818.** Zekioglu O, Ozdemir N, Terek C, et al. Clinicopathological and immunohistochemical analysis of sclerosing stromal tumours of the ovary. Arch Gynecol Obstet. 2010 Dec;282(6):671–6. PMID:20135135

**7819.** Zelaya G, López Marti JM, Marino R, et al. Gonadoblastoma in patients with Ullrich-Turner syndrome. Pediatr Dev Pathol. 2015 Mar-Apr;18(2):117–21. PMID:25535833

**7820.** Zembowicz A. Blue nevi and related tumors. Clin Lab Med. 2017 Sep;37(3):401–15. PMID:28802492

**7821.** Zembowicz A, Mandal RV, Choopong P. Melanocytic lesions of the conjunctiva. Arch Pathol Lab Med. 2010 Dec;134(12):1785–92. PMID:21128776

**7822.** Zembowicz A, Phadke PA. Blue nevi and variants: an update. Arch Pathol Lab Med. 2011 Mar;135(3):327–36. PMID:21366456

**7823.** Zembowicz A, Scolyer RA. Nevus/melanocytoma/melanoma: an emerging paradigm for classification of melanocytic neoplasms? Arch Pathol Lab Med. 2011 Mar;135(3):300–6. PMID:21366452

**7824.** Zen Y, Vara R, Portmann B, et al. Childhood hepatocellular carcinoma: a clinicopathological study of 12 cases with special reference to EpCAM. Histopathology. 2014 Apr;64(5):671–82. PMID:24138022

**7825.** Zenner K, Jensen DM, Dmyterko V, et al. Somatic activating BRAF variants cause isolated lymphatic malformations. HGG Adv. 2022 Mar 15;3(2):100101. PMID:35373151

**7826.** Zeybek AC, Kiykim E, Soyucen E, et al. Hereditary tyrosinemia type 1 in Turkey: twenty year single-center experience. Pediatr Int. 2015 Apr;57(2):281–9. PMID:25223216

**7827.** Zhang C, Berney DM, Hirsch MS, et al. Evidence supporting the existence of benign teratomas of the postpubertal testis: a clinical, histopathologic, and molecular genetic analysis of 25 cases. Am J Surg Pathol. 2013 Jun;37(6):827–35. PMID:23598964

**7828.** Zhang C, Morimoto LM, de Smith AJ, et al. Genetic determinants of childhood and adult height associated with osteosarcoma risk. Cancer. 2018 Sep 15;124(18):3742–52. PMID:30311632

**7829.** Zhang C, Ostrom QT, Hansen HM, et al. European genetic ancestry associated with risk of childhood ependymoma. Neuro Oncol. 2020 Nov 26;22(11):1637–46. PMID:32607579

**7830.** Zhang C, Ulbright TM. Nuclear localization of β-catenin in Sertoli cell tumors and other sex cord-stromal tumors of the testis: an immunohistochemical study of 87 cases. Am J Surg Pathol. 2015 Oct;39(10):1390–4. PMID:26034868

**7831.** Zhang HL, Wu BQ, Zhang WG. [The expression of 67-KD laminin receptor (LN-R) gene in PG tumor cells with high metastatic potential]. Zhonghua Zhong Liu Za Zhi. 1994 Nov;16(6):403–6. Chinese. PMID:7720491

**7832.** Zhang J, Benavente CA, McEvoy J, et al. A novel retinoblastoma therapy from genomic and epigenetic analyses. Nature. 2012 Jan 11;481(7381):329–34. PMID:22237022

**7833.** Zhang J, Ding L, Holmfeldt L, et al. The genetic basis of early T-cell precursor acute lymphoblastic leukaemia. Nature. 2012 Jan 11;481(7380):157–63. PMID:22237106

**7834.** Zhang J, Walsh MF, Wu G, et al. Germline mutations in predisposition genes in pediatric cancer. N Engl J Med. 2015 Dec 10;373(24):2336–46. PMID:26580448

**7835.** Zhang J, Wu G, Miller CP, et al. Whole-genome sequencing identifies genetic alterations in pediatric low-grade gliomas. Nat Genet. 2013 Jun;45(6):602–12. PMID:23583981

**7836.** Zhang L, Hwang S, Benayed R, et al. Myositis ossificans-like soft tissue aneurysmal bone cyst: a clinical, radiological, and pathological study of seven cases with COL1A1-USP6 fusion and a novel ANGPTL2-USP6 fusion. Mod Pathol. 2020 Aug;33(8):1492–504. PMID:32157177

**7837.** Zhang L, Smyrk TC, Young WF Jr, et al. Gastric stromal tumors in Carney triad are different clinically, pathologically, and behaviorally from sporadic gastric gastrointestinal stromal tumors: findings in 104 cases. Am J Surg Pathol. 2010 Jan;34(1):53–64. PMID:19935059

**7838.** Zhang LY, Smith ML, Schultheis B, et al. A novel K509I mutation of KIT identified in familial mastocytosis-in vitro and in vivo responsiveness to imatinib therapy. Leuk Res. 2006 Apr;30(4):373–8. PMID:16183119

**7839.** Zhang M, Wang Y, Jones S, et al. Somatic mutations of SUZ12 in malignant peripheral nerve sheath tumors. Nat Genet. 2014 Nov;46(11):1170–2. PMID:25305755

**7840.** Zhang MY, Churpek JE, Keel SB, et al. Germline ETV6 mutations in familial thrombocytopenia and hematologic malignancy. Nat Genet. 2015 Feb;47(2):180–5. PMID:25581430

**7841.** Zhang MY, Keel SB, Walsh T, et al. Genomic analysis of bone marrow failure and myelodysplastic syndromes reveals phenotypic and diagnostic complexity. Haematologica. 2015 Jan;100(1):42–8. PMID:25239263

**7842.** Zhang Q, Jing W, Ouyang J, et al. Six cases of aggressive natural killer-cell leukemia in a Chinese population. Int J Clin Exp Pathol. 2014 May 15;7(6):3423–31. PMID:25031771

**7843.** Zhang S, Wilson D, Czader M. Pediatric B-cell lymphoma, unclassifiable, with intermediate features between those of diffuse large B-cell lymphoma and Burkitt lymphoma: a report of two cases. Ann Lab Med. 2015 Mar;35(2):254–6. PMID:25729731

**7844.** Zhang Y, Shan CM, Wang J, et al. Molecular basis for the role of oncogenic histone mutations in modulating H3K36 methylation. Sci Rep. 2017 Mar 3;7:43906. PMID:28256625

**7845.** Zhao B, Zhou Y, Zhao Y, et al. Co-occurrence of pheochromocytoma-paraganglioma and cyanotic congenital heart disease: a case report and literature review. Front Endocrinol (Lausanne). 2018 Apr 17;9:165. PMID:29719528

**7846.** Zhao C, Vinh TN, McManus K, et al. Identification of the most sensitive and robust immunohistochemical markers in different categories of ovarian sex cord-stromal tumors. Am J Surg Pathol. 2009 Mar;33(3):354–66. PMID:19033865

**7847.** Zhao F, Li C, Zhou Q, et al. Distinctive localization and MRI features correlate of molecular subgroups in adult medulloblastoma. J Neurooncol. 2017 Nov;135(2):353–60. PMID:28808827

**7848.** Zhao M, Yin M, Kuick CH, et al. Congenital mesoblastic nephroma is characterised by kinase mutations including EGFR internal tandem duplications, the ETV6-NTRK3 fusion, and the rare KLHL7-BRAF fusion. Histopathology. 2020 Oct;77(4):611–21. PMID:32590884

**7849.** Zhao Z, Paquette C, Shah AA, et al. Fine needle aspiration cytology of diffuse-type tenosynovial giant cell tumors. Acta Cytol. 2017;61(2):160–4. PMID:28324880

**7850.** Zhao Z, Yin Y, Zhang J, et al. Spindle cell/sclerosing rhabdomyosarcoma: case series from a single institution emphasizing morphology, immunohistochemistry and follow-up. Int J Clin Exp Pathol. 2015 Nov 1;8(11):13814–20. PMID:26823695

**7851.** Zheng L, Tang H, Chen X, et al. Paratesticular fetal-type rhabdomyoma in a 12-year-old boy: a case report and literature review. Urology. 2013 Nov;82(5):1150–2. PMID:23768526

**7852.** Zhong M, De Angelo P, Osborne L, et al. Dual-color, break-apart FISH assay on paraffin-embedded tissues as an adjunct to diagnosis of Xp11 translocation renal cell carcinoma and alveolar soft part sarcoma. Am J Surg Pathol. 2010 Jun;34(6):757–66. PMID:20421778

**7853.** Zhou J, Shrikhande G, Xu J, et al. Tsc1 mutant neural stem/progenitor cells exhibit migration deficits and give rise to subependymal lesions in the lateral ventricle. Genes Dev. 2011 Aug 1;25(15):1595–600. PMID:21828270

**7854.** Zhou M, Epstein JI, Young RH. Paraganglioma of the urinary bladder: a lesion that may be misdiagnosed as urothelial carcinoma in transurethral resection specimens. Am J Surg Pathol. 2004 Jan;28(1):94–100. PMID:14707870

**7855.** Zhou S, Hertel PM, Finegold MJ, et al. Hepatocellular carcinoma associated with tight-junction protein 2 deficiency. Hepatology. 2015 Dec;62(6):1914–6. PMID:25921221

**7856.** Zhou S, Venkatramani R, Gupta S, et al. Hepatocellular malignant neoplasm, NOS: a clinicopathological study of 11 cases from a single institution. Histopathology. 2017 Nov;71(5):813–22. PMID:28660626

**7857.** Zhou T, Bloomquist MS, Ferguson LS, et al. Pediatric myeloid sarcoma: a single institution clinicopathologic and molecular analysis. Pediatr Hematol Oncol. 2020 Feb;37(1):76–89. PMID:31682773

**7858.** Zhou Y, Fan X, Routbort M, et al. Absence of terminal deoxynucleotidyl transferase expression identifies a subset of high-risk adult T-lymphoblastic leukemia/lymphoma. Mod Pathol. 2013 Oct;26(10):1338–45. PMID:23702731

**7859.** Zhou YX, Flint NC, Murtie JC, et al. Retroviral lineage analysis of fibroblast growth factor receptor signaling in FGF2 inhibition of oligodendrocyte progenitor differentiation. Glia. 2006 Nov 1;54(6):578–90. PMID:16921523

**7860.** Zhou YY, Coffey M, Mansur D, et al. Images in endocrine pathology: progressive loss of sustentacular cells in a case of recurrent jugulotympanic paraganglioma over a span of 5 years. Endocr Pathol. 2020 Sep;31(3):310–4. PMID:32548761

**7861.** Zhu B, Laskin W, Chen Y, et al. NUT midline carcinoma: a neoplasm with diagnostic challenges in cytology. Cytopathology. 2011 Dec;22(6):414–7. PMID:21210877

**7862.** Zhu G, Benayed R, Ho C, et al. Diagnosis of known sarcoma fusions and novel fusion partners by targeted RNA sequencing with identification of a recurrent ACTB-FOSB fusion in pseudomyogenic hemangioendothelioma. Mod Pathol. 2019 May;32(5):609–20. PMID:30459475

**7863.** Zhu S, Lee JS, Guo F, et al. Activated ALK collaborates with MYCN in neuroblastoma pathogenesis. Cancer Cell. 2012 Mar 20;21(3):362–73. PMID:22439933

**7864.** Zhu X, Mao X, Hurren R, et al. Deoxyribonucleic acid methyltransferase 3B promotes epigenetic silencing through histone 3 chromatin modifications in pituitary cells. J Clin Endocrinol Metab. 2008 Sep;93(9):3610–7. PMID:18544619

**7865.** Zhu Y, Ren C, Yang L, et al. Performance of p16/Ki67 immunostaining, HPV E6/E7 mRNA testing, and HPV DNA assay to detect high-grade cervical dysplasia in women with ASCUS. BMC Cancer. 2019 Mar 27;19(1):271. PMID:30917784

**7866.** Zhuang Z, Devouassoux-Shisheboran M, Lubensky IA, et al. Premeiotic origin of teratomas: Is meiosis required for differentiation into mature tissues? Cell Cycle. 2005 Nov;4(11):1683–7. PMID:16258281

**7867.** Zhuge Y, Cheung MC, Yang R, et al. Pediatric intestinal foregut and small bowel solid tumors: a review of 105 cases. J Surg Res. 2009 Sep;156(1):95–102. PMID:19560163

**7868.** Zhukova N, Ramaswamy V, Remke M, et al. Subgroup-specific prognostic implications of TP53 mutation in medulloblastoma. J Clin Oncol. 2013 Aug 10;31(23):2927–35. PMID:23835706

**7869.** Ziegler DS, Wong M, Mayoh C, et al. Brief report: Potent clinical and radiological response to larotrectinib in TRK fusion-driven high-grade glioma. Br J Cancer. 2018 Sep;119(6):693–6. PMID:30220707

**7870.** Ziemer M, Diaz-Cascajo C, Köhler G, et al. "Tubular Spitz's nevus" an artifact of fixation? J Cutan Pathol. 2000 Nov;27(10):500–4. PMID:11100809

**7871.** Zietz C, Rössle M, Haas C, et al. MDM-2 oncoprotein overexpression, p53 gene mutation, and VEGF up-regulation in angiosarcomas. Am J Pathol. 1998 Nov;153(5):1425–33. PMID:9811333

**7872.** Zillmer DA, Dorfman HD. Chondromyxoid fibroma of bone: thirty-six cases with clinicopathologic correlation. Hum Pathol. 1989 Oct;20(10):952–64. PMID:2793160

**7873.** Zils K, Ebner F, Ott M, et al. Extraskeletal osteosarcoma of the breast in an adolescent girl. J Pediatr Hematol Oncol. 2012 Aug;34(6):e261–3. PMID:22246152

**7874.** Zimmerman LE. Phakomatous choristoma of the eyelid. A tumor of lenticular anlage. Am J Ophthalmol. 1971 Jan;71(1 Pt 2):169–77. PMID:5542122

**7875.** Zimmerman MW, Liu Y, He S, et al. MYC drives a subset of high-risk pediatric neuroblastomas and is activated through mechanisms including enhancer hijacking and focal enhancer amplification. Cancer Discov. 2018 Mar;8(3):320–35. PMID:29284669

**7876.** Ziogas IA, Benedetti DJ, Matsuoka LK, et al. Surgical management of pediatric hepatocellular carcinoma: an analysis of the National Cancer Database. J Pediatr Surg. 2021 Apr;56(4):772–7. PMID:32660779

**7877.** Zipursky A. Transient leukaemia–a benign form of leukaemia in newborn infants with trisomy 21. Br J Haematol. 2003 Mar;120(6):930–8. PMID:12648061

**7878.** Zizic M, Faquin W, Stephen AE, et al. Upper neck papillary thyroid cancer (UPTC): a new proposed term for the composite of thyroglossal duct cyst-associated papillary thyroid cancer, pyramidal lobe papillary thyroid cancer, and Delphian node papillary thyroid cancer. J Pediatr Surg. 2016 Jul;126(7):1709–14. PMID:26691539

**7879.** Zmora O, Klin B, Iacob C, et al. Characterizing excised breast masses in children and adolescents-Can a more aggressive pathology be predicted? J Pediatr Surg. 2020 Oct;55(10):2197–200. PMID:32061367

**7880.** Znaor A, Lortet-Tieulent J, Laversanne M, et al. International variations and trends in renal cell carcinoma incidence and mortality. Eur Urol. 2015 Mar;67(3):519–30. PMID:25449206

**7881.** Zöllner S, Dirksen U, Jürgens H, et al. Renal Ewing tumors. Ann Oncol. 2013 Sep;24(9):2455–61. PMID:23761687

**7882.** Zou H, Duan Y, Wei D, et al. Molecular features of pleomorphic xanthoastrocytoma. Hum Pathol. 2019 Apr;86:38–48. PMID:30496796

**7883.** Zou Y, Huang MZ, Liu FY, et al. Absence of DICER1, CTCF, RPL22, DNMT3A, TRRAP, IDH1 and IDH2 hotspot mutations in patients with various subtypes of ovarian carcinomas. Biomed Rep. 2015 Jan;3(1):33–7. PMID:25469243

**7884.** Zreik RT, Meyer RG, Jenkins RB, et al. A rare pediatric example of subcutaneous extraskeletal osteosarcoma: a case report and review of the morphologic differential diagnosis. Am J Dermatopathol. 2016 Apr;38(4):e44–8. PMID:26460626

**7885.** Zuccaro G, Taratuto AL, Monges J. Intracranial neoplasms during the first year of life. Surg Neurol. 1986 Jul;26(1):29–36. PMID:3715697

**7886.** Zuckerman T, Rowe JM. Pathogenesis and prognostication in acute lymphoblastic leukemia. F1000Prime Rep. 2014 Jul 8;6:59. PMID:25184049

**7887.** Zucman J, Delattre O, Desmaze C, et al. EWS and ATF-1 gene fusion induced by t(12;22) translocation in malignant melanoma of soft parts. Nat Genet. 1993 Aug;4(4):341–5. PMID:8401579

**7888.** Zugor V, Labanaris AP, Witt J, et al. Congenital juvenile granulosa cell tumor of the testis in newborns. Anticancer Res. 2010 May;30(5):1731–4. PMID:20592370

**7889.** Zukerberg LR, Nickoloff BJ, Weiss SW. Kaposiform hemangioendothelioma of infancy and childhood. An aggressive neoplasm associated with Kasabach-Merritt syndrome and lymphangiomatosis. Am J Surg Pathol. 1993 Apr;17(4):321–8. PMID:8494101

**7890.** Zunino V, Catalano MG, Zenga F, et al. Benzene affects the response to octreotide treatment of growth hormone secreting pituitary adenoma cells. Environ Res. 2019 Jun;173:489–96. PMID:30986651

**7891.** Zuntini M, Pedrini E, Parra A, et al. Genetic models of osteochondroma onset and neoplastic progression: evidence for mechanisms alternative to EXT genes inactivation. Oncogene. 2010 Jul 1;29(26):3827–34. PMID:20418910

**7892.** Zuurbier L, Gutierrez A, Mullighan CG, et al. Immature MEF2C-dysregulated T-cell leukemia patients have an early T-cell precursor acute lymphoblastic leukemia gene signature and typically have non-rearranged T-cell receptors. Haematologica. 2014 Jan;99(1):94–102. PMID:23975177

**7893.** Zvizdić Z, Karavdić K. Spleen-preserving surgery in treatment of large mesothelial splenic cyst in children–a case report and review of the literature. Bosn J Basic Med Sci. 2013 May;13(2):126–8. PMID:23725510

**7894.** Zvulunov A, Rotem A, Merlob P, et al. Congenital smooth muscle hamartoma. Prevalence, clinical findings, and follow-up in 15 patients. Am J Dis Child. 1990 Jul;144(7):782–4. PMID:2356798

**7895.** Zwaan CM, Kaspers GJ, Pieters R, et al. Different drug sensitivity profiles of acute myeloid and lymphoblastic leukemia and normal peripheral blood mononuclear cells in children with and without Down syndrome. Blood. 2002 Jan 1;99(1):245–51. PMID:11756178

**7896.** Zwaan CM, Kolb EA, Reinhardt D, et al. Collaborative efforts driving progress in pediatric acute myeloid leukemia. J Clin Oncol. 2015 Sep 20;33(27):2949–62. PMID:26304895

**7897.** Zwick DL, Livingston K, Clapp L, et al. Intracranial trigeminal nerve rhabdomyoma/choristoma in a child: a case report and discussion of possible histogenesis. Hum Pathol. 1989 Apr;20(4):390–2. PMID:2703230

**7898.** Zynger DL, Dimov ND, Luan C, et al. Glypican 3: a novel marker in testicular germ cell tumors. Am J Surg Pathol. 2006 Dec;30(12):1570–5. PMID:17122513

# Subject index

Bold page numbers indicate the main discussion(s) of the topic.

Please note: The pages of this volume have been divided between the two print books as follows:

    Part A: pages 1–646

    Part B: pages 647 and above

## Numbers and symbols

2-succinocysteine   863

3-methoxytyramine   854, 859

4E-BP1   973

5A4   455

34βE12   346, 836

α1-antitrypsin   783, 796, 902

α-inhibin   747, 848, 863

α-internexin   246, 973

α-Klotho   572

α-naphthyl acetate esterase   46

α-naphthyl butyrate esterase   46

α-SMA   508

β-catenin   286, 289, 292, 294, 300, 344-345, 347, 419, 432-435, 441-443, 457, 540, 733, 777-780, 787, 791, 793, 807, 810, 813-815, 834-836, 850, 884, 890, 897-898, 903, 938-939, 968, 992-993, 995

βF1   126

β-hCG   656, 659-660, 679, 686-687, 812

β-Klotho   572

## A

A2M   915-916

ABCB1   133

ABCC6   928

ABCC8   869

ABI1   60

ABL1   41-43, 56, 78

ABL1b   41

ABL2   77

ACD   63

acinic cell carcinoma   873-874, **901-902**

ACO1 (IRP1)   862

ACTB   488, 495

ACTH   335-336, 339, 341-343, 805, 809-810, 837, 839, 867, 872

actin   150, 560, 791, 923, 968

activation-induced cytidine deaminase   110

acute myeloid leukaemias (AMLs) defined by differentiation   **53-55**, 56-57, 61

acute myeloid leukaemias (AMLs) defined by differentiation   53

acute myeloid leukaemias (AMLs) with defining genetic abnormalities   **56-61**

ACVR1   189, 415-416

ACVRL1   472-473

adamantinoma   398, **640-641**, 643

adamantinomatous craniopharyngioma   168, 331, **343-348**

adenosine deaminase   103, 155-156, 438

adrenal cortical tumours   821, **846-850**, 863

AE1/AE3   659

AFDN (MLLT4)   60

AFF1   60

AFF3   60

AFP   656, 659, 666, 671-672, 675, 679-683, 687, 689, 732, 774-775, 777-778, 781, 783-785, 790, 795-796, 803, 805-807, 809-810, 812, 903, 908, 910

aggrecan   583-584

aggressive NK-cell leukaemia   39, **117-118**, 137

AGR2   783

AICDA   156

AIP   335-336

AKT   81, 100, 127, 142, 159, 163, 227, 329, 357, 404, 422, 466, 469, 472, 475, 478, 509, 525, 679, 687, 741, 749, 770, 777, 803, 861, 963, 968, 973

AKT1   741, 749, 770, 803

albumin   783

aldosterone   846

ALK   99-100, 104-105, 107, 116, 124, 129-132, 151-153, 197, 200-201, 232-233, 357-359, 361-362, 449, 454-456, 459-461, 514, 551, 706-707, 710, 829, 914-915, 948-949, 953

ALK1   152

alkaline phosphatase   630, 651

ALK-positive anaplastic large cell lymphoma   39-40, 115, **129-132**

ALK-positive large B-cell lymphoma   39, **99-100**, 104

ALK-rearranged renal cell carcinoma   691, **706-707**

Alpha   See MALAT1

alveolar soft part sarcoma   398, 400, **554-555**, 560, 702

AMACR   713

AMER1   786

amylase   810, 902

amyloid   837, 839-840, 842, 886, 906

ANAPC1   1002-1004

anaplastic sarcoma of the kidney   691, **727-728**, 1008, 1011

androgen   650, 652-653, 846

aneurysmal bone cyst   398, 411-412, 465, 573, 594, 598, 601, 609, 614, **628-629**, 644, 881, 889, 895

angiocentric glioma   167, 176, **177-179**, 227

angiokeratoma   925, **932-933**

angiomatoid fibrous histiocytoma   398, 459, **550-551**

angiosarcoma   397, 492-493, 497, **502-503**, 524, 773, 801-803

ANKRD26   64

ANO1   520

ANTXR2 (CMG2)   426

AP-2β   515

AP-2γ   651

AP2S1   843

APC   282, 285, 287, 297, 344-345, 419, 435, 441, 780, 786, 806-808, 810, 813-814, 834-836, 991-995, 1003

APC1   1003

APC/C   1003

appendiceal neuroendocrine tumours   773, **818-819**, 822

AR   155-156, 303, 432-434, 634, 801, 813-814, 891, 903, 958-961, 1017

ARAP1   60

ARG1   783, 787

arginase   778

ARHGEF37   60

ARID1A   214, 286, 522

ARID1B   522

ARPP21   77

ARTEMIS   See DCLRE1C

arteriovenous malformations   397, **471-473**

ASAP1   628

ASCL1   307, 575

ASPL   See ASPSCR1

ASPSCR1 (ASPL)   554, 702

astroblastoma, MN1-altered   167, **222-224**

ASXL1   42, 50, 1013

ASXL2   1013

ATF1   550-553, 570

ATIC   454

ATM   146, 180, 182, 189

ATP2A2   935

ATP2C1   935

ATP6AP1   534

ATP6AP2   534

ATRX   175, 179, 181-182, 190, 194, 206-
207, 209, 211, 214, 233, 357, 359, 361-
362, 603, 786, 847-848, 850, 861, 864,
963-964

atypical choroid plexus papilloma   167,
**277-278**

atypical teratoid/rhabdoid tumour   168, 190,
215-216, 299, 302, **303-307,** 308, 313,
316, 321, 324, 677, 725, 1017

AXIN1   834

AXIN2   345, 993


**B**

B2M   142, 144

BAIAP3   575

BAK1   682

BAP1   327, 759, 861, 926, 946, 953, 957,
1012-1013

BAP1 tumour predisposition syndrome   926,
953, 957, **1012-1013**

Bartonella   498

B-cell receptor   110, 141

BCL2   84-87, 90-95, 97, 110-113, 117, 159,
164-165, 563, 700, 723, 796, 938

BCL2L14   77

BCL6   84-87, 90-95, 97-98, 104, 107, 110,
112-113, 143, 145-147, 159, 164-165, 214

BCL10   97, 807, 810-811, 814

BCL11A   83, 145

BCOR   168, 214, 250, 302, 317-319, 398,
579, 586-589, 606, 716, 722-724

BCR   41-43, 56, 78

BDNF   987-988

Beckwith–Wiedemann and related overgrowth
syndromes   957, **989-990**

benign triton tumour / neuromuscular
choristoma   398, **539-540**

BerH2   658

biotin   807, 835

bizarre parosteal osteochondromatous
proliferation   398, **592-593**

Blimp1   91-92, 100, 104-105

BLM (RECQL3)   603

blue naevus   374, 925, **945-946,** 952

B-lymphoblastic leukaemia/lymphoma   39,
60, **75-79,** 80, 111, 155-156

BMP   305, 415, 650

BOB1   85, 90, 100, 107-108, 143-144, 146

BOC   405

BORCS5   77

BPTF   61

brachyury   635-636

BRAF   81, 105, 149-153, 178, 180-186, 189-
190, 197, 202-204, 206-207, 211, 213-217,
220, 224, 226-229, 232-236, 241-244,
246-247, 329, 347, 373, 376, 396, 446-448,
450, 472-473, 478, 486, 508, 520, 641,
669, 694, 713-717, 786, 810, 829-832, 836,
884, 910, 926, 942-945, 948, 953, 996-998,
1010, 1013

BRCA1   736, 1012-1013

BRCA2 (FANCD1)   282, 284, 293-294, 297,
736, 786, 869, 959

BRD3   908

BRD4   321, 908

breakpoint cluster region   41-42

BRIP1 (FANCJ)   959

BRWD3   61

BSEP   785-788

BTBD12   *See* SLX4

BTG1   77

BUB1   993, 998

BUB3   998

Burkitt lymphoma   39, 87-88, **109-112,** 113-
114, 155-156, 163-164


**C**

CAIX   863

calcifying aponeurotic fibroma   397, 423,
**430-431,** 435

calcifying nested stromal-epithelial
tumour   773, **793-794**

calcitonin   825, 830, 835, 837-840, 842, 857,
869, 871

caldesmon   425, 443

calponin   425, 455, 457, 560, 570, 898, 903

calretinin   534, 555, 653-654, 732-733, 738,
740-741, 743, 745, 747, 752-753, 759, 817

CAM5.2   272, 817, 830, 898

CAMTA1   500, 626-627

capillary malformations   397, **466-467,** 471

carboxyl ester lipase   810

CARD11   145

cardiac rhabdomyoma   913, **922-924**

CARMIL2   509

carnitine palmitoyltransferase 1A   982-983

CARS1 (CARS)   454

CASR   843

cathepsin K   555, 560, 703-705, 709

CBFA2T3   55-56, 60

CBFB   56

CBL   45, 47, 63-65, 649

CCDC6   829

CCDC88C   47

CCN2   575

CCNB3   587-589, 606, 722-724

CCND1   374, 807, 844, 1018

CCND2   195, 586, 679, 687

CCND3   110, 112, 114

CCNJL   60

CD1a   81, 116, 150-152

CD2   40, 68, 73-74, 78, 81-85, 87-88, 90-91,
95, 97-98, 100, 102-103, 105-108, 110-111,
118, 121-122, 124, 134, 137, 143-144, 146-
147, 150-152, 155, 164-165, 376, 451, 576

CD3   39, 42, 46, 52, 55, 60, 68, 73-74, 78,
81-82, 84-85, 90, 100, 102, 104, 107-108,
111, 113, 116, 118, 121-125, 127, 129,
131-132, 134, 137, 143-144, 146, 150, 154-
155, 161, 164-165, 175, 180-182, 185, 205,
214-215, 221, 226-227, 235-236, 246, 376,
406, 419, 421-422, 439, 443, 446-447, 449-
450, 452, 461, 478, 484, 486, 488, 491,
493, 496, 498, 500, 502-503, 520, 523-524,
527-528, 530, 532, 546-547, 549, 551, 563,
567, 583, 627, 659, 680, 700, 714, 716,
723, 791, 798, 801, 804, 817, 908, 933

CD3ε   118

CD4   49, 53, 68, 79, 81, 85, 97-98, 100, 103,
107, 111, 121-122, 124, 127, 134, 137,
139, 142-144, 146, 154, 163-165, 278, 376,
465, 660, 783

CD5   60, 68, 81-82, 91, 100, 104, 113, 118,
122, 124, 127-128, 131, 134, 137, 139,
146-147, 154, 272, 299, 319, 359, 406,
573, 669, 700, 713, 738, 741, 743, 783,
793, 796, 814, 817, 825, 830, 836, 842

CD7   42, 46, 68, 81-82, 85, 87, 90-91, 95,
100, 103, 105, 107-108, 110, 116, 121-122,
124, 134, 143, 146-147

CD8   81, 102, 111, 113, 121-122, 124, 127-
128, 134, 137, 139, 146-147, 154

CD9   81, 272, 313, 431, 551, 557, 563, 580-
581, 583, 586, 589, 624, 669, 729-730,
741, 814, 911

CD10   42, 78, 81, 84, 87, 90-91, 93, 95, 97-
98, 104, 107, 110-113, 146, 164-165, 743,
745, 752-753, 814, 817, 836

CD11b   81, 134

CD11c   54

CD13   46, 81, 100, 104-105, 143, 583, 801

CD14   150, 153, 554-555

CD15   42, 90, 102, 107-108, 131, 143-144,
146-147, 164

CD16   46, 113, 118, 134, 150, 153, 465

CD19   42, 55, 78, 84-85, 87, 91, 98, 100,
107-108, 110-111, 143, 164

CD20   84-85, 87, 90-91, 95, 98, 100, 102-
103, 105, 107-108, 110-111, 143-144, 146-
147, 150-152, 155, 164-165, 376, 576

CD21   88

CD22   78, 110

CD23   68, 84-85, 107
CD24   451
CD25   73-74
CD27   83, 85, 106, 146, 576
CD30   73-74, 84-85, 90, 100, 102, 104, 107-
    108, 116, 121-122, 124-125, 127, 131-132,
    143-144, 146, 154-155, 161, 164-165, 659,
    680
CD31   478, 484, 486, 488, 491, 493, 496,
    498, 500, 502-503, 627, 791, 798, 801,
    804, 933
CD33   46, 68, 81
CD34   42, 52, 68, 78, 81, 116, 150, 175,
    180-182, 185, 205, 214-215, 221, 226-
    227, 235-236, 246, 406, 422, 439, 443,
    446-447, 449-450, 452, 461, 478, 484, 486,
    488, 491, 493, 496, 498, 500, 502, 520,
    523-524, 528, 530, 532, 546-547, 549, 551,
    563, 567, 583, 627, 700, 714, 716, 723,
    791, 798, 801, 804, 817, 908
CD36   68, 81
CD38   60, 104, 111
CD41   49, 53, 68
CD42   66
CD43   98, 100, 111
CD44   111, 278, 783
CD45   79, 85, 100, 103, 143-144, 165, 376,
    465
CD45RO   154
CD56   60, 68, 81-82, 104, 113, 118, 127-128,
    131, 134, 137, 272, 299, 319, 359, 406,
    573, 669, 700, 738, 741, 743, 783, 793,
    796, 814, 817, 825, 830
CD57   100, 134, 146-147, 154, 700, 713
CD61   49, 53
CD63   534
CD64   54, 58-59
CD65   81
CD68   150, 153, 465, 534, 551, 783, 879
CD68R   46
CD70   156
CD71   54
CD79   90, 100
CD79a, CD79A   58, 78, 81, 85, 87, 91, 95,
    100, 103, 105, 107-108, 110, 116, 143,
    146-147
CD79B   105
CD81   111
CD99   81, 272, 313, 431, 551, 557, 563,
    580-581, 583, 586, 589, 624, 669, 729-730,
    741, 814, 911
CD113   783
CD123   127
CD133   801
CD138   100, 104-105, 143, 583

CD147   554-555
CD163   150, 153, 465
CD200   84-85, 576
CD207   150-152
CD235a   68
CD274   83, 85, 106, 146
CD276   576
CD371   76
CDC73   844, 888
CDH11   628
CDK4   195, 209, 211, 409, 578, 603, 606
CDKN1B   336, 843, 868, 960
CDKN1C   514, 989-990
CDKN2A (P16INK4A)   786
CDKN2B   81, 173, 191, 197, 207, 209-211,
    213, 215-217, 224, 233, 243, 254, 526,
    528, 542, 577, 905, 963
CDX2   836, 870-871
CEA   710, 783, 793, 812, 830, 837-839, 842,
    857, 869, 900
CEBPA   56, 60-61, 63-65
CEBPE   77
central giant cell granuloma   873, **881-882**
CGRP   839, 869
CHCHD7   897
CHD8   110, 768
CHEK2   829
childhood myelodysplastic neoplasm with
    increased blasts   See myelodysplastic
    syndrome with excess blasts
childhood myelodysplastic neoplasm with
    low blasts   See refractory cytopenia of
    childhood
chondroblastoma   398, 605, **608-610**
chondromesenchymal hamartoma of the
    chest wall   398, **598-599**
chondromyxoid fibroma   398, 573, 609,
    **613-615**
chondrosarcoma   398-399, 515, 609, 612,
    617, **618-622**, 623-624, 636, 676, 918
choriocarcinoma (non-gestational)   647,
    **686-687**
choroid plexus carcinoma   167, 277-278,
    **279-281**, 309, 1017
choroid plexus papilloma   167, **274-276**,
    277-278, 328, 983
CHRND   517
chromogranin   181, 205, 226, 235, 243, 246,
    324, 339, 344, 359, 393, 517, 788, 793,
    807, 810, 814, 818-819, 848, 856, 859,
    863, 870, 872, 908, 911, 985
chronic myeloid leukaemia   39-40, **41-44**, 45
chymotrypsin   807, 810-811
CIC   502, 585-586
CIC-rearranged sarcoma   398, 579, **585-586**

CIITA   83, 85
CITED1   505, 830
CITED2   505, 514
CK1   347, 394, 567, 641-642, 787-788, 791,
    810, 830-831, 902-903
CK5   272, 346, 567, 641-642, 759, 771, 836,
    898, 900, 903
CK5/6   272, 346, 567, 759, 771, 898, 900,
    903
CK7   258, 272, 347, 394, 709-710, 713,
    745, 747, 783, 788, 791, 810, 830, 898,
    902-903
CK8   347, 567, 902
CK8/18   902
CK14   641-642
CK17   347, 641-642
CK18   394
CK19   347, 567, 641-642, 787-788, 791, 810,
    830-831, 902-903
CK20   258, 272, 347, 394, 708-710, 791,
    830, 835
class III β-tubulin   214, 220, 973
classic Hodgkin lymphoma   39, 83, 106,
    **141-144,** 145, 155-156, 161, 163-164
claudin-1   452, 530-532, 535
CLC1B   490
clear cell sarcoma of soft tissue   398, 550,
    **552-553,** 560
clear cell sarcoma of the kidney   552, 560,
    587-589, 691, 716-717, **722-724**
CLTC   100, 454, 495, 702
clusterin   131, 465
c-Met   554-555
CMG2   See ANTXR2
CMV   98
CNBP (ZNF9)   628
CNS embryonal tumour NEC/NOS   168,
    **320-321**
CNS neuroblastoma, FOXR2-activated   168,
    **314-316**
CNS tumour with BCOR internal tandem
    duplication   168, 302, **317-319**
cohesin   67
COL1A1   412, 438-439, 628
COL1A2   405
COL3A1   405
COL6A3   438-439
COL12A1   590
collagen IV   508, 527, 839
collagen VI   426
composite phaeochromocytoma/
    paraganglioma   821, 864, **865-866**
condyloma acuminatum   735, **757-758,** 875
congenital granular cell epulis   873-874,
    **879-880**

congenital haemangioma   397, 472, **479-480,** 502, 773, 797, 800-801, 804

congenital naevi   328, 925, **940-942,** 952-954

congenital peribronchial myofibroblastic tumour   913, **916-917,** 920

conjunctival junctional, compound, and subepithelial naevi   365, **372-374**

connexin 26   973

connexin 32   973

constitutional mismatch repair deficiency syndrome   196, 199, 285, 297, 957, 991, 993-994, **1014-1016**

COX-2   486, 597

CPS1   793

CREB1   550-552

CREB3L1   451-452

CREB3L2   451-452

CREB3L3   452

CREBBP   56, 59, 117, 145, 282, 289, 293, 321

CREM   452, 550

CRH   335, 837

cribriform morular thyroid carcinoma   821, **834-836**

cribriform neuroepithelial tumour   168-169, 302, **308-309**

CRLF2   64, 76

CRTC1   899

CRTC3   899

CRX   325, 392

CSDE1   861

CSF1   465

CSF1R   151, 153, 465

CTC1   63

CTCF   519

CTCL   See TSPYL2

CTLA4   156

CTNNB1   283, 285-287, 311, 343-345, 347-348, 432, 435, 441-442, 539-540, 628, 701, 733, 777, 779-780, 783, 786-787, 793, 806-807, 810, 813-814, 847, 897, 938, 995-996

CTPS1   156

cullin-2   982

cyclin B3   588-589, 723

cyclin D1   589, 720, 723-724, 807, 814, 830

CYSLTR2   327, 945

cytokeratin   100, 336-339, 344, 347, 500, 503, 576, 609, 636, 641-642, 659, 680, 700, 710, 796, 817, 848

**D**

D2-40   223, 469-470, 478, 480, 492-493, 659, 687, 791, 933

D-2-HG   617

D3   533, 800

D5F3   455

DAB   376

DAXX   357

DBH   863

DCLRE1C (ARTEMIS)   155

DCTN1   454

DDB2   1000-1001

DDIT3   409

DDR1   522

DDX3X   117, 286, 289

DDX6   405

DDX10   61

deep angiomyxoma   398, **548-549**

DEK   56

dentin   884-885

dermatofibrosarcoma protuberans   397, **437-440**

desmin   406, 413, 443, 447, 455, 457-458, 461, 465, 506, 510, 512, 515, 517, 520, 540, 543, 549, 551, 555, 560, 563, 570, 576, 583, 624, 700, 716, 720, 723, 729, 791, 793, 796, 817, 911, 915, 917, 923

desmoid fibromatosis   397, 419, **441-442,** 539-540, 991

desmoplastic infantile ganglioglioma / desmoplastic infantile astrocytoma   167, **230-233**

desmoplastic small round cell tumour   398, **574-576**

DHH   977

DICER1   302, 310-311, 313, 322-325, 331, 341-342, 366, 392-393, 399, 514-515, 543, 695-697, 727-728, 741, 743, 746-750, 792, 822, 824, 828-829, 833, 874, 894-895, 918-920, 938, 957-958, 1008-1011

DICER1 syndrome   366, 399, 514-515, 695, 697, 741, 746-748, 792, 822, 824, 828, 833, 874, 918-919, 938, 957-958, **1008-1011**

diffuse astrocytoma, MYB- or MYBL1-altered   167, 172, **174-176,** 178-179, 236

diffuse choroidal neurofibroma and ganglioneuroma   365, 378

diffuse glioneuronal tumour with oligodendroglioma-like features and nuclear clusters   167, 169, 172-173, **238-240**

diffuse hemispheric glioma, H3 G34–mutant   167, 172, **193-195**

diffuse large B-cell lymphoma   39, 83-85, **86-88,** 89, 91, 93, 95, 97, 102, 104, 106, 110, 145, 155-156, 161, 163-164

diffuse leptomeningeal glioneuronal tumour   167, 207, 227, **241-244**

diffuse low-grade glioma, MAPK pathway–altered   167, 172, **183-186**

diffuse meningeal melanocytic neoplasms: melanocytosis and melanomatosis   168, **328-330**

diffuse midline glioma, H3 K27–altered   167, **187-192**

diffuse paediatric-type high-grade glioma, H3-wildtype and IDH-wildtype   167, 172, **196-199**

DKC1   63

DLG2   603

DLST   861

DMD   452

DMRT1   658

DNAH11   768

DNAJB1   774, 782-783

DNAJC21   63

DNMT3A   50, 52-53, 861

DOCK8   155

DOG1   520, 609, 902

dopamine   340, 854, 984

DUSP2   123-124, 145

DUSP22   123-124

DUX4   585-586

DYNC2H1   768

dysembryoplastic neuroepithelial tumour   167, 180, 185, 207, 227, **234-237,** 243, 402

**E**

E2F   679, 687

EBER   90, 102, 104, 116, 118, 137, 139-140, 144, 157, 159, 161-162, 164-165, 498, 510, 906-907

EBF1   77

EBNA1   164-165

EBNA2   90, 509

EBNA3   509

EBV   40, 88-90, 97-98, 100-102, 106-110, 116-117, 127-128, 131, 133-139, 141-142, 144, 146, 154-155, 157-165, 399, 433, 504, 509-510, 905

EBV-associated smooth muscle tumour   **509-510**

EBV-positive diffuse large B-cell lymphoma   39, **89-90,** 106, 161

E-cadherin   814, 836

ectomesenchymoma   398, **517-518**

ectopic meningioma and meningothelial hamartoma   398, **537-538**

EED   528, 542

EEF1G   131

EFL1   63

EGF   422-423, 430-431

EGFR (HER1)   335, 422, 431, 635, 777

EGLN1 (PHD2)   861

EGLN2 (PHD1)   861
EIF1   628
EIF1AX   327, 829
ELANE   63, 65
ELL   60
elongin B   982
elongin C   982
EMA   100, 131-132, 146, 179, 181, 223, 243,
    250, 255, 258, 266, 269, 272, 275, 280,
    306, 309, 313, 341, 394, 452, 488, 503,
    523, 530, 532, 535-536, 538, 540, 551,
    557, 563, 567, 570-571, 576, 606, 627,
    636, 659, 676, 700, 704, 710, 713, 718,
    723, 740-741, 743, 747, 793, 835, 900
embryonal carcinoma   647, 650-651, 659,
    **679-680,** 681-682, 688-690
embryonal sarcoma of the liver   773, **795-
    796**
embryonal tumour with multilayered
    rosettes   168, 190, 302, **310-313,** 316,
    324, 1008, 1011
EMILIN2   438-439
EML4   100, 446, 454, 456, 707
enchondroma and enchondromatosis   398,
    **616-617**
ENG   472-473
eosinophilic solid and cystic renal cell
    carcinoma   691, **708-709**
EP300   59, 81, 105, 318
EP400   406
EPAS1 (HIF2A)   861-862
EpCAM, EPCAM   783, 786-787, 959, 995,
    997
EPHB4   472-473, 475-476, 478, 641
epibulbar choristoma   365, **367-368,** 369
epibulbar osseous choristoma   365, **369**
epidermal naevi   403, 466, 925-926, **934-937**
epinephrine   855, 984
epithelioid haemangioendothelioma   397,
    **500-501,** 625
epithelioid haemangioma   397, **487-488,** 625
epithelioid sarcoma   398, 494, **565-568,**
    577, 1017
EPO   982
EPOR   77
EPS15   60
ER   336, 338-340, 375, 513, 517, 569, 696,
    745, 753, 759, 771, 835-836
ERBB2   531-532
ERBB4   948
ERCC1   1001
ERCC2   1000-1001
ERCC3   1000-1001
ERCC4   1000-1001
ERCC5   1000-1001

ERG   60, 443-444, 478, 486, 488, 491, 493,
    496, 498, 500, 502-503, 567, 573, 580-581,
    627, 730, 804, 933
ERK   100, 151-152, 329, 469, 473, 525, 786,
    803, 829, 963
erythropoietin   712, 862, 982
estrogen   762, 846
ETS   53, 401, 579-582, 729-730
ETV1   581, 730
ETV4   581, 586
ETV6   56-58, 76, 81, 445-447, 716, 720-721,
    763, 916-917
EVI1   See MECOM
Ewing sarcoma   60, 386, 398-399, 401, **579-
    581,** 584, 586, 588-589, 602, 605, 624,
    669, 691, 729-730, 763, 903, 908-909, 911
EWSR1 (EWS)   224, 400, 409, 443-444, 451-
    452, 514, 550-553, 569-571, 574-576, 579,
    581-584, 948
EWSR1::SMAD3-rearranged fibroblastic
    tumour   397, **443-444**
EXT1   612, 619
EXT2   612, 619
extragonadal teratoma   647, **666-667**
extrarenal rhabdoid tumour   398, **556-558**
EZH1   824
EZH2   81, 188, 260, 393, 566, 1018
ezrin   968

## F

factor XIIIa   150, 153, 461
FAK   968
familial adenomatous polyposis   282, 323,
    344, 418, 432, 441, 540, 806-807, 809,
    813, 834, 884, 938-939, 957-958, **991-993,**
    994
FAN1   993
FANCA   214
FANCB   959
FANCC   62, 959
FANCD1   See BRCA2
FANCD2   214
FANCE   959
FANCF   959
FANCG   62, 959
FANCI   214
FANCJ   See BRIP1
FANCL   959
FANCM   214
FANCW   See RFWD3
FAS (TNFRSF6)   156
fasciitis/myositis   397, **411-414,** 417, 457,
    506
fascin   143, 150-151
FASL   117-118

FAT1   628
FBXW7   81
fetal lung interstitial tumour   913, **914-915,**
    916-917, 920
fetus in fetu   647, **684-685**
FEV   581, 730
FGD6   406
FGF   344, 519, 572-573, 644, 801
FGF1   573
FGF4   519
FGF23   572-573, 644
FGFR1   183-186, 189, 203-206, 211, 227-228,
    233-236, 242, 404, 514, 572-573, 603,
    632-633, 881
FGFR2   182, 185, 227-228, 236, 247, 884
FGFR3   182, 227, 236, 937
FGFR4   514, 576
FH   459-461, 861
FHL2   739
fibrin   545, 605
fibrinogen   783
fibrodysplasia ossificans progressiva   397, 415
fibroepithelial tumours   761, **764-766**
fibrolamellar variant of hepatocellular
    carcinoma   773, **781-783,** 787
fibroma of tendon sheath   397, 412, **417**
fibromatosis colli   397, **428-429**
fibronectin   830
fibrous dysplasia   398, 545, 573, 606, 642-
    643, **644-645,** 888
fibrous hamartoma of infancy   397, **420-421,**
    463
fibrous histiocytoma   397-398, **459-461,** 550,
    577, 630, 632
FIP1L1   47
FLCN   511
FLI1   478, 496, 580-581, 627, 669, 729-730
FLNA   768
FLT3   53, 60, 81
FLT4   486, 502
FMC7   111
FN1   422-423, 430-431, 443, 454, 572-573
FNBP1   60
follicular adenoma of the thyroid   821, **823-
    826**
FOS   488, 495, 594-595, 597, 606, 626-627
FOSB   488, 495-496, 594-595, 626-627
FOSL2   628
FOXA1   768
FOXA2   801
FOXK1   1013
FOXK2   1013
FOXL2   653-654, 732-733, 738, 740-741,
    743, 746-747, 750
FOXO1   514-516

FOXO4   514, 586
FOXP1   97
FSIP2   768
fumarate hydratase   693, 863
FUS   60, 409, 451-452, 514, 550-551, 570, 581-584, 730

G
GABBR1   905
galectin-3   341, 825, 830
ganglioglioma   167, 182, 185, 190, 197, 201, 205, 207, 215, **225-229,** 230, 232-233, 235-236, 243, 395-396
ganglioneuroblastoma, intermixed   349-350, **353-355**
ganglioneuroblastoma, nodular   349-350, **363-364**
ganglioneuroma   349-350, **351-352,** 353, 358, 361, 363-365, 378, 380, 517, 527, 865-866
GAP   525, 959, 963
Gardner fibroma   397, **418-419,** 441
gastrin   867, 869, 871
gastroblastoma   773-774, **816-817**
GATA1   66-68
GATA1s   67
GATA2   49-52, 63-65, 509
GATA3   81, 143, 333, 336, 338-340, 687, 753, 844, 856-857, 863, 985
GCGR   868
GCK   869
G-CSF   63-64
GDF2   472-473
GDF3   687
GDNF   838
germinoma/dysgerminoma/seminoma   647, 654, **655-660**
GFAP   175, 179, 181, 185, 189, 194, 197, 201, 205, 214, 220, 223, 226, 232, 235, 243, 246, 250, 258, 266, 269, 272, 275, 299, 306, 309, 313, 315, 319-320, 394, 452, 523, 530, 570-571, 583, 716, 857, 866, 898, 967, 973
giant cell tumour of bone   398, 605, 609, **630-631,** 881
GJB2   936
GLI   289, 291, 739, 801, 816-817, 977
GLI1   289, 816-817
GLI2   289, 291, 739, 801
glicentin   870
GLIS2   55-56, 60
GLMN   508
glomus tumour and glomuvenous malformation   397, **507-508**
GLP-1   870
GLP-2   870

glucagon   870
GLUD1   869
GLUT1   469-470, 482, 484, 502, 530-532, 535-536, 798, 800-801, 804
GLUT2   See SLC2A2
glycogen   659, 710, 785-786, 796, 902, 915, 923
glycophorin A   54
GNA11   327, 479-480, 798, 945, 953
GNA14   490
GNAQ   327, 373, 466-467, 479-480, 798, 945, 953
GNAS (GNAS1)   888
gonadoblastoma   647-648, **652-654,** 657, 987
Gorlin syndrome   See naevoid basal cell carcinoma syndrome
GOT2   861
GPC3   557, 658-659, 672, 683, 687, 732, 778-779, 783, 787, 791, 796, 798, 801
GPR101   334, 336
GPR161   288-289, 292, 297, 976-977
G$_q\alpha$   953
granular cell tumour   331, 398, **533-534,** 879
granulocyte–macrophage colony–stimulating factor   45
granzyme   124, 127, 131, 134, 139
GRIPAP1   704
GRM1   614-615
growth hormone   333, 337, 341, 343
GRP   839
GS   644, 778-779, 814
GSK3B
G$_s\alpha$   644
GTF2I   842
gynandroblastoma   735, 749, 1010

H
H19   483, 514, 989-990
H3.3   187-191, 193-194, 608-610
H3-3A (H3F3A)   194, 630
H3-3B (H3F3B)   609
HADH   869
haemangioma of placenta   397, **483-484**
haemoglobin   45, 47-48, 710
Haemophilus influenzae   98
haemosiderin   272, 345, 347, 463-465, 479, 484, 498, 545, 550-551, 614, 629, 631, 633, 639, 778, 798
hamartin   219, 221, 559, 923, 972-974
hamartomas   365-366, 399, 403, 481, 537-538, 883, 894-895, 925, **927-931,** 962, 964, 966-967, 971
HAS2   405
HAVCR2   127-128

HAX1   63
HBEGF   422
HBME1   825, 830-831
HBV   774, 785-786
h-caldesmon   457, 506, 508, 510
HCFC1   1013
hCG   344, 675-676, 680, 683, 689, 905
HCG9   905
HCV   774
HDC   869
head and neck paraganglioma   See parasympathetic paraganglioma
hedgehog   274, 280, 282, 284, 286, 288, 291, 293, 295, 344, 511, 777, 801, 816-817, 975, 977, 1006
heparan sulfate   612
hepatic angiosarcoma   773, **803-804**
hepatic congenital haemangioma   773, **797-799,** 800-801, 804
hepatic infantile haemangioma   773, **800-802,** 803
hepatoblastoma   773-774, **775-781,** 783, 785, 787, 790-791, 801, 806, 835, 903, 919, 989-992
hepatosplenic T-cell lymphoma   39, **133-134**
HER1   See EGFR
hereditary phaeochromocytoma–paraganglioma syndromes   957, **984-986**
HERPUD1   810
HEY1   623-624
HGAL   110
HHV6   47
HIF1α   482, 801, 982
HIF2α   862, 982
HIF2A   See EPAS1
HIFα   861
high-grade astrocytoma with piloid features   167, 172, 207, 209-211
high-grade B-cell lymphoma with 11q aberration   39, 87, 111-112, **113-114**
high-molecular-weight cytokeratin   710
HIV   89, 103, 109, 144, 157, 163-165, 402, 497, 758
HIV-associated lymphoproliferative disorders   39, **163-165**
HLA-DR   42, 46, 60, 81
HLF   7
HMB45   374, 376, 394, 524, 534, 553, 560, 704-705, 911, 948, 953
HMGA2   404, 406-407, 515, 548, 777, 897-898
HMGB3   61
HNF1α   777
HNF4A   869
HNRNPA1   454

HOOK1 707

HOXA13 61

HOXA9 61

HOXB7 526

HOXD13 61

hPL 659, 687

HPS 943-944

HPV 736, 755, 757-758, 875-876

HPV1 875-876

HPV6 875

HPV11 875-876

HPV16 875

HPV18 875

HRAS 472-473, 478, 513-514, 517, 669, 803, 884, 948, 953

hSNF5 *See* SMARCB1

HTN3 901

HTRA1 522

hyaline fibromatosis syndrome *See* juvenile hyaline fibromatosis

hyaluronidase 384

hybrid nerve sheath tumour 398, **531-532**

hydroa vacciniforme lymphoproliferative disorder 39, **138-140**

**I**

ID2 115, 197

ID3 110, 112-114

IDH1 175, 179, 181, 191, 194, 196, 198, 205, 211, 228, 235, 242-244, 609, 617, 619, 621, 624, 737, 741

IDH2 179, 191, 194, 196, 198, 228, 242, 244, 609, 617, 619, 621, 624, 741

IDH3B 861

IFNGR1 497

IgA 100

IgD 98, 146-147

IGF1 332, 334, 337

IGF1R (IGFIR) 575, 590, 603

IGF2 482, 514, 576, 701, 801, 806-807, 847, 862, 989-990

IgG 100, 147, 151, 376-377

IgG4 147

IGH 91-92, 94-95, 97-98, 112, 165

IGHV 97

IGK 91-92, 95, 98, 112, 165

IGL 91, 112, 165

IgM 136

IHH 977

IKZF1 64, 76, 81

IKZF2 77

IKZF3 77

IL2RB 575

IL3 7

IL-7 81

IL7R 81

IL-10, IL10 117, 142, 486

IL-17 376

IL17RB 968

immature teratoma (female gonadal) 647, **671-672**

inclusion body infantile digital fibromatosis 397, **424-425**

infantile fibrosarcoma 397, 400, 423, **445-447,** 448-450, 506, 589, 721, 916-917

infantile haemangioma 397, **481-482,** 773, 790-791, 797-798, 800-801, 803

infant-type hemispheric glioma 167, 172, 197, **200-201,** 232-233

inflamed juvenile conjunctival naevus 365, **375-377**

inflammatory myofibroblastic tumour 397, 449-450, **454-456,** 914, 916

inhibin 534, 653-654, 687, 732-733, 738, 740-741, 743, 752

INI1 *See* SMARCB1

INO80D 514

INSM1 856, 863, 868

insulin 590, 870-871

insulin receptor 590

interferon 83, 140, 802

intramuscular vascular anomalies 397, **474-476**

intramuscular/juxta-articular myxoma 397-398, 403, 411-412, 414, 474-475, 494, 534, **545-546,** 554, 644

intratubular germ cell neoplasia (male gonadal) 647, **649-651,** 657, 677, 679-683, 686-687, 689-690

IPMK 869

IRF4 39-40, 84, 88, 90-95, 100, 103, 105, 107, 124, 143, 146, 164

IRF8 94, 97

iris hamartoma *See* Lisch nodule

IRP1 *See* ACO1

IRS4 590

ISL1 871

ITGB6 905

ITK 155-156

**J**

JADE2 (PHF15) 61

JAK1 81

JAK2 83, 106, 145, 641, 862

JAK3 81

JMJD1C 689

JNK 968

JUNB 145

junctional, compound, and dermal naevi 925, **943-944**

juvenile fibroadenoma 761, **767-769**

juvenile granulosa cell tumour of the ovary 735, **741-742**

juvenile granulosa cell tumour of the testis 691, **732-733**

juvenile hyaline fibromatosis (hyaline fibromatosis syndrome) 397, **426-427**

juvenile myelomonocytic leukaemia 39, **45-47,** 62, 958-961, 963

juvenile papillomatosis 761-762, **770-772,** 875

**K**

KANK1 713

KANSL1L 405

Kaposi sarcoma 397, 399, **497-499**

KAT6A 56, 59

KAT7 61

KCNJ11 869

KCNQ1OT1 989-990

KDM5A 55, 60

KDM6A 293

KDR 502, 803

keratin 343, 345, 347, 455, 488, 571, 583-584, 586, 606, 627, 664, 687, 729, 778, 836, 842, 864, 877, 885, 891, 911, 935, 939

Ki-67 87-88, 104, 111-113, 127-128, 164-165, 175, 179, 181, 194, 205, 214, 220, 223, 227, 232, 243-244, 272, 275, 278, 280, 299, 309, 312, 315, 319-320, 324, 340-341, 347, 374, 376, 384, 523, 528, 677, 804, 831, 836, 849-850, 857, 863-864, 868-870, 872, 904, 944

KIAA1549 202-204, 207, 211, 216, 226, 233, 241-244, 396

KIT 67, 70, 72-74, 81, 519-520, 649-653, 659, 679, 683, 687, 709, 793, 817, 898, 903

KITLG 650, 653

KLF10 405

KLF15 570

KLF17 570

KLLN 959

KMT2A (MLL) 83

KMT2C 97, 293, 768, 835, 841

KMT2D 86, 286, 289, 293, 392-393, 452, 768, 835, 861

KMT3D *See* SMYD1

KRAS (KRAS2) 803

KRT1 877

KRT4 877

KRT10 935

KRT13 877

KSHV/HHV8 100, 104-105, 165, 399, 433, 497-499

**L**

L   78, 145, 451-452, 454, 514-515, 562-563, 842, 875, 940

lactoferrin   902

LANA   498

Langerhans cell histiocytosis and related disorders   39, **148-153**

large B-cell lymphoma with IRF4 rearrangement   39-40, 88, **91-92,** 93-94

LASP1   60

LATS1   522

LATS2   522

LDH   94, 96, 117, 136, 656, 679

lectin   490

LEF1   111, 345, 807, 814

LEMD3   930

let-7   777, 919

LEUTX   586

LIFR   570, 897

Li–Fraumeni syndrome   64, 76, 188, 196, 280, 282, 284, 291-292, 297, 299, 399, 408, 514, 603, 697, 822, 847, 874, 957-958, **1005-1007**

LIG4   49

LIN28A   313, 324, 392, 394, 651, 680, 683

LIN28B   777

lipase   807, 809-810

lipoblastoma/lipoblastomatosis   397, **405-407**

lipofibromatosis   397, **422-423,** 449

lipomatosis   203, 397, **402-404**

liposarcoma   397, 406-407, **408-410**

Lisch nodule (iris hamartoma)   365, **381-382**

LKB1   *See* STK11

LMNA   454, 488, 626

LMO1   81

LMO2   81, 110, 113

LMO3   81

LMP   90, 104, 139, 141, 144, 161, 164-165, 509

LMP1, LMP-1   89-90, 104, 136-137, 139, 141, 144, 161, 164, 165, 509

LMP2   141, 164-165

lobular capillary haemangioma (pyogenic granuloma)   397, 472, **485-486,** 952

low-grade fibromyxoid sarcoma / sclerosing epithelioid fibrosarcoma   397, 406, **451-453**

low-grade myofibroblastic sarcoma   397, 413, **457-458**

LRBA   156

LRRC15   575

LRRFIP2   995-996

LYL1   81

lymphatic anomalies   397, 477

lymphomatoid granulomatosis   39, **101-102**

LYN   60, 77

Lynch syndrome   196-198, 736, 809, 813, 822, 957-958, 991, **994-998,** 1014-1015

lysozyme   46, 902

LYVE1   491, 498, 801

LZTR1   523, 966

**M**

M2A   658

MAFA   868

MAGEA4   658

MAGT1   155-156, 497

MAL   84-85

MALAT1 (Alpha)   702, 705

malignant mixed germ cell tumours   647, **688-690**

malignant peripheral nerve sheath tumour   398, 449, 523-524, 526, 529, **541-544,** 563, 866, 962

malignant rhabdoid tumour of the kidney   691, **725-726**

MALT1   97

MAML2   176, 899-900

MAML3   861, 864

MAP2   175, 189, 194, 214, 226, 235, 239, 243, 246, 299, 309, 973

MAP2K1   94, 97, 185, 227, 236, 246-247, 469-470, 472-473, 475-476

MAP3K1   768

MAP3K3   469

MAP3K8   948

MAP4K5   768

MAPK1   786

MARCHF10 (MARCH10)   641

mastocytosis   39-40, 69-70, 72-74

mature cystic teratoma   647, **663-665,** 669, 671

MAX   861-863, 866

MBNL1   488, 626

MCT1   554-555

MDH2   861

MDM2   195, 280, 409, 578, 603, 606-607, 888

MDR3   785

MECOM (EVI1)   53, 56, 58, 64, 905

MED12   765, 768

MED15   702

mediastinal grey zone lymphoma   39, 84, **106-108**

medullary thyroid carcinoma   821-822, **837-840,** 857

medulloblastoma, histologically defined   167, 283, **295-301**

medulloblastoma, non-WNT/non-SHH   167, **293-294**

medulloblastoma, SHH-activated and TP53-mutant   167, **291-292**

medulloblastoma, SHH-activated and TP53-wildtype   167, **288-290,** 292

medulloblastoma, WNT-activated   167, **285-287**

medulloepithelioma   310, 312-313, 365-366, 388, **392-394,** 669, 1008, 1010-1011

MEF2C   81

MEF2D   76-77

MEIS1   514

melan-A   374, 382, 534, 543, 553, 560, 704-705, 709, 747, 848, 911, 948

melanin   312, 328-330, 527, 553, 559-560, 704, 738, 755, 778, 910-911, 941, 946, 950, 953, 1003

melanoma   131, 327-330, 366, 372-374, 376-378, 543, 552-553, 560, 578, 669, 704, 763, 911, 925-926, 941-942, 944, 946-947, 949-950, **952-955,** 980, 989, 999-1000, 1002, 1012-1013

melanotic neuroectodermal tumour of infancy   324, 873-874, **910-911**

MEN1   822, 844, 861, 869, 871

menin   868

merlin (NF2)   967-968

MERRF   *See* MT-TK

mesenchymal chondrosarcoma   398, **623-624**

mesenchymal hamartoma   773-774, **790-792,** 795-796, 801, 894

mesoblastic nephroma   445-446, 691-693, 716-717, **720-721,** 916-917

mesonephric remnants and hyperplasia   735, **753-754**

MET   185, 197, 200, 204, 232-233, 446-447, 449, 642, 692, 694, 787, 829, 948, 953

metanephric adenofibroma   691, 694, **714-715,** 716

metanephric adenoma   691, 694, 707, **712-713,** 714-715

metanephric stromal tumour   691, 694, 714-715, **716-717**

metanephrine   855, 859

MFN2   404

MHC   83, 104

MIB1   220, 309, 863-864, 948

MIR143   508

miR-210   861

MIST1   902

MITF   374, 534, 552-553, 583, 703, 948

MK2   357

MKL1   *See* MRTFA

MLF1   575

MLH1   994-998, 1014-1016

MLL See KMT2A

MLLT1 53, 57

MLLT3 57

MLLT4 See AFDN

MLLT10 53, 57

MLLT11 60

MNX1 56-57

MOC31 778-779

moesin 968

monodermal teratomas (female gonadal) 647, **668-670**

MRLN 517

MRTFA (MKL1) 56, 59-60

MSA 413, 431, 455, 484, 508, 512, 517, 543, 557, 895, 898

MSANTD3 901

MSH2 340, 994-997, 1014-1016

MSH3 993, 996

MSH6 340, 994-997, 1014-1016

MSN 131

MST1R 905

mTOR, MTOR 127, 129, 142, 159, 169, 218-219, 221, 227, 329, 422, 466, 469, 472, 475, 478, 499, 509, 525, 559, 561, 603, 679, 687, 709, 861, 924, 963, 968, 972-973

mTORC1 404, 559, 923

mTORC2 72

MT-TK (MERRF) 403-404

MUC4 443, 451-452

MUC5AC 586

mucicarmine 900

mucoepidermoid carcinoma 873-874, **899-900**

Müllerian papilloma 735, **755-756**

multinodular and vacuolating neuronal tumour 167, 172, 227, **245-247**

MUTYH 994

MVD 935

MVK 935

MYB 81, 174-179, 185, 227-228, 236, 374

MYC (MYCC) 77, 81, 85, 87-88, 90, 92-94, 104-105, 109-114, 118, 145, 159, 164-165, 195, 268, 283-284, 293-294, 301, 303, 305, 307, 322-325, 357-359, 361-362, 374, 502-503, 509, 586, 603, 803, 810, 1019

MYCN 190, 194-199, 248, 265, 267-269, 289-293, 353, 357-362, 364, 386-387, 389, 701, 866

mycosis fungoides 39, **119-122,** 125

myelin 530, 973

myelodysplastic syndrome with excess blasts (childhood myelodysplastic neoplasm with increased blasts) **51-52**

myeloid neoplasms associated with germline predisposition 39, 49, 51, 55, 61, **62-65**

myeloid proliferations associated with Down syndrome 39, 63, **66-68**

myeloperoxidase 42, 81-82, 116

MYH9 411

MYH11 56

MYO1F 60

MYOD1 512, 514-517, 543, 551, 576, 583, 796

myoepithelial tumours of soft tissue 398, 569, 571

myofibroma and myopericytoma 397, **504-506**

MYOG 517

myogenin 512, 515-517, 540, 543, 551, 576, 583, 624, 796

myoglobin 923

myxopapillary ependymoma 167, 248, 265, 267, **271-273**

N

naevoid basal cell carcinoma syndrome (Gorlin syndrome) 284, 288, 957, **975-978**

NAF1 63

NANOG 651

NAP 42

NAPEPLD 61

naphthol AS-D chloroacetate esterase 46

nasal chondromesenchymal hamartoma 873-874, **894-895,** 1008, 1011

nasal dermoid cyst 873-874, **891-892**

nasopharyngeal carcinoma 873-874, **905-907**

nasopharyngeal dermoid 873, **893**

NB84 359, 729

NBN (NBS1) 282

NBS1 See NBN

NCOA1 514

NCOA2 505, 514-516, 623-624

NCOA4 829

NCOR1 768

NDRG4 505

NEK9 935

nephroblastoma 691-692, 694, 696, **697-701,** 713-714, 721-723, 988-989, 1005

nestin 221, 312, 534, 973

NeuN 181, 205, 221, 226-227, 232, 235, 239, 243, 246, 299, 313, 319, 392

neuroblastoma 13, 33, 168, 227, 239, 269, 295, 302, 314-316, 321, 340, 349-353, 355, **356-362,** 363-364, 388, 399, 517, 559, 708, 729, 736, 763, 865-866, 919, 958, 989-990, 1005

neurofibroma 17-18, 365, 378-379, 398, 463, **525-528,** 531-532, 543-544, 962-964, 969

neurofibromatosis type 1 45, 63, 177, 183, 202-203, 209, 213, 220, 225, 234, 378, 381, 395, 399, 513, 522, 525, 529, 531, 534, 541, 543, 632, 716, 866, 881, 957, **962-965,** 967, 994, 1014

neurofibromatosis type 2 265, 268, 381, 522, 531, 957, **966-970**

neurofibromin (NF1) 525, 963

neurofilament 189, 214, 220, 226, 232, 243, 359

neuromelanin 778

neurotensin 781, 839

NF1 45-47, 63-64, 183, 198, 202-203, 206, 209, 211, 216, 225-226, 228, 234, 378, 380-381, 395-396, 507, 513-514, 520, 525-529, 541-544, 632, 861-862, 866, 945, 962-965

NF2 265-268, 522-524, 529, 966-970

NFATC2 582-584

NFE2L2 777, 780, 786

NFKB1 156

NFKBIA 145

NFKBIE 505

NFP 205, 246, 306, 313, 324, 523, 527, 535-536

NF-κB 72, 90-91, 122, 142, 145, 253, 906

NG2 57-58, 75

NHP2 63

NID1 77

NIPAL1 905

NKX2-1 81, 219

NKX2-2 81, 580, 583, 586, 624, 729, 813

NKX2-5 81

NKX3-1 583-584

NMDAR 663-664

nodular lymphocyte-predominant Hodgkin lymphoma 39, 88, 144, **145-147,** 155-156, 164

NONO (P54NRB) 702

non-ossifying fibroma 398, **632-633**

nonspecific esterase 54

NOP10 63

norepinephrine 854, 984

normetanephrine 854, 859

NOS2 660

NOTCH1 81-82, 508

NOTCH2 97, 214, 508, 768

NOTCH3 214, 505, 508

notochordal tumours 398, **634-637**

NPM1 56, 60, 100, 129, 131-132

NR4A2 902

NR4A3 901-902

NR5A1 652

NRAS 45, 47, 81, 329-330, 373, 376, 478, 514, 649, 659, 841, 884, 942, 944-945, 953, 1010

NSD1   60
NSD2 (WHSC1)   77, 609
NSD3   908
NSDHL   935
NSE   299, 324, 389, 393, 534, 669, 793, 879
NTHL1   869, 993, 997
NTRK1   185, 200, 216, 232-233, 242, 446-448, 450, 829, 831, 948, 953
NTRK2   182, 185, 200, 216, 232-233, 242, 446-448, 450
NTRK3   185, 200, 216, 232-233, 242, 321, 445-448, 450, 454, 456, 713, 716, 720-721, 763, 829, 831, 916-917, 948, 950, 953
NUP214   56
NUP98   55-56, 60-61
NUT   586, 873-874, 908-909
NUT carcinoma   873-874, **908-909**
NUTM1   585-586, 908-909
NUTM2A   586
NUTM2B   588

O

OCT2   85, 90, 100, 107-108, 143-144, 146-147
OCT3/4   652-654, 657-659, 680, 687, 710, 752
OCT4   357, 650-651
odontogenic tumours   344, 873, 881, **883-887**
OLIG2   81, 175, 181, 185, 189, 194, 197-198, 205, 223, 226-227, 235, 243, 246, 250, 258, 266, 269, 272, 315, 319-320
OMD   628
OPA1   768
ORF73   497
ossifying fibroma   642, 644, 873-874, **888-889**
ossifying renal tumour of infancy   691, 717, **718-719**
osteoblastoma   398, **594-595,** 605
osteochondroma   398, **611-612,** 618-619
osteofibrous dysplasia   398, 640, **642-643**
osteoid osteoma   398, 594, **596-597**
osteosarcoma   398-400, 413, 515, 579, 595, **600-607,** 609, 620-621, 624, 629, 631, 755, 889, 1002-1004, 1006-1007
ovarian fibroma   735, **737-738,** 976

P

P2RY8   77
p14ARF   526
p15   60, 514, 526, 701, 806-808, 847, 868-869, 989-990
p16   83, 106, 205, 384, 406, 523, 526-528, 753, 757, 759, 862, 944, 948, 953, 964, 997, 1015

P16INK4a   *See* CDKN2A
p17   163
p27   830
p40   842, 898, 900, 906, 908
p53   189-190, 194, 215, 280, 289, 292, 299-300, 341, 384, 409, 527, 710, 796, 803, 847, 849-850, 1006
P54NRB   *See* NONO
p63   346, 538, 570, 641-642, 687, 771, 842, 898, 900, 903, 906, 908
p75-NGFR   299-300, 723
p130   384
PABPC1   131
paediatric cystic nephroma   691, **695-696,** 1008
paediatric gastrointestinal stromal tumour   398, **519-521**
paediatric hepatocellular carcinoma   773, **784-789**
paediatric nodal marginal zone lymphoma   39, 95, **96-98**
paediatric NTRK-rearranged spindle cell neoplasm   397, 446, **448-450**
paediatric-type follicular lymphoma   39-40, 88, 91, **93-95,** 97-98
PAFAH1B1   628
PAK   968
PALB2   282, 293-294, 297, 404
pancreatic acinar cell carcinoma   773, **809-811**
pancreatoblastoma   773-774, **805-808,** 814, 871, 989
pancytokeratin   272, 394, 747, 804, 830, 836, 842, 898, 906, 908, 911
pankeratin   523
pan-TRK   152, 447, 450, 720
PAP   870
papillary cystadenoma   735, **745**
papillary intralymphatic angioendothelioma and retiform haemangioendothelioma   397, **492-493**
papillary thyroid carcinoma   821-826, **827-833,** 834-835, 840
parafibromin   844
parasympathetic paraganglioma (head and neck paraganglioma)   821, **854-857**
parathyroid adenoma   821-822, **843-845**
PARN   63
parvovirus B19   47
PATZ1   582-584
PAX2   745
PAX3   514-516
PAX5   76, 78, 90-91, 95, 100, 103, 107-108, 110, 131, 143-147, 452
PAX6   871, 987-988

PAX7   514-516
PAX8   669, 700, 704, 709-710, 716, 729, 745, 753, 759, 825, 829-831, 836, 839, 871
PBX1   570
PBX3   570
P-cadherin   515
PD1   98, 142, 146-147, 154, 998
PDGF   505
PDGFA   575
PDGFB   437-439, 982
PDGFD   437-439
PDGFRA   189, 195, 198-199, 234-236, 519-520
PDGFRB   422, 455, 504-506
PDL1   83-85, 104, 106, 146, 347, 998
PDL2   83-85, 106, 146
PDX1   810, 813-814, 871
PEComa   398, **559-561,** 704
perforin   100, 127, 131-132, 134, 139
perineurioma   398, 404, **529-530,** 531-532
peripheral T-cell lymphoma   39, **115-116,** 131, 146, 155-156
peritoneal inclusion cysts   735, **759**
PGE2   597
PGI2   597
PGM1   54, 151
PGP9.5   359
phaeochromocytoma   821-822, 837, 851-853, 855-856, **858-864,** 865-866, 957-958, 963, 981, 984, 989-990
phakomatous choristoma   365, **370-371**
PHD1   *See* EGLN2
PHD2   *See* EGLN1
PHF15   *See* JADE2
PHF23   61
PHF6   77
phosphaturic mesenchymal tumour   398, **572-573**
phosphorylated ERK   151-152
phosphorylated STAT3   100, 104
PHOX2B   356-357, 359, 729
PI3K   72, 81, 98, 100, 112, 127, 130, 142, 145, 154, 159, 163, 189, 197, 200, 227, 235, 329, 357, 404, 422, 469, 472, 475, 478, 525, 603, 679, 687, 777, 838, 861, 906, 936, 968, 973
PICALM   53
pigmented spindle cell naevus (Reed naevus)   925, **950-951**
PIK3CA   151, 189, 286, 404, 466-467, 469-470, 475-476, 478, 768, 770, 798, 803, 829, 835
PIK3CD   156
PIK3R1   189

pilocytic astrocytoma 14, 167, 169, 185, 190, **202-208,** 209, 211-212, 217, 226, 242-244, 266, 347, 365, 395, 402, 962-963

pilocytic astrocytoma and other gliomas of the optic nerve 365, **395-396**

pilomatricoma 925, **938-939**

PIM1 145

pineoblastoma 168, 316, 322, **325-326,** 385-386, 390, 980, 1008, 1011

pituitary adenoma / pituitary neuroendocrine tumour 168, **332-340**

pituitary blastoma 168, 331, **341-342,** 1008, 1011

PKA 335, 774, 782-783

PKC 72, 76, 460

PKCδ 72

PKCμ 76

PKD1 972

PLAG1 405-407, 409, 570-571, 897-898

plantar/palmar fibromatoses 397, 403-404, 430, **435-436,** 930, 975

PLAP 651, 653-654, 659, 676, 679, 683, 687

plasmablastic lymphoma 39, 100, **103-105,** 165

Plasmodium falciparum 110

PLCγ 129

PLCB4 327, 945

PLCG1 502

pleomorphic adenoma 406, 570, 873, **896-898,** 900

pleomorphic xanthoastrocytoma 167, 185, 197, 207, 210-211, **213-217,** 226-228, 232-233

pleuropulmonary blastoma 392-393, 695, 727, 894, 913, 915, 917, **918-921,** 1008, 1010-1011

plexiform fibrohistiocytic tumour 397, **462-463**

PMEL 77

PML 56

PMS2 994-997, 1014-1016

PMVK 935

podoplanin 223, 490-492, 498, 500, 651, 653-654, 659

POLD1 998, 1015

POLE 997-998, 1014-1015

POLH 1001

polycomb 304, 964, 1018

polymorphous low-grade neuroepithelial tumour of the young 167, 172, **180-182,** 185, 227, 236

posterior fossa ependymoma 167, 248, **257-259**

posterior fossa group A (PFA) ependymoma 167, 172, **260-262**

posterior fossa group B (PFB) ependymoma 167, 172, **263-264**

postpubertal-type teratoma 647, 663-665, **675-678**

posttransplant lymphoproliferative disorders 39, 158-159

POT1 63

POU5F1 570, 652

PP 868-871

PPARG 669

PPFIBP1 454

PPP6R3 412

PR 696, 745, 753, 759, 793, 813-814, 835-836

PRC1.1 722

PRC2 188, 260, 304, 542, 566, 963, 1018

PRCC 692, 702, 705

PRDM1 91, 100, 104-105, 679, 687

PRDM14 679, 687

prepubertal-type testicular teratoma 647, **673-674,** 731

PRF1 156

primary cutaneous CD30-positive T-cell lymphoproliferative disorders 39, **123-125**

primary immunodeficiency–associated lymphoproliferative disorders 39, **154-157**

primary mediastinal large B-cell lymphoma 39, **83-85,** 106

PRKACA 774, 781-783

PRKAR1A 454, 524, 774, 783

progesterone 538, 743

prolactin 333, 337-339

proteoglycan 886, 930

PROX1 469, 478, 491-493, 933

PRRX1 452

pseudomyogenic haemangioendothelioma 397, **494-496,** 567

PSF See SFPQ

PTCH1 282-283, 288-289, 292, 299, 301, 511-512, 737, 884, 975-978

PTCH2 288, 884, 975

PTEN 15-16, 182, 189, 214, 378, 380, 402-404, 474-476, 534, 537, 577, 741, 803, 822, 824-825, 828-829, 833, 989

PTF1A 813

PTH 825-826, 844-845

PTK2B 77

PTPN11 45, 47, 203, 881

PTPRB 502

PTPRG 505

PU.1 85, 143

pyogenic granuloma See lobular capillary haemangioma

PYY 870

R

RAB2A 405

RAC 968

RAD21 50

RAD51B 405-406

RAD51C 959

radixin 968

RAF1 203, 216, 226, 228, 232-233, 242, 446, 448-450, 810, 942

RAG1 155-156

RAG2 155-156

RANBP2 100, 454

RANK 631

RAP1GAP 972

RARA 56

RASA1 472-473, 475-476, 478

RASAL1 888

RAS-GAP 525

RASGRF1 948

RASGRP1 156

RB1 (RB) 77, 182, 322-325, 383-384, 386, 389-390, 394, 399, 577, 603, 679, 687, 787, 961, 979-980, 1018

RBM10 702, 704

RBM15 56, 59-60

RBMX 704

RBX1 982

receptor tyrosine kinase 200, 203, 232-233, 357, 446-448, 450, 572, 642, 829, 838

RECQL2 See WRN

RECQL3 See BLM

RECQL4 603, 1002-1004

Reed naevus See pigmented spindle cell naevus

refractory cytopenia of childhood (childhood myelodysplastic neoplasm with low blasts) 39, **48-50,** 52

REL 83, 106, 145

RELA 252-255, 505

renal cell carcinoma with MiT translocations 691, **702-705**

renal Ewing sarcoma 691, **729-730**

RET 422, 446-450, 455, 669, 810, 829, 831, 835, 838-840, 861-863, 948, 953

reticulin 49, 52, 67, 213-215, 226-227, 272, 298-299, 340, 787, 848

retinoblastoma 14, 32, 209, 322-323, 325-326, 365-366, 383-384, **385-391,** 393-394, 399, 404, 602-603, 874, 957-958, 979-980

retinoblastoma syndrome 326, 386, 390-391, 957, **979-980**

retinocytoma 365-366, **383-384,** 388

rhabdoid tumour predisposition syndrome 302, 304, 556, 725, 751, 957, **1017-1019** rhabdomyoma 398, **511-512,** 539, 913, 922-923

rhabdomyosarcomas 398, **513-516,** 677, 1006

RHOA 115

RHOH 145

RIT1 45, 47

RMRP 155

ROS1 197, 200-201, 232-233, 422, 449, 454, 456, 768, 803, 948, 953

Rothmund–Thomson syndrome 603, 957-958, **1002-1004**

round cell sarcoma with EWSR1::non-ETS fusions 398, **582-584**

RPS6KA3 787

RRAS 45

RRBP1 454

RREB1 374

RTEL1 63

RUNX1 6-7, 49-50, 56, 63-64, 81

RUNX1T1 56

RUNX2 628, 630

S

S100 150-152, 189, 205, 214, 220, 235, 243, 250, 258, 266, 272, 275, 278, 280, 309, 319, 355, 359, 371, 374, 382, 394, 406, 421, 431, 443, 446-447, 449-450, 452, 512, 520, 523-524, 527-528, 530, 532, 534-536, 543-544, 551, 553, 557, 563, 570-571, 580, 586, 609, 615, 636, 642, 716, 723, 817, 842, 853, 857, 863, 866, 879-880, 895, 898, 900, 911, 917, 948, 964, 967, 985

S100A4 830

S100A6 948

S100P 583

S6K1 973

SALL4 557, 659, 672, 680, 683, 687, 732, 752, 777

SAMD9 49-50, 64

SAMD9L 49-50, 64

SAP See SH2D1A

SAR1A 628

sarcoma with BCOR genetic alterations 398, 579, **587-589**

SARNP 60

SATB2 573, 589, 606, 630, 723, 870

SBDS 63

schwannoma 17-18, 266, 398, **522-524,** 527, 531-533, 541, 543-544, 966-967, 969

sclerosing stromal tumour 735, **739-740**

SDHA 519-520, 861-863, 984-985

SDHAF2 861, 984-985

SDHB 519-520, 822, 851, 853, 855-857, 861-864, 866, 984-986

SDHC 519-520, 822, 855, 861-862, 984-985

SDHD 519, 822, 855-856, 861-862, 984-985

SEC31A (SEC31L1) 454

SEPTIN6 60

SEPTIN9 60

serotonin 818-819, 869-871

SERPINE1 495

Sertoli–Leydig cell tumour **746-748,** 749-750, 918, 1008-1010

SET 61

SETBP1 50, 64

SETD1B 77

SETD2 81, 133, 194, 609, 864

sex cord tumour with annular tubules 735, **743-744**

SF1 335-336, 339-340, 654, 732-733, 738, 741, 743, 747, 848, 863

SFPQ (PSF) 702

SGK1 145

SH2B3 81

SH2D1A (SAP) 156

SH3BP2 881

SH3PXD2A 522

SHOC2 960

sialoblastoma 873-874, **903-904**

simple bone cyst 398, **638-639**

sinonasal angiofibroma 397, **432-434**

sinonasal tract myxoma 873, **890**

SLC2A2 (GLUT2) 786

SLC16A1 869

SLC17A9 935

SLC25A11 861

SLX4 (BTBD12) 959

SMA 306, 413, 421-422, 425, 431, 433, 441, 443, 447, 455, 457-458, 461, 463, 493, 500, 506, 508, 510, 512, 520, 546, 549, 563, 570, 576, 720, 793, 796, 817, 890, 895, 898, 903, 915, 917

SMAD3 443-444

SMAD4 472-473, 768, 808, 813, 992

small cell carcinoma of the ovary, hypercalcaemic type 735, **751-752**

SMARCA2 318, 526, 752, 963

SMARCA4 114, 280, 286, 293, 299, 302-304, 306, 324, 556, 558, 566, 725-726, 736, 751-752, 1017-1018

SMARCB1 (hSNF5, INI1, SNF5) 170, 214-215, 280, 299-300, 302-309, 313, 322, 324-325, 496, 523-524, 542-544, 556-558, 563-567, 570, 635-637, 677, 693, 707, 710-711, 725-726, 729, 736, 752, 774-775, 778, 869, 966, 968-969, 1017-1019

SMARCB1-deficient renal medullary carcinoma 691, **710-711**

SMARCC1 566

SMARCC2 566

SMC1A 58

SMC3 58

SMMHC 898

SMO 289, 292, 884, 977

SMYD1 (KMT3D) 841

SND1 810

SNF5 See SMARCB1

SOCS1 86, 145

solid pseudopapillary neoplasm 773, **812-815,** 871

solitary circumscribed neuroma 398, **535-536**

somatostatin 340, 839, 870

sonic hedgehog 274, 280, 282, 284, 286, 288, 291, 293, 295, 344, 777, 801, 975, 977, 1006

SOS1 960

SOX2 221, 347, 650, 659, 672, 680

SOX9 347, 551, 609, 652-654, 732, 813, 895

SOX10 189, 205, 266, 374, 382, 443, 523-524, 527, 530, 532, 534, 543-544, 553, 570-571, 583-584, 857, 863, 879, 898, 900, 902-903, 948, 964, 985

SOX11 111, 814

SOX17 650-651, 659

SP7 transcription factor 630

SPARC 628

spinal ependymoma 167, 172, 248, **265-267,** 268-270

spinal ependymoma, MYCN-amplified 167, 172, **268-270**

spindle epithelial tumour with thymus-like elements 821, **841-842**

Spitz naevus 925, **947-949,** 950, 953-954

SPRED1 963

SPT24 835, 869

SQSTM1 100

squamous papilloma and papillomatosis 873, **875-876**

SRC 968

SRF 505-506, 514

SRP54 63

SRY 652-653

SS18 (SYT) 920

SS18L1 562-563, 842

SSTR2A 538, 573

SSX1 562-563

SSX2 562-563

SSX4 562-563

STAG2 318, 580-581

STAT1 145

STAT3 100, 104-105, 117-118, 122, 133, 628, 768

STAT4 497

STAT5 72, 117

STAT5B 133

STIM1   497
STK4   155
STK11 (LKB1)   737, 743, 960
STN1   63
STRN   707
subcutaneous panniculitis-like T-cell
   lymphoma   39, **126-128,** 139, 165
subependymal giant cell astrocytoma   167,
   169, **218-221,** 972
substance P   870
subungual exostosis   398, **590-591**
succinate   519, 693, 829, 859, 984
succinate dehydrogenase   519, 693, 829, 984
SUFU   282, 288-289, 292, 301, 737, 884,
   975-978
superficial angiomyxoma   398, **547**
supratentorial ependymoma   167, 172, 248,
   **249-251,** 252, 254-256
supratentorial ependymoma, YAP1 fusion–
   positive   167, 172, **255-256**
supratentorial ependymoma, ZFTA fusion–
   positive   167, **252-254**
SUZ12   81, 528, 542-543, 964
SWI/SNF   286, 299, 304, 556, 562, 566, 725,
   752, 1018
sympathetic paraganglioma   821, **851-853,**
   855, 858
synaptophysin   181, 189, 205, 214, 221, 226,
   232, 239, 243, 246, 299, 306, 309, 313,
   315, 320, 324, 355, 359, 389, 393, 517,
   557, 669, 788, 793, 807, 814, 818-819,
   839, 848, 856, 863, 868, 908, 911, 985
synovial sarcoma   398, 400, 543, **562-564,**
   589, 842, 920
systemic EBV-positive T-cell lymphoma of
   childhood   39, **135-137**
SYT   See SS18


**T**
T- and NK-lymphoblastic leukaemia/
   lymphoma   39, **80-82**
TAF15   581
TAL1   81
TAL2   81
TALLA-1   See TSPAN7
TBC1D7   973
TBL1XR1   77
TBX3   768
TBXT   635
TCEA1   897
T-cell receptor   50, 118, 139
TCF/LEF proteins   110, 112-114, 835
TCF3   110, 112-114
TCF4   110
TCL1   111

TCN1   781
TCRαβ   134
TCRβ   127
TCRγ   127, 134
TCRγδ   127, 134
TCRδ   127
TdT   42, 78, 81, 87, 110-111, 116
TEAD1   514
TEF3   See TRIM37
TEK (TIE2)   469
telomerase   357, 786, 795
tenosynovial giant cell tumour   397, **464-465**
TERC   63
TERT   63, 173, 191, 198, 209, 211, 213,
   216-217, 224, 289, 357, 359, 361-362, 765,
   768, 777, 779-780, 786, 829, 835, 864,
   944, 949, 953-954
TET2   50, 52-53, 115, 117
TFCP2   514
TFE3   500, 534, 554-555, 560-561, 626-627,
   702-705, 707, 814
TFEB   702-705
TFG   454
TGF-β   142, 344, 443, 977
TGFA   422, 982
THADA   833
THRAP3 (TRAP150)   628
thyroglobulin   669, 825-826, 830, 836, 842
thyroid hormone   800
thyroperoxidase   830
thyroxine   332, 337
TIA1   124, 127, 131-132, 134, 137, 139, 147
TIE1   502, 803
TIE2   See TEK
Tinea capitis   828
TINF2   63
TJP2   785, 787
TLE1   563-564, 589, 723
TLX1   81
TLX3   81
TMEM127   861
TNC   628
TNF   133
TNFAIP3   145
TNFRSF4   497
TNFRSF6   See FAS
TNFRSF9   156
TNFRSF14   94, 97
TNFRSF19   905
TOP1   61
TP53   50, 52, 64, 76, 78, 115, 117, 165, 179,
   182, 189-191, 194, 197-198, 213, 233, 275,
   280-282, 284, 286-289, 291-292, 299, 301,
   311, 335, 399, 514, 542, 577, 580-581,
   603, 641, 701, 741, 783, 786, 795-796,

   803, 810, 847-849, 899, 919, 963, 992,
   1005-1007, 1010, 1015
TP63   124
TPM3   129, 454, 707
TPM4   454
TPR   446
TRA   81
TRAF1   131
TRAF7   529
TRAP150   See THRAP3
TRB   81
TRD   81
TRG   82, 102
TRIM37 (TEF3)   737
TRPV4   881
trypsin   807, 810-811, 814
tryptase   70, 73-74
TSC1   219, 221, 559, 635, 704, 708-709,
   923, 971-974
TSC2   219, 221, 559-561, 635, 704, 708-709,
   923, 971-974
TSH   337-339, 343, 829
TSHR   824, 829
TSPAN7 (TALLA-1)   575
TSPY   649-650, 652-653
TSPY1   649, 652
TSPYL2 (CTCL)   99
TTF1   219, 221, 331, 340, 669, 752-753, 825,
   830-831, 835-836, 839, 842, 857, 869,
   908-909
tuberin   219, 221, 559-560, 923, 972-974
tuberous sclerosis   218-219, 402, 420, 560-
   561, 635, 704, 708-709, 741, 822, 922-924,
   930, 957, **971-974**
tufted angioma and kaposiform
   haemangioendothelioma   397, **489-491**
tyrosinase   305, 307-309, 543, 948
tyrosine hydroxylase   340, 359, 856-857,
   863, 985
tyrosine kinase   42, 58, 75-76, 129-130, 183,
   191, 200, 203, 232-233, 236, 357, 438, 445-
   448, 450, 505, 521, 555, 572, 642, 829, 838


**U**
undifferentiated sarcomas   398, **577-578,**
   587, 589, 677, 1006
UNG   156
USP2   60
USP6   411-412, 414, 417, 465, 628-629
USP7   80
USP9X   628


**V**
vascular tumours of bone   398, **625-627**
V-ATPase   534

VCA   136

VCL   706-707, 710

VE1   152, 215, 227-228, 232, 694, 713, 830

VEGF   376, 801, 804

VEGF-A, VEGFA   482, 801, 982

VEGFR   492-493, 502, 801, 803

VEGFR2   492, 502, 803

VEGFR3   492-493, 502

venous malformations   397, **468-470**

VGLL2   514-516

VHL   692, 745, 813, 851, 860-863, 981-983

VIM   488, 626

vimentin   266, 275, 306, 309, 312, 315, 319-
320, 371, 393, 508, 538, 560, 567, 700,
710, 718, 723, 747, 791, 796, 817, 866,
879, 911, 915, 923, 973

VIP   356, 865-866, 871

VMAT1   870

VMAT2   869

von Hippel–Lindau syndrome   745, 822, 860,
871, 874, 957, 958, **981-983**

von Willebrand factor   484, 804

VPREB1   77

VS38   100

VS38c   104

**W**

WAGR syndrome   697, 957-961, **987-988**

WAS (WASP)   155, 497, 961

white sponge naevus   873-874, **877-878**

WHSC1   *See* NSD2

WRAP53   63

WRN (RECQL2)   603

WT1   53, 60, 574-576, 586, 652-653, 692,
698, 700-701, 713, 729, 732, 738, 741,
743, 745, 747, 752, 793, 798, 835, 933,
987-988

WWTR1   488, 495, 500, 626-627

**X**

XBP1   100

XBP1s   104

xeroderma pigmentosum   502, 953, 957-958,
**999-1001**

XIAP   156

XPA   999-1001

XPB   999-1000

XPC   999-1001

XPD   999-1000

XPE   999-1000

XPF   999-1000

XPG   999-1000

XPO1   144

**Y**

YAP1   17, 167, 172, 248-250, 255-256, 289,
292, 294, 299-300, 319, 452, 466, 479,
500, 626-627, 777, 1018

yolk sac tumour   647-648, 656, 666, 671,
675, 677, **681-683,** 685, 688, 690, 731-
732, 752

YWHAE   588, 722, 724

YY1   1013

**Z**

ZEB2   77

ZFP36   488, 626

ZFP36L1   145

ZNF9   *See* CNBP

ZNF384   7

ZNF444   570

ZNF532   908

ZNF592   908

zymogen   810, 901

# The World Health Organization Classification of Tumours

## Head and neck
El-Naggar AK, Chan JKC, Grandis JR, et al., editors. WHO classification of head and neck tumours. Lyon (France): International Agency for Research on Cancer; 2017. (WHO classification of tumours series, 4th ed.; vol. 9). https://publications.iarc.fr/548.

## Endocrine organs
Lloyd RV, Osamura RY, Klöppel G, et al., editors. WHO classification of tumours of endocrine organs. Lyon (France): International Agency for Research on Cancer; 2017. (WHO classification of tumours series, 4th ed.; vol. 10). https://publications.iarc.fr/554.

## Haematopoietic and lymphoid tissues
Swerdlow SH, Campo E, Harris NL, et al., editors. WHO classification of tumours of haematopoietic and lymphoid tissues. Lyon (France): International Agency for Research on Cancer; 2017. (WHO classification of tumours series, 4th rev. ed.; vol. 2). https://publications.iarc.fr/556.

## Skin
Elder DE, Massi D, Scolyer RA, et al., editors. WHO classification of skin tumours. Lyon (France): International Agency for Research on Cancer; 2018. (WHO classification of tumours series, 4th ed.; vol. 11). https://publications.iarc.fr/560.

## Eye
Grossniklaus HE, Eberhart CG, Kivelä TT, editors. WHO classification of tumours of the eye. Lyon (France): International Agency for Research on Cancer; 2018. (WHO classification of tumours series, 4th ed.; vol. 12). https://publications.iarc.fr/561.

## Digestive system
WHO Classification of Tumours Editorial Board. Digestive system tumours. Lyon (France): International Agency for Research on Cancer; 2019. (WHO classification of tumours series, 5th ed.; vol. 1). https://publications.iarc.fr/579.

## Breast
WHO Classification of Tumours Editorial Board. Breast tumours. Lyon (France): International Agency for Research on Cancer; 2019. (WHO classification of tumours series, 5th ed.; vol. 2). https://publications.iarc.fr/581.

## Soft tissue and bone
WHO Classification of Tumours Editorial Board. Soft tissue and bone tumours. Lyon (France): International Agency for Research on Cancer; 2020. (WHO classification of tumours series, 5th ed.; vol. 3). https://publications.iarc.fr/588.

## Female genital tract
WHO Classification of Tumours Editorial Board. Female genital tumours. Lyon (France): International Agency for Research on Cancer; 2020. (WHO classification of tumours series, 5th ed.; vol. 4). https://publications.iarc.fr/592.

## Thorax
WHO Classification of Tumours Editorial Board. Thoracic tumours. Lyon (France): International Agency for Research on Cancer; 2021. (WHO classification of tumours series, 5th ed.; vol. 5). https://publications.iarc.fr/595.

## Central nervous system
WHO Classification of Tumours Editorial Board. Central nervous system tumours. Lyon (France): International Agency for Research on Cancer; 2021. (WHO classification of tumours series, 5th ed.; vol. 6). https://publications.iarc.fr/601.

## Paediatric tumours
WHO Classification of Tumours Editorial Board. Paediatric tumours. Lyon (France): International Agency for Research on Cancer; forthcoming. (WHO classification of tumours series, 5th ed.; vol. 7). https://publications.iarc.fr/608.

## Urinary and male genital tracts
WHO Classification of Tumours Editorial Board. Urinary and male genital tumours. Lyon (France): International Agency for Research on Cancer; 2022. (WHO classification of tumours series, 5th ed.; vol. 8). https://publications.iarc.fr/610.

## WHO Classification of Tumours Online
The content of this renowned classification series is now also available in a convenient digital format: https://tumourclassification.iarc.who.int